MW01055563

Veterinary Dentistry
Principles and Practice

Veterinary Dentistry
Principles and Practice

Editors

Robert B. Wiggs, D.V.M.

Diplomate, American Veterinary Dental College
Adjunct Assistant Professor
Baylor College of Dentistry, Texas A&M University Systems
Coit Road Animal Hospital
Dallas, Texas

Heidi B. Lobprise, D.V.M.

Diplomate, American Veterinary Dental College
Coit Road Animal Hospital
Dallas, Texas

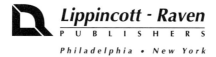

Lippincott · Raven
PUBLISHERS
Philadelphia · New York

Acquisitions Editor: Paula Callaghan
Developmental Editor: Julia Benson
Manufacturing Manager: Dennis Teston
Production Manager: Lawrence Bernstein
Production Editor: Loretta Cummings
Cover Designer: Doug Smock
Indexer: Jayne Percy
Compositor: Lippincott–Raven Electronic Production
Printer: Maple Press

© 1997 by Lippincott-Raven Publishers. All rights reserved. This book is protected by copyright. No part of it may be reproduced, stored in a retrieval system, or transmitted, in any form or by any means—electronic, mechanical, photocopy, recording, or otherwise—without the prior written consent of the publisher, except for brief quotations embodied in critical articles and reviews. For information write **Lippincott-Raven Publishers, 227 East Washington Square, Philadelphia, PA 19106-3780.**

Materials appearing in this book prepared by individuals as part of their official duties as U.S. Government employees are not covered by the above-mentioned copyright.

Printed in the United States of America

9 8 7 6 5 4 3 2 1

Library of Congress Cataloging-in-Publication Data
Veterinary dentistry: principles and practice / editors, Robert B. Wiggs, Heidi B. Lobprise.
    p.   cm.
Includes bibliographical references and indexes.
ISBN 0-397-51385-2
1. Veterinary dentistry   I. Wiggs, Robert B.   II. Lobprise, Heidi B.
SF867.V47   1997
636.089′76—dc20   96-43290
                                                                                          CIP

Care has been taken to confirm the accuracy of the information presented and to describe generally accepted practices. However, the authors, editors, and publisher are not responsible for errors or omissions or for any consequences from application of the information in this book and make no warranty, express or implied, with respect to the contents of the publication.

The authors, editors, and publisher have exerted every effort to ensure that drug selection and dosage set forth in this text are in accordance with current recommendations and practice at the time of publication. However, in view of ongoing research, changes in government regulations, and the constant flow of information relating to drug therapy and drug reactions, the reader is urged to check the package insert for each drug for any change in indications and dosage and for added warnings and precautions. This is particularly important when the recommended agent is a new or infrequently employed drug.

Some drugs and medical devices presented in this publication have Food and Drug Administration (FDA) clearance for limited use in restricted research settings. It is the responsibility of the health care provider to ascertain the FDA status of each drug or device planned for use in their clinical practice.

To our families and friends

Contents

Contributing Authors ix

Preface xi

1. Dental Equipment 1
    Robert B. Wiggs and Heidi B. Lobprise

2. Basic Materials and Supplies 29
    Robert B. Wiggs, Heidi B. Lobprise, and John J. Hefferren

3. Oral Anatomy and Physiology 55
    Robert B. Wiggs and Heidi B. Lobprise

4. Oral Examination and Diagnosis 87
    Robert B. Wiggs and Heidi B. Lobprise

5. Clinical Oral Pathology 104
    Robert B. Wiggs and Heidi B. Lobprise

6. Dental and Oral Radiology 140
    Robert B. Wiggs and Heidi B. Lobprise

7. Pedodontics 167
    Robert B. Wiggs and Heidi B. Lobprise

8. Periodontology 186
    Robert B. Wiggs and Heidi B. Lobprise

9. Oral Surgery 232
    Robert B. Wiggs and Heidi B. Lobprise

10. Oral Fracture Repair 259
    Robert B. Wiggs and Heidi B. Lobprise

11. Basic Endodontic Therapy 280
    Robert B. Wiggs and Heidi B. Lobprise

12. Advanced Endodontic Therapies 325
    Robert B. Wiggs and Heidi B. Lobprise

13. Operative and Restorative Dentistry 351
    Robert B. Wiggs and Heidi B. Lobprise

14. Operative Dentistry: Crowns and Prosthodontics 395
    Robert B. Wiggs and Heidi B. Lobprise

15. Basics of Orthodontics 435
    Robert B. Wiggs and Heidi B. Lobprise

16. Domestic Feline Oral and Dental Disease 482
    Robert B. Wiggs and Heidi B. Lobprise

17. Dental and Oral Disease in Rodents and Lagomorphs 518
    Robert B. Wiggs and Heidi B. Lobprise

18. Exotic Animal Oral Disease and Dentistry 538
    Robert B. Wiggs and Heidi B. Lobprise

19. Oral and Dental Disease in Large Animals 559
    Peter Emily, Paul G. Orsini, Heidi B. Lobprise, and Robert B. Wiggs

20. Marketing Veterinary Dentistry 580
    Steven E. Holmstrom

21. Behavioral Problems Associated with the Oral Cavity 598
    Janine Charboneau McInnis

Glossary of Terms 628

Abbreviations, Dental and Oral Indices, International System of Units,
Conversion Tables, and American National Standard and American Dental
Association Specifications 677

Index to Manufacturers and Distributors 697

Subject Index 719

Contributing Authors

Peter Emily, D.D.S. *Dental Faculty, Colorado State University School of Veterinary Medicine; Dental Faculty, University of Missouri School of Veterinary Medicine; Honorary Diplomate of the College of Veterinary Dentistry, Academy of Veterinary Dentistry; and Past President of the American Veterinary Dental Society, Lakewood, Colorado*

John J. Hefferren, Ph.D. *Research Professor, Center for Biomedical Research, Higuchi Biosciences Center, University of Kansas, Lawrence, Kansas*

Steven E. Holmstrom, D.V.M. *Diplomate, American Veterinary Dental College; Instructor, Foothill College, Los Altos, California; and Private Practice, Companion Animal Hospital, Belmont, California*

Heidi B. Lobprise, D.V.M. *Diplomate, American Veterinary Dental College and Coit Road Animal Hospital, Dallas, Texas*

Janine Charboneau McInnis, D.V.M. *Behavioral Veterinary Consultants of Dallas, Dallas, Texas*

Paul G. Orsini, D.V.M. *Diplomate, American Veterinary Dental College; Diplomate, American College of Veterinary Surgeons; and Assistant Professor of Veterinary Dentistry and Anatomy, University of Pennsylvania School of Veterinary Medicine, Veterinary Hospital of the University of Pennsylvania, Philadelphia, Pennsylvania*

Robert B. Wiggs, D.V.M. *Diplomate, American Veterinary Dental College; Adjunct Assistant Professor, Baylor College of Dentistry, Texas A&M University Systems; and Coit Road Animal Hospital, Dallas, Texas*

Preface

Dentistry has emerged over the last twenty years as a distinct and significant part of clinical veterinary medicine. This emergence as a prominent and accepted science has not come easily nor without controversy in the modality of treatments and in organization. The veterinary dental pioneers faced numerous scientific and technical barriers, as well as lack of acceptance on occasion, by colleagues. However, science embraces and accepts science, and as research continues to link oral health with general health, dentistry is becoming more widely appraised and appreciated.

The birthing pains and evolution of modern veterinary dentistry moved slowly through the 1970s, gained momentum in the 1980s and has been surging in the 1990s. Veterinary dental gurus came and went in the developing years as the focus was on instruments, materials, and clinical techniques with little attention to the physiology and biological implications of the equipment, instruments, materials, and techniques promoted. Today, the profession finds itself entangled in an attempt to make use of the latest technical, scientific, and manufacturing discoveries, many times without adequate knowledge of their mechanism of action or appropriate use. Additionally, it is easy to become overwhelmed by the plethora of new information, fancy gadgets, and high-tech devices.

Within the past few years, quality research has delved into the anatomical and physiological soundness of procedures, response to treatment, and development of the associated diseases. Only through an understanding of anatomical function, the development of oral diseases, and response to therapies can valid clinical concepts for materials and techniques be developed and safely advocated. Of particular importance is the assessment of short- and long-term responses to certain concepts and techniques.

Animals, both pets and wild, are cherished and respected for their nature and individuality. Their care and health are an important and accepted responsibility. Nevertheless, oral and dental disease have continued in an unaltered, ever-growing, upward spiral, and research has begun to link many serious diseases, as well as overall health, to that of oral cavity.

This book was written to assess, integrate, and consolidate the growing body of clinical and scientific literature related to veterinary dentistry. We have approached this task in a systematic, categorical, and thorough manner to provide the reader with a broad spectrum of essential tools for veterinary dentistry. These are addressed beginning with the currently accepted biological foundations for the advocation of the concepts and clinical techniques. The reader will find some archaic concepts identified and refuted, dogma challenged, and many additional questions raised indicating the need for further investigation and research. We acknowledge and embrace the fact that by the time this book is published there will be components already requiring revision and updating, as changes and improvements in this field occur constantly.

This text will provide the necessary foundation that will enable all who aspire to work within this unique part of our medical profession to meet the professional challenges of modern veterinary dental care in a knowledgeable manner and with a clinical perspective.

Robert B. Wiggs, D.V.M.
Heidi B. Lobprise, D.V.M.

Veterinary Dentistry

Principles and Practice

1

Dental Equipment

Robert B. Wiggs and Heidi B. Lobprise

Veterinary dentistry has experienced significant growth in the last decade or so, certainly because of the benefits it can provide. The background of knowledge and equipment adopted from the human dental field, with some variations, has greatly enhanced this area also. The fact that specific dental instruments and equipment can be added as slowly or as quickly to a practice as the need arises, from simple hand instruments to sophisticated power equipment, may also contribute to dentistry's popularity.

PERIODONTAL EQUIPMENT

Hand Equipment

When considering veterinary dental equipment, many individuals may start by thinking about power equipment, particularly ultrasonic scalers. While these are extremely important and widely used by many veterinarians, in the decision on how to supplement your dental armamentarium, certain hand instruments are indispensable for accurate assessment and treatment of dental disease. Hand instruments have three basic parts: the *handle (shaft)*, *shank*, and *working end*. The working end can be a *blade*, *point*, or *nib*. Double-ended instruments will have two working ends. On scalers and curettes, the surface between the two blades is known as the *face*, the opposite side is the *back*, and where the shank ends and the working end begins, the outside curve is called the *heel* (Figs. 1 and 2) (1–3). Handles come as solid or hollow. Solid handles give a firmer grip; however, the hollow handles conduct vibrations better, giving enhanced tactile sensitivity (2). The angle of the shank dictates areas of best use, for anterior or posterior teeth, lingual, buccal, mesial or distal surface. The working end determines the instrument use: probe, explorer, curette, explorer, etc.

Instrument Grasps

Generally, the palm grasp and the modified pen grasp are good and effective ways to hold and use most hand instruments (3,4). These increase control and tactile sense, while reducing hand and finger fatigue. With the *palm-grasp technique*, the instrument is held in the palm at the base of the fingers. The working end extends out from the hand in front of the thumb. This is similar to the grasp used in carving with a knife. The thumb is rested

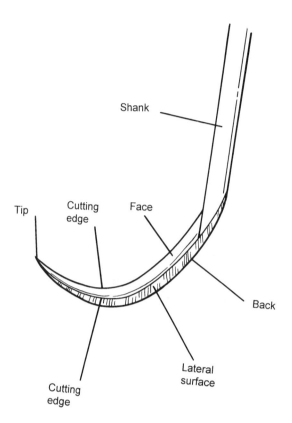

Shank

Tip   Cutting   Face
       edge

Back

Cutting   Lateral
edge   surface

FIG. 1. Illustration of curved scaler showing shank, face, back, tip and cutting edges.

in the mouth on a tooth and used as a fulcrum, as well as to stabilize the hand. It is the finger rest that stabilizes the hand and instrument, allowing them to act as a single unit, while helping to protect the patient's soft tissues. The palm-grasp technique increases strength of grasp and control, but the range of movement is limited and tactile sense may be reduced. It is used more commonly with rubber dam forceps, Porte polishers, and air/water syringes. Modifications of this grasp are used for holding forceps, with the instrument beak being the fulcrum. Another variation, sometimes called the *palm and thumb grasp*, can be used to instrument and to sharpen instruments. In this modification, the thumb is placed on the back of the shaft for additional pressure to the working end, while a finger knuckle acts as the fulcrum (2,5).

With the *modified pen grasp*, the instrument handle is held between the thumb and index fingers, and the middle finger is placed on the shank (Fig. 3). The thumb should be slightly bent, not straight, or some loss of control will result. The ring finger is used in the patient's mouth on a tooth as the fulcrum, as well as to stabilize the hand. It is the most commonly used grasp for mirrors, probes, explorers, curettes, and scalers. The modified pen grasp gives excellent control, stabilization, range of movement, and tactile sense (2,3).

Motion of activation is the way in which scalers and curettes are used in the hand to effect proficient work. The way in which the instrument contacts the intended surface is known as *instrument adaptation*. There are three basic motions of activation for proper instrument adaptation: rotary, wrist, and digital. *Rotary* motion is when the wrist and arm act as a single unit in a twisting or rotating motion similar to that of opening a door. *Wrist* motion is when the hand and wrist act as two separate units, as the wrist and hand artic-

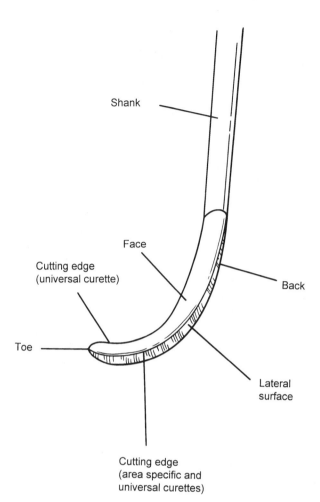

Shank

Face

Cutting edge
(universal curette)

Back

Toe

Lateral
surface

Cutting edge
(area specific and
universal curettes)

FIG. 2. Illustration of curette showing shank, face, back, toe, lateral surfaces, and cutting edges (two for universal curettes, and one for area-specific curettes).

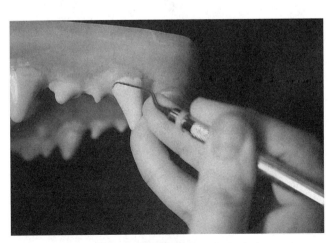

FIG. 3. Modified pen grasp.

ulate or bend in an up and down action. The hand, wrist, and arm are held parallel to each other with the middle finger acting as a finger rest. The wrist is then pushed forward and back. *Digital* motion is used with the palm-grasp technique, where the fingers are used to push the instrument in an up and down movement. Digital motion causes rapid hand and finger fatigue (2).

Dental Mirrors

Dental mirrors are used for indirect visualization of teeth, illumination, transillumination, and retraction. Some areas are difficult to visualize directly, such as the distal and lingual aspects of the maxillary molars. Mirrors can also be used to illuminate areas by reflecting light onto the teeth or to transilluminate them by reflecting light from the lingual side through the teeth for examination on the facial surface. This allows checking for tooth discoloration (internal hemorrhage), opacity (possible nonvital tooth), areas of greater translucency (possible resorptive activity), and dental caries.

The mirrors come in various sizes and surfaces. There are basically three surface types of mirrors: plane flat, front, and concave. *Plane flat-surface* mirrors have the reflective surface on the back surface. This protects the reflective surface from scratching but sometimes causes ghost or double images to appear. *Front-surface* mirrors eliminate double images and provide a clearer image but are susceptible to surface scratching. *Concave-surfaces* produce a magnified image but distort features. The front-surface mirror is the most commonly used.

Periodontal Probes

Periodontal probes are flat- or round-tipped instruments that have various lengths in millimeters marked on them (Fig. 4). They should be slender enough to easily insert into the patient's sulcus. These probes are typically either indented or color-coded in bands to assess the amount of attachment loss at various points around each tooth. The *Marquis* probe is color-coded with alternating bands at 3, 6, 9 and 12 mm. The *Williams* probe is

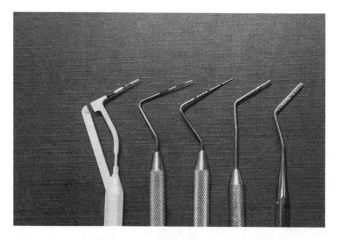

FIG. 4. Periodontal probes: flat or round with indentations or color-banded.

usually indented with lines marking 1, 2, 3, 5, 7, 8, 9, and 10 mm. The *Michigan-O* probe is customarily marked at 3, 6, and 8 mm. The *Nabors No.2* probe has no calibration markings and is curved. It is used for probing and examination of furcations (2,3).

The probe is gently inserted into the gingival sulcus to the depth of the epithelial attachment, without force that might damage the epithelial attachment, and several measurements are made. The depth of the actual pocket from the epithelial attachment to the gingival margin can be compared with the level of the cementoenamel junction (neck) to assess soft and/or hard tissue loss, root exposure, or gingival overgrowth. Taking measurements at the six line angles (mesiobuccal, distolingual, etc.) gives a more accurate representation than checking just one point.

Periodontal Explorers

Often a periodontal probe has an *explorer* on the opposite end, although double-ended probes and explorers are available in a multitude of configurations. The explorer end has a sharp, pointed tip at the end of a thin, almost wire-like semicircle, or angulated head (Fig. 5). The explorer is designed to provide maximum tactile sensitivity and is used to delicately detect debris and calculus on subgingival root surfaces, explore the furcation, detect softened tooth structure, and check margins on restorations. If used carelessly, the sharp point can damage the soft tissue and epithelial attachment. The fine tip of some explorers is used extensively in human dentistry to detect softened areas of enamel that might indicate decalcification and potential decay. The tip is pressed into the suspect area, then pulled back. If a slight tug-back is felt, the enamel may be softened, indicating that incipient caries or external resorption is possibly developing. Some explorers have gentle curves that can be used subgingivally to explore furcations for indications of attachment loss, calculus, or structural defects. They can also be used to explore fractured tooth surfaces for evidence of exposed pulp chambers or canals and to assess the smoothness of a metal crown–tooth interface.

Explorers must be selected for the intended use, such as detection of subgingival calculus or tooth lesions. The *Hu-Friedy No.3A* explorer has a gentle long curve that makes it excellent for examination of furcations for calculus or carious lesions. The *No.17* is

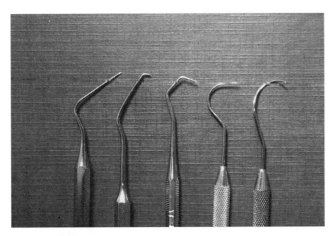

FIG. 5. Periodontal explorers.

designed for detection of subgingival calculus and examination of restorative margins, not caries. The *No. 23*, or classic *Shepherd's hook*, explorer is designed for detection of tooth caries or lesions above the gingival margin. It is heavy and thick for occlusal caries detection. It should generally not be used below the gingival margin as the design results in the point and tip being aimed directly down into the sulcus, and as it is advanced, it is likely to penetrate the epithelial attachment (2,3).

Scalers, Curettes, Hoes, Chisels, and Files

The *sickle scaler* is used for the removal of supragingival calculus. Its design allows subgingival use only in special circumstances of heavy calculus buildup with gingival margin distention that would allow easy entry, and even then the contours do not allow for safe and effective use. The classic configuration of this scaler is of a triangular cross-section with a sharp back (although some have a rounded back), two straight cutting edges, and a pointed tip (Figs. 2 and 6). This gives it outstanding strength, but when used subgingivally, it can result in gouged tooth surfaces and damage to the epithelial attachment and other soft tissues. The two basic designs are the *curved sickle* and the *straight sickle* scalers. The straight is also known as a *Jacquette* scaler.

The *curette* is the instrument of choice for removal of light subgingival calculus, root planning, and gingival and subgingival curettage. In comparison with the scaler's sharp tip, it is designed with two cutting edges and a rounded back and toe (see Figs. 1 and 2). These contours allow it to be introduced gently into the sulcus, with the face "closed," so the cutting edge does not engage the tooth surface. On reaching the depth of the sulcus, the curette is angled to bring the working edge into contact with the surface, and a pull stroke is used to dislodge the calculus and debris and bring it out of the canal. These pull strokes can be combined in vertical, horizontal, and oblique directions to provide a smooth, clean surface, in a procedure called root planing. The instrument may also be slightly angled, bringing the other working edge against the soft tissue, with gentle digital pressure on the external gingival surface to debride any diseased tissue, bacteria, or debris, known as gingival or subgingival curettage. True subgingival curettage, by defin-

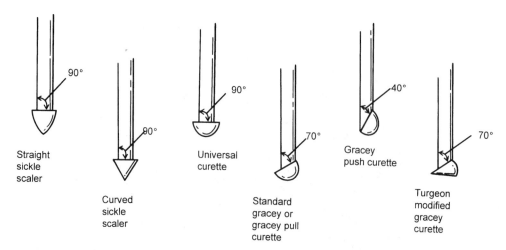

FIG. 6. Cross-sections and angulations of instrument working ends.

ition, refers to an intentional introduction of the curette below the epithelial attachment, but for all practical purposes, this is seldom done.

Curettes are divided into three types: universal (Columbia, Goldman, Langer, etc.), area-specific pull (Gracey, Demarco, Turgeon Modified, Furcation, etc.), and area-specific push (Gracey) (2). The major difference between the three is the working head angulation to the shaft. *Universal* curettes generally have two cutting blades and a 90° blade angulation to the shaft, although some have an 80° blade angle (see Fig. 6). Proper working angulation of the blade against the tooth is 45–90°; therefore, the shaft is angled to the handle to obtain the appropriate angle. This allows the handle to be parallel to the working surface for orientation below the gum line, which is known as *handle parallelism*. Both blades can be used for curetting, although using the second blade requires moving the handle to an angle perpendicular to the working surface for proper working angulation. The blade curves in only one direction, up from heel to toe, which can be seen when viewing it from the side. No curvature can be seen from a perpendicular view above the face. Each universal curette is double-ended with mirror images on opposite ends. From the midline of each tooth, the toe should be aimed at the proximal surface. This means that both ends are used on each facial and each lingual surface. Universal curettes can be used on any area or tooth surface.

Of the *area-specific* curettes, the Graceys are the most commonly used. They were designed by Dr. Clayton H. Gracey of Michigan in the late 1930s. In the early 1940s, he collaborated with Hugo Friedman, founder of the Hu-Friedy Company, to produced the first complete set of Gracey curettes. Each instrument was developed for a specific area of the human oral cavity, and some were developed for specific surfaces of the teeth (see Table 1).

The Gracey curettes have an offset blade with only one cutting edge. The blade is curved in two planes, which means from heel to toe the blade can be seen to curve from above and from the side. The shanks can be obtained in two types: rigid and flexible. The rigid shank gives good strength for heavier calculus work, while the flexible shank provides more tactile sensitivity.

Additionally, there are two types of blade angulation for the Gracey curettes: 70° and 40° of the instrument face to the shank (see Fig. 6). The original Gracey curettes had a 40° angle and were used only in a push stroke. These are known as *area-specific push* curettes or *Gracey push* curettes. They are still made by some manufacturers but are no longer common.

The *area-specific pull* curette or *Gracey pull* curette has a 70° angulation of the face to the shaft (see Fig. 6). This angle provides effective calculus removal and root planing primarily on the pull stroke. Because of the altered angulations of the shaft and handles of Gracey curettes, they are oriented to the working surface of the tooth with *shaft parallelism*, as compared with handle parallelism for the universal curettes.

TABLE 1. Gracey curette numbering nomenclature

Gracey 1-2	Anterior teeth
Gracey 3-4	Anterior teeth
Gracey 5-6	Anterior and premolar teeth
Gracey 7-8 surfaces	Posterior teeth: buccal and lingual
Gracey 9-10 surfaces	Posterior teeth: buccal and lingual

There are also *prophylactic* (or *"P"*) *series* Gracey curettes. These were originally developed for dental hygienists at a time when their role was limited primarily to supragingival scaling. There is a set of four pairs of these curettes, which are designed with slightly heavier shanks (3). They have had limited popularity in routine use, as most hygienists prefer the standard series of Gracey curettes.

The *Turgeon Modified* Gracey curettes have a more triangular cross-section. This is due to the lower lateral surface's being flat instead of rounded. This provides a more acute active cutting blade angle that may furnish a superior cutting effect. The dual flat surfaces (face and lower lateral surfaces) forming the active blade result in ease of sharpening.

The *hoe* is used to remove large deposits of supragingival calculus in a pull stroke. It has one cutting edge, usually at a 99–100° angle to the shank. Although it has no pointed tip to lacerate the soft tissues, its overall bulk and size do not readily lend it to subgingival work. When the gingival margin is distended and the sulcus sufficiently open, it can be used carefully below the gum line.

The *chisel*, which has limited use in veterinary dental prophylaxis, has a heavy shank and one straight cutting edge on the leading surface. Designed for removal of heavy supragingival calculus from the facial surface of the anterior teeth, chisels can also be used to some extent in the interproximal spaces. They are used in a pushing horizontal stroke across the teeth. They should never be used subgingivally or with vertical strokes toward the gingiva, as a slipped movement can seriously lacerate the soft tissues.

The *periodontal file* also has a limited usage. It is designed to fragment large supragingival calculus deposits by crushing them. It can also be used to smooth exposed root surfaces, but its size usually prohibits its use subgingivally. It has multiple cutting blades angled at 90–105° to the shank.

With both curettes and scalers, it is essential to keep the working edge clean and sharpened. Carbide instruments tend to sharpen more easily and have a better cutting edge, but they do not maintain the edge as well a stainless steel does, due to corrosion if not well maintained. Stainless steel varieties resist rusting better, maintaining their edge longer than carbide steel, but do sharpen well. After each use, the instrument should be rinsed, scrubbed, dried, sharpened, and sterilized appropriately.

Sharpening

Sharpening hand instruments is an art unto itself but, once mastered, provides the optimum working conditions, since a dull instrument tends to burnish calculus, not remove it, and will result in greater operator fatigue (6,7).

The devices used for sharpening are either natural or artificial, and mounted or unmounted (8). The Arkansas oilstone is a fine-textured natural stone. Aloxite, India, ruby, and diamond are artificial stones that typically have a coarse texture. Ceramic stones (not actually stones) are artificial, consisting of a metal alloy (aluminum oxide) with a relatively fine surface texture. The coarser stones are used to recontour very dull instruments, with the finer stones used for the final smooth cutting edge of the instruments.

Stones come in numerous styles: unmounted flat and conical, and mounted conical and wheels. The mounted stones are on mandrels, used on a slow-speed handpiece for rapid recontouring. Unmounted stones are customarily preferred, as they are kinder to the instrument by removing less metal in the sharpening process.

The most commonly used stone for sharpening is Arkansas stone with fine grit that produces a smooth finish (9). India stone may be either fine or medium, the latter being used only for very dull instruments because it will wear away excessive amounts of metal. Once the stone is lightly oiled and wiped, the cutting edge of the curette is held to form an angle of approximately 100–110° between the face of the instrument and the stone, to conform to the curve where the back meets the face. Either the instrument or the stone can be moved; in effect the instrument may be drawn back and forth in short strokes, rocking from the portion of the head closest to the shank on through to the toe. At that point, the angulation of the instrument should be at about 45°, with gentle contouring of the toe with the final strokes. With universal curettes, where the face is perpendicular to the shank and both edges can be used, both should be sharpened (10).

A scaler is sharpened in basically the same fashion, but sharpening ends instead at the sharp tip, without changing the angulation. To remove any spurs that might have formed on the edges, a conical stone may be lightly rotated along the face of the instrument by holding the toe or tip away from your body and rolling the stone toward you on the face. Except for this and for quick touch-ups during an actual procedure, or if no other method is known, face sharpening should generally not be used as the primary maintenance. Rotating the conical stone on the face removes too much of the instrument, weakening it prematurely and even changing the angle of the curette edge.

Periodontal files are most often sharpened with a jeweler's tang file. Each of the multiple blades must be sharpened individually. The tang file is used with horizontal reciprocal strokes.

To examine blade sharpness, there are two basic clinical criteria: the shave test and the visual test. With the shave test, the blade is engaged with light pressure on an acrylic test stick. Sharp instruments will either bite into the stick or shave a thin slice off it, while dull instruments will do neither. The use of a fingernail as a test stick should be discouraged, for hygienic reasons. The visual test involves examining the blade's reflectivity to light. Sharp instrument blades do not reflect light, while dull edges do. Magnification can be used to improve the visual inspection.

Explorers can be sharpened with an unmounted conical or flat stone, or a mounted hollow conical stone (Getz Explorer Sharpener, Teledyne, Elk Grove Village, Illinois). With the conical stone, the explorer is held steady and the stone is twirled around the tip at a slight angle. With the flat stone, the tip is placed against the surface at a 15° angle and drawn across the stone, while it is rotated to assure an even sharpening. The mounted sharpeners are placed on the slow-speed straight dental handpiece. It is then rotated at <5000 revolutions per minute (rpm), and the explorer tip is inserted into the hollow tip at a slight angle. Their sharpness can be assessed by gently pressing the point into the flat end of an acrylic stick to see if it sinks into it slightly.

Oral Irrigators

Oral irrigators have been used and recommended for over a century in various forms. There is little evidence indicating these are effective in reducing plaque, calculus, gingivitis, or periodontal disease, when used with water only (11,12). When used with other chemicals and medicaments, they can be of benefit. Water and saline irrigation of the sulcus in the presence of established periodontal infection has been shown to stimulate bacterial migration into the bordering bloodstream. Therefore, they should be used with care in patients with advanced periodontal disease and predisposition to bacteremia, especially those with cardiac conditions (13).

OPERATIVE HAND INSTRUMENTS

These are the hand-held instruments used in cavity preparation, placement of restoratives, and finishing restoratives (14). They are typically explorers, gauges, and cutting and smoothing tools, generally available in single- and double-ended types. They have a handle, shank, and working end, as most other hand-held instruments. The working end on cutting instruments is called the *blade*, while on restorative tools used to place, compact, or smooth materials, it is called the *nib* (15). *Dr. Black's instrument numbering formula* is a universally accepted three- or four-number formula for identification of cutting instrument. For an instrument labeled 10-7-14, the first number indicates the width of the blade in tenths of a millimeter (10 = 1.0 mm), the second number represents the blade length in whole millimeters (7 mm), and the third number designates the angle the blade forms to the long axis of the handle or shaft in degrees centigrade (14°C). When a fourth number is used, eg 10-95-7-14, it is placed between the first and second numbers. This usage is applied to instruments, such as margin trimmers, on which the cutting edge does not form a right angle (eg, 25°C). This number represents the angle of the cutting edge of the blade to the long axis of the handle (95°C) (14,15). Operative instruments include chisels, hoes, hatchets, margin trimmers, angle formers, excavators, condensers, burnishers, and carving instruments. The shaft angulation of these may be straight, bayonet, monangle, binangle, or triple-angled (16).

Dental operative cutting instruments are usually classified according to shape and function. *Discoid* indicates a disc-shaped excavator used to cut or dig out diseased dentin in a cavity preparation. *Cleoid* denotes a claw-shaped instrument used to form corners in a cavity preparation. Discoid and cleoid nibs are commonly on opposite ends of the same instrument. *Spoons* are designed like an ordinary kitchen spoon, but the entire margin is sharp and used to cut and remove dentin. *Hatchets* are used to cut grooves in dentin for restorative retention. *Chisels* are used only in a push motion and can be used on dentin or enamel that is undermined, such as the Wedelstaedt (curved) chisel. *Angle formers* are used to emphasize line and point angles in internal form of the cavity preparation. *Hoes* are used only on the pull stroke to cut dentin in the axial wall of the preparation. *Gingival margin trimmers* are modified hatchets used in a sideways motion to bevel the cervical cavosurface for inlays or amalgam preparations (17).

RESTORATIVE INSTRUMENTS AND EQUIPMENT

While extractions are certainly warranted in many cases, the ability to preserve teeth and restore them to a relatively normal structure and function is a growing discipline. Instruments for restorative procedures vary from those that remove or recontour dental structure to those that handle, mix, and even cure restorative materials.

In some restorative attempts, such as upper fourth premolar slab fracture or cuspid buildup, retention must be provided in order to keep the material in place. Placement of pins and posts will be discussed in the restorative chapter.

While the use of amalgam is not as popular as it has been in years past or as it is in human dentistry, with the proper skills and tools it can be beneficial. *Amalgamators* that accomplish the rapid mixing of the alloy should be fairly recent models to adapt to the newer materials, including some encapsulated glass ionomers. Any discrepancy in mixing speed or timing will produce an inferior product, so instructions should be followed closely. Once triturated, the amalgam is placed in an *amalgam well*, where the alloy is picked up by an *amalgam carrier* for transfer to the prepared site. Amalgam should be carefully introduced into the carrier and not condensed; otherwise, it will not be easily extruded when the plunger is depressed. Carriers should be thoroughly cleaned with cotton swabs or paper points to avoid residual debris being trapped, and tips should be replaced when needed. Plastic-tipped carriers can also be used to transport difficult to handle composites, powders (calcium hydroxide), and semisolids (calcium hydroxide mixed in saline). *Retrograde carriers* with small tips are helpful in the placement of apex closure materials in the restricted spaces of a surgical or retrograde endodontic procedure. The long, narrow delivery system of the Messing root canal gun may provide for the introduction of amalgam through the coronal aspect to fill the entire length of the canal; however, this practice is no longer common. A plastic, "no-plug" carrier is also available (17).

Once placed in the defect, amalgam must be condensed to force it into voids and internal line angles, as well as to remove excess mercury. The different sizes and shapes of *condensers* can adapt to various needs; a large size is used for spherical alloys. Once condensed, *amalgam carvers* help to shape and trim the amalgam of any excess material, especially on the margins. Depending on the product, use of *amalgam burnishers* must sometimes be delayed until the "set" is completed. By providing a very smooth surface, however, appropriate use of burnishers can help slow down plaque accumulation that would be more rapid with a rougher surface.

Other dental materials such as composites and glass ionomers have specific instruments to be worked with. *Plastics-filling* or *-working instruments* allow some shaping of the material before curing, as can mylar strips, to minimize the amount of contouring necessary after curing. Products can be mixed on disposable paper pads or on glass slabs, which are helpful with certain cements, especially if the slab is cooled (eg, zinc phosphates). Delivery systems such as Jiffy Tubes (Teledyne Getz, Elk Grove Village, Illinois) and curved tip syringes may facilitate the placement of materials in or on teeth.

Many dental materials have the capacity to be light cured, and except for the expense of the light gun, the advantages of allowing ample time to work with the material before curing and yet having a very rapid curing time with reduced polymerization shrinkage make them indispensable in a busy practice. Older lights are in the ultraviolet range of 325–350 nanometers (nm), but most guns are now in the visible or near-red range of 400–450 nm (18,19). They can come as pistol-type models or with a fiberoptic cord that allows a larger fan in the handle, decreasing the likelihood of bulb burnout. The fiberoptic cord is thicker but the fibers are delicate, and breakage can lead to a diminished light output. Some have adjustable time exposure with a one-button touch, continuous "on" cycle, but others must have the button depressed for the entire curing time. Those with a higher energy output have better penetration with a deeper cure, but the safety concern of limiting retinal exposure, important in every model, is even more crucial with this type. The small shield tips help block out the light and are not cumbersome, but some light can still shine out, so using larger shields with protective eyewear is a good idea. When curing the material, the filter should never touch the material; otherwise, material will cure onto the filter and is very difficult to remove without damaging the filter. Regular filter inspection (with the light off, of course) is important, and it should look like a little purple mirror. If any holes are present, the filter should be replaced. A yearly inspection with a light-analysis tool to evaluate the light's intensity is ideal, but the equipment to do so is expensive.

MODELS AND IMPRESSIONS

Using the proper impression materials is always important, but appropriate trays also make a difference. Ideally, a tray should be rather rigid and just large enough to fit the width and depth of the oral structures to be examined. No teeth should touch the sides or bottom of the tray, yet there should not be excessive spaces that the impression material should have to fill. Keeping the amount of impression material to a relative minimum is especially important for the alginates because extra material may lead to excessive instability or shrinkage (17). Tray rigidity will also decrease distortion of the impression, as will vents or holes in the tray to allow for outflow extrusion, which helps lock the impression in place in the tray. There are a number of varieties of specially designed veterinary trays that approximate the majority of mouth sizes that may be encountered. For unusually shaped mouths, a custom tray material, such as tray acrylics and malleable plastics, may be needed to fabricate a tray for that particular instance. Some human trays can be used for limited impression areas and are generally less expensive. The lack of commercial trays for individual crown impressions of large cuspids has resulted in syringe casing and other materials being used. Individual tooth and full-mouth impression of exotic and large animals requires even more ingenuity and imagination for success.

For the mixing of both alginate and even dental stone, the flexible bowls are indispensable for proper spatulation and ease of cleaning. A variety of spatulas may be used depending on operator preference, from the highly flexible plastic spatulas to those made of metal with varying degrees of stiffness. For delivery of the material into trays (alginate) or into the impression (stone), these spatulas may also be used, but smaller dental spatulas work best when stone is first poured in small amounts to fill in individual teeth.

With the pouring of stone into impressions, it is virtually impossible to avoid large bubbles and voids if a *vibrator* is not used. This is especially important when the teeth are initially filled. The vibration effect also helps with the "flowability" of the stone as it is placed in small increments on the impressions and allowed to flow into the depressions.

Once poured and set, the model can be released from the impression (and the impressions from the tray) with the spatulas or impression knives. Plaster nippers can help remove some of the excess stone material, but care must be taken not to break the model. An *electric model trimmer* with a grinding disc and water flow can provide a cosmetically pleasing, articulating, and mountable model, but the plaster traps must catch the slurry water to prevent blockage of drain pipes. If used properly, the trimmer may also be used to block off the model at its caudal extent, with both halves in proper articulation. Heavy curettes are useful in removing and popping off small accumulations of stone that may have filled bubbles in the impression material.

Proper articulation for an individual can be marked with ink on the models, or a bite registration may be taken with softened wax or rapid-setting impression material after extubation; but the patient's air intake should never be compromised. Once correctly marked, the two models can be positioned on an articulator, a hinged device that can hold the models in alignment to verify crown and appliance fit.

ORTHODONTICS

In the making of some devices, with the proper skills and soldering units and welders, a practitioner may design custom appliances. While this takes a lot of time to become proficient, the ability to control the quality of the product and to make on-site adjustments is advantageous (9).

In *bracket* or *button* application, bracket holders allow manipulation of the device, while limiting digital contact, particularly in hard-to-reach areas. On small or conical teeth, the *three-prong (triple-beak) pliers*, which are normally used to adjust heavy wires, can also be carefully used to put a slight curvature on the bracket to maximize contact with the tooth. Other wire-bending instruments include *Howe pliers* for holding wires or making freeform bends, and *bird-beak pliers* with one round tip and one flat tip to make round and angular bends, respectively. *Tweed loop-forming pliers* also can make round bends of various diameters depending on which area of the tip is used. Heavier laboratory work with arch wires may require *Tweed arch-adjusting pliers*. Appliances can be removed with special pliers that have protective nylon caps on the larger beak or crown pullers that utilize tapping vibrations to loosen the cement's hold. Care must always be taken not to injure any teeth or soft tissue. Other necessary equipment includes wire cutters, crown calipers, and sticky wax (17).

SURGICAL INSTRUMENTS

With all the power instruments available, a veterinary dentist still relies on many other hand-held instruments and equipment in other disciplines. Surgical procedures in the oral cavity often involve some of the tough, fibrous tissues and even bone. Standard scalpel blades, especially ones with smaller, thinner cutting edges (No.11, No.12B, No.15, and No.15C), are useful to trim and contour small amounts of tissue. Often, specific surgical knives with various angulations can be used, such as an Orban knife for cutting periodontal tissues and surgical hoes used to detach gingival collars incised by the knives. *Periodontal pocket markers* are frequently used to mark sulcal depth prior to gingivectomies. These look similar to college pliers except that the tips have an inwardly directed point. They are inserted to the bottom of a gingival pocket and then pinched together, leaving an indentation in the gingival tissue externally indicating the pocket depth. These can then be used to guide the appropriate depth for gingivectomies.

For contouring thick, cut edges or trimming smaller areas, fluted burs and diamond points on a high-speed handpiece can provide a smooth finish, with a variety of bur and point shapes. With any gingival trimming, applying a topical anesthetic or gingival dressing (tincture of myrrh and benzoin) is recommended to diminish discomfort.

Surgical scissors of various types are useful in the oral cavity, including the sharp-sharp, slightly curved blade of the Goldman-Fox No.15. Working with oral tissues can often dull the cutting edges, so regular maintenance and sharpening of the scissors and gingival knives will be necessary.

In procedures that require the lifting or manipulation of gingival flaps, the sharp, broad, thin blades of periosteal elevators or surgical curettes are functional in reflecting the mucoperiosteum while preserving the soft tissue with the convex side. The blade or working end of the elevator may vary in size to accommodate different needs, but they should be kept sharpened to be most effective.

When the term *elevator* is used in dentistry, the instruments that usually first come to mind are dental elevators used during exodontia. The function of an elevator is exactly as the name implies—to elevate the tooth or root section out of the alveolus during extraction. Once the epithelial attachment is severed with a blade, elevators are used as levers or wedges between tooth and bone or adjacent teeth or teeth segments to fatigue the periodontal ligament and its connection to the tooth. The concave edges are kept sharp with conical stones to facilitate their placement in the periodontal space between the tooth and alveolus. In human dentistry, there are as many elevator shapes as there are tooth surfaces (and people to design them), but staying with a smaller number with moderate-size variations (small, medium, large) will usually suffice. *Dental luxators* have a wider, more delicate blade than elevators and are also used in the periodontal space to sever the periodontal ligament attachment. It is used in a light rocking motion, while being pushed apically; however, it should never be used with any force in a lever or wedge action, as this can result in bending or fracturing of the instrument's working head.

Specialized elevators, such as the narrow, sharp *root tip picks* can be introduced into the alveolus to carefully loosen retained or broken root tips. They are much more delicate and should be used with a very light touch, particularly avoiding excessive apical pressure that could force the sharp tips beyond the alveolus.

Once tooth sections are loosened, they can be gently grasped by *extraction forceps* specifically designed for veterinary use. Human dental extraction forceps come in many configurations but are usually concave in design for grasping the neck of the tooth below the bulge of the crown; therefore, they do not fit well with animals' conically shaped teeth. Some of the smaller veterinary models ("cat forceps") might be preferable, because the operator is less likely to try to use excessive force on teeth that are not yet loosened sufficiently.

Electrosurgery, Electrocautery, and Radiosurgery Units

These units are designed to produce a high-frequency electrical current to cut or destroy tissue (frequencies >10,000 hertz [Hz] or 10 kHz). Use of frequencies <10,000 Hz can be dangerous to the patient. Most units currently in use work in the 2–4 million-Hz range (2–4 MHz) on a electromagnetic radiofrequency. The term *radiosurgery* is usually reserved for units in which the ground acts as an antenna, meaning that the ground antenna does not always need to be in contact with the patient to provide a functional grounding effect. Grounding can come from the table, as the ground lead simply provides a more efficient passage of current through the patient. The grounding can be between the instrument tip and patient (unipolar) and the two parts of the instrument tip (bipolar).

The degree of desiccation of tissues is determined by power settings and the type of tip used. The units are very effective in controlling many hemorrhage problems. Care must be exerted not to overcauterize the tissue, causing thermal injury to adjacent soft and hard tissues. With electrosurgical units, interference with fulguration effect and dissemination of large amounts of heat to adjacent tissues can occur when attempts are made for use on larger tumors close to hard tissue. Therefore, electrosurgical units are best used in periodontal surgeries of smaller lesions, such as fibrous epulides, and slight-to-mild gingival hyperplasia. Damage to the periodontal ligament and burning of dental cementum can be avoided by attention being paid to maintaining appropriate unit settings, probing depth, biological width (1–2 mm), and attached gingiva (2 mm). Dental electrosurgical units are currently evaluated by ANSI/ADA Specification No.44, which is helps to assure both safety and efficiency (18).

Electrosurgical Currents

There are presently four different current types commercially available. Not all electrosurgical units are capable of producing all four current types.

Fully Rectified Current. The mode of action of this current provides easy cutting of most oral soft tissues, while providing a good degree of hemostasis. It is used for the following procedures:

A. Gingivectomy
B. Gingivoplasty
C. Palatal soft tissue surgery
D. Frenectomy
E. Fibrous epulis removal.

Fully Filtered Current. This current, the least traumatic of the four currents, is used for delicate cutting but provides little hemostasis or coagulation effect. It is used for the following:

A. Widening of the gingival sulcus for crowns, etc.
B. Gingival grafting
C. Biopsy specimens
D. Any surgery close to cementum or bone.

Partially Rectified Current. This is used to coagulate tissues for hemostasis, as well as for electrophoresis effects to stimulate solutions to penetrate hard tissues. It is useful for the following:

A. Coagulation of soft tissue bleeding problems
B. Bleaching of endodontically treated teeth
C. Desensitizing dentin and cementum.

Fulgurating Current (Sparking Current). This is a spark-gap technique used at high-power settings. It is the most destructive of the four current types described. It may be used for the following:

A. Hemostasis involving osseous surgical sites
B. Destruction of cyst remnants
C. Destruction of fistulous tract linings.

Advantages and Disadvantages. The main advantages of fulgurating current are speed, hemostasis, good healing, and improved clear field. Its disadvantages are odor, shock hazards, and restricted use around flammable products.

Contraindications. The use of fulgurating current is contraindicated in the following situations:

1. Operation within 16 feet of certain pacemakers. The radiofrequency wave can interfere with the frequency output of unshielded pacemakers of not only the patient but also the operator, assistants, and spectators.
2. Previous radiation therapy to the area. In patients who have had radiation therapy in the area to be worked on (head and neck for dentistry), the decreased vascularization in the area can easily lead to radionecrosis.
3. Use in the presence of flammable or explosive chemicals or materials (ie, ether, alcohols, etc.).

Harmonic Scalpels

Harmonic scales are ultrasonic units operating usually at or above 45 kHz. Most have titanium blades that cut by the use of kinetic energy. They provide a highly controllable depth of tissue kill that presently can only be matched by certain lasers. However, they are currently cost prohibitive.

POWER EQUIPMENT

While hand instruments typically cause the least amount of damage to the teeth, their use is often slow in all but the most experienced hands. The development of mechanized, power dental instruments is constantly advancing, making instrumentation easier, quicker, and more precise in most cases.

Scalers

Powered scalers are the most common powered dental equipment used by veterinarians. They are used either parallel to the tooth or at an angle of <15° to it (8). The ADA Council on Dental Materials, Instruments, and Equipment has grouped these into three major categories: type A, type B, and type C (19). Type A powered scalers are the ultrasonics, either magnetostrictive or piezoelectric. Type B scalers are the mechanical scalers, either sonics (Titan-S, Star Dental, Valley Forge, Pennsylvania) or rotary (Roto-Pro™, Ellman Co., Hewlett, New York). Type C scalers are hydraulic (Prophy-Jet™, Dentsply International, York, Pennsylvania) (19,20).

Ultrasonic Scalers

Ultrasonic dental scalers generally function at >20 kHz. The terms *ultrasonic* and *supersonic* are scientifically somewhat synonymous, meaning "beyond or above sound." However, supersonic is customarily used to denote speeds greater than the speed of sound (738 mph), while ultrasonic is most commonly used to denote vibration frequencies (sound) beyond those audible by the human ear, such as frequencies of 20 kHz or greater. Ultrasonic scalers work by two basic principles: mechanical kick and cavitation. The mechanical kick is the actual effect of the metal tip contacting the calculus, while the water spray hitting the vibrating tip is energized to cavitate or clean the tooth surface—and possibly affecting bacterial integrity as well. There are two varieties of ultrasonic scalers, the *magnetostrictive* and the *piezoelectric.* Two types of magnetostrictive units are available: ferromagnetic stack and ferrite rod. Ferromagnetic stacks are strips of laminated nickel that shorten and lengthen approximately 0.001 inch when stimulated by alternating current electromagnetic energy (19). This vibration or oscillation moves the tip in an elliptoid, figure-8 pattern, which sometimes results in the tip not contacting the tooth completely. The ferrite rod ultrasonic scalers use a titanium tip and produce an elliptical circular pattern. It is generally considered that the more elliptical the tip pattern, the fewer potentially unstruck or dead-zones in the movement. Ultrasonics generally work with frequencies that often range from 20 kHz to 45 kHz, with stacks averaging 25 kHz (9) and rods 42 kHz. Both types generate heat that may harm the tooth (21), so water irrigation as a coolant is always necessary. This energized water spray provides the cavitation effect, but the aerosolization of debris and bacteria necessitates protection for both the patient (cuffed endotracheal tube) and operator (face shield, mask, gloves). In most models, the area of maximum vibration and the spot where the water exits (point of frequency) is about one inch from the tip, but newer models have water exiting from the tip. Ultrasonic scalers should be used with care and with appropriate tips subgingivally due to heat generation and lack of irrigation at the tip of the majority of scalers. Newer improved units with slim-line design and coolant liquid better directed to the tip lessen the chance of damage in the sulcus and provide sulcal irrigation with water or special medicaments.

For maintenance, all manufacturers' recommendations should be followed closely. The removable tips must be replaced at times, and regular inspection of the stack will show any bulging and splaying of the strips, or even a break in the soldering, which would warrant replacement of the entire stack (Fig. 7). Additionally, many companies imprint the date of manufacture on the stack, which aids in determining its useful life.

Another variety of ultrasonic scaler, the piezoelectric, utilizes the expansion and contraction of quartz crystals to commonly provide frequencies of 20–45 kHz, with a curved linear tip movement (20). Units developed before the mid-1970s had crystal failure problems due to design problems. Newer versions protect the crystals by silver coating and sandwiching them between pieces of stainless steel separated with thick aluminum spacers (22). The optional water flow to cool the tooth surface exits at the focal point of frequency about 1–5 mm from the tip, so the spray is generally directed in a subgingival direction.

Sonic Scalers

Sonic or, more correctly, *subsonic* scalers operate when pressurized air passes through the shaft and out a hole, causing a metal sleeve (rotor) that encircles the shaft to spin, creating a oval–elliptical tip oscillation generally at much less than 20 kHz. Very little heat is produced at these frequencies, and since there is minimal cavitation effect as well (10), water is delivered primarily for irrigation, not cooling. The cost of these scalers is one drawback, and this pertains not only to the handpiece itself but also to the air-delivery unit of the high-speed handpiece that must provide a minimum of 30–40 pounds per square inch (psi) to the scaler in order for it to be effective (22). The psi requirement may be one reason studies vary on the reported effectiveness of such models (21,23), but if used correctly, they can be very effective and potentially less damaging to the tooth structure. Daily lubrication is important, and while broken rotors are easily replaced, the tip must not be tightened with anything but fingers; otherwise, the shaft may break and its replacement is costly.

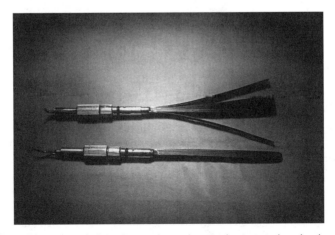

FIG. 7. Magnetostrictive ultrasonic scaler stacks: normal and splayed.

Rotary Scalers

Another form of scaling that utilizes the high-speed handpiece on an air-driven unit is the rotary bur, a six-sided, noncutting soft-steel bur. At a speed of 300,000 rpm with six sides hitting during each rotation, this translates into a frequency similar to ultrasonic units (about 30 kHz) (20). With a very light touch, and a nondulled bur, these impacts help to rapidly vibrate the calculus loose. Even with water for cooling, however, this is potentially the most damaging scaling method (24). Minimizing the amount of time spent on a tooth at any one time (10–12 seconds maximum) and avoiding direct contact of the bur with the tooth surface will help limit the harm done. Teeth that are small (feline) or have enamel deficits (hypocalcification/hypoplasia) should not be cleaned with this instrument; otherwise, excessive amounts of dental tissue can be removed. At this practice, rotary burs are only used to carefully help remove deposits of orthodontic bonding materials. If the burs are not changed regularly, they will tend only to burnish the calculus, even with increased working pressure from the operator. Therefore, with the switch to a new, sharp bur, great care must be taken to decrease the force with which the instrument had been previously used. This system must only be used by experienced operators with an extremely delicate touch.

Hydraulic Scalers

Hydraulic scalers work as a water and abrasive stream on the tooth to "sandblast" the tooth clean. Many are handpieces that accept a cartridge of a fine baking soda power. They may attach to the high-speed air and water line of the dental unit. Water funneled through a jet pulls the baking soda crystals into the water stream to abrade debris from the tooth surface. Care should be taken, as baking soda crystal can be blown into the soft tissues, causing irritation and swelling, or even into salivary ducts where more serious inflammatory responses can be expected. Baking soda (sodium bicarbonate) is contraindicated in patients who need to restrict sodium intake. The stream should be directed away from the soft tissues and kept on the tooth (19).

All of the aforementioned scaling methods, from hand to rotary scaling, cause some degree of damage to the enamel surface, so light polishing scaling is usually recommended.

Dental Power and Handpieces

Electric Motor Units

Some of the earliest dental machines had bands driven by electric motors. While fairly inexpensive, small, and portable, they are slow and have no water source for cooling, and the belts tend to break. At 3–30,000 rpm, they are currently usually only used for lab work. Cable-driven handpieces have the same advantages and disadvantages and, at speeds of <3,000 rpm, are typically useful only for polishing.

A moderately heavier dental case load will require slightly more advanced equipment. One step up from the bench motors are the handpieces with micromotors built in. A little more expensive (yet less than an air-driven unit), this type of handpiece provides speeds in the range of 3,000–35,000 rpm with a control unit that is small and portable and requires little maintenance. Some models incorporate an ultrasonic scaler along with the micromotor to allow routine use for scaling and polishing combined. For heavy work, such as cutting teeth, it is slow, and water must be provided from an external source for cooling and lubrication. With excessive use, breakdowns can be a problem, and the handpiece can become difficult to hold due to heat and weight in the worker's hands. With the vibration and higher torque (the ability to continue rotating even when pressed against a firm surface) experienced, the bur can tend to "walk off" the tooth if not held firmly (10). Newer versions can go up to 100,000 rpm, but with more torque than air-driven models and no water source, the generated heat can be a factor for concern. Handpieces with the high torque are less likely to stall under load. Using steel burs, they are too slow to cut enamel efficiently and can cause chipping of tooth structure (9). Some of these problems can be overcome with the use of diamond-coated burs or points.

Air-Driven Units

The air-driven units are the fastest and most effective of the dental-drive types. Basically, such a unit takes air either from a compressor or pressurized tank and delivers it through tubing into handpieces. The air, along with water, also acts as a coolant for the handpiece and the bur or instrument tip making contact with the tooth surface. Compressed-gas drives are more versatile and have the high-speed capability that makes many procedures quicker and easier. Their biggest disadvantages are cost, size, and in some models noise. Additionally, the aerosolization of the water (and bacteria) may also be a potential problem.

Units powered by compressors vary according to their size and form. They are generally rated by horsepower (hp) but should attain a minimum of 30–40 psi, at 3 cubic feet per minute at the handpiece level. Many types of compressors are available, each varying in size, cost, output, and noise. Less expensive compressors are frequently as effective as their more expensive counterparts, but commonly produce excessive noise. If they can be isolated away from the practitioner and the patient, they can work satisfactorily. However, if the unit is to be close to the operator, a quiet-type compressor should be used. Many of the smaller quiet models ($^1/_2$-hp refrigerator compressor) do not hold up well to heavy use, having problems with overheating. Some smaller models have an on/off electric foot switch to activate the compressor as needed chairside but have no air storage. Most medium-powered compressors ($^3/_4$ hp) have rheostats, and a preset pressure switch allows the tank to fill to a pressure level of approximately 80–120 psi. Regulators allow delivery of a measured 30–40 psi to the handpieces and can be adjusted. In heavy use, these units can also have problems with overheating.

Larger heavy-duty compressors can be very effective but require a location with adequate ventilation to store the louder compressors connected with tubing to the units. Such compressors provide few limits to the amount of work that can be done, but it should be noted that the requirements of multiple sonic scalers used simultaneously may be too much for all but the largest of units. Additionally, compressor units housed outside with lines running inside have more moisture condensation problems due to the temperature variation. To provide larger volumes of compressed air without the noise problem, many manufacturers have begun using two or three of the smaller quiet compressors mounted on a manifold system to provide for one larger storage tank.

There are many other variations in compressor operation and maintenance to choose from. Many models contain oil for lubrication and therefore require regular checking of oil levels, either through a dipstick method or with view ports for level indication. Oil filters and special synthetic oils are often required, so always follow the manufacturer's recommendations carefully, especially with some that state that they are "oil-less" and yet still have some oil requirements. Even with careful use, oil can enter the air delivery system, damaging the air lines and turbines (22), so in-line filters should be employed here as well. True oil-free compressors that are air-cooled frequently involve less maintenance but generally are more expensive and often noisier.

Water may also collect in the compressed air, especially with reserve tanks, and therefore in-line filters should be used to remove moisture as well. Related condensation tends to build up and must be drained periodically. Automatic drain valves require less "hands-on" maintenance and may decrease the chance for internal tank corrosion, but they can breakdown as well. Desiccant canisters and/or beads may be used with larger storage tanks to help remove excess moisture.

In larger systems, the water source for high-speed handpiece irrigation and the three-way water/air syringe is typically from the local water source. With these units, water filters should be used and changed regularly to minimize the amount of minerals and debris moving through the system. Adequate filtration of the air supply should keep water and oil contamination to a minimum in the three-way syringe as well.

Units using compressed nitrogen instead of a compressor will not have the oil/moisture contamination problems. Although the initial purchase cost is less than a compressor, the cost of additional nitrogen tanks will eventually exceed the start-up costs of a compressor. For limited use, however, compressed nitrogen can be very reasonable, and its portability and independence from an electric source make it ideal for some large and exotic animal field work.

The assembly delivery system or control panel of most units is basically the same. While the minimum of three ports—for a high-speed handpiece, slow-speed handpiece, and three-way syringe—is met in almost every model, quite often one or two additional outlets may be available. Additional high-speed handpieces or sonic scalers are often added, as well as suction units and light-curing units. These accessories may be switched on and off mechanically with a switch, or automatic switching devices may be activated when the handpiece is removed from its stand.

Handpieces

Dental handpieces are designed to hold and provide rotary power to instruments such as dental burs. They are precision instruments usually powered by compressed gases or electric motors (25). Handpieces should be cleaned, lubricated, and sterilized after each use to prolong instrument life and prevent future patient contamination. Almost all handpieces are now constructed of materials that can withstand autoclaving, but the manufacturers' recommendations should be followed concerning sterilization procedures. The *high-speed handpieces* provide greater speed of operation but less tactile sense than the slow-speed units. High speeds can be used for efficient removal of enamel and dentinal, bone, and other hard tissues, while slow speeds are better suited for dentinal tissues when good tactile sense is required for finishing and polishing, placement of certain pins, and laboratory procedures. *Slow-speed handpieces,* when used with burs, produce a more perceptible vibrational effect than the high-speed units, which may cause more pulpal concussion (26). All handpieces commonly produce high-frequency noises, but for hearing safety, they should not be used if the noise level approaches or exceeds 75 decibels (19). Out of concern for the hearing of patient and operator, many of the newer handpieces have improved noise reduction. Regular lubrication is required, and the manufacturers' recommendations should be followed at all times on types of lubrication, locations, and times. Handpieces are currently classified according to speed by the ADA (Table 2).

Handpieces come in three basic types: straight, slow-speed angled, and high-speed angled. *Straight* handpieces used in standard dental procedures usually generate 6000 rpm; however, laboratory models can produce in excess of 100,0000 rpm. Straight handpieces use burs and mandrels placed directly in the nose cone by twisting the locking collar to open the chuck, inserting the instrument shank, and then closing the collar to lock it in place. Many types of dental and surgical cutting and finishing burs, often long models up to 40 mm, can be used in this fashion. Both forward and reverse movements are possible, as indicated by either dots or the letters *R* and *F* marked on the base. Moving the screwhead or dot to the right for forward movement switches the head to counterclockwise rotation (as you look into the bur). The neutral position is in the middle.

The *slow-speed angled handpieces* actually attach to the straight handpiece and are driven by its chucking device. The *contra-angles* (CA) and *right-angles* (RA) change the straight handpiece into an angled handpiece, and their gear systems will change the rpm up or down, typically from between 3,000 rpm and 40,000 rpm. Most of these either have a latch attachment to lock instruments in place or use screw-on or snap-on instruments. *Prophylaxis angles* (right angles) are commonly used on slow-speed handpieces; the head is angled at 90°. There are three main types of angles used for polishing: CA latch, RA snap-on, and RA screw-on. The RA prophylaxis angles are available with either a full 360° continual rotation or an oscillating 90° back-and-forth motion (Prophymatic™, Micro-Mega®, Zurich, Switzerland). The former type is much less expensive, but the unsealed units require regular cleaning and lubrication, with removal of the head and/or cap portions. Disposable plastic and sealed angles are also available. The oscillating-angles type needs no lubrication, reduces the throwing of prophylaxis paste, and does not catch the patient's hair (winding it up on the prophylaxis cup); however, this type is more expensive. Prophylaxis angles may use snap-on, screw-on, or latch-on prophylaxis cups, which come in a variety of shapes and degrees of stiffness. The softer gray cups allow a moderate splaying of the cup foot with minimal pressure.

Contra-angles change the angulation of the handpiece with an initial 25° bend followed by a 90° reverse bend for a net 65° redirection that facilitates access to hard-to-reach areas (120). Speeds can be increased or decreased with selection of the type of CA and desired use. Angles used at <10,000 rpm are typically used for restorative pin placement and polishing; at approximately 20,000 rpm, they are customarily used for sectioning of teeth; and at 30,000 rpm and greater, they are used most commonly for laboratory work. Special CAs known as minimizers or reduction angles are available, the most common of which is the 10:1 reduction angle used in endodontics with spiral

TABLE 2. Handpiece classification by speeds

High speed
    Type I (high speed): 100,000–800,000 rpm
      Class A: >160,000 rpm
      Class B: 100,000–160,000 rpm
Slow speed
    Type II (midspeed): 20,000–100,000 rpm
    Type III (low speed): <20,000 rpm

fillers and Gates-Glidden and Peeso burs or in restorative work with certain drilling burs for pins and self-seating pins. These fillers, burs, and pins have a notched end of the shank to fit into the angle and are secured by the handle's fitting into the latch locking device. Some CAs are adapted to accept the lower-friction grip burs but have no water source for cooling when used for cutting. Some friction grip burs may also be used with a slow-speed/high-speed handpiece adapter that holds the bur in a latch-type CA.

Air-Driven Handpieces

Air-driven units have the ability to act as the drive for either slow- or high-speed handpieces. The slow-speed units can make use of RA and CA handpieces, as well as handpiece burs and instruments. But if there is a need for speed in order to cut teeth and bone more efficiently, the high-speed handpiece with speeds in excess of 400,000 rpm and water cooling is the instrument of choice. Those running between 500,000 rpm and 800,000 rpm are high-speed but are sometimes referred to as ultra-speed handpieces. On standard angled high-speeds, the angulation of the handpiece is changed, with an initial 25° bend followed by a 90° reverse bend for a net 65° redirection. Surgical angled handpieces have a 45° angulation of the head that allows them to be used in a flatter approach to the back of the mouth. These are available in both mid-speed type II (30,000–50,000 rpm) and high-speed type I (400,000 rpm).

The free-running speed of most high-speed handpieces is usually reduced up to 40% under load of cutting, due to their low torque. This is advantageous in that the bur will usually stall when excessive pressure is applied while under load (27). A water flow is used to help dissipate the frictional heat generated by burs in contact with hard tissues at high speeds (25). Seldom is water not used, but the aerosolization of bacteria should be addressed with patient and operator protection, as stated earlier. Without a light touch, continued stalling and thermal damage is distinctly possible. The high-speed handpiece holds friction grip burs (in its turbine) that are changed either with a chuck key in the back of the handpiece head or, in wrenchless models, by depressing the back cap on the head or pressing a lever lightly sideways to release the instrument shaft. Running the handpiece without a bur or blank can cause the turbine shaft grips to totally close down, preventing instrument insertion and ruining the turbine, which may then need repair or replacement. Signs of defective turbines include increased noise or vibration, failure of the chuck to tighten, or complete failure with freeze-up of turbine. Replacement of the turbine is relatively easy to accomplish by loosening the cap-back and pressing on the inserted blank to remove the cartridge and replacing it with a new one. If the turbine housing has been damaged by the defective turbine, the entire handpiece may need replacing. Failure of a replacement turbine to easily slip in place may be an indication of severe scarring of the internal surface or warping of the housing.

Fiberoptic Handpieces

The additional expense of a fiberoptic option for the handpiece may be offset by the enhanced visualization of the working areas; however, potential breakdown of the light source and costly repairs are not unusual. Handpieces with small or mini-heads can be used in areas with limited space.

TABLE 3. Bur shapes and sizes

Shapes	Size numbers
Round (plain or crosscut)	$^1/_4$–11
Wheel	$11^1/_2$–16
Inverted cone	$31^1/_2$–40
Straight fissure, plain	$55^1/_2$–62
Tapered fissure, noncrosscut	169–171
Pear shape	330–333
Rounded crosscut	502–504
Straight fissure, crosscut	556–563
Tapered fissure, crosscut	700–703
End and side cutting	901–903
End cutting	957–959

Burs

Rotary dental instruments with cutting blades as active parts of the operative head are known as burs. All dental burs were made of carbon steel prior to the 1940s. The general availability of tungsten carbide steel burs around 1947 was a major factor in making high-speed dental handpieces practical. Carbon steel burs are initially sharper, but also softer, than carbide steel burs. This makes (carbon) steel burs the preferred type for dentinal work, but their soft metal structure is virtually useless on enamel when used with high-speed handpieces. When applied to enamel, the steel ball disintegrates into a burnt-match-tip appearance almost instantaneously. Only carbide steel holds up well to enamel when used with high speed and maintains its sharpness when doing so. Dental burs are used for excavating dental tissues, occlusal adjustments, bone removal, adjustment of prosthetic appliances, and the shaping and finishing of dental restorations. ADA Specification No.23 covers the size, shape, strength, dimensions, performance characteristics, testing, and evaluation of dental burs, both carbon and carbide (28). Because of the continual development of new bur types, not all are covered in this document. General shapes and sizes of dental burs are recognized by the ADA (Tables 3 and 4).

The friction-grip (FG) high-speed handpiece burs come in standard (FG), short shank (S or SS), miniature (M), long-operating head (L), and surgical-length (SU or SL) shanks, while CA burs come in right-angle slot-locks (RA) and surgical length (SL or SU) and the straight handpiece bur comes in a large straight shank (SH or HP) (Fig. 8). Many of the bur head types are available in each of the bur shank types. Cutting burs have blades and valleys or flutes between each blade. The blade provides the cutting action, while the flutes act as carriers to remove the cut material. Six-fluted burs are used for

TABLE 4. Bur guide

Shank type	Shank diameter (in.)	Shank length (in.)
FG (friction grip)	0.0630	0.768
FG: L (long FG)	0.0630	0.847
FG: SS (short shank FG)	0.0630	0.670
FG: SL or SU (surgical FG)	0.0630	1.004
RA (right angle)	0.0925	0.886
RA: SL or SU (surgical RA)	0.0925	1.023
HP or SH (handpiece)	0.0925	1.772

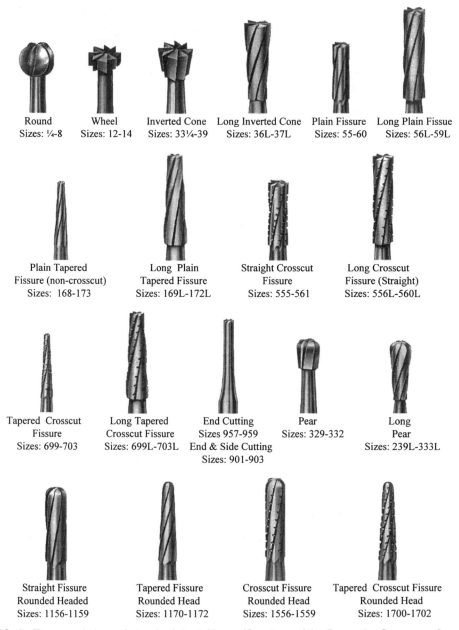

Round   Wheel   Inverted Cone   Long Inverted Cone   Plain Fissure   Long Plain Fissue
Sizes: ¼-8   Sizes: 12-14   Sizes: 33¼-39   Sizes: 36L-37L   Sizes: 55-60   Sizes: 56L-59L

Plain Tapered   Long Plain   Straight Crosscut   Long Crosscut
Fissure (non-crosscut)   Tapered Fissure   Fissure   Fissure (Straight)
Sizes: 168-173   Sizes: 169L-172L   Sizes: 555-561   Sizes: 556L-560L

Tapered Crosscut   Long Tapered   End Cutting   Pear   Long
Fissure   Crosscut Fissure   Sizes 957-959   Sizes: 329-332   Pear
Sizes: 699-703   Sizes: 699L-703L   End & Side Cutting   Sizes: 239L-333L
                                        Sizes: 901-903

Straight Fissure   Tapered Fissure   Crosscut Fissure   Tapered Crosscut Fissure
Rounded Headed   Rounded Head   Rounded Head   Rounded Head
Sizes: 1156-1159   Sizes: 1170-1172   Sizes: 1556-1559   Sizes: 1700-1702

FIG. 8. Types and sizes of standard dental burs. (Courtesy of the Brasseler Company, Savannah, Georgia.)

their rapid cutting action, while ten or more flutes are used for finishing (Fig. 9), with the greater number of flutes providing a smoother finish. Fluted burs with notches cut into them are referred to as crosscut, and studies have shown that crosscut fissure burs are more efficient at removing hard tissue compared with plain-fissure burs (29,30). The shape of the bur determines its optimum function and the type of defect it will create, as does the structure on the tip (9). If the tip of the bur is flat or noncutting, as in fissure and tapered-fissure burs, only the sides do the cutting, and the floor of the preparation is spared. Rounded bur tips result in smoothly rounded internal line angles at the depth of a preparation, while square tips make 90° angles at the junction of the preparation wall and floor, a configuration that is more difficult to fill completely. Internal line angles >90° are formed when tapered burs are used, and angles of <90° result when "undercut" (inverted cone) burs are used.

More specifically, small round burs (size $^1/_4, ^1/_2$) can make marks, undercuts, retention grooves, and cavity preparations in small animals, while larger sizes (1,2,4,6,8) can begin cavity preparations and bulk removal and can even delineate the appropriate depth for a crown-preparation reduction. The inverted cone ($33^1/_2$, 34–39) is wider at the tip but has a flat end that allows undercutting in cavity preparations. The parallel sides of a straight-fissure bur (plain $55^1/_2$–62 and crosscut 556–563) are used for sectioning teeth and will create a cavity preparation with parallel walls. The tapered-fissure burs, whether plain (169–171) or crosscut (699–703L), will produce a cavity preparation without undercuts if used perpendicular to the preparation floor with their narrower tip. They can also be used for tooth sectioning and bulk tissue removal. Pear-shaped burs (330–333) can be used for endodontic access, undercuts, and rounded internal line angles of cavity preparations. Flame or perio-pointed six-sided rotary scaling burs are used to vibrate calculus off, but they can also cut tooth structure if used improperly (see Rotary Scalers above). Electroplating diamond grit onto burs with nickel or chromium provides a superior cutting instrument. While other burs can be cleaned with a special brush, diamond burs need to be run over a wet diamond-cleaning block or stone to remove debris.

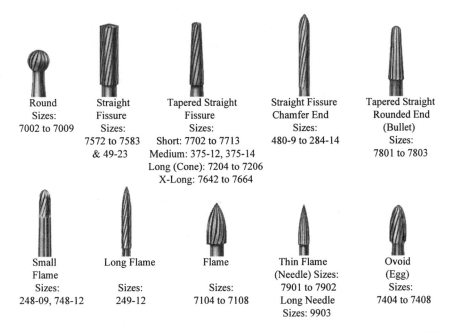

Round	Straight	Tapered Straight	Straight Fissure	Tapered Straight
Sizes:	Fissure	Fissure	Chamfer End	Rounded End
7002 to 7009	Sizes:	Sizes:	Sizes:	(Bullet)
	7572 to 7583	Short: 7702 to 7713	480-9 to 284-14	Sizes:
	& 49-23	Medium: 375-12, 375-14		7801 to 7803
		Long (Cone): 7204 to 7206		
		X-Long: 7642 to 7664		

Small	Long Flame	Flame	Thin Flame	Ovoid
Flame			(Needle) Sizes:	(Egg)
Sizes:	Sizes:	Sizes:	7901 to 7902	Sizes:
248-09, 748-12	249-12	7104 to 7108	Long Needle	7404 to 7408
			Sizes: 9903	

Not Shown: * T-Series: Concave Tapered Flames, Sizes: 7114-T1, 7214-T2, 7714-T3, 7610 to 7613.
* Concave Tapered Blunt Tip, Sizes: 7606.
* Inverted Tapered Cone, Sizes: 7304.

FIG. 9. Types and sizes of 12-bladed finishing burs. (Courtesy of the Brasseler Company, Savannah, Georgia.)

Gates-Glidden drills have a long shaft and flame head to open coronal endodontic access sites. Peeso reamers have a larger torpedo head, and while best used to widen a prepared canal to accept a post, they can make their own path because they do not necessarily follow a preexisting hole, as do Gates-Glidden drills.

Abrasive Points

Abrasive points are rotary instruments that have an abrasive coating on the operative head (Fig. 10). Materials used as abrasives include Carborundum stones, white stones or points, and diamonds.

Silicon carbide (or *green stone*) helps remove rough, bulky areas of a restoration, followed by *white stone* (dense, micrograined aluminum oxide bonded to a shape and mounted on a mandrel) to provide a smooth final surface. These abrasives are very useful for finishing and polishing work on porcelain, metal, enamel, and composites. Discs of flexible molded or cut rubber, plastic, paper, stone, or metal materials can finish restorations, cut teeth, and even adjust occlusional surfaces. These can be on their own straight shafts or can be attached by pop-on or screw-on method to a mandrel that can be used in straight, latch-type, or friction-grip attachments to the slow-speed handpiece. Various rubber or phenolic-resin molded abrasive wheels, sometimes used on mandrels, help in finishing and polishing, particularly with laboratory procedures (9).

Diamond rotary instruments are provided in many of the same shapes and designs as steel burs. The major difference between the steel burs and diamond points concerns the cutting efficiency and heat generated. The diamond is more aggressive and faster than carbon or carbide steel burs. At the same time, the diamond has greater continuous surface contact, thereby generating greater heat, and this increases the potential of frictionally induced thermal pulpitis in the vital tooth (31). Both steel and diamond produce heat, and for this reason, no matter which is used on the high-speed handpiece, adequate air/water spray is mandatory. Furthermore, clean, sharp burs are essential for efficient structural removal expeditiously with the least thermal insult.

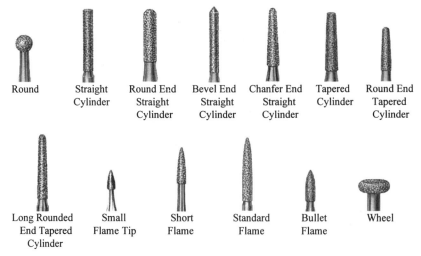

FIG. 10. General shapes of diamond and abrasive points. (Courtesy of the Brasseler Company, Savannah, Georgia.)

Diamond rotary instruments have defied normal classification in the past, with well over 400 types currently available. There is an endless potential variety of shapes, sizes, and coarseness that can be manufactured based on demand. A proposed ADA Specification No.36 for rotary diamonds has been under development by ANSC MD 156 (19). Diamond rotary instruments are available in friction-grip, latch-attachment, and the standard straight handpiece shanks. The diamond grit is applied to the operative head in one to three layers, these being electroplated to the bur blanks with either nickel or chromium bonding material. The classification of fineness to coarseness of the bur is determined by the mesh size of the diamond particles, and in the finer sizes the mesh size is commonly given (eg, 20 mm). Both natural and synthetic diamonds are used, with manufacturers touting the supposed advantages of each. Instruments with extracoarse particles are generally used for removal of connective tissues or bone, as in crown-lengthening procedures. Coarse-grit burs are primarily for the bulk removal of tooth structure. The medium grit, sometimes called regular grit, is the more common type used in routine tooth preparations involving dentin and enamel. The fine-grit instruments are ordinarily used for wall finishing and margin preparation. Extrafine, very fine, and superfine rotary diamond instruments were developed for composite finishing and, if used for crown-preparation work, frequently do not leave a rough enough finish on the tooth for good cementation adherence. A good water flow is recommended to prevent thermal problems with vital teeth and to avoid clogging of the diamond grit bed of the instrument. Diamond burs must be cleaned on a diamond bur cleaning block, while rotating on the handpiece.

Abrasive Strips

These are typically 1–3 mm in width and of various lengths. The strips are commonly made of extremely thin metal and coated with an abrasive material such as sand, garnet, cuttlefish bone, or diamond dust. They are used for interproximal reduction or finishing of restoratives. Lubrication of the strips with petroleum jelly facilitates their placement and ease of movement.

Other Abrasive Materials

Pumice, silex, tin oxide, aluminum oxide, and ferrous oxide are all abrasive materials used in dentistry. Flour of pumice is used to polish teeth, restorations, and acrylics. It commonly has fluoride incorporated into it in prophylaxis pastes. Coarser pumices are sometimes used in stain removal, but they should be used with care as dental structure can rapidly be removed. Silex is a refined silica powder. It is mixed with water and used to reduce scratches on metal castings. Aluminum oxide is used for polishing and finishing restoratives and for air-abrading the internal surface of crowns to enhance bonding strength. Tin oxide is mixed with water and used to produce a high polish in metal restorations. Ferrous oxide (Tripoli or Jeweler's Rouge) is used dry on cloth buffer wheels to place a high-luster finish on metal castings.

REFERENCES

1. Black GV. *Operative Dentistry,* vol II. 8th ed. Woodstock, IL: Medico-Dental Publishing Co; 1947:85.
2. Pattison G, Pattison AM. *Periodontal Instrumentation: A Clinical Manual.* Reston, VA: Reston Publishing Co;1979:17.

3. Nield JS, O'Connor GH. *Fundamentals of Dental Hygiene Instrumentation.* Philadelphia: WB Saunders Co;1983.
4. Stone S, Kalis PJ. Periodontics. In: Dunn MJ, ed. *Dental Auxiliary Practice.* Baltimore:Williams & Wilkins; 1975:126.
5. Simon WJ. *Clinical Dental Assisting.* Hagerstown, MD: Harper & Row Publishing; 1973:200.
6. *Smarten Up, Sharpen Up: A Practical Workbook on Sharpening Dental Curets and Scalers.* Hu-Friedy Department of Professsional Education Chicago, IL; 1982.
7. Aller S. Restore DS-01: Small Animal Dental Instrument Sharpening Kit. Harbor City, CA: VRx Products; 1992.
8. Steele PF. *Dimensions of Dental Hygiene.* 3rd ed. Philadelphia: Lea & Febiger; 1982:143.
9. Holmstrom SE, Frost P, Gammon RL. Dental equipment and care. In: *Veterinary Dental Techniques.* Philadelphia: WB Saunders Co; 1993:23.
10. Harvey CE, Emily PP. Small animal dental equipment and materials. In: *Small Animal Dentistry.* St. Louis, MO: Mosby Yearbook; 1993:378.
11. Krajewski JJ, Giblin J, Gargiulo AW. Evaluation of a water pressure cleaning device as an adjunct to periodontal treatment. *J Periodontics* 1964;2:76.
12. Krajewski JJ, Rubach WC, Pope JW. The effects of water pressure cleaning on the clinically normal gingival crevice. *J So Calif Dent Assoc* 1967;43:452.
13. Feliz JE, Rosen S, App GR. Detection of bacteremia after the use of an oral irrigating device in subjects with periodontitis. *J Periodontol* 1971;42:785.
14. Howard WW, Moller RC. *Atlas of Operative Dentistry.* St Louis, MO: CV Mosby Co; 1981:10.
15. Bell B, Grainger D. *Basic Operative Dentistry Procedures.* 2nd ed. Philadelphia: Lea & Febiger; 1971.
16. Council on Dental Materials and Devices. New American Dental Association Specification No.29: General specification for hand instruments. *JADA* 1976;93:818.
17. Torres HO, Ehrlich A. *Modern Dental Assisting.* 2nd ed. Philadelphia: WB Saunders Co; 1980:403,735.
18. Council on Dental Materials, Instruments and Equipment, American National Standards Institute. American Dental Association Specification No.44 for dental electrosurgical equipment. *JADA* 1980;100:410.
19. *Dentist's Desk Reference: Materials, Instruments, and Equipment.* 2nd ed. Chicago: American Dental Association; 1983:361.
20. *Guide to Dental Materials and Devices.* 6th ed. Chicago: American Dental Association; 1972.
21. Bojrab MJ, Tholen M. *Small Animal Oral Medicine and Surgery.* Philadelphia: Lea & Febiger; 1990:56.
22. Floyd M. Dental operatory design and equipment. In: Spondnick GJ, ed. *Seminars in Veterinary Medicine and Surgery (Small Animal).* Philadelphia: WB Saunders Co; 1993;8(3):129.
23. Grant DA, Stern IB, Listgarten MA. *Periodontics in the Tradition of Gottlieb and Orban.* St.Louis, MO: CV Mosby; 1988:552.
24. Wiggs RB, Lobprise HB. Oral disease. In: Norsworthy GD ed. *Feline Practice.* Philadelphia: J. B. Lippincott Co.; 1993:438.
25. Peyton FA. Status report on dental operating handpieces. *JADA* 1974;89:1162.
26. Walsh JP, Symmons HF. Vibration perception and frequencies. *N Z Dent J* 1949;45:106.
27. Taylor DF, Perkins RR, Kumpula JW. Characteristics of some air-turbine handpieces. *JADA* 1974;89:1162.
28. Council on Dental Materials and Devices. Revised ADA Specification No.23 for dental burs. *JADA* 1975;90:459.
29. Eames WB, Nale JL. A comparison of cutting efficiency of air drive burs. *JADA* 1973;86:412.
30. Luebke NH, Chan KC, Bramson JB. The cutting effectiveness of carbide fissure burs on teeth. *J Prosthet Dent* 1980;43:42.
31. Reder BS, Eames WB. The cutting rates and durability of diamond stones. *J Dent Res* 1976;55(B):B186. Abstract 499.

2

Basic Materials and Supplies

Robert B. Wiggs, Heidi B. Lobprise, and John J. Hefferren

Veterinary dentistry requires scientific knowledge and skills, but also involves some artistic abilities using various dental materials as the medium. An entire listing of individual dental materials is nearly impossible to compile because practically every day new or changed products are being introduced. This chapter will discuss basic categories of materials, including the composition, properties, and usage of individual products where applicable.

ENDODONTIC MATERIALS

While the most common supplies used during endodontic therapy may be instruments, such as files and reamers, there are many products that are necessary in the preparation, sterilization, and obturation of the pulp cavity.

In preparation and sterilization, lubricants, inorganic chelators, organic dissolvers, and antibacterials are used. Various products can be used as lubricants, such as KY-Jelly™ (Johnson & Johnson). These act not only as a lubricant but also as an emulsifier of pulpal tissues. The chelating agent most commonly used is ethylenediaminetetraacetic acid (EDTA) in a solution, paste, or gel. Some of the more common are Glycoxide™, a gel-paste; REDTA™ (Roth Drug, Chicago, Illinois), a solution; and RC Prep™(Premier Dental, Norristown, Pennsylvania). All of these chelate or soften inorganic structures. RC Prep™ also facilitates the file placement and motion within the canal by lubrication, as well as softening the internal dentinal surface, so the files can remove the innermost layers that might harbor bacteria. Chelators should not be left in contact with the canal wall for long periods of time to avoid excessive inorganic dissolution. RC Prep additionally contains urea peroxidase, which aids in dissolution of organic debris, while providing some antibacterial activity as well, by destroying many forms of bacteria (1,2).

The effects of EDTA on inorganic compounds is complemented by dissolving organic debris with one of the frequently used endodontic irrigants, 5.25% sodium hypochlorite (NaClO$_3$; bleach). At either full or half strength, sodium hypochlorite is a vital part of the sterilization of the root canal spaces. Care must be taken not to use the solution in teeth with open apices or those suspected of having excessive erosive or perforating lesions. Even in a seemingly intact apex, if a standard injection needle, and not an endodontic irrigating or side-slotted needle is used, the canal can be occluded by the needle, and the

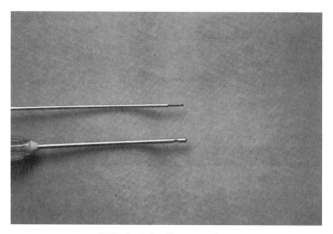

FIG. 1. Irrigation needles.

material can be forcefully injected into periapical tissue (Fig. 1). This can cause extreme irritation and severe pain (2,3). If this occurs, attempts should be made at flushing the areas, and injection with a local anesthetic and anti-inflammatory agent may be necessary. Any solution that comes into contact with other oral tissues should be rinsed off thoroughly. Hydrogen peroxide can also be used as an irrigant, with its abilities to help flush out debris. If it is used, again, care should be taken not to extrude the solution into the periapical tissues, to avoid formation of gas bubbles in the area. Copious flushing with saline after both hydrogen peroxide and sodium hypochlorite is always required, and in cases where apical pathology is severe, sterile saline alone used in large amounts can provide sufficient cleansing of the canal system.

Once the canal is filed and flushed, sterile paper points are used to dry the canal before it is obturated (Fig. 2). A sealer cement in the root canal is almost always recommended

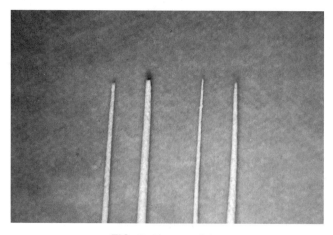

FIG. 2. Paper points.

in combination with the core-filling material to enhance the apical hermetic seal. The sealer cement has two interfaces: a nonadhesive one with the core material and an adhesive one to the apical dentin (4,5). Most sealer cements fit into one of four general generic categories: eugenol types, noneugenol types, therapeutic sealer cements, and temporary canal dressings.

One of the simplest and most commonly used cements is a combination of zinc oxide powder and liquid eugenol (ZOE) (6,7). It is relatively inexpensive and easy to work with, the powder and liquid being spatulated on a glass slab until a thread of the paste can be drawn up 1–2 cm from the slab (8,9). The paste can be injected or placed with a spiral filler or on a file into the canal. Extrusion may cause mild irritation to the periapical tissues, but it is usually not a severe problem. One problem is that ZOE can be resorbed over time (7), but with the limited life span of most veterinary patients, the significance of this is questionable, especially if a denser core-filling material such as gutta-percha is also used. Unless it is used as the sole canal filler, this does not seem to pose a major problem for the dog. Initially, most ZOE sealer cements expand slightly to enhance the apical seal. Composites cannot be used directly over eugenol products because of interference with the setting time. There are many variations of the basic ZOE mixture available, including reinforced products and specific endodontic fillers. They have variable setting times according to the product used (10).

For the reasons that ZOE may eventually disintegrate and can be cytotoxic and antigenic to living tissues, noneugenol sealer cements have been advocated by some authors (11). The three most commonly used of this category are Diaket (Premier Dental, Norristown, Pennsylvania), a polyvinyl resin; AH26 (Caulk, Milford, Delaware), an epoxy resin; and No-genol™ (Coe Laboratories, Chicago, Illinois). Other noneugenol products, such as N2 or RC2B pastes, have highly toxic additives such as paraformaldehyde and lead tetroxide and should be avoided because any extrusion could cause severe complications. One of the newer noneugenol cements is a glass ionomer product. One advantage of such a sealer is that it has a long-term adhesion to the enamel and dentin with or without removal of the smear layer, even if slightly moist (12), providing a superior apical seal. A glass ionomer product such as Ketac Endo® (ESPE-Premier, Norristown, Pennsylvania) has an adequate setting time and radiopacity and helps prevent bacterial penetration and percolation. Even if the cement is extruded apically, the inflammation typically resolves quickly with new bone formation on the material (13). Its one major disadvantage is the great difficulty encountered in its removal should complications ever arise.

Therapeutic sealer cements are those that are classified as biologically active. These usually incorporate calcium hydroxide to promote periapical healing or partial apical closure (14). The two most common are CRCS™ (Hygenic, Akron, Ohio), and Sealapex™ (Kerr Manufacturing, Romulus, Michigan).

Calcium hydroxide is used extensively as a temporary canal dressing, particularly when there is a need for stimulation of a hard-tissue closure associated with open apices (apexification) or with perforations. Since the calcium hydroxide resorbs over time, it is not permanent and must be replaced if additional closure is required after its influence has subsided (15). Endodontically, calcium hydroxide can also be placed on coronal pulpal tissue to stimulate reparative dentinal closure (see Chapter 12).

Once the sealer cement is placed, the majority of the canal system should be obturated with the appropriate filling material. One of the prime objectives in endodontics is to maximize core material in comparison with sealer, since it is generally the more stable of the two. While silver points may inhibit bacterial growth and can be sterilized, their potential for corrosion, lack of ability to conform to a canal, especially if narrow or curved, and staining do not help their popularity.

The viscoelastic properties of *gutta-percha*, which is about 60% crystalline and slightly flexible, make it a desirable filling agent. It meets many of the requirements for an ideal filling material: It is nonirritating, impervious to moisture, and radiopaque (due to its barium content); and it can be condensed laterally and apically (although it does not seal) and be easily removed, and does not stain or encourage bacterial growth (16).

Gutta-percha cones or points are provided in two types. Type I are standard points and come in sizes approximately equal to standard file sizes. Type II cones are known as auxiliary or accessory cones and are more tapered (Fig. 3). While standard cones can be condensed with additional auxiliary cones placed to help complete the fill, use of solvents or heat can facilitate a more complete obturation. Chloroform can be used to form several gutta-percha cones into a customized master point, or a paste can be formed and placed into the canal. This can help to fill fine, tortuous canals, but the potential carcinogenic properties of chloroform and shrinkage of the material after placement are causes for concern (8). Gutta-percha is less soluble in oil of eucalyptus, but this is can also be used.

Gutta-percha softens when exposed to heat, whether heated by an endodontic instrument or warmed in cannulas, on files, or in syringes, for application into the canal. Most of the warm gutta-percha techniques have their own advantages and disadvantages (see Chapter 11).

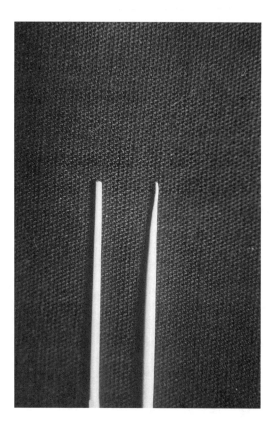

FIG. 3. Gutta-percha points type I and II.

RESTORATIVES

Many dental materials are used in a restorative capacity to "restore" the structure and function of the tooth as close to normal as possible (17). There are myriad products available, each with its own indications. Ideally, a restorative material should chemically bind to dentin and enamel, not break, fatigue, or distort after placement, have the coefficient of expansion as teeth, have high impact strength, and wear at the same rate as teeth (18). Porcelains have tremendous hardness, which may result in attritional wear of opposing teeth, while acrylics are generally softer than dental structure and are worn down easily by the opposing teeth (7).

Plastics/Resins

One large group of dental materials includes plastic materials consisting of polymer/monomer combinations with a large assortment of uses.

Acrylics

The *acrylic* plastics, basically methyl methacrylate, mixed from a powder (polymer) and liquid (monomer), were once used more extensively as restoratives. Their use is not as popular currently, due to high shrinkage during polymerization and lack of resistance to wear. They are extremely useful in other areas of dentistry such as intraoral splints, orthodontic appliances, temporary crowns, denture bases, and custom trays (7).

Acrylics have an initiator, benzoyl peroxide $[(C_6H_5CO)_2O_2]$, which, when activated by heat or an amine activator, results in polymerization. There are basically two types of acrylics: cold cured and heat cured (19). Cold-cured acrylics are the self- or auto-curing acrylics. An amine in the monomer activates the initiator to simulate polymerization. The term *cold curing* can be misleading in that all cold-cure acrylics liberate heat to some degree during the curing process. If the acrylic is formed directly in the mouth, the heat and vapors can be a problem for the patient. Most orthodontic acrylics do not generate excessive amounts of heat, while those used for impression trays can generate considerably more. With the addition of small increments of liquid, powder, and then liquid again, the heat, bubble formation, and volume contraction can be minimized. Protecting the gingiva with wax or petroleum jelly and irrigating with water can also help prevent problems. Additionally, when used to fabricate an appliance on a stone model, a separator must be used to prevent the acrylic from bonding to the model (9).

Heat-cured acrylics are those in which the activator of the initiator is actually externally applied heat. When heated to approximately 60°C or 140°F, the initiator is activated and polymerization occurs, and then maintained at approximately 74°C. If heated too quickly, the monomer may vaporize prior to the complete polymerization and the acrylic will be porous and of poor quality. These acrylics are primarily used in dental laboratories for denture bases (19).

Composite Resins

Composite restoratives are typically composed of an organic polymer matrix of high molecular weight (20,21), usually a bisphenol A-glycidyl methacrylate (Bis-GMA) resin, with or without fillers. Unfilled resins are used to coat or line the area to be filled and to help decrease microleakage that could otherwise lead to shrinkage, lack of bonding, and even sensitivity if vital teeth are involved. It is best to acid-etch the enamel to create microporosities that the unfilled resin can flow into, while keeping a very thin film of the material to which the filled resin will bind.

Fillers are added to increase hardness, strength, resistance to temperature, ability to withstand wear, and control of shrinkage during polymerization (22). Fillers can also provide a lower coefficient of thermal expansion, lower water absorption, and greater wear resistance; they also alter polishability and, depending on the material, come in a variety of colors (23). The inorganic filler portion is typically 70–80% of the material by weight, primarily in the form of crystal quartz, silica, lithium, and other particles (7). One newer product incorporates fibers as well as particles to enhance the strength of the final restoration.

The size of the particles determines most of the compound's characteristics. Microfill composites have particles ≤0.04 µm, usually a colloidal silica. The filler content may be only 35–50%, so there will be a higher coefficient of thermal expansion and potentially increased shrinkage during polymerization (making acid-etching and dentinal bonding vital); it may also absorb more water (24) and is less fracture- and wear-resistant. With the small particle size, however, it is extremely polishable, so it is esthetically advantageous in nonstressed areas.

Conventional fill composites may have particles up to 20–35 µm, similar to the macro- or coarse fill with particulate size >1 µm, and averaging 15–25 µm. These materials are more resistant to fracture and wear and tear, but have a rough surface that does not polish readily (17) and will accumulate plaque more easily (25). Intermediate composites have particles at 1–5 µm and so provide a more esthetic finish than the macrofill but are sturdier than the microfill (23). Hybrid products combine different sizes of particles, averaging 1.5 µm, to integrate the advantages of the macrofill with the polishability of the microfill.

While the actual polymerization continues throughout the life of the material, the initiation of the process is typically by either chemical (self-cure) or light (photo-cure) means. The self-, or chemical, cure starts when the two compounds are mixed together and catalyzed by the benzoyl peroxide combining with the amine. When mixing is adequate, this allows for a more uniform cure, especially in thick applications such as crown or core buildups. Light-cure products are more homogeneous, being a single material with fewer bubbles because no mixing is necessary, and have a longer working time and yet faster curing time. The greatest advantage of light-cure composites is operator control of the polymerization. But they can only be placed in 1–2 mm increments due to the limits of light penetration, and the cure may not be as uniform in deeper preparations. Products that use ultraviolet light in the 320–365-nm range have a benzoin catalyst, and a camphor quinone/amine catalyst is incorporated into materials using a visible-light range of 450–500 nm (7). Some products in the latter category can provide a greater depth of polymerization, up to 4.5–5.5 mm, even through shallow depths of tooth structures encountered with undercuts. Any time curing lights are used, adequate protection in the form of shields or glasses must be used to eliminate exposure of the operator's eyes to the light. Self-cure products may need more mechanical retention such as undercuts and even pins. Acid-etching of the enamel (as discussed previously) creates microporosities for the unfilled resin or dentinal bonding agent to flow into, enhancing the bonding and increasing retention and the resistance to microleakage at the margins (21).

Bonding Agents

Various bonding agents are available, although some, like polyurethanes with a weak tensile strength, are not used extensively. Polyacrylic acids, the liquid component of some glass ionomers, bond better to dentin than composites do. Specialized *dentinal bonding agents* provide nearly as much bonding capacity as can be provided by acid-etching enamel. By decreasing the shrinkage that can be seen during polymerization, marginal leakage can be reduced, and the light-cure capability of some products, along with usually good biocompatability, makes these agents very useful.

Other similar materials include some of the newer *pit-and-fissure sealants* that are similar to composite resins (Bis-GMA) and are available with fluorides that are slowly released in small amounts. When placed on occlusal tables and other high-risk areas, they can provide a temporary barrier to cariogenic influences in those individuals deemed at greater susceptibility to caries. The complete role of fluoride additives in dental materials has always been debated; they probably do not do any harm or a great amount of good. There are also powder–liquid mix composites that can be painted on with a small brush, such as Brush Technique™ (Dorby Dental, Rockville Center, New York), which can provide a thin protective layer or even a thicker buildup.

Glass Ionomers

While *glass ionomer* products typically do not bear up to stress or wear as well as composites or amalgam, in nonocclusal areas (class V, Modified Black Classification) these compounds can be very useful. They chemically bind to enamel and dentin by ions forming salts that bond to the calcium in the tooth (26), even if slight moisture is present. This can be an advantage, especially when mechanical retention procedures of undercutting and acid-etching are best avoided in small or delicate teeth. Some of the glass ionomers use either a mild citric or polyacrylic acid to prepare the lesion by removing the smear layer, potentially enhancing the bonding. Generally, the manufacturers' recommendations should be followed concerning cavity preparation.

Another supposed advantage of glass ionomers is that they slowly release fluoride over time, helping to retard decay and decrease sensitivity, while being biologically compatible with the pulp, negating the need for cavity liners in most cases (24,27). However, it must be understood that this is associated with a chemical change in the glass or a degradation process. The *coefficient of thermal expansion* closely approximates that of the tooth structure, so a tight marginal seal is maintained. Some products have silver added to enhance the strength, with decreased setting time, but the darker color is not as esthetically pleasing.

The longer setting time of some glass ionomer products, along with moisture restrictions in the area (should not be desiccated, but not moist), makes them very technique-sensitive at times (27). Products with more rapid setting times, such as Ketac Bond® (ESPE-Premier), and even combination products that allow for light-curing (eg, Vitrebond™, 3M Dental Products, St. Paul, Minnesota) are sometimes preferred.

The basic composition of glass ionomers is an aluminosilicate glass powder mixed with a polyacrylic acid or a powder with water (24). If finely grained, glass ionomers can be classified as type I and used for luting and cementation for crowns and bridges. Type II glass ionomers, which are coarser, represent the esthetic restorative group, while type

III agents are the base and liner materials. As a thin liner, a glass ionomer agent can be used as a foundation for other material. It can be acid-etched, and a composite can then be bonded to it for a sandwich effect (26). Using the glass ionomer under a composite can separate it from zinc oxide–eugenol cement (ZOE), if present, and help minimize the amount of polymerization shrinkage by decreasing the amount of composite used. The type III products are also sometimes used as a restorative material in treatment of feline dental disease. Type IV is the admixture group. Products in this group have metal admixtures added to them, such as silver, amalgam, gold, and titanium. These metallic additions do not increase the materials' resistance to wear or add strength, unless the metal is sintered to the glass component. These type IV materials are sometimes used for cores and buildups, but they are still much weaker than more conventional materials used for restorations and cores.

Amalgam

In contrast to glass ionomers, *amalgam* strength and resistance to wear and fracture are extremely good. In fact, the surrounding tooth structure might wear faster than the restorative, leaving a "button" of it protruding. This is due to the fact that amalgam is an alloy or combination of finely powdered metals that are mixed, or triturated, with mercury, a liquid at room temperatures (28), to "wet" the particles and form a condensable mass (7). Of the metals potentially used, silver is commonly found, and it increases the strength and expansion of the material. Tin is used to decrease setting expansion and to assist in the amalgamation. Silver and tin combine (Ag_3Sn) to form the gamma phase, which is the strongest component of the mixture. In fact, the earliest alloys used were made of about two-thirds silver and one-third tin (28). Tin, however, is susceptible to corrosion, and the final gamma-2 (Sn_8Hg) phase decreases the corrosive resistance and strength of the restorative.

Copper in the alloy, like silver, increases the product's setting expansion, strength, and hardness and, when present in high amounts of 13–30%, helps eliminate the weak gamma-2 phase by binding with the tin instead of letting it combine with the mercury (18).

Zinc in the alloy provides a scavenging service to produce clean ingot castings (24). To be considered a zinc-containing product, at least 0.01% zinc is necessary. Less than 0.01% zinc is required to be a nonzinc amalgam, which would be preferred over the zinc product in the case of retrofill of an apicoectomy site. If a zinc amalgam is brought into contact with periapical tissues, the zinc reacts with the moisture at the site to form bubbles of hydrogen gas. Gas bubbles in the preparation cause excessive expansion, then strength reduction, excessive corrosion, leakage around the margins, and sensitivity (19).

Amalgam particles originally were produced by lathe-cut methods, which makes for a material that compacts well but has an irregular, rough surface and requires more mercury for trituration (24). Firm condensation of these products is necessary to remove as much of the mercury as possible. Spherical alloys are produced by "atomizing" molten metals (7,28). These do not require as much mercury and can result in a smoother, more polishable surface with reduced cracking and crevicing (margin breakdown) (7) and decreased surface deterioration. Higher copper content can be found in these unicompositional spherical alloys, and often high compressive strength is experienced within an hour, an advantage with patients who may not pay close attention to postoperative instructions. They are more difficult to condense, especially if small-tipped condensers are used that might penetrate into the amalgam as the spheres roll over on top of each other. All types of alloys are seen, from lathe-cut, low-copper alloy to admixed (spherical and lathe-cut particles) or unicompositional (spherical) types with high copper content.

One of the disadvantages of amalgam is the preparation considerations, especially that of mercury contamination. Using preencapsulated products, with the "mortar and pestle" effect of the capsule and enclosed ball, can help avoid dermal contact with the alloy. Principles of proper ventilation protection (use of masks and gloves) and disposal procedures should be observed. These capsules should be mixed in the appropriate amalgamator with a frequency >3000 cycles per minute. It is also important to triturate for the correct amount of time (10–30 seconds, according to manufacturers' recommendations), because undermixing will result in a grainy, dull material with a roughened, weakened surface and potentially more exposed mercury (28). Overmixing is not the answer either, because it will cause the alloy to set up too quickly.

Amalgam does not chemically bond to dentin and enamel, nor can it flow into the microporosities formed during enamel acid-etching, although some bonding agents are now available. Accordingly, an amalgam restorative relies on undercuts for mechanical retention, which is inadvisable in small teeth. Amalgam initially does have some marginal leakage, which leads to corrosion. Corrosional products, such as tin and silver sulfides, accumulate to eventually minimize or even eliminate microleakage. This will lead to an expected "black line" edge, but proper placement of a cavity varnish will minimize the discoloration (19). With proper technique, an excellent restorative effect can be accomplished.

Varnishes, Liners, Bases, and Cements

With many of the restoratives previously described, quite often a practitioner should use additional materials to obtain the best treatment possible. The protective capabilities of a *varnish* to keep chemical irritants from the pulp, as well as providing marginal seals to reduce microleakage, can be attained with both natural (copal gum) and synthetic (nitrated cellulose) resins. Varnish on dentinal tubules and sealing the margins will also reduce the seepage of corrosive amalgam that causes discoloration (7).

Cavity varnishes can dissolve if left exposed on the margins to the moist oral cavity. They are contraindicated for placement under composites because the varnish solvent may soften the resin and the residual monomer of the resin may dissolve the varnish. The varnish, furthermore, will act as a separator preventing direct bonding of the resin to the tooth (29).

Waterproof varnishes help contain moisture contamination during glass ionomer restoration by first protecting the material from excessive moisture during its set-up time, then protecting the completed restoration from dehydration (24,30). Some varnishes with fluoride have been reported to be used on feline resorptive lesions to reduce sensitivity. Varnishes do not provide thermal insulation, nor can they stimulate the production of reparative dentin.

There are several different types of materials that can be used as *liners*, *bases*, or *cements*, depending on the formulation, thickness, and application (7). Cavity liners help protect the pulp and decrease dentinal sensitivity like varnishes, but they can also provide other advantages, especially if the pulp is exposed or near exposure. While providing a physical support for the final restoration when replacing structural loss, bases can also help protect the pulp from irritating substances and thermal changes. Liners, listed earlier, may be placed in several layers to achieve the same bulk, but they do not have the strength of some materials specifically used as bases, such as reinforced ZOE products and other cements. Cements are used to apply orthodontic brackets, appliances, crowns, or other prosthodontics devices.

Calcium hydroxide liners are used primarily to induce (actually by irritating the odontoblasts) reparative dentin bridge formation that will protect the pulp. This is important especially where 0.5 mm or less of dentin is left. They cannot withstand occlusive forces, however, and if exposed to oral fluids at margins, they will dissolve. In deep preparations, an additional cement base may also be needed.

ZOE products can be used as liners to protect the dentinal surfaces from sensitivity, as the pH of 7–8, even of the reinforced ZOE cements, helps sedate the pulp, in contrast to zinc phosphate or other restoratives. Direct placement over exposed pulp can cause inflammation, so with exposed pulp or near exposure, it is still recommended to use a calcium hydroxide liner under the ZOE base. Contraindications to using it under composites or with cavity varnishes are some disadvantages, and it does not have the strength of the zinc phosphates, although the reinforced products are useful as intermediate or temporary restoratives.

Type II glass ionomers can be used as liners, particularly some of the newer light-cured products. The benefits of bonding to the dentin and releasing fluoride are complemented by the fact that type II glass ionomers have greater tensile and compressive strength than calcium hydroxide (31) and even comparable to or higher than zinc phosphate, making them very useful bases. Placed over an endodontically treated tooth, the liner bonds to the internal dentin and can be acid-etched to facilitate the placement of composites (31). The cariostatic effects of its fluoride are also good when it is used to cement on orthodontic brackets and bands. All these advantages, plus the low viscosity of type I, or luting, glass ionomers, make them good for post and crown cementation, too. Generally, they have been found to retain complete coverage castings better than zinc phosphates or polycarboxylates (32). Some sensitivity may be experienced after crown cementation, for various reasons, and of course any near-pulpal exposure should be treated appropriately. Removal of the smear layer has been debated (increased binding vs. potential sensitivity), and dentinal desiccation should be avoided.

Zinc phosphate cement has been regulated by American Dental Association (ADA) Specification No.8 since 1935 (24). It is sometimes incorrectly termed zinc oxyphosphate cement, but no study has proven oxyphosphate formation during setting. It is supplied in powder/liquid kits for mixing. Type I zinc phosphate cements have a fine particle size (25 μm) and are used for seating precision appliances and crowns. Type II cements are of a medium particle size (40 μm) and used as a cement for orthodontic bands.

The high compressive strength and thermal insulation of zinc phosphate cements are useful both under composites and over gutta-percha. When placed in the canal, even if the final restoration is lost, the zinc phosphate can still protect the underlying fill, yet it can be removed easily with a bur on a high-speed handpiece, should the need arise. In vital teeth, without two thin coats of varnish over the dentin, placement of phosphoric acid cements such as zinc phosphate can result in the acid's penetrating through the dentinal tubules into the pulp, causing irritation or death of the pulp (22,33). Calcium hydroxide can be used if there is any near exposure of the pulp, but the final preparation of the tooth should not be polished, as a rougher surface provides enhanced mechanical interlock and a greater surface area for cement adhesion. A frozen glass slab can be used to increase the amount of powder in the mix, thereby decreasing its water solubility. This solubility can be addressed also by placing a varnish on the margins. If it does dissolve at the margins or the mechanical bond breaks exposing the tooth, the area can decalcify and progress to a carious lesion (24).

The polycarboxylate cements are regulated by the ADA under Specification No.61 (7). They form a good adhesive bond to enamel, dentin, and stainless steel, but a very weak bonding to gold and almost negligible attachment to porcelains. Studies show poor solubility values, and the short working time and thickness of the material are all disadvantages. Recently, some of these cements have had fluoride salts added to their composition. With these, fluoride release similar to that of glass ionomers occurs, which exerts an anticariogenic effect helping to control the onset of carious lesions. In crowning of vital teeth, although acidic, it is potentially less irritating to the pulp than zinc phosphates, due to the weaker acidity of the acrylic acids as compared with the phosphoric acids, and the larger molecular chain sizes reduce penetration into the dentinal tubules. Still, all marginal surfaces should be cleaned and polished with pumice to reduce the potential of acid effects, and there should be no oil, moisture, or varnish on the tooth surfaces, to enhance the cement's bond to enamel and even dentinal surfaces.

Cements made either of composites or acrylic resins are useful in bracket cementation due to their lack of solubility in water. Whether a two-paste system or a single filled resin is used with a liquid activation on the bracket, the tooth should first be cleaned, polished with a flour pumice, rinsed, dried, and acid-etched. These cements tend to be thinner preparations than the typical restorative composites, to allow a minimal thickness of the material to obtain better retention. With posts and crowns, use of a light-cured bonding agent will also increase adherence. Newer products that bond to sandblasted base or noble metals are extremely useful in crowns, though oxygen inhibition is necessary for the chemical cure and it is an expensive material.

Materials used in the construction of crowns and other prosthetic devices will be discussed in the restorative chapter (see Chapter 13).

IMPRESSION MATERIALS

Most dental appliances, whether orthodontic or prosthodontic, are fabricated outside the patient's mouth on models. How functional and how well the appliance fits in the mouth is directly related to how successfully the models replicate the oral tissues. The accuracy of the model depends on the accuracy of the *impression* and the care in pouring up the models. A good impression material must have many features. The material used must be nontoxic, nonirritating, clean to use, and acceptable in taste and odor. It must also have a good shelf life and be economical, and have ease of manipulation and placement, plasticity when placed, flowability to enter and record fine details, and reasonable working and setting times. Finally, it must allow for draw or have a degree of elasticity for removal of the model, and retain good dimensional stability to produce a model of sufficient detail for the use intended. Impression materials fall generally into two major categories: nonelastic and elastic materials. There are advantages and disadvantages of each product that make it suitable for specific uses.

Nonelastic Impression Materials

There are four main groups in this category: impression plaster, impression compound, impression ZOE, and impression waxes. *Impression plaster*, or *type I gypsum*, is similar to dental plasters used for some models, except it has a fine grain and a higher water:mix ratio to allow recording of fine details (7). Because of its high flowability, it cannot be used in standard impression trays, as it quickly leaks out. It is very brittle when set and is generally used for edentulous areas or single-tooth crown preparations. If undercuts are encountered, the material is commonly fractured in removal and then reconstructed, unless excessive damage has occurred.

Impression compound is a rigid plastic used in sticks or sheets. It is typically referred to as a *thermalplastic*, as it softens when heated and becomes rigid again as it cools. ADA Specification No.3 divides these compounds into type I, low fusing, and type II, high fusing (34). Type I compound is used as an impression material and type II for fabrication of impression trays. Type I sheets are heated with a water bath and at 55–60°C. If underheated, it will not flow or record details well, and if overheated, it becomes tacky, sticky, too liquefied, and unmanageable. The sticks are commonly heated with an alcohol lamp or Bunsen burner. Skill is needed to heat the material to soften it to the right consistency, without its becoming too fluid or igniting. Copper bands are usually placed around an individual tooth, and then the softened stick is added to obtain an impression. If undercuts are present, problems in removal can be expected. The sheets are primarily used on edentulous areas.

ZOE impression materials typically come as two pastes—a base and a catalyst—that are mixed together. It is used for obtaining impressions over large edentulous areas (7). Fractures of the impressions or distortions occur when the material is removed from areas of undercuts. Small defects can usually be corrected with impression waxes. Noneugenol–zinc oxide impression materials are also available for those patients with allergies or sensitivities to eugenol.

Impression waxes are customarily a combination of low-melting paraffin wax and beeswax in about a 3:1 ratio (7). They are rarely used to obtain actual impressions for pouring models, although they can be used in small or restricted areas. Most frequently, they are used for bite registration in combination with other impression materials.

Elastic Impression Materials

Elastic impression materials are more commonly used for models and bite registrations (34). This category is further broken down into the hydrocolloids and synthetic elastomers. The hydrocolloids include alginate (irreversible hydrocolloids) and agar (reversible). The synthetic elastomers include polysulfides, polyethers, and silicones.

Hydrocolloids

Hydrocolloid impression material is based on colloid suspensions of polysaccharides in water. When water is used as the fluid medium of colloids, it is referred to as a *hydrocolloid*. These exist in two forms a *sol* and a *gel* (34). The sol form is the form derived when water is first added to alginates or agars are heated, and the material takes on a fluid state with low viscosity. The gel form is the gelatinized stage that occurs as the material sets up into the stable impression.

Alginate, an irreversible hydrocolloid, is used quite frequently in veterinary dentistry, especially when partial- or full-mouth models are needed that require decent, yet not excellent detail. The dimensional stability of alginate is not good, especially if too much moisture is lost or taken up, so the stone model should be poured as soon as possible. The characteristics of alginates are defined in ADA Specification No.18 (7). Alginates are grouped into two types. Type I alginates are fast-setting, gelling in 1–2 minutes after beginning of mixing. Type II materials are regular-set and should gel within 2–4.5 minutes.

The alginate powder should be gently "fluffed" by inverting the can several times and then allowed to settle before its airtight container is opened. While most products are nontoxic to ingest, inhalation of the silica particle dust should certainly be avoided. Precise measurement of the powder (no packing, straight-edge removal of overflow contents) and water is important in determining its setting characteristics. Regular- or fast-setting products are both available, and by using cool or slightly increased amounts of water, the gelation time can be extended. Accurate mixing, with a figure-8 spatulation using the side of the flex bowl, will provide a material with minimal bubbles and maximum strength. Once placed in the mouth, the material sets in 2–3 minutes, after which the tray and material should be removed from the mouth in a firm, quick motion. Pouring of the models will be discussed in the orthodontics chapter (see Chapter 15).

Reversible colloids (*agar*) are supplied in tubes of gel. When heated, agar material converts to the sol state to obtain an impression and then back to the gel state on cooling, for a stable impression (34). The accuracy of the impression is extremely good, but it has a poor tear resistance. Special thermostat-controlled hot-water-bath equipment is needed to accurately soften the material, and water-cooled trays can be used to accelerate the setting. The material can be used by itself or in combination with alginates to record fine details for crown work (35,36). Their characteristics are delineated under ADA Specification No.11 (37).

Synthetic Elastomers

Synthetic elastomers are rubber-like, composed of large molecules joined with weak interactions at certain points in a three-dimensional network (18). They provide better tear resistance and dimensional stability than the hydrocolloids do (34) but are also more expensive, and so in veterinary dentistry are typically used for limited-area impressions rather than full-mouth. Within this category are four groups in fairly common use: the polysulfides, the polyethers, and the silicones (silicone rubber and polysiloxane). Most are supplied as a two-paste system for mixing catalyst and base in tubs, tubes, or cartridges. The tube and cartridges are usually available in a light body and a regular body, while the tubs are generally a heavy-body material. Typically, two types are used for taking the impression, with a regular or heavy body placed in the tray and the light body placed directly on the tooth as a wash and pressed down on the tooth by the heavier-body material in the tray to record fine details.

Polysulfide rubber impression materials have good accuracy and a tear resistance of about 700% tensile strain before tearing (34). Although setting commences immediately on mixing of the base and catalyst, total setting time is a little long, up to 10 minutes or more for the light-bodied material. Additionally, these materials are odorous and can cause dental staining, and most have lead compounds in them. The short duration of exposure and the hydrophobic state of the lead compounds make it unlikely that these impression materials will cause harmful effects to the patient. However, more lead-free polysulfides are being developed due to concerns. Some shrinkage occurs, and while one authors states it should be poured anytime after 15 minutes up to 72 hours (26), other references say it should be less than 1 hour (34,38).

Polyether rubber materials have a shorter working time, good dimensional stability, and less shrinkage compared with polysulfides. Their tear resistance approaches that of the silicones (39). They are usually available in only one viscosity (regular body); however, a diluent oil is available that can produce a paste similar to the light-bodied products (40).

These materials can absorb water and so should be stored dry (7). Their stiffness can be improved by adding body modifiers to the mixture of base and catalyst. Some patients may exhibit a hypersensitivity to the product, but its modest price is an advantage.

The *silicone* impression materials are available in two forms: condensation curing (silicone rubber) and addition curing (polysiloxanes). Their tear resistance is about 300% tensile strain (34). The *silicone rubber* (*condensation-curing silicone*) material has many limitations in comparison with the other elastomers. It has significant shrinkage, requiring special custom trays (41) and a short working time, and the preparation area must be dry and free of moisture or its physical properties will be altered (42).

Siloxane polymers (*polysiloxane* or *addition-curing silicone*) for crown and bridge impressions provide accurate detailing, but the lack of flowability of dental stone into the impression can be a problem. Some of the newer polymerizing vinyl polysiloxanes have improved wetting characteristics, no odor, easy mixability, and a short working time. They have excellent dimensional stability up to 2 weeks and provide superior detail, especially with the light-bodied materials (34). However, either the powder of vinyl gloves or the vinyl itself has been shown to inhibit setting of the polysiloxanes, and therefore should not be used. Plastic gloves have not demonstrated this problem. While the two-putty method of mixing the heavier-body compound (clean hands, no rubber gloves) can cover large areas, the syringe method with automatic mixing can form a more uniform, bubble-free material. The light material can be applied directly onto the tooth with a syringe and blown into the sulcus for better detail, with the regular-body material placed over it in a tray. The two mixtures then crosslink to become an elastic solid as the material sets up in 5–8 minutes. Its resistance to tear allows the impression to be removed even if small undercuts are present, without damaging the impression. The model should not be poured until at least 1 hour has passed to allow the dissipation of hydrogen gas released during polymerization (34). The main disadvantage of this material is its cost.

MODEL AND CAST MATERIALS

Models are generally of two types: those for demonstrational use (plastics, acrylics, silicones, urethanes, polyvinyls) and those for construction of dental appliances (primarily gypsum). Demonstration models are typically made from various plastics and acrylics. White-tooth shade *acrylics* can be used for teeth and pink-fibered acrylics for the base and gingival structures. The techniques for their construction have been described (43). Work models for construction of dental appliances are typically made from gypsum, although some are made from epoxy die materials (44). The *epoxy* materials are usually in the form of a paste with an activator added to initiate hardening. Many of the activators are toxic compounds and should not be allowed to contact skin during mixing or manipulation of the unset material. The set epoxy models are stronger and more resist to abrasion than gypsum models. However, many cannot be used with alginate or agar impressions, as the water content retards polymerization, and some cannot be used with polysulfide (rubber-base) materials. Always check manufacturers' recommendations. The viscosity of the materials can make them difficult to introduce into some small impressions, and sometimes fine details are not replicated (45). Additionally, they are cost-prohibitive.

Gypsum is a naturally occurring chalky, porous white mineral, chemically known as *calcium sulfate dihydrate*. Plaster of Paris is a gypsum, so named because the mines where it was obtained for centuries were near Paris, France. The dental-powder product used to make models is calcium sulfate hemihydrate. When mixed with water to form the stable, structured model, it once again becomes calcium sulfate dihydrate and releases some exothermic heat (34):

$$(CaSO_4)2 - H_2O + 3H_2O = 2CaSO_4 - 2H_2 + Heat$$
(gypsum dental powder plus water equals model plus heat)

The properties of dental gypsum are regulated by ADA Specification No.25 (7). Type I dental gypsum products are impression plasters, type II model plasters, type III unimproved dental stones, and type IV improved dental stones. Type I dental plaster is used for impressions, primarily for dentures. Type II dental plaster is used for model fabrication and study and reference casts, as well as for flasking dentures. Type III unimproved dental stones are well suited for casts to construct dentures. Type IV improved dental stones, because of their accuracy and strength, are used extensively for crown and bridgework casts (37).

Type II dental plaster, produced by baking the mineral in open air to 110–120°C, is known as *beta-calcium sulfate hemihydrate*. *Type III unimproved dental stone* is developed by heating the mineral to 125°C under pressure and in the presence of water vapor and is known as *alpha-calcium sulfate hemihydrate*. *Type IV improved dental stone* is produced by removing the crystallization water with boiling in a 30% calcium chloride solution, and the chlorides are then removed by washing in 100°C water. This is the most dense of the four types and is usually referred to as *high-strength dental stone*. Synthetic calcium sulfate hemihydrates have been developed to replace natural gypsum; currently, however, production expenses have made them cost-prohibitive (7).

The handling characteristics of the gypsum can be altered with the addition of certain chemicals. Potassium sulfate, terra alba, and sodium chloride are all effective setting-time accelerators; however, the sodium chloride also causes expansion problems. Borax has been demonstrated to retard setting time. Terra alba is finely ground calcium sulfate dihydrate added in very small amounts to calcium sulfate hemihydrate to act as foci for neocrystal formation to speed setting. Calcium oxide and gum arabic in small amounts reduces the amount of water required for mixing and improves some properties (7).

The main difference in the dental plasters and stones is the shape of the calcium sulfate crystals. Plasters have irregularly shaped crystals, which are weak and require more water to return to the dihydrate form. The stones have well formed, dense crystals. Dental plaster requires approximately 45 mL of water per 100 g of powder to mix properly; unimproved dental stone requires about 30 mL and improved dental stone only 19–24 mL. The less water required to form the dihydrate crystals, the denser and heavier the material is and the greater the compressive strength and the resistance to abrasion (34).

The powder is mixed with water and spatulated until smooth, sometimes under vacuum to reduce gas or air bubbles in the mix. Increasing spatulation, either in speed, time, or a combination of the two, will decrease the setting time by fracturing the dihydrate crystals to form more nuclei for increased spread of the setting reaction. The proper ratio of water to powder should be used when mixing for best results. Adding the powder to the water, instead of the water to the powder, can help reduce air-bubble formation; however, this can only be done when powder and water ratios are premeasured. By using flexible bowls and proper stone mixing spatulas, improved and easier spatulation ensues. Initially, place the stone into the impression in small increments using a vibrator to minimize bubbles and related voids. Once surface details are covered, larger amounts of the mix can be added to enhance pouring. Place a damp cloth or paper towel over the model, while setting up in the impression. Once the model or cast is removed from the impression, do not use for at least 45 minutes to 1 hour to allow for dimensional stabilization and water loss from sweating. Keep in mind that most plasters and stones do not reach their full compressive strength until about 24 hours after pouring (7).

When waxes, other gypsums, or acrylics are to be worked on gypsum models, casts, or dies, a *separating agent* must be used to prevent the materials from adhering or locking together. With waxes used for crowns, various oils, liquid soaps, detergents, and numerous commercial products can be used as a separator or die lubricant. However, some oils act as a solvent on wax and cannot be used. With gypsum (type III) models poured into gypsum (type I) impressions, liquid waxes and thin varnishes that are applied and allowed to dry work well as separating agents, although some fine detail may be lost. Acrylic oils, dental tinfoil, tinfoil substitutes, and many other commercial products are available. With the oils, the acrylic can be applied immediately, while with some of the tinfoil substitutes they must be painted on and allowed to dry for several hours (34).

Dental Waxes

There are numerous types of dental waxes used in veterinary dentistry. Some of the more common dental waxes are inlay, casting, sticky, boxing, carding, utility, and bite-registration waxes. Each type has specific physical and mechanical properties resulting from variations in its compositional components. Most are a combination of animal, plant, mineral, and synthetic waxes with the addition of some resins and occasionally metallic fillers. Mineral waxes are paraffin and microcrystalline waxes, both of which come from petroleum distillation. The animal wax is usually beeswax, used to reduce the brittleness and flow of paraffin when under stress or pressure. The plant waxes most commonly used are carnauba and candelilla, which modify paraffin properties and control the softening temperature. Any group can form the major component of dental waxes, but the minerals normally perform that function (7,34,47).

Inlay waxes are used to make wax patterns for crowns, bridges, and some other dental appliances. These waxes must provide exact and well fitting appliances, which requires their properties be more precise and have better control than the other dental waxes. Under ADA Specification No.4, inlay waxes are divided into type I direct and type II indirect (37). Type I waxes are used to fabricate the wax model directly in the mouth on the patient. This requires that they be a hard wax with a lower flow value to compensate for the patient body temperature and greater temperature variation when removed. Type II (indirect) inlay waxes are used to construct appliances outside the mouth on the patient's dental models. They are softer waxes with higher flow values than type I. The low flow of type I and the ease of carving of type II are both desirable characteristics. Once the wax pattern is created, it is used in a lost-wax technique to fabricate the actual restoration or appliance in both inlay and casting waxes (7).

Casting waxes are used to produce the patterns for the metallic framework of removable partial dentures, some orthodontic frames, and other similar structures (7). These are available in bulk, sheets, and ready-made shapes for rapid adaptation. They provide similar function to inlay waxes in producing patterns but have different physical properties. They are generally a little more tacky, which helps them maintain their position on the pattern during assembly. Additionally, they have a greater ductility for pliability or bending without breaking, when properly handled. Federal Specification U-W-140 defines their properties, as there is no ADA specification (46).

Sticky wax is used to temporarily stick or fix various metallic, resin, or wax assembly parts of dental appliances to stone or plaster dental models (7). The material is sticky when melted but at room temperature is firm, brittle, and nontacky. There is no ADA specification on this material, but Federal Specification U-W-00149a (DSA-DM) does regulate many of its properties (46).

Boxing wax is flat sheets of wax used to form a box around an impression to hold freshly mixed plaster or stone solution in and on the impression when poured (7). Occasionally, boxing wax is referred to as *carding wax*. However, carding wax was originally used as a card or sheet of wax to mount porcelain teeth when shipped from the manufacturer, but resourceful practitioners began reusing it for boxing. The terms are frequently considered interchangeable, but boxing is more appropriate for the use described here. A narrow stick of utility wax is first placed around the entire impression just below its peripheral height, followed by a sheet of the boxing wax. Federal Specification U-W-138 regulates some of its properties, but there is no ADA specification (46).

Utility wax is used for many purposes, but increasing impression-tray height is the most common. It is available in both sheets and sticks, being both adhesive and pliable for easy adaptation for various uses. Some products are made specifically for orthodontic use, having mint flavors, and are used both for elevating tray height and for covering brackets and rough edges on appliances in the mouth to protectant mucous membranes. There is no ADA specification, but Federal Specification U-W-156 governs some of its properties (46).

Bite-registration wax is used to orient opposing dental models for articulation (34). Some of these waxes contain aluminum or copper particles to give additional strength and to reduce distortion problems from heat. In the dog, a rolled sheet is typically placed behind the first premolars, and the bite is closed to imprint a dental registration on the wax. The registration can then be placed in the same location on the models to obtain a precise articulation or fitting together of the models. This allows inlays, crowns, and appliances to be manufactured to fit properly in the mouth without occlusal interference. Care must be taken in handling, as temperature variations can distort wax bite registrations. There are no ADA or Federal specifications currently concerning bite-registration waxes (7).

PERIODONTAL MATERIALS

There are a large number of periodontal materials available in dentistry. Some of the more common are the protectants, barriers or perio-packs, topical hemostatic-type agents, and topical antimicrobial agents (7,33). More detail about materials used for regenerative therapy will be given in the periodontal chapters (see Chapters 8 and 9).

The *protectants* are various topically applied medicaments that form a thin coating on the periodontal tissue. These are used either to prevent moisture and other contamination from entering, to seal in medicaments against the tissues or in the sulcus, or to provide some discomfort control. Two of the more common products are Orabase™ (Hoyt Laboratories, Needham, Massachusetts) and Tincture of Myrrh and Benzoin (Sultan Chemicals, Englewood, New Jersey) (Fig. 4) (47). Orabase™ is a combination of sodium carboxymethylcellulose, sodium, pectin, and gelatin in a base of polyethylene resin and mineral oil. It is used as a topically applied protective coating of the gingiva, and sometimes as a vehicle for carrying other drugs, such as anti-inflammatories, it can be applied to the moist surface of mucous membranes.

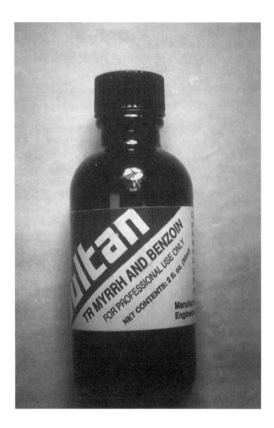

FIG. 4. Tincture of myrrh and benzoin.

Tincture of Myrrh and Benzoin is simply an alcohol suspension of myrrh and benzoin. On drying, it provides a thin protective barrier, while acting as a soothing agent on the mucous membranes. Additionally, it has been used for sealing medicaments in the gingival sulcus (37).

Periodontal packs are adhesive putties applied over periodontal surgery sites. Typically, they comprise a liquid portion of eugenol or noneugenol substitutes and oils that are combinations with a powder containing zinc oxide and usually rosin, tannic acid, binders, soluble salts, and oils. At one time, asbestos fibers were used as a binder but have been removed from most products due to health concerns (48). Antibiotics are sometimes incorporated into them. The packs reduce pain, hemorrhage, trauma, and debris package due to mastication, while acting as a barrier to bacteria and support for mobile teeth, all to promote healing. The liquid and powder are mixed together to a homogenous heavy putty. Its adhesive properties help to hold it in place when it is worked into the interdental spaces, but it can still be cracked and broken loose after short periods of time.

Hemorrhage control and retraction of the periodontal tissues in various procedures is important for the health of the tissues, visualization during procedures, and retraction of tissues for placement of many cements and restoratives without contamination. Topical pressure, astringents, vasoconstrictors, and hemostatics either by themselves or in coordination with *retraction cords* are commonly used for these purposes. Digital pressure with a sterile gauze or unmedicated retraction cord is still one of the simplest yet very effective means for controlling most slight-to-mild hemorrhage problems. Mild-to-moderate bleeding problems can usually be treated with topical astringents, vasoconstrictors, and hemostatic agents. More serious hemorrhaging should be handled with perio-packs and/or suturing.

Topical astringents, vasoconstrictors, and *hemostatic agents* are usually of three basic types: epinephrine and epinephrine-like drugs, epinephrine combinations, and non-epinephrine. Epinephrine constricts the gingival vasculature to shrink tissues and reduce or prevent hemorrhage. In retraction cords, string-like cords, are used to be packed in the gingival sulcus (Fig. 5), with racemic epinephrine as high as 8%, that is, several hundred times more concentrated than that in local anesthetics with 1:100,000 epinephrine combination. An undetermined amount of the solution will be absorbed systemically, a situation that can be accelerated greatly in lacerated or injured tissues. Therefore, patients with contraindications to the use of epinephrine (cardiac disease, natural or induced hyperthyroidism, certain other endocrine disorders, and halothane use) should not be exposed to this type of agent (49,50). Additionally, epinephrine can result in localized tissue destruction due to ischemia (50). With tissue injury, a pressor response should be expected. For these reasons, products containing epinephrine generally should be used only on healthy tissues in healthy patients, as in retraction cords prior to crown preparation or in anticipation or prevention of problems. Those wishing to make use of the advantages of epinephrine, but with reduced risk, usually use the combination products. In these, the amount of epinephrine has usually been significantly reduced, and zinc phenolsulfonate, a gentle astringent, has been added to improve the effect. Another similar product is 4% levoepinephrine with 9% potassium alum. The most common non-epinephrine solution is aluminum chloride, which works by an astringent action to produce shrinkage or contraction of the tissues and reduce sulcal secretions and minor hemorrhage. It is commonly available in 5% solutions but can be used in higher concentrations of 25% (Hemodent™, Premier Dental) when properly buffered. Some other products used are 100% alum solution, 20% tannic acid, 8% zinc chloride, ferric subsulfate (Monsel's solution), and 13.3% ferric sulfate (Astringedent™, Ultradent Products, Salt Lake City, Utah) (47,51–52).

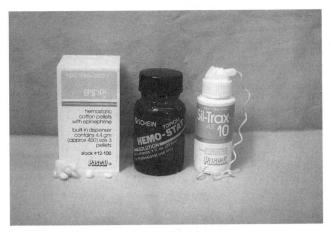

FIG. 5. Retraction cord or hemol sol.

Fluoride—Systemic and Topical Considerations

Fluoride in human dentistry is available in systemic (dietary) and topical dosage forms. Fluoride in water and foods (53,54) is absorbed from the gastrointestinal tract and is distributed throughout the body to exert a systemic effect. This systemically absorbed fluoride is recycled to the saliva to provide low-level topical delivery that can effectively repair acidic demineralized tooth surfaces (55). Since fluoride is readily absorbed, there is the potential for toxicity from both dietary and topical fluoride preparations, as well as simple overdoses taken from fluoride product containers. The fatal human oral dose of fluoride has been estimated at 2.5–5 g, or about 50 mg/kg body weight (56). The Council on Dental Therapeutics of the American Dental Association recommends that no more than 120 mg of fluoride be dispensed in any human fluoride product (57). Any professionally or owner-applied topical fluoride has the potential to exert systemic toxicity, since animals will not normally expectorate the fluoride. For this reason, it is important to apply the higher concentration of fluoride directly to isolated teeth, thereby minimizing soft tissue absorption. Application with a small brush or cotton swab and cotton-roll isolation can minimize oral soft tissue contact and thus absorption. Since there does not appear at the moment to be supporting data for the use of dietary or systemic fluorides with companion animals, the remainder of the fluoride section will focus on topical fluoride use.

Topical fluorides are commonly used in human dental offices and have had a growing popularity in veterinary dentistry. There is reliable evidence in man and animals that it has adverse affects on some of the types of bacteria that are found in root caries, coronal caries, and periodontal lesions (58–60) and can inhibit plaque formation and reduce dental sensitivity (61–63).

The most common topical fluorides used in veterinary dentistry are sodium fluoride, acidulated phosphate fluoride, stannous fluoride (SnF_2), hydrogen fluoride, and sodium monofluorophosphate. For initial treatments, the teeth are cleaned, dried, and isolated with cotton rolls, and the teeth are coated with the fluoride by brush or in trays for 3–5 minutes. The material is then removed by vacuum, blown free with air, or gently wiped clean, but not rinsed off with water.

Neutral sodium fluoride (pH 7.0) is one of the most common topical preparations (47). Sodium fluoride (NaF; molecular weight 42.00; F 45.2%; Na 54.8%) is freely soluble in water with a resultant neutral pH. It is typically used as a 2% sodium fluoride (10,000 ppm F) topical solution or thickened gel with an agent such as carboxymethylcellulose. Neutral fluoride is passively absorbed into enamel primarily at partially demineralized areas, whereas acidic fluoride preparations react with enamel to create a light demineralization and thereby increase the fluoride concentrations in the tooth surface area. It is available in gels or solutions of 0.01–2.0%. PreviDent Plus® (Colgate-Hoyt Laboratories, Canton, Massachusetts) is a 2.0% neutral sodium fluoride gel of this category designed for professional use. Varnishes such as Copanol-F™ (Sultan Chemicals) are copal gum with fluoride (derived from sodium fluoride) 0.055%. These are painted onto the dry tooth surface and allowed to dry, in hopes of attaining a longer duration of tooth contact and a slow release of the fluoride (64). C.E.T®. Oral Hygiene Spray with Fluoride (St. Jon Laboratories, Harbor City, CA) is a 0.02% sodium fluoride solution (100 ppm F) for home care with dogs and cats.

Acidic fluorides such as acidulated phosphate fluoride (APF) is most commonly available as Brudevold's Solution. The original APF solution was prepared with sodium fluoride, hydrogen fluoride (hydrofluoric acid in water) to 1.23% fluoride in 0.1 mol/L phosphoric acid to a final pH of 3.0 (65). This APF solution is very difficult to prepare, and manufacturers therefore have not used the hydrogen fluoride, thus giving a final solution pH of about 5. The fluoride uptake levels of acetic solutions at pH 3 and pH 5 are considerably different. The fluoride uptake of higher pH solutions are more comparable with neutral fluoride solutions than APF solutions. On the other hand, both neutral and acetic solutions at 1.23% have been found to be clinically effective in reducing human dental caries. The question remains whether an aggressive fluoride uptake solution might be more effective in reducing the special tooth demineralization occurring in cats. APF is used in solutions and gels. It is a combination of sodium fluoride 1.23% and orthophosphoric acid 1.0% usually with a pH between 3.0 and 3.4 (33). The acid may allow greater penetration and remineralization of the tooth surface with a fluoride-rich superficial zone. C.E.T®. Oral Hygiene Spray with Fluoride is an APF oral rinse for use in dogs, cats, and horses.

Stannous fluoride is a tin–fluoride compound (SnF_2; molecular weight 156.70; F 24.2%; Sn 75.8%), as the stannous ion is freely soluble in solution to give an acetic pH (66). The pH of stannous fluoride solutions depends on the concentration, eg, 8%, pH 2.3; 0.4%, pH 3.2. The fluoride of stannous fluoride exists in stannous fluoride solutions as a complex that stabilizes both the stannous and fluoride ions. In an aqueous solution of 8.0%, it is fairly acidic in nature (pH 3) and rapidly deteriorates within a few hours by being hydrolyzed into the insoluble stannous hydroxide that precipitates as a flocculent white precipitate (50). Because of its instability in water, fresh solution must be mixed immediately prior to use. To overcome this problem, many manufacturers have prepared 0.4% gels with glycerin that are stable for prolonged periods of time, although always imprinted with an expiration date (47). Stannous fluoride is more stable in a nonaqueous solution such as glycerine, but such solutions need to be hydrated to provide maximum fluoride activity. The stannous ion of stannous fluoride exerts a modest antimicrobial effect that can be demonstrated by plaque reduction (67,68). Typical of chemical antimicrobial agents such as chlorhexidine (69), stannous fluoride stains dental enamel. The stain is superficial and can be removed by simple abrasion with a rubber cup and prophylaxis paste. Stannous fluoride has been used in human dentistry as a professionally applied topical solution at an 8% solution or as a home-use regular rinse solution or dentifrice at 0.4% stannous fluoride, or 1000 ppm fluoride. QyGel™ (Veterinary Products Labs, Phoenix, Arizona) is a 0.4% stannous fluoride gel developed for used in dogs and cats.

Sodium monofluorophosphate (MFP) is a relatively stable inorganic salt that allows its combining with dentifrices and other compounds that have long shelf lives (50). The MFP ion is obtained with sodium monofluorophosphate (Na_2PFO_3; molecular weight 143.95; F 13.2%; P 21.5%; O 33.3%; Na 32.0%); it is absorbed by enamel as such and slowly releases fluoride ion. The same reaction occurs in a calcium-containing product such as a dentifrice. For this reason, sodium MFP is the preferred fluoride source if a calcium-containing system is used, eg, dentifrice with a calcium carbonate abrasive cleansing system (70). Although the release of fluoride from the fluorophosphate ion is slower than from sodium fluoride, the clinical anticarious activity of fluoride from both sources at 1000 ppm in dentifrice formulations is comparable. Sodium MFP has been used in human dentistry primarily in dentifrice formulations at 0.76% (1000 ppm F), rather than topical solutions. C.E.T®. toothpaste (VRx Products, Division of St. Jon Laboratories, Harbor City, California) is a dog and cat dentifrice with 250 ppm fluoride.

Other miscellaneous fluoride compounds are used or are being tested for use. Among these are hydrogen fluoride 0.14%, ammonium fluoride 0.1–1.23%, sodium silicofluoride 2.0% , and titanium tetrafluoride 1.0% (71–74).

Fluorides have been used for treatment of sensitive teeth for many years, although the mechanism by which they work is not fully understood (62,63). DentinBloc® (Gel Kam International, Dallas, Texas), a combination of sodium fluoride 1.09%, stannous fluoride 0.40%, and hydrogen fluoride 0.14% is a solution that is painted on sensitive root structures. Sodium Fluoride Paste™ (Sultan Chemicals) contains kaolin, glycerine, and 33⅓% sodium fluoride and is placed on teeth to help desensitize them. Another desensitizing fluoride is 2% sodium silicofluoride.

Use of in-office topical applications has been considered relatively safe and effective. However, with home-care products, more care should be taken as safety and health issues have not been well explored. Fluorides are generally not meant to be taken in large amounts orally, as they may have an adverse effect on calcium metabolism and the gastrointestinal system, nephrotoxic, as well as possibly being genotoxic; and animals will typically swallow any product placed in the mouth (75). Routine or daily home use of fluoride-containing dentifrices or gels in young animals in which teeth have not erupted should be done carefully to reduce the risk of dental fluorosis through unintentional ingestion, however uncommon.

Their use for controlling sensitivity in dogs has been observed by these authors, and since carious lesions are not uncommon in the dog and the fluorides have a distinct effect on their progression, they may be beneficial. Fluorides have been used for slowing the progression and reducing the sensitivity of resorptive lesions in the dog and cat, but no studies have proven a beneficial effect to date.

Chlorhexidine digluconate solutions of 0.1–0.2% have been used in the treatment of periodontal disease. It is a diguanidohexane and has shown abilities to inhibit the development of plaque and calculus and the onset of gingivitis in humans (76). It is available in solutions, gels, and dentifrices. It does have a bitter taste and has been reported to cause severe skin and mucosal irritations on occasions when it is used in high concentration or left on tissues for too long a time. It also has been reported occasionally to stain teeth, restorations, tongue, and oral mucosa brown. It can be irritating to the eyes and is ototoxic, and if it makes contact with the middle ear, deafness has been reported (77,78). CHX™ (VRx Products) is a 0.12% chlorhexidine gluconate tooth-brushing gel for dogs, cats, and horses, and is also available in a oral cleansing solution. *Chlorhexidine acetate* is also used in animals for a similar effect as the gluconate form. Oral Fresh™ is one such cleansing solution (Cislak®, Burbank, Illinois). Although little actual research information is available on the effectiveness of the acetate form in animals, it is reasonable to expect a similar mode of effect.

Zinc ascorbate solutions have been shown to support collagen synthesis (61) and generally reduce bad breath for a short period of time. Maxiguard™ Oral Cleansing Gel (Addison Biological Laboratory, Fayette, Missouri) is a gel developed for dog and cat use. It is generally used to aid in control of oral-related malodor and to stimulate healing following surgery.

Stabilized chlorine dioxide is a chemical used in various products to reduce odor. It is available in a toothpaste and mouth rinse as Oxyfresh™ (Oxyfresh USA, Spokane, Washington) for use in humans. It is being used in veterinary dentistry, but no research is available on its safety or effectiveness in animals.

Lactoperoxidase and *glucose oxidase* are enzymes used to augment normal salivary peroxidase production for a mild antiplaque and antibacterial effect (61). The enzymatics are used to improve dentifrice performance with less actual mechanical action. C.E.T® Enzymatic Dentifrice (St. Jon Laboratories) has both chemicals present in it and was designed for companion animals. C.E.T.® Oral Hygiene Spray (St. Jon Laboratories), used in dogs, cats and horses, has zinc gluconate, citric acid, and glucose oxidase as active ingredients.

Hydrogen peroxide in a 3% solution is a mild oxidizing agent that kills certain anaerobic bacteria (79). Its germicidal effect is considerably diminished when in contact with tissues, as it rapidly deteriorates in the presence of organic matter. It is used to some degree in cleansing of periodontal lesions and irrigation of a root canal. It should be used with care in deep periodontal pockets and deep dental lesions, as gas is liberated and must have a route of escape (47).

Bleaching agents are typically hydrogen peroxide or complexes of it such as *urea peroxide* (*carbamide peroxide*) (50). Hydrogen peroxide in 29–39% concentrations (Superoxol™, Union Broach, Monrovia, California) is used for in-office bleaching of vital and nonvital teeth, frequently with the aid of a strong light source or a heating unit to enhance its effect. It is a strong oxidizing agent and all tissues except the teeth being treated should be protected against its highly irritational action (47). Storage should only be in the original container in a cool, dark, secured location. It should not be stored near other products that are easily oxidized. Carbimide (urea) peroxide is used for some office and many home tooth-bleaching products. It is usually provided in 10–16% gels (Rembrandt Lighten™ Bleaching Gel, Den-Mat® Corporation, Santa Maria, California) that use glycerin as a base to improve its adherence to the dental tissues.

Pumice is an abrasive formed from a mixture of complex aluminum, potassium, and sodium silicates. Flour of pumice is used to polish teeth following prophylaxis, as well as in laboratory work to polish restorations and acrylics. It commonly has fluoride incorporated with it in prophylaxis pastes. Coarser pumices are sometimes used in stain removal, but they should be used with care, as dental structure can rapidly be removed (47). Pumice should not be used in dentifrices for routine use, as it is too abrasive and can cause excessive abrasion of dental tissues. Even after prophylaxis, it should be used carefully and with a light touch. In human dentistry, at times teeth are not polished to prevent additional wear and sensitivity problems.

Disclosing agents are solutions or wafers that are effective in staining plaque, calculus, and bacterial deposits on the teeth, tongue, and gingiva (Fig. 6). Three types of disclosing agents are available: one stage, two stage, and fluorescein (80–82). The one-stage

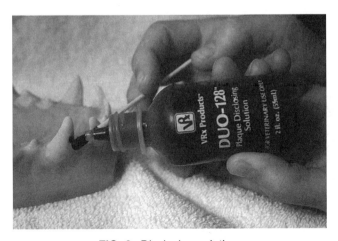

FIG. 6. Disclosing solution.

agent, usually erythrosine (FD&C Red No.3) or Bismark Brown, discolor plaque and calculus the same color. The two-stage agents, a mixture of two dyes (FD&C Green No.3 and FD&C Red No.3), discolor new deposits and old deposits different colors. The fluorescein-disclosing agent (FD&C Yellow No.8) requires an ultraviolet-light source in the 380-nm range for discernible observations (82). The wafers are seldom useful for animals, but the solutions provide a quality-control check following prophylaxis. The agent is applied to a cotton tip applicator, then applied to the teeth. The mouth is rinsed with water to remove excess agent, and stained areas are examined for. It can also be used on patients in front of clients as a motivational tool to encourage home care and professional dental cleanings. However, these products can cause staining to hair, oral tissues, hands, clothing, sinks, tables, etc. and must be used cautiously, as they can be a client irritator rather than a motivator at times (83).

REFERENCES

1. Buchanan LS. Cleaning and shaping the root canal system. In: Cohen S, Burns RC, eds. *Pathways to the Pulp.* 5th ed. St. Louis, MO: Mosby-Year Book; 1991:166.
2. Wiggs RB. Endodontic instrumentation. *J Vet Dent* 1991;8(4):4.
3. Becker GL, Cohen S, Borer R. The sequelae of accidentally injected sodium hypochlorite beyond the root apex. *J Oral Surg, Oral Med, Oral Pathol* 1974;38:633.
4. Bernatti O, Stolf WC, Ruhnke LA. Verification of the consistency, setting times, and dimensional changes of root canal filling materials. *J Oral Surg, Oral Med, Oral Pathol* 1987;46:107.
5. Brayton SM, Davis SR, Goldman M. Gutta-percha root canal fillings: An in vitro analysis. I. *Oral Surg* 1973;35:226.
6. Schindler W. Nonsurgical endodontic therapy on the canine tooth of the dog. *J Endod* 1986;12:573.
7. *Dentists' Desk Reference: Materials, Instruments and Equipment.* 2nd ed. Chicago: American Dental Association; 1983.
8. Grossman LI. Physical properties of root canal cements. *J Endod* 1976;2:166.
9. Wiggs RB. *Orthodontics in the Canine. AVDS Proceedings.* St. Louis, MO: 17;1989.
10. Copeland HI, Brauer GM, Forziati A. The setting mechanism of zinc oxide and eugenol mixtures. *J Dent Res* 1955;34:740.
11. Crane D, et al. Biological and physical properties of experimental non-eugenol endodontic sealers. *J Dent Res* 1975;54(A):L40.
12. Pawes DR, Folleras T, Merson SA, Wilson AD. Improved adhesion of a glass ionomer cement to dentin and enamel. *J Dent Res* 1982;61:1416.
13. Blackman R, Gross M, Seltzer S. An evaluation of the biocompatability of a glass ionomer-silver cement in rat connective tissue. *J Endod* 1989;12:76.
14. Cacedo R, Von Fraunhofer JA. The properties of endodontic sealer cements. *J Endod* 1988;14:527.
15. Cohen T, Gutmann JL, Wagner M. An assessment in vitro of sealing properties of calciobiotic root canal sealer. *Int Endod J* 1985;18:172.
16. Grossman L. Obturation of the canal. In: *Endodontic Practice.* 9th ed. Philadelphia: Lea & Febiger; 1978:277.
17. Holmstrom SE. Restorative materials. *J Vet Dent* 1991;8:12.
18. Phillips RW. *Skinner's Science of Dental Materials.* 8th ed. Philadelphia: WB Saunders Co; 1982:28,195.
19. Phillips RW. *Elements of Dental Materials.* 2nd ed. Philadelphia: WB Saunders Co; 1971:96.
20. Craig RG. Chemistry, composition, and properties of composite resins. *Dent Clin North Am* 1981;25:345.
21. Macchi RL, Craig RG. Physical and mechanical properties of composite restorative materials. *JADA* 1969;78:328.
22. Zwemer TJ. *Boucher's Clinical Dental Terminology.* 3rd ed. St.Louis, MO: CV Mosby Co; 1982:228.
23. Wiggs RB, Lobprise HB. *Dental Materials.* AVDC/AVD Forum Proceedings. New Orleans, Louisiana. 1991:27.
24. Craig RG, ed. *Restorative Dental Materials.* 7th ed. St Louis, MO: CV Mosby Co; 1985:198,232,249.
25. Braswell LD, Smith JS. Veterinary dental materials. *J Vet Dent* 1989;6:8.
26. Oilo G. Bond strength of new glass ionomer cements to dentin. *Scand J Dent Res* 1981;89:344.
27. Mount GJ. Restoration with glass ionome cement: Requirements for clinical success. *Oper Dent.* 1981;6:59.
28. Holmstrom SE, Gammon RL. Amalgam. *J Vet Dent* 1988;5:6.
29. Going RE. Status report on cavity liners, varnishes, primers and cleansers. *JADA* 1972;85:654.
30. Phillips S, Bishop BM. An in vitro study of the effect of moisture on glass ionomer cement. *Quint Int* 1985;16:175.
31. Garcia-Godoy F, Malone W. The effect of acid etching on two glass ionomer lining cements. *Quint Int* 1986;17:621.

32. Omar R. A comparative study of the retentive capacity of dental cementing agents. *J Prosthet Dent* 1988;60:35.
33. *Accepted Dental Therapeutics*. 40th ed. Chicago: American Dental Association; 1984:259.
34. McCabe JF. *Anderson's Applied Dental Materials*. 6th ed. Boston: Blackwell Scientific Publishing; 1985:111.
35. Appleby DC, Pameijer CH, Boffa J. The combined reversible hydrocolloidal/irreversible hydrocolloidal impression system. *J Prosthet Dent* 1980;44:72.
36. Appleby DC, Cohen SR, Racowsky LP, Mingledroff EB. The combined reversible hydrocolloidal/irreversible hydrocolloidal impression system: Clinical application. *J Prosthet Dent* 1981;46:48.
37. *Guide to Dental Materials and Devices*. 7th ed. Chicago: American Dental Association; 1974:197.
38. Strassler H. Impression materials duplicate oral tissues. *Dentist* 1987;65(4):15.
39. Hertfort TW, et al. Viscosity of elastomeric impression materials. *J Prosthet Dent* 1977;38:396.
40. Council on Dental Materials and Devices. Status report on polyether impression materials. *JADA* 1977;95:126.
41. Fusayama T, et al. Accuracy of the laminated single impression technique with silicone materials. *J Prosthet Dent* 1974;53:1033.
42. Hembree JH Jr, et al. Effects of moisture on silicone impression materials. *JADA* 1974;89:1134.
43. Wiggs RB, Lobprise HB. Veterinary dental demonstration models. *J Vet Dent* 1992;9:19.
44. Lyon K. Using epoxy for dental castings. *J Vet Dent* 1992;9:4.
45. Luria MA, Dennison JB. A comparison of epoxy resin, dental stone, and silver plated dies for cast gold restorations. *Mich Dent Assoc J* 1981;63:17.
46. United States General Services Administration, Federal Supply Service. Federal Specifications, U-W-138, U-W-140, U-W-00149a (DSA-DM), U-W-156. Washington DC, National Bureau of Standards.
47. *Accepted Dental Therapeutics*. 38th ed. Chicago: American Dental Association; 1979:277.
48. Otterson EJ, Arra MC. Potential hazards of asbestos in periodontal packs. *J Wis State Dent Assoc* 1974;50:435.
49. Nicholson RJ, et al. The detection of C14 labeled epinephrine in the blood stream of a Rhesus monkey following gingival retraction cord. *Journal of Dental Research*. Reprinted Abstracts. 1966:317.
50. *Accepted Dental Therapeutics*. 37th ed. Chicago: American Dental Association; 1977:220.
51. Woycheshin FF. An evaluation of the drugs used for gingival retraction. *J Prosthet Dent* 1964;14:769.
52. Harrison JD. Effects of retraction materials on the gingival sulcus epithelium. *J Prosthet Dent* 1961;11:514.
53. Council on Dental Therapeutics. *Physiology of Fluorides: Accepted Dental Therapeutics*. Chicago: American Dental Association; 1984:395.
54. Mellberg JR, Ripa LW, Leske GS. Fluoride metabolism. In: *Fluoride in Preventive Dentistry*. Chicago: Quintessence Publishing Co; 1983:81.
55. Mellberg JR, et al. Salivary fluoride in remineralization. In: *Fluoride in Preventive Dentistry*. Chicago: Quintessence Publishing Co; 1983:30.
56. Hodge HC, Smith FA. *Biological Effects of Inorganic Fluorides in Fluoride Chemistry*. New York: Academic Press; 1965:4.
57. Council on Dental Therapeutics. *Maximum Amount of Fluoride to Be Dispensed*. Accepted Dental Therapeutics. Chicago: American Dental Association; 1984:401.
58. Bibby BG, Van Kesteren M. The effect of fluorine on mouth bacteria. *J Dent Res* 1940;19:391.
59. Keyes PH. Evaluation of two topical application methods to assess the anticaries potential of drugs in hamsters. *J Oral Ther Pharm* 1966;2:285.
60. Tinanoff N. Review of the antimicrobial action of stannous fluoride. *J Clin Dent* 1990;II(1):22.
61. Holmstrom SE, Frost P, Gammon RL. *Veterinary Dental Techniques for the Small Animal Practitioner*. Philadelphia: WB Saunders Co; 1992:134.
62. Lukomsky EH. Fluorine therapy for exposed dental and alveolar atrophy. *J Dent Res* 1941;20:649.
63. Newman MG, Carranza FA Jr, Mazza JE. Fluorides in periodontal therapy. Clinical Uses of Fluoride. Philadelphia: Lea and Febiger; 1985.
64. Seppa T, Leppanen T, Hansen H. Fluoride varnish versus acidulated phosphate fluoride gel: A three-year clinical trial. *Caries Res* 1995;29:327.
65. Council on Dental Therapeutics. *Acidulated Phosphate Fluoride Formulas*. Accepted Dental Therapeutics. Chicago: American Dental Association; 1984:402.
66. Hefferren JJ. Qualitative and quantitative test for stannous fluoride. *J Pharm Chemistry* 1963;52:1090.
67. Addy M, Moran J. Extrinsic tooth discolouration by metal and chlorhexidine: Clinical staining produced by chlorhexidine, iron and tea. *Br Dent J* 1985;159:331.
68. Tinanoff N. Review of the antimicrobial action of stannous fluoride. *J Clin Dent* 1990;11:24.
69. Boyce EN, Logan EI. Oral health assessment in dogs: Study design and results. *J Vet Dent* 1994;11:64.
70. Council on Dental Therapeutics. *Sodium Monofluorophosphate Dentifrices*. Accepted Dental Therapeutics. Chicago: American Dental Association; 1984:410.
71. DePaola PF, et al. Effects of high-concentrations ammonium and sodium fluoride rinses on dental caries in school children. *Community Dent Oral Epidemiol* 1977;5:7.
72. Shern RJ, et al. Clinical study of an amine fluoride gel and acidulated phosphate gel. *Community Dent Oral Epidemiol* 1976;4:133.
73. Reed AJ, Bibby BG. Preliminary report on effect of topical applications of titanium tetrafluoride on dental caries. *J Dent Res* 1976;55:357.
74. Hunter GC Jr, Barringer M, Spooner G. Analysis of desensitization of dentin by sodium silicofluoride. *J Periodontol* 1961;32:333.

75. Dietrich UB. No justification for fluoride use in dogs. *Vet Forum* 1992;7:96.
76. Loe H, ed. Symposium on chlorhexidine in the prophylaxis of dental disease. *J Periodontal Res* 1973; (suppl 12):12;5–6.
77. Gjermo P. Chlorhexidine in dental practice. *J Clin Periodontol* 1974;1:143.
78. Birdwood G. Reactions to chlorhexidine and cetrimide. *Lancet* 1965;1:651. Letters to the Editor.
79. Knighton HT. The effect of oxidizing agents on certain non-spore-forming anaerobes. *J Dent Res* 1940;19:429.
80. Arnim SS. The use of disclosing agents for measuring tooth cleanliness. *J Periodontol* 1963;34:227.
81. Block PL Lobene RR, Desdivonis JA. Two-tone dye test for dental plaque. *J Periodontol* 1972;43:423.
82. Lang NP, Ostergaard S, Loe H. A fluorescent plaque disclosing agent. *J Peridontal Res* 1972;7:59.
83. Cohen DW, et al. A comparison of bacterial plaque disclosants in periodontal disease. *J Periodontol* 1972; 43:333.

3

Oral Anatomy and Physiology

Robert B. Wiggs and Heidi B. Lobprise

The dog will be primarily discussed in this chapter, although some comparative information will be covered. Related anatomy and variations for other species will be discussed within chapters covering those matters. This chapter is intended to provide the foundation knowledge for the chapters that follow. The practice of veterinary dentistry is concerned with the conservation, reestablishment, and/or treatment of dental, paradental, and oral structures. In dealing with their associated problems, a fundamental awareness of anatomy and physiology is essential for an understanding of the presence or absence of the abnormal or pathologic structure. Anatomy and physiology are acutely interactive, with anatomy considered to be the study of structure and with physiology the study of function. These deal with bones, muscles, vascularity, nerves, teeth, and periodontium, as well as general oral functions and their development.

GENERAL TERMS

Dentes decidui—deciduous teeth
Dentes permanentes—permanent teeth
Dentes incisivi—incisor teeth
Dentes canini—canine, cuspid, eye, and fang teeth
Dentes premolares—premolar teeth
Dentes molares—molar teeth

Three Basic Types of Tooth Development

Monophyodont. In this type of tooth development, only one set of teeth will erupt and remain in function throughout life; there are no deciduous teeth. As currently accepted, most rodents (heterodont) and the dolphins (homodont) are in this group.

Polyphyodont. Most of the animals in which many sets of teeth are continually replaced are homodonts. In fish, such as the shark, the replacement is generally of a horizontal nature, with new teeth developing caudally and moving forward. In the amphibians, such as the crocodile, the replacement is generally of a vertical nature, with new teeth developing immediately below the teeth in current occlusion and replacing them when lost.

Diphyodont. Most domesticated animals (cat, dog, cow, horse, etc.) and humans are diphyodonts, having two sets of teeth, one designated deciduous or primary and one permanent.

Common Terms Used with Diphyodont Tooth Development

Deciduous Teeth (Dentes Decidui). These are considered to be the first set of teeth that are shed at some point and replaced by permanent teeth. Some distractors feel the term is not totally correct in that *deciduous* indicates something that is shed and replaced on regular basis, such as the leaves of deciduous trees.

Primary Teeth (Dentes Primarii). Like deciduous teeth, primary teeth are considered to be the first set of teeth that are shed at some point and replaced by permanent teeth. Some distractors feel this term is not totally correct because in some species primary teeth are also their permanent teeth and even in diphyodonts some permanent teeth (eg, the first premolar and molars in the dog) may theoretically also be classified as primary, since all teeth may eventually be exfoliated.

Temporary Teeth (Dentes Temporarii). Like the previous two terms, these are considered to be the first set of temporary teeth that are shed at some point and replaced by permanent teeth.

Note: The terms *deciduous* and *primary* are generally more accepted than the terms *temporary, baby,* or *milk* teeth.

Permanent Teeth (Dentes Permanentes). The final or lasting set of teeth are typically of a very durable and lasting nature (opposite of deciduous).

Nonsuccessional Teeth (Dentes Nonsuccedaneous). These are permanent teeth, classically molars, that do not succeed a deciduous counterpart.

Successional Teeth (Dentes Succedaneous). Permanent teeth, typically certain diphyodont incisors, cuspids, or premolars, that replace or succeed a deciduous counterpart are successional teeth.

Mixed Dentition. A combination of erupted deciduous and permanent teeth may develop within the same oral cavity. It is commonly seen in diphyodonts during the early stages of permanent tooth eruption, until all deciduous teeth have been exfoliated.

Two Basic Categories of Tooth Types or Shapes

Homodont. All teeth are of the same general shape or type, although size may vary, as in fish, reptiles, and sharks.

Heterodont. Several types of teeth are represented in the dentition, including incisors, cuspids, premolars, and molars. The domestic dog and cat have heterodont dentition.

Three Common Types of Vertebrate Tooth Anchorage

Thecodont. Teeth are firmly set in sockets, typically using gomphosis, as in dogs, cats, and humans. Gomphosis is a type of fibrous joint, in which a conical object is inserted into a socket and held in place.

Acrodont. In acrodonts, such as the agomid and turatara, teeth are not set in sockets and there is no true root structure. Teeth instead are ankylosed directly to underlying bone.

Pleurodont. Teeth are not set in sockets but, as in most lizards and snakes except the agomid, grow from pockets inside the jaw.

Two Basic Tooth Crown Types

Brachyodont. Dogs, cats, primates, and carnivores in general have dentition with a shorter crown:root ratio.

Hypsodont. In this crown type, dentition has a submerged, longer anatomical or reserved crown and comparatively short roots. As the crown wears down, additional submerged crown erupts. As in the horse and cow, these are continually erupting teeth.

Radicular Hypsodont. In this subdivision of the hypsodont type, dentition has true roots (sometimes called *closed rooted*) and erupts additional crown through most of life. These teeth eventually close their root apices and cease growth. As teeth are worn down, new crown emerges from the reserve or submerged crown of the teeth, as in the cheek teeth of the horse and cow. These are also known as continually erupting closed-rooted teeth.

Aradicular Hypsodont. This other subdivision of the hypsodont crown type is marked by the absence of true roots (some times called *open rooted*). In this type, additional crown is produced throughout life. As teeth are worn down, new crown emerges from the continually growing teeth, as in the lagomorphs and the incisors of rodents. These are known as continually growing teeth or open-rooted teeth.

General Crown Cusp Terms of Cheek Teeth

Secodont Dentition. In this type of dentition, cheek teeth have cutting tubercles or cusps arranged to provide a cutting or shearing interaction. This is especially notable in the carnassial teeth, such as the premolars in most carnivores (eg, the dog and cat).

Bunodont Dentition. Low, rounded cusps on the occlusal surface of the crown mark this form of cheek teeth. Cusps are commonly arranged side by side on the occlusal surface for crushing and grinding, such as the molars in primates (including man), bears, and swine, the first maxillary molar in the cat, and the first and second maxillary and second and third mandibular molars in the dog.

Lophodont Dentition. This type is marked by cheek teeth having cusps that connect to form ridges, as in the rhinoceros and elephant.

Selenodont Dentition. Cheek teeth with cusps that connect may also form a crescentic outline, with a quarter-moon or concavoconvex ridge pattern, as in the artiodactyls, except swine.

Bunolophodont Dentition. In this form of dentition, cheek teeth have both rounded cusps and transverse ridges on the occlusal surface of the crown.

Bunoselenodont Dentition. In this type, cheek teeth have both rounded cusps and crescentic ridges on the occlusal surface of the crown.

Two Types of Jaw Occlusal Overlay

Isognathous. With equal jaws, the premolars and molars of opposing jaws align with the occlusal surfaces facing each other, forming an occlusal plane. Man is an imperfect isognathic, having nearly equal jaws.

Anisognathous. In unequal jaws, the mandibular molar occlusal zone is narrower than the maxillary counterpart, as in the cat, dog, cow, horse, etc.

Description of the Oral Anatomy of the Dog and Cat

The dog and cat have diphyodont tooth development with heterodont tooth-type variation; their jaws are anisognathic. Tooth anchorage is thecodont, and crowns are of the brachyodont type, with secodont premolars and bunodont molars.

DEVELOPMENT

Development of the gastrointestinal tract begins early in embryonic formation. The roof of the entodermal yolk sac enfolds into a tubular tract forming the gut tube that will become the *digestive tract*. It is initially a blind tract, being closed at both the upper and bottom ends. The bottom ultimately becomes the anal opening (cloaca), and the upper portion connects with the primitive oral cavity (*stomodeum* or *ectodermal mouth*). The stomodeum and foregut are at this time separated by a common wall known as the *buccopharyngeal membrane*. It is located at a level that will become the *oropharynx*, a section between the tonsils and base of the tongue. This pharyngeal membrane eventually disappears, establishing a shared connection between the oral cavity and the digestive tract.

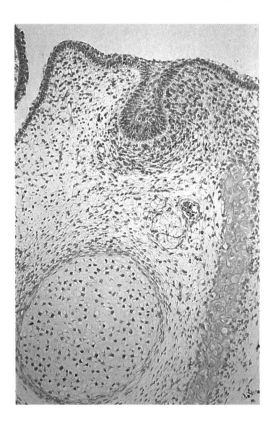

FIG. 1. Enamel organ development: bud stage of tooth germ in 16-mm, 24-day-old cat embryo. Bone formation of mandible can be found beside the Meckel's cartilage. Infra-alveolar artery and nerve are present between the tooth germ and the cartilage. (Courtesy of Dr. Ayako Okuda, Tokyo, Japan.)

Around day 21 of development, *branchial arches I* and *II* are present. By day 23, the paired *maxillary* and *mandibular processes of branchial arch I* have become distinct. The mandibular processes grow forward, forming the *mandible* and merging at the *mandibular symphysis*, which in the dog and cat normally remains a fibrous union throughout life. The paired maxillary processes form most of the *maxillae, incisal* and *palatine bones* of the roof of the mouth.

Initial development of the dental structures occurs during embryonic formation. Rudimentary signs of tooth development occur approximately at the 25th day of development when the *embryonic oral (stratified squamous) epithelium* begins to thicken. This thickening, known as the *dental lamina*, forms two U-shaped structures that eventually become the *upper* and *lower dental arches*. The *enamel organ* arises from a series of invaginations of the dental lamina. The oral epithelium, dental lamina, and enamel organ originate from the outer embryonic germ layer known as *ectoderm*. The *dental papilla* and *sac* appear in coordination with the enamel but originate from *mesoderm*.

The enamel organ develops through a series of stages known as the *bud, cap,* and *bell* (Figs. 1–3). The first, known as the bud stage, is the initial budding off from the dental lamina at the areas corresponding to the deciduous dentition. The bud eventual develops a concavity at the deepest portion, marking the start of the cap stage. As the enamel organ enters this stage, it is composed of three parts: the *outer enamel epithelium (OEE)* on the outer portion of the cap, the *inner enamel epithelium (IEE)* lining the concavity, and the *stellate reticulum* within the cap. The onset of the bell stage occurs as a fourth layer to

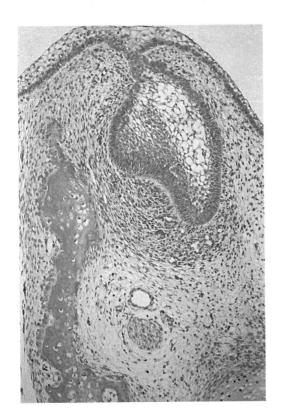

FIG. 2. Enamel organ development: cap stage of tooth germ in 24-mm, 28-day-old cat embryo. The enamel organ, outer enamel epithelium, stellate reticulum, and inner enamel epithelium are covering the dental papilla, mesenchymal. (Courtesy of Dr. Ayako Okuda, Tokyo, Japan.)

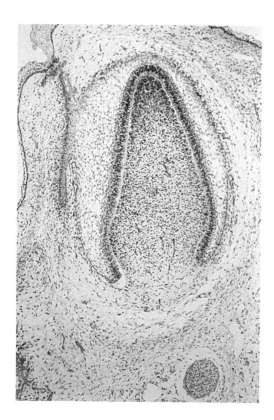

FIG. 3. Enamel organ development: bell stage of tooth germ in 40-mm, 33-day-old cat embryo. The enamel organ is shaped in the complete contour of the tooth. Inner enamel epithelial cells are elongated with nuclear polarization, called ameloblasts. Once odontoblasts (differentiated from mesenchymal cells at the outer cell layer of the dental papilla) form dentin, ameloblasts start enamel formation. (Courtesy of Dr. Ayako Okuda, Tokyo, Japan.)

the enamel organ, the stratum intermedium, emerges between the IEE and the stellate reticulum (Fig. 4).

Each layer of the enamel organ is thought to have a specific functions to perform. The OEE acts as a protective layer for the entire organ. Stellate reticulum works as a cushion for protection of the IEE and allows vascular fluids to percolate between cells and reach the stratum intermedium. The stratum intermedium apparently converts the vascular fluids to usable nourishment for the IEE. The IEE goes through numerous changes, ultimately being responsible for actual enamel formation.

The dental lamina buds that form the primary dentition develop lingual extensions referred to as *successional lamina*. The successional lamina progresses through bud, cap, and bell stages to eventually form the successional permanent dentition. The *nonsuccessional teeth* (those permanents not succeeding deciduous counterparts) develop directly from the dental lamina in the posterior portion of the arch.

During late bud stage, embryonic connective tissue known as *mesenchymal cells* begins development of the dental papilla and dental sac from an area adjacent to the IEE. The mesodermal cells of the dental papilla form the dentinal and pulpal tissues of the forming tooth. The dental sac is composed of several rows of flattened mesodermal cells covering the dental papilla and attaching part of the way up the OEE of the bud. It gives rise to cementum, periodontal ligament, and some alveolar bone.

The *frontal prominence*, the forehead area of the embryo, occurs in coordination with the stomodeum and mandibular processes. *Nasal pits*, the beginning of the nasal cavities,

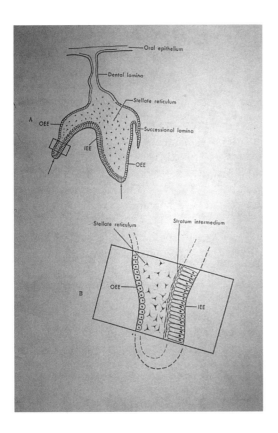

FIG. 4. At the bell stage, onset of enamel organ development. **(A)** Concavity of inner enamel epithelium cells has increased. Successional lamina can be seen developing to lingual side of primary tooth. **(B)** Enlargement of outline section of part A. There are several layers of flattened cells: stratum intermedium, as well as IEE, OEE, and stellate reticulum. (Reproduced with permission from Brand RW, Isselhard DE. *Anatomy of Orofacial Structures.* 4th ed. St Louis, MO: CV Mosby Co; 1994:49.)

are first revealed by two small depressions found low on the frontal prominence. On either side of the nasal pits are the *medial* and *lateral nasal processes*. The two medial nasal and the two maxillary processes form the upper lip. The groove between the two fills with connective tissue in a process known as *migration*. If migration fails to occur, the tissues will be stretched thin and will tear. This results in a separation between the medial nasal and maxillary process, causing a *cleft lip*.

The left and right maxillary processes and the single medial nasal processes also form the *palate*. The incisal portion (maxilla) of the hard palate is the part from the maxillary incisal teeth back to the incisive foramen. The area of the *incisal bone* (the premaxilla in some species and formerly in the dog) is also known as the *primary palate* and is formed solely by the medial nasal process. At this stage, the oral and nasal cavities communicate with each other. The medial nasal process forms the *philtrum* and helps form the *nasal septum*. The left and right maxillary processes form two palatal shelves that grow inward toward the midline, beginning rostrally and then attaching to the primary palate and growing together. This is known as the *secondary palate*.

Cleft lips and *palates* are not uncommon. Clefts are generally designated as unilateral or bilateral and may occur at days 24–27 of gestation. A unilateral cleft lip occurs when migration fails to occur between one of the maxillary processes and the medial nasal process. A bilateral cleft lip occurs when both maxillary processes fail to migrate. A unilateral cleft palate occurs when only one of the palatal plates of the maxillary processes fuses with the nasal septum. A bilateral cleft palate occurs when both palatal plates of the maxillary processes fail to fuse with the opposite plates at the nasal septum. Clefts of hard or soft palates develop in a wide range of varying degrees of severity.

Enamel, Dentin, and Pulp

Enamel, dentin, and pulp are three structures that have an intimate relationship during early development, although they do not all develop from the same foundation cells. Enamel is produced by the enamel organ, which is derived from ectoderm. In contrast, the dentin and pulp develop from the dental papilla, which is derived from mesoderm.

During the bell stage, the IEE cells evolve into a taller form and become known as *pre-ameloblasts*. The peripheral cells of the dental papilla bordering the preameloblasts transform into low-columnar or cuboidal shapes and are referred to as *odontoblasts*. As the newly formed odontoblasts move toward the center of the dental papilla and away from the preameloblasts, they leave behind a secreted *matrix* of mucopolysaccharide ground substance and collagen fibers. This substance appears to stimulate a polarity shift in the preameloblasts of the nucleus from the center of the cell toward the stratum intermedium. It is thought that this shift in polarity is caused by an alteration in the nutritional supply route to the cells. With this shift in polarity, the cells are now termed *ameloblasts*, signifying their ability to begin secretion of enamel matrix. As this enamel matrix (mucopolysaccharide ground substance and organic fiber) is laid down next to the dentinal matrix, the *dentinoenamel junction (DEJ)* is formed. As the ameloblasts lay down matrix, it moves away from the dentin and toward the OEE. Both the dentin and enamel begin to lay down crystal and mineralize into hard tissue at this point.

Enamel is the hardest and most dense known structure in the body. It has a translucent white color, although it may appear other colors due to the refraction of the underlying dentin. Staining and color changes of the enamel can occur with age. Enamel is approximately 96% inorganic in composition. This inorganic portion is formed by millions of *hydroxyapatite* crystals, as well as magnesium and other ions. The remaining 4% of enamel composition is principally water and fibrous organic material. Enamel is thickest at the cusp, or point, of the tooth. Despite its hardness, enamel is subject to attrition, or wear, from friction of use. Fluorinated enamel has an improved resistance to degradation by acids generated from bacterial activity. Enamel has no capability to regenerate itself when damaged.

The basic building block of enamel is the *enamel rod*. Each rod is a column of enamel that extends from the DEJ to the coronal surface of the tooth. These rods are generally perpendicular both to the DEJ and the surface. In primates, enamel rods are keyhole-shaped in cross-section and fit tightly together. The carnivores have straight Schreger's bands with the enamel rods being more polygonal in shape. The development of this shape is not well understood, since the ameloblasts that secrete them are round to hexagonal in cross-section. Each rod is composed of two parts. The *rod core* and the *rod sheath*. The rod core is composed of hydroxyapatite crystals. The rod sheath, surrounding the columnar side of the rod core, is composed mostly of the organic fibrous substance.

The enamel matrix is laid down at the end of the bell stage. All of the crystal placed within the rods is laid down at this time. This is known as the *mineralization stage of calcification* of the enamel rod. The next is the *maturation stage of calcification*. It is during this stage that the crystals grow in size, becoming tightly packed together within the enamel rod. Should the crystals fail to grow to full size, the rods will be poorly calcified and have less than 96% inorganic composition. This results in a condition known as *hypocalcification.* The *striae* or *stripes of Retzius* are darker lines in the enamel that radiate out in a curve from the DEJ. These are areas of slight variation in the crystal content of the rods. In humans, it appears that at approximately every fourth day of the ameloblast cycle, there is a change in the rod development or cycle of rest that results in these lines or striae. As these Retzius' striae are visible on the exposed surface enamel, they cause slight horizontal lines or ripples in the enamel. Known as *imbrication* or *perikymata lines*, they have not been distinctly described in dog or cat teeth.

As enamel is produced by the ameloblasts, a change occurs in the enamel organ. The ameloblasts gradually begin to compress the two middle layers of the organ, the stratum intermedium and the stellate reticulum. The middle layers are eventually lost, and the ameloblasts make contact with the OEE. This activates the final two functions of the ameloblasts to commence. First, a protective layer is laid down on top of the enamel, known as the *primary enamel cuticle* or *Nasmyth's membrane.* This cuticle remains on the teeth for weeks to months, until it is worn away by abrasion. It is laid down on the crown from the tip toward the cementoenamel junction. Once the cuticle is formed, the ameloblasts merge with the OEE to form the *reduced enamel epithelium.* The reduced enamel epithelium is produced on adhesive-like secretion known as the *secondary enamel cuticle* or *epithelial attachment.* The epithelial attachment functions to hold the gingiva and tooth together at the bottom of the gingival sulcus.

During enamel development, several abnormalities may develop. These are sometimes found on clinical, radiologic, or histologic examination. *Hypoplastic enamel* is marked by generally normal density or calcification, but the enamel is thinner than normal. With *enamel hypocalcification*, spots or areas of the teeth are poorly mineralized, resulting in white, yellow, or brown spots in the enamel. These teeth, being undermineralized, may be soft and wear faster than normal teeth. This condition has frequently been mislabeled as *enamel hypoplasia* but is more correctly characterized as hypocalcification. *Enamel tufts* are small areas of hypocalcification found at the DEJ and extending a quarter to a third of the way toward the surfaces. These have no known clinical significance but are commonly found on histologic sectioning. Odontoblastic processes occasionally become entrapped between ameloblasts during development and become embedded in the enamel, being referred to as *enamel spindles.* They are typically found histologically and have no known clinical significance. Cracks in enamel caused by either developmental problems or trauma are known as *enamel lamellae.* The most common form is that caused by trauma resulting in hairline cracks in the enamel. These can be of clinical significance depending on their number and severity,.

Dentin is the hard yellow substance covered by the enamel and cementum. It is approximately 70% inorganic hydroxyapatite crystal and about 30% organic (collagen fibers, mucopolysaccharide substance, and water). Dentin grossly appears to be a solid structure but in reality is perforated by a multitude of openings. In microscopic cross-section, it has three distinct structures. The first is the *dentinal tubule,* a tube extending from the DEJ to the pulp (Fig. 5). The *odontoblastic process* or *Tomes fiber* is a cellular extension of the odontoblast that runs the length of the dentinal tubule. The tubule is surrounded by the *peritubular dentin,* which has a higher crystalline content than the intertubular dentin. The intertubular dentin constitutes the bulk of the dentinal substance.

There are seven basic classifications of dentin: two basic and five variations. Of the two basic types of dentin that develop, *primary dentin* is the first. Primary dentin forms before eruption of the tooth, and *secondary dentin* forms after eruption. Dentin is laid down in layers within the pulp cavity as long as the tooth is vital, resulting in the pulp cavity's gradually decreasing in diameter with age. Secondary dentin begins forming at

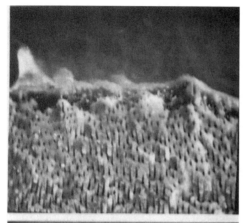
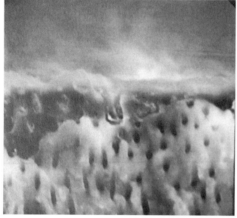

FIG. 5. Scanning electron micrograph cross-section of dentin showing dentinal tubules. (Reproduced with permission from Seltzer S, Bender IB. *The Dental Pulp: Biologic Consideration in Dental Procedures*. 3rd ed. St. Louis, Missouri: Ishiyahu Euroamerica; 51.)

about the same time that root formation is nearing completion. It is formed by the same odontoblasts that formed the primary dentin.

The five variations of dentin types are reparative, interglobular, granular layer of Tomes, dead tract, and sclerotic. *Reparative dentin*, sometimes called *tertiary dentin*, is formed due to trauma of the odontoblasts. This trauma may be thermal, mechanical, occlusal, or chemical. This type of dentin differs histologically from the normal dentin in that it generally has few, if any, dentinal tubules present and appears to be very dense and unorganized. It forms immediately below the cause of the irritation and can result in alteration of normal pulp cavity anatomy. Occlusal trauma subjects the tooth to stresses that cause pressure trauma to the odontoblastic processes, thus stimulating the rapid production of unorganized tertiary dentin. Mechanical trauma is typically the result of cavity preparations in the tooth. These preparations normally extend through the enamel and into the dentin. There are approximately 30,000–40,000 odontoblastic processes damaged for every square millimeter of dentin cut. Many of these injured odontoblasts may die. The adjacent pulp tissue replaces these with reserve mesenchymal cells that differentiate into odontoblasts and immediately begin producing reparative dentin. Thermal damage from polishing, scaling, and other causes can result in the death of odontoblastic processes and the same general effect as mechanical trauma. Chemical trauma is classically the result of acids produced by carious action, but it can result from various substances used to treat or fill teeth.

Interglobular dentin represents areas of dentin found next to the DEJ. It is hypocalci-fied dentin that occurred during formation. *Granular layers of Tomes dentin* is the same as interglobular, except that it is found next to the cementodentinal junction (CDJ). *Dead-tract dentin* is simply an area of dentin in which the dentinal tubules are empty. This typ-ically occurs due to some form of trauma that kills the odontoblasts. These dead tracts or open tubules are easy pathways for bacteria and other substances to make rapid access deep within the tooth. *Sclerotic dentin*, also called *transparent* dentin because of its visual appearance, is made of tubules that have been vacated by the odontoblastic processes and filled with dentinal matrix material. This occurs when traumatized processes begin to secrete matrix substance as they retreat from the tubule.

Mesodermal tissue from the dental papilla forms the *pulp*. Once developed, the pulp consists of blood vessels, lymphatic vessels, nerves, fibroblasts, collagen fibers, undif-ferentiated reserve mesenchymal cells, other cells of connective tissue, and odontoblasts. Odontoblasts are not only an integral part of the dentin but also the peripheral cells of the pulp. The nerves are primarily sensory and transmit only the sensation of pain. There are some motor nerves that innervate the smooth muscles within the blood vessels. These result in constriction of the vessels in response to irritation. Young pulps have a large vol-ume, which is considered primarily cellular, with a small concentration of fibers. The large number of cells allows for repair from trauma. As the pulp ages, it loses volume and reserve mesenchymal cell capacity. This loss of reserve cells is thought to be the reason that older patients are more susceptible to permanent pulpal damage.

The only abnormality of the vital pulp of any consequence is *pulp stones*. These are small calcifications, generally circular in shape. They are commonly found in older humans but do not appear to affect the health of the pulp directly. However, they can pose a problem for teeth being treated endodontically.

Root Formation

Formation of the *root* begins after the general form of the crown has developed but before it completely calcifies. At the junction of the outer enamel epithelium (OEE) and the inner enamel epithelium (IEE), the stellate reticulum and stratum intermedium are missing from the enamel organ at this deepest point, referred to as the *cervical loop*. These two layers of cells become the *epithelial root sheath* or *Hertwig's epithelial root sheath* (Fig. 6). This sheath begins to grow into the underlying connective tissue by rapid mitotic division. This is the initiation of root formation. This growth continues deep into this tissue but at some point angles back toward the center of the forming tooth. The por-tion of the sheath that turns back in is known as the *epithelial diaphragm*. The growth pattern of the epithelial diaphragm determines the number of roots a tooth develops. The point at which the epithelial diaphragm meets will be the apex of a single-rooted tooth but the furcation in multirooted teeth. As the root sheath makes contact with the dental papilla, the epithelial cells stimulate the peripheral contact cells to differentiate into odontoblasts. Once the odontoblasts begin to produce dentin, the root sheath trapped between the dental sac and the dentin begins to break up. As Hertwig's epithelial root sheath dissolves, the dental sac comes into direct contact with the newly formed dentin. Some of the dental sac cells differentiate into cementoblasts and initiate cementum for-mation, while some may differentiate into odontoblasts. The cementum that contacts the dentin becomes the *dentinocemental junction (DCJ)*.

The epithelial root sheath cells that move away from the dentin but fail to dissolve become entrapped in the periodontal ligament and are referred to as *epithelial rests* or

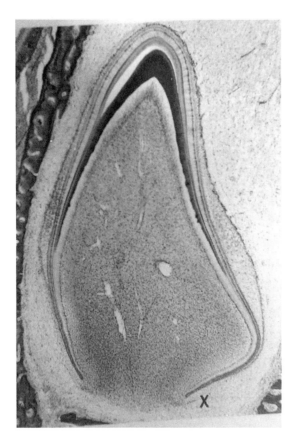

FIG. 6. In the appositional stage of development of premolar teeth, the dentinoenamel and cementoenamel junctions are demarcated, and crown form is apparent (*X*, Hertwig's epithelial Root sheath. (Reproduced with permission from Grant D, Bernick S. Morphodifferentiation and structure of Hertwig's root sheath in the cat. *J Dent Res* 1971;50:1580. Copyright by the American Dental Association.)

epithelial rests of Malassez. These are a normal finding, but should these cells be stimulated to begin dividing again later in life, cysts will develop in the jaws. When epithelial root sheath cells fail to dissolve and remain in contact with the dentin, they typically convert to ameloblasts. These will secrete enamel on the roots, forming what is known as *enamel pearls*. If the root sheath's epithelial diaphragm malfunctions, accessory roots may be formed.

Cementum is an off-white or ivory-colored hard substance that covers the root surface. Its composition is approximately 45–50% inorganic and 50–55% organic materials and water. The inorganic portion is primarily hydroxyapatite crystals, and the organic part primarily collagen fibers and mucopolysaccharide ground substance.

Cementum formation begins at the neck or cervical circumference of the tooth forming the *cementoenamel junction (CEJ)*. This junction is generally one of three types formed: cementum slightly overlapping the enamel, cementum meeting enamel evenly, and cementum failing to meet the enamel. In this third category, a cervical exposure of dentin occurs, which may result in tooth sensitivity problems, should gingival recession occur.

Cementoblasts secrete cementum as they move away from the DCJ. In the cervical one-half to two-thirds of the root, the cementoblasts remain on the surface as the cementum is deposited, and few, if any, of these cells become entrapped in the cementum, which is referred to as the *acellular cementum*. In the apical third, cementoblasts commonly surround themselves with cementum and become trapped. These trapped cells are referred to as *cementocytes*, and this portion of the cementum is identified as *cellular cementum*.

The cementoblast on the surface of the cementum deposits cementum around the ends of the periodontal ligament making contact with them, attaching them to the tooth. These fibers trapped within the cementum are known as *Sharpey's fibers*. The ends of the fibers entrapped in the alveolar bone are also known as Sharpey's fibers.

The cellular cementum of the root apex typically increases with time due to occlusal stresses of the tooth. This thickening is known as *hypercementosis*. Should this become excessive, a bulbous apex may form, which can impede extraction attempts.

Cementum is vital and has the ability to repair itself when injured. The cementoblasts on the surface and the embedded cementocytes receive nourishment from blood vessels of the periodontal ligament.

The bone of the jaws that forms the socket support for the teeth is known as the *alveolar bone*. In the mature animal, this bone, which is mesodermal in origin, is approximately 65% inorganic and 35% organic in composition. The *alveolus* is composed of three distinct layers. The compact bone on the inside of the socket next to the tooth is known as the *cribriform plate* and, radiographically, is termed the *lamina dura*. It has no periosteal covering, being covered instead by the periodontal ligament. The fibers of the periodontal ligament embedded in the cribriform plate are called Sharpey's fibers. The compact bone rises to the top of the socket, where the *cortical* and cribriform plates meet at the *alveolar crest*. The cortical plates are covered with periosteum. Between the two plates is spongy, cancellous, or trabecular bone, a form of bone marrow. The cribriform plate is constantly undergoing remodeling due to occlusal stresses. This may lead to additional bone being laid down on the plate, referred to as *bundle bone*.

The *periodontal ligament* is derived from the mesodermal cells of the dental sac. This formation begins after cementum deposition has been initiated. The dental sac on contact with the cementum forms fibroblasts that produce collagen fibers at the same time other components of the periodontal ligament are developing. These are blood vessels, lymphatic vessels, nerves, and various types of connective tissue cells. The nerves of the periodontal ligament are quite important in that they provide additional senses to the tooth. It has pain fibers, which the pulp has, but also pressure, heat, and cold fibers, which the pulp does not.

As the fibers of the periodontal ligament form, they begin to arrange themselves into three distinct categories: *gingival*, *trans-septal*, and *alveolodental*. There are three types of gingival fibers: dentogingival, alveologingival and circular gingival. *Dentogingival fibers* run from the cementum to either attached or free gingiva, providing a firm support for these tissues. *Alveologingival fibers* run from the alveolar bone to either attached or free gingiva, providing further support for these tissues. The *circular gingival fibers* are found in the free gingiva running in a circular pattern around the tooth, providing additional support to hold it firmly against the tooth. *Trans-septal fibers* extend from the cementum of one tooth across the interproximal area to the cementum of an adjacent tooth. *Alveolodental fibers* run from alveolar bone to the cementum and are typically divided into five types: alveolar crest, horizontal, oblique, apical, and interradicular. *Alveolar crest fibers* run from the crest in an apico-oblique direction to the cementum. These aid in resistance to extrusion and horizontal movement of the tooth. The *horizontal fibers* also run from the cementum to the alveolar crest, but they run horizontally to resist horizontal tooth movements. *Oblique fibers* extend from the cementum in a coronal-oblique pattern to the alveolar bone and resist occlusal stresses. *Apical fibers* run from the apex to the alveolar bone and resist extrusional forces. The *interradicular fibers* are found only in multirooted teeth and go from the interradicular crestal bone to cementum, counteracting various types of movement according to their direction of attachment.

Tooth Eruption

The emergence and movement of the crown of the tooth into the oral cavity is typically termed *tooth eruption*. The eruption process is generally considered a lifelong process beginning with crown development and progressing until the tooth is exfoliated or the individual dies. The eruptive sequence is generally divided into three stages. The *preeruptive stage* commences with crown development and the formation of the dental lamina. With the onset of root development, the *eruptive stage* begins; this is also sometimes referred to as the *prefunctional* eruptive stage. When the teeth move into actual occlusion, it is termed *posteruptive stage* or *functional* eruptive stage. This stage is considered to continue until tooth loss or death occurs. This stage functions to serve occlusion in several ways. As the jaws grow, the spatial relationship of the mandible and maxilla changes; they move further apart, and the teeth continue to erupt to maintain occlusion. With time, attrition results in loss of dental occlusal contacts, and it is this further eruption that maintains the occlusal balance. In some cases, this can cause an imbalance in occlusion when teeth are lost and *supraeruption* of the opposing teeth occur. Supraeruption is when teeth erupt beyond the normal occlusal line.

Four major theories for eruption have been expounded in the literature. Most likely, none is totally correct in itself, and the most accurate picture is probably a combination of them. The *theory of root growth* is the belief that root growth pushes the crown into the oral cavity. Experiments involving removing Hertwig's epithelial root sheath on developing teeth have stopped root formation. However, these rootless teeth still erupt, thus disproving this as a major factor in eruption. The *theory of growth of pulpal tissue* is the thought that continued growth of the pulp tissue while the hard sides of the tooth were forming provided apical propulsion. Yet developing teeth in which the pulp dies or is removed still erupt, also disproving this as a major factor in eruption. The *theory of bone deposition in the alveolar crypt* is the precept that bone deposition within the alveolar crypt forces the tooth to erupt. This deposition is not constant, and even when the crypt undergoes resorption due to various factors, teeth generally still erupt, making this theory a dubious major factor. The *theory of periodontal ligament force* is the hypothesis that it is the periodontal ligament's driving force that maintains occlusal contact also

TABLE 1. *Eruption times of deciduous and permanent teeth in the dog and cat*

	Deciduous teeth (wk)	Permanent teeth (mo)
Dog		
Incisors	3–4	3–5
Canines (cuspids)	3	4–6
Premolars	4–12	4–6
Molars		5–7
Cat		
Incisors	2–3	3–4
Canine (cuspids)	3–4	4–5
Premolars	3–6	4–6
Molars		4–5

thrusts the tooth into the oral cavity. This is the most plausible postulate, although the exact mechanism is unknown. Eruption times are variable not only with size and breed, but within the breeds themselves. Table 1 shows the general time tables for the dog and cat, respectively.

Exfoliation of deciduous dentition is a complex function and not fully understood. It is believed that as the root of the permanent tooth begins to develop, the crown makes contact with the deciduous tooth root structure. The pressure of the crown on the root and possibly the contact of the permanent tooth's dental sac or the outer enamel epithelium with the root stimulate the resorptive process of the root of the deciduous tooth. Deciduous root resorption is not constant, occurring in cycles or stages. Once sufficient root support is lost, the crown is *shed* or *exfoliated*. Although it is common for deciduous teeth to be retained when a permanent successor does not develop, this is not always the case, indicating that other factors may play a part in root resorption.

Retained (persistent) deciduous teeth are commonly attributed to four causes. The first is lack of a permanent successor. Second is *ankylosis* of the tooth to the alveolus. This occurs during root resorption when holes in Hertwig's root sheath develop and the tooth's cementum makes contact with the alveolar bone and fuses to it. In these cases, it is common to find teeth with almost the entire root structure dissolved, but the crown still firmly in place. Once the ankylosis is relieved, typically the crown rapidly exfoliates. The third reason is failure of the permanent crown to make contact with the deciduous root during eruption. This occurs if either tooth is in an improper position in comparison with the other. The fourth reason is hormonal influences that can effect growth or metabolism.

DENTAL FORMULAS

The currently accepted designations of the dental formula for the dog are as follows:

Deciduous teeth: 2 × (3/3 i, 1/1 c, 3/3 pm) = 28
Permanent teeth: 2 × (3/3 I, 1/1 C, 4/4 PM, 2/3 M) = 42

The currently accepted designations of the dental formula for the cat are as follows:

Deciduous teeth: 2 × (3/3 i, 1/1 c, 3/2 pm) = 26
Permanent teeth: 2 × (3/3 I, 1/1 C, 3/2 PM, 1/1 M) = 30

Additional dental-formula information for the dog and cat can be found in the oral examination chapter (see Chapter 4). Similar information for other species can be found in other chapters (see Chapters 16–19).

DIRECTIONAL, SURFACE, AND RIDGE NOMENCLATURE

Before discussion of dental anatomy, a general understanding of directional, surface, and ridge nomenclature is required (Fig. 7).

First, it must be understood that it is common for ridges to sometimes be referred to as a surface rather than a ridge. Incisors and canine teeth have four exposed surfaces and a ridge or cusp, or five surfaces. Premolars in the dog have four exposed surfaces and a ridge, or five surfaces. Molars have five exposed surfaces.

In the incisor and canine teeth, the surface directed toward the lips is called the *labial surface*. With premolars and molars, the surface facing the cheek is known as the *buccal*

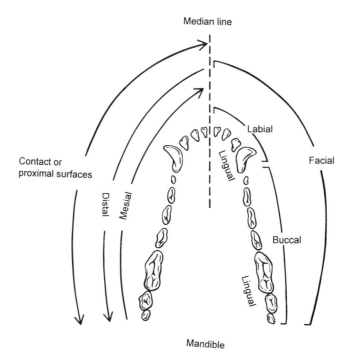

FIG. 7. Directional nomenclature.

surface. The buccal and labial surfaces are known collectively as the *facial surfaces*. All surfaces facing the tongue are described as *lingual*, although in the maxillae this surface is sometimes described as the *palatal surface*. In premolars and molars, the surface making contact with the teeth in the opposite jaw during closure is known as the *occlusal surface*. The ridge of the premolars that does not make contact with opposing teeth is typically referred to as the *occlusal ridge*. In the incisors, the ridge along the most coronal aspect is referred to as the *incisal ridge*. In the canine or cuspid tooth, the cusp is generally called *cusp surface*. Surfaces facing toward adjoining teeth within the same jaw quadrant or dental arch are collectively called the *contact* or *proximal surface*. Proximal surfaces may be either distal or mesial. The term *distal* indicates a proximal surface facing away from the median line of the face. In contrast, the term *mesial* designates the proximal surface facing toward the median line. The space between two facing proximal surfaces is known as the *interproximal space*. *Apical* is a term used to denote a direction toward the root tip or away from the incisal or occlusal surface. The *cusp* is the point or tip of the crown of a tooth. *Coronal* is a term used to indicate a direction toward the crown tip or occlusal surface. The terms *incisal* for incisors and *occlusal* for premolars and molars is also used to indicate the coronal direction. The term *cervical* either means the juncture of the tooth crown and root or a direction toward that point.

Division into Thirds

To further break down tooth locations, for purposes of description and comparison, combinations of the above terms are sometimes used, with one additional term, *middle*

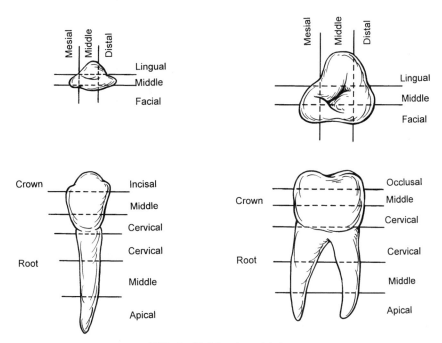

FIG. 8. Division into thirds.

(Fig. 8). The term *middle* means at or toward the middle of a designated portion of the tooth and can indicate either a horizontal, vertical, or occlusal middle area.

Crown Line and Point Angles

For purposes of identifying and classifying distinct areas on teeth in operative dental procedures, the coronal surfaces can be divided and classified by eight line angles and four point angles. These lines and points are also sometimes used for identification of cavity preparation areas.

The *line angles* are simply the dividing lines formed between the surface areas. They are named from the two of the five surfaces that divide them (facial, lingual, mesial, distal, and occlusal, coronal, or incisal). Where the surface terms are joined the *-al* ending is dropped and *o* is added. The eight line angles are (a) mesiofacial (mesiolabial, mesiobuccal); (b) mesiolingual; (c) mesioincisal (mesiocoronal, mesio-occlusal); (d) distofacial (distobuccal, distolabial); (e) distolingual; (f) distoincisal (distocoronal, disto-occlusal); (g) linguoincisal (linguocoronal, linguo-occlusal); and (h) facioincisal (facio-coronal, facio-occlusal).

The *point angles* are the junctures of three of the line angles. There are four coronal point angles, each named for the three surfaces that acutally make the juncture or point. The four point angles are (a) mesiofacioincisal (mesiofaciocoronal, mesiofacio-occlusal, mesiolabioincisal, mesiobuccocoronal, mesiobucco-occusal); (b) mesiolinguoincisal (mesiolinguocoronal, mesiolinguo-occlusal); (c) distofacioincisal (distofaciocoronal, distofacio-occlusal, distolabioincisal, distobuccocoronal, distobucco-occlusal); and (d) distolinguoincisal (distolinguocoronal, distolinguo-occlusal).

Contact Points and Areas

Contact points or areas are the sites where adjacent or opposing teeth make contact. The term *contact area* is frequently considered a more correct term than contact point, since an area is typically making contact rather than a specific point. Adjacent teeth have proximal contact areas, whereas opposing teeth have occusal contact areas.

Embrasures

Projecting away from the proximal contact areas are V-shaped areas termed *embrasures*, named for the surface from which they are derived and the direction they radiate toward. There are theoretically four embrasures between each tooth with proximal contacts. The embrasures are the (a) faciogingival (labiogingival, buccogingival); (b) facioincisal (faciocoronal, facio-occlusal, labioincisal, buccocoronal, bucco-occlusal); (c) linguogingival; and (d) linguoincisal (linguocoronal, linguo-occlusal).

Tooth Function and Terms

Teeth are multifunctional organs that play an important part in overall animal health and activity. Their shape aids physiologically in protection of the oral mucosa and reduction of stress forces on the teeth and the alveolar process. Teeth are used to catch, hold, carry, cut, shear, crush, and grind sustenance. Besides their masticatory functions, they are used in protection, aggression, and sexual attraction. *Sexual dimorphism*, such as length of tooth, may play a part in sexual attraction, as well as social behavior for defense.

Each tooth has a *crown* and a *root*, except for aradicular hypsodonts (see Chapter 17). Generally, the crown is covered with enamel and the root with cementum (Fig. 9). Where the enamel of the crown and cementum of root meet is known as the *cementoenamel junction (CEJ)*. The line formed by the CEJ is commonly called the *neck, cervix,* or *cervical line*. In many cases, especially during eruption and hypsodonts in general, not all of the crown may be fully exposed. The entire crown, whether exposed or not, is the *anatomic crown*. The portion of the crown above the gum line is the *clinical crown* and that below, the *reserved crown*. The reserved crown is occasionally referred to as the *clinical root* as compared with the *anatomic* or *true root*. Teeth may have single or multiple roots. The point at which roots diverge is the *furcation*, and this can be a *bifurcation, trifurcation,* and so on. The termination or apical end of the root is the *apex*. The apex can have a single-opening *apical foramen* or a multiple-opening *apical delta*, through which vessels, nerves, and other structures may pass into the tooth to merge with the pulp (Fig. 10).

The tooth is made up of basically four tissues: three hard and one soft. The *hard tissues* are enamel, cementum, and dentin; the *soft tissue* is the pulp. The pulp tissue occupies the cavern within the tooth known as the *pulp cavity*, which is occasionally improperly referred to as the *root canal system* in some endodontic texts. This cavity is further divided into *pulp chamber* (portion in the crown) and *root canal* (portion within the root). The bottom of the pulp chamber is referred to as the *chamber floor*, and the most coronal part as the *chamber horns*, in which the pulp horns reside.

The *incisor teeth* are designed to cut, scoop, pick at or up, and groom. The term incisor means "that which cuts." The actual biting edge of the incisor is the *incisal edge* or *ridge*. The incisal edge pick up and cuts food, grooms the hair, and is used to catch parasites. The concave lingual surface acts as a scoop and, along with the tongue, aids in carrying

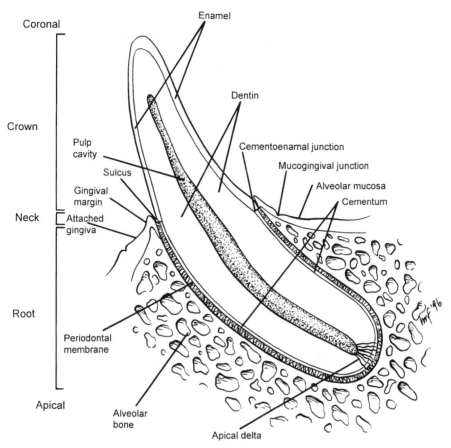

FIG. 9. Normal dental and paradental anatomy.

food into the oral cavity. The *canine* or *cuspid* teeth are designed to pierce and hold a victim. They can also be used to slash and tear, when used as weapons in fighting. In the carnivores, these are the longest crowned and longest rooted teeth. The large roots make them very stable and good anchorage points. *Premolars*, sometimes called *bicuspids*, are actually a cross between cuspids and molars. They are not as long as cuspids but generally have multiple functional cusps. The term *bicuspid* comes from the fact that in some species the premolars have two functional cusps. Being a cross between a cuspid and a molar, they are designed to function in a manner similar to both. They help to hold and carry, while also helping to break food down into smaller pieces. *Molars* have an occlusal surface that can be used to grind food or break it down into smaller pieces. The incisors and canine teeth are referred to as anterior teeth, while the premolars and molars are posterior teeth. The *carnassial* teeth are considered to be the largest shearing teeth in the upper and lower jaws. In the dog and cat, they are the maxillary fourth premolars and the first molars in the mandibles. The term *carnassial* means "flesh cutting."

Crown formation generally occurs from four or more growth centers known as *lobes*. Their fusion, termed *coalescence*, can result in various depth grooves known as *developmental grooves*. Most incisors, cuspids, and premolars develop from four lobes: three facial and one lingual. The two developmental grooves on the facial surface of the

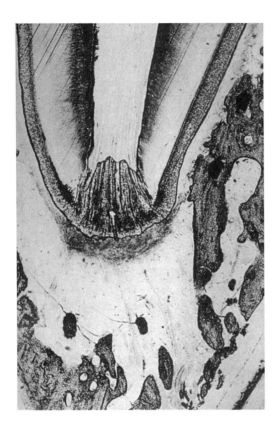

FIG. 10. Structure of the apex with an apical delta and periapical inflammatory reaction. (Reproduced with permission from Zetner K. *J Vet Dent* 1992;9(3): cover photo.)

incisors are the coalescence or fusion points of the three facial lobes. The three protrusions along the incisal edge formed by the developmental grooves are the *mamelons*. The deep developmental grooves in many carnivores and some primates appear to help in cutting the flesh as it slides up the tooth, and act as *bleeding grooves* allowing blood to escape from the punctures in the victim while it is still held in a firm grasp. The fourth lobe on the lingual surface typically forms the majority of the tooth bulk at the lingual cervical third and is called the *cingulum*. Just above this on the incisor, customarily, there is a slight concavity known as the *lingual fossa*.

The *proximal contacts* are the points at which adjacent teeth make contact. These contacts aid in preventing food from being packed between the teeth from above, while the gingival papillae serve the same purpose from the facial and lingual surfaces. The contacts of the anterior teeth are located close to the incisal ridge, whereas they are located more apically in the posterior teeth. With the diastema and tooth spacings in the canine and posterior teeth in the dog, contacts do not always make contact with the adjacent teeth. The bulge, curvature, or contour of the tooth aids in directing food away from the gingival sulcus, while using the food's frictional movement to clean the gingivae, cheeks, and lips.

MOUTH

The mouth (*os*) is the entrance of the oral cavity. It is solely the opening between the lips, designating the beginning of the digestive tract. The most rostral extent of the oral cavity is secured by the lips (*labia oris*). The upper lip (*labium superius*) and lower lip (*labium inferius*) converge at the angles of the mouth (*anguli oris*), forming the commissures of the lip.

Oral Mucous Membrane

The stratified squamous epithelium that runs from the margins of the lips to the area of the tonsils and lines the oral cavity is known as the *oral mucosa* or *oral mucous membrane*. The epithelium does extend past the tonsils into the pharynx and beyond, but it is not considered part of the oral cavity. These oral mucous membranes are divided into three categories. The first is the *specialized mucosa*, found on the dorsum of the tongue. The exception to this is the hyperkeratinized filiform papillae of the cat. Second is the *masticatory mucosa*, which undergoes routine masticatory trauma and stress, and is generally parakeratinized or keratinized. This is the tissue of the hard palate and gingivae. The third is the *general* or *lining mucosa* that constitutes the remaining oral mucosa. It is nonkeratinized to parakeratinized, with an underlying connective tissue containing fairly well developed collagen fibers that provide support but still allow substantial movement of the overlying epithelium.

An interdigitation exists between the epithelium and the underlying connective tissue (Fig. 11). The interdigitation of the submucosal connective tissue into the epithelium is termed the *dermal papilla*. The pegs of epithelium that insert into the connective tissue are known as *rete ridges* or *pegs* and cause small dimples in the ginigival tissue known as *gingival stippling*. Stippling can be present or absent in healthy or diseased gingival tissue and therefore is not a reliable indication of gingival health; it is also less prominent

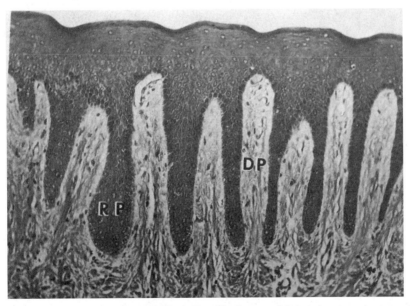

FIG. 11. Interdigitation between oral gingival epithelium and the submucosal connective tissue dermal papilla (RP, rete pegs of the epithelium). Indentations on epithelial surface represent stippling. (Reproduced with permission from Baer PN, Morris ML. *Textbook of Periodontics*. Philadelphia: JB Lippincott Co; 1977:6.)

in the cat. Its reduction or loss may be an indicator of disease but does not automatically signify it (1–4). The length of the pegs determines how tight or mobile the attachment of the epithelium is to the underlying connective tissue. The lining mucosa has poorly developed pegs and is therefore fairly movable above the connective tissue. In comparison, the masticatory mucosa has well developed rete pegs and consequently a tighter attachment.

The gingival masticatory mucosa is one of the most important support structures for the tooth. It is divided into two major parts: the *free gingiva (marginal gingiva)* and the *attached gingiva*. The two combine to form a peak of gingiva known as the *interdental papilla* between teeth that are closely adjacent. The interdental papilla plays an important part in maintenance of gingival health by preventing food and debris from being impacted between the teeth. Between the facial and lingual interdental papillae between two adjacent teeth may be found a valley of gingiva known as the *col*. Between the tooth and the free gingiva, there can typically be found a shallow groove known as the *gingival sulcus*. The epithelium lining the sulcus and the col is among the very few areas of masticatory gingiva that are nonkeratinized. At the bottom of the sulcus is the *epithelial attachment* or the *junctional epithelium*, which directly attaches the gingiva to the tooth. In periodontal disease, it is common for the sulcus depth to increase as attachment is lost. The remaining gingiva is the attached gingiva.

On the facial surfaces of the teeth, there is a distinct demarcation, the *mucogingival junction* or *line*, that separates this attached gingiva from the alveolar mucosa, which is part of the general or lining mucosa. The transition from attached gingiva to general mucosa is less apparent on lingual and palatal surfaces.

ORAL CAVITY

The oral cavity (*cavum oris*) is typically considered to be the area extending from the lips to the oral pharynx at the level of the palatine tonsils. Anteriorly, it is bound by the lips, laterally by the cheeks (*buccae*), above by the hard and soft palates, and below by the floor of the mouth. The oral pharynx is also the location where the digestive and respiratory tracts share a common, intersecting pathway.

The oral cavity is generally subdivided into two parts: the vestibule (*vestibulum oris*) and the oral cavity proper (*cavum oris proprium*). The vestibule is the theoretical space between the lips or cheeks and the teeth, gums, and alveolar ridges. The oral cavity proper extends from the alveolar ridge and teeth to the oral pharynx. It is additionally defined by the roof and floor of the mouth and is generally filled by the tongue.

Vestibule

The lips comprise three components, one of which is the facial stratified squamous epithelium portion. The vestibular component is covered with oral mucosa that is nonkeratinized to parakeratinized squamous epithelium. The transitional zone between facial and vestibular components is the vermilion zone of the lip in humans. The facial or skin part of the upper lip at the midline has an indentation known as the *philtrum*. Cleft lips are most commonly seen to occur off-center, and not directly at the philtrum. The point at which the oral mucosa and the top or bottom of the vestibule turn toward the alveolar ridge is known as the *mucobuccal* or *mucolabial fold*. The attachment of the mucosa to the alveolar bone is loose and movable, and the point where it becomes tightly attached is the beginning of the gingiva. The line formed by the junction of the mucosa and the alveolar mucosa is known as the *mucogingival margin* or *mucogingival junction*.

Within the vestibule is also contained the *frenula*, which are areas where folds of alveolar mucosa form a noticeable ridge of attachment between the lips and the gum. The dog has three primary frenula: one upper and two lower. The upper frenulum extends from the midline of the lip to the gingiva immediately below the two central incisors. The lower two frenula extend from the lip to the level of the mandibular canine teeth.

Oral Cavity Proper

Within the oral cavity proper is contained a multitude of structures. Among those are the hard and soft palate, tongue, and floor of the mouth.

The hard palate (*palatum durum*) is the soft tissue–covered, bony vault of the oral cavity proper. It has a *median raphe* dividing the left and the right sides. The transverse epithelial ridges that radiate out from the median raphe are known as *rugae*. The rugae should meet symmetrically at the median raphe. Asymmetrical junctures of the rugae at the raphe may be an indication of poor migration of the left and right maxillary processes and a tendency toward cleft palate formation. It is not uncommon to find this asymmetrical rugal pattern in parents of cleft palate puppies. At the beginning of the raphe, immediately behind the two central incisor teeth, is a single rounded elevation of tissue known as the incisive papilla (*papilla incisiva*). The incisive ducts (*ductus incisivus*) open either lateral side of the papilla. The ducts travels caudodorsally, communicating with the cavity of the vomeronasal organ and leaving the oral cavity through the palatine fissures to open into the floor of the nasal fossa. Beneath the papilla is the incisive foramen, through which the nasopalatine nerve travels to the soft tissue lingual to the anterior maxillary teeth.

Soft Palate

The soft palate (*palatum molle* or *velum palatinum*) is the unsupported soft tissue that extends back from the hard palate free of the support of the palatine bone. It is relatively thick at its attachment to the hard palate and thins at the margins. In a relaxed state it typically makes contact with the oral surface of the epiglottis but may make contact with the respiratory surface of the epiglottis. The hard and soft palates serve to separate the oral cavity from the nasal cavity.

OSSEOUS TISSUE

The head consisting of the *skull* and *mandible* support all the teeth (Fig. 12). The *incisive bone* (formerly premaxillae in the dog and still considered such in some species), *maxillae*, and *mandibular bones* have sockets, in which the teeth are seated. This firm attachment of teeth to support is termed *thecodontia*. The alveolar process is that portion of these bones that encompasses and supports the tooth structure. It is composed of a cortical plate, trabecular bone, and the cribriform plate. The *cortical plate* is the outside wall of the process. The *cribriform plate*, known radiologically as the *lamina dura*, is the thin layer of bone within the tooth socket. *Trabecular bone* acts as the support between the cortical plate and the lamina dura. The *alveolar crest* is the occlusal portion of the alve-

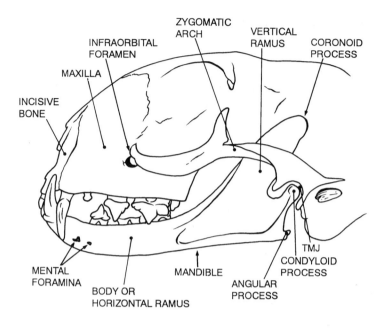

NORMAL SKULL AND MANDIBULAR ANATOMY

FIG. 12. Normal skull and mandibular anatomy of the cat.

olar process near the neck of the tooth. The mandibles and maxillae containing the teeth are known as the *jaws*.

The *incisive bone (premaxillae)* accommodates the six upper incisor teeth. They articulate with the maxillae at the *incisivomaxillary suture*. Both *oval palatine fissures* are situated in this bone directly behind the incisal teeth. The palatine vessels pass through these fissures. The maxillae act as the mooring for the remainder of the upper dentition. This includes the canine (cuspid), four premolars, and two molars in each maxilla. The lateral wall of the maxilla is relatively thin, resulting in prominences in the alveolar bone lateral to many of the tooth roots. These prominences, called *alveolar juga*, act as landmarks in certain surgical endodontic procedures. The bony partitions between adjacent teeth are referred to as *interalveolar septa*. Partitions between roots of an individual tooth are known as *interradicular septa*.

The *mandible* consists of two bilateral bones attached rostrally at the midline by a strong fibrous joint referred to as the *mandibular symphysis*. The mandible comprises two major sections: the horizontal and vertical rami. The *horizontal ramus* is composed of the body and symphysial area of the mandible, in which the teeth are contained. The *vertical ramus* constitutes the coronoid process, the articular or condyloid process, and the angular process. The *temporomandibular joint (TMJ)* is formed by the *mandibular articular process* and the *mandibular fossa* of the temporal bone. This joint is sometimes referred to as the *craniomandibular articulation (CMA)*. Depending on the species, this joint has both translational and rotational movement capabilities, which allows a degree of both rostral and lateral movement, as well as rotational hinge action. The joint is separated by an articular disc into two compartments: the dorsal (temporal) and ventral (mandibular). Fibrous tissue surrounds the joint capsule, which forms its lateral ligament.

The mandible and skull together can form various head types or shapes. Brachycephalic, mesaticephalic, and dolichocephalic are the three most common terms used to describe head shape. *Brachycephalic* indicates a short, wide head. The shortness of the head commonly results in rotation of premolar teeth. Boxers, Boston terriers, Chinese pugs, bulldogs, and Pekingese are some of the breeds commonly called brachycephalic. *Mesaticephalic* designates a head shape of medium proportions. Beagles, German shepherds, Labrador retrievers, and poodles are typical examples. *Dolichocephalic* refers to a long, narrow head shape. The collie, borzoi, and Russian wolfhound are representative of this head type. Posterior cross-bites, in which the upper fourth premolar is in linguoversion (lingual) to the lower first molar, are more common in these breeds.

MUSCLES AND RELATED NERVES OF MASTICATION

The majority of the muscles associated with the masticatory action act to close the mandible (5). Of this group the *temporalis muscle* is the largest and most powerful, occupying the temporal fossa and extending to the coronoid process of the mandible. The *masseter muscle* arises from the zygomatic arch and inserts on the lateral ramus of the mandible, while the *lateral* and *medial pterygoid muscles* extend from the sphenoid bone and surrounding areas to the condyle and articular process, respectively. These muscles are all innervated by the mandibular branch of the *trigeminal (fifth cranial) nerve*. Only the *rostral belly of the digastric muscle* is stimulated by the trigeminal nerve, as the *caudal belly* is innervated by the *facial (seventh cranial) nerve*. The digastric muscle, responsible for opening the jaws, arises from the jugular process of the occipital bone and inserts on the mandible along the ventral border.

These muscles, in coordination with the teeth, have a tremendous biting-force potential. *Biting force* is the pressure, typically measured in pounds per sqaure inch (psi), exerted by the teeth when engaged by the muscles of mastication. In humans, they have been shown to have about 250–300 psi of passive biting force (6). Additionally, in humans, the abrupt closing or snapping shut of the jaws on the few millimeters of tooth-cusp contact can reach a *sudden localized biting force* of 25,000–30,000 psi, which can easily result in tooth fractures or injury to the periodontal structures (6). In the dog, the passive biting force has been estimated to be possibly much greater than in humans, reaching the 300–800-psi range (7). This could place the sudden localized biting-force potential in an extremely high range, possibly as high as 30,000–80,000 psi if the force is at 100 times the strength of passive biting force, as in humans.

TONGUE

The tongue (*lingua*) is a mobile prehensile structure of the oral cavity used for grooming and the intake of food and fluids. It is formed primarily of skeletal muscle covered by a mucosal membrane. Its actions are controlled by both *intrinsic* and *extrinsic* muscles of the tongue (*musculi linguae*). The intrinsic muscle of the tongue (*m. lingualis proprius*) contains superficial longitudinal, deep longitudinal, perpendicular, and transverse muscle fibers. As a unit, these produce the complicated protrusion and prehensile movements of the tongue and prevent trauma from teeth. The intrinsic lingual muscle is innervated by the hypoglossus (twelfth cranial) nerve. The extrinsic lingual muscles are the styloglossus, hypoglossus, and genioglossus muscles. The styloglossus draws the tongue caudally, the hypoglossus retracts and depresses it, and the genioglossus depresses and protrudes the tongue. All three of the extrinsic muscles are also innervated by the hypoglossus nerve. The total innervation of the tongue is by the lingual (fifth cranial), chorda tympani (seventh cranial), glossopharyngeal (ninth cranial), and hypoglossal nerves. The afferent activities of touch, pain, heat, and taste and the efferent activities of tongue gland innervation are controlled by the lingual, chorda tympani, and glossopharyngeal nerves.

The tongue is divided into an tip (*apex linguae*), margin (*margo linguae*), body (*corpus linguae*), and a root (*radix linguae*). It is wide and thin at the two lateral margins that meet at the tip or most rostral portion of the margins, but it becomes thicker toward the body and root. The dorsum is covered with a thick rough cornified mucous membrane known as the lingual mucosa (*tunica mucosa linguae*). The ventral surface is covered with a smooth, thinner, and less cornified surface. The thicker dorsal mucosa forms into papillae of various shape and function. The rostral two-thirds is thickly covered with short, pointed, filiform papillae (*papillae filiformes*), with their tips directed caudally, which may aid in grooming. In the root area are found soft, long, conical papillae (*papillae conicae*) pointing caudally; these probably have a mechanical function. Fungiform papillae (*papillae fungiformes*) are mushroom-shaped and scattered along the dorsal sides and the anterior portion of the tongue. Each contains up to eight taste pores, although some have none. A small number of vallate papillae (*papillae vallate*) are found at the posterior border of the tongue, where the conical papillae begin. There are three to six vallate papillae in the dog, with four being the most common. These may be simple or complex and contain taste buds. The foliate papillae (*papillae foliatae*) are immediately rostral to the palatoglossal fold, located on the dorsolateral aspect of the caudal third of the tongue, and contain taste buds. Marginal papillae (*papillae marginales*) are present at birth along the margins of the rostral half of the tongue in the dog. They are mechanical in nature, aiding in nursing by sealing the lips to the nipple for suction and reducing milk spillage around the tongue. These normally disappear as puppies progress to more solid foods. The taste buds (*caliculus gustatorius*) are pear-shaped organs located in the gustatory papillae: the fungiform, vallate, and foliate papillae. The filiform, conical, and marginal papillae are mechanical papillae containing no taste buds. There is an extensive number of lingual salivary glands (*glandulae linguales*) in the surface of the tongue. The dorsum of the tongue is divided by a median groove in the anterior portion.

The ventral part of the tongue is covered by smooth mucous membrane. Extending from the floor of the mouth to the anterior ventral base is a fold of tissue known as the lingual frenulum (*frenulum linguae*). Within the ventral portion of the tip, along the midline, is a fusiform cord known as the *lyssa* composed of fat, muscle, and occasionally islands of cartilage and fibrous sheath tissue. The lyssa, formerly known as the lytta, is typically about 4 cm in a medium-sized dog and may act as a stretch receptor for the rostral portion of the tongue. Beneath the smooth mucosa of the underside of the tongue is a highly vascular network. The primary blood supply to the tongue is through the paired lingual arteries (*arteria linguales*) with return via the lingual veins.

The base of the lingual frenulum rests in the floor of the mouth. To either side of this base are small elevations of tissue known as the sublingual caruncle (*caruncula sublingualis*). These serve as the anatomic locations of the duct openings for the sublingual and mandibular salivary glands. A fold of tissue known as the sublingual fold (*plica sublingualis*) extends back from the sublingual caruncle along the floor of the mouth with the side of the tongue. This fold marks the path of numerous structures that run across the floor of the mouth, including the ducts for the sublingual and mandibular salivary glands.

SALIVARY GLANDS

Submerged beneath the mucous membranes of the oral cavity exists a complex system of salivary tissues. These salivary tissues secrete saliva, a serous and mucous fluid that contains a complex mixture of inorganic and organic substances such as electrolytes, proteins, hormones, minerals, bactericidal substances, vitamins, and, in some species, enzymes. In most animals, a relatively high concentration of amylase is found in saliva from the parotid and slightly lower levels in mandibular secretions. The concentrations of amylase, however, are relatively low in the domestic dog and cat. Fluid formation in the salivary tissue occurs in the acini.

Isotonic water transport is an acinar secretory process in which the main active step is a sodium transport system from the intracellular to the intercellular space. The duct epithelium can secrete and absorb water, as well as the basic electrolytes: calcium, chloride, bicarbonate, sodium, and potassium. It is also involved with the concentration of iodide and thiocyanate. The concentrations of some salivary constituents such as iodide, calcium, and bicarbonate are dependent on their blood plasma levels; therefore, the saliva:plasma ratio of these electrolytes remains relatively constant.

Regulation of saliva secretions is controlled by the autonomic nervous system. The centers for saliva secretion are located on the salivary nuclei in the medulla oblongata. The salivary glands are regulated by a double efferent pathway via the parasympathetic and sympathetic portions of the autonomic nervous system. A basal flow of saliva is continuously stimulated by the parasympathetic system's efferent impulses from the salivary nuclei. Sight, taste, and olfactory stimulation initiate afferent impulses to the nuclei, which in turn release efferent impulses to the parasympathetic system to increase salivation. Sympathetic stimulation may increase salivary flow to the mouth due to contraction on the myoepithelial cells by constriction of the lumen of both the acini and the ducts. Sympathetic stimulation actually increases salivary secretion by the acinar cells of some salivary glands in the cat.

Saliva has both qualitative and quantitative aspects. The quantitative properties are twofold: the basal and surge flow rates. The basal production level maintains the protective moist mucoid layer environment for the teeth and mucous membranes. This layer possibly aids in protecting the mucosa from the detrimental effects of bacterial and other toxins, as well as minor traumas. The flow rate aids in mechanically flushing and cleansing the teeth and mucous membranes of the oral cavity, possibly limiting the microbial population in the oral environment. The elevated surge flow rates aid in flushing mucoid trapped bacteria and foreign materials from the mouth and into the acidic gastric system for destruction. Additionally, the mucus coats foodstuffs to lubricate, while the serous volume acts to carry the material through the tract with the aid of muscular activity.

Qualitatively, it is a complex combination of organic and inorganic substances, with a pH component. In broad groups, these can be classified as minerals and electrolytes, enzymes and other proteins, low molecular weight compounds, and vitamins. The ultimate composition is generally regulated by the autonomic nervous system, the serum level of systemic counterparts, and humoral activity. The qualitative portion contains a potent antimicrobial component consisting of mucous and pH factors, lysosomes, immunoglobulins, fluoride, and antilactobacillus thiocyanate-dependent and many other possible factors. The teeth are theoretically affected by saliva by reduction of tooth solubility, buffering acids, remineralization, antimicrobial actions, and mechanical cleansing. Enzymes, such as amylase, aid in initiation of digestion while food is still in the mouth. The mixed pH of saliva varies widely even in individuals. It is affected by numerous factors, but flow rate and duration appear to be the most important. Starr (8) shows a slightly acidic average pH of 6.6 for humans. Most domestic animals demonstrate a slight alkaline pH, except ruminants whose saliva is distinctively alkaline. Schwarte (9) obtained the following pH values: dog and cat, 7.5; swine, 7.37; horse, 7.42; and ox, 8.23. Schwatz and Hermann (10) obtained the following mean pH values: dog and horse, 7.56; swine 7.32; and ox, 8.1.

There is a large assortment of salivary glands and tissue in and emptying into the oral cavity. The lingual, labial, buccal, and palatine salivary glands represent a large number of very small disseminated glands that secrete minute amounts of serous or mucus fluid into the oral cavity. The *lingual salivary glands* are located in the submucosa and muscles of the tongue in its caudal third, with numerous small excretory ducts. The *labial glands* are found scattered throughout the submucosa of the lips, with numerous small excretory ducts. The *buccal glands* are situated in the submucosa of the buccal cavity, with numerous small excretory ducts. The *palatine glands* are located in the submucosa of the ventral surface of the soft palate. There are four or five larger glands that are more clinically significant in disease and saliva production. In the dog these are the parotid, mandibular, sublingual, and zygomatic (Fig. 13). In the cat the two molar salivary glands are also of clinical importance (Fig. 14).

The parotid salivary gland (*glandula parotis*) is divided into a superficial portion (*pars superficialis*) and a deep portion (*pars profunda*). The gland is generally V-shaped and located beneath the ear and behind the posterior border of the mandible and the temporomandibular joint. Although a part of the gland is superficial in location, its blending

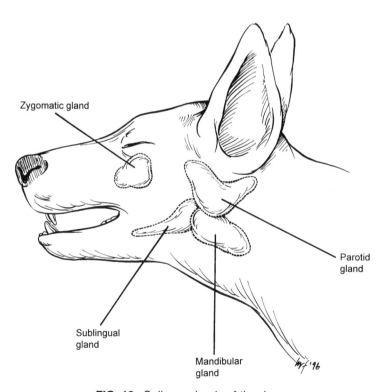

FIG. 13. Salivary glands of the dog.

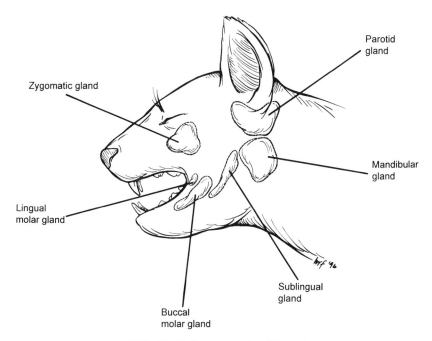

FIG. 14. Salivary glands of the cat.

with the surrounding anatomy makes its typically difficult to palpate. The *parotid lymph nodes* usually lie under the rostroventral border of the parotid salivary gland.

The parotid duct (*ductus parotideus*) is formed by the union, a few millimeters from the gland, of two or three tributaries originating from the ventral third of the rostral border of the gland. It proceeds rostrally and toward the cheek along the lateral surface of the masseter muscle, closely paralleling the muscle fibers. Near the terminal end, the duct generally makes two slight right-angle turns, one medially and one vertically, before passing through the buccal mucosa and opening into the buccal vestibule. The opening is at the *parotid papilla* located at the rostral end of a blunt ridge of mucosa superficial to the distal root of the upper fourth premolar. For catheterization of the ducts, the terminal angulations can be relatively straightened by lightly retracting the papilla rostrally. The gland produces a primarily serous-type saliva.

Accessory parotid glands (*glandulae parotis accessoria*) are typically present in the dog. These are usually located bilaterally above the duct and range from single, small lobules to glandular masses over a centimeter in length. These each have small ducts that empty into the main parotid duct.

The mandibular gland (*glandula mandibularis*) is an ovoid, compact, yellow-to-buff-colored gland. In the dog, cat, and most domestic animals, the gland is located just caudal to the angle of the jaw and is easily palpable. In most primates, however, it is located beneath the mandible and is referred to as the submandibular salivary gland. The gland shares a connective tissue capsule with a portion of the sublingual gland. In the dog, it rests between the linguofacial and maxillary veins, while in the cat these veins may unite over the lateral surface. It is classified as a mixed gland in the dog.

The mandibular duct (*ductus mandibularis*) emerges from the deep or medial surface of the gland. It courses rostromedially between the mylohyoid and styloglossus muscles medially to the mandible. The duct emerges from the sublingual mucosa into the oral cavity proper below the tongue on the small sublingual papilla or caruncle, near the rostral attachment of the lingual frenulum. The small opening of the duct appears as a small red slit along the frenulum's ventral surface. Approximately 30% of dogs have a shared or common opening with the sublingual duct.

The sublingual salivary gland (*glandula sublingualis*), slightly darker pink than the mandibular gland, is the smallest of the four major salivary gland pairs in the dog. The gland is divided into a monostomatic (*pars monostomatica*) and polystomatic (*pars polystomatica*) portions. The monostomatic part consists of the portion contained within the mandibular gland capsule and a group of loose lobules that cluster close to the sublingual and mandibular ducts near the root of the tongue. These all discharge into the major sublingual duct (*ductus sublingualis major*), which typically travels just dorsal to the mandibular duct, opening 1–2 mm caudal to or in common with it on the sublingual caruncle.

The polystomatic portion is a group of 6–12 small, scattered lobules of sublingual salivary tissue. These do not communicate with the major sublingual duct but empty into the several minor sublingual ducts (*ductus sublingualis minores*). These empty into the oral cavity between the tongue and mandible in the lateral sublingual recess. The sublingual gland is smaller in the cat, with the polystomatic portion sometimes absent.

The zygomatic gland (*glandula zygomatica*), an enlarged member of the dorsal buccal gland group, was formerly known as the *orbital gland*. It is located ventral to the rostral end of the zygomatic arch, making access relatively difficult. It is well developed in most

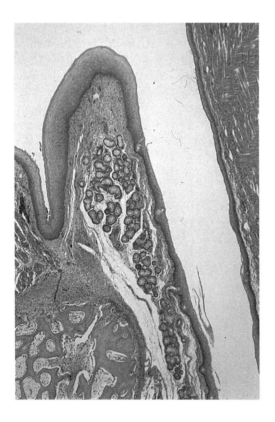

FIG. 15. Minor lingual molar salivary gland in membranous bulge lingual to the lower molar of the cat. (Courtesy of Dr. Ayako Okuda, Tokyo, Japan.)

carnivores and found only in the dog and cat among domestic mammals. There is one major duct (*ductus glandulae zygomaticae major*) and up to four minor ducts (*ductus glandulae zygomaticae minores*) that travel from the gland to the caudal part of the buccal vestibule. The major duct opens caudal to the parotid papillae and caudal to the last upper molar on a ridge of mucosa at the zygomatic papilla (*papilla zygomatica*). The minor ducts open caudal to the major ducts and appear as a line of small red dots on the mucosa.

There are two well developed molar salivary glands in the cat. The buccal molar salivary gland (*glandula molaris buccalis*), previously known just as the molar gland (*glandula molaris*), is a modified ventral buccal gland located between the orbicularis oris muscle and the mucous membrane of the lower lip at the angle of the mouth. It empties into the buccal cavity by several small ducts. The second gland is the lingual molar salivary gland (*glandula molaris lingualis*), a small salivary gland recently demonstrated in the membranous molar pad just lingual to the lower molar. It is primarily composed of mixed predominant mucous acini with semilunar serous gland cells (Fig. 15). Numerous small openings of this lingual molar salivary gland open in a direction toward the tongue and do not have a common transportation duct.

REFERENCES

1. King JD. Gingival disease in Dundee. *J Dent Res* 1945;65:9.
2. Orban B. Clinical and histological study of surface characteristics of the gingiva. *Oral Surg* 1948;1:827.
3. Greene AH. Study of the characteristics of stippling and its relation to gingival health. *J Periodontol* 1962; 33:176.
4. Hurt WC. *Periodontics in General Practice*. Springfield, IL: Charles C Thomas; 1976:9.
5. Evans HE. *Miller's Anatomy of the Dog*. Philadelphia: WB Saunders Co; 1993:258.
6. Fagan DA. Diagnosis and treatment planning. In: Frost P, ed. *Veterinary Clinics of North America*. 1986; 16(5):789.
7. Tholen MA. *Concepts in Veterinary Dentistry*. Edwardsville, KS: Veterinary Medicine Publishing Co; 1983:135.
8. Starr AW. *J Biol Chem* 1922;54–55.
9. Schwarte C. Digestion in the mouth. In: Duke H. H., *The Physiology of Domestic Animals*. Ithaca, New York: Comstock Publishing Co; 1942:245.
10. Schwarz C, Hermann B. Mean pH values in animals, *Pflüger's Archiv für die Gesamte Physiologie*. 1924;202:475.

BIBLIOGRAPHY

Arnall L. Some aspects of dental development in the dog: Calcification of crown and root of the deciduous dentitions. *J Small Anin Pract* 1961;1:169.
Avery LB. *Developmental Anatomy*. 7th ed. Philadelphia: WB Saunders Co; 1966:199.
Bennett GA, Hutchinson RC. Experimental studies on the movements of the mammalian tongue; protrusion mechanism of the tongue (dog). *Anat Rec* 1946;94:57.
Bojrab MJ, Tholen MT. *Small Animal Oral Medicine and Surgery*. Philadelphia: Lea & Febiger; 1990.
Boucher CO. *Current Clinical Dental Terminology*. St Louis, MO: CV Mosby Co; 1963.
Brand RW, Isselhard DE. *Anatomy of Orofacial Structures*. St Louis, MO: CV Mosby Co; 1986:3,46,209,270.
Ciancio SC, Neiders ME, Hazen SP. The principal fibers of the periodontal ligament. *J Periodontics* 1967;5:76.
Colyer JF. Variations and diseases of the teeth of animals. In: Miles AEW, Grigson C, eds, Cambridge: Cambridge University Press; 1990:62.
Compton AW, Parker P. Evolution of the mammalian masticatory, apparatus. *Am Scientist* 1978;66:377.
Dorland's Medical Dictionary. 24th Ed. Philadelphia; WB Saunders Co; 1969.
Dox I, Melloni BJ, Eisner GM. *Melloni's Illustrated Medical Dictionary*. Baltimore: Williams & Wilkins; 1979.
Eastoe J, Eastoe B. The organic constituents of mammalian compact bone. *Biochem J* 1954;57:453.
Eisenmenger E, Zetner K. *Veterinary Dentistry*. Philadelphia: Lea & Febiger; 1985:2.
Fearnhead RW, Suga S. *Tooth Enamel IV*. New York: Elsevier Science Publishing; 1984.
Gier HT. Early embryology of the dog. *Anat Rec* 1950;108:561.
Glock GE, Mellanby H, Mellanby M, Murry MM, Thewlis J. A study of the development of dental enamel in dogs. *J Dent Res* 1942;21:183.

The Academy of Denture Prosthetics, the Journal of Prosthetic Dentistry. *Glossary of Prosthodontic Terms*. 5th ed. St Louis, MO: CV Mosby Co; 1987.

Grandage J. In: Slatter DH, ed. *Textbook of Small Animal Surgery*. Philadelphia: WB Saunders Co; 1985:606.

Grandage J. The salivary glands anatomy. In: Slatter DH, ed. *Textbook of Small Animal Surgery*. Philadelphia: WB Saunders Co; 1985:644.

Kent CK. Comparative anatomy of the vertebrates. St Louis, MO: CV Mosby Co; 1965:244.

Kornfeld R. *Dental Histology and Comparative Anatomy*. Philadelphia: Lea & Febiger; 1937.

Kraus BS, Jordan RE, Abrams L. *A Study of the Masticatory System Dental Anatomy*. Baltimore: Williams and Wilkins; 1969:1, 263.

Kremenak CR Jr. Dental exfoliation and eruption chronology in Beagles. *J Dent Res* 1967;46:686.

Leahy JR. *Muscles of the Head, Neck, Shoulder and Forelimb of the Dog*. Ithaca, NY: University of Cornell; 1949. Thesis.

Lobprise HB, Wiggs RB. Anatomy, diagnosis, and management of disorders of the tongue. *J Vet Dent* 1993;10:16.

Major MA. *Wheeler's Dental Anatomy, Physiology and Occlusion*. 7th ed. Philadelphia: WB Saunders Co; 1993: 24,89.

Miller ME. *Anatomy of the Dog*. Philadelphia: WB Saunders Co; 1969:27.

Nomina Anatomica Veterinaria. 3rd ed.: Published by International Committee on Veterinary Gross Anatomical Nomenclature under the World Association of Veterinary Anatomists; 1983.

Nomina Histologica. 2nd ed.: Published by International Committee on Veterinary Gross Anatomical Nomenclature under the World Association of Veterinary Anatomists; 1983.

Perman D. *Oral Embryology and Microscopic Anatomy*. 4th ed. Philadelphia: Lea & Febiger; 1969:44,128.

Revell DG. The pancreatic ducts of the dog. *Am J Anat* 1902;1:443.

Roth GI, Calmes R. *Oral Biology*. St Louis, MO: CV Mosby Co; 1972:119.

St Clair LE, Jones ND. Observations on the cheek teeth of the dog. *JAVMA* 1957;130:275.

Schour I, Hoffman MM. The rate of apposition of enamel and dentin in man and other animals. *J Dent Res* 1939; 18:161.

Secord AC. Small animal dentistry. *JAVMA* 1941;98:470.

Sicher H, Bhaskar SN. *Orban's Oral Histology and Embryology*. 17th ed. Philadelphia: Lea & Febiger; 1972:38,33.

Sisson S, Grossman JD. *The Anatomy of the Domestic Animals*. 4th ed. Philadelphia: WB Saunders Co; 1969:45,140, 157,174,189,219,257,387.

Stack MV. Organic constituents of enamel. *JADA* 1954;48:297.

Walker WF. *Vertebrate Dissection*. 7th ed. Ft Worth, TX; Saunders College Publishing; 1986:62,172,268,324.

Wheeler RC. *Dental Anatomy Physiology and Occlusion*. Philadelphia: WB Saunders Co; 1974:7,9.

Wiggs RB. Canine oral anatomy and physiology. *Compendium on Continuing Education for the Practicing Veterinarian* 1989;11(12):1475.

Williams RC. *Observations on the Chronology of Deciduous Dental Development in the Dog*. Ithaca, NY; Cornell University; 1961. Thesis.

Williams RC, Evans HE. Prenatal dental development in the dog, *Canis familiaris*: Chronology of tooth germ formation and calcification of deciduous teeth. *Zentalbl Veterinarmed C: Anat Histol Embryol* 1978;7:152.

Wodsedalek JE. The digestive system and nutrition of man. In: *General Zoology*. Dubuque, IA: Wm C Brown Co; 1963:366.

Zander HA, Hurzder B. Continuous cementum deposition. *J Periodontol Res* 1958;37:1035.

Zwarych PD, Quigley MB. The intermediate plexus of the periodontal ligament: History and further observations. *J Dent Res* 1965;44:383.

4

Oral Examination and Diagnosis

Robert B. Wiggs and Heidi B. Lobprise

Oral and dental pathology is not an uncommon finding in most animals. In many cases, when detected by the owner, the disease will be well advanced and obvious at presentation, while other cases are more obscure requiring in-depth diagnostics. Signs and symptoms may indicate oral disease to be primary or secondary in nature (1). A thorough examination in coordination with a suitable knowledge of anatomy and function is the basis for diagnostic ability. Proper examination and accurate diagnosis are the key to appropriate treatment planning. Clinically, oral diagnosis is a six-part interactive process of history, physical examination, initial oral survey, preanesthesia diagnostic testing, in-depth oral examination, and oral diagnostic testing (2).

HISTORY

The gathering of history is the foundation of a proper examination. It relies on the owner's direct personal involvement and provides information that can be an invaluable aid in directing the full examination. In addition, the history is the link between all other parts of the physical, oral, and laboratory examination. A complete history should provide vaccination status, details of diet, levels of professional and home dental care, past disease problems and treatments, current problems and treatments in progress, exposure to infectious diseases, traumatic incidents, and behavioral changes—all of which may help the clinician fully evaluate every aspect of the animal's general health. Signalment of age, breed, and sex is always the starting point. History encompasses past and present information concerning the individual, family line, other household pets, and breed characteristics. Additionally, drugs previously and currently being taken should be recorded, both for general information and avoiding adverse reaction problems (3–5).

Once significant general data are obtained, information more specific to oral and dental pathology should be given close attention. Information of actual oral symptoms should include onset, duration, degree of severity, and recurrence profile (6). Details of type of diet, chew toys, chewing, and eating habits should be scrutinized. Additionally, history of chronic cough, regurgitation, vomiting, and skin allergies can all produce effects on the oral cavity.

Questions with respect to the patient's hesitancy to pick up, chew, or swallow food can provide significant information. Has the animal been observed to drop food, toys, or training articles from the mouth? Has quivering of the jaw or chattering of the teeth been noticed, especially while training articles are in the mouth? What are the training articles and what are they made of? Sensitive teeth more commonly react to metals, from both thermal and galvanic stimulus. Food shifted to or chewed primarily on one side or a preference for soft food may be a sign of periodontal or endodontic disease. Hesitancy in swallowing food can be due to oral inflammations, ulcers, sensitive teeth, tonsillitis, and foreign bodies. In the cat, the most common causes of these symptoms are feline dental resorption (FDR) or cervical line lesions (CLL) of the teeth and lymphocytic plasmocytic stomatitis (LPS).

Inappetence and anorexia can both be associated with general disease processes, but can commonly be indications of ulcerations, inflammation, and pulp exposure within the oral cavity (6). True anorexia is uncommon in oral disease, except in cases of severe pain. In such cases, all indications of systemic disease should first be ruled out. Oral pain can additionally cause pawing at, tilting, bobbing, shaking, and sliding of the head and mouth along the floor. Differential diagnosis would include problems with the skin, lips, ears, eyes, salivary glands, and central nervous system.

One of the most commonly reported symptoms is simply *bad breath* or *halitosis*. This condition is reported more frequently in house pets, probably due to their close contact with owners. Orally, periodontal disease is the most common cause of halitosis (7). This occurs due to the bacterial breakdown of food and other materials on the crown surfaces, but more importantly on the root structure. Other causes of oral malodor are stomatitis, tumors, cleft palates, cleft lips, oronasal and oroantral fistulas, and foreign bodies. Differential diagnosis concerns are uremia, sinusitis, gastrointestinal problems, respiratory diseases, nasal disorders, diet, lip-fold pyoderma, and lesions such as abscesses or infected anal glands being licked or chewed at.

Clicking or popping noises noticed during jaw movement are typically associated with problems with the temporomandibular joint (TMJ) or the coronoid process and zygomatic arch (8–10). Differential diagnoses can be dental, jaw, or palatal fractures.

Indications of acute or chronic oral pain associated with mandibular movement, or open-mouth behavior, can be related to numerous oral problems. Differential diagnoses can be dental, jaw or palatal fractures, myositis, foreign bodies, mandibular neuropraxia, salivary gland disease, craniomandibular osteopathy, severe stomatitis, acute necrotizing ulcerative gingivitis, chronic ulcerative paradental stomatitis or kissing ulcers, tumors, TMJ disease, or coronoid process problems with the zygomatic arch (6,8–10).

Chronic ptyalism or drooling is most commonly caused by a reluctance or inability to swallow rather than increased salivary flow or production (6). Acute endodontic exposure, severe inflammatory disease, ulceration of any of the oral mucosae, and foreign bodies are the more common oral causes. Other causes can be systemic bacterial infections such as leptospirosis and viral diseases such as rabies and the feline upper respiratory tract infections. Toxins, such as man-made organophosphates and animal toxins like those found on many toads, can also result in acute excessive salivation. Heat and excitement can result in ptyalism, but this is generally acute in onset with other obvious symptoms.

Facial swellings, edema, draining tracts, sores, or bleeding from the mouth, nose, or facial area can have oral origins. Endodontic, periodontal, or salivary disease or trauma can result in these symptoms. Differential problems are insect and snake bites, allergic reactions, tumors, hematomas, and subcutaneous air (2,6).

GENERAL PHYSICAL EXAMINATION

The external physical examination should never be overlooked in the attempt to press on to more obvious oral problems. Skin allergies may lead to hair chewing, which can cause attrition of the incisors with loose hair tangled around teeth, acting to retain debris and to enhance an environment for periodontitis (2). Observe the entire animal in general, but concentrate on the respiratory and cardiovascular soundness, as these are the most common areas to result in complicating factors associated with sedation or anesthesia used in the in-depth oral examination, dental prophylaxis, and oral treatments (2).

Closely observe the face, mandible, and head for swellings that can indicate neoplastic enlargements, cellulitis, or abscesses (2,7,11–16). Cellulitis and abscess formation can be due to foreign bodies, fight wounds, periodontal disease, or periapical disorders. Fistulous tracts may be present with or without serous or purulent drainage according to the cycle of disease. Neoplasia and eosinophilic granuloma complexes may result in raised ulcerative lesions of the lip and gingiva or enlargement of the mandibular lymph nodes (6). Always palpate the lymph nodes and salivary glands in the head and neck region for enlargement or indications of pain.

Asymmetry of the face or head can be seen in hereditary or congenital abnormalities, inflammatory disease, neoplasia, dislocations, fractures, and nerve damage. Some of the more common of these in the cat are dislocation of the TMJ and maxillary or mandibular fractures, and in the dog, allergic responses and wry mouth (8,9). Open mouth disorders are usually a result of trauma to the TMJ, maxillary or mandibular bones (fractures), or nerve damage or disease (8–10).

INITIAL ORAL SURVEY

The initial oral survey is generally performed in the examination room following the physical examination and normally without the aid of sedation or anesthesia. Correct assessment of an animal's oral and dental health relies on familiarity with normal anatomy. The amount of information that can be obtained varies greatly from individual to individual based on the animal's temperament and the owner's ability to properly and adequately restrain the pet. A well trained technician can many times facilitate this process better than the owner, although the owner will typically need to be present to elaborate on the primary complaint. A detailed, systematic approach is necessary for a complete oral examination (17,18). Head type and symmetry, swellings, draining sores, and occlusion or malocclusion are always the beginning point of the oral examination. Examine the lips and commissures for lesions, pyoderma, or tumors.

Next lift the lips with the thumb and forefinger and examine the exposed teeth and mucosae (Fig. 1); then progress to an open mouth examination if possible. There are several ways to adequately open and examine the mouth. The most common is an overhand technique with the palm over the bridge of the nose and the thumb behind the canine tooth on one side and the index finger behind the canine tooth on the opposite side. The opposite hand grasps the mandible from below, with the forefinger and thumb to either side and the index finger placed on the incisors and used to lever the mouth open. Care should be exerted in trauma and severe periodontal cases, as the jaws in such circumstances can be easily fractured. Evaluate the mucous membranes for color, moistness, ulcerations, lacerations, and swellings. Examine the gingivae for color, inflammation, hyperplasia, recession, sulcal exudate, sulcal bleeding, normal architecture, and the presence of swellings or tumors. Inspect the teeth for occlusion, fractures, discoloration, calculus, plaque, mobility, caries, cervical line lesions, and developmental defects. The buccal surfaces can generally be examined on the alert pet and the lingual surfaces under sedation. The roof of the mouth should the be examined for swellings, defects, foreign bodies, and rugae symmetry (Fig. 2). The tongue should be mobile and have good strength. Inspection of

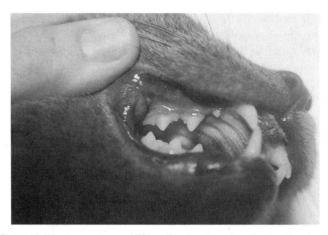

FIG. 1. Holding muzzle and lifting lips to examine the teeth, gingiva.

the ventral tongue can be facilitated by pushing a finger up into the ventral inter-mandibular space (6) (Fig. 3). Always check under the tongue for tumors, lacerations, ulcerations, and foreign bodies. The salivary papillae should be free of inflammation and patent. Patency can sometimes be difficult to assess without passing a catheter, but in some cases saliva may be expressed by placing light pressure caudal to the papilla and rolling the finger toward the duct. Observe also for halitosis, oral bleeding, epistaxis, and rhinitis, as well as the condition and strength of the masticatory muscles.

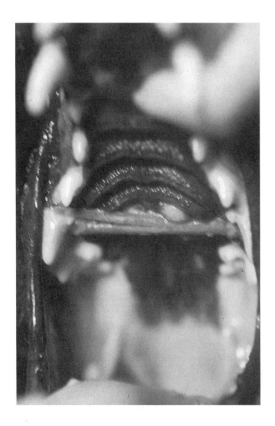

FIG. 2. Examination of the palate may reveal imbedded foreign objects, such as this rib bone.

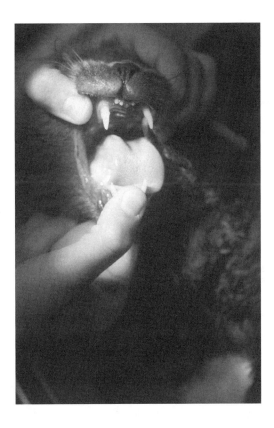

FIG. 3. Pushing a finger up into the intermandibular space allows better visualization of the ventral tongue.

PREANESTHESIA DIAGNOSTIC TESTS

The preanesthesia diagnostic testing is performed in order to reduce the risk of pathophysiologic complications during or after induction (2,6). Testing emphasis should be directed by the history, physical examination, and the initial oral survey. The minimum data base for most individuals would generally be considered to include a hematocrit (HCT) and blood urea nitrogen (BUN) level, while a complete blood count (CBC) and chemical profile would be preferred. Special tests are based on the clinician's assessment of the individual. In cases where cardiovascular, respiratory, or neoplastic disease is suspected, radiographic surveys are indicated. An electrocardiogram (ECG) may also be suggested based on similar criteria. In questionable cases, it is very wise to consult specialists in internal medicine or the most appropriate field before proceeding.

IN-DEPTH ORAL EXAMINATION

Once all available information has been correlated, the in-depth oral examination can begin. A complete in-depth oral examination can only be performed on a patient highly sedated or under general anesthesia. All information discussed within the initial oral survey that was not obtained in full detail should be acquired at this time. This should incorporate the oral examination, periodontal examination, dental examination, and the charting process (19).

Periodontal disease is initiated when the bacteria in the mouth collect with a matrix of salivary glycoproteins and extracellular polysaccharides to form *plaque* that adheres to the tooth surface (11). After a time, the plaque will mineralize to form calculus (7,11–13). As the plaque contacts the attached gingiva, the bacteria and byproducts, joined later by the body's own immune response, can cause inflammation, infection, and eventually destruction of tissues (20,21). At first, the supragingival plaque bacteria are gram-positive, nonmotile, aerobic cocci, but as the infection progresses deeper into the sulcus, gram-negative, motile, anaerobic rods predominate. The signs of periodontal disease include edema and inflammation of the gums, plaque and calculus deposition, halitosis, gingival bleeding with probing, ulceration, gum recession, bone loss, mobile teeth, and tooth loss (22,23).

The *gingival sulcus* should be examined with a periodontal probe for abnormal pocket depths and with an explorer for indication of cervical line lesions, subgingival plaque, and calculus. Limited direct observation in the sulcus can be obtained by using a three-way air/water syringe. The air can be used to gently blow the sulcus open for a look inside. Additionally, even thin unnoticeable pieces of calculus usually show up as chalky white areas when the air is blown across them. The gingival sulcus is a groove or space between the gingival margin and the tooth and can be up to 1–3 mm in depth in the normal dog (Fig. 4). The gingival margin of a cat is usually so closely associated with the tooth that any sulcus deeper than 0.5 mm may be considered abnormal (24). The sulcus depth should be checked at four to six sites around the tooth, and variations from the norm should be recorded on the animal's chart (see Oral and Dental Charting below). In periodontal disease, radiographs can show signs of subgingival calculus, loss of crestal bone, widening or loss of the periodontal ligament, root ankylosis, and loss of lamina dura; however, most of this information can be determined by visual inspection, probing, and palpation for mobility. Radiographs provide a good monitor for control of attachment loss, but only if the same exposure and angulation technique are repeated exactly.

The *furcation* is a site were two roots separate from the body of the tooth. In multi-rooted teeth, furcations are common areas of attachment loss and periodontal disease occurrence. Exposure of furcations (Fig. 5) and degree of exposure should be recorded (see Chapters 7 and 8).

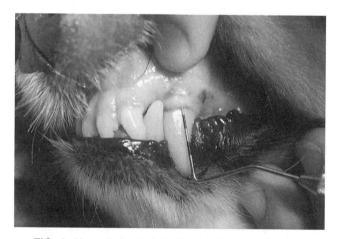

FIG. 4. Normal gingival depth of 1–3 mm in the dog.

Endodontic disease, although not as common as periodontal disease, is common in the dog and cat (14). While some manifestations are significant indications of pulpal pathology, other endodontically compromised teeth are less obvious in their symptoms. A complete endodontic examination includes visual inspection, palpation, and radiographic assessment. This assists in the diagnosis of the lesion and its localization to the area of origin (25,26). As in all veterinary cases, a thorough medical and dental history is needed to assess both the localized problem and the overall health of the patient. Specifically, any previous indication of oral discomfort, possible dental abscess, or facial trauma may warrant further investigation.

The crucial tools necessary for the complete assessment of endodontic lesions are the actual oral examination, including visual inspection, palpation, sensitivity testing, and radiographs (25–28). The most obvious sign seen by the owner or the veterinarian will be a fractured tooth, whether just a crack or split, or up to partial loss of the crown with exposed canal. If the fracture is recent, the exposed pulp may appear pink or edematous, or hemorrhage may be present. These teeth can be painful, so palpation should be attempted with care. Once the pulp has necrosed and the nerve has died, the tooth should not be acutely sensitive, and a dark spot will indicate the canal opening. Teeth that have sustained enough trauma to disrupt the apical blood supply or cause *irreversible pulpitis* appear intact, but discolored, as the inflammatory byproducts leach into the dentinal tubules. An injured tooth that initially appears pink will turn purple to gray or beige later on. As the pathology of the infection progresses, various indications of abscessation may become apparent. Mucosal swelling or discoloration, discharge through the gingiva and even out through the skin, facial swelling, and fistulous tracts may appear, depending on the site of the problem.

Palpating the defect with an endodontic explorer or pathfinder is sometimes possible in the awake patient, but full assessment will usually require general anesthesia. Checking for mobility of teeth fragments and even loose teeth, as well as gently spreading the cracks to see if they extend vertically, are helpful palpation practices. Placing a cold material in contact with various teeth to elicit an exaggerated response is one further test, but it is most reliable in a calm, awake patient or one mildly sedated. Water or gelatin from a freezer bag can be frozen in a tuberculin syringe with the tip cut off to make a cold tester.

No endodontic examination can be complete without proper radiographs for valid diagnosis (Fig. 6). Assessment of open canals and cracks to determine the extent of struc-

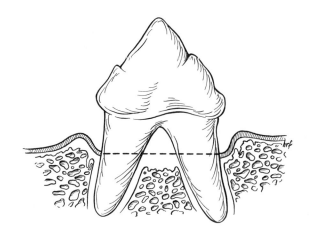

FIG. 5. Furcation exposure due to attachment loss.

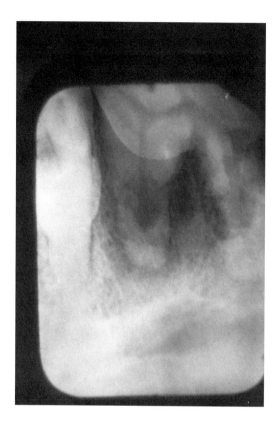

FIG. 6. Radiograph showing root re-sorption. This tooth would not be a good candidate for endodontic therapy.

tural damage, including fractured roots, can reveal tooth injuries that would make successful endodontics dubious. Questionable teeth are radiographed to look for periapical lucency, an indication of possible pathology such as apical granulomas, abscesses, or periapical cysts. Additional lesions of periodontal ligament space widening and external or internal resorption lesions, as well as endoliths and other anatomic anomalies, should be considered to make the prognosis worse (25–28).

Problems with the temporomandibular joint (TMJ) can be difficult to assess at times (8–10). Radiographs can give much information, if the suitable positioning can be attained (see Chapter 6). Palpation during manipulation of the joint may produce crepitus. A stethoscope can be placed over the TMJ during manipulation to listen for this. Also palpate the zygomatic arch area during manipulation to evaluate if the coronoid process is flaring across, causing locking, popping, or inflammatory trauma to the area. Always palpate the borders of the mandible for enlargements or swellings.

ORAL DIAGNOSTIC TESTING

Based on this information, additional oral diagnostic tests may be considered. Among these are cultures and sensitivities, biopsy and histopathology, transillumination, thermal tests, electronic vitality testing, oral and intraoral radiographs, and gingival crevicular fluid tests. Oral and intraoral radiographs and techniques are addressed in detail in the chapter on radiology (see Chapter 6) and will be addressed only lightly here.

To date, *oral cultures and sensitivities* have not been shown to be of significant importance in the dog and cat (27). It is rare that sensitivities are called for in endodontic infections, as exodontics (extraction) and standard endodontics (root canal therapy) are generally curative. For stomatitis and periodontitis, multiple bacterial isolates are common and expected, even in healthy animals, as a large and diverse flora is always present (29–36). Little research has been performed on the pathogenicity of oral flora in the dog and cat. Bacteria are commonly found on the dorsum of the tongue shortly after birth. As teeth erupt, bacteria will be found colonizing tooth plaque, with the largest populations typically located in the sulcus (37). It is believed that the most pathogenic bacteria in the oral cavity are motile flagellates and anaerobes, which are rarely detected by routine culture techniques. Small amounts of gingival crevicular fluid (GCF) can be placed on a slide and observed under a phase-contrast microscope to estimate the percentage of motile bacteria (38). In most cases, normal GCF has a low number of motile bacteria, while in active disease (periodontitis), the GCF typically reveals higher counts. One problem with this is that periodontal disease, even advanced disease (degree of attachment loss), is cyclic in activity, and the infection may be inactive at the time of sampling. Oral fungal cultures can be useful in confirming *Monilia albicans* and occasionally in disclosing the presence of various systemic mycoses contributing to oral lesions. Viral isolate techniques require active viral shedding and can give useful information in some cases, but little data are available on the normal oral viral flora of the dog or cat. A degree of research has been performed on rhinotracheitis and calicivirus infections and oral lesions in cats (39–41).

Thermal tests are typically used for location of sensitive and endodontically compromised teeth (25). Heat or cold is applied directly to the tooth without making contact with any other oral structures. The main problem with these tests is the reliance on a reaction by the patient, which is not dependable. This also requires the tests to be performed on an unanesthetized individual. Reaction to cold may suggest a sensitive or compromised tooth. Sensitivity to heat generally indicates a more serious problem of irreversible pulpitis and impending devitalization of the tooth.

Transillumination is the use of light to examine the reflectivity of the internal tooth structures (42) (Fig. 7). In healthy teeth, light passes through fairly well, while in devitalized teeth a more opaque effect may be seen. It is best to compare teeth within the same

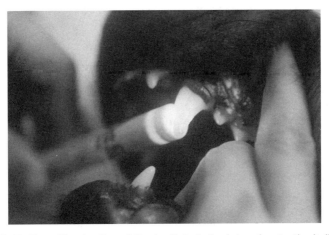

FIG. 7. Transillumination of the tooth to help determine tooth vitality.

mouth as control guides. Electronic pulp testers have not at this time shown a great deal of reliability in the dog and cat, but new developments in electrical resistance testing may provide precise and reliable instruments in the very near future.

Gingival crevicular fluid (GCF) tests make use of sulcal fluid samples. Many are currently in use in humans and include elastase, aspartate aminotransferase (AST), alanine aminotransferase (ALT), and cellular identification studies (41–48). To date, of these tests only GCF/AST has shown any indication of being a reliable indicator of periodontitis in the dog and cat (38,49–54). Additional research will be necessary to determine the clinical practicality of any of these tests.

Biopsy information frequently is one of the most reliable and informative diagnostic tools available, whether cytologic, incisional, or excisional (55). Cytology can be helpful in differential diagnosis between eosinophilic granuloma and squamous cell carcinoma. Many times this can be done with little or no sedation, with a scalpel blade used to lightly scrape the lesions; the cells are then placed on a slide to air-dry and to be stained.

Incisional biopsy allows for diagnosis prior to complete lesion removal. This allows for determination of the necessity for more radical treatment (maxillectomies, mandibulectomies, radiation therapy, chemotherapy, etc.) before therapy is addressed. Such procedures may irritate some lesions, stimulating them to grow, spread, or metastasize (6). Therefore, incisional biopsy should be selected in those cases where such occurrence would hopefully not be of serious significance. For this reason, many practitioners will elect to proceed with excisional biopsy. In these cases, the lesion is removed to well beyond its margins in hopes of total removal. All, or a representative portion, of the tumor is then submitted for histopathology and determination of the need for additional surgery or therapy.

With most lesions, the biopsy should be full-depth and catch some of the normal margin for reliability. Some lesions such as fibrosarcoma may extend below apparently normal structures, and failure to penetrate these may lead to misdiagnosis. As in all procedures, thought should be given to the tissues, vessels, ducts, canals, nerves, and organs that may run through or deep to lesions, and every precaution should be taken to avoid unnecessary complications. Biopsy punches are helpful in many cases of incisional biopsy to obtain samples of good depth. Routine tissues collected should be placed in 10% neutral buffered formalin solution for proper fixing. If too large a specimen is placed in the formalin solution, cells deep within the sample may not be properly fixed.

In lesions suspected of autoimmune involvement, Michel's solution rather than formalin should be used to preserve the sample. These biopsy samples should be selected for the most active and intact epithelial vesiculation or pocketed serum-like lesions. The margins should also include apparently normal adjacent tissue for comparative histology.

The pathologist can frequently provide a more reliable diagnosis and prognosis when relevant clinical data are provided with the specimen. Standard signalment should be provided plus location, duration, symptoms, previous biopsy information, and other pertinent history. Most pathologists can be directly contacted for supplementary consultation on cases, which can be in many cases be informative and educational.

ORAL AND DENTAL CHARTING

Charting is the process of recording the state of health or disease of the teeth and oral cavity. It is an integral part of diagnosis, treatment planning, and monitoring. There are many forms of abbreviations and charting.

Palatal—surface of tooth toward the palate (upper)
Lingual—surface of tooth toward the tongue (lower or upper)
Labial—surface of tooth toward the lips
Buccal—surface of tooth toward the cheek
Facial—labial or buccal surface
Occlusal—surface of tooth facing a tooth in opposite jaw
Interproximal—surface between two teeth
Mesial:—surface of tooth toward the front midline
Distal—surface of tooth away from the front midline
Apical—toward the apex (root)
Coronal—toward the crown

Knowing the correct dental formulas (56) of both deciduous and permanent teeth as well as eruption times will help one recognize abnormalities such as missing teeth, supernumerary (extra) teeth, and even retained deciduous teeth (which generally should be extracted) (56,57) (Table 1). The term *mixed dentition* simply refers to a normal mixture of both deciduous and permanent teeth in the same dentition. This is common finding between 3 months and 7 months of age in the dog and cat. Identifying the tooth type is essential for good charting:

I: incisor; *dI* or *i:* deciduous incisor
C: canine or cuspid; *dC* or *c:* deciduous canine/cuspid
P: premolar; *dP* or *p:* deciduous premolar
M: molar; *dM* or *m:* deciduous molar
S: supernumerary

The currently accepted designations of the dental formula for the cat are as follows:

Deciduous: 2 × (Id 3/3, Cd 1/1, Pd 3/2) = 26
Permanent: 2 × (I 3/3, C 1/1, P 3/2, M 1/1) = 30

The currently accepted designations of the dental formula for the dog are as follows:

Deciduous: 2 × (Id 3/3, Cd 1/1, Pd 3/3) = 28
Permanent: 2 × (I 3/3, C 1/1, P 4/4, M 2/3) = 42

Note: The actual numbering of the individual deciduous teeth in the dog and cat and of the permanent teeth in the cat is currently disagreed on by various authors and groups

TABLE I. *Eruption times of deciduous and permanent teeth in the dog and cat*

	Deciduous teeth (wk)	Permanent teeth (mo)
Dog		
Incisors	3–5	3–5
Canines (cuspids)	3–6	3.5–6
Premolars	4–10	3.5–6
Molars		3.5–7
Cat		
Incisors	2–3	3–4
Canines (cuspids)	3–4	4–5
Premolars	3–6	4–6
Molars		4–6

(20,58,59). Under currently accepted scientific anatomic nomenclature, there are no molars in deciduous teeth, and it is always the most rostral premolars and most caudal molars that are missing in normal dental formulas. In both the dog and cat, the lower last, and in the dog the upper last, deciduous cheek teeth are noted as deciduous premolar number 4. Yet even a casual examination reveals that these teeth are almost identical in shape and structure to lower and upper 1st permanent molars, and they function in a similar fashion to the permanent molar teeth. Clinically, these are deciduous molars. However, the successional teeth that replace these are premolars, which can be confirmed radiographically. Additionally, in the permanent dentition of the cat, it is currently considered that the "missing" premolars are actually those in front, based on scientific methodology; that is, the upper premolars should be numbered from 2 to 4, and the lower premolars should be numbered 3 and 4 (56–63). The lower numbering system appears grossly correct, but clinical examinations of the first upper cheek teeth typically show a single-rooted tooth with a small diastema between it and the next cheek tooth. Normally, it is the first premolars and last molars that are single-rooted, and with the gap or diastema behind the first upper cheek tooth, this would indicate that the tooth missing is not the 1st premolar but the 2nd. Currently, most clinically based authors accept the present scientific system for simple consistency, although at some juncture an opened-minded systematic reevaluation may be advisable.

The current scientifically accepted numbering systems for the dog and cat are the following (counting from the most rostral or mesial tooth):

Dog Primary or Deciduous Teeth (Repeated Left and Right)

Maxillary:	Incisors 1–3	Canine 1	Premolars 2–4
Mandibular:	Incisors 1–3	Canine 1	Premolars 2–4

Dog Permanent Teeth (Repeated Left and Right)

Maxillary:	Incisors 1–3	Canine 1	Premolars 1–4	Molars 1–2
Mandibular:	Incisors 1–3	Canine 1	Premolars 1–4	Molars 1–3

Cat Primary or Deciduous Teeth (Repeated Left and Right)

Maxillary:	Incisors 1–3	Canine 1	Premolars 2–4
Mandibular:	Incisors 1–3	Canine 1	Premolars 3–4

Cat Permanent Teeth (Repeated Left and Right)

Maxillary:	Incisors 1–3	Canine 1	Premolars 2–4	Molars 1
Mandibular:	Incisors 1–3	Canine 1	Premolars 3–4	Molars 1

There are numerous tooth-naming and coding systems in current use, and all have advantages and disadvantages (3,4,40,64). This makes it essential that the practitioner be familiar with some of the more commonly used systems, although for ease of clinic charting one should be selected and used consistently.

The first item to correctly understand is the proper identification sequence. This is simply dentition, arch, quadrant—and tooth in that order (64). *Dentition* refers to differentiation between deciduous and permanent dentition. *Arch* is in notation of maxillary or mandibular. *Quadrant* implies right or left side of the individual. *Tooth* pertains to incisor, cuspid, premolar, or molar, and its number or identification, eg: 1st incisor, 4th premolar, 1st molar, etc:

Deciduous	Maxillary	Right	1st Incisor
(DENTITION)	(ARCH)	(QUADRANT)	(TOOTH)
Permanent	Mandibular	Left	4th Premolar

Therefore, the proper sequence of identification would be: permanent maxillary right 4th premolar—not: right permanent maxillary 4th premolar.

One of the simpler systems is to indicate the tooth type by the previously described abbreviations, and then indicate the position and number by super- and subscripts:

^1C: Permanent maxillary left canine or cuspid
dP_3: Deciduous mandibular right 3rd premolar
SP^1: Supernumerary permanent maxillary right 1st premolar

The American Veterinary Dental College Nomenclature and Classification Committee has suggested the use of the *Triadan* tooth numbering system employing three-digit numbers without commas, although not officially accepted at this date. The first numeral designates the quadrant location and whether a tooth is primary or secondary. The number sequence is upper right, upper left, lower left and lower right. The adult dentition utilizes numbers 1–4, and primary dentition uses numbers 5–8. In each quadrant, the 1st incisor is always 1, with incisors numbered 1–3, cuspids numbered 4, premolars numbered 5–8 (except when not present), and molars numbered 9–11 (except when not present) (15,16). This numbering is based on a fully phenotypic dentition—(I 3/3, C 1/1, P 4/4, M 3/3) × 2 = 44, as in swine. The cat's reduced dentition numbering is appropriately altered:

Upper right 1/5	Upper left 2/6
Lower right 4/8	Lower left 3/7

Examples:

101 = Permanent maxillary right 1st or central incisor
204 = Permanent maxillary left canine or cuspid
308 = Permanent mandibular left 4th premolar
409 = Permanent mandibular right 1st molar
604 = Deciduous maxillary left canine or cuspid
807 = Deciduous Mandibular Right Third Premolar

The number of root tips is also important, particularly in exodontia (extractions) and endodontics (root canal procedure).

Root Tips of Teeth in the Dog

One root:	All incisors, canines, commonly 1st premolars
Three roots:	Upper 4th premolars, upper 1st and 2nd molars
Two roots:	All others

Root Tips of Teeth in the Cat

One root:	All incisors, canines, upper 2nd premolars
Three roots:	Upper 4th premolars
Two roots:	All others

It is also useful to have a dental chart on the permanent record, either a stamped impression, sticker, or separate sheet. One chart can be used for recording the examina-

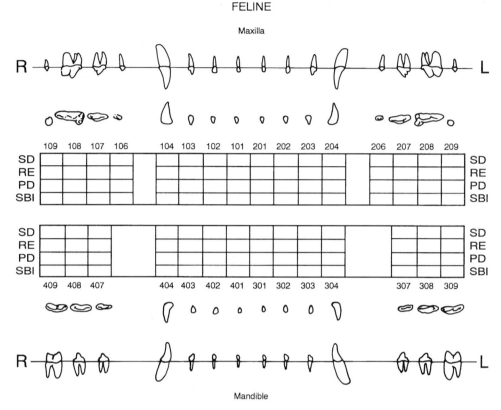

FIG. 8. Dental chart for record.

tion, assessment, and pathology, with a second to denote the specific treatment; otherwise, a single diagram may be used as a combined report form (Fig. 8).

Some Common Dental Abbreviations (65–70)

For a more detailed list, see the abbreviations in Chapter 23.

AL = attachment loss   E = enamel lesion
AT = attrition   EP = epulis
BL = bone loss   FE = furcation exposure[c]
BKT = orthodontic bracket   Fx = fracture
CA = cavity   GCF = gingival crevicular fluid
CI = calculus index[a]   GP = gingivoplasty
CR = crown restoration[b]   GV = gingivectomy
CU = contact ulcer   GI = gingivitis index[d]

---

[a] CI: rate, 0–3: none, slight, moderate, abundant (67).
[b] CR: CRC-composite, CM-metal, PFM-porcelain (68).
[c] FE: rate, 1–3: 1, exposed; 2, undermined; 3, through-and-through communication. Additionally, facial (F), lingual (L), mesial (M) and distal (D) can be used to denote furcation, eg, F2-F, furcation exposure and undermined on facial surface of tooth (70).
[d] GI: rate, 0–3: none, mild, moderate, severe (65)

GH = gingival hyperplasia
GR = gingival recession
GTR = guided tissue regeneration
LPS = lymphocytic plasmocytic stomatitis
M = mobile tooth[e]
O = missing tooth
OA = orthodontic appliance
ONF = oronasal fistula
PDI = periodontal disease index[f]
PE = pulp exposure
PI = plaque index[g]
PP = periodontal pocket

R = restoration
R/A = restoration amalgam
R/C = restoration composite
R/I = restoration glass ionomer
RC = root canal therapy
RD = retained deciduous tooth
ROT = rotation
RE = root exposure
RL = resorptive lesion[h]
RR = root resorption
SBI = sulcus bleeding index[i]
VP = vital pulpotomy
X = extraction

REFERENCES

1. Thoma KH, Robinson HBG. *Oral and Dental Diagnosis*. 4th ed. Philadelphia: WB Saunders Co; 1956:3.
2. Wiggs RB. Oral diagnosis and treatment planning. In: Low D, ed. *The Friskies Symposium on Veterinary Dentistry*. Davis, California;1993:32.
3. Torres HO, Ehrlich A. *Modern Dental Assisting*. 2nd ed. Philadelphia: WB Saunders Co; 1980:481.
4. Treatment considerations of dental patients. In: *Accepted Dental Therapeutic*. 38th ed. Chicago: American Dental Association; 1979:3.
5. Black GV. *Operative Dentistry*, vol 1. 7th ed. Chicago: Medico-Dental Publishing Co; 1936:16.
6. Burrows CF, Harvey CE. Oral examination and diagnostic techniques. In: Harvey CE, ed. *Veterinary Dentistry*. Philadelphia: WB Saunders Co; 1985:23.
7. Goodson JM, Tanner AC, Haffajee AD, Sornberger GC, Socransky SS. Patterns of progression and regression of advanced destructive periodontal disease. *J Clin Periodontol* 1982;9:472.
8. Lobprise HB, Wiggs RB. Modified surgical treatment of intermittent open-mouth mandibular locking in a cat. *J Vet Dent* 1992;9:8.
9. Robins G, Grandage J. Temporomandibular joint dysplasia and open mouthed jaw locking in the dog. *JAVMA* 1977;171:1072.
10. Lantz GC, Cantwell HD. Intermittent open-mouth lower jaw locking in five dogs. *JAVMA* 1986;188:1403.
11. Socransky SS, Haffajee AD, Goodson JM, Lindhe J. New concepts of destructive periodontal disease. *J Clin Periodontol* 1984;11:21.
12. Page RC, Schroeder HE. Pathogenesis of inflammatory periodontal disease. A summary of current work. *Lab Invest* 1976;33:235.
13. Page RC, Schroeder HE. *Periodontitis in Man and Other Animals: A Comparative Review*. Basel: Karger; 1982:251;265.
14. Wiggs RB. Is periodontal disease a measurement of a pet's general health? *Vet Forum* 1995:2;66.
15. Floyd MR. The modified Triadan system: Nomenclature for veterinary dentistry. *J Vet Dent* 1991;8(4):18.
16. Schumacher CB. Charting and the oral examination. *J Vet Dent* 1993;10(3):9.
17. Gruffydd-Jones, Evans RJ, Gaskell CJ. The alimentary system. In: Pratt PW, ed. *Feline Medicine*. Santa Barbara, CA: American Veterinary Publishers; 1983:202.
18. Holzworth J, Stein BS. The sick cat. In: Holzworth J, ed. *Diseases of the Cat*. Philadelphia: WB Saunders Co; 1987:4.
19. Eversole LR. Clinical outline of oral pathology: Diagnosis and treatment. Philadelphia: Lea & Fibger; 1978:20.
20. Ranney RR. Classification of periodontal diseases. *Periodontology 2000* 1993;2:13.
21. Page RC. Gingivitis. *J Clin Periodontol* 1986;13:345.
22. Theilade E. The non-specific theory in microbial etiology of inflammatory periodontal disease. *J Clin Periodontol* 1986;13:905.

---

[e] M: rate, 0–3: none, slight, moderate, severe (70).

[f] PDI: rate, 1–4: gingivitis 0% AL; early <25% AL; moderate <50% AL; severe >50% AL (20).

[g] PI: rate, 0–3: none, slight, moderate, severe (66).

[h] Feline dental resorptive lesions (FDR, resorptive lesion, cervical neck lesion, cervical line lesions): rated as stage 1–5: RL1, into enamel only; RL2, into dentin; RL3, into pulp; RL4, extensive structural damage; RL5, crown lost, only roots remain (20,68).

[i] SBI: rate, 0–5: 0, none on probing to 5, spontaneous bleeding (69).

23. Rateitschak KH. *Periodontology.* 2nd ed. New York: Thieme Medical Publishers; 1989:130.
24. Wiggs RB, Lobprise HB. Dental disease, In: Norsworthy GD, ed. *Feline Practice.* Philadelphia: JB Lippincott Co; 1993:290.
25. Cohen S. Diagnostic procedures. In: Cohen S, Burns R, eds. *Pathways to the Pulp.* 15th ed. St. Louis: Mosby-Year Book; 1991:2.
26. Chambers IG. The role and method of pulp testing: A review. *Int Endod J* 1982;15:10.
27. Kaufman AY. An enigmatic sinus tract origin. *Endod Dent Trauma* 1989;5:159.
28. Samulson MH. Classification and diagnosis of pulp pathosis. *Dent Clin North Am* 1984;28:699.
29. Harvey CE, Emily PP. *Small Animal Dentistry.* St. Louis: Mosby-Year Book; 1993:35.
30. Saphir DA, Carter CR. Gingival flora of the dog with special reference to bacteria associated with bites. *J Clin Microbiol* 1976;3:344.
31. Clapper WE, Meade GH. Normal flora of the nose, throat, and lower intestine of dogs. *J Bacteriol* 1963;85:643.
32. Smith JE. The aerobic flora of the nose and tonsils of healthy dogs. *J Comp Pathol* 1961;71:428.
33. Hani M. Characteristics of coagulase-positive staphylococci from the nose and tonsils of apparently healthy dogs. *J Comp Pathol* 1977;87:(2)311.
34. Syed SA, Svanberg M, Svanberg G. The predominant cultivable dental plaque flora of beagle dogs with gingivitis. *J Periodont Res* 1980;15:123.
35. Syed SA, Svanberg M, Svanberg G. The predominant cultivable dental plaque flora of beagle dogs with periodontitis. *J Periodontal Res* 1981;16:45.
36. Theilade E, Wright WH, Jensen SD, Loe H. Experimental gingivitis in man. *J Periodontal Res* 1966;1:13.
37. Burrows CF, Harvey CE. Oral examination and diagnostic techniques. In: Harvey CE, ed. *Veterinary Dentistry.* Philadelphia: WB Saunders Co; 1985:27.
38. Armitage GC. Periodontal diagnostic aids. *Calif Dent Assoc J* 1993;21(11):35.
39. Johnson RP, Povey RC. Effect of diet on oral lesions of feline calicivirus infection. *Vet Rec* 1982;110:106.
40. Gaskell RM, Wardley RC. Feline viral respiratory disease: A review with particular references to its epizootiology and control. *J Small Anim Pract* 1978;19:1.
41. Thompson RR, Wilcox GE, Clark WT, Jansen KL. Association of calicivirus infection with chronic gingivitis and pharyngitis in cats. *J Small Anim Pract* 1984;25:207.
42. Goerig AC. Endodontic emergencies. In: Cohen S, Burns R, eds. *Pathways to the Pulp.* 5th ed. Baltimore: Mosby-Year Book; 1991:31.
43. Wiggs RB, Lobprise HB. Assessment of GCF/ALT (SGPT) in fifteen dogs as a marker of active periodontal disease and response to therapy. Dallas Dental Service Animal Clinic Clinical Study; 1993; unpublished.
44. Lamster IB, Vogel RJ, Hartley LJ, DeGorge CA, Gordon JM. Lactate dehydrogenase, beta-glucuronidase and arylsulfatase in gingival crevicular fluid associated with experimental gingivitis in man. *J Periodontol* 1985;56:130.
45. Last KS, Stanbury JB, Emberg G. Glycosaminoglycans in human crevicular fluid as indicators of active periodontal disease. *Arch Oral Biol* 1985;30:275.
46. Golub LM, Siegal K, Ramamurthy NS, Mandel ID. Some characteristics of collagenase activity in gingival crevicular fluid and its relationship to gingival diseases in humans. *J Dent Res* 1976;55:1049.
47. Offenbacher S, Odle BM, Van Dyke TE. The use of crevicular fluid prostaglandin E_2 levels as predictor of periodontal attachment loss. *J Periodontal Res* 1986;21:101.
48. Palcanis KG, Larjava IK, Wells BR, Suggs KA, Landis JR, Chadwick DE, Jeffcoat MK. Elastase as an indicator of periodontal disease progression. *J Periodontol* 1992;63:237.
49. Chambers DA, Crawford JM, Mukherjee S, Cohen RL. Aspartate aminotransferase increases in crevicular fluid during experimental periodontitis in beagle dogs. *J Periodontol* 1984;55:526.
50. Chambers DA, Imrey PB, Cohen RL, Crawford JM, Alves MEAF, McSwiggin TA. A longitudinal study of aspartate aminotransferase in human gingival crevicular fluid. *J Periodontal Res* 1991;26:65.
51. Imrey PB, Crawford JM, Cohen RL, Alves MEAF, McSwiggin TA, Chambers DA. A cross-sectional analysis of aspartate aminotransferase in human crevicular fluid. *J Periodontal Res* 1991;26:75.
52. Wiggs RB, Lobprise HB, Holmstrom SE. Clinical evaluations of gingival crevicular fluid aspartate aminotransferase (GCF/AST) in relationship to serum alanine aminotransferase (SALT), and serum AST (SAST) in the dog. 1994; submitted for publication.
53. Wiggs RB, Lobprise HB, Holmstrom SE. Gingival crevicular fluid aspartate aminotransferase (GCF/AST) as a marker of naturally occurring active periodontitis in the dog. 1994; submitted for publication.
54. Wiggs RB, Capron K, Lobprise HB. Gingival crevicular fluid aspartate aminotransferase (GCF/AST) as a marker of naturally occurring periodontitis in the cat. 1994; submitted for publication.
55. Arens DE. Surgical endodontics. In: Cohen S, Burns R, eds. *Pathways to the Pulp.* 5th ed. Baltimore: Mosby-Year Book; 1991:582.
56. Frost P. Feline dentistry. In: *Canine Dentistry.* 3rd ed. Nabisco Compendium; Mount Kisco, New York: Day Communications; 1990:60.
57. Lyons KF. An approach to feline dentistry. *Compend Cont Educ Dent* 1990;12:493.
58. Eisner E, et al. *Tooth Designation of the Reduced Dentition of the Domestic Cat.* Report of the Committee of Veterinary Dental Nomenclature and Classification; March 10, 1992.
59. Westhyde L. The enigma of feline dentition. *J Vet Dent* 1990;7(3):16.
60. de Lahunta A, Habel RE. Teeth. In: *Applied Veterinary Anatomy.* Philadelphia: WB Saunders Co; 1986:5.

61. Peyer B. Teeth and dentition in different groups of vertebrates. In: Zangeri R, trans-ed. Comparative Odontology. Chicago: University of Chicago Press; 1968:244.
62. Gaunt W. The development of the deciduous teeth of the cat. *Acta Anat* 1959;38:187.
63. Williams R. *Observations on the Chronology of Deciduous Development in the Dog.* Ithaca, NY: Cornell University; 1961. PhD thesis.
64. Brand WB, Isselhard DE. *Anatomy of Orofacial Structures.* 3rd ed. St Louis, MO: CV Mosby Co; 1986:237.
65. Silness J, Loe H. Periodontal disease in pregnancy. II. Correlation between oral hygiene and periodontal conditions. *Acta Odontol Scand* 1964;22:121.
66. Loe H, Silness J. Periodontal disease in pregnancy. I. Prevalence and severity. *Acta Odontol Scand* 1963;21:533.
67. Ramfjord SP. The periodontal disease index (PDI). *J Periodontol* 1967;38:602.
68. *Veterinary Dental Abbreviations.* American Veterinary Dental College, Residency Tracking Committee, 1994; Supplement to the American Veterinary Dental College Residency Tracking Requirements.
69. Muhlemann HR, Son S. Gingival sulcus bleeding—a leading symptom in initial gingivitis. *Helv Odontol Acta* 1971;15:107.
70. Diagnosis, prognosis and treatment planning. In: *Periodontic Syllabus.* Naval Graduate Dental School: Bureau of Medicine and Surgery; Bethesda, Maryland: 1975:35.

5

Clinical Oral Pathology

Robert B. Wiggs and Heidi B. Lobprise

Oral and dental lesions are common in most animals (1,2,3). *Clinical oral pathology* is concerned with the symptoms, signs, diagnosis, changes in structure and function, causes, progression, and prognosis of oral lesions. The principle function of the study of pathology is to assist the clinician in the correct diagnosis of abnormalities, specifically to aid in determining the appropriate treatment, whose success is dependent on accurate diagnosis.

Oral pathology, the study of oral cavity disease, is considered present when a departure from normal sufficient to cause signs or symptoms occurs. *Symptoms* are the abnormalities detected by the patient or owner, while *signs* are those noted by the clinician (4). A *syndrome* is a defined group of signs or symptoms, but with the syndrome not always resulting from the same specifically defined cause. *Etiology* is the theory of the cause of the disease, and the *DAMNIT* approach can offer a systematic review of potential causes:

D   degenerative, developmental
A   autoimmune, allergic
M   metabolic, mechanical
N   nutritional, neoplastic
I   infectious, immune-mediated
T   toxic, traumatic

When there is no acceptable theory as to etiology available, a disease is called *idiopathic*.

This chapter will cover developmental problems encountered, divided into different areas of the oral cavity. This developmental category will deal with anomalies due to a specific inherited cause (genetic), with probable genetic etiologies with a familial tendency, and with anomalies that occur due to congenital influences. *Genetic* describes conditions that are hereditary. *Congenital* describes abnormalities present at birth, either inherited or due to conditions that occurred during pregnancy (eg, infection, drugs, injury). *Familial* describes conditions that affect a family to an extent that is considered greater than expected by random or chance circumstance. The remainder of acquired (problems) will be divided by tissue area and then categorized within that field by the DAMNIT scheme, as applicable. Lesions found specifically in feline patients are discussed in more detail in the feline chapter (see Chapter 16).

DEVELOPMENTAL PATHOLOGY

Dental Tissues

Just like a fetus in utero, the forming tooth is very susceptible to various influences during periods of rapid growth and change. Many variations of normal tooth structure, number, and size are possible.

Variation in tooth size may be exhibited as macrodontia, microdontia, taurodontia, peg teeth, dilacerations, and so forth. *Macrodontia* is the condition in which the crown of the tooth is oversized but the root and pulp cavity are near normal. While macrodontia could lead to tooth overcrowding and periodontal disease, crowding is generally caused by reduction in jaw size (select breeding) unaccompanied by similar tooth-size reduction. *Taurodontia* is present when the crown and pulp chamber are enlarged and the root is typically small. The condition is considered hereditary in humans and has been seen in the boxer. Treatment is generally similar to that for macrodontia. *Peg teeth* are small conical or cone-shaped teeth with a single cusp (Fig. 1). They may be genetic or congenital, being seen in ectodermal dysplasia and other conditions. *Microdontia* describes when the crown of the tooth is normal in general shape, but reduced in size. It is most commonly seen in the maxillary corner incisors in the dog. Other than esthetics and some loss of function, it typically causes no problems and requires no treatment. *Dilacerated teeth* are those that have a distorted development; dilacerations can involve either the crown or the root. This condition may be hereditary or a congenital disorder, or it may be caused by an injury, infection, or inflammation. Treatment is typically symptomatic.

Dens in dente (tooth within a tooth) is formed when the top of the tooth bud folds onto itself, producing additional layers of enamel, cementum, dentin, or pulp tissue inside the tooth as it develops (5). These invaginations may be in the crown or the root. Root invaginations are typically found radiographically or at the time of extraction (6). Coronal invaginations may be simple shallow lesions that may increase the susceptibility to fracture or carious lesions (7), lesions that extend from crown to apex, and variations in

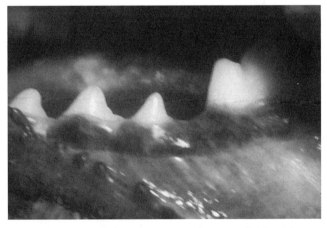

FIG. 1. One-year-old female Doberman pinscher with a mandibular 4th premolar peg tooth.

between these (8). This formation typically results in exposure of the pulp with eventual abscess formation. Depending on the severity of the lesions, endodontics can sometimes be performed to save the tooth, but the treatment can be complicated (9). Incisor teeth with deep coronal lesions can be lost fairly quickly to disease following eruption and exposure of the invagination to the oral flora. Treatment typically consists of extraction, but conventional or apical surgical root canal therapy can be very successful in preserving affected teeth (10). The terms *dens in dente* and *dens invaginatus* are sometimes used interchangeably; however, dens invaginatus has classically been considered a developmental anomaly of an invagination on the lingual or palatal surface of an incisor (11).

Enamel pearls or *enamelomas* are small beads of enamel found apical to the cementoenamel junction, and not uncommonly in the furcational areas (5). The periodontal ligament does not attach well to the tooth at these sites, resulting in a long junctional epithelium within the sulcus, fenestrations, and inflammation of the periodontium. Food and plaque can more easily accumulate at the deceased locations, encouraging the development of periodontal disease (5,12).

A *fusion tooth* is the result of two separate tooth buds joined at the crown by enamel and possibly dentin (5,12,13). There will be a reduced number of teeth, and the fused tooth will be smaller than the two separate teeth would have been. Unless there is communication of the junction groove of the two teeth that extends to or below the gingival margin to trap food and contribute to periodontal disease, few problems should be seen with these teeth (5). There appears to be a familial tendency in dogs with fused incisors due to abnormal interdental laminar growth. *Concrescence* is a fusion of the cementum and sometimes the dentin of two teeth only along their roots. Conditions encountered and treatment are similar to routine fusion.

A *gemination tooth* is one in which the developing bud attempted to split but failed to do so completely (5,12,13). The actual number of teeth is not altered in this condition. However, the structure will generally be larger than normal, which may result in tooth crowding. The condition is common in the maxillary incisors of the boxer without crowding.

Twinning occurs when there has been a complete cleavage of the splitting gemination bud, with the extra tooth being a mirror image of the original. This is a type of supernumerary tooth that does not arise from a separate tooth bud (13).

Shell teeth describes a disorder of teeth, in which there is little-to-no root development but there is a crown. The condition can be hereditary or congenital, or due to certain infections that affect Hertwig's epithelial root sheath during root formation (13). Due to the poor root:crown ratio, the teeth are more easily avulsed. Additionally, due to the short or nonexistent root depth, bacteria from the oral cavity can rapidly invade the pulp tissue via the sulcus, resulting in devitalization and rapid loss of the teeth. Unless a reasonable amount of root structure develops, there is no suitable treatment.

A hereditary reduction in the amount of enamel matrix laid down during its formation causes a condition called *amelogenesis imperfecta* (13). *Dentinogenesis imperfecta*, considered to be hereditary, can be found in both deciduous and permanent teeth (13). The teeth, though normal in shape, appear opalescent and nearly amber. The enamel on these teeth chips away easily, followed by extreme wear. Congenital ectodermal defects may combine deformed teeth with partial or total baldness in a hereditary etiology as well.

In comparison with these genetic causes of enamel changes, it is more common to see acquired changes in the enamel due to stimuli affecting it during critical times in its development. Whether a local inflammation affecting one tooth or a systemic virus or fever affecting several to all teeth, these episodes can cause a disturbance in enamel development that manifests itself in macroscopic changes. While commonly called *enamel hypoplasia* (meaning thin enamel), the true process is more properly termed *enamel hypocalcification* with resultant changes of enamel pitting and discoloration (13). Canine distemper has been reported as one cause of enamel "hypoplasia," with one individual also experiencing microdontia and root dysplasia of some teeth, as well as missing teeth and eruption abnormalities (14). Depending on which point in time the stimulus occurs, different teeth can be affected, as well as their roots. Radiographs should always be taken to assess total tooth structure whenever any abnormality is found.

The presence of certain compounds and chemicals during the time of development can affect the tooth. Excessive fluoride intake will result in enamel dental fluorosis marked by opaque, white, lusterless patches in a mottled, striated, and pitted enamel. These patches may later pick up stain or decay, making it difficult to distinguish from enamel hypocalcification, except with detailed history (12,13). Intrinsic dental staining can be caused by tetracycline compounds, which can cause discoloration ranging from yellow to orange or gray to blue as the drug is absorbed into and binds with tissue undergoing calcification (12). The color and intensity of staining depends on which tetracycline, the amount used, and the age of the individual (12).

Radiographs are also important to take with any variation in the number of teeth. The terms *hypodontia* and *oligodontia* imply that some teeth are missing, while *anodontia* signifies that all teeth are missing, unless qualified as *partial* anodontia. Missing teeth are most commonly seen in small dogs, and in some larger breeds can be considered a serious fault. Permanent teeth are more frequently missing, and if a deciduous tooth is genetically not present, the permanent analog that arises from the primary should also be absent (12,15). Generally, a tooth that is truly missing can only be distinguished from a unerupted or impacted tooth by obtaining radiographs of the site.

Missing and extra (*supernumerary*) teeth alike share a familial tendency and may even be hereditary in some cases and acquired in others (see also "twinning" above) (14). Supernumerary incisors are not uncommon in bull dogs (15) and boxers, and some individuals have extra premolars or cuspids, at times with multiple supernumerary teeth that may be visible only on radiographs. It is not uncommon in the boxer to find supernumerary maxillary incisors without crowding due to their wide brachycephalic bite. However, it is also not uncommon to find boxers with supernumerary 1st or 2nd premolars associated with crowding and rotations of the cheek teeth. If the extra teeth are not causing any crowding or periodontal disease, they may be left in, but extraction may be necessary if the tooth contributes to such problems (16).

Even if all development of the structure of the tooth occurs normally, disruption in the patterns of eruption can also cause major problems. A partially or even fully erupted tooth may be covered by thick, fibrous gingiva known as an *operculum* that can be excised (operculectomy) to release the impediment. A tooth that remains unerupted beyond its normal time is considered to be impacted (13). This is sometimes due to a mechanical interference (eg, lack of space, fibrous gingiva), although delayed eruption has been seen in Tibetan and Wheaton terriers (15). If diagnosed at an early age when root maturation is not complete, the physical barrier can be removed to assist the tooth in finishing eruption on its own. *Impaction* of a tooth can lead to dentigerous cyst formation, with a radiolucent cyst originating from the remnant enamel organ at the neck of the tooth (2). The forces of impaction may even cause an abnormal bending or dilaceration of the roots (15). Impacted maxillary teeth may occasionally be found in the nasal cavity. When impacted teeth are totally encased by bone, they stand little chance of moving into normal location without oral surgery and orthodontics; therefore, extraction is the most common treatment of choice to avoid cyst formation (2).

Retained or persistent deciduous teeth can also delay the eruption of the permanent teeth, particularly if the deciduous teeth are ankylosed (13). Even if the permanent tooth is not delayed in eruption, it may be deflected if the deciduous analog is still present. Deflection may occur lingually, mesially, distally, or facially, but most commonly lingually or mesially. Any of these deflections can contribute to malocclusion (see Chapter 15).

Soft Tissue

Periodontal Gingiva

Gingival tissue seldom shows distinct signs of developmental problems by itself, but there are some conditions that can be found in the oral cavity of young animals. As discussed previously with tooth eruption problems, a thick, fibrous gingival covering can either inhibit full eruption or prevent the erupted tooth from being fully exposed. Although there may be familial tendencies to develop an operculum, such tissues can be treated by excision to expose the underlying tooth.

Along similar lines, *pericoronitis* may develop as food, debris, and bacteria accumulate in gingival flaps that are created during the eruption process, resulting in inflammation (4). Debridement and antibiotics are the treatment of choice.

Periodontal disease typically begins at a young age but is not clinically detectable in most individuals unless there is an underlying problem associated with an abnormal immune system (see Chapters 8 and 16). A young cat presented with hypertrophic gingival margins that were easily excised, yet they showed no evidence of extension of the inflammation into the attached gingiva or alveolar mucosa. Histopathologic diagnosis was fibropapillomatosis of unknown etiology. This form of hypertrophy in a young cat differs from the typical picture of familial gingival hypertrophy often seen in mature boxers.

Oral Cavity

Generalized developmental syndromes can be found that affect more of the soft tissues of the oral cavity than just the gingiva. Bleeding disorders of a congenital nature, such as *von Willebrand's disease*, may first be manifested in the oral tissues (4). *Gray collie syndrome*, a simple autosomal-recessive disease, produces a cyclic neutropenia that exhibits stomatitis and pharyngitis with associated fever. The Maltese breed shows an increased incidence of ulcerative stomatitis (4,15), to be differentiated from a local, acquired ulceration that may be seen in a patient that chewed on an electrical cord (18). Severe ulcerative stomatitis with lesions on the buccal mucosa and palate were reported in a 5-month-old Labrador retriever due to renal hyperparathyroidism that also resulted in a "rubber jaw" syndrome (19). Though not a primary oral development, this congenital kidney defect was first detected by the oral lesions.

Palate

The most common developmental defect seen in the palate is some type of *cleft* (*palatoschisis*), as either an inherited or congenital problem, due to influences during the fusion of the parts of the oral cavity. A *primary cleft* refers to a defect between the incisal bone and maxilla, resulting in an anterior lesion lateral to the midline (see Chapter 3). This type of cleft is often associated with *harelip* or *cleft lip* (*cheiloschisis*), considered to be familial. Defects in the maxilla are considered to be *secondary palatal clefts* and can cause more severe problems involving aspiration, particularly in the newborn. A congenital hard cleft palatal usually extends into the soft palatal. Soft palate clefts may be midline or unilateral. The soft palate may also be abnormal in length and either soft or long, the latter of which is frequently seen in brachycephalic individuals. Cysts can also be found, including median palatine, bronchial cleft, and lymphoepithelial cysts, though they are uncommon (15). On oral examination, the soft palate may appear swollen and distended in a young animal, with a nasopharyngeal polyp arising from the auditory canal area occupying the space above the palate. Although it is typically found in cats, one case in a dog has been reported (20).

Tongue

The most significant developmental tongue lesion is a simple autosomal-recessive lethal glossopharyngeal defect called *microglossia*, or *"bird tongue"* (21,22). The tongue is small, narrow, and fimbriated and does not allow for proper nursing, so the puppies often do poorly (possibly one variation of "fading puppy" syndrome). This lesion is the earliest, most visible symptom of a more extensive syndrome of multisystemic signs.

Less serious problems in the tongue may include a *lateral protrusion* due to hypoglossal nerve damage (which may be managed with plication), *macroglossia* (which can be partially resected), or a *short frenulum ("tongue tie")* (which can be incised to release the tongue). A *median rhomboid glossitis* can be found, as can ectopic thyroid tissue and abnormal formations, such as *bifid* or *fissure tongue* or *"hairy tongue"* with long filiform papillae that resemble hair and can stain darkly (20).

Salivary Gland

A congenital atresia of a salivary duct or the absence of one gland is unlikely to make a difference due to the presence of the other glands (1). *Hyperptyalism* (excessive drooling) has been seen in cases with congenitally enlarged parotid ducts, but these are rare primary salivary gland abnormalities, which can be managed well by ligating the duct. Sialadenitis, of probable immune-mediated causes, was described in a young golden retriever that presented with epiphora and facial swelling extending from the inflamed submucosal glands; the condition responded to anti-inflammatory treatment (23).

Lips

The most obvious abnormality affecting the lips is cheiloschisis or cleft lip (discussed earlier in relation to the palate). The failure of two sides of the primary palate to fuse results in a defect that can be caused by intrauterine stress, although a familial tendency is sometimes apparent.

Lip-fold abnormalities may be even more frequent than clefts, particularly in breeds like spaniels. Resecting the fold to obliterate the channel formed will help with maintenance in the area. *Microcheilia* (literally, "small lips") is actually seen as a small oral

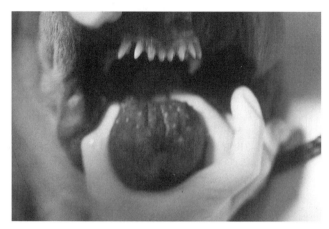

FIG. 2. Seven-month-old male Shar-Pei with tight-lip syndrome. Notice that the lower lip covers all the mandibular incisor and canine teeth.

opening. Found in many breeds but most commonly in schnauzers, this condition predisposes the lips to trauma and food accumulation with resultant cheilitis (4). Areas of pigmentation loss can also be present on the lips, whether the spontaneous vitiligo seen in Belgian terriers or rottweilers with no other signs, or vitiligo seen in the probably autoimmune Vogt-Koyanagi-Harada syndrome in huskies, Akitas, and Samoyeds with accompanying uveitis. The vitiligo in these latter cases responds to corticosteroids.

With the introduction of the Chinese Shar-Pei, practitioners have become familiar with many of the breed's problems, including *tight-lip* (Fig. 2). In this syndrome, there is typically little or no lower lip anterior vestibule, leading to the lip's curling up and lingually over the mandibular incisors and even the cuspids. This often results in lingual or distal displacement of the teeth and inhibits the full growth potential of the mandible, possibly causing a class II malocclusion. If resected early enough to create a vestibule and release tension, the mandible and teeth may not be as severely affected.

Skeletal

With the multitude of genes that affect the growth of each jaw quadrant, the possibility of getting abnormalities is great. Many such abnormalities are covered in the orthodontics chapter (see Chapter 15).

Other developmental skeletal problems can be found, as in many small or medium-size breeds that can carry a gene for *achondroplasia* (15). With a deficiency in the growth of cartilage (24) due to an autosomal-dominant gene with variable penetrance, individuals with this disorder can have an underdeveloped midface and short legs. Consistent occlusal abnormalities are also seen with hypothyroid cretinism, a hereditary metabolic disorder.

Another problem, *cartilaginous perisymphysis*, involves deficient ossification of the rostral angle of the mandible. In this disorder, which may be inherited and is sometimes seen in newborn puppies (25), the mandible on either side of the normally fibrous symphysis is cartilaginous or fibrous. While this condition does not affect overall function,

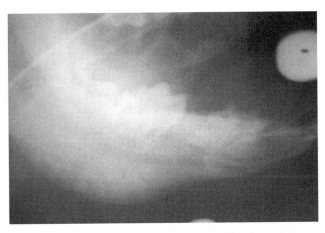

FIG. 3. Radiograph demonstrating classic periosteal proliferation of the mandible of a 10-month-old female bull terrier with craniomandibular osteopathy.

the associated teeth may be slightly mobile and even malocclusive. Orthodontic treatment of these teeth is generally unrewarding, as they cannot typically be retained in their new locations easily due to their lack of osseous support. If not closely monitored and treated as needed, they are sometimes lost to secondary periodontal disease due to their poor-quality periodontium.

West Highland white, Scottish, and Cairn terriers are the breeds most frequently affected by craniomandibular osteopathy, although other breeds have been reported with this possibly genetic condition (26). *Craniomandibular osteopathy* is generally a condition of the horizontal ramus (26,27). Clinically, the jaw may appear swollen, with bilateral mandibular enlargement due to periosteal proliferation along the body of the mandible, incorporating the tympanic bullae or temporomandibular joint in extreme cases (see Chapter 6) (26) (Fig. 3). With more severe signs, discomfort, inability to open the mouth fully, and inappetence may be seen. Treatment involving anti-inflammatory agents may help discomfort but will not change the disease development. This condition usually regresses at 11–13 months of age, corresponding with the completion of regular endochondral bone growth and ossification (26). If the temporomandibular joints or tympanic bullae have been extensively involved, the regression may not allow complete recovery (28). A familial jaw panosteitis may produce inflammation of the jaw bones as a potential differential diagnosis for craniomandibular osteopathy (29).

Disease associated with congenital renal dysplasias, as well as secondary renal hyperparathyroidism, can result in severe bilateral mandibular and maxillary swelling that may yield a flexible "rubber jaw" on palpation (19,30,31). Renal dysplasias in older animals, such as interstitial nephritis, glomerulonephritis, nephrosclerosis, or amyloidosis, and congenital renal dysplasias in younger pets result in inappropriate renal function (30). Secondary hyperparathyroidism of renal origin is a problem of chronic renal failure, associated with progressive loss of glomerular and tubular function. The reduction in glomerular filtration can result in a hyperphosphatemia, leading to hypocalcemia and the stimulation of the release of parathyroid hormone (31). The resulting hyperparathyroidism can cause facial and jaw abnormalities from bony changes. Generalized osteodystrophy that causes "rubber jaw" is more common in older animals, whereas hyperostotic osteodystrophy is more common in younger animals (32). These conditions occur in cats, but are more common in the dog (30). The long-term prognosis is poor due to the progressive nature of most kidney dysfunctions encountered.

Although dysplasia of the temporomandibular joints has some developmental basis, as it affects the structure, specific problems in this area will be discussed later in this chapter.

ACQUIRED DISORDERS

Dental Tissue

A great number of structural abnormalities of teeth have already been described pertaining to development. Although changes occur as a vital tooth matures (eg, reduced pulp cavity, apical cemental deposits, etc.), the external shape of the adult tooth is relatively static, barring external physical forces that come into play. With few exceptions, inflammatory, immune, metabolic, and toxic forces cause changes in tissue around the tooth with secondary effects on the tooth or root structure, as in resorptive lesions (see Chapters 6 and 16).

Hypercementosis is an increase in the layering of cementum, customarily in the apical third of the root structure. It typically appears as an bulbous enlargement of the root tip, as compared with the normal tapering contour (see Chapter 6). *Cementomas (fibro-osteoma)* are generally benign proliferations of the connective tissues in the jaws that produce cementum or cementum-like tissue (see Odontogenic Tumors on page 130).

There can be an expected level of physiologic attrition or wear seen as teeth gradually lose substance due to normal masticatory forces, and even the force of tooth against tooth (13). With malocclusions, an increased amount of wear of a single tooth or confined area is termed *dental attrition*, which can also occur from chewing hair. If the process is gradual enough, once the enamel is gone, reparative dentin, often brown in color, will be deposited to help protect the pulp from being exposed. With long-term influences, the crown may become level with the gingiva, yet the canal may still be closed, the retreating pulp being protected by the dentinal deposition. Attrition by external objects, particularly chewing metal bowls or bars, may also cause staining of the tooth surface. Excessive wear may also be apparent from the friction of an externally applied force, such as brushing or flossing; this is termed *dental abrasion*.

Erosion is the external loss of tooth hard tissue due to a chemical process without active bacterial involvement (11). Dental erosion may be caused by either extrinsic or intrinsic factors. Some of the more common extrinsic factors that may come in contact with the teeth are airborne acids, acidic fluids (eg, chlorinated pool water, some fruit juices, etc.), acidic foods, and some medicines, such as chewable vitamin C, iron tonics, and hydrochloric acid replacements. Erosional lesions from ingestion of acidic liquids are most often found on the gingival half of a facial surface of the posterior teeth. With the ingestion of acidic foods, the lesions are more commonly located on the facial surfaces of the anterior teeth. Intrinsic factors are vomiting, gastric reflux, and saliva quality and quantity. Dental erosions associated with vomiting and gastric reflux are usually found on the lingual surfaces of the anterior maxillary teeth.

External resorption, particularly seen on radiographs of the roots, may at times have a traumatic cause, whether mechanical, chemical, or thermal. Mechanical forces of mastication, especially when exaggerated, may result in loss of the periodontal ligament and ankylosis of the cementum to the alveolar bone, which may eventually result in external

TABLE 1. *Dental resorptive lesions*[a]

Stage	Lesion extent
1	Into enamel only
2	Into dentin
3	Into pulp
4	Extensive structural damage
5	Crown lost, only roots remain

[a] Feline dental resorption (FDR), resorptive lesion (RL), cervical line lesion (CLL), and cervical neck lesion (CNL)(129,130). These are generally referred to as stages and used in combination with Black's Modified Classification of tooth lesion locations.

root resorption. Additionally, mastication may cause flexure of the tooth near the cementoenamel junction in imperceptible cracks or chips of the cementum or enamel, known as *abfraction.* The small tooth fragments from abfraction may impale the periodontal ligament and stimulate an external resorption at the site. These lesions are most commonly seen in the dog at the gum line on the facial surface of the maxillary 4th premolars and at the gum line of the lingual surface of the mandibular 1st molar. *Bruxing* is the state of excessive occlusional pressures due to clenching the teeth together. In humans who brux, abnormal wear patterns are evident on the teeth, and dental resorptive problems have been shown to be more common. External resorption has also been observed to occur on some teeth following heavy-force orthodontic movements (Table 1) and at the sites of material wedged onto the periodontal ligament to hold or force a movement. If there is resorption, it is usually caused by an inflammatory response of the surrounding alveolar bone and/or periodontal ligament, as compared with *internal resorption.* When there is loss of the dentinal structure from the inside, inflammation is typically in the pulpal tissue. Radiographically, these lesions appear as areas of lucency (see Chapter 6).

While bacteria may or may not play a causative role in these resorptive lesions, they are the certainly the primary initiator of carious dental lesions (13). The process first begins as a decalcification of inorganic material by acids formed when bacterial enzymes ferment carbohydrates (13), often in sheltered areas between teeth or in pits and fissures. While more common in humans, these lesions are sometimes found on the occlusal surface of maxillary molars in dogs. A chalky white spot known as an *incipient caries* is the first indication of enamel demineralization, which progresses relatively slowly. In contrast, carious caries are produced by bacteria invading the dental tissues, causing the classic black cavity, with a more rapid demineralization of dentin once the lesion reaches the dentinoenamel junction and sometimes mushrooming to undermine the enamel. More advanced lesions will present as brown to black in color and soft, so a sharp explorer will often stick into the material. Without intervention, the decay can extend into the pulp cavity itself, resulting in infection and eventual pulp necrosis. These lesion are classically staged by the G.V. Black classification (Table 2).

Some of the most common problems encountered with teeth are related to trauma other than gradual wear. Tooth fractures may occur from an animal's chewing on hard objects or from external sources of trauma. Classification of fractures can also be done using the G.V. Black classification (see Table 2), and further classification can be made according to the degree of damage (Table 3).

Superficial fractures, especially in older dogs, may just result in the loss of enamel and some dentin without pulp exposure. With more extensive tooth loss, near or complete

TABLE 2. *G.V. Black modified cavity preparation classification system*

Class	Tooth type	Characteristics
1	I,PM,M	Beginning in structural defects, such as pit or fissure, commonly found on occlusal surfaces
2	PM,M	Proximal surfaces; when a tooth with a class 2 lesion includes a class 1 lesion, it is still considered class 2
3	I,C	Proximal surfaces; incisal angle not included
4	I,C	Proximal surfaces; incisal angle included
5	I,C,PM,M	Facial or lingual, gingival third; excluding pit or fissure lesions
6	I,C,PM,M	Defect of incisal edge or cusp; not included in Black's original classification

I, incisor; C, canine or cuspid; M, molar; PM, premolar.
(Adapted from ref. 131.)

exposure of the pulp may occur, necessitating appropriate treatment. Repeated blunt trauma may not grossly break the tooth but may cause structural weakening or even pulpal inflammation without exposure (see Pulp below). A crown may remain intact, but the root may be fractured or fracture lines may extend from the crown into the root structure (see Table 3). The type of fracture, its location, and its nearness to the gingival sulcus all play a part in prognosis (see Chapters 11 and 12).

Teeth may also be avulsed, often with concurrent bone trauma, or even invulsed or intruded, particularly if periodontal disease has compromised the supporting structures (see Chapters 11 and 12).

Pulp

Pulpitis is the inflammation of the pulp that clinically expresses itself as dental pain (see Chapters 11 and 12). Pulpitis can be reversible with the tooth's maintaining its vitality, or irreversible, eventually resulting in pulpal death and a nonvital tooth. The pathogenesis of pulpitis depends on many factors, including type and extent of stimuli, integrity of the pulp cavity (open or not), maturity of the tooth, and interventive measures.

The inflammation of the pulp in response to any of these factors is typically from tubular hydraulics and pulpal edema with an inflammatory cell component. Increased blood flow and even pressure by hyperemia, or an increase of blood in the small arteries, can

TABLE 3. *Staging of tooth injuries*[a]

Stage	Injury extent
1	Simple fracture of the enamel
2	Fracture extending into dentin
3	Fracture extending into pulp chamber; pulp vital
4	Fracture extending into pulp chamber; pulp nonvital
5	Tooth displaced
6	Tooth avulsed
7	Root fracture; no coronal involvement; tooth stable
8	Root fracture; combined with stage 1–2 coronal fracture; tooth stable.
9	Root fracture; combined with stage 3 coronal fracture; tooth stable.
10	Root fracture; in combination with stage 1–4; unstable tooth

[a] (129,132,133). These are generally referred to as stages and used in combination with Black's Modified Classification of tooth lesion locations.

cause an increased pressure that stimulates pain receptors. The size of the pulp chamber and vascularity (both greater in the immature tooth) can influence how pulpitis will progress. If the stimulus is temporary and minor (without exposure to infection), the pulpitis can be reversible, especially in the young patient. With older, more constricted pulp cavities, there is less space to accommodate the edema and pressure, so pulpal death and necrosis may occur more easily. The pain experienced with pulpitis of a closed tooth system is often more intense than that felt in an open-canal tooth, due to the pressure buildup. The increased vascularity and cellularity of immature teeth are sometimes beneficial in bacterial contamination of fractured teeth, as the pulp may respond by becoming hyperplastic (13). Typically, however, bacterial infection of the pulp, if untreated, will often lead to pulpal death. The initial severe, pulsating pain experienced in bacterial pulpitis may diminish, once the nerves become devitalized.

Direct exposure to bacteria occurs when a fracture breaks off a significant portion of the crown to open the pulp cavity, but bacteria may also enter through dead tracts or open tubules in the dentin from the death of odontoblastic processes. The pulp can also be exposed to bacteria by caries or through a hematogenous route (*anachoresis*) (34,35). Pulpitis may develop when chemical agents such as etching acids and bleaching agents affect odontoblastic processes or when they travel through exposed dentinal tubules. Pulpitis may occur in intact teeth due to hyperthermia from improper scaling or polishing or due to concussive shock from repeated blunt trauma (excessive biting or chewing exercise) that can cause edema and even disruption of the periapical blood supply (13).

If changes in the pulp were limited to its own tissues, there would be few problems experienced with pulpitis. With mild, intermittent stimuli, or even in older teeth, an excess of dentin deposition may lead to pulp calcification that can obliterate portions of the lumen of the pulp cavity. An internal resorption, particularly in cats, may be the first indication of ongoing pathology, and should be treated promptly. More often, the internal canal experiences few changes, but the inflammation ordinarily extends into the periapical tissues through vascular channels. Periapical tissue response may also vary, often influenced by the extent and duration of pulpal pathology. Radiographic evidence of periapical involvement is seen by a variable radiolucency in the area. This is often not detectable until osseous changes occur months after the initial pulpal insult. Diagnosis of the true nature of the lesion is possible only by histopathology. Using the term *periapical abscess* to describe a "halo" of bone loss around the apex is not necessarily correct. Abscess formation may be an acute or chronic form of suppuration, often developing from periapical granulomas or cysts (36). A *periapical granuloma* seldom demonstrates bacteria, and a chronic granuloma may encompass epithelial cells from the rests of Malassez. This epithelium, when stimulated by inflammation, can result in the formation of a *periapical cyst*. Cysts or granulomas can convert to an active abscess, and extension of the infection into the bone can lead to osteomyelitis. Extension of the abscess into soft tissue can result in fistulation, which allows pressure release and decreased pain. A more distinct description of periapical pathology is described in the chapter on basic endodontics (see Chapter 11).

In cases of dental lesions seen externally (fractures, cavities, resorptions, etc.), radiographs should generally be taken, not only to assess any root damage present but also to examine for any signs of pulpal reaction, such as internal resorption, discrepancies in the pulp cavity dimensions, and apical or periapical changes. Though externally a tooth does not substantially change once eruption is complete, it is a living, dynamic, and evolving organ, particularly as related to the pulp cavity and pulpal function. The odontoblasts in a vital tooth continue to produce secondary, tertiary, and other forms of dentin throughout the tooth's vital existence (primary dentin is only that which is present at eruption). These resultant changes provide a means for assisting in the assessment of pulp vitality. As the tooth matures, additional secondary dentin is deposited, resulting in a thickening of the dentinal wall and a diminished pulp cavity. In pulpal response to irritation, tertiary or reparative dentin is deposited, which is useful in therapy to encourage dentinal bridge formation and maintenance of tooth vitality in pulp-capping procedures. Cessation of normal dentinal deposition due to pulpal death will halt dentinal production, and the pulp cavity will become static in its dimensions, indicating a nonvital state.

SOFT TISSUE PATHOLOGY

Gingiva and Oral Mucosa

Although teeth are the primary structures of function in the oral cavity, they cannot remain healthy without the supporting tissues of the periodontium. The most visible of these tissues is the gingival tissue. The most common problem seen in the soft tissue, and even all structures of the oral cavity, is periodontal disease, which is the most frequently seen infectious disease in dogs and cats (37). Since periodontal disease is covered in great detail in periodontology chapter (see Chapter 8), other lesions seen on the gingival and soft tissues of the oral cavity will be discussed here.

There are a few problems seen that may be limited to the attached gingiva, one of which is *gingival hyperplasia*. This proliferation of the attached gingiva in some cases is due to a chronic inflammatory response to the bacteria in plaque (1,2) and often results in deep *pseudopockets* formed by the excessive amounts of gingiva and initially not due to attachment loss. Such deep pockets can predispose the individual to ongoing periodontal problems and eventual loss of the periodontal ligament and bone. Though sometimes quite focal, these lesions often are fairly well generalized, particularly in breeds that show a familial tendency, such as boxers, Great Danes, collies, Doberman pinschers, and dalmatians (38). Individuals on diphenytoin therapy may show similar signs. Although gingival hyperplasia is known as a nonneoplastic lesion, unusual areas should be biopsied to determine its true nature. Treatment aims to reduce the gingiva to a more normal height and contour and to minimize the pocket depth.

Irritation at a specific site may give rise to a granulomatous reaction or *pyogenic granuloma*. This proliferation of the gingival margin is usually red and friable and can typically be excised, along with dealing with the instigating cause. Attached gingiva may also be the site of fistulation or fenestration from a periodontal abscess or chronic infection caused by retained calculus or debris in a sulcus. While this can only be confirmed by radiographs, in a mature animal a fistula opening coronal to the mucogingival line is more likely to be due to a periodontal abscess, while one draining apical to the mucogingival junction is more likely to be traced to an endodontic periapical lesion. Use of a contrast fistulogram can often confirm the origin of the problem.

While the attached gingiva is histologically a different tissue from other oral mucosa, often gingival lesions are not confined to the area and instead lead to more generalized stomatitis problems. Like the term hepatitis, stomatitis refers to a broad group of inflammatory diseases, and not a single syndrome. With the tremendous vascularity and potential for external exposure of the oral cavity, examination will often reveal things about the entire patient. A change in mucosal color may indicate anemia (pale), shock (white), cyanosis (blue), bleeding disorders (petechiae), or uremic ulcers. Though an inflammatory response is expected in the typical pathogenesis of periodontal disease, there are many factors that can contribute to excessive levels of inflammation.

Infectious agents, such as bacteria, viruses, protozoans, and fungi can elicit tremendous response from healthy individuals, and in hyperresponsive or immunosuppressed animals, even normally innocuous agents may elicit substantial soft tissue changes. Ulceromembranous stomatitis, also known as necrotizing ulcerative gingivitis, *Vincent's stomatitis*, or *trench mouth*, occurs when spirochetes and fusiform bacteria, normally opportunistic oral flora, synergistically act in the presence of some oral insult (4,39) or poor oral hygiene (13). The classic initial lesion is ulceration of the interdental papillae (15) or marginal gingiva that may remain focal or progress to a generalized extent, often with a rapid onset. This can evolve to necrotic, gray-to-yellow, bleeding ulcers of the gingiva and tongue (4), at times covered by a thin, grayish pseudomembranous membrane (13). The *aphthous* ("to set on fire") *ulcers* that may develop can be extremely painful and stimulate copious amounts of ropy saliva.

Mycotic stomatitis may be initiated in the presence of immunodeficiency, systemic disease, or antibiotic administration (4). Primarily seen on the tongue and at the mucocutaneous margins, the ulcers can also be seen throughout the oropharynx, coated with a white plaque.

Occasionally, extension of a nasal aspergillosis infection through the nasopalatine ducts may lead to hyperemia or ulceration at the incisive papilla (15). The tongue can rarely be the site of lesions related to a systemic histoplasmosis or blastomycosis.

Systemic bacterial infections, which are considered to be more of an exogenous type of infection as related to the oral cavity, may also exhibit lesions. *Leptospira canicola* can cause severe oral mucous membrane congestions, hemorrhage, oral ulceration secondary to uremia, and glossitis that can progress to necrosis of the tip of the tongue (40). Severe congestion of the oral mucous membranes may also be seen with infections with *L. icterohaemorrhagiae*, as well as petechiae and hemorrhage associated with the thrombocytopenia. In cats, infection with *Mycobacterium lepraemurium*, or feline leprosy, can cause one or more raised, plaque-like lesions on the lips and/or the tongue, but these are generally not painful.

With a few exceptions, primary oral viral disease is fairly uncommon. Cats may experience calicivirus or herpesvirus infections with ulceration of the tongue, pharynx, and sometimes the glossopalatine folds (15). They may also have nasal discharge and sneezing. Calicivirus in the dog is often confined to the tongue, presenting as 1–2 mm vesicles on its dorsal surface. Distinct, wart-like growths on the buccal mucosa, lips, and tongue are generally self-limiting lesions in dogs, caused by exposure to a papillomavirus. Lesions on the mucous membrane of the tongue and oral cavity may be an uncommon presentation of canine visceral leishmaniasis, and they often must be biopsied to be differentiated from other oral tumors.

Other viruses in the cat that are more systemic and affect the immune system, such as feline leukemia virus (FeLV) and feline immunodeficiency virus (FIV), hyperptyalism may predispose the individual to secondary oral infections (15). Distemper in the dog may exhibit oral signs of hyperemia and ulceration with increased salivation (41), and hepatitis may show hyperemia and petechiae (15).

There are many means by which an abnormality in the body's immune system can have an effect on the oral cavity. While certain viruses, stress, and corticosteroids may lead to a decreased immune response that predisposes to opportunistic infections, the response may at times be an exaggerated one to relatively normal stimuli. An increase in immunoglobulin G and immune complex deposition in a syndrome of ulcerative stomatitis in

Maltese dogs, particularly males, may explain an excessive host response (increased gingival index) in the presence of minimal stimuli (low plaque and calculus indices). Other breeds, such as Cavalier King Charles spaniels, may show similar syndromes, (42). There may be a marked ulceration of buccal mucosa that contacts a tooth/calculus surface, similar to the lesions of *chronic ulcerative paradental stomatitis* (*CUPS* or *"kissing lesions"*) in other patients (43). These animals appear to develop a plaque intolerance and consequently exhibit an excessive immune response to any deposition. The condition is typically in localized areas of the canine and carnassial teeth initially, but it may progress to a more general condition in the mouth. If effective plaque control cannot be maintained, extractions are often necessary, as anti-inflammatory agents provide only transitory relief. Additionally, selective extractions customarily provide only temporary relief, as the condition has a tendency to recur at new sites adjacent to the teeth.

While distinct autoimmune syndromes can at times be confined to the dermal tissues, up to 90% of patients with *pemphigus vulgaris* and half of those with *bullous pemphigoid* will have oral lesions, frequently at the mucocutaneous junctions, with some mucous membrane ulceration (4) (Fig. 4). These two entities can only be distinguished histologically, although they are treated similarly with corticosteroids (44). Any refractory oral ulceration should be biopsied if unresponsive to standard treatment.

Even less common in the dog, and not reported in the cat (45), are the oral sequelae of *systemic lupus erythematosus*, which may appear as shallow areas of ulceration with erythematous, painful margins (46). *Discoid lupus erythematosus* in dogs can potentially ulcerate the tongue or cause hypopigmentation of the nasal planum, gums, and lips (47).

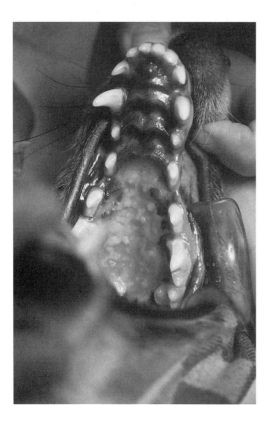

FIG. 4. Palate of a 5-year-old male sheltie with pemphigus vulgaris. Note the loss of pigment and widespread ulceration.

The immune system also plays a part in acute hypersensitivity reactions to drugs (eg, systemic penicillins, chloramphenicol, tetracyclines, etc., or topical agents such as chlorhexidine) (48). What can start out as ulceration and hemorrhage may progress to a more extreme drug eruption with edema and massive tissue destruction and necrosis. *Toxic epidermal necrolysis*, as this condition is called, is uncommon, but patients will be febrile, depressed, and anorectic (15,49).

Eosinophilic Lesions

The *eosinophilic granuloma complex in cats* is a group of similar lesions, often with an eosinophilic component, with possible immune ramifications (50,51). These lesions are also known as *indolent ulcers* and *rodent ulcers*, and are discussed in more detail in Chapter 16. The eosinophilic or indolent (literally, "painless") ulcer is typically a well circumscribed, ulcerated, red-to-brown lesion, usually on the upper lip and more often (3:1 ratio) found in females (52,53). Collagenolytic granulomas on the caudal surface of the rear limbs, again found more commonly in females, can at times be accompanied by multiple smooth, glistening nodules in the pharynx or tongue. If severe enough, these lesion can result in dysphagia. Eosinophilic plaques on the medial thigh or ventral abdomen will occasionally be accompanied by lesions as well.

Oral eosinophilic granuloma in dogs is found in young animals, usually 1–7 years of age. It is most common in Siberian huskies, in which it may be hereditary (38,54). In this condition, the lateral margins and frenulum of the tongue may be involved with raised, firm, yellow-brown to pink lesions that are sometimes ulcerated (4) Histologically, this lesion is similar to that in the feline disease complex, demonstrating eosinophils and granulomatous inflammation. Treatment with corticosteroids or surgical excision is customarily curative, although on occasion recurrences may occur (38,54).

Viral Papillomatosis

Viral papillomatosis, caused by a papovavirus, is a disease resulting in wart-like lesions. It is most common in young animals and appears to spread by horizontal transmission, from animal to animal. There may be multiple lesions, and the lesions may be multilobular. They can be found almost anywhere in the oral cavity, but the lips, palate, and tongue are possibly the most common sites. Most lesions are self-limiting and undergo spontaneous regression requiring no treatment (55). Occasionally, due to masticatory trauma or other reasons, surgical debulking may be desirable. In highly resistant cases, lesion crushing (to stimulate an immune response), autogenous vaccines, and chemotherapy have been attempted (56). The lesions are considered benign, but there have been a few reported cases in which squamous cell carcinomas developed later at these sites (57).

Metabolism

There are many systemic conditions, such as uremic ulceration, that will manifest themselves in the oral cavity. As ammonia levels in the saliva rise, irritation, dehydration, and clotting abnormalities may develop, as the normal mucosal protection is compromised (4,15). The hemorrhagic ulceration of the dorsum of the tongue can lead to necrosis and sloughing. Vasculitis and xerostomia seen with diabetes mellitus can enhance the progression of periodontitis if untreated. The decreased calcium in hypoparathyroidism can interfere with enamel calcification early on in development and contribute to later ulceration of the tongue margin and mucocutaneous junctions (15). Hypothyroidism can hinder the development and eruption of teeth, while macroglossia and puffy lips are sometimes seen as well (15).

Although not caused by any known systemic problem, the idiopathic deposition of amorphous calcified tissue, or calcinosis circumscripta, may be identified by white, chalky, gritty nodules in the tongue and buccal mucosa. These are typically found in young, large breeds and can progress to shallow ulceration.

Hematology

With the excellent vascularity of the oral cavity, abnormalities in the blood components will often show early oral lesions. Anemia due to an iron deficiency will cause a pale mucous membrane that is slow to heal. If the pallor is accompanied by gingival bleeding, petechiae, purpura, or ulcers with a surrounding erythema, an aplastic anemia should be considered. A decrease in the neutrophils, or neutropenia, or may lead to large, deep, irregular or mucosal irritation that can be painful. These lesions may become necrotic, but they will typically lack a surrounding inflammatory response (4,15). There are many things that can contribute to neutropenia, including viral diseases, chemo- or radiation therapy, estrogens, or chloromphenicol or phenylbutazone toxicity. In gray collies, a simple autosomal-recessive disorder called cyclic neutropenia can cause stomatitis and pharyngitis with fever (17). These individuals will often have recurrent large, deep, scarring ulcers associated with periodontal disease. Leukemia and other myeloproliferative diseases (4) in humans have contributed to gingival ulceration and necrosis, even gingival hypertrophy with myelocytic leukemia (58). The tonsils and pharynx may also be involved, so dysphagia may be a problem as well.

Systemic treatments may give rise to oral lesions. Chemotherapy may result in ulcers that are large, irregular, and foul-smelling, at times with concurrent anemia, as evident in the pale mucous membranes. A neutropenia can allow bacterial infections to flourish and can explain the lack of inflammatory zone around ulcerations (15). Subsequent to radiation therapy, erythema and mucositis start as a granular inflammatory reaction that progresses to a nodular, white, keratotic layer that can slough (13). There may also be a reduction in salivary flow, an increase in its viscosity, or xerostomia that can contribute to periodontal disease and caries formation. Severe damage by radiation may lead to a later osteonecrosis (59).

Chrysotherapy may cause secondary stomatitis with a peripheral eosinophilia, especially during the initial treatment (4,15). Ingestion of warfarin and indanedione may lead to various degrees of clotting abnormalities, while doses of thallium can cause erythema and inflammation of the oral epithelium and lips, as well as other tissues. Horseshoe or linear ulcers on the tongue and/or palate are seen after ingestion of caustic chemicals.

Nutrition

Nutritional deficiencies or excesses are often manifested in the oral cavity, particularly the tongue, which has the highest rate of cell turnover in the mouth (60). A protein-calorie malnutrition, as seen in a protein-losing enteropathy or a nephropathy, contributes to a decrease in cell-mediated immunity and shows a linear ulceration on the dorsum of the tongue (15,61). Chronic niacin deficiency, if severe, leads to red ulceration of the mucous membranes or to "black tongue." Decreases in biotin result in hypersalivation and scaling of the skin around the lips (15), while riboflavin deficiencies exhibit an angular stomatitis/cheilosis with initial pallor, then sloughing. *Pellagra* is a term used for a severe lack of several of the B vitamins, in which early tenderness progresses to a scarlet-to-beefy red ulceration of the lips and lateral margins of the tongue.

Deficiencies of vitamin C lead to scurvy lesions primarily in animals unable to store the nutrient, mainly humans and guinea pigs. It is an important component in maintaining the health of the gingiva and mucous membranes.

Low calcium intake can directly affect the periodontium and all calcified tissues during formative stages. More important, if a decreased calcium intake leads to a secondary hyperparathyroidism (or due to renal causes), there will be resorption of calcium from alveolar bones, leaving them soft and contributing to tooth mobility and "rubber jaw" (62) (Fig. 5).

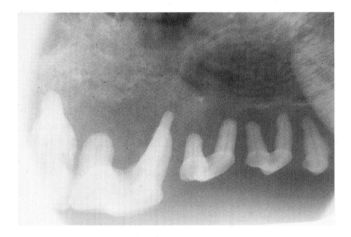

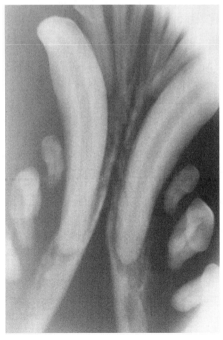

FIG. 5. Radiograph of "rubber jaw" syndrome in a 3-year-old male Labrador retriever with renal secondary hyperparathyroidism.

One nutrient in particular that should be avoided in excessive amounts is vitamin A, found in raw liver in large amounts. The gingiva may become proliferative, and in young cats there may be retarded development or early loss of incisors.

Trauma

Particularly in young animals that tend to explore their environment on an oral level, certain traumas to the mouth can cause serious problems. Laceration from licking or chewing on sharp objects may be very obvious around the lips and commissures, the dorsum of the tongue, and the gums, but it may also be hidden, especially under the tongue. If appliance power cords are chewed on, electrical shocks, tissue burns, or electrocution may result (18,63). In areas using 110–140-volt power systems, burns are often found at the lips, gums, tongue, and palate, varying from superficial to deep wounds that compromise even the underlying bone or teeth. The circumscribed areas with tan-to-gray surfaces often heal well with conservative therapy, occasionally needing reconstructive surgery later (64). Patients with such injuries should always be fully evaluated for dyspnea and pulmonary edema, which can be life-threatening (18). In areas where 210–240-volt standard power systems are used, the electrical shock is typically fatal.

Chemical burns from ingestion are less common and appear as acute ulcers covered by necrotic debris (15). Dysphagia or acute, rapid jaw movements may be a clue that a foreign object is present in the mouth. The entire oral cavity, including the palate, pharyngeal walls, and floor of the mouth should be examined carefully, as well as the root of the tongue, particularly for linear foreign bodies such as string. The tongue and lips can be penetrated by burdock burs that cause small papules that slough at the center and then coalesce to form an ulcer with a granular center.

External traumatic sources such as bite wounds and hit-by-car (HBC) lesions can be quite variable and require thorough assessment. A snake bite in the facial area can be quite progressive, with local edema, petechiae, and even ecchymosis.

Self-trauma to the buccal mucosa and tongue from chewing on the tissues, "gum-chewer's" syndrome, can cause proliferative, cauliflower-like lesions (65). Unless they lead to obvious inflammation or discomfort, excision may not be necessary, but any persistent lesions should be biopsied.

Soft Palate

Though many problems that can affect the palate have already been discussed either in the developmental section or in the soft tissue section above, the palate should always be closely examined for specific lesions that might be confined to the area. Fibrosarcomas are frequently located in the palate, and it will occasionally be the site of an extension of a malignant melanoma or other tumor. Infectious diseases affecting both the oral (FeLV,FIV) and nasal cavities (eg, extension of nasal aspergillosis through the incisive papilla) can have extensive palatal lesions, as can autoimmune diseases such as pemphigus vulgaris or bullous pemphigoid. The roof of the mouth can be a common site for foreign objects, such as rib bones and tacks, and is often affected by chemical ingestion or electric cord burns. The palatal mucosa and bone can be compromised severely enough during periodontal disease to cause fistulation into the nasal cavity or sinuses (oronasal or oroantral fistulas). The palate can also be injured by malocclusion of mandibular teeth that are in linguoversion (base narrow). Ventral displacement of the caudal soft palate may result from the presence of a retropharyngeal abscess or tumor, or even a nasopharyngeal polyp. The latter, seen usually in young cats that demonstrate dysphagia and nasal discharge (66), are protruding, pedunculated growths from the mucous membranes of the auditory canal as a response to chronic inflammation. While not a distinct oral process, it is part of a differential diagnoses list, a factor to be ruled out. Often the soft palate has to be gently retracted to visualize a polyp, whose treatment sometimes also requires a ventral tympanic bullae osteotomy in addition to the polyp removal.

At the back of the pharynx on either side, the tonsils will often not be normally visible in their crypts. An increase in the size or redness of a tonsil may indicate an inflammatory process or even a cyst formation (67), but any lesion that does not respond well to conservative therapy such as antibiotics should be biopsied. This will be further discussed in the section on neoplasia below.

Tongue

Like the palate, many problems of the tongue are extensions of oral problems, such as ulcerative stomatitis. Due to the high cell turnover rate of the lingual mucosa, it may exhibit changes, especially nutritional, more quickly than elsewhere in the oral cavity.

Infectious agents that have a particular predilection for the tongue include calicivirus, herpesvirus, and rhinotracheitis virus in the cat with ulceration, and a vesicular glossitis associated with calicivirus in the dog (68). *Leptospira canicola* infection leads to severe congestion with a glossitis related to uremia that can eventually necrose the tongue tip. Opportunistic infections such as Vincent's stomatitis, or trench mouth, may exhibit necrotic bleeding ulcers, and candidiasis may stimulate a diffuse inflammation with a whitish plaque coating of the surface (4).

Metabolic uremia (as described earlier) demonstrates distinct lingual signs, including hemorrhagic, brownish ulcers of the dorsal tongue with potential necrosis and sloughing. Hypothyroidism in earlier stages of development may result in a macroglossia, while hypoparathyroidism can contribute to ulceration and necrosis of the tongue tip. Calcinosis circumscripta refers to the idiopathic deposition of calcified, amorphous, chalky nodules on the surface or in the sublingual area. Occasionally, these can be seen in conjunction with a glossitis secondary to bite wounds contaminated with *Pasteurella multocida* (69). Other traumas to the mouth may cause inflammation, including foreign body penetration such as embedded burdock burs (*Arctium lappa*) with small papules that coalesce into a deep necrotic center on the dorsum and edges of the tongue (70). Chewing on electric cords can cause a host of problems, locally and systemically. Immediately after the injury, it is sometimes difficult to assess the potential viability of different areas, so conservative debridement with frequent monitoring and retreatment is often required (71). Severe injury of any type with loss of a substantial portion of the tongue (or due to surgery) requires management of the animal's diet, as its prehension and swallowing capabilities may change (72). In cats, it is also important to consider its ability to groom itself.

Ingestion of caustic chemicals tends to leave an ulcerated area on the dorsum of the tongue in a horseshoe or linear pattern. A redness or loss of papillae on the rostral third of the tongue's dorsal surface was a problem experienced by military dogs in South Vietnam. A combination of exposure to sunlight with high temperatures and humidity is thought to contribute to the pathology, leading to signs of excessive salivation, a decrease in appetite, and "bird-drinking" (4).

At the base of the tongue, entrapment of a string or other linear foreign bodies can cause laceration or granulation tissue, not to mention the consequences that the remainder of the string can cause to the rest of the gastrointestinal system. A proliferative or hyperplastic granuloma in the sublingual area may result from the self-trauma of accidentally chewing the tissue in the area, or "gum-chewer's" syndrome, as can also be seen in the buccal mucosa (65).

Iatrogenic trauma can occur due to a lack of control of dental instruments, such as elevators, during procedures. Slipping of the device into the soft tissue of the sublingual space can lead to edema, hemorrhage, and the introduction of air.

The sublingual area can be swollen or distended due to a number of other reasons as well. Unilaterally, a soft, fluctuant swelling may be indicative of an extravasation of saliva into the area, or a ranula (15). Sublingual edema may be secondary to venous obstruction in the pharyngeal region due to abscess formation or surgery (15). The tongue can also have papillomatosis lesions.

Nutritional

Nutritional deficiencies that are manifested distinctly on the tongue include protein-calorie malnutrition and niacin deficiency. A protein-losing hepatopathy or nephropathy may be the contributing factor that results in a decrease in the cell-mediated immunity, as well as immunoglobulin A, making the individual more susceptible to pathogens (15). A linear ulceration of the tongue's dorsal surface is a typical finding (59). *"Black tongue"* is the term used for the red, ulcerated lesion seen with severe niacin deficiency (73).

Tumors

Masses on the tongue frequently require biopsy to arrive at a definitive diagnosis, as an eosinophilic granuloma on the lateral surface of the tongue of a Siberian husky or the dorsal tongue of a cat may not be distinguishable from a squamous cell carcinoma. Squamous cell carcinoma is probably most frequently seen on the dorsal surface or lateral margins of a dog's tongue, but more typically at the root or base of a cat's tongue. Other tumors are not commonly found on the tongue, but melanomas have been reported in older dogs, and sometimes in smaller breeds (4), although it is not confined to these. Myoblastoma may present in the dog as a red, elevated granulomatous mass on its dorsolateral tongue surface.

Miscellaneous

There are several conditions of the tongue that may be encountered, with variable consequences. As covered in the development section above, discovery of "bird-tongue," or microglossia, in the newborn can only bring a recommendation of euthanasia. On a less serious note, a condition called "hairy tongue," in which filiform papillae are elongated to resemble hairs and often stain darkly, are typically an incidental finding during oral examination. Rarely will a glossitis be present, and though "epilation" through electrocautery may be considered, it should be done with care.

A large, firm, symmetrical lesion or granuloma known as lingual myositis has not been connected yet with a known etiology, but it may be secondary to trauma. In humans, zones of desquamation of filiform papillae in well demarcated but irregularly shaped areas are known as *geographic tongue* (13).

Salivary Glands

The overall incidence of salivary gland disease in dogs and cats has been reported to be very low: 0.3% (74). Malignancies accounted for only 30% of this overall low rate, generally as adenocarcinoma but with some secondary lymphosarcomas (75). However, primary salivary gland cancer in the dog and cat is considered rare (75–77). The mandibular gland was most frequently affected, followed by the parotid gland (74). These lesions are invariably invasive, and metastasis to regional lymph nodes is common. Although typically slow to develop, distant metastasis has been reported and is more common in the cat than in the dog (78). Symptoms are principally firm, nonpainful enlargements in the areas of primary or accessory salivary gland tissues. Aggressive surgical excision is the treatment of choice. However, due to the numerous vital structures in the area and the tendency for these tumors to become extracapsular and spread out in the region, other therapies in addition to surgery may be required. Radiation therapy following surgery has shown benefits in good local control and prolonged survival rates, although little has been reported on chemotherapy potentials (79). Prognosis is highly variable with the type of tumor, its duration, and therapies attempted. Some of the more common differential diagnoses would be sialoliths, mucoceles, lymphoma, abscesses, reactive lymphadenopathy, infarction of the salivary gland, and sialadenitis (74,75).

Sialadenitis represented 26% of the overall incidence rate of salivary disease, both as primary and secondary disease, and was seen more often in males (74). Another case reported episodic acute facial swelling ventral to the right eye that would resolve the next day; eventual progression lead to swelling of the hard and soft palate due to suppurative sialadenitis of the palatal submucosal salivary tissue (23). The pain on opening the mouth and inability to close the mouth resolved with antibiotics and corticosteroids, but recurred when the latter was discontinued, leading to suspicion of possibly bacterial and/or immune etiologies.

Sialoceles are retention cysts of salivary fluids and may constitute up to 9% of all salivary gland disease (74). Their presentation can be variable, depending on the gland affected. *Ranulas* are salivary retention cysts (sialoceles, salivary mucoceles), typically located under the tongue; they occur when the sublingual gland or duct is blocked by mucus, sialoliths, inflammation, or injury. *Mandibular salivary mucoceles* generally produce an enlargement under the mandible or near the throat area.

Craniofacial trauma, as reported in one dog, resulted in a painful mass over the frontal sinus that was filled with a reddish-brown fluid that put pressure on the cranial vault and caused an exophthalmos. Repeated surgeries did not work until the sinus was obliterated (80). Any treatment of salivary glands must take the gland and duct location into account.

Infarction of portions of a salivary gland, usually the mandibular, can result in an acute coagulation necrosis, possibly due to trauma. This firm, discrete swelling will often resolve within 7–10 days. This is similar to a syndrome seen in the minor palatine glands in humans that includes a metaplastic proliferation of the salivary ducts but is generally self-limiting. The canine form of necrotizing sialometaplasia as seen in terriers and other breeds can be associated with extreme pain and vomiting.

Salivary glands may also be affected by radiation therapy of the head and neck. While some saliva will still be produced, it is thick and ropy, causing a dry mouth. This can pre-

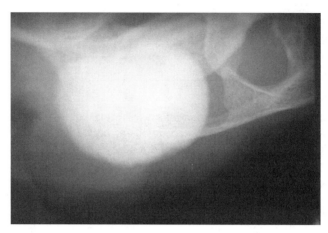

FIG. 6. Sialolith (salivary stone) near the mandibular gland in a 5-year-old male domestic short-haired cat.

dispose the patient to oral infections, even leading to postirradiation caries in 2–10 months if quality oral hygiene is not maintained. The patient's teeth may also be more sensitive to hot and cold.

Salivary stones (*sialoliths*) are calcifications found in salivary glands or ducts. Radiographically, they may appear as radiopaque objects in the oral soft tissues. Most commonly, they are found in the mandibular ducts causing obstruction of salivary flow, but they may be found in association with any of the salivary glands and sometimes attain substantial size (35,36,55) (Fig. 6). If they are within the duct, pressure placed behind the sialolith and quickly moved forward along the duct may force expulsion of the stones; if they cannot be expelled, surgery may be required.

Lips

Particularly in fractious patients, lesions on the lips may be the only oral-related problems that some owners will ever notice. Cheilitis, or lip inflammation, may occur as a secondary bacterial infection after some irritant (plastic bowl) or trauma (electric cord) has injured the lips. Severe trauma may cause the avulsion of the soft tissue of the lower lip from the mandible, as can be seen in cats hit by a car (81). Spaniels and other breeds with pendulous lips can get lip-fold dermatitis, as saliva drains into the folds, keeping them moist and readily susceptible to infection. Any inflammatory lesion that does not respond to routine treatment should always be biopsied. While neoplasia is fairly uncommon at this site, histopathology may reveal an autoimmune disorder (systemic or discoid lupus erythematosus), particularly as related to the mucocutaneous margins.

Shar-Peis may exhibit the tight-lip syndrome, with the lower lip folding in over the mandibular incisors and even canines. Not only do maxillary teeth then traumatize the lip, but the interference can alter the normal growth pattern of the mandible. A similar term may be used to describe animals with limited commissure opening. Schnauzers with microcheilia will experience repeated trauma to the lips and will accumulate saliva and food in the lip folds.

Nutritional deficiencies are usually seen in the lips only in the presence of a severe lack of niacin. Patients with this deficiency will salivate excessively and develop a scaliness of the skin at the lips.

Skeletomuscular

Without the proper action of the muscles of mastication, all oral function would cease. One particularly painful problem seen in dogs is *masticatory muscle myositis*, an inflammatory and possibly immune-mediated disease that affects the muscles of mastication innervated by the trigeminal nerve, sometimes with a local or systemic peripheral eosinophilia (82,83). This inflammation can progress to necrosis and even atrophy and fibrosis in a chronic state, as well as the inability to open the mouth easily (15). The presence of autoantibodies to type 2M muscle fibers indicate a selective immune-mediated response (84) and dictate an immunosuppressive treatment regimen to reduce the pain on opening the mouth. Identification of these autoantibodies is diagnostic of the disease.

The inability to open the mouth is also present with a tetanus infection, but this is primarily due to the spasms of the masticatory and facial muscles. While dogs may be less susceptible to *Clostridium tetani* than other species, such as horses and humans, the characteristic grimace of the lips being pulled back and the overall weakness may lead a clinician to suspect this infection.

In comparison, if a dog presents with a dropped-open mouth that can be closed passively with little effort, mandibular neuropraxia may be suspected. If the animal has a history of carrying heavy or large objects in its mouth, it is possible that the branches of the nerves supplying the masticatory muscles have been stressed or stretched (15). Recovery usually occurs in 2–4 weeks with rest and conservative support.

Temporomandibular Joint

There are numerous pathologies of the *temporomandibular joint (TMJ)* or *craniomandibular articulation (CMA)*, all of which vary in radiographic signs according to the problem (85,86) (see Chapter 6). Problems in opening or closing the mouth may also occur with many skeletal abnormalities, particularly those involving the TMJ. Dysplasia of the joint may lead to laxity and excessive lateral movement of the mandible. With wide opening of the mouth during vocalization or yawning, this movement can allow the contralateral coronoid process of the mandibula to slip under and lateral to the zygomatic arch and remain locked in that position (87). While basset hounds are a breed typically considered to have a predilection for this condition, cases in Irish setters, spaniels, and even cats have been reported (87). Correction lies in removing the ventral portion of the zygomatic bone and/or dorsal coronoid process to prevent the interlocking from recurring. Typically, no treatment is performed to the TMJ, unless ongoing problems contribute to severe arthritic changes. There are times when sufficient bony alterations or even fractures in the area necessitate condylectomy to diminish a patient's pain and restore reasonable function. Fractures of this area are typically due to trauma, and other traumatic consequences might cause a *luxation* of the joint. This is more frequently seen in cats experiencing head trauma and will present with an open-mouth appearance like the open-mouth locking situation. Depending on the location of the luxation, use of a dowel as a fulcrum in the mouth can help facilitate reduction of the problem.

Surgery is not an option with patients experiencing craniomandibular osteopathy, where the caudal mandible and base of the skull are enlarged by the deposition of excessive periosteal new bone formation (15). This disorder typically affects young West Highland white terriers and other terrier breeds, and occasionally enough new bone will be present to prevent the mouth from opening fully. Symptomatic treatment to reduce discomfort is recommended.

The jaws may also appear swollen in cases of hyperparathyroidism, whether primary or secondary to dietary calcium deficiency or renal failure (15). The resulting resorption of calcium from calcified tissues generally begins with the mandible, progressing to the maxilla, and skull, and then to the axial and long bones. The decalcified bones become soft ("rubber jaw"), with radiographic densities, affected first with the loss of definition of the lamina dura, then of the trabecular and cortical bone regions. Tooth loss will be accelerated due to loss of bony support. Since the mandible may be the first indication of a problem, it is very important to investigate the primary cause and, if dietary or renal, take steps for correction where possible.

Osteomyelitis

There are many routes for an infection to start in the bones of the oral cavity. Extensions from periodontal and periapical infections and retained roots, as well as exposure to pathogens from trauma, bite wounds, or penetrating foreign objects, can set up an active infection, as can a hematogenous or systemic source, including fungal infections (88). In one study of cats and dogs with anaerobic osteomyelitis, the mandible was the third most common site, outranked by the radius and ulna (89). The swelling associated with the lesion can get large and firm and is often painful on palpation. Radiographically, there may be a zone of bony destruction surrounded by a region of increased density or sclerosis. Additionally, a periosteal reaction may be present and sequestration may be noted (53). Osteomyelitis of the jaws is typically seen as a proliferative reaction of the periosteum at the periphery of the lesion with lysis of the associated cortical and alveolar bone. The bone lysis may give the appearance that teeth are supported primarily by soft tissue, but seldom are the teeth displaced (as is seen with many cysts and tumors). In the oral region, fractures and tooth infections are commonly an initiating force. Any lesion that does not respond to treatment with curettage and appropriate antibiotic therapy (sometimes extensive) should be biopsied. Of a group of mandibular swellings in cats, about half were osteomyelitis and the other half were malignant tumors (squamous cell carcinoma, lymphosarcoma, melanosarcoma) (90).

Neoplasia or Tumors

A *neoplasia* is a new growth or tumor, which may be benign or malignant, slow- or fast-growing, and metastatic or nonmetastatic (Table 4). Treatments usually involve radiotherapy, chemotherapy, surgical excision, cryosurgery, diathermy, or a combination of these. Neoplasias are customarily classified according to tissue of origin and the lesion's behavior (11).

In the oral tissues, both cysts and tumors may occasionally be found (27,91,92). In the initial stages, oral tumors can be misdiagnosed as abscesses, gingivitis, stomatitis, gingival hyperplasia, cheilitis, tonsillitis, sialadenitis, salivary mucoceles, ranulas, or osteo-

TABLE 4. *General findings of some common oral tumors in the dog*

Feature	MM	SCC	FSC	Dental tumors Crown cysts Ameloblastomas Odontomas	Root cysts Epulidies Cementomas
Av. age (yr)	11	7 (tonsillar) 9 (gingival) <5 (papillary)	7	<1	8
Frequency (%)	30–40	20–30	10–20	5–10	
Sexual predilection	Male>female	Equal	Male>female	Male<female	
Size predilection	Small to medium	Medium to Large	Medium to large	None observed	
Site predilection	Rostral mandible	Buccal mucosa	Palate	Rostral mandible	
Local metastasis to regional lymph nodes	Common	Tonsillar: common Nontonsillar: rare	Rare	Not observed	
Distant metastasis	Common	Tonsillar: common Nontonsillar: rare	Occasional	Not observed	
Gross appearance	Ulcerated; raised; majority pigmented black	Ulcerated; raised; cauliflower; pink to red	Ulcerated; flat; firm; no typical color change	Smooth; raised; soft to firm; blue to red	

MM, malignant melanoma; SCC, squamous cell carcinoma; FSC, fibrosarcoma.
(Adapted from ref. 76.)

myelitis. In the early stages, most oral tumors do not cause substantial clinical signs or symptoms. As the disease advances through increased mass, invasiveness, or metastasis, signs of halitosis, dysphagia, oral pain, excessive salivation, oral bleeding, facial swelling, facial asymmetry, mobile or displaced teeth, lethargy, respiratory distress, or weight loss may be seen (see Table 4) (93).

Once a neoplasia is suspected or detected, the examination may need to include a history, physical examination, blood work, oral examination, radiographs, biopsies, and cytology. A good-quality oral examination will most times necessitate sedation or anesthesia, before which blood and other workups should be carried out. Biopsies should include a portion of healthy margin and be made to a depth that obtains a representative sample of diseased tissue. Regional lymph nodes should be examined, and if enlargement or asymmetry is detected, cytologic examination of needle aspirates should be considered.

Radiographically, cysts appear as radiolucencies, while tumors may present as radiopacities or radiolucencies. The radiolucency of cysts or tumors indicates the loss or destruction of the normal tissues and replacement by cyst or tumor tissue. The more aggressive neoplasias commonly displace adjacent structures, causing destructive damage. Several times previously in this text biopsy has been recommended for any lesion that does not respond to conventional therapy or that looks suspicious. Even with a mass fitting the description of what a specific tumor would look like, histopathology is necessary for the most accurate assessment. In general, oral malignancies account for 5.3% of all malignancies found in the dog, and 6.7% of those in the cat (2). Thoracic radiographs should also be taken if metastasis is suspected; however, tumor masses <0.5–1.0 cm in diameter are below the radiographic diagnostic threshold for most standard radiographic detection (93).

Benign

Benign tumors are considered to be nonmalignant, in that they do not destroy the tissues from which they originate or spread to other parts of the body (metastasize). Generally, surgical removal is curative in the majority of cases. With the exception of papillomas and odontogenic tumors, benign masses in the mouth are relatively uncommon, but they may include adenomas, fibromas, hemangiomas, and lipomas. As distinct from malignancies, they generally are slow-growing, well encapsulated (may or may not be pedunculated), and typically not painful; there is no metastasis.

Oral papillomas, caused by a canine virus in dogs, are self-limiting and generally left untreated. They may be present as multiple, gray-to-white, small, pedunculated masses on the oral mucosa, lips, tongue, and even esophagus. Surgery may be done in areas of occlusal or masticatory interference. The tumors are classified as benign, but cancers have been reported to occur at these lesion sites on rare occasion (57).

Odontogenic tumors and *cysts* are not uncommon in domestic animals, arising from cellular components of the developing tooth structure (2). There are several classification systems of odontogenic tumors, a situation that can at times lead to confusion in com-

---

TABLE 5. *Classification of tumors and cysts of odontogenic origin*

I. Odontogenic epithelial tumors or cysts
    Fibrous epulis (peripheral odontogenic fibroma)
    Ossifying epulis (calcifying epithelial odontogenic tumor)
    Giant cell epulis
    Acanthomatous epulis (acanthomatous ameloblastoma)
    Ameloblastoma
    Ameloblastic carcinoma
    Squamous odontogenic tumor
    Primordial cyst
    Dentigerous cyst
      Follicular
      Eruption
    Periodontal ligament cysts
    Gingival cysts
      Newborn
      Adult odontogenic
    Benign odontogenic epithelial tumors
II. Mesenchymal tumors
    Cementoma
    Cementoblastoma
    Benign odontogenic mesenchymal tumors
III. Mixed tumors
    Odontoma
      Compound odontoma
      Complex odontoma
    Ameloblastic fibroma
    Ameloblastic odontoma
    Ameloblastic fibro-odontoma

---

parison of information. For that reason, a short schematic and some definitions are listed here for the classification system used in this portion of the text. The tumors are divided into three basic categories according to the type or combination of types of tissue found within the tumor: epithelial, mesenchymal, and mixed (containing both epithelial and mesenchymal) (Table 5).

Primordial cysts are the result of degeneration of the stellate reticulum of the enamel organ (94). They are found in place of a tooth and generally occur early in life. Surgical removal and curettage is the treatment of choice in most cases, with a low incidence of recurrence.

There are two basic types of *dentigerous cysts*: eruption and follicular (94). *Eruption cysts* are a dilation of the normal follicular space surrounding a tooth crown during eruption. Treatment is generally not required, although incision to ease eruption is sometimes performed. *Follicular cysts* are dilations of the follicular space around the crown of a tooth that is unerupted or impacted. A distinct radiolucent area around the crown of an embedded tooth is a diagnostic sign of a dentigerous cyst. The cystic structure arises from all or a remnant of the developing dental follicle at the neck of the tooth, which is typically lost at the time of eruption. If the tooth fails to erupt, the follicle remains and produces the sac lined by stratified mucous or cutaneous epithelium (13). This cyst can be very invasive and expansile, even into bone, and requires thorough surgical removal and curettage (95).

There are two basic forms of gingival cysts: newborn and adult (94). *Newborn gingival cysts* arise from the remnants of dental lamina in newborn animals. The are usually multiple, nonpainful swellings along the alveolar ridge. *Adult odontogenic gingival cysts* may arise from remnants of dental lamina, enamel organ, or epithelium associated with the periodontal ligament (96) (Fig. 7). Surgical excision is normally curative. There are also *adult nonodontogenic gingival cysts*. These generally result from the traumatic implantation of gingival epithelium into the gingival connective tissues.

An *epulis* arises from the periodontal ligament around a tooth and is the most common type of benign growth found in the oral cavity (53,97). The classification of epulides changes on a regular basis. One common means of distinguishing them is grouping them according to histologic characteristics: fibromatous, ossifying, acanthomatous, and giant cell. Surgery is generally the treatment of choice for epulides.

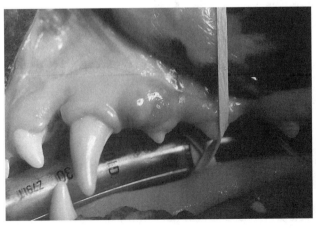

FIG. 7. Adult gingival cyst immediately apical to the crown of the maxillary 1st premolar.

A *fibromatous epulis* may be single or multiple and pedunculated or sessile, and usually has a smooth, pink surface (53). If large enough, it can interfere with mastication (97) and should be differentiated from gingival hyperplasia, particularly in boxers (98).

An *ossifying epulis* is similar to the fibromatous version but is composed of an osteoid matrix. Another term used to describe both of these tissue types is *peripheral odontogenic fibroma* (99).

The *acanthomatous epulis* (97) has been given many names: adamantinoma (100), basal cell carcinoma (101), and acanthomatous ameloblastoma (102). Although this neoplasia is considered benign, it can be locally aggressive, even infiltrating into bone, and is considered the most common invasive tumor of the dog jaw (97). It is often located at the rostral mandible and can be treated with surgical excision, radiation, or a combination of the two (Fig. 8). The recurrence rate following aggressive surgical resection has been reported to be less than 5% (103,104). Radiation therapy has been shown to control well over 90% of these tumors (105,106), but there have been reports of malignant tumor formation at previously irradiated sites in 20% of the cases (107). A *giant cell epulis* appears similar to the acanthomatous type, except it is not quite as aggressive and can only be differentiated by histopathologic examination.

The *ameloblastoma* is the most common tumor of the dental laminar epithelium (108). Grossly, it may appear soft and fleshy on its gingival surface, but it may extend much deeper into the bone. It is a slow-growing epithelial tumor that may be solid but often

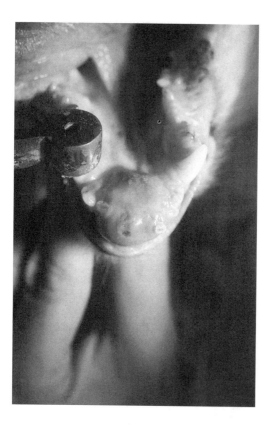

FIG. 8. Acanthomatous epulis in the rostral mandible of an 8-year-old female springer spaniel.

TABLE 6. *Radiographic staging of cementomas*

Stage	Signs
1	Radiolucency around the root apex appears
2	Some radiopaque densities within the radiolucency
3	Entire lesion becomes radiopaque

(Reproduced from ref. 134.)

shows a multiple cystic structure (108,109); teeth at the site may be mobile, moved, or absent (110). Although locally aggressive, it does not tend to metastasize, so complete resection generally carries a good prognosis. Radiation may be used for nonresectable or recurring tumors (53).

Cementomas (fibro-osteoma) are generally benign proliferations of the connective tissues in the jaws that produce cementum or cementum-like tissue. It is occasionally found on oral radiographs, most often associated with the root apex. It is ordinarily asymptomatic and self-limiting, and requires no direct treatment. It typically develops in a three-stage sequence (Table 6) (33). In the first stage, it appears as a radiolucency around the root apex, appearing identical to periapical disease, but the tooth is still vital. In the second stage, some radiopaque densities occur within the radiolucency. In the third stage, the entire lesion becomes radiopaque.

An *odontoma* biologically behaves similarly to the ameloblastoma (111), but it is a mixed odontogenic tissue tumor, containing both epithelial and mesenchymal cells. This lesion generally occurs in young animals, with the exception of rats (112). The two common forms are the compound and complex odontomas. The *complex odontoma* is a disorganized mass that contains no tooth-like structures. The *compound odontoma* has the characteristic of containing small tooth-like structures (denticles). These denticles will have various levels of differentiation and shapes and are often associated with radiolucent areas (2).

Malignant

Malignant tumors show an uncontrollable growth and destructive growth pattern of the tissues of origin and may exhibit a metastasis, or dissemination to other parts of the body. Most tumors seen in the oral cavity are malignant, and many have grown to a significant size before their discovery. Because early detection is unusual and possibly because the oral cavity is highly vascular, most oral tumors have a guarded-to-poor prognosis. Malignant tumors exhibit rapid, diffuse growth, local infiltration, possible pain, ulceration, and metastasis to distant sites, depending on tumor type and location. In dogs, the prevalence of incidence of malignancies ranges from melanosarcoma (most common), to squamous cell carcinoma, and fibrosarcoma. The most common sites affected are the gingiva, followed by the buccal mucosa, palate, and tongue (113–115). In cats, squamous cell carcinoma is the most common, with some occurrence of fibrosarcoma and rarely malignant melanoma; the gingiva and tongue are the sites most frequently affected in the cat.

Oral *melanosarcoma* is the most assertive oral tumor, with aggressive invasion and recurrence and a high rate of early metastasis to the lungs, lymph nodes, and bones (Fig. 9). Older (>11 years), dark-pigmented dogs are most commonly affected, with a higher

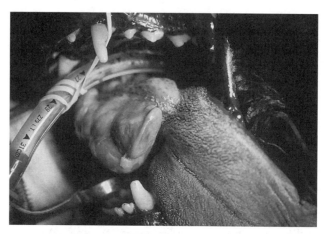

FIG. 9. Melanoscarcoma on the dorsal base of the tongue in an 11-year-old male chow chow.

incidence in males (2). Smaller dogs (116), particularly cocker spaniels, have frequently been reported to be affected, but so have German shepherds (117,118). Melanosarcoma is rarely found in cats (118). The gingiva is the most common site affected, but lesions may appear in the buccal or labial mucosa, hard and soft palate, or tongue (113,118,119). They may or may not be pigmented and can be firm initially, but they tend to ulcerate and become necrotic later on. Even with aggressive surgical treatment and ancillary therapy, the prognosis is poor and survival time is limited. Each year, new combinations of surgery, radiation therapy, and chemotherapy have produced some encouraging results, but there is still no definitive cure.

Squamous cell carcinoma can have a variable presentation in the oral cavity, depending on its location. It is the most common tumor in cats (69%) and the second most common in dogs (20%). There are two distinct forms: nontonsillar and tonsillar. *Nontonsillar squamous cell carcinoma* carries the better prognosis, and while locally invasive, it is slow to metastasize (119). It is most commonly located on the gingiva of the rostral portion of the oral cavity but may also be found on the lips, hard and soft palate, buccal mucosa, and tongue. Nodular and gray to pink, the mass is often irregular and ulcerated; 77% of cases show local infiltration into bone (4). Most squamous cell tumors are sensitive to radiation or may be resectable, but the success of therapy decreases, the further caudally the tumor is located, particularly behind the cuspids. *Papillary squamous cell carcinoma* is a form of nontonsillar gingival squamous cell carcinoma reported in the dog in 1988 (120). It occurs primarily in young animals, in the papillary gingiva, and is rapid-growing; however, there have been no reported cases of metastasis. It appears to respond well to excision.

The most aggressive form is *tonsillar squamous cell carcinoma* (Fig. 10). This is typically unilateral and appears as a firm, irregular gray-to-pink enlargement of the tissue. About 98% of these tumors metastasize early to the regional lymph nodes, with distant metastases in 63% (121) carrying a grave prognosis, even with tonsillectomy and cervical radiation (122). Tonsillar enlargement and swelling may lead to pharyngeal obstruction, if left untreated.

The third most common tumor in dogs (second in cats) is *fibrosarcoma*, which has a predilection for larger (>23 kg), male dogs over 7.5 years of age. It has rapid local invasion, including into bone (68%), and high recurrence rate, although it metastasizes late

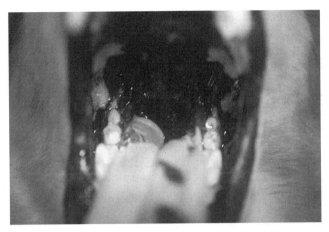

FIG. 10. Tonsillar squamous cell carcinoma in an 8-year-old female German shepherd.

(119,123). The gingiva, particularly in the maxillary region from the canine to 4th pre-molar, is the most common site, followed by the hard and soft palate and oral mucosa (119). It is typically firm and fleshy and may be mistaken for a benign growth early on, but it may progress to an irregular, friable, or ulcerated mass. In fact, in humans, some fibrosarcomas appear benign at the first biopsy with a low histologic grade yet biologi-cally high-grade characteristics (123). Early aggressive resection is the only hope for effective treatment, but the prognosis still is generally poor due to the rate of occurrence and occasional metastasis, because lesions are seldom found extremely early.

Of all *osteosarcomas* in dogs, the maxilla and mandible are the site of 3% each. The tumor may initially appear as a bony swelling but then starts to invade and destroy nor-mal bone structure. At these sites, there tends to be less vascular invasion by the cells and a lower percentage of pulmonary metastasis than tumors of the appendicular skeleton (91). Therefore, the biological activity of being locally invasive but slow to metastasize makes it possible to have a better prognosis with early detection and wide resection (124). In one reported case, the histopathology of osteogenic sarcoma was not given until a third biopsy, being initially read as a fibromatous epulis and then as an acanthomatous epulis; however, it did respond to aggressive surgical therapy (125).

Other malignancies may be seen infrequently in the oral cavity. *Lymphosarcoma* may be noted in the tonsils as part of a generalized lymphadenopathy, but it may be present as a primary focal lesion as well on the lips or gingiva. A more diffuse presentation of an ulcerative or proliferative stomatitis may require a combination of chemo- and/or radia-tion therapy (53).

Mastocytoma may be present on the upper lip, gingival or buccal mucosa, or palate, typically in males. Though it may be dormant for years, it is frequently malignant, with rapid growth and metastasis. Excision may be accompanied by corticosteroids and irra-diation (127).

Hemangiosarcoma presents as a red, raised, friable nodule. It has a poor prognosis with a high malignancy and early metastasis. The chest and abdomen should always be checked for metastases. Lingual myoblastoma in the dog (74), which is unlikely to metas-tasize, appears as a red, ulcerated granulomatous mass on the dorsolateral surface of the tongue.

Transmissible venereal tumor (TVT) is usually transmitted sexually, and the lips, buccal mucosa, and tonsils are considered aberrant sites. It can be variable in appearance on the lips, appearing cauliflower-like, peduncular, nodular, papillary, or multilobular with a variation of size, color, and degree of ulceration (121). Intraoral lesions are diffusely red with a raised hyperemic border; most regress spontaneously.

A similar clinical appearance may be seen in dogs with *leishmanial stomatitis*, which results from an infection with the protozoan *Leishmania donovani infantum* or *Leishmania tropica*. While typically found in Mediterranean areas, cases have been reported in the United States. The usual skin lesions involving alopecia, seborrhea, and nonpainful ulcers may be accompanied by cutaneous nodules. In four cases reported in United States, there were proliferative lesions on the mucosa of the penis, tongue, oral cavity, prepuce, or nose. Histopathology with special stains may reveal amastigotes in macrophages (128).

REFERENCES

1. Burrows CF, Miller WH, Harvey CE. Oral medicine. In: Harvey CE, ed. *Veterinary Dentistry*. Philadelphia: WB Saunders Co; 1985:23.
2. Tholen MJ, Hoft RF. Oral pathology. In: Bojrab MJ, Tholen MT, eds. *Small Animal Oral Medicine and Surgery*. Philadelphia: Lea & Febiger; 1990:42.
3. Bhaskor SN. *Synposis of Oral Pathology*. St Louis, MO: CV Mosby Co; 1961:122.
4. Anderson J. Approach to diagnosis of canine oral lesions. *Compend Cont Educ Dent* 1991;13:1215.
5. Ross D. Evaluation of dental abnormalities. American Animal Hospital Association Annual Meeting. Salt Lake City, Utah: 1978:78.
6. Lee MP, Bedi R, O'Donnell D. Bilateral double dens invaginatus of maxillary incisors in a young Chinese girl. *Aust Dent J* 1988;33:310.
7. Payne M, Craig GT. A radicular dens invagination. *Br Dent J* 1969;123:94.
8. Vajrabhaya L. Non-surgical endodontic treatment of a tooth with double dens en dente. *J Endod* 1989; 15:323.
9. DeForge DH. Dens-en-dente in a six-year-old Doberman Pinscher. *J Vet Dent* 1992;9:9.
10. Hata Gin-ichrio, Toda Todao. Treatment of dens invagination by endodontic therapy, apicocurettage and retrograde filling. *J Endod* 1987;13:469
11. Harty FJ. *Concise Illustrated Dental Dictionary*. 2nd ed. Boston: Wright Co; 1994.
12. Rossman LE, Garber DA, Harvey CE. Disorders of teeth. In: Harvey CE, ed. *Veterinary Dentistry*. Philadelphia: WB Saunders Co; 1985:79.
13. Bhaskor SN. *Synopsis of Oral Pathology*. St Louis, MO: CV Mosby Co; 1961:129.
14. Bittegeko SBPR, Arnbjerg J, Nkya R, Asborn T. Multiple dental abnormalities following canine distemper infection. *JAAHA* 1995;31:42.
15. Harvey CE, Emily PP. Occlusion, occlusive abnormalities and orthodontic treatment. In: *Small Animal Dentistry*. St.Louis, MO: Mosby-Year Book; 1993:266.
16. Skrabalak DS, Looney AL. Supernumerary tooth associated with facial swelling in a dog. *JAVMA* 203(2):266.
17. Cherville N. The gray collie syndrome. *JAVMA* 1968;152:620.
18. Kolata RT, Burrows CF. The clinical features of injury by chewing electrical cords in dogs and cats. *JAAHA* 1981;17:219.
19. Sarkiala EM, Dambach D, Harvey CE. Jaw lesions resulting from renal hyperparathyroidism in a young dog—a case report. *J Vet Dent* 1994;11(4):121.
20. Fingland RB, Gratzek A, Vorhies MW, Kirpensteijn J. Nasopharyngeal polyp in a dog. *JAAHA* 1993;29:311.
21. Hutt FB, deLaHunta A. A lethal glossopharyngeal defect in the dog. *J Hered* 1971;62:291.
22. Wiggs RB, Lobprise HB, deLaHunta A. Microglossia in three littermate pups. *J Vet Dent* 1994;11(4):129.
23. Simison WG. Sialadenitis associated with periorbital disease in dogs. *JAVMA* 1993;202(12):1983.
24. Emily P. The genetics of malocclusion. *Vet Forum* 1990;6:22.
25. Ross DL. Veterinary dentistry. In: Ettinger SJ, ed. *Textbook in Veterinary Internal Medicine*. Philadelphia: WB Saunders Co; 1975:1047.
26. Riser WH, Parkes LJ, Shirer JF. Canine craniomandibular osteopathy. *J Am Vet Radiol Soc* 1967;8:23.
27. Lee R. Radiographic examination of localized and diffuse tissue swellings in the mandibular and pharyngeal area. *Vet Clin North Am Small Anim Pract* 1974;4:723.
28. Pool RR, Leighton RL. Craniomandibular osteopathy in a dog. *JAVMA* 1969;154:657.
29. Robinson R. Genetic abnormalities in dogs. *Canine Pract* 1991;16:29.

30. Capen CC, Martin SL. Calcium metabolism and disorders of parathyroid glands. *Vet Clin North Am Small Anim Pract* 1977;7:513.
31. Chew DJ, DiBartola SP. Diagnosis and pathophysiology of renal disease. In: Ettinger SJ, ed. *Textbook of Veterinary Internal Medicine*. Philadelphia: WB Saunders; 1989:1893.
32. Hazewinkel HAW. Nutrition in relation to skeletal growth deformities. *J Small Anim Pract* 1989;30:625.
33. Frommer HH. *Radiology for Dental Auxiliaries*. 3rd ed. St.Louis, MO: CV Mosby Co; 1983:281.
34. Robinson HBG, Boling LR. Diagnosis and pathology of anachoretic pulpitis. I. Bacteriologic studies. *Arch Pathol* 1941;28:268.
35. Boling LR, Robinson HBG. The anachorectic effect in pulpitis. II. Histological study. *Arch Pathol* 1942;33:477.
36. Gorrel C, Robinson J. Endodontics in small carnivores. In: Crossley DA, Penman S, eds. *Manual of Small Animal Dentistry*. 2nd ed. Gloucestershire, UK: British Small Animal Association; 1995:168.
37. Wiggs RB. Is periodontal disease a measure of a pet's general health? *Vet Forum* 1995;2:66.
38. Madewell BR, Stannard AA, Pulley LT, Nelson VG. Oral eosiniophilic granuloma in Siberian Husky dogs. *JAVMA* 1980;177:701.
39. Ribbie J. Fusospirochetal infections. In: Wintrobe M, et al, eds. *Harrison's Principles of Internal Medicine*. 7th ed. New York: McGraw-Hill Book Co; 1974.
40. Innes J. The pathophysiology and pathogenesis of tuberculosis in domesticated animals compared with man. *Br Vet J* 1940;96:96.
41. Farrow B, Lane D. Bacterial, viral and other infectious problems. In: Ettinger SJ, ed. *Textbook of Veterinary Internal Medicine*. 2nd ed. Philadelphia: WB Saunders Co; 1983:269.
42. Joffe DJ, Allen AL. Ulcerative eosinophilic stomatitis in three Cavalier King Charles spaniels. *JAAHA* 1995;31:34.
43. Wiggs RB. Periodontal disease and its multifactorial causes. Osaka Japanese Veterinary Group Proceedings. Osaka, Japan: June 23, 1995.
44. Halliwell REW. Skin disease associated with autoimmunity. Part I: The bullous autoimmune disease. *Compend Contin Ed*. 1980;2:911.
45. Scott D, Haupt K, Knowlton B, et al. A glucocorticoid-responsive dermatitis in cats resembling systemic lupus erythematosus in man. *JAAHA* 1979;15:157.
46. Matus R, Scott R, Saal S, et al. Plasmaphoresis-immunoadsorption for treatment of systemic lupus erythematosus in a dog. *JAVMA* 1983;182:499.
47. Griffin G, Stannard A, Ihrke P, et al. Canine discoid lupus erythematosus. *Vet Immun Immunopathol* 1979;1:79.
48. Scott D. Immunologic skin disorders in the dog and cat. *Vet Clin North Am Small Anim Pract* 1978;8:641.
49. Scott D, Halliwell R, Goldschmidt M, et al. Toxic epidermal necrolysis in two dogs and a cat. *JAAHA* 1979;15:271.
50. Reed JH. The digestive system. In: Catcott EJ, ed. *Feline Medicine and Surgery*. 2nd ed. Santa Barbara, CA: American Veterinary Publications; 1975:154.
51. Hess PW, MacEwen EG. Feline eosinophilic granuloma. In: Kirk RW, ed. *Current Veterinary Therapy—VI*. Philadelphia: WB Saunders Co; 1977:534.
52. Song MD. Diagnosing and treating feline eosinophilic granuloma complex. *Vet Med* 1994;89(12):1141.
53. Manfra-Marretta S, Matheissen D, Matus R, Patniak A. Surgical management of oral neoplasia. In: Bojrab MJ, Tholen MT, eds. *Small Animal Oral Medicine and Surgery*. Philadelphia: Lea & Febiger; 1990:96.
54. Potter KA, Tucker RD, Carpenter JL. Oral eosinophilic granuloma in Siberian huskies. *JAAHA* 1980;16:595.
55. Norris AM, Withrow SJ, Dubielzig RR. Oropharyngeal neoplasia. In: Harvey CE, ed. *Veterinary Dentistry*. Philadelphia: WB Saunders Co; 1985:123.
56. Calvert CA. Canine viral transmissable neoplasias. In: Greene CE, ed. *Clinical Microbiology and Infectious diseases of the Dog and Cat*. Philadelphia: WB Saunders Co; 1984:461.
57. Watrach AM, Small E, Case MT. Canine papilloma: Progression of oral papilloma to carcinoma. *J Natl Cancer Inst* 1970;45:915.
58. Boggs D, Wintrobe M, Cartwright G. The acute leukemias. *Medicine* 1962;41:163.
59. Spodnick G. Oral complications of cancer therapy and their management. In: Spodnick G, ed. *Dentistry: Seminars in Veterinary Medicine and Surgery*. Philadelphia: WB Saunders Co; 1993:8(3):213.
60. Cutright D, Baver H. Cell renewal in the oral mucosa and skin of the rat, part I: Turnover time. *Oral Surg* 1967;23:249.
61. Sheffy B, Williams A. Nutrition and the immune response. *JAVMA* 1982;180:1073.
62. Saville P, Krook L, Gustafsson P, et al. Nutritional secondary hyperparathyroidism in the dog: Morphological and radioisotope studies with treatment. *Cornell Vet* 1969;59:155.
63. Harvey CE. Oral Surgery. In: Harvey CE, ed. *Veterinary Dentistry*. Philadelphia: Lea and Febiger; 1985:157.
64. Legendre LFJ. Management and long-term effects of electrocution in a cat's mouth. *J Vet Dent* 1993;10(3):6.
65. Hawkins BJ. Gum-chewer's syndrome: Self-inflicted sublingual and self-inflicted buccal trauma. *Compend Cont Educ Dent* 1992;14:219.
66. Bradley RL, Noone KE, Saunders GK, Patnaik AK. Nasopharyngeal and middle ear polypoid masses in five cats. *Vet Surg* 1985;14:141.
67. Degner DA, Bauer MS, Ehrhart EJ. Palatine tonsil cyst in a dog. *JAVMA* 1994;204:1041.
68. Evermann J. Isolation of calicivirus from a case of canine glossitis. *Canine Pract* 1981;8:36.

69. Arnbjerg J. *Pasteurella* glossitis in a dog. *Nord Vet Med* 1972;30:332.
70. Thivierge G. Granular stomatitis in dogs due to burdock. *Can Vet J* 1973;14:96.
71. Monasterio F. Early definitive treatment of electric burns of the mouth. *Plast Reconstr Surg* 1980.
72. Head KW. Tumors of the alimentary tract. In: Moulton JE, ed. *Tumors in Domestic Animals*. 3rd ed. Berkeley, CA: University of California Press; 1980:348.
73. Kallfelz FA. Skeletal and neuromuscular diseases. In: Lewis LD, Morris ML, Hand MS eds. *Small Animals Clinical Nutrition III*, 3rd ed; Topeka, Kansas: Mark Morris and Associates; 1987:12–14.
74. Spangler WL, Culbertson MR. Salivary gland disease in dogs and cats: 245 cases (1985-1988). *JAVMA* 1991;198:465.
75. Koestner A, Buerger L. Primary neoplasms of the salivary gland in animals as compared to similar tumors in man. *Vet Pathol* 1965;2:201.
76. Withrow SJ, MacEwen EG. *Small Animal Clinical Oncology*. 2nd ed. Philadelphia: WB Saunders Co; 1996:240.
77. Carberry CA, Glanders JA, Harvey HJ, Ryan AM. Salivary tumors in the dog and cat: A literature and case review. *JAAHA* 1988;24:561.
78. Hammer AS. Interim analysis of 90 dogs and cats with salivary gland tumors. *Vet Coop Oncol Group* 1994.
79. Evan SM, Thrall DE. Postoperative orthovoltage radiation therapy of parotid salivary gland adenocarcinoma in three dogs. *JAVMA* 1983;182:993.
80. Gilson SD, Stone EA. Sinus mucocele secondary to craniofacial trauma in a dog. *JAVMA* 1991;198:2100.
81. Masztiz P. Repair of labial avulsion in a cat. *J Vet Dent* 1993;10(1):4.
82. Brogdon JD, Brightman AH, McLaughlin SA. Diagnosing and treating masticatory myositis. *Vet Med* 1991;86(12):1164.
83. Gilmour MA, Morgan RB, Moore FM. Masticatory myopathy in the dog: A retrospective study of 18 cases. *JAAHA* 1992;28:300.
84. Anderson JG, Harvey CE. Masticatory muscle myositis. *J Vet Dent* 1993;10(1):6.
85. Ticer JW, Spencer CP. Injury of the feline temporomandibular joint: Radiographic signs. *J Am Vet Radiol Soc* 1978;19:146.
86. Morris E, Smallwood JE. The temporomandibular joints and tympanic bullae of the dog. In: *Radiographic Aids*. Chicago: The Quaker Oats Co; 1979; Series II, spring:1.
87. Lobprise HB, Wiggs RB. Modified surgical treatment of intermittent open-mouth mandibular locking in a cat. *J Vet Dent* 1992;9(1):8.
88. Lyon KF, Bard RA. Mandibular osteomyelitis caused by *Coccidiodes immitis*. *J Vet Dent* 1988;5(2):5.
89. Johnson KA. Osteomyelitis in dogs and cats. *JAVMA* 1994;205:1882.
90. Manfra-Marretta S. Feline mandibular swellings. American Veterinary Dental College/Academy of Veterinary Dentistry Proceedings. New Orleans, Louisiana: December 1989:77.
91. Hardy WD, Brodey RS, Riser WH. Osteosarcoma of the canine skull. *J Am Vet Radiol Soc* 1967;8:5.
92. Farrow CS. Radiographic characterization of an intermandibular mass in a dog. *J Mod Vet Pract* 1985;6:386.
93. Rochitz I. Oropharyngeal neoplasia in the cat. *J Feline Advis Bureau* 1993;30(1):22.
94. Anderson JG, Harvey CE. Odontogenic cysts. *J Vet Dent* 1993;10(4):5.
95. Lobprise HB, Wiggs RB. Dentigerous cyst in a dog. *J Vet Dent* 1992;9(1):13.
96. Ritchey B, Orban B. Cysts of the gingiva. *Oral Surg* 1953;6:765.
97. Dubielzig R, Goldschmidt M, Brodey R. The nomenclature of periodontal epulides in dogs. *Vet Pathol* 1979; 16:209.
98. Burstone MS, Bond E, Little R. Familial gingival hypertrophy in the dog (Boxer breed). *Am Med Assoc Arch Pathol* 1952;54:208.
99. Holmstrom SE. Canine oral diagnosis. In: Crossley DA, Penman S, eds. *Manual of Small Animal Dentistry*. 2nd ed. Gloucestershire, UK: British Small Animal Association; 1995:114.
100. Langham RF, Keathy KK, Mostosky UV, Schirmer RG. Oral adamantinoma in the dog. *JAVMA* 1965;146:474.
101. Bostock DE, White RAS. Classification and behavior after surgery of canine epulides. *J Comp Pathol* 1987;97:196.
102. Reichart PA, Philipson HP, Durr WN. Epulides in dogs. *J Oral Pathol Med* 1987;18:92.
103. Bjorling DE, Chambers JN, Mahaffey EA. Surgical treatment of epulides in dogs: 25 cases (1974-1984). *JAVMA* 1977;190:1315.
104. White RAS, Gorman NT. Wide local excision of acanthomatous epulides in dogs. *Vet Surg* 1989;18:12.
105. Thrall DE. Orthovoltage radiotherapy of acanthomatous epulides in 39 dogs. *JAVMA* 1984;184:826.
106. Langham RF, Mostosky UV, Schirmer RG. X-ray therapy of selected odontogenic neoplasms in the dog. *JAVMA* 1977;170:820.
107. Thrall DE, Goldschmidtt MH. Malignant tumor formation at the site of previously irradiated acanthomatous epulides in four dogs. *JAVMA* 1981;178:127.
108. Dubielzig RR. Proliferative dental and gingival disease of dog and cats. *JAAHA* 1982;18:566.
109. Dorn DR, et al. Survey of animal neoplasms in Alameda and Contra Counties, California—I. Methodology and description of cases. *J Natl Cancer Inst* 1968;40:295.
110. Dubielzig RR, Thrall DE. Ameloblastoma and keratinizing ameloblastomas in dogs. *Vet Pathol* 1982;19:596.
111. Figueiredo C, Alvares LC, Damante JH. Composed complex odontoma in the dog. *Vet Med Small Anim Clin* 1974;69:268.
112. Fitzgerald JE. Ameloblastoma odontoma in the Wistar rat. *Tox Pathol* 1987;15:479.

113. Hoyt RF Jr, Withrow SJ. Oral malignancy in the dog. *JAAHA* 1984;20:83.
114. Cohen D, et al. Epidemiologic aspects of oral and pharyngeal neoplasms in the dog. *Am J Vet Res* 1964; 25:1776.
115. Colmery BH. Dentistry. In: Bojrab MJ, ed. *Pathophysiology in Small Animal Surgery*. Philadelphia: Lea & Febiger; 1981.
116. Todoroff RJ, Brodey RS. Oral and pharyngeal neoplasia in the dog: A retrospective study of 361 cases. *JAVMA* 1979;176:561.
117. Dorn CR, et al. Survey of animal neoplasms in Alameda and Contra Counties, California—II. Cancer morbidity in dogs and cats from Alameda County. *J Natl Cancer Inst* 1968;40:307.
118. Dorn DR, Priester WA. Epidemiologic analysis of oral and pharyngeal cancer in dogs, cats, horses and cattle. *JAVMA* 1976;169:1202.
119. Brodey RS. A clinical and pathologic study of 130 neoplasms of the mouth and pharynx in the dog. *Am J Vet Res* 1960;21:787.
120. Ogilvie GK, Sundberg JP, O'Banion K, Badertscher RR, Wheaton LG, Reichmann ME. Papillary squamous cell carcinoma in three young dogs. *JAVMA* 1988;192:933.
121. Head KW. Tumors of the alimentary tract. In: Mouton J, ed. *Tumors in Domestic Animals*, 3rd ed. Berkeley, California: University of California Press; 1990:352.
122. MacMillan R, Withrow SJ, Gillette EL. Surgery and regional irradiation for treatment of canine tonsillar squamous cell carcinoma: Retrospective review of eight cases. *JAAHA* 1982;18:311.
123. Gorlin RJ, et al. The oral and pharyngeal pathology of domestic animals: A study of 487 cases. *Am J Vet Res* 1959;20:1032.
124. Cielot PA, Powers BE, Withrow SJ, et al. Histologically low-grade, yet biologically high-grade fibrosarcomas of the mandible and maxilla in dogs: 25 cases (1982-1991). *JAVMA* 1994;204:60.
125. Bradley RL, Sponenberg DP, Martin RA. Oral neoplasia in 15 dog and 14 cats. *Semin Vet Med Surg (Small Anim)* 1986;1:33.
126. Yovich JC, Reed RA, Huxtable CR. Mandibular osteosarcoma of possible odontogenic origin in a dog. *Aust Vet Pract* 1994;24:186.
127. Thrall DE, Dewhirst MW. Use of radiation and/or hyperthermia for treatment of mast cell tumors and lymphosarcomas in dogs. *Vet Clin North Am Small Anim Pract* 1985;15:835.
128. Font A, Roura X, Fondevila D, et al. Canine mucosal leishmaniasis. *JAAHA* 1996;32:131.
129. Veterinary Dental Abbreviations. American Veterinary Dental College, Residency Tracking Committee, Dallas, Texas: 1994; suppl.
130. Wiggs RB, Lobprise HB. Dental disease. In: Norsworthy GD, ed. *Feline Practice*. Philadelphia: JB Lippincott Co; 1993:290.
131. Howard WW, Moller RF. *Atlas of Operative Dentistry*. 3rd ed. St.Louis, MO: CV Mosby Co; 1981:4.
132. Robinowich BZ. The fractured incisor. *Pediatr Clin North Am* 1956;3:979.
133. Torres, HO, Ehrlich A. Pedodontics. In: *Modern Dental Assisting*. Philadelphia: W. B. Saunders Co. 1980:725.
135. Frommer HH. *Radiology for Dental Auxiliaries*. 3rd ed. St. Louis, MO: CV Mosby Co;1983:307.
136. Brodey RS. A clinico-pathological study of 200 cases of oral and pharyngeal cancer in the dog. In: *New Knowledge about Dogs*. New York: Gaines Dog Research Center;1961:5.

6

Dental and Oral Radiology

Robert B. Wiggs and Heidi B. Lobprise

Radiology is a vital tool in veterinary dentistry, assisting in diagnosis, treatment planning, and monitoring of oral disease, as well as being a integral part of the patient record. Diagnostically, being able to assess normal anatomy helps determine whether abnormalities exist, including variations in development (eg, missing or aberrant teeth) and acquired diseases that may affect the bone and tooth structure (eg, craniomandibular osteopathy, hyperparathyroidism, neoplasia). In the planning of possible treatment for problems such as feline cervical line lesions, endodontically compromised teeth, or periodontal disease, radiology assists the practitioner in making a more accurate assessment. Preoperative radiographs can help monitor extractions by revealing abnormal root structures, impacted teeth, and ankylosed roots, and postoperative films are helpful for monitoring for treatment success. Endodontics requires multiple films during the procedure to evaluate routine treatment and reveal complications.

X-RADIATION

Dental x-ray machines are used to generate x-radiation, which is the emission and propagation of energy through space or substance in the form of waves or particles. *X-rays* are a form of wave energy that belongs to the electromagnetic spectrum, the same as radio, television, radar, micro-, infrared, visible-light, and ultraviolet waves. *Gamma radiation* is also within this spectrum and has the same approximate wavelengths as x-radiation, but it is naturally occurring rather than man-made. The various wavelengths of this spectrum overlap, and there is no clear-cut delineation between them. These waves have electric and magnetic fields associated them, hence the name *electromagnetic spectrum*. The electrical field is at right angles to the waves' path of travel, and the magnetic field at right angles to the electric. These radiations are odorless, invisible to the naked eye, and composed of pure energy known as photons or quanta that have no mass or weight. This differs from corpuscular or particulate radiations that consist of bits of matter or subatomic particles that have weight and mass. The electromagnetic spectrum is a group of energy waves that have in common their weightlessness and the fact that they travel at an equivalent speed of light (186,000 miles per second in a vacuum). Frequency and wavelength are the differences between the various radiations within this spectrum. The *frequency* is the number of oscillations per second in the wave. The distance from the crest of one wave to that of the next is the *wavelength*, which is usually abbreviated with

TABLE 1. *X-ray wavelengths and use*

Ray type	Wavelength (Å)	Use
Grenz rays	5.00–0.60	Superficial therapy
Soft x-rays	0.60–0.30	Radiography of thin tissue sections for research
Diagnostic x-rays	0.30–0.10	Diagnostic radiographs, most dental and medical units
Deep x-rays	0.10–0.06	Deep therapy

the Greek letter *lambda* (λ) The height of the waves is known as the *crest*, while the depth is designated the *trough*. These wavelengths are measured in angstroms (Å). One Å is 0.0000000001 m or 0.00000001 cm, which is occasionally expressed as 10^{-8} cm. Long wavelength equates with low frequency, and short wavelength with high frequency. The shorter the wavelength and the higher the frequency are, the greater are the photon energy of these radiations and the penetrating ability of the wave. Waves travel through space as transverse waves. American Dental Association (ADA) Specifications No.26 and No.31 specify the important features for dental x-ray generators (1). The x-radiation wavelengths are divided in to four basic categories according to use,: *grenz, soft, diagnostic,* and *deep* (16) (Table 1).

X-rays can be directed and energized by frequency or wavelength to penetrate through opaque tissues or structures and affect a photographic emulsion on an acetate film (2,3). The film can be processed or developed to provide a visible two-dimensional black-and-white image or negative shadow of the tissues penetrated. Because of this effect, at one time, the film exposed by x-radiation was commonly referred to as a shadow graph. Later, for a period, it was known as a skiagraph or skiagram, which was derived from the Greek term *skia* (shadow). X-rays react with certain chemical crystals, resulting in energy in the form of light being given off. It is this ability that lead to the development of intensifying screens in panoramic and other radiographic cassettes.

X-rays, gamma rays, and some particulate radiation are known as *ionizing radiations* (4,5). Ionization occurs when an orbiting electron is ejected, or ionized, from its place in an electrically stable or neutral atom. The atom has been converted into two ions. The original ion now caries a positive charge, and the ejected electron ion a negative charge. It is this ionization process that is the basis for the biological effects of electromagnetic radiation. Ionization occurs when the radiation transfers sufficient energy to the atom to result in the ejection of electrons. Radiations may react with atoms in which part or all of the energy is transferred to the atom. It is also possible for the atom to return to a stable state by the release of excess energy in the form of long-wave radiation, which may demonstrate itself as visible light. This effect is seen in the intensifying screens used in many film cassettes (6).

HISTORY

The discovery of x-radiation is generally attributed to Wilhelm Conrad Roentgen, a professor of physics at the University of Würzburg in Germany (7–10). On November 8th, 1895, Roentgen was experimenting with a "gas tube" (Crookes' tube) that was covered in black paper. In a darkened room, he had observed a greenish glow from a cardboard plate across the room that had been painted with a fluorescent material (barium platinocyanide), when electrical current was passed through the covered tube. Shadows of varying density could be seen of objects placed between the tube and plate, and when a photographic film was substituted, the shadow could be recorded. He was quick to realize that an unknown radiation being produced by the Crookes' tube was responsible for the effect. He named the radiation *x* from the algebraic designation for an unknown. Roentgen presented his first paper on the subject on December 28, 1895. At that time, he exhibited a radiograph of his wife's hand, which he had earlier produced. Great interest with x-radiation and radiographs ensued in the science fields throughout the world. In 1901, Roentgen was presented with the first Nobel Prize awarded in physics, in recognition of his discovery. In actuality, a Professor Goodspeed in Philadelphia may have made the discovery of the unknown radiation and made radiographs much earlier, on February 22, 1890, but he had failed to recognize the significance of the discovery and had filed it away (11). Attempts to attach Roentgen's name to his discovery have not been popularized. Although the use of roentgenogram, roentgenology, and roentgenography is considered proper, the simpler term *x-ray* has been most widely accepted.

In January 1896, less than a month after the publication of Roentgen's papers, Dr. Otto Walkhoff, a German dentist made the first known dental radiograph of a lower premolar (10). He used an intraoral technique with a small glass photographic plate wrapped in black paper to block light and covered in rubber to prevent contamination by saliva. His experiments required an exposure time of 25 minutes to provide a suitable dental radiograph.

The first intraoral radiograph in the United States was most probably made by either Dr. William Rollins, Dr. William James Morton, or Dr. C. Edmund Kells in early 1896 (11). Generally, credit has been given to Dr. C. Edmund Kells, a progressive New Orleans dentist (9–11). Another leader in the field of intraoral radiology was Dr. William Rollins, who possibly developed the first dental x-ray unit in 1896 (10). He was also the first to recommend use of lead aprons and lead lining of the glass tube, and warned about the risks of x-rays on pregnant women. Failure of many of these early pioneers to realize the hazards and biological effects of x-radiation resulted in many grave medical side effects. Dr. Kells eventually died from complications of radiation exposure (8,9). The hot cathode x-ray tube, which was the forerunner and prototype of today's x-ray tubes, was developed in 1913 by William Coolidge (Coolidge tube) (10). It was also in this year that the first American commercially manufactured dental x-ray machine was produced by the Victor X-ray Corporation, later known as General Electric X-ray Corporation. In 1914, dental radiology was first added to dental school curriculum in America (10). During this time, radiology was primitive, dangerous, and considered by many as quackery. This was the result of the use of radiology units in many circuses and carnivals as forms of sideshow entertainment ("The Mr. Bones Show"). It would take many years for x-ray generators and radiology to be accepted and practiced on a regular basis in dentistry. One of the first important achievements occurred in 1920 when Franklin McCormack formulated the right-angle or paralleling technique, which greatly diminished dimensional distortion. Dr. G.M. Fitzgerald and Dr. William J. Upgrave further refined the technique and made it more practical for the dental practitioner (11).

X-RAY MACHINES OR GENERATORS

X-ray generators take the kinetic energy of accelerated electrons and convert it into x-ray photons by colliding them with a target in a controlled fashion (3). The dental x-ray machine comprises two basic components: a control unit and a tube head. The *control unit* consists of a control panel with an on/off switch, a meter or light indicator, a timer dial, a *kilovoltage (kVp) selector*, a *milliampere (mA) selector*, and an exposure button with an indicator meter or light. The tube head consists primarily of the x-ray tube, the tube housing, cooling devices, tube circuits, and the *position-indicating device (PID, cone)* (6).

The exposure button is typically attached with a six-foot cord or linked to a remote station for the safety of the operator. All dental x-ray units have a "dead-man" type exposure switch, which will automatically terminate the x-ray exposure when pressure on the button is released. This makes it necessary to maintain a positive pressure on the exposure button throughout the entire exposure cycle. Additionally, most current dental units have an audible sound or noise alert that activates at the time of an actual exposure when x-rays are produced. The timer controls the overall length of time during which x-radiation is produced. Direct-current generators have time exposures listed in seconds; alternating-current generators may have timers with the exposures listed in seconds or pulses. In the United States, alternating current (AC) is supplied in 60 cycles per second (hertz, Hz). Each cycle results in one positive pulse. Each pulse lasts a $1/60$th of a second, although x-radiation is emitted for only $1/120$th of a second during the positive half of the pulse cycle, because no radiation is produced during the negative half of the pulse. A pulse timer set to six pulses is the equivalent of $6/60$ths or $1/10$th of a second. Generators operating at frequencies greater than 60 Hz typically have their timers expressed in 60-Hz equivalents.

Newer units have milliampere selection of between 5 mA and 20 mA, and most are between 7 mA and 15 mA. Many of these units have preset fixed milliampere selections of 8, 10, or 15 mA, or a combination of these. The kilovoltage options may be fixed or have a range from 50 kVp to 120 kVp, with 65–90 kVp being the most common. The tube head is supported by extension arms of various lengths, which allow vertical, horizontal, and rotational movements of the tube head. The longer, 74-inch extension arms are the most versatile and useful for most veterinary dentistry practitioners. This permits mobility of the PID to aim the useful primary beam for the radiographic technique desired.

Most dental x-ray units make use of 110 V, 60 Hz, AC electricity, although some use 220 V and AC. Direct-current (DC) generating units are also available, although they do not provide the same wave pattern or x-ray spectrum as AC units. When an AC unit is set at 70 kVp, the alternating cycle results in the unit's tube potential varying from 0 kVp to 70 kVp. A DC unit set at 70 kVp essentially maintains a constant 70 kVp. For this reason, some generators are constructed to convert the AC power supply to DC in order to maintain a constant kVp. These are generally referred to as DC generators or constant-potential (CP) generators. Additionally, the AC units can be made to approach the spectrum generated by DC units by electrically altering the waveform to be more square than sinusoidal. One advantage to the AC generators is that AC results in less heat production within the tube and less chance of tube burn-out. The power supply is activated by the on/off or master switch. Power is then provided to the two major circuits: the filament circuit and high voltage circuit. Each makes use of transformers to alter the electrical current levels. The filament circuit uses a step-down transformer to reduce the 110-V line current to the 3–5 V needed to warm the filament in the tube head. It is regulated by a rheostat, which is controlled by the milliamperage selector. Milliamperage regulates the quantity of x-radiation produced. It is multiplied by the exposure time in seconds to provide the milliamperage per second (mA/sec). The kilovoltage selector controls the high voltage circuit, which requires a step-up transformer to increase the 110-V line to 55,000–120,000 V. This corresponds to 55–120 kVp. Kilovoltage determines the quality of the x-radiation produced. The higher the kVp setting, the greater the acceleration of the electrons. The greater the force with which the electrons strike the target, the shorter the x-ray wavelengths and the greater their penetration potential. Fluctuations in line voltage entering the system is corrected by an autotransformer in the circuit that acts as a line compensator.

X-ray generators produce x-radiation by bombardment of a target with a focused electron beam within a vacuum tube. For x-radiation to be produced, three things must be present: a source of free electrons, high voltage acceleration for the free electrons, and a target to bring them to a stop. Typically, a tungsten filament is used to generate the electron beam. The target is generally also made of tungsten. The exact location at which the electron beam strikes the target is the focal spot, and the region of the target that effectively produces the x-radiation. The smaller the focal-spot size, the higher the resolution is of the projected image. However, the smaller the focal spot, the more intense is the heat generation to a smaller portion of the target, increasing the risk of target melt down and tube failure. Rotating targets are used in larger generators to prevent the electron beam from bombarding the same region of the target unceasingly. Normally, the filament and the target rotate between being the anode and cathode 120 times per second, because of the change in polarity from the alternating current. But the filament is commonly referred to as the cathode and the target as the anode, because x-radiation is produced only when they are in this configuration. This pattern of the tube's producing x-radiation only when the filament is the cathode is known as self-rectification; it is also the reason for the tube's being known as a cathode ray tube. All AC dental x-ray machines are self-rectifying.

Unfortunately, even with today's improvements in x-ray generators, they are very inefficient: Less than 1% of the energy activated is converted into a useful form of x-ray photons, and the remaining 99% is lost as useless heat in the tube. The radiation produced is polychromatic, meaning that it consists of x-ray photons of various wavelengths and frequencies. Filtration is used to alter the spectrum emitted from the PID. This is done to selectively inhibit the longer-wavelength, low-frequency, low-energy portion of the spectrum that would be almost totally absorbed by the patient, thereby adding to the patient's radiation dose without contributing to the actual film image. Typically, aluminum and in some cases copper have been the accepted materials used for filtration. The tube potential, waveform, and filtration all interact to determine the x-ray spectrum emitted from an x-ray machine. Once the primary beam has been filtered and collimated, it is known as the *useful beam*. Federal requirements regulate the amount of filtration based upon the kVp operating levels of individual dental x-ray generators (4–6).

Collimation of the x-ray beam is the restriction of the size and shape of the beam as it exits the tube head. This reduces the amount of scatter radiation and the radiational dose to the patient. A lead diaphragm with a circular aperture within the PID is most commonly used as the collimating device in dental x-ray machines. Open-ended PIDs, if lead-lined or made of metal, work as an additional collimating mechanism. Metallic film-holding shields with a film-shaped opening provide even more collimation and patient protection. Closed-end and pointed-cone PIDs were designed to aid in aiming the useful beam. Unfortunately, even the plastic of the closed cone results in secondary radiation from reaction with the primary beam. This secondary radiation increases the long-wave radiational dose to the patient, while degrading the quality of the image on the film. For these reason, the open-end PIDs are preferable to the closed-end cone-type PIDs (10).

FOCAL–FILM DISTANCE AND OBJECT–FILM DISTANCE

Focal–film distance (FFD) and *object–film distance (OFD)* directly affect image magnification and distortion of detail on the film. FFD is the distance from the focal spot on the tube's target to the film. OFD is the distance from the object being x-rayed to the film. Three premises aid in the control of magnification: These are to (a) use as great an FFD as feasible, (b) have the minimal OFD as possible, and (c) place the film and object parallel to each other's long axis and perpendicular to the central useful primary beam. These goals are ideal in theory, but in veterinary oral radiography can seldom be strictly adhered to.

In dental radiology, the most common FFDs used are 8, 12, and 16 inches. Generally, an 8-inch FFD as a short-cone technique and a 16-inch FFD as a long-cone technique are utilized. One important factor in choosing an FFD is the *inverse square law*. This law states that the intensity of radiation required varies inversely with the square of the distance from the source. This implies that if the FFD is doubled, with the milliamperage and kilovoltage remaining the same, the exposure time should be quadrupled to maintain the same effect. Preferably, the milliamperage and kilovoltage would be adjusted to prevent excessive exposure times when the FFD is increased.

RADIATION BIOLOGY

The science dealing with the effects of radiation on living tissues is known as *radiation biology* (8). Of the useful beam generated for a film exposure, a portion passes through the patient, part is halted within the body's cells, some is stopped by the film, and part interacts with the film to cause secondary radiation that is passed on to the cells in the form of longwaves (4,7,8). Organ functions, tissues, and cells of the body are based on ionic activity. Normal ions are present in the body in a finely balanced state that allows precise control of cell function and body activity. X-rays, being a form of ionizing radiation, can interact with living cells, resulting in tissue damage. These effects can be either somatic (general body cells) or genetic (hereditary). Reproductive cells, lymphatic tissues, young bone cells, skin, and blood-forming tissues are among the more radiosensitive of the body. Immature cells, rapidly reproducing cells, and those in increased metabolism are also more sensitive.

Radiation exposure and *radiational dose* are distinct terms used when discussing radiation safety. The measurement of ionization in the air produced by gamma and x-radiation to which a patient is exposed is known as radiation exposure. The unit most commonly used to measure exposure is termed *roentgen* (R) or milliroentgen (mR) (1000 mR = 1 R). A roentgen is the unit of exposure dose needed to produce one electrostatic charge in 1 cm of air. The radiational dose is usually expressed in *radiation absorbed dose (rad)* or *roentgen equivalents man (rem)*. The rad is defined as 100 ergs of energy per gram of absorber. One R of exposure is approximately equal to 1 rad of absorbed dose in dental x-rays. Dose radiation expressed in rem is the rad dose with certain qualifying factors (QF) (rem = rad × QF). The rem takes into consideration that different types of radiation will have different effects on human tissue.

Personal Safety and Protection

Use of x-ray machines can be simple and safe when appropriate radiation safety practices are strictly observed with a comprehension of the sources of exposure (5). Generally, there are three sources of possible radiation exposure (12): the primary beam, scatter radiation, and radiation leakage from the machine head. To minimize these risks, staff personnel should follow the following guidelines: Avoid the primary beam by not standing in its path or holding films in the patient's mouth. Films can be held in the mouth by closing the occlusion or with the help of plastic holders, hemostats, rubber bands, or malleable materials (modeling clay) in plastic bags. Scatter radiation can be minimized by standing at least 6 feet from the source, maintaining a 90–135° angle from the path of the primary beam, and not touching the PID, head, or housing during exposures. Leakage radiation should be tested for on a regularly scheduled basis by a licensed technician. Film badges are the only efficient monitor for exposures and provide legal documentation of safety policy.

Use a short-cone technique when possible. Based on the inverse square law an 8-inch cone requires only one-fourth the exposure time of the long 16-inch cones (example: 0.1 second vs. 0.4 second). Additionally, the use of E-speed film can reduce exposure time requirements by approximately another 40–50%, in comparison with D-speed film. This reduces radiational dose to the patient and scatter potential to staff. Although some detail is lost with E-speed film when inspected under high magnification, clinically no difference in detail is ordinarily observed (12,13).

DENTAL FILMS

Dental x-ray films are used to capture the image exposed by the useful primary beam. Dental radiographic films are composed of a transparent polyester sheet core with a base coating of a predominantly silver halide emulsion suspended in a gelatin and covered with a clear protective coating. Typically, these halides are principally silver bromide with some silver iodide and small amounts of silver sulfide present. Today's high-speed dental films (D and E) have silver halide emulsion covering both sides of the film and are known as double-emulsified. This allows the film to be read or interpreted from either side or direction, contrary to the older slow films (A and B) and intermediate-speed films (C) that typically had a single coating and could be easily read from only one side.

The film is further encased in a protective packet (Fig. 1). The packets are designed to be light-tight and resistant to saliva and moisture and allow a degree of flexibility for oral

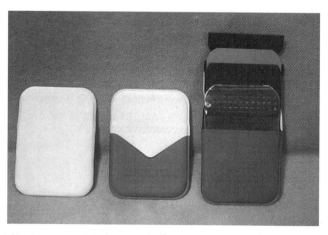

FIG. 1. Intraoral film is encased in a protective packet enveloped in front and back by black paper and backed by a thin sheet of lead foil. From left to right are shown the front of and unopened film, the back of an opened film, and the back of and opened film showing contents.

placement. Within the film packet, the film is enveloped in front and back by black paper, and backed by a thin sheet of lead foil. The black paper provides additional light protection, and the lead backing aids in reducing film fog from backscatter. The *backscatter* radiation originates from x-rays interacting with the patient's tissues, producing scatter radiation that may bounce back through the reverse side of the film. Backscatter fogging results in higher radiograph exposure and an increase in density or darkening of the film. This increase in density can obscure the film image and decrease the film's diagnostic quality. The lead backing generally has a pattern imprinted into it, commonly called the *stipple*. Should the film be exposed from the back side, the lead will result in a decrease in density and possibly a stipple pattern will be apparent on the developed film (Fig. 2). The film and packet are embossed with a dot or button, visible on the outside of the packet, for orientation during exposure and after development. This embossing results in a concave *dimple* on the back side of the film and a convex dot or button on the font. Intraoral packets are available with one or two films in the packet. Double-film packets are generally used when duplicate radiographs are desired for the client and referring doctor, or for sending to a specialist for consultation.

There are basically two types of radiographic films: those sensitive primarily to x-radiation and those sensitive primarily to light. Those sensitive primarily to light require fluorescent intensification for proper exposure. Dental radiography uses films that are sensitive primarily to the photons of x-radiation and do not use intensifying screens. For this reason, dental films are called *nonscreen films*. Dental films are light-sensitive to a

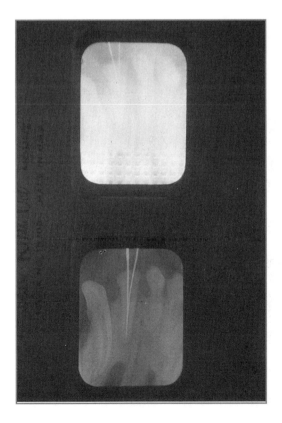

FIG. 2. Stipple pattern apparent on a developed radiographic film due to incorrect placement of film in the mouth.

degree and therefore must still be protected from light until the development process is completed. Some research has been directed toward the implementation of intraoral screen films (14).

Film Storage

Light, heat, chemicals, strong aromatic substances, humidity, and radiation can detrimentally affect undeveloped films. Unexposed dental x-ray film should be stored in a light-retardant location that is cool, dry, and radiation-safe. Within the operatory area, a lead or metal storage box should be used to protect unexposed films from scatter radiation. Exposed films kept within the operatory during a series of exposures should temporarily be placed in a similar receptacle until the studies are completed and the films are removed for development.

Film Sizes

Currently, intraoral nonscreen films are available in five basic sizes: 0, 1, 2, 3, and 4 (Fig. 3). Size 0 film measures 0.875×1.375 ($^7/_8$×1$^3/_8$) inches or 22×35 mm. Size 1 film measures 0.938×1.562 ($^{15}/_{16}$×1$^9/_{16}$) inches or 24×40 mm. Size 2 measures 1.219×1.609 (1$^1/_4$×1$^9/_{16}$) inches or 31×41 mm. Size 2 film is commonly referred to as standard size or

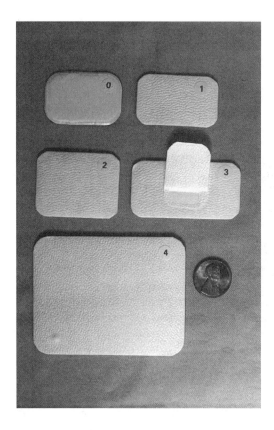

FIG. 3. Intraoral films: sizes 0, 1, 2, 3, and 4.

standard film. Sizes 0, 1, and 2 are considered *periapical films*. Size 3 film measures 2.109×1.047 (1$\frac{1}{16}$×2$\frac{1}{8}$) inches or 27×54 mm. Size 4 film measures 2.250×3.000 (2$\frac{1}{4}$×3) inches or 57×76 mm. The number 4 film is referred to as an *occlusal film* because, in humans, it is typically positioned in the occlusal plane of the patient. Film sizes 1, 2, and 3 are available in bitewings. The number 3 film is available only in *bitewing* packets. The bitewing film or packet has a tab or wing across the center of the packet front that allows the human patient to bite on the wing with the film in a lingual position to hold it in place for exposure. This allows x-rays to be taken of both the upper and lower tooth crowns while they are in normal occlusion or contact. Bitewing loops are available that fit over periapical packets to convert them into bitewing service.

Views of supporting tissues and the apices of the tooth can be produced with periapical radiographs. Bitewing films are used to provide views of the crowns and proximal surfaces of teeth, thus providing information about the extent of fractures, caries, and cervical line lesions. Occlusal films are used in surveys of the mandible and maxilla to search for and locate various normal or abnormal anatomy and pathologic conditions. Panoramic films in primates have been used for dentitional surveys for orthodontics and oral surgery procedures.

Extraoral films, both screen and nonscreen, are also used in dentistry. Extraoral studies may be used, in parallel or bisecting techniques, for survey films to assess massive oral injuries, fractures, neoplasia, or temporomandibular studies. They can also be used for actual dental studies when good technique is followed. For these studies, the most commonly used nonscreen films are the 5-×-7-inch and 8-×-10-inch sizes. These extraoral nonscreen films are very similar to the intraoral films in that they are x-radiation-sensitive and can be obtained in large individually sealed film packets, although they do not have the embossed dimple/dot. This means they must have a lead marker attached prior to exposure for orientation following development. Additionally, these films and their packets can be custom-cut to almost any desired size or shape in the darkroom. While still in the darkroom, the exposed edges must be sealed and made light-tight with black plastic tape.

Film Speed

Dental film speeds are defined in ADA Specification No.22 (Table 2). Films are designated with the letters *A*, *B*, *C*, *D*, *E*, and *F*, with the slowest-speed film being A and the fastest-speed F. Currently, only D- and E-speed films are marketed to general dental practices. The use of the slow A and B films and the intermediate-speed C speed films is discouraged because of movement blurring and increased health hazards to the patient from the increased exposure times. Film speed is generally determined by the size of the sil-

TABLE 2. *Radiographic film speeds*

Speed group	Speed range[a] in reciprocal roentgens
C	6.0–12.0
D	12.0–24.0
E	24.0–48.0
F	48.0–96.0

[a] The upper limit of each speed range shall be excluded from that range.

ver bromide (halide) crystals in the film emulsion: the larger the crystals, the faster the film. In addition, the larger the crystals are, the coarser is the fine detail in the image. This means a trade-off is made of increased speed for a slight loss of fine detail.

INTRAORAL RADIOGRAPHIC TECHNIQUES

Intraoral radiology makes use of two basic techniques to attain accurate film images: paralleling and bisecting-angle techniques. A basic knowledge of regional anatomy is necessary to appropriately position films and aim the position-indicating device (PID) for either of these techniques.

Common terminology used to describe PID position in relation to the image is vertical and horizontal angulation. *Vertical angulation* is the degree of angulation above or below the neutral line (0°), a line perpendicular to the long axis of the tooth. A negative (–) degree is below the neutral line and a positive (+) degree is above it. *Foreshortened* images result from excessive vertical angulation and *elongated* images from too little. Vertical angulation is intentionally used in bisecting-angle techniques.

Movement of the PID in a direction mesial or distal from the center of the object is known as *horizontal angulation*. Horizontal angulation is used primarily for two reasons. The first of these is to avoid overlapping of structures, sometimes referred to as oblique technique. The second use of horizontal angulation is discussed later as a tube-shift procedure (see Localization Techniques below).

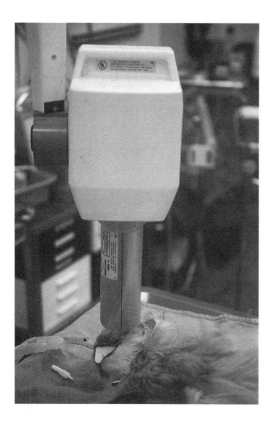

FIG. 4. Parallel technique: film and tooth parallel and primary beam perpendicular.

Paralleling Technique

This technique requires that the film and the long axis of the tooth or object be relatively parallel to each other and that the primary beam be directed perpendicular to these (Fig. 4). To prevent magnification and distortion, the film should be adjacent to the tooth or object. When properly executed, the films are linearly and dimensionally accurate. Unfortunately, the palatal vault and floor of the mouth do not always allow for such close proximity of film and object, while maintaining the paralleling. In these cases, an increase in the object-to-film distance (OFD) is required. Increasing the OFD results in distortion and magnification. An increase in the focal–film distance (FFD) or source-to-film distance (SFD) can dramatically reduce the distortions. Typically, an FFD or SFD increase from 8 inches to 14–18 inches is used, resulting in paralleling technique sometimes being called *long-cone technique*. In the dog, this technique is used most frequently for the mandibular cheek teeth.

Bisecting-Angle Technique

In animals, the restrictions of the palatal vault and floor of the mouth many times do not allow for paralleling technique to adequately demonstrate periapical structures. In these cases, a bisecting-angle technique is utilized. The film is placed as close as possible to the tooth or object, without bending the film. The angle between the tooth's long axis and film is then bisected, and the primary beam is directed perpendicular to the bisecting line (Fig. 5). When appropriately performed, the technique yields film images that are linearly correct, although some slight dimensional distortion of the image on the portion of the film most distant from the tooth will be present. The precept of the bisecting-angle technique is based on the geometric theory of isometric triangles. Image reproduction is good even with the shorter 8-inch cones; this has caused some people to refer to bisecting angle as *short-cone technique*. This usage is improper, however, because both bisecting-angle and paralleling techniques can be performed with either long or short

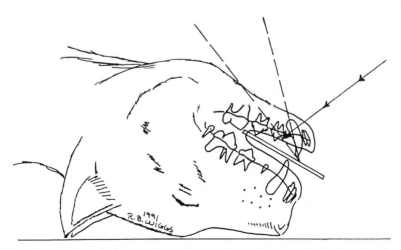

FIG. 5. Bisecting-angle technique: primary beam directed perpendicular to a line that bisects the angle formed by the long axis of the tooth and the film.

cones. Use of the shorter cone does allow for reduction in exposure times, based on the inverse square law. This means the short 8-inch cones require only one-quarter of the exposure time of the long 16-inch cones.

Localization Techniques

Standard dental radiography depicts teeth, bone, and structures in a two-dimensional aspect, which does not distinguish well between the buccolingual planes. Clinically, it is often necessary to radiographically establish the buccal or lingual position of objects or structures in the dental arcade. There are three basic localization techniques available to the veterinarian to establish this information: definition evaluation, right-angle technique, and tube shift.

Definition evaluation is a simple premise that structures lying closest to the x-ray film will show better definition than those farther from the film. This indicates that with standard intraoral radiology, the lingually established structures should demonstrate a higher degree of definition. Although it takes time and practice to be skilled at this technique, it has the advantage of not requiring additional exposures.

Right-angle technique requires two radiographs to be taken, one with the standard paralleling or bisecting-angle technique. The second film is usually placed in the occlusal plane, and the exposure is made perpendicular to the film and at a 90° vertical angulation from the first exposure. The two films are compared, which allows for localization of structures. This technique is primarily used for the mandible, as the complexity of structures in the maxilla causes excessive superimposition on the radiographs. Occasionally, the technique can be modified for the maxilla by reducing the vertical angle to 60–80°, allowing suitable results.

Tube-shift technique is used when two roots or objects are overlapping on a radiograph or are so close that it cannot be determined which is lingual or buccal, so a second radiograph can be taken with an adjustment in the horizontal angulation. The mesial or distal tube shift produces a film in which the images of the overlapped objects will be moved apart. When the tube head is shifted, the lingual object will shift toward the tube head and the buccal object will move away from the tube head. This is known as the *"SLOB"* rule, signifying "same—lingual; opposite—buccal." This technique has also been referred to as the *buccal object rule* and *Clark's rule* (10–12).

Extraoral Techniques

Extraoral radiology has basically three indications for use. The first indication is for the novice veterinary dentist who does not have intraoral films or a dental x-ray machine but does have access to a standard veterinary unit and screen film with cassettes. It should be kept in mind that the smaller intraoral films can be used with standard x-ray units. Although positioning is a little challenging, it is not as awkward as cassette film for dental isolations. In dealing with select structures and teeth, extraoral radiology often cannot provide sufficient detail or accuracy due to superimposition of structures or distortion. The intraoral films are relatively inexpensive and can be developed quickly in rapid dental developer/fixer solutions. The following can be used as a starting point by the practitioner for developing a technique chart for his or her specific equipment. Intraoral films (D speed) can be used with a standard x-ray machine using a technique of 100 mA and a focal distance of 12 inches (0.067–0.1 second) or 36–42 inches (0.4–0.6 seconds). The kilovoltage will vary from 65 kVp for a cat or toy dog, to 70 kVp for a small dog, 75 kVp for a medium-size dog, 80 kVp for a large dog, and up to 85 kVp for a giant breed. With the use of E-speed film, the exposure time can typically be reduced by half.

The second indication for extraoral radiology involves the patient whose mouth cannot be sufficiently opened for placement of intraoral films, even under sedation. Certain myositis diseases (eosinophilic myositis) result in masticatory muscle contractions that restrict or totally prevent opening of the occlusion for intraoral film placement. In temporomandibular joint (TMJ) disease, problems are also encountered. Ankylosis of the TMJ may greatly restrict opening of the mouth. In addition, some patients have histories of TMJ dysfunction and can have ensuing difficulties with oral pain and mastication following oral manipulations. Care must be taken in selecting mouth props to prevent stress or tension on the TMJ and minimization of oral manipulation; otherwise, extraoral radiographic techniques must be used.

The third indication is when the area to be studied is too large to permit adequate use of even the occlusal No.4 intraoral films and still capture an image of the entire lesion. Some portions of the mandible and maxilla cannot be properly radiographed with intraoral technique. Massive injuries are often best studied with the larger extraoral films so that the full extent of pathology can be adequately assessed.

A standard x-ray unit is used at an FFD of 36–42 inches in most cases. Nonscreen 5×7-inch or 8×10-inch films, or 8×10-inch or 10×12-inch screen film with cassettes, may be used. Bisecting-angle and oblique techniques generally provide suitable imaging (15–22).

FILM PROCESSING

After radiographs have been properly exposed and before development, they are said to contain a *latent image*. This means that for the image on the film to be seen, it must be processed or developed. Two basic techniques are used for development: time-temperature technique and sight technique. *Time-temperature development* is based on the manufacturer's recommendations for a specific film and type of developer at time intervals based on the temperature of the solutions. This is the most scientifically correct technique. *Sight development* is the observation by the operator through the safe-light transparent top of a developer box that the film image has emerged, with no specific predetermined time.

Development can be performed in a conventional darkroom or in a chairside developer (Fig. 6). The chairside developer is a light-safe box with a light-selective see-through cover. Hands with film packets and hangers are inserted through light-retardant opening in the front, and the packets are opened and moved through the various solutions with the visual aid of being able to see through the light-retardant transparent top. This allows for processing at or near chairside, which is a tremendous time saver.

Equipment that the veterinarian already has on hand for standard x-ray development may be employed. The standard hand-developing tank may be slow, while automatic processors, with the dental film taped to a "leader" standard film, are not as cost-effective, and films may be lost. A relatively inexpensive and simpler method is the use of dental rapid developers and fixers. These solutions may be placed in small containers in the existing darkroom or in a chairside developer. The film packet is opened under appropriate light restrictions, and the film is attached to a film hanger (either metal or plastic) or a hemostat. After being immersed in water for 5 seconds to hydrate the emulsion, the film

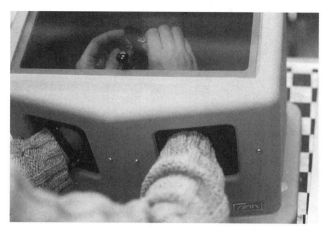

FIG. 6. Chairside developer.

is place in the developer with initial agitation for 15–60 seconds (depending on solution and temperature). Following a water rinse, the film is then placed in the fixer solution with intermittent agitation for approximately twice the developing time. After a final water rinse, initial assessment can be made. The film holders may be suspended for drying or placed in a film-drying stand. Rapid-drying or fix-off products may be used to enhance finishing. Film identification can be facilitated by the used of radiopaque ID numbers placed on the film before the exposure or with marking pens after drying. Films may be displayed in cardboard or plastic mounts, or stored in dental envelopes.

Developer

The *developer solution* makes the latent image visible. This solution classically contains water as a vehicle and five active chemical types. Sodium carbonate is used as an activator to act as an alkaline medium and to soften the gelatin emulsion. There are two developer chemicals, one that quickly develops the image (elon or metol) and a second (hydroquinone) that works slower to develop the contrast. The restrainer (potassium bromide) is a solution to prevent chemical fogging. The last is the preservative (sodium sulfite) to slow oxidation of the developer chemicals and prolong their useful life. The film is then rinsed in a water, sometimes called a stop bath, to remove the developer chemicals and stop the development process. Should the alkaline developer chemical be carried into the acid fixer chemicals, it will weaken the fixer solution.

Fixer

Fixer solutions preserve and enhance the latent image on the film. It is routinely composed of a water vehicle and four active agent groups. An acidifier (acetic acid) provides the needed acid medium for the fixing process. The fixing agent (sodium thiosulfate), sometimes called "hypo," removes the unexposed or undeveloped silver bromide crystals in the gelatin emulsion. A hardening agent (potassium alum) then shrinks and hardens the gelatin emulsion. A preservative (sodium sulfite) slows oxidation of the fixer chemicals to delay their weakening. Once properly fixed, the film is washed in a water bath to remove all fixer solution and then allowed to dry. The processed film is now a radiograph.

Film Identification

Film identification is an extremely important part of film processing. The small intra-oral films do not lend themselves to the normal patient ID tags. Stick-on lead-coated numbers are available for application to the film packet prior to exposure. Once the patient ID number is recorded, the stick-on number can be moved from film to film as additional exposures are taken. To prevent confusion, most developer film hangers come with a white reusable plastic tab, where patient information can be recorded to maintain identity. Once films are dry, white-ink x-ray marker pins can be used to permanently iden-tify films. X-ray envelopes can also be used for both identification and storage of films.

Film Mounts

A large selection of types and sizes of mounts for intraoral films is available. The majority are made from either pressboard, (usually gray in color) or plastic (usually opaque colors or transparent). The clear plastic mounts allow full view of the entire film, but they are more difficult for viewing because they do not block light around the film. Opaque pressboard and plastics improve viewing by blocking light immediately around the film, but at the mount sites a 1-mm margin around the edges of the film is typically lost from view and this may obscure important details. Some newer opaque plastic mounts have a clear plastic pocket for the film that allows full-film viewing.

Film Mounting

Mounting films makes it easier to view, diagnose, chart, and store radiographs. It is a simple procedure, and when radiographs are systematically placed, they are easier to view and review than films on hangers or those loose in envelopes. An understanding of basic oral anatomy is required to appropriately mount, as identification of tooth and tooth area is required.

Films have an embossed, raised dot or button that aids in orientation for mounting. In standard techniques, the film is in the mouth with the dot aimed toward the tooth and toward the radiographic source. If films are mounted with the raised dot toward you, then you are looking at the films as if you were looking into the patient's mouth. This means that the radiographic patient's right is your left. This is known as *labial mounting*. If the films are mounted with the dimple toward you and the dot away, you are viewing the films as though you were looking out of the patient's mouth. This means that the patient's radiographic right is the same as your right. This is known as *lingual mounting*. Both sys-tems are used, and each has its advantages and disadvantages. Labial mounting appears to be slightly more popular, but each clinic should adopt one system or the other accord-ing to personal preference, and stay consistent.

The first step is to arrange all films with the dot in the same direction, according to whether labial or lingual mounting is to be used. Next the films are sorted as to mandib-ular or maxillary. Maxillary teeth typically show radiolucent areas beyond tooth apices representing the nasal cavity or a sinus. Mandibular teeth usually show cortical plates, mental foramina, mandibular canal, or the mandibular symphysis beyond the tooth apices. After this, the teeth must be identified as the patient's right or left side. A basic knowledge of tooth anatomy and the progression of incisor, cuspid, premolar, and molar are usually sufficient to make this identification. With the films now sorted, they are ready to be slipped into the mounts. The patient's name and other information is then recorded on the mount prior to filing.

FILM QUALITY

The diagnostic quality of x-ray film is primarily determined by density, contrast, and definition. The *definition* or *detail* of a film is its inherent ability to reproduce sharp lines of detail. This is dependent on the size of silver halide crystals in the film emulsion. The smaller the crystals are, the finer the detail is, but also the longer the exposure time required. *Density* is the amount of light restriction through the developed film when placed on an illuminator. This is determined by the total radiation exposure that is controlled by the kilovoltage, milliamperage, and exposure time. An increase in any of these factors or a combination of them can increase density. *Contrast* relates to the variation of density on areas of the film—the variation of black and white, or radiolucency and radiopacity. This variation of contrast allows for differentiation between structures and is sometimes referred to as the gray scale. Higher kilovoltage settings (90 kVp) produce a longer gray scale or low contrast. A low kilovoltage setting (70 kVp) at the same milliamperage produces a shorter gray scale or high-contrast film with more black and white rather than grays. Short-scale high-contrast films are preferred by some dentists for detection of interproximal caries. Long-scale low-contrast films show subtle changes in tooth, bone, and cementum, and are preferred by some periodontists. Many of the fixed kilovoltage units are preset to 80 kVp as a compromise between low and high contrast.

Film Faults and Artifacts

Film quality and diagnostic value can be detrimentally affected by various film faults and artifacts (Table 3). The most common faults are incorrect vertical angulation, imprecise horizontal angulation, curving of films, cone cutting, and improper exposure. Inaccurate angulation results in foreshortening, elongation, or overlapping of structures. Curving of films to fit the palatal vault or other restricted areas produces distortion of structures. Cone cutting is the circular pattern of development resulting from improper alignment of position-indicating device (PID) and film.

Film fogging describes when part or all of the developed x-ray film is darkened by sources other than the useful primary beam. This loss of contrast can obscure or hide details on the film, reducing its diagnostic value. *Chemical fogging* occurs when improperly mixed or exhausted processing solutions are used. *Light fogging* results when the film is exposed to a light source before or during processing. *Radiation fogging* follows exposure of the film to radiation other than the useful primary beam. This is typically from scatter or backscatter of radiation off the patient's tissues.

Static electricity can produce artifacts of characteristic dark streaks on the processed radiograph. Generally, this occurs when very dry room air and too forceful opening of the film packet combine to generate a static charge. Pressure from teeth or fingernails sometimes result in light or dark crescent-shaped artifacts. Acute bending of the film results

TABLE 3. *Radiographic and processing faults*

Problem	Possible cause(s)

Dark film	1. Overexposure
	2. Overdevelopment
	   A. Too much time
	   B. Too high a temperature
	   C. Too strong a developer mix
	3. Fog (see "Fogged film" below)

Light film	1. Underexposure
	2. Underdevelopment
	   A. Too little time
	   B. Too cold a temperature
	   C. Exhausted developer
	   D. Contaminated developer
	3. Film exposed through back of packet
	4. Overfixed

Stipple pattern	1. Film exposed through back of packet

Blurred image	1. Movement
	   A. Patient
	   B. Tube head

Magnification	1. Object-to-film distance too long 2. Focal–film distance too short
Distortion	1. Incorrect positioning of primary beam

Fogged film	1. Light-leak fog
	   A. Packet leak
	   B. Darkroom leak
	   C. Defective safe-light
	   D. Loose lid on chairside developer
	   E. Use of wrong lid filter on chairside developer
	      a. Orange (D speed)
	      b. Red (E speed)
	2. Chemical fog
	   A. Overprocessing (developer or fixer)
	      a. Time too long
	      b. Mix too strong
	      c. Temperature too high
	   B. Exhausted chemicals
	3. Radiation fog
	   A. Overexposure
	   B. Scatter
	   C. Backscatter
	4. Storage fog
	   A. Out-of-date films
	   B. Moisture or vapor contamination
	   C. Exposure to heat

Finger prints	1. Improper handling of films; fingers contaminated with chemicals
	   A. White: fixer
	   B. Dark: fluorides (stannous) or developer

Frosty appearance of films	1. Inadequate processing 2. Inadequate fixing 3. Exhausted solutions 4. Inadequate washing
Yellow or brown film staining	1. Inadequate processing 2. Inadequate fixing 3. Exhausted solutions 4. Inadequate washing 5. Contaminated water bath
Green or unprocessed areas	1. Inadequate processing 2. Films touching in processor
Black spots	1. Developer contamination or splash prior to processing
White spots	1. Fixer contamination or splash prior to processing

TABLE 3. *Continued*

Problem	Possible cause(s)
White half-moons or crescents	1. Focal pressure to film prior to exposure
Dark half-moons or crescents	1. Focal pressure to film after exposure and prior to processing
Black or white fine lines	1. Bending or crimping of films—white prior to exposure, black after
Irregular white or clear lines	1. Emulsion scratches or tears
Black marks or black lightening	1. Static electrical charge
Small white or clear circular marks	1. Air bubbles on films during processing
Clear upper portion of film	1. Processing solutions too low
Clear area around circular developed section (cone cutting)	1. Film and position-indicating device not properly aligned
Films clear after processing	1. Films left in water bath for 12–48 hours; emulsion soaks off exposing transparent film base
Film streaks	1. Inadequate processing 2. Contaminated solutions 3. Inadequate washing 4. Contaminated water bath
Reticulation or wrinkled films	1. Developer too hot or water bath too cold
Lost films (fishing for films)	1. Film hangers need replacing, clips worn

in crease artifacts that can be either white or black lines. Finger prints typically result from fixer solution or fluorides on the hands during handling of the film as it is placed in the developer solution (Fig. 7). Film hangers may result in scratches and irregular clear or white-line artifacts. *Reticulation* describes the classic wrinkled appearance that occurs when moving the film from warm developer solution to a cold-water bath causes shrinking of the emulsion. Air bubbles create clear or white spots on the films and are a con-

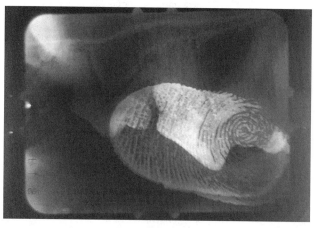

FIG. 7. White finger print on a developed film from fixer solution contamination.

sequence of inadequate agitation of the film to remove air bubbles as it is placed in the developer solution. Delayed clearing of films occurs when developed films are left in water baths in excess of 24 hours, which soaks off the emulsion from the transparent film base. Frosty-appearing films evolve from poor fixation from either too weak a fixer solution or too short a time in the solution. Yellow-to-brown spots or entire films occur from inadequate fixation or washing. Streaks are commonly the outcome of inadequate washing or contaminated water bath. Green areas generally indicate inadequate processing time. White spots are frequently fixer splash or contamination prior to processing; dark spots reflect developer contamination.

RADIOGRAPHIC VIEWING

Systematic viewing procedures must be adhered to in order to derive the maximum quantity of information from each radiograph. An appropriate-size viewbox with uniform light intensity is the first requirement. Use of alternate viewing lights (overhead and surgical lights) is acceptable. Subdued background lighting is preferred to normal room light or total darkness. Light blockers that only allow light to pan through the film and obstruct the remaining viewbox noticeably improve readability. A *"hot light"* should be available for films displaying marginally excessive density or darkness. A magnifying glass is useful for close examination of small detail (12,23,24).

The first step is to examine the radiograph for quality of exposure, processing, and artifacts. It is hazardous to attempt diagnosis from assessments of substandard radiographs. The film should be examined systematically, as though a document were being read, from left to right and top to bottom; every detail should be checked, even on small dental films. Jumping ahead to obvious pathologies can result in missing subtle anomalies.

RADIOGRAPHIC INTERPRETATION

Interpretation starts with three basic steps. First is the identification of the location and structures. Next is the recognition of normal from the abnormal. Finally, there is the diagnosis, or classification of pathology is performed. All of these steps are based on the use of a three-dimensional imagination on a two-dimensional radiographic film. Therefore, multiple views may be necessary for a rational diagnosis.

Proper mounting of the films in association with a basic knowledge of oral anatomy will facilitate identification of location and structures. The assessment of normal from abnormal anatomy requires the recognition of variations in the structures examined. Inspect the structures' contour, internal detail, variation of density, and displacement. When possible, examine two or more views of areas of suspected pathology. This will assist in a better three-dimensional perception of the area. When there is doubt as to normalcy, radiograph the same structures of the opposite arcade for comparison. In some cases, a series of radiographs over a period of time is necessary to determine whether pathology is in a static, active, or regressive stage. Finally, the radiographic findings must correlate with the history, clinical examination, and other diagnostic information before a diagnostic judgment is made.

Preeruption examination of permanent tooth buds is not an uncommon request for certain breeds that require a full complement of 42 teeth for show (Doberman pinscher, German shepherd, rottweiler, etc.) (25). The permanent tooth buds for the cheek teeth are generally found just apical to the deciduous, the incisors and mandibular cuspids apical and slightly lingual, and the maxillary cuspids apical and slightly rostral. It is common to have mixed dentition (combination of permanent and deciduous teeth) in the mouth at one time (see Chapter 7).

Some radiographic changes are due to normal physiologic maturation. There are many *radiographic signs of aging*, both in the teeth and the adjacent support structures (15,26). One of the first recognized in healthy young teeth is closure of apices to form an apical delta. The tooth is a dynamic and vital structure that continues to lay new layers of secondary dentin within the pulp cavity, resulting in its progressive narrowing (see Chapter 7). The alveolus shows increased density and coarseness of the trabecular bone pattern, and the radicular cortical plate or lamina dura becomes less distinct with age. Additionally, the alveolar crest may demonstrate signs of regression, or slight cupping (concavitation) between teeth.

When teeth are missing, radiographs are the primary diagnostic tool for determining whether the tooth is congenitally missing or impacted (27). *Impacted teeth* usually have a slight lucency around the crown. They may be covered with a cortical plate cap and be *bony impactions* or by a gingival cap and be known as a *soft tissue impaction*.

Supernumerary teeth and *roots* are sometimes found on radiographs. Supernumerary impacted teeth may need extraction if in tight contact with the root structure of adjacent teeth, as root resorption may occur. Supernumerary roots are primarily of importance in endodontic and exodontic treatments (10).

Enamel pearls or *enamelomas* are small enamel spheres found on the root structure. Radiographically, they appear as areas that are more radiopaque on the root structure. They may cause periodontal inflammation and require surgical removal (28).

Determination between *gemination* and *fusion teeth* can sometimes be made easier with radiographs. Gemination teeth typically have two crowns, each with a separate pulp chamber merging into a common root canal system. Fusion teeth also have two crowns, but with two distinct root canal and root systems.

Concrescence is when the cementum of two teeth is joined. *Dens invaginatus* is an invagination of the enamel organ back into the tooth. This results in exposed dentin or pulp and the rapid devitalization of the tooth upon eruption. The term *dens in dente* (tooth within a tooth) is also used for this condition, but this is a misnomer as dens invaginatus is truly an invagination and not a tooth within a tooth.

Dilaceration is simply a permanent distortion of the crown or root structure. Dilacerated crowns can pose esthetic problems, and dilacerated roots may complicate endodontic and exodontic difficulty.

Taurodontia is a condition of an enlarged crown and pulp cavity in association with reduced root structure. Suspected cases can be confirmed radiographically.

Caries and *resorptive lesions* are visualized on radiographs as radiolucencies in the crown, cervical area, or roots. The demineralization of hard tooth tissue results in decreased density. Radiographs are often used to aid in determining the stage of destruction and the prognosis for treatment (29–31).

Ankylosis occurs when the periodontal ligament that separates the root cementum and alveolar bone is lost and the two hard structures merge (Fig. 8). Radiographically, this is seen as a loss of the lamina dura and loss of root detail in the alveolar bone. These findings are common sequelae of developing feline resorptive lesions and occlusal trauma.

Periodontal disease is accompanied by a combination of hard and soft tissue changes (10). It must be understood that various stages of periodontal disease can exist in the same mouth at the same time. Early periodontal disease is marked by interproximal crestal bone changes (resorption) and triangulation of the crestal periodontal ligament. The

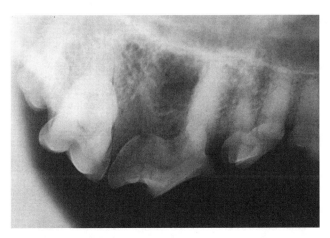

FIG. 8. Radiograph showing ankylosis of the root to the surrounding alveolar bone, indicated by radiographic loss of the lamina dura and root detail.

interproximal crestal bone should show a straight and level radiopaque line running from 1–2 mm below the cemenoenamel junction (CEJ) of one tooth to that of the proximal CEJ of the adjacent tooth. Loss of density of these septa and cup-like depressions are signs of early periodontal disease. Additionally, triangulation or a slight widening of the periodontal ligament at the crestal margin is sometimes observed. In *moderate periodontal disease*, additional bone loss up to 50% occurs. Both horizontal and vertical bone loss can be seen, as well as loss of bone in the furcation areas. With vertical bone loss, infrabony pockets may develop. In *advanced periodontal disease*, a loss of greater than 50% of the bone attachment has occurred, furcation involvement is common, and the periodontal ligament space may widen, indicating tooth movement or mobility.

Periapical lesions are generally associated with endodontic devitalization. This lesion appears as a radiolucency surrounding the tooth apex with loss of the lamina dura in the immediate area (Fig. 9). Fistulous tracts from these are seldom observed on radiographs, unless a fistulogram is taken. This requires the injection of radiopaque material into the fistula to trace its path and a radiograph is then taken.

Periodontal abscesses can occur in any stage of periodontal disease and vary radiographically in signs from none in acute episodes to extensive bone loss in semiacute and chronic cases. These typically occur from occlusion of a deep pocket, with rampant production of toxins, fragments of calculus, or other debris impaling the periodontal structures.

Pulp changes and lesions can also be found on radiographs. *Pulp stones* (*endoliths*) or *calcifications* may appear as radiopacities within the pulp cavity. Clinically, they do not appear to cause pathosis. Endodontic instrumentation appears to be the main problem concerning endoliths. Those found in the chamber can usually be worked around or removed, but those in the root canal can prevent proper instrumentation.

Pulpitis does not show radiographic signs, except when *internal resorption* is occurring. This can present itself as a well defined radiolucency spreading into the dentin from the pulp cavity or as an irregular widening of the canal or chamber. *External resorption* appears as an irregular loss of root structure. Loss of the lamina dura is also common in these lesions. In many cases, external resorptive lesions may appear to be internal, as they lay on the root over the canal. A second radiograph at a more mesial or distal angle will usually move external lesions, aiding in their differential diagnosis.

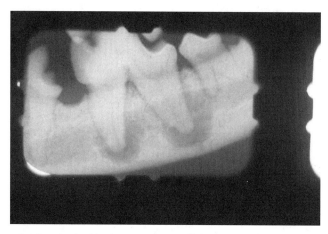

FIG. 9. Radiograph of periapical lesion seen as radiolucency around apex and loss of lamina dura, generally associated with endodontic pathology.

Hypercementosis is the increased layering of cementum in the apical third of the root structure. Radiographically, it appears as a club-like root tip, instead of a tapering contour. *Cementomas* (fibro-osteoma) are occasionally found on radiographs. They are generally asymptomatic and self-limiting, and require no treatment. They typically develop in a three-stage sequence (10). In the first stage, the lesion appears as a radiolucency around the root apex, appearing identical to periapical disease, but the tooth is still vital. In the second stage, some radiopaque densities occur within the radiolucency. In the third stage, the entire lesion becomes radiopaque.

In *traumatic injuries* of teeth or bone, fractures are the most common symptom. They appear as radiolucent lines across the hard tissues. Jaw and crown fractures are easier to detect than those of roots. The superimposition of alveolar bone can aid in concealing true root fractures and sometimes, due to anatomic shadows, can give the false appearance of fractures that are not present. Multiple views are always prudent in suspected cases.

Salivary stones (*sialoliths*) are calcifications found in salivary glands or ducts. Appearing as radiopaque objects in the oral soft tissues, they most commonly involve the mandibular ducts, causing obstruction of salivary flow; however, they can be found in association with any of the salivary glands (32–34).

Imaging of the salivary glands is occasionally needed for diagnosis of pathology or identification of involved gland. *Saliograms* can be made by isolating the papilla to the duct of a gland. A small-gauge catheter is manipulated into the duct and 0.5–1.5 mL of a radiopaque contrast solution injected to delineate the duct and gland. A radiography is then immediately taken for the actual sialogram.

Pathologies of the *temporomandibular joint (TMJ)* or *craniomandibular articulation (CMA)* vary in radiographic signs according to the problem (35,36). Luxations are fairly obvious because of the separation of the joint. Dysplasias may show no signs, widening of the joint, ankylosis, joint mouse, irregular articular surface, or variations in bone density. The major problem is obtaining diagnostic-quality radiographs because of the superimposition of other complex structures in the area. In many cases, multiple views are required to obtain even minimal information. Both ventrodorsal (VD) and dorsoventral (DV) extraoral techniques can provide some information. A lateral oblique view with the head slightly rotated (nose pointing up—sagittal view) and the primary beam aimed at the TMJ just below the ear can also provide information. The lateral oblique can be taken in open- and closed-mouth positions for slightly varying views. With a dental x-ray unit, the small-tube position-indicating device can sometimes be positioned in the mouth, with the film extraoral, to better isolate the TMJ.

Craniomandibular osteopathy is generally a condition of the horizontal ramus (37,38). Clinically, a swelling of either or both posterior jaws, together with pain and malaise, may be associated with the disease. Radiographically, a proliferative periosteal reaction with bone deposition occurs. In some cases, the reaction also occurs in the temporal bone, causing pain, dysphagia, and atrophy of the temporal musculature.

The most notable signs of *osteomyelitis* of the jaws is proliferative reaction of the periosteum at the periphery of the lesion with lysis of the associated cortical and alveolar bone. In the oral region, fractures and tooth infections are commonly an initiating force. The bone lysis may give the appearance that teeth are supported primarily by soft tissue, but seldom are the teeth displaced as is seen with many cysts and tumors.

In the oral tissues, both cysts and tumors may occasionally be found (37,39,40). *Cysts* appear as radiolucencies, while *tumors* may present as radiopacities or radiolucencies. The radiolucency of cysts or tumors indicates the loss or destruction of the normal tissues and replacement by cyst or tumor tissue. These lesions commonly displace adjacent structures causing serious destructive damage.

REVIEW QUESTIONS

1. X-radiation
   A. Travels at 186,000 mph in a vacuum.
   B. Has no mass.
   C. Is in the electromagnetic spectrum.
   D. Is composed of photon energy.
   E. All of the above.
2. X-radiation is measured in
   A. Angstrom (Å).
   B. Frequency.
   C. Wavelength.
   D. Lambda (λ) units.
   E. All of the above.
3. The person who is given credit for having discovered x-radiation and received the first Noble Prize in physics is
   A. L.H. Crooke.
   B. P.E. Coolidge.
   C. Otto Walkhoff.
   D. W.C. Roentgen.
   E. C. Edmund Kells.
4. The person given credit for having produced the first dental radiograph is
   A. C. Edmund Kells.
   B. Otto Walkhoff.
   C. William Rollins.
   D. William J. Morton.
   E. W.C. Roentgen.

5. A 110 volt, 60 Hz, AC dental unit with a pulse timer set to 24 will have a _____ second exposure.
   A. 0.1
   B. 0.2
   C. 0.4
   D. 0.6
   E. 0.8

6. The distance from the film to the focal spot of the tube head is the
   A. FFD.
   B. MFP.
   C. OFD.
   D. FOD.
   E. FFA.

7. Radiation biology is significant in radiology because of
   A. Kilovoltage (kVp).
   B. Milliamperage per second (mA/sec).
   C. Ionization.
   D. Milliampere (mA).
   E. Atomization.

8. The five common intraoral dental film sizes are
   A. A, B, C, D, E.
   B. 1, 2, 3, 4, 5.
   C. VS, S, I, U, E.
   D. 0, 1, 2, 3, 4.
   E. A, E, I, O, U.

9. Current ADA intraoral film speeds are
   A. A, B, C, D, E, F.
   B. 1, 2, 3, 4, 5, 6.
   C. VS, S, I, U, E, L.
   D. 0, 1, 2, 3, 4, 5.
   E. A, E, I, O, U, W.

10. The technique of placement of the film as close to the tooth as possible and then dividing the angle between the two and directing the primary beam perpendicular to this angle is known as
   A. Paralleling technique.
   B. Bisecting-angle technique.
   C. Localization technique.
   D. Tube-shift technique.
   E. Right-angle technique.

11. The "SLOB" rule means
   A. So long ole boy.
   B. Slide lateral object back.
   C. Same lingual original back.
   D. Slow lingual original buccal.
   E. Same lingual opposite buccal.

12. Film fog can be caused by
   A. Chemicals.
   B. Storage.
   C. Radiation.

D. Light leaks.
E. All of the above.

Answers

1. E; 2. E; 3. D; 4. B; 5. C; 6. A; 7. B; 8. D; 9. A; 10. B; 11. E; 12. E

REFERENCES

1. *Dentists' Desk Reference*. 2nd ed. American Dental Association; Chicago, Illinois: 1983:269;367.
2. Ter-Pogossian MM. *The Physical Aspects of Diagnostic Radiography*. New York: Hoeber Co; 1976.
3. Johns HE, Cunningham JR. *The Physics of Radiology*. Springfield IL: Charles C Thomas; 1974:557.
4. National Council on Radiation Protection and Measurements. *Ionizing Radiation Exposure of the Population of the United States*. NCRP Report No.93; Washington, DC: 1987.
5. National Council on Radiation Protection and Measurements. *Recommendations on Limits for Exposure to Ionizing Radiation*. NCRP Report No.91; Washington, DC: 1987.
6. Performance standards for electronic products: Diagnostic x-ray systems and their major components. *Federal Register* 1972;37:16461.
7. Wilkins EM. *Clinical Practice for the Dental Hygienist*. 5th ed. Philadelphia: Lea & Febiger; 1983:131.
8. Richardson RE, Barton RE. *The Dental Assistant*. 5th ed. New York: McGraw-Hill Book Co; 1978:341.
9. Torres HO, Ehrlich A. *Modern Dental Assisting*. 2nd ed. Philadelphia: WB Saunders Co; 1980:515.
10. Frommer HH. *Radiology for Dental Auxiliaries*. 3rd ed. St Louis, MO: CV Mosby Co; 1983:1,168,268.
11. Wolf RDL, Johnson ON. *Essentials of Dental Radiology for Dental Assistants and Hygienists*. 4th ed. Norwalk CT: Appleton and Lange; 1990:1.
12. Miles DA, Van Dis ML, Razmus TF. *Basic Principles of Oral and Maxillofacial Radiology*. Philadelphia: WB Saunders Co; 1992:37.
13. Silha RE. Methods for reducing patient exposure combined with Kodak Ekta-speed dental x-ray film. *Dent Radiogr Photogr* 1981;54:80.
14. Dawood FF, Manson-Hing LR. Evaluation of new radiographic screens for intraoral radiography. *Oral Surg Oral Med Oral Pathol* 1979;48:178.
15. Zontine WJ. Dental radiographic technique and interpretation. *Vet Clin North Am* 1974;4(4):741.
16. Morgan JP, Silverman S, Zontine WJ. *Techniques of Veterinary Radiography*. Davis CA: The Printer, Davis, California;1975:120.
17. Morris E, Smallwood JE. The inferior teeth of the dog. In: *Radiographic Aids*. Chicago: The Quaker Oats Co; 1978. Series 10, fall.
18. Morris E, Smallwood JE. The superior teeth of the dog. In: *Radiographic Aids*. Chicago: The Quaker Oats Co; 1978. Series 10, spring.
19. Morris E, Smallwood JE. The canine skull. In: *Radiographic Aids*. Chicago: The Quaker Oats Co; 1977. Series 10, summer.
20. Morris E, Smallwood JE. The dolichocephalic skull. In: *Radiographic Aids*. Chicago: The Quaker Oats Co; 1979. Series 11, winter.
21. Morris E, Smallwood JE. The brachycephalic skull. In: *Radiographic Aids*. Chicago: The Quaker Oats Co; 1980. Series 12, summer.
22. Morris E, Smallwood JE. The head of the cat. In: *Radiographic Aids*. Chicago: The Quaker Oats Co; 1979. Series 11, fall.
23. Douglas SW, Williamson HD. *Veterinary Radiological Interpretation*. Philadelphia: Lea & Febiger; 1970:14.
24. Carlson, WD. *Veterinary Radiology*. 2nd ed. Philadephia: Lea & Febiger; 1971:11.
25. Wiggs RB. Intraoral radiology: Basic technique and equipment. Cent Vet Conf Proceedings. Kansas City, Missouri: Sept. 26–29, 1992:115.
26. Zontine WJ. Canine dental radiology: Radiographic technic, development, and anatomy of teeth. *J Am Vet Radiol Soc* 1975;16(3):75.
27. Eisner ER. Intraoral radiography: An indispensable diagnostic aid. *J Vet Med* 1988;88:1131.
28. Ross DL. Dental diagnostic and therapeutic techniques. *JAVMA* 1972;161:1426.
29. Gardner AF, Drake BH, Keary GT. Dental caries in the domesticated dogs. *JAVMA* 1962;140:433.
30. Kaplan B. Root resorption of the permanent teeth of a dog. *JAVMA* 1967;151:708.
31. Lewis TM. Resistance of dogs to caries: A two-year study. *J Dent Res* 1965;44:1354.
32. Glen JB. Salivary cysts in the dog: Identification of sublingual defects by sialography. *Vet Rec* 1966;78:488.
33. Harvey CE. Sialography in the dog. *J Am Vet Radiol Soc* 1969;10:18.
34. Karbe E, Nielsen SW. Canine ranulas, salivary mucoceles and branchial cysts. *J Small Anim Pract* 1966;7:625.

35. Ticer JW, Spencer CP. Injury of the feline temporomandibular joint: Radiographic signs. *J Am Vet Radiol Soc* 1978;19:146.
36. Morris E, Smallwood JE. The temporomandibular joints and tympanic bullae of the dog. In: *Radiographic Aids.* Chicago: The Quaker Oats Co; 1979. Series 11, spring.
37. Lee R. Radiographic examination of localized and diffuse tissue swellings in the mandibular and pharyngeal area. *Vet Clin North Am* 1974;4:723.
38. Riser WH, Parkes LJ, Shirer JF. Canine craniomandibular osteopathy. *J Am Vet Radiol Soc* 1967;8:23.
39. Hardy WD, Brodey RS, Riser WH. Osteosarcoma of the canine skull. *J Am Vet Radiol Soc* 1967;8:5.
40. Farrow CS. Radiographic characterization of an intermandibular mass in a dog. *J Mod Vet Pract* 1985;6:386.

7

Pedodontics

Robert B. Wiggs and Heidi B. Lobprise

Pedodontics is the branch of dentistry that deals with the care of oral or dental structures of immature individuals or mature individuals with immature structures. Endodontics, orthodontics, oral surgery, and possibly prosthodontics are a few of the branches of dentistry that may be involved with the pedodontic patient. Because the deciduous teeth are replaced somewhat quickly in cats and dogs, many problems they experience are sometimes misunderstood, overlooked, or disregarded. Even with young permanent teeth, dental problems are usually not anticipated, since the prevalence of periodontal disease seen in older patients is typically not realized. These teeth have their own unique set of potential problems, and failure to address them properly may eventually lead to detrimental effects on them and systemic health.

DEVELOPMENT

Similar to a developing fetus in the uterus, developing, rapidly changing tooth precursors exist in a very delicate balance (1–3). The longitudinal *dental lamina* is formed when the ectodermal epithelium pushes into the mesodermal tissues underneath. The tooth buds are formed, with the deciduous and permanent buds beginning near the same time (4). The permanent bud will stay quiescent for a while as the primary bud, or enamel organ, begins to differentiate into the formative layers of the tooth (see Chapter 3). The sequence of this delay allows for the increase in jaw length and width that will be necessary to accommodate the permanent teeth.

During tooth development, whether deciduous or primary, various stimuli can cause disruptions that can be grossly manifested in the erupted tooth (5,6). Inflammation, trauma, infection, systemic disease, and endocrine activity can all adversely affect the proper formation of enamel, dentin, cementum, roots, pulp, and bone (7). Additionally, during development of dental tissues, the presence of certain compounds, such as tetracycline or fluoride, can cause their excessive accumulation and affect mineralization (eg, fluorosis). While discoloration may be the only problem with tetracyclines, fluorosis and inflammatory disruptions of tooth development may result in a weaker tooth with a reduced percentage of inorganic matrix, or *hypocalcification*. Much research on fluorosis in animals has been performed (8). Hypocalcification of the enamel is probably the most common sequela seen from many of the above mentioned influences, which will result in a softer, discolored, chalky, pitted-enamel surface, often mistermed hypoplasia

(9,10). *Enamel hypoplasia* actually means a thin or reduced enamel layer on an area of a tooth either from reduced production or pressure on an enamel bud during development, causing a spreading or thinning of the enamel in an area. Hypoplastic enamel can be fully mineralized, not soft or discolored, just thin. However, enamel hypoplasia is commonly found in association with enamel hypocalcification.

While these influences are often systemic, as mentioned previously, the close proximity of the primary teeth to their permanent tooth-bud counterparts may induce problems with the underlying buds ranging from structural and positional problems to eruption abnormalities (5). Additionally, facial trauma has been found to result in enamel defects in animals with developing teeth (6).

Development of Other Oral Structures

Other areas of development that can play significant roles in oral health are the closures of the soft and hard tissues of the palate in the fetus and the growth of jaw length in the young animal. In forming the palate, the maxillary processes do not join at the midline at their most rostral aspect. Instead, they join to the *incisal area*, formally termed the *premaxilla*, forming a Y-shaped fusion. This central rostral portion is termed the *primary palate*, while the two maxillary sides that join at the midline caudal to this are called the *secondary palate*. Complete development in this area is susceptible to outside stimuli, and abnormalities are not extremely uncommon.

Another complex process is the growth of the maxillae and mandibles. The development of each of the four jaw quadrants is genetically determined independently of others (11), as is tooth form, which is the least likely feature to change (11). While most of the time this process is well coordinated, many factors may influence bone growth, including genetics, hormones, tooth development, and soft tissues (muscles and lips) (12). This is particularly evident in the Shar-Pei breed, which has a high incidence of mandibular tight-lip syndrome in which the lip can cover and interfere with occlusion of the lower incisors and canines (Fig. 1). Experimental extraction of deciduous teeth and/or permanent tooth buds has been shown to effect jaw development (13), and injuries to the region can cause severe abnormalities. Even the normal interlock of a dog's teeth in the closed-mouth position contributes to functional influences.

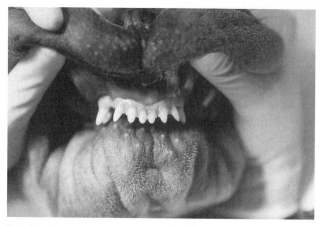

FIG. 1. Shar-Pei tight lip with mandibular lip folded back over the canines and incisors.

ERUPTION OF TEETH

Eruption is classically thought of as the appearance of the tooth through the oral mucosa. However, in reality, it is a continuous process that begins with the formation of the tooth bud and stops only when the tooth is lost or the host dies (7). The rapidity of tooth eruption and movement in relationship to the jaws varies greatly due to many physiologic and pathologic stimuli, but teeth are always in a state of eruption or movement, unless ankylosed, impacted, cystic, or lost.

Eruption can be classified as to movement and eruptive stages (7). As the tooth germ develops from the dental lamina, the jaws are also rapidly growing. The dental germ must therefore move as it grows to keep position in the developing jaws; this movement activity is known as the *preeruptive phase*. Once the crown has formed and root formation begins, the *prefunctional phase* of eruption begins. The *functional phase* initiates when a tooth comes into occlusion and ends when that tooth is ankylosed or lost, or shortly after an animal becomes deceased.

The crown structure's formation is typically well underway or even complete before that of the root (4). The specific mechanism of eruption is not fully known, but it is probably initiated and driven by multiple complex factors (see Chapter 3).

The eruptional pressures of the permanent successional tooth in association with physiologic activity of the periodontal ligament of the primary tooth play an integral role in the dissolution of the root and eventual exfoliation of the deciduous precursors (14). Many influences play a role in the loss of deciduous teeth, including genetic, hormonal and nutritional (14–16). Even if the root is completely resorbed, any type of ankylosis of the crown to alveolar bone can result in its remaining solidly in place (14). Any delay in the *exfoliation* of the primary teeth will typically cause the permanent teeth to be deflected or delayed in their eruption. The majority of the teeth will erupt in a more lingual position, although in animals such as the canine and feline families in which a diastema is present between the maxillary cuspids and incisors, the maxillary cuspids will erupt rostrally to the persistent or retained deciduous tooth (9,17). Eruption sequences for the deciduous and permanent teeth of the dog and cat are given in Table 1.

TABLE 1. *Eruption sequence of the deciduous and permanent teeth of the dog and cat*

	Deciduous (wk)	Permanent (mo)
Dog		
Incisors	3–4	3–4
Canines (cuspids)	3	4–6
Premolars	4–12	4–6
Molars		5–7
Cat		
Incisors	2–3	3–4
Canines (cuspids)	3–4	4–5
Premolars	3–6	4–6
Molars		4–5
Deciduous dental formulas[a]		
Dog: 2 × (Id 3/3; Cd 1/1; Pd 3/3) = 28		
Cat: 2 × (Id 3/3; Cd 1/1; Pd 3/2) = 26		

[a]Identification of deciduous teeth in the Triadan system uses the 500 sequence for right maxillary, 600 for left maxillary, 700 for left mandibular, and 800 for right mandibular (18,19) (see Chapter 4).

Anomalies of Tooth Eruption

Retarded eruption of teeth may effect either or both the primary and permanent dentition. Imbalances of the endocrine system, such as those associated with hypothyroidism, cretinism, hypogonadism, mongolism, and hypopituitarism, can cause retarded tooth eruption in primates (7), and similar disturbances in the dog and cat are assumed to cause a similar effect. Single-tooth retarded eruption is generally due to local factors and is more commonly seen in association with the permanent dentition. Early loss of a primary tooth and closure of the space occupied by it can occasionally retard eruption of a successional tooth (7). Additionally, retained deciduous teeth can also delay successional tooth eruption (see Immature Permanent Tooth Pathology below for a discussion of treatment).

Failure of tooth eruption can be seen in primary or permanent teeth, involving individual teeth, multiples of teeth, or all teeth. Failure of tooth eruption can be caused by many complications, including partial or total absence of tooth development (anodontia), abnormalities in tooth development (cyst formation), and tooth malpositioning (ankylosis or impaction).

Total anodontia indicates the total absence of teeth due to a failure in development. *Partial anodontia* is also the result of a failure in development; however, only a portion of the dentition is involved. Both conditions are typically hereditary and may be associated with ectodermal dysplasia (14,18). Individual tooth germs may also fail to develop, but they are seldom associated with generalized anomalies. In the dog, individual missing teeth are seen in all tooth categories, but premolars appear to be the most commonly affected group. In primates, missing maxillary lateral incisors and 3rd molars are more commonplace (7).

Abnormalities in tooth development can affect the eruption process (7). Tooth buds or germs may fail to grow in a normal sequence, resulting in incomplete or abnormal tooth development and failure of eruption. These problems are seen in association with primary and permanent teeth. Radiographs are typically used to identify incomplete, abnormal, or cystic dental development. If the tooth germ develops but undergoes cystic degeneration prior to the apposition of enamel or dentin, it is identified as a *primordial cyst*. The space for these teeth are edentulous with cysts. Tooth formation may also develop to the stage of apposition of enamel and dentin, and then the enamel organ can undergo cystic transformation. These cysts, called *dentigerous cysts*, typically surround the crown of an incompletely formed or erupted tooth. Disturbances in the morphogenic development of the tooth enamel, dentin, or cementum may result in teeth that form but are irregularly mixed in a mineralized mass. These masses are called *odontomas*. Each of these entities can radically effect jaw symmetry, result in a failure to erupt, and require surgical intervention (see Chapter 5). Treatments are addressed later in in this chapter (see Immature Permanent Tooth Pathology below).

Tooth malpositioning can also result in eruption disturbances due to the abnormal location in the jaws (7,14). In humans, horizontal impaction of the 3rd molars and maxillary cuspids are common examples of this form of eruptive failure (7). In the dog, horizontal impaction of the maxillary or mandibular cuspids is the most common example seen by these authors. This is generally considered to result from failure of the tooth to undergo normal preeruptive movements (7,14).

Submerged teeth are those that are covered by bone and may also be ankylosed. *Shortened teeth* are those that are lower than expected in the occlusal plane. Submerged and shortened teeth may occur in either primary or permanent teeth. Shortened teeth typically result from one of two factors. The first is traumatic injury to the root area resulting in root ankylosis prior to full eruption. The second is traumatic impaction, as is seen in base-narrow canine teeth that make traumatic contact with the roof of the mouth. Even when orthodontics moves these teeth labially out from the traumatic restriction, they commonly fail to erupt further without orthodontic extrusion, if the condition has persisted for several months before correction. An *operculum*, or tough fibrous gingival covering, may persist over the crown of a tooth that has erupted to nearly full height, giving the appearance of an unemerged tooth.

DECIDUOUS TOOTH PATHOLOGY

Deciduous Tooth Anomalies

With the limited number of deciduous teeth as compared with permanent teeth in the dog (not as much of a discrepancy in the cat), some young animals may be presented for missing teeth, when in fact the whole complement may be there. If deciduous teeth are missing (*oligodontia* or *partial anodontia*) it may be due to tooth loss from normal exfoliation or to trauma, neither of which is a serious clinical problem. However, there can be some correlation to missing deciduous teeth and their permanent successional counterparts. Since the dental lamina of the successional tooth normally splits off from the deciduous lamina, should the deciduous tooth be missing due to failure of lamina development, theoretically the permanent tooth cannot develop. However, a missing deciduous tooth may have been lost to trauma or resorptive action, in which case a permanent successional tooth would most likely develop (7,10) (see Anomalies of Tooth Eruption above).

Radiographs to check for retained roots or nonerupted teeth may be warranted. Surveys done at 8–12 weeks will also allow the practitioner to assess the presence of the permanent tooth buds as well. At times, supernumerary, peg, gemination, or fusion deciduous teeth may be seen, but if there is no problem such as a compromised endodontic system, crowding, malocclusion, or periodontal disease, monitoring until exfoliation is generally acceptable.

Deciduous Endodontics

If the crown of a deciduous tooth is broken off, it should be determined whether or not the pulp has been exposed; pulp exposure is highly likely, given the large size of the pulp chambers of these teeth. Extraction is generally the treatment of choice to remove any chance of a periapical infection that could damage the underlying permanent tooth bud. However, by releasing dental interlocks, extraction may allow potential malocclusions to progress or develop. In these cases, endodontic treatment of the primary tooth may be selected, possibly *pulp capping* with calcium hydroxide to stimulate the formation of a dentinal bridge in minimally contaminated or injured pulp that has been recently exposed. If pulpal exposure is more extensive with moderate hemorrhage and some contamination, *pulpotomy*, or the removal of a portion of the exposed pulp, is followed by the calcium hydroxide application and closure. Complete *pulpectomy* is reserved for an infected or nonvital pulp. This procedure involves removing all pulpal debris, flushing copiously with sterile saline, and filling with either zinc oxide–eugenol paste or calcium hydroxide if resorption has already started, together with access closure with either a permanent or temporary filling material (20). Such treatment should not alter the normal exfoliation process, but the tooth is best monitored during the anticipated eruption time of the permanent. With the limited life span of these teeth in most animals, extraction is the most commonly selected treatment plan; however, it must be properly performed to reduce the chances of injury to the unerupted permanent teeth in close proximity. It must also be understood that any "presumed" deciduous tooth fracture or loss during permanent eruption times may actually be normal exfoliation, and confirmation with radiographs may be required to make that determination.

Deciduous Malocclusions and Orthodontics

Malocclusions in young dogs and cats with deciduous dentitions, which are best termed *deciduous malocclusions*, are not unusual. A fairly mild malpositioning of the jaw positions could be due to a temporary disproportionate relationship caused by an independent jaw growth surge (21). If left on its own, there is a chance that the opposing jaw will soon experience its own surge in growth to return it to the correct relationship, if genetically coded to do so. Maturation usually evens out this unique growth pattern between the jaws, with the mandible typically experiencing the later growth of the two. One problem that can result in the interim, however, is the abnormal or malignant interlocking of deciduous teeth in a relationship opposite to their norm or impinging on soft tissue. One of the most common deciduous malocclusions involves excessive growth mandible with the incisors becoming rostral (labial) to the maxillary incisors. While this is certainly anticipated in brachycephalic breeds, in others, this interlock may have serious consequences. With mechanical interference such as this, maxillary growth could be hindered, keeping the jaw relationship abnormal. If still in this position when the permanent maxillary incisors begin to erupt, affected teeth will come in even further lingually, especially if the maxillary deciduous incisors are retained.

One possible option in handling this situation is a procedure termed *interceptive orthodontics*, which is the selective extraction, usually of deciduous teeth, to attempt to help resolve a potential permanent malalignment or malocclusion (21,22). This is done by removing the teeth that are causing the unfavorable mechanical interlock, so the animal may have the possibility of realizing its true genetic potential of jaw growth (hopefully, a normal pattern), time allowing. An owner must understand that if the patient's genetic tendency is for an abnormal jaw-length relationship (eg, brachygnathism, prognathism, or brachycephaly), interceptive extractions will not alter the outcome. In addition, the extractions ideally are done as soon as possible between 4–8 weeks of age (no later than 12 weeks) to allow any potential normalization of the growth pattern before eruption of the successional teeth and reinterlocking of the bite pattern. In individual cases, extractions later than 12 weeks may yield successful results, but this is the exception.

While some advocate the removal of the cuspids and incisors of the "shorter" jaw, there are many instances in which this could be a detriment. Therefore, each case should be evaluated individually by trying to determine the ultimate effect of each extraction. In *deciduous class III malocclusions* or the prognathic-like patient (mandibular jaw longer than maxillary) with the mandibular incisors in labioversion to the maxillary incisors, the mandibular cuspids are often close to or touching the maxillary corner (3rd) incisors. If this is the case, the interlock formed by these two teeth on both sides may be the only reason the mandible has not grown out further, and this interlock should be preserved (9). Thus, the maxillary central and intermediate incisors should be extracted bilaterally, as well as possibly the mandibular corner incisors if their interlock is not required.

In *deciduous class II malocclusions* or the brachygnathic-like patient (mandibular jaw shorter than maxillary), any mandibular incisors or cuspids that are contacting or indenting into the palate or other soft tissue should ordinarily be extracted, or have crown amputation and pulp capping performed. It is most important with the mandibular cuspids, whether displaced distally and/or medially (*base narrow*), that treatment be undertaken as soon as the condition is identified (Fig.2). With a firm-holding indentation into the palate, not only can these teeth interfere with the forward growth of the mandible (even to the point of mandibular downward bowing), but they can also disrupt the normal lateral growth, exacerbating the width-discrepancy problem. If the teeth are lightly contacting the edge of the gingiva, causing a slight indentation, gingivoplasty to remove the indentation (creating a gingival incline plane) and gentle digital pressure of the mandibular cuspids outward (labially) may improve or even correct the problem. However, should extractions be necessary, early initiation of therapy to release the interlock and, hopefully, avoid further medial deflection of the permanent teeth as they erupt is crucial to the chances of success (23).

Grossly abnormal dentitions, such as wry bite, may require exodontia, just to provide the patient with a functional or comfortable malocclusion. *Wry mouth* describes when one of the four jaw quadrants is grossly out of proportion to the others, causing a facial deviation from the midline (22). This is typically either genetic in origin or the result of facial trauma affecting bone growth. Trauma problems vary greatly, but facial bites by the mother or litter mates have been seen to cause wry mouth. Genetic wry bites may cause either a shortening or elongation of one of the jaw quadrants, although elongation may be more prevalent. While traumatically acquired, wry mouth almost always results from a shortening of one quadrant due to effects from reduced or anomalous bone growth.

Retained deciduous teeth following initiation of eruption of the successional permanent tooth, as a rule, necessitates the extraction of the deciduous tooth. The factors influencing exfoliation are numerous (see Chapter 3). The *rule of dental succession* is simple: No successional and deciduous precursor teeth should be erupted simultaneously or in competition for the same dental arcade space at any time. Most of the permanent teeth will be erupting lingually to the primary tooth, with two exceptions: the maxillary cuspids and

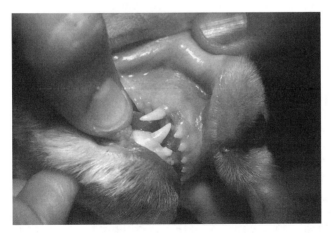

FIG. 2. Base-narrow deciduous canines with linguoversion (no distal deviation), hitting the palate.

the 4th premolars. The permanent maxillary cuspids erupt rostrally to their deciduous precursors in species with an associated diastema. The permanent maxillary 4th premolar erupts buccally and slightly distally to the last deciduous cheek tooth—the opposite of the eruption pattern of most of the other permanent teeth. However, if there is any doubt whatsoever, radiographs should be taken for confirmation. For the most accurate documentation, pre- and postoperative radiographs can be taken to confirm extraction of the correct teeth and presence of the permanent teeth and/or buds in any suspicious areas. If a deciduous tooth fails to develop its normal permanent successor, it does not necessarily have to be extracted, but the owner must be aware that it is a primary tooth and probably will eventually be lost. Such teeth can occasionally remain reasonably functional for many years. However, in show animals, this may lead to the unintentionally deceptive appearance of a full or satisfactory dentition. Impacted or intruded deciduous teeth should generally be extracted to reduce the likelihood of pathologic injury or changes from inflammation or infection that may occur near the permanent tooth buds (24).

Deciduous Tooth Extraction

While already discussed as a treatment alternative for several conditions, the actual procedure for extracting deciduous teeth demands special consideration. Particularly in younger animals, the process of exodontia should be carried out with extreme caution to minimize the potential damage to the adjacent permanent tooth buds. Preoperative antibiotics are warranted if any signs of infection are present, and submucosal infiltration of a local anesthetic (lidocaine with 1:100,000 epinephrine—barring any contraindications) will help alleviate discomfort and reduce hemorrhage. With immature tooth buds, excess accumulation of pigments from red blood cells during tooth crown development may produce discoloration of teeth and should be minimized (7,21). Gingival flaps or epithelial-attachment severing are best performed gently. Elevators used to fatigue the periodontal ligament should be small and delicate, and utilized with minimal pressure, preferably on the sides of the tooth that are furthest from the permanent bud. Excessive force or gouging should be avoided, and extraction forceps should only be used to remove an extremely loose tooth from its attachment. Any fractured or retained roots tips should be retrieved, if possible, especially in interceptive orthodontic cases, as the root can still deflect the permanent tooth's eruption. A retained root fragment may be treated as a foreign body by the patient and cause significant inflammation (25). Use of gingival flaps and careful alveoloplasty may be necessary, with reasonable care not to damage any tooth buds. Extraction of retained deciduous teeth usually occurs once the permanent tooth has begun eruption, so damage to its formative stages is less likely. Once the tooth is extracted, the alveolus can be flushed with a solution containing a local anesthetic and a mild anti-inflammatory agent and treated with a topical antibiotic. Postoperative antibiotics can be used to combat infections, and if excessive trauma or inflammation is noted, an anti-inflammatory drug may also be considered, if not otherwise contraindicated. Any reasonable steps to eliminate possible damage to the buds should be taken.

When considering deciduous extraction, the owner should always be informed that while reasonable precautions are being taken to minimize potential damage to the developing permanent teeth, problems may still occur. These vary from minimal pitting of the enamel, to major structural defects (eg, gouging, disruption of the crown–root junction), to complete relocation of the tooth (26) (Fig. 3). With skillful care and appropriate protocol, the risk and degree of complications can be greatly reduced.

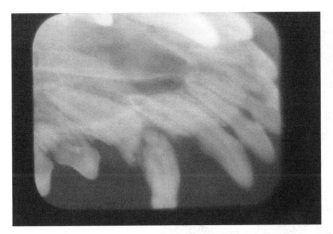

FIG. 3. Radiograph of abnormal cuspid development (disruption of the junction of the crown and the root). The deciduous tooth had been extracted at the site prior to the permanent tooth eruption; no other sites were affected.

Other Oral Abnormalities

While problems with the teeth can certainly be significant, abnormalities in the rest of the oral cavity can sometimes determine whether or not the neonatal animal will survive. With the complicated and multistaged process of development, abnormalities of the palate are sometimes experienced. A *primary palatal cleft* (failure to close) is located at the junction of the incisal area (premaxilla) with one or both of the maxillary processes (Fig. 4). It may even be present with a *cleft lip*. A defect on the midline of the palate behind the incisal area involving the hard and/or the soft palate is a *secondary cleft palate*. Secondary clefts can also be *unilateral* (one side of the nasal passage exposed) or *bilateral* (both sides of the nasal passage exposed). With either of these two situations, a newborn cannot nurse because an effective vacuum cannot be attained. What milk

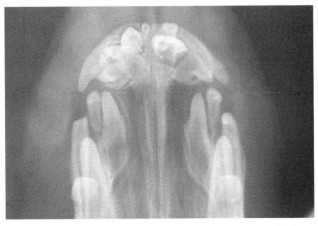

FIG. 4. Radiograph of bilateral primary palate cleft (palatoschisis) at the junctions of the incisive bone and maxillary processes.

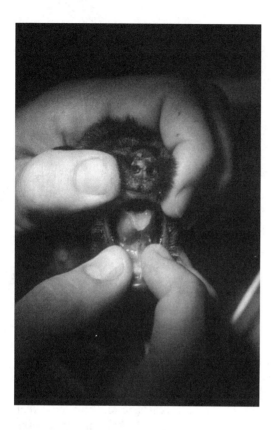

FIG. 5. Microglossia ("bird tongue") with a short, narrow pointed tongue tip.

reaches the oral cavity is often aspirated into the lungs, some coming out of the nose. This is one of the first conditions checked for at birth, and unless it is very minor, euthanasia is the treatment of choice, except in special cases. Tube feeding is generally necessary to keep affected animals alive to an age at which surgery might be an option, but even then, potential complications are numerous, and long term management is often needed. Surviving animals should not be used for breeding purposes due to the possibility of hereditary involvement.

Another condition that can be found in newborn puppies, but possibly unrecognized or lumped into the "fading puppy" syndrome, is *microglossia*, an abnormality of the tongue sometimes referred to as *"bird tongue"* (27,28) Individuals with this condition have much narrower and shorter tongues than normal, often with fimbriated edges (Fig. 5). The first indication of a problem may be the total lack of interest or the inability of these patients to nurse. Whether correctly diagnosed or not, they typically die or are euthanized. In one litter, three abnormal puppies were tube-fed and cared for to monitor their development. The abnormalities encountered as they aged went far beyond the tongue problem, including neural, musculoskeletal, cranial, and ocular manifestations (27). The initial diagnosis of the tongue abnormality is only part of a complicated, multisystem syndrome.

IMMATURE PERMANENT TOOTH PATHOLOGY

Some of the more obvious abnormalities in the oral cavity are missing and extra teeth and abnormal tooth shape and structure. As discussed earlier, while missing deciduous teeth are not always clinically important, they may be an indication that the permanent teeth are also missing. For the pet animal, a missing tooth or even several may be no cause for alarm; however, in breeding stock, particularly in the conformation-showing classes of the working breeds such as Doberman pinschers, German shepherds, and rottweilers, a missing tooth can be considered a serious fault (29). In an individual, one missing tooth may be the result of an abnormality in a developmental stage; but if there is a familial tendency or there are multiple missing teeth, especially in a bilateral pattern, some genetic influences are probably involved. Full-mouth radiographs can be taken of puppies at 8–12 weeks of age, even as a prepurchase evaluation to determine the presence or absence of each tooth bud (9). Under anesthesia, the rostral maxillary and mandibular regions (incisors and cuspids) can be radiographed using an occlusal film for each (periapical in small dogs). In short-faced dogs, a single periapical film (size 2 or 3) may be sufficient in each of the four quadrants to reveal all the premolar and molar tooth buds, but additional films to visualize the distal most molars may be necessary. A total of 6–10 films may be taken, depending on the mouth size. Teeth or tooth buds found to be missing, either visually or radiographically, should be documented on the patient record. If a tooth had been present, then lost, the empty alveolus could be detected on radiographs possibly for up to 4 weeks after the loss (25).

Areas where the tooth is not visible above the gum line generally should be radiographed, as the tooth may be present and unerupted or impacted (see Anomalies of Tooth Eruption above). If radiographs reveal abnormal dental structure, the tooth may need surgical extraction; however, if a tough gingival covering (operculum) appears to be the only obstacle to simple eruption (Fig. 6), the soft tissue should be excised to remove the restraint and encourage further eruption. If the tooth is normal and the apex is fully closed, the chances of continued timely eruption are poor, and orthodontic extrusion may be warranted, if the tooth is to be preserved and made functional. If no additional eruption is experienced in an expendable tooth, it is best extracted, for if it is left buried, a dentigerous cyst may develop (30). Occasionally, unerupted teeth may suddenly erupt after many years. It is not uncommon for the enamel to have pitted areas that are discolored from light to dark brown, showing indications of demineralization—findings that probably the result of the body's immune system attacking the buried enamel.

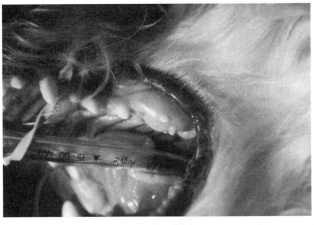

FIG. 6. Operculum (tough gingival covering) over partially erupted maxillary 4th premolars (bilateral).

During the development of teeth, even where the dental lamina forms the buds, stimuli can cause extra bud formation, resulting in supernumerary (extra) teeth or gemination teeth (from a partially split tooth bud). If crowding or tooth deflection is apparent, the supernumerary tooth or teeth should be considered for extraction to help avoid future malocclusion and/or periodontal problems. If no complications are currently being experienced or can be predictably foreseen, the teeth can often be left undisturbed.

Other abnormalities in tooth development such as fusion, gemination, dens in dente, concrescence, and so on are discussed in more detail in the pathology chapter (see Chapter 5). As a general rule, any tooth that will be predisposed to future problems (eg, exposed canal systems, grooves extending to the gingival margin) should be considered for extraction.

Even if the proper number of teeth is present, harmful stimuli experienced during tooth development can cause a variety of changes. Enamel hypocalcification may be evident in mild or early lesions as a chalky-white to a brown-yellow region or shallow pitting (10). With more generalized lesions or those that have already experienced an increased attritional rate, large areas of discolored, rough, or missing enamel may be present, with regions of exposed dentin. The extent of the damage may include the majority of the teeth, indicating a stimulus of longer duration. If the problem is focal and limited to specific areas or specific teeth, the inflammation or influence probably occurred as a finite episode during a distinct phase of tooth development.

Treatment will often depend on the extent of the lesions and the level of discomfort the animal may be experiencing. Very small or shallow lesions can be gently smoothed, and any rough or discolored enamel removed, usually with a 12-fluted bur or white stone. Care must always be taken not to damage the tooth structurally or with hyperthermia. Application of a fluoride varnish or sealant can help decrease potential sensitivity and very slightly strengthen the tooth. However, the use of a good-quality dentinal bonding agent to better seal the tubules is probably superior to the use of varnishes, especially if the bonding agent incorporates a slow fluoride release. Regular home care to reduce plaque buildup on roughened tooth surfaces, and weekly stannous fluoride applications are helpful.

With more extensive lesions on a limited number of teeth, an attempt at restoration may be made after removal of the diseased enamel. Some lesions may be broad, shallow areas, some may look like bands encircling the cuspids, and others may be relatively deep. Some teeth will show striated gradation of lesions circling the tooth, which give a stair-stepping appearance known as *telescoping hypocalcification*. It is sometimes difficult to get adequate retention in such lesions because techniques such as undercuts and pin placement are usually not possible with the thin dentinal walls of immature teeth. Paying close attention to gently curetting the areas, making an external bevel on the margin of the enamel, carefully acid-etching the enamel and the dentin if called for by the product used, and using a good dentinal bonding agent can increase the chances of success. The paint-on or brush-on technique of applying a thin layer of certain composites (Brush-Technique™, Rugby Laboratories, a division of Darby Dental, Rockville Centre, New York) with a small brush has proven to be relatively easy, while other tooth-colored composites may be used. The owner must realize that these products can also be worn or broken off and that the remaining enamel should be closely monitored for any signs of continuing degradation, which would necessitate retreatment. Porcelain crowns or veneers may also be considered, but their cost is usually prohibitive even for a few teeth. Again, regular home care, prophylaxis, and fluoride applications are helpful.

With severe or generalized hypocalcification problems, treatment planning is limited to crown restoration or enamel scrubbing, scaling, and sealing. An enamel scrub and sealing in many cases is esthetically pleasing and not as financially burdensome to the client as full crown restorations. The removal of large amounts of diseased enamel can be hastened by the use of a 12-fluted bur and white stone: however, care should be taken to use adequate water as coolant to prevent thermal pulpitis. Once the abnormal enamel is removed, the remaining tooth structure may appear diminutive, with a yellowish color due to the exposed dentin, but this is generally acceptable to most clients. It is probably best not to leave large exposed slabs of unaffected enamel, particularly as a bulb on the tip of cuspids, so the edge should be gently tapered to provide a smoother finish. Placement of multiple layers of a dentinal sealant or bonding agent can greatly reduce sensitivity and enhance tooth smoothness. Regular oral care is important, and should indications of sensitivity occur, the dentin should be resealed. Some of the diseased enamel may appear chalky-white or so close to normal that it is not detected initially as diseased. With time, these areas may change to a more brown-to-yellow color. In case all enamel is not removed at the initial visit, the owner should be instructed to examine the teeth on a regular basis for signs of the residual hypocalcified enamel's becoming evident.

Application of opaque pit and fissures sealants has also been used in cooperation with dentinal bonding agents in the treatment of hypocalcified and hypoplastic enamel, following enamel scrubbing to remove diseased enamel. However, color matching is typically a problem with most of these products because they are generally of too white a shade. Some chipping and loss of materials occur over time, and this typically requires reapplication of the pit and fissure sealant material.

Orthodontics (Immature Permanent Teeth)

While orthodontic abnormalities are generally detected and evaluated in immature animals, a more complete discussion on the subject can be found in the chapter on orthodontics (see Chapter 15). While hereditary factors may be the primary reason for many malocclusions, particularly those with disproportionate jaw growth (classes II and III and some class I), various influences that may be developmental in the neonate and young animal may also result in the malpositioning of individual teeth where the jaws are in correct alignment (22,31). Some of the more common problems occur when retained deciduous teeth cause deflection of the permanent teeth into an abnormal position during eruption. Although some genetic factors may play a role in the retention of deciduous teeth, if all other orthodontic parameters are normal, retained deciduous teeth in many breeds and lines may be more of a focal, developmental problem and may not necessarily translate into aberrations in their offspring (22). An *anterior crossbite* having one or more maxillary incisors lingual to their mandibular counterparts may not have serious consequences if left alone. To restore these teeth to a more comfortable bite, however, orthodontic brackets and power chains can be used in a tipping movement to pull the mandibular incisors lingually, or a maxillary arch bar or wire with elastics may be employed to tip the maxillary incisors labially (32). Additionally, maxillary expansion devices—a kick spring or a combination of several of these—can be used. With a single-tooth misalignment or extremely rotated teeth, extraction to provide a more comfortable bite is a viable option. Extractions can also be performed in situations such as *lance teeth*, in which one or both of the maxillary cuspids are in significant rostroversional tipping, thus pushing out the mandibular cuspid from the space it should customarily occupy (22). Lance teeth are most common in Shetland sheepdogs (shelties) and Italian greyhounds, indicating a possible hereditary involvement. In other malocclusions, such as the cuspids' making physical contact with other teeth and pressuring them out of position, extraction of the smaller, nonstrategic tooth may provide substantial relief.

Base-narrow mandibular cuspids is a condition in which one or both of the lower canine teeth are tipped too far lingually, resulting in the cusp tip's making contact with the palate (32). This can result in palatal defects, oronasal fistulas, dental wear, and periodontal disease. This condition is sometimes caused by lingual deflection of the permanent tooth by retained deciduous cuspids. Once the palatal trauma is relieved, the patient's comfort is greatly improved. These teeth can be moved orthodontically with *incline planes* or *mandibular expansion devices*, provided there is enough room in between the maxillary cuspid and corner incisor to accept the tooth. An alternative to orthodontics or extraction would be sufficient coronal height reduction with vital pulpotomy and pulp capping to remove the trauma and yet retain the large root structure (see Chapter 12).

With conventional orthodontic therapy, movement should ordinarily not be attempted until the animal's teeth are fully erupted and the roots are well on their way to maturity, unless oral discomfort is severe enough to warrant early intervention. Any orthodontic force should be relatively light to avoid potential tooth complications such as pulpitis, cervical resorption, and reduced root structure (33–39). Reduced root-structure development can arise from one of two causes (33,39): either early closure of the root apex due to pressure, or resorption of actual root structure. Principal periodontal ligaments fibers are not well organized until occlusal contact has been established (40). When possible, light digital pressure by the owner at an early age may even be helpful.

Endodontics (Immature Permanent Teeth)

Any time the endodontic system of a tooth is exposed, inflamed, infected, or injured, whether in a primary or permanent, or mature or immature tooth, it requires appropriate treatment. While extraction is always an option for removing the potential source of chronic infection, in young permanent teeth the alternative selected depends principally on the viability of the pulp, attempts to keep it vital if possible, and the extent of root maturation. The location and stage of progression of dental disease can be important in treatment planning and prognosis (41–46) (see Chapter 5 and the Dental and Oral Indices in the Appendix).

If a canal of a permanent tooth is exposed by fracture in a dog under 18 months of age, radiographs should be obtained to evaluate the apical root-structure development and ascertain the vitality of the pulp, if maintaining the tooth is desired. If the apical structure is closed and the root walls sufficiently matured, then a standard root canal procedure can be performed. If the apex has not closed, then treatment to stimulate apexogenesis for a vital tooth or apexification for a nonvital one can be attempted (see Chapter 12).

If the tooth is still vital but the apex has not yet closed, an attempt can be made to remove the inflamed pulp at the coronal extent of the tooth (vital pulpotomy) and, after hemorrhage is controlled, place calcium hydroxide on the pulp (pulp capping) to encourage the stimulation of a dentinal bridge closure, with a permanent restoration placed at the access. While not every procedure will be completely successful, within reason, efforts should be made to maintain the tooth vitality to encourage continued root maturation and closure (*apexogenesis*). Young permanent teeth, as compared with those that are older, have a larger open canal system with an excellent blood supply and a large reserve of undifferentiated mesenchymal precursor cells, all of which enhance the ability to withstand moderate amounts of trauma and inflammation, particularly if no infection is present (47,48). While keeping the pulp viable for the life of the tooth is the ideal objective in performing a vital pulpotomy and pulp capping, it should be noted that a certain percentage of teeth treated in this manner will ultimately fail. These will require additional endodontic therapy or extraction.

If the pulp of an immature permanent tooth is nonvital or necrotic and the apex is not sufficiently closed to allow a standard endodontic procedure, the canal should be thoroughly cleaned and flushed, and a calcium hydroxide paste used to fill the canal. This procedure is typically designated *apexification*, although the term actually refers to the physiologic process apex closure with a hard tissue closure by action of cementoblasts and odontoblasts that are already present (40) (see Chapter 12). Surgical endodontics with apicoectomy is frequently not an option in such immature teeth due to the large size of the apex and the thin dentinal walls. The minimum goals of both these procedures is to attain an apical closure firm enough to maintain an effective seal for an eventual endodontic filling or root canal, and a root structure sufficiently developed to support crown function.

If a horizontal root fracture should occur, particularly in a tooth before the completion of root formation, the chance of recovery in children is up to 77% (49). The fracture should be reduced, and to minimize mobility, the tooth should be stabilized with a tooth splint, possibly made with an acrylic or composite. Such a device should not be left on indefinitely in young animals (usually less than 3–4 weeks) to prevent interference with jaw growth. For the classification of fracture location and extent, see Chapter 22.

Periodontics Allied with Deciduous and Immature Permanent Teeth

Although periodontal disease is not uncommon in young animals, it is generally poorly recognized, with the exception of transient eruption gingivitis. The use of periodontal probes and conventional intraoral radiographs aid in the assessment of attachment loss over a period of time, but they are not always applicable for discriminating areas of active disease from inactive locations or detecting the early rudimentary signs of adult periodontitis found in most young animals (50,51). Staging of gingivitis and periodontitis can aid in treatment planning (45,52,53) (see Chapter 5 and the Dental and Oral Indices in the Appendix). However, without a doubt, the process leading to periodontal disease begins shortly after eruption, when the tooth is initially exposed to oral flora. For this reason, the need for oral home care should be properly emphasized when a puppy or kitten is first examined (see Chapter 21).

Many forms of periodontitis exist, each progressing to cause attachment loss at variable rates (54–56). The five current common international pathobiologic classifications of periodontitis in humans include adult periodontitis, rapidly progressive periodontitis (RPP), localized juvenile periodontitis, prepubertal periodontitis, and refractory rapidly progressive periodontitis, a subform of RPP (57–63).

All of these forms are discussed in more detail in the chapter on periodontal disease (see Chapter 8). Adult periodontitis (AP) will be discussed here only to reemphasize that it is initiated shortly after tooth eruption in young animals; however, because of its slow progression, AP typically does not demonstrate itself overtly until the animal is an adult. RPP is a rapidly progressive and generalized form of periodontitis seen mostly in young adult animals such as the greyhound, the Maltese, and the Shih Tzu. In RPP, it is typical to see highly inflamed gingival tissue and rapid attachment loss. Localized juvenile periodontitis (LJP) is a rapidly progressive localized periodontitis seen to develop in young animals; for example, it is commonly seen in the mandibular or maxillary incisors of the miniature schnauzer. Prepubertal periodontitis (PP) is a very rapidly progressing periodontitis found in association with deciduous dentition. PP may later progress into RPP or refractory rapidly progressive periodontitis (RRPP). This condition is possibly most commonly seen in young Somali and Abyssinian cats demonstrating lymphocytic plasmocytic stomatitis (LPS) (64). RRPP, a therapy-resistant periodontitis subform of RPP, may be seen in young or old animals (57–63).

Many of the forms of periodontitis actually begin in the young or juvenile animal (64). In cats with RPP/LPS, the severe gingivitis/periodontitis may give rise to the secondary development of cervical line lesions (CLLs) or feline dental resorptive (FDR) lesions due to inflammatory resorption. These forms of periodontitis occur in many young animals without appreciable plaque or calculus accumulations. With these patients, every attempt should be made to keep the oral cavity as free from plaque as possible, with a professional prophylaxis every few months or as required and rigorous home care. This is done to minimize attachment loss in the hope that the animal will eventually stabilize or recover from the disease with treatment and maturity. Of course, cats with feline leukemia virus (FeLV), feline immunodeficiency virus (FIV), or calicivirus, among other organisms, tend to have more extensive gingival lesions than the typical patient. Young cats (negative for FeLV and FIV) exhibiting a proliferative gingival margin (fibrous papillomatosis) that comes close to covering the tooth crowns have responded well to excision in some cases. A syndrome in young dogs approximates that of the juvenile forms of periodontitis in man, with a potential defect in the defense capabilities of the polymorphonuclear cells (65). Rigorous home care and professional cleaning with appropriate antibiotics and immunomodulators may help decrease the signs of disease.

Considering the dire consequences that can arise from periodontal disease (66–69), its early control and prevention are extremely important. Since young animals are very impressionable and more readily accept training, it is at this stage of life that it is best to get both the owner and the pet introduced to the concept of good oral health care. This can be done by starting with a strong foundation for the need for oral care and progressing from there to routine oral examination of the pet by the owner, home dental care (including brushing), and regular prophylaxis for the early detection and treatment of problems. With this approach, the animal can experience the best oral health possible.

Preventive Dentistry

Fluoride Topical Application

In human dentistry, the topical use of fluorides in children has been advocated for many years (70,71). Fluorides are commonly used in human dental offices and have had a growing popularity in veterinary dentistry. There is evidence in humans and animals that it affects some bacterial strains found in root caries, coronal caries, and periodontal lesions (72–74) and helps inhibit plaque formation and to a slight degree reduce dental sensitivity (75–77). At least one study of the responses of aging animals to chronic fluoride exposure has not demonstrated any physiologic or genotoxic effects due to increased fluoride levels of clinically monitored "wellness" markers (78). Although little specific research has been performed in dogs (79,80) and even less in cats, the use of in-office topical applications has generally been considered to be safe, while providing some beneficial effects. However, with home-care products, more care should be taken, as safety and health issues have been poorly defined in most animals. Fluorides are generally not meant to be ingested in large quantities, as they may have an adverse effect on calcium metabolism and the gastrointestinal system, as well as possibly being genotoxic (81). It must be kept in mind that typically most animals will swallow any product placed in the mouth. Routine or daily home use of fluoride-containing dentifrices or gels in young animals whose teeth have not erupted should be done carefully in order to reduce the risk of dental fluorosis through unintentional ingestion.

Research has indicated that most fluorides are more effective when placed on clean dry teeth (82). Selection of the type of fluoride used depends on the clinician's personal preference and knowledge of the products available (see Chapter 2). The most common topical fluorides used in veterinary dentistry are sodium fluoride, acidulated phosphate fluoride (APF), stannous fluoride (SnF_2), hydrogen fluoride, and sodium monofluorophosphate (MFP). In young animals, the neutral sodium fluoride will penetrate the tooth reasonably well due to the young tooth's early developmental stage and greater porosity. However, in older individuals, mature enamel is less porous and the use of APF will be needed to enhance dental penetration. Stannous fluoride, a tin fluoride compound, is naturally fairly acidic in nature, allowing reasonable tooth penetration (83).

For initial treatments, the teeth are first cleaned and/or polished. In many young animals, a simple polishing with a flour of pumice will suitably prepare the tooth. After the removal of any debris, the teeth are dried, isolated with cotton rolls, and coated with the fluoride by brush or in trays for 3–5 minutes. Strive to keep the material principally on the tooth surfaces. A saliva ejector, oral vacuum, or a three-way syringe may be used to blow excess material from the teeth—it can also be gently wiped from the teeth—once the manufacturer's recommended time of treatment has been attained (usually 3–5 minutes). Do not use water to rinse the material off the tooth, as this will possibly inactivate the fluoride's progressive effect, at least until the animal drinks water.

Application of pit and fissures sealants, a common practice in children, may help prevent caries formation. Unless there is specific indication of an individual predisposition to problems, such sealants are infrequently used in animals. However, they have been used together with dentinal bonding agents in treatment of hypocalcified and hypoplastic enamel (see "Immature permanent tooth pathology" earlier in this chapter).

Home Care

Instruction to owners for beginning home dental care early in a pet's life can alert them to the importance of good hygiene from the start. As with any individual, starting out slow and making the experience relatively pleasant at first can turn the process into an uncomplicated routine. The use of fluoride home-care products should be done under supervision (see "Fluoride topical application" earlier in this chapter). Smaller, softer toothbrushes or gauze with flavored products can make the animal look forward to the brushing sessions, or at least be more tolerant (see Chapter 21).

REFERENCES

1. Avery LB. *Developmental Anatomy: A Textbook and Laboratory Manual of Embryology.* 5th ed. Philadelphia: WB Saunders Co; 1947:217.
2. Jennings HS. Hereditary and environment in pediatrics. In: Brennemann J, ed. *Practice of Pediatrics.* Hagerstown, MD: WF Prior Co; 1945;1(3):63.

3. Warkany J. Congenital malformations. In: Levine SZ, ed. *Advances in Pediatrics*. Chicago: Year Book; 1947:2:1.
4. Harvey CE. Function and formation of the oral cavity. In: Harvey CE, ed. *Veterinary Dentistry*. Philadelphia: WB Saunders Co; 1985:5.
5. Bhaskar SN. *Synopsis of Oral Pathology*. St Louis, MO: CV Mosby Co; 1961:110.
6. Suckling GW. Defects of enamel in sheep resulting from trauma during development. *J Dent Res* 1980;59:1541.
7. Cohen MM. *Pediatric Dentistry*. 12nd ed. St Louis, MO: CV Mosby Co; 1961:416.
8. Richards A. Nature and mechanism of dental fluorosis in animals. *J Dent Res* 1990;69(spec issue):701.
9. Clarke CE, Lobprise HB. Some aspects of clinical paedodontics in dogs and cats. *Aust Vet Pract* 1994;24:203.
10. Andreasen JO, Ravn JJ. Enamel changes in permanent teeth after trauma to their primary predecessors. *Scand J Dent Res* 1973;81:203.
11. Stockard CR. *The Genetic and Endocrinic Basis for Differences in Form and Behavior*. Philadelphia: The Wistar Institute of Anatomy and Biology; 1941. The American Anatomical Memoirs, Number 19.
12. Hennet PR, Harvey CE. Craniofacial development and growth in the dog. *J Vet Dent* 1992;9(2):11.
13. Baker LW. The influence of the forces of occlusion on the development of bones of the skull. *Int J Orthod Oral Surg Radiol* 1922;53(5):259.
14. Wheeler RC. *Dental Anatomy, Physiology, and Occlusion*. Philadelphia: WB Saunders Co; 1974:24.
15. Williams RC. *Observations on the Chronology of Deciduous Dental Development in the Dog*. Ithaca, NY: Cornell University; 1961. Thesis.
16. Williams RC, Evans HE. Prenatal dental development in the dog, *Canis familiaris*: Chronology of tooth germ formation and calcification of deciduous teeth. *Zentralbl Veterinarmed C: Anat Histol Embryol* 1978;7:152.
17. Wiggs RB. Canine oral anatomy and physiology. *Comp Cont Ed* 1989;11:1475.
18. Floyd MR. The modified Triadan system: Nomenclature for veterinary dentistry. *J Vet Dent* 1991;8(4):18.
19. Schumacher CB. Charting and the oral examination. *J Vet Dent* 1993;10(3):9.
20. Carmichael D. Crown amputation and vital pulpotomy. World Veterinary Dental Congress Proceedings, Philadelphia; 1994:110.
21. Wiggs RB. Basics of orthodontics. AVDS Proceedings. Seattle, WA. 1993:15.
22. Harvey CE, Emily PP. *Small Animal Dentistry*. St.Louis, MO: Mosby-Year Book; 1993:4, 278.
23. Emily P. Adolescent dentistry. AVDC/AVD Proceedings; 1991.
24. Andreasen JO. The influence of traumatic intrusion of primary teeth on their permanent successors: A radiographic and histologic study in monkeys. *Int J Oral Surg* 1976;5:207.
25. Eisenmenger E, Zetner K. Abnormalities in dentition and change in teeth. In: *Veterinary Dentistry*. Philadelphia: Lea & Febiger; 1985:48.
26. Manfra-Marretta S, Patnaik AK, Schloss AJ, Kapatkin A. An iatrogenic dentigerous cyst in a dog. *J Vet Dent* 1989;6(2):11.
27. Wiggs RB, Lobprise HB. Microglossia in three littermate puppies. *J Vet Dent* 1994;11(4):129.
28. Hutt FB, de LaHunta A. A lethal glossopharyngeal defect in the dog. *J Hered* 1971;62:291.
29. *The Complete Dog Book: An Official Publication of The American Kennel Club*. New York: Howell Book House; 1973: 252, 256, 304.
30. Lobprise HB, Wiggs RB. Dentigerous cyst in a dog. *J Vet Dent* 1992;9(1):13.
31. Richardson RE, Barton RE. *The Dental Assistant*. 5th ed. St.Louis, MO: McGraw-Hill Book Co; 1978:527.
32. Holmstrom SE, Frost P, Gammon RL. *Veterinary Dental Techniques for the Small Animal Practitioner*. Philadelphia: WB Saunders Co; 1992:339.
33. Dewey M, Anderson GM. *Practical Orthodontics*. St.Louis, MO: CV Mosby Co; 1942:262.
34. Simonton FV, Jones MR. Mineral metabolism in relation to alveolar atropy in dogs. *JADA* 1928;15:881.
35. Becks H, Weber M. The influence of diet on the bone system with special reference to the alveolar process and labyrinthine capsule. *JADA* 1931;18:197.
36. Becks H. Root resorptions and their relation to pathologic bone formation following orthodontic treatment. *Orthodia Oral Surg Int J* 1936;12:445.
37. Ketcham A. A progress report on an investigation of apical root resorption of vital permanent teeth. *Int J Orthod* 1929;15:310.
38. Selhorst F. Orthodontische Behandlungen an Hunden. *Tierartz Umschau* 1965;20:166.
39. Goldman HM, Gianelly AA. Histology of tooth movement. *Dent Clin North Am* 1972;16:439.
40. Torneck CD. Effects and clinical significance of trauma to the developing permanent dentition. *Dent Clin North Am* 1982;26:481.
41. Howard WW, Moller RC. *Atlas of Operative Dentistry*. 3rd ed. St.Louis, MO; CV Mosby Co; 1981:4.
42. *Veterinary Dental Abbreviations*. American Veterinary Dental College, Residency Tracking Committee, suppl; 1994 University of California, Davis.
43. Wiggs RB, Lobprise HB. Dental disease. In: Norsworthy GD, ed. *Feline Practice*. Philadelphia: JB Lippincott Co; 1993:290.
44. Robinowich BZ. The fractured incisor. *Pediatr Clin North Am* 1956;3:979.
45. Torres HO, Ehrlich A. Pedodontics. In: *Modern Dental Assisting*. 2nd ed. Philadelphia: WB Saunders Co; 1980:725.
46. Ellis RG, Davey KW. *Classification and Treatment of Injuries to the Teeth of Children*. 5th ed. Chicago: Year Book Medical Publishers; 1970:285.

47. Andreasen JO, Hjorting-Hansen E. Replantation of teeth. II. Histological study of 22 replanted teeth in humans. *Acta Odontol Scand* 1966;24:257.
48. Maltz J, Torneck CD. Orthodontic treatment of teeth with fractured roots: A case report. *Ont Dent* 1980;57:12.
49. Torneck CD. The dentin-pulp complex. In: Ten Cate AR, ed. *Oral Histology*. St Louis, MO: CV Mosby Co; 1980.
50. Armitage GC. Periodontal diagnostic aids. *Calif Dent Assoc J* 1993;21(11):35.
51. Wiggs RB, Lobprise HB, Capron CM, Bellinger LL. Gingival crevicular fluid aspartate aminotransferase as a marker of naturally occurring active periodontal disease in the cat. 1994; submitted for publication.
52. Loe H, Silness J. Periodontal disease in pregnancy. I. Prevalence and severity. *Acta Odontol Scand* 1963;21:533.
53. Wiggs RB, Lobprise HB. Oral disease. In: Norsworthy GD, ed. *Feline Practice*. Philadelphia: JB Lippincott Co; 1993:438.
54. Reddy MS, Jeffcoat MK. Periodontal disease progression. *Curr Op Periodontol* Philadelphia: 1993:52.
55. Ranney RR. Classification of periodontal diseases. *Periodontology 2000* 1993;2:13.
56. Page RC. Gingivitis. *J Clin Periodontol* 1986;13:345.
57. Loe H, Theilade E, Jensen S. Experimental gingivitis in man. *J Periodontol* 1965;36:177.
58. Page RC, Schroeder HE. Pathogenesis of inflammatory periodontal disease. A summary of current work. *Lab Invest* 1976;33:235.
59. Page RC, Schroeder HE. *Periodontitis in Man and Other Animals: A Comparative Review*. Basel: Karger; 1982:53, 226.
60. American Academy of Periodontology. Glossary of Periodontic Terms. *J Periodontol* November 1986;(suppl).
61. *Current Procedural Terminology for Periodontics and Insurance Reporting Manual*. 5th ed. American Academy of Periodontology; Chicago 1986:(2)40.
62. Deutsche Gesellschaft für Parodontologie: Neue PAR-Nomenklatur. *DGP-Nachrichten* 1987;1:1.
63. Schroeder HE. Klinik und Pathologie verschiedender Formen von Parodontitis. *Dtsch zahnarztl Z* 1987;42:417.
64. Williams CA, Aller MS. Feline stomatology. AVDC/AVD Proceedings. 1991:101.
65. Guilford GW. Primary immunodeficiency diseases of dogs and cats. *Friskes Res Dig* 1988;24(1):1.
66. Debowes L. Systemic effects of oral disease. AVDC/AVD Proceedings. 1992:65.
67. Mattila KJ, Nieminen MS, Valtonen VV, et al. Association between dental health and acute myocardial infarction. *Br Med J* 1989;298:779.
68. Syrjanen J, Peltola J, Valtonen V, et al. Dental infections in association with cerebral infarction in young and middle-aged men. *J Intern Med* 1989;225:179.
69. DeStefano F, Andra RF, Kahn HS, et al. Dental disease and risk of coronary heart disease and mortality. *Br Med J* 1993;306:688.
70. Knutson JW, Armstrong WD. Effect of topically applied sodium fluoride on dental caries experience. *Public Health Report* 1943;8:1701.
71. Muhler JC. Topical application of stannous fluoride. *JADA* 1957;54:352.
72. Bibby BG, Van Kesteren M. The effect of fluorine on mouth bacteria. *J Dent Res* 1940;19:391.
73. Keyes PH. Evaluation of two topical application methods to assess the anticaries potential of drugs in hamsters. *J Oral Ther Pharm* 1966;2:285.
74. Tinanoff N. Review of the antimicrobial action of stannous fluoride. *J Clin Dent* 1990;II(1):22.
75. Holmstrom SE, Frost P, Gammon RL. *Veterinary Dental Techniques for the Small Animal Practitioner*. Philadelphia: WB Saunders Co; 1992:134.
76. Lukomsky EH. Fluorine therapy for exposed dental and alveolar atrophy. *J Dent Res* 1941;20:649.
77. Newman MG, Carranza FA Jr, Mazza JE. Fluorides in periodontal therapy. Clinical Uses of Fluoride. 1984:83.
78. Dunipace AJ, Brizendine EJ, Zhang W, et al. Effect of aging on animal response to chronic fluoride exposure. *J Dent Res* 1995;74:358.
79. Ekstrand J, Whitford T. Fluoride metabolism: Longitudinal study in growing dogs. *J Dent Res* 1984;63:206. Abstract.
80. Whitford GM, Pashley DH. Plasma fluoride levels in the dog as a function of age. *Caries Res* 1983;17:561. Abstract.
81. Dietrich UB. No justification for fluoride use in dogs. *Vet Forum* July 1992:96.
82. Knutson JW. Sodium fluoride solutions; technic for application to teeth. *JADA* 1948;36:37.
83. *Accepted Dental Therapeutics*. 37th ed. Chicago: American Dental Association, 1977.220.

8

Periodontology

Robert B. Wiggs and Heidi B. Lobprise

Periodontology is the study of the periodontium in health and disease, as well as the study of its treatment to maintain or reestablish health. *Periodontium* comes from Latin and Greek, meaning "around the tooth." The true anatomic periodontium is restricted to the connective tissue between the teeth and the bony sockets (periosteum alveolare) and to the periodontal ligament (1). However, clinically and more practically, the periodontium is considered those tissues that immediately support and invest the teeth such as the alveolus, cementum, periodontal membrane or ligament, and the gingivae (2).

Periodontal disease is the process consisting of stages of progressive attachment loss. This is seen in a cyclic process of recurring intervals of active destruction (periodontitis) and inactive dormancy; it is not a linearly continuous sequence (3–5). *Gingivitis* is considered to be the inflammation of the gingiva, which typically begins along the margin (6–12). The term *periodontal disease* refers to the inflammation of the gingiva or periodontium, their active recessive alteration, or their alteration state with or without active disease (6–12). *Periodontitis* is defined as an active disease state of the periodontium (6,12). This means that an animal may be in a stage III periodontal disease, but if the active disease has been controlled or is dormant, gingivitis or periodontitis may not be present.

Periodontitis occurs in many forms and is driven by many different causes, each developing and inducing attachment loss at variable rates according to host and other factors (13,15). Periodontitis usually develops from gingivitis, but not all untreated gingivitis develops into periodontitis, nor does all periodontitis progress to initiate attachment loss (15). As periodontitis occurs, the body reacts to the insult to ordinarily control the condition and avoid loss of attachment. Eventually, repeated assaults of periodontitis in association with the body's defenses may result in loss of periodontal attachment and progression of the stages of periodontal disease.

PERIODONTAL DISEASE AND GENERAL HEALTH

Research has begun to link numerous serious diseases to periodontal disease in both in humans and animals (16). A group at the University of Michigan has described some research work on the potential influence of periodontal infection on cardiovascular disease in humans (17). Finnish researchers have presented data linking dental infections with cerebral infarction (18) and acute myocardial infarction (19). A United Kingdom study involving close to 10,000 human patients supports the Finnish study results and also the association of poor oral health with general mortality (20). people with periodontal disease in this study, including those who were edentulous due to periodontal or dental disease, were 2.6 times more likely to die before their tenth year in the study as compared with those with good oral health.

Similar effects have long been suspected in dogs, but these remain unproven. Research done at the Kansas State University's Department of Veterinary Medicine has described investigations into similar implications for the relationship of periodontal disease to heart, liver, and kidney disease in the dog (21). In a six-state study, early results from several hundred randomly selected animals found approximately 80% of the dogs and 70% of the cats aged 20–27 months (average, 2 years) demonstrated signs or positive tests for periodontal disease (22). Additionally, a National Companion Animal Study of 39,556 dogs and 13,924 cats divided up animals into three categories according to age (0–7, 7–10, and 10–25 years) to show that dental disease was the number one diagnosed disease in both species in all age categories (23). These studies indicate that periodontal disease is the most common disease of adult dogs and cats, while suggesting that poor oral health may directly affect an animal's overall general health (16).

Another serious concern has to do with the possibility of humans and animals' acting as reservoirs for each other for the pathogens that cause periodontal disease (24). In at least one case, there has been reasonable indication of the possible infection of a child with a rapidly destructive form of periodontal disease from a dog source (25). Additionally, there is no reason not to assume the infectious process cannot also be passed from human to animal. For this reason, it should be kept in mind that periodontal disease is an infectious disease, whose spread and reservoir system are not fully understood. This would indicate that treatment of suspected reservoirs (humans or other animals in the household) may be required to control the condition.

Common Signs and Symptoms
Associated with Periodontal Disease

Edema and inflammation of gums (gingivitis)
Plaque and calculus deposition
Debris accumulation around teeth
Purulent exudate
Halitosis
Ulcerations
Gums that bleed easily when probed
Loss of gingival stippling
Change in architecture of gingival papillae
Loss of bone around teeth
Gum recession
Pocket formation around teeth
Tooth mobility
Tooth migration or new diastema formations
Tooth extrusion
Tooth loss

ANATOMY

To recognize and understand periodontal disease and its treatment require a familiarity with the normal anatomy and physiology of the periodontium (see Chapter 3). The following is a list of anatomic and descriptive terms that will help build an understanding of basic periodontal structures:

Subgingival–below the gum line; in the sulcus
Supragingival–above the gum line; on the crown
Sulcus–the normal crevicular groove between the tooth and gum
Pocket–an abnormal depth of the crevicular groove between the tooth and gum.
Epithelial attachment or *junctional epithelium*–base of the crevicular groove formed by the tooth and gingiva (26).

The gingival masticatory mucosa is one of the most important support structures for the tooth. It is divided into two major parts: the *free gingiva* (marginal gingiva) and the *attached gingiva*. The free gingival margin is that unattached portion that lies coronal to the junctional epithelium, serving to form the outer extent of the gingival sulcus. The attached gingiva is not mobile upon the underlying structures and is firm. The two combine to form a peak of gingiva known as the *interdental papilla* between teeth that are closely adjacent. The interdental papilla plays an important part in maintenance of gingival health by preventing food and debris from being impacted between the teeth.

Between the facial and lingual interdental papilla and two closely adjacent teeth may be found a valley of gingiva known as the *col* (Fig. 1). This interpapillary saddle is covered with a thin layer of nonkeratinized epithelium between the junctional epithelium of two adjacent teeth and will vary with tooth morphology, crown width, and tooth position (27). This thin epithelium can be easily irritated, and with the tooth morphology, food debris and plaque can easily accumulate to cause gingivitis (28). In the dog, the most common area for col involvement is between the maxillary 4th premolar and 1st molar, between the mandibular 1st and 2nd molar, and occasionally between incisors.

Between the tooth and the free gingiva can typically be found a shallow groove known as the *gingival sulcus* (Fig. 2). The epithelium lining the sulcus and the col is among the very few areas of masticatory gingiva that is nonkeratinized. At the bottom of the sulcus is the *epithelial attachment* or the *junctional epithelium*, which directly attaches the gingiva to the tooth. In periodontal disease, it is common for the sulcus depth to increase as attachment is lost. The remaining gingiva is the attached gingiva.

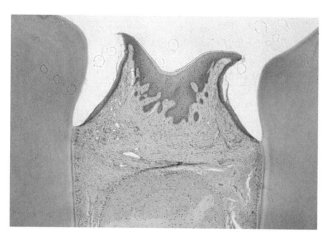

FIG. 1. Interdental gingival tissue (col) between mandibular 4th premolar and 1st molar. (Courtesy of Dr. Ayako Okuda, Tokyo, Japan.)

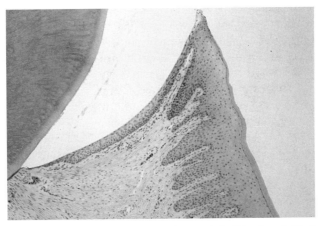

FIG. 2. Marginal area of gingiva and gingival sulcus in a cat. In this decalicified section, free gingiva exhibits deep epithelial rete pegs *(right)*, while none are observed in junctional epithelium or epithelial attachment facing the sulcus. (Courtesy of Dr. Ayako Okuda, Tokyo, Japan.)

On the facial surfaces of the teeth, there is a distinct demarcation, the *mucogingival junction* or *line*, that separates this attached gingiva from the alveolar mucosa, which is part of the general or lining mucosa. The transition from attached gingiva to general mucosa is less apparent on the palatal surfaces. There is variability in gingival width, and while it is optimum to maintain sufficient attached gingiva (2 mm) (29), this minimum standard has been questioned by some authors (30–33).

The gingivae and hard palate, which undergoes routine masticatory trauma and stress, is generally parakeratinized or keratinized. An interdigitation exists between the epithelium and the underlying connective tissue (see Fig. 2). The interdigitation of the submucosal connective tissue into the epithelium is termed the *dermal papilla*. The pegs of epithelium, known as *rete ridges* or *pegs*, that insert into the connective tissue may cause small dimples in the gingival tissue known as *gingival stippling*. Stippling can be present or absent in healthy or diseased gingival tissue and therefore is not a reliable indication of gingival health; it is also less prominent in the cat. Its reduction or loss may be an indicator but does not automatically signify disease (34–36). The length of the pegs determines how tightly or mobilely the epithelium is attached to the underlying connective tissue. The alveolar mucosa, which has poorly developed pegs, is somewhat movable above the connective tissue. In comparison, the gingival masticatory mucosa has well developed rete pegs and, logically, has a firm attachment.

The *cementum* is an anatomic part of the tooth; however, since periodontal and gingival fiber bundles anchor in it, it is also a functional part of the periodontium. Cementum is approximately 50% inorganic material, similar in structure to bone, and has regenerative capabilities due to viable cells in its apical third and sometimes in furcation areas (27). In the dog, it is generally thicker at its apical extent as compared with areas more coronal (37). There are two basic types of collagen fibers in cementum: Sharpey's fibers (entering the cementum perpendicular to the root surface) and collagen fibers (originating from within the cementum and running parallel to the cemental surface) (38).

The *tooth roots* are encased in the alveolar processes of the maxillae, mandibles, and incisal bone (37). The *alveolar process* is composed of the alveolar bone proper, trabecular bone, and compact bone. The compact bone covers the outer surface of the processes, blending into the alveolar bone at the entrance to the alveoli. The alveolar (wall) bone lines the alveoli or sockets, and being more dense than the trabecular bone that lies between it and the compact (cortical) bone, it is seen radiographically as the *lamina dura* (27). The alveolar bone is sometimes referred to as the *cribriform plate*. The trabecular bone is less dense and contains marrow spaces, as it supports the compact and alveolar bone. The alveolar crest is the thinnest portion of the alveolar process, especially facially, as there is no underlying trabecular bone supporting it. In the maxilla of the dog, this facial surface closely follows the contour of the roots, forming palpably distinct juga over the roots (37).

The *periodontal ligament* or *membrane* is made of collagen fibrils arranged parallel in fibers and grouped to form fiber bundles. These bundles insert into the cementum on one end and the alveolar bone on the other, as Sharpey's fibers (37,39). In rodent and immature human teeth, an interdigitating rather than solid fiber arrangement, called the *intermediate plexus*, has been demonstrated traversing the periodontal space (40). This intermediate plexus is found in association with most hypsodont teeth, which allows for their continual growth or eruption. The periodontal ligament also contains nerves and vessels, ground substance, and various cells such as surface osteoblasts, cementoblasts, and fibroblasts interspersed with the fiber bundles. These fibers serve to support and protect the teeth by absorbing forces applied to the teeth. In Chapter 3, a more complete discussion is given on fibers and their physiology.

These connective tissue attachments work with the *epithelial attachment*, specialized junctional epithelium of the free gingival margin. The *junctional epithelium* is vital in maintaining periodontal health by its tooth attachment and role in diapedesis and providing for transmigration of polymorphonuclear granulocytes (PMNs) toward the sulcus in response to metabolic products of plaque bacteria (41). Surrounding the neck of each tooth and at about 2 mm in depth in humans and dogs, this epithelium is only a few cell-layers thick (0.15 mm wide) at its apical extent and up to 15–30 cell layers coronally (2). This tissue is continuously renewed throughout life (42) with a high cell-turnover rate (junctional epithelium, 4–6 days) (43) as compared with other oral epithelium (6–12 days) (44,45).

The actual attachment to the tooth surface can occur on enamel, cementum, or dentin with an *internal basal lamina (IBL)* of the hard tissue (made up of the lamina densa and the lamina lucida) and a 0.5–1.0-mcm thick dental cuticle between the IBL and tooth surface, probably synthesized by junctional epithelial cells (46). Hemidesmosomes are found in cells adjacent to the tooth and lamina lucida to allow attachment to the IBL. The *external basal lamina* (EBL), running external to the basal layer of cells, joins the IBL at the apical extent of the epithelium. Hemidesmosomes of the basal cell lining interface through the EBL to the adjacent connective tissue (1,27).

In young healthy periodontal tissues, the apical boundary of the junctional epithelium ends at the cementoenamel junction. The basal cells produce offspring cells that continually migrate coronally. For those cells contacting the tooth surface, the hemidesmosomal attachments are constantly dissolved and reformed. Once the cells reach the bottom of the gingival sulcus, they are sloughed. The sulcus is a narrow groove formed by the tooth on one side and the nonkeratinized oral sulcal epithelium on the other (47). It should only be 0.5 mm deep in cats and 2 mm in most dogs, although the size or diameter of the probe and the degree of pressure during insertion can affect depth readings even in healthy tissues.

The blood supply to the periodontium is generous both for the high metabolic rate of related tissue and for the fluid dynamics (hydraulic pressure distribution, dampening) that come into play in order for the periodontal ligament to resist occlusal forces. The main vascular sources include the anterior and posterior alveolar, intraorbital, and palatine arteries for the maxilla, and the sublingual, mental, buccal, and facial arteries for the mandible. There are substantial anastomoses, with a dense network of vessels in the periodontal ligament. The vessels also form a compact plexus in the region of the junctional epithelium, probably to assist in inflammatory cell–host response. Capillary loops travel into the rete ridges or pegs that interdigitate into the oral epithelium to the underlying connective tissue (1).

PERIODONTAL DISEASE AND SUSPECTED CAUSATIVE FACTORS

Periodontal disease has been described as a multifactorial infection (48). Plaque, microflora, calculus, species, breed, genetics, general health, age, home dental care, chewing behavior, salvia, and local irritants are some of the more common general factors thought to be involved with susceptibility to and progression of periodontitis (49). However, while there may be many factors that influence the scope of periodontal disease, the primary etiology of the process is perceived to be plaque bacteria (41). Epidemiologic studies have indicated that the etiologic factors of periodontal disease in dogs are similar to those in humans (50–52).

Plaque is an organic matrix of salivary glycoproteins, oral bacteria, and extracellular polysaccharides that adheres to the tooth surface. It is thought that the glycoproteins and polysaccharides provide the adherence for the bacteria to the tooth surface (53). In primates, the extracellular organic matrix of supragingival plaque consists of approximately 30% carbohydrates, 30% proteins, 15% lipids, with the nature of the remaining 25% being variable and undefined. The components are derived from ingested foodstuff, salivary glycoproteins, and bacterial byproducts. The principal carbohydrate is dextran, a polysaccharide produced by plaque bacteria, representing approximately 9.5% of the total plaque. Other matrix carbohydrates are levan, galactose, and methylpentose in the form of rhamnose. Another common extracellular carbohydrate is mutan, which is found when plaque is colonized by *Streptococcus mutans*. Bacterial remnants provide muramic acid and lipids, as well as part of the matrix proteins.

The inorganic components of the supragingival plaque matrix are provided principally by foodstuff and saliva. These are calcium and phosphorus, with small amounts of magnesium, potassium, and sodium. The total inorganic content of early plaque is very low, but it gradually increases as plaque is converted into calculus. Fluoride from drinking water, food, toothpastes, gels, and oral solutions also become incorporated into plaque. Fluoride may act to deter plaque bacterial metabolism, kill bacteria, and aid in the remineralization of enamel and dentin.

Teeth form a suitable surface for bacteria to accumulate. Within minutes after cleaning, a thin pellicle (0.1–0.8 mm) of salivary glycoprotein covers the tooth (1). This is the beginning matrix for plaque formation as gram-positive, colony-forming bacteria (*Streptococcus sanguis* and *Actinomyces viscosus*) adhere to the pellicle and become established within 24 hours. With the addition of extracellular polysaccharides (bacterial byproduct), plaque takes on its classic ivory-to-yellow-to-grayish appearance.

Dental plaque is not a food residue. It actually forms more readily during sleep, when there is no food taken in or when tube feeding is being performed (54). The mechanical action of food and the saliva it stimulates appear to deter plaque formation. Dietary increases in sucrose increase formation of supragingival plaque and have an influence on its bacterial composition.

Supragingival plaque probably strongly affects the growth, accumulation, and pathogenicity of subgingival plaque in the early stages of periodontal disease. It does this by providing protection to the subgingival plaque and by reducing the oxygen available deeper in the plaque matrix. The noxious agents released by the bacteria are likely the initial insult to stimulate gingival reaction. Once pocket formation occurs, the influence of supragingival plaque on subgingival plaque is minimal and only occurs where the two make contact. It is evident that supragingival and subgingival plaque in unison are directly responsible for the initiation and progression of periodontal disease.

Initially, there is little difference between the *microflora* of supragingival and subgingival plaque at healthy gingival sites. *Aerobic bacteria* are those that thrive in the presence of oxygen, but most can usually live in anaerobic conditions. *Strict anaerobic bacteria* live in a relatively oxygen-free environment. *Facultative anaerobic bacteria* can live in either aerobic or anaerobic conditions. In clinically healthy gingiva of dogs and cats, the microflora is composed primarily of aerobic and facultative anaerobic bacteria (55). The greater part of these bacteria are gram-positive, nonmotile, aerobic cocci. However, as bacteria continue to accumulate, there will be a change in the flora to more gram-negatives, anaerobes, rods, filamentous, and motile organisms (56,57). In dogs, anaerobes constitute only about 25% of the culturable subgingival flora in healthy gingiva, but they becomes approximately 95% of the flora in dogs with periodontitis (55). The aerobic populations do not actually decrease in most cases, but rather an extensive increase in anaerobes occurs that changes the ratio dramatically.

Aerobes and Facultative Anaerobes (55,58)

Gram-positive	
Streptococcus sp.	Coccus
Actinomyces sp.	Bacillus
Lactobacillus sp.	Bacillus
Gram-negative	
Neisseria sp.	Coccus
Coliforms	Bacillus
Campylobacter sp.	Bacillus
Capnocytophaga sp.	Bacillus
Eikenella sp.	Bacillus
Actinobacillus sp.	Bacillus

Strict Anaerobes (55,59,60)

Gram-positive	
Peptostreptococcus sp.	Coccus
Actinomyces sp.	Bacillus
Eubacterium sp.	Bacillus
Clostridium sp.	Bacillus
Gram-negative	
Veillonella sp.	Coccus
Fusobacterium sp.	Bacillus
Wolinella sp.	Bacillus
Bacteroides sp.	Bacillus
Prevotella sp.	Bacillus
Prophyromonas sp.	Bacillus
Spirochetes sp.	Bacillus

As the virulence of the bacteria increases, so does the effect of bacterial byproducts that elicit inflammation, including chemotoxins, mitogens, antigens, and enzymes such as hyaluronidase, chondroitin sulfate, and proteolytic enzymes. Cytotoxins (ammonia, hydrogen sulfide, and organic acids), as well as bacterial endotoxins, can invade tissue on their own. In fact, the early effect of bacteria is due to the diffusion of these products into the tissue, increasing exudation and polymorphonuclear granulocyte migration response. The toxins can likely cause direct tissue destruction and injury in the absence of a host response. It is the combination of the virulence of the bacterial flora and the host response that is a major factor influencing whether or not gingivitis will actually progress into periodontitis in an individual animal. The host immune response generally plays an important role in the progression of periodontal disease. However, as long as the bacteria and their byproducts can be minimized, and as long as the type remains less virulent, a normal host can provide suitable defense to maintain the integrity of the periodontium (41). In gingivitis and periodontitis, the development of attachment loss depends on the interaction between the resident microflora and the host immune response. Although inflammation is a host defense response to localize and destroy foreign materials, the host's own tissues may be destroyed in the process.

Subgingivally, as the disease progresses, a layer of filaments and gram-positive cocci forms an adherent plaque layer that can become mineralized to form calculus. Motile and nonmotile gram-negative anaerobes can be found in nonadherent accumulations of bacteria near the soft tissue. In acute inflammatory lesions, these bacteria increase dramatically in number and appear to have a role in periodontitis progression (8,57,61). Within the depth of the pocket, if protective leukotoxins are secreted, bacteria can sometimes escape the marginal accumulation of inflammatory infiltrate and invade the subepithelial connective tissue (1). This may be seen in rapidly progressive periodontitis (RPP) and localized juvenile periodontitis (LJP), or a purulent abscess with drainage may result (62–65).

Opportunistic infections are possible when reduced host resistance allows facultative pathogens that are normally innocuous and found in the normal oral flora to proliferate (37). There can be pathogenic bacteria in low levels in normal plaque that become destructive if their numbers increase dramatically in acutely diseased pockets. The *specific plaque hypothesis* that explains this process states that periodontitis is caused by these specific strains of virulent bacteria. This type of hypothesis could explain the nature of certain forms of RPP. Adult periodontitis is more likely to be caused by an etiology of a *nonspecific plaque hypothesis*, where there is a superinfection of a mixed bacterial population from subgingival plaque (1). Lack of an effective host response allows these bacterial groups (gram-negative) to influence the disease process.

In the dog, over 700 representative anaerobes have been isolated from subgingival plaque, with species of black-pigmented anaerobes (*Prevotella* and *Porphyromonas* spp.) exhibiting possible periodontopathic characteristics (66,67). Some forms of black-pigmented anaerobes can not only colonize root surfaces and survive in pockets but also have the ability to circumvent host defenses (leukotoxins) and directly damage tissue (endotoxins) (1). These studies reinforce the current belief in veterinary dentistry (59) that black-pigmented and related organisms probably directly contribute to the histopathologic changes seen in canine periodontitis. As a rule, periodontal disease is caused by an infection of a mixture of varying bacteria (68); however, there are always exceptions to any rule. In primates, it is common to find *Actinobacillus actinomycetemcomitans* and spirochetes in some forms of LJP, as well as the combination of *Fusobacterium*, *Bacteroides intermedius*, and *Selemonas* in certain cases of ulcerative gingivitis (69,70). However, in the dog and cat, *A. actinomycetemcomitans* is not a common pathogen, as it is in primates (55).

Typically, even without culturing each form of periodontal disease, there is a tendency to have a certain group of bacteria being associated with various stages (1). Usually, only a thin layer of gram-positive plaque is present when the gingiva is healthy, but with a heavier plaque accumulation comes the appearance of gram-negative bacteria as gingivitis develops. Without cessation of the process or even exacerbation, this will typically progress into adult periodontitis (AP). In contrast to the LJP or RPP, which tend to involve specific gram-negative anaerobes, AP will be relatively quiescent. The nonadherent subgingival plaque in RPP may be similar to that found in an active phase of AP, but the supragingival plaque is typically minimal and similar to that found in gingivitis.

Calculus is mineralized dental plaque that adheres to tooth surfaces and prosthetic dental materials. Plaque and calculus accumulate more significantly on the buccal surface of the maxillary teeth, with the carnassials being the worst effected (55). Its primary effect on periodontal disease is aiding in plaque and bacterial adherence near the gingival margin (71–73). This allows for the continued close contact of plaque in a protected environment. Calculus itself also provides a local irritant effect, but this is a passive, not an active, mechanism. Subsequently, when calculus is present, gingival inflammation normally occurs, and when calculus occurs subgingivally, healing of the tissues is not possible. Therefore, the complete removal of all supra- and subgingival calculus is of great importance in the control of periodontal disease.

Concerning the *breeds of dogs and cats*, there has been a general trend in the general public toward ownership of smaller breeds of dogs. Many of the smaller breeds have a predilection toward crowding of the teeth and malocclusions, both of which predispose to the development of periodontal disease (73). In the cat, the Somali and Abyssinian both are well known for their predilection for LJP, RPP, and refractory RPP (RRPP) forms of periodontal disease. Additionally, many lines of miniature schnauzers and greyhounds have a similar propensity for LJP, RPP, and RRPP. Genetics of course can also predispose to oral disease by affecting structure, size, immune system, organ health, and numerous other body systems (74).

General health becomes an integral part of the pathogenesis of periodontal disease for numerous reasons. Animals in poor health are more susceptible to disease, and periodontitis is the most common infectious disease of the adult dog (2). Animals with underlying systemic problems such as diabetes mellitus, hepatitis, nephritis, and immunosuppressant diseases can be expected to have more oral problems. *Home dental care* can dramatically affect the development and control of periodontal disease. Home care encompasses diet, chew toys, chewable dental abrasives and chemicals, hygiene solutions and gels, and brushing (75–83). With improved diets and medical care, animals are living longer, healthier lives. Unfortunately, it has also been demonstrated that as animals age, dental and periodontal disease increases (73,84,85). This could be one of the factors in the increase of periodontal disease over the last few decades, as increasing life expectancy with good health care has been realized.

Although pet foods have been involved with the changes in general health and longer life expectancies, the factors of chewing behavior, nutrition, and diet have been altered to an even greater degree. *Chewing behavior* affects the oral cavity in two ways: with normal chewing and abnormal chewing activity (75). First, normal chewing activity has been modified in that the food textures of most commercial diets have generally reduced the need for functional dentition, and the need to chew. This has altered the normal physiologic cleaning of both the teeth and gingiva. This has been further complicated by the rapid growth of the use of various chew products and toys. Some of these help reduce calculus and plaque that can lead to periodontal disease (75,80,82). However, many others make little to no difference, while some actually cause additional problems or even broken teeth. Abnormal chewing habits are those that occur due to nervous or dermatologic problems (49). Many pets have anxiety attacks when owners are not present or when storms and thunder occur. During these nervous episodes, animals may chew various articles or attempt to chew out of confining areas, causing damage to the teeth and periodontium. During dermatologic problems, animals may groom or chew at their skin excessively. The chewing of hair causes two serious problems. First it can cause a gradual attrition, or wearing down, of the teeth, at times exposing the pulp canal. This can result in endodontic problems that may eventually disseminate to the periodontal structures through the apical delta, causing an endodontic–periodontic type of disease. Secondly, hair wrapped around teeth or even small pieces caught in the gingival sulcus act as a local irritant, leading to gingivitis, and later progress into periodontitis. Certain individuals can build up a large amount of matted hair that can completely cover the incisors, if not removed on a regular basis.

Pet food *nutrients and food components* have been involved with the changes in general health and longer life expectancies (76). Normal chewing activity has been modified by the food textures now provided. These have generally required less chewing, thereby reducing the need for a functional dentition. This has altered the normal physiologic cleaning of both the teeth and gingiva (48).

Diet is concerned with the foods fed to the pet. This deals with the actual products from which a food is made and how they are treated, which greatly influences food texture, pH, and taste appeal. It has been shown that alteration of textures can greatly affect the natural cleansing effects of the gingiva and teeth, as wells as the development of gingivitis and periodontal disease (81). Textures deal not only with the coarseness of a food but also its compressibility and resistance to tearing. When all other factors are equal, studies in the dog and cat have indicated that a greater plaque and calculus accumulation and associated gingivitis occurred in animals fed a soft diet in comparison with a hard diet (86,87). The pH of a food or diet has been shown in humans to influence the dental oral health through the development of cervical line lesions (88–90). The development of these lesions can then act as a local irritant to initiate periodontal disease.

Nutrition is concerned with what a food is composed of that actually nourishes the body: vitamins, minerals, carbohydrates, sugars, fats, etc. Variations in vitamin and mineral content can produce numerous tooth, alveolar-bone, and periodontium problems (74). Vitamin C and selenium deficiencies have both been shown to result in a weak periodontal ligament that is easily damaged. Increases in sugars, decreased minerals, and increased pH can all have effects on coronal and root caries development. Since many of these food changes have occurred gradually over the last 30–50 years–the same general time frame as the increase in periodontal disease–they may correlate to some degree.

Saliva quality and *quantity* are major ecologic influences on supragingival plaque for mation (13,91). Individuals with reduced salivary flow ("dry mouth") have a higher rate of supragingival plaque development. Additionally, animals on soft diets may accumulate plaque more readily than those on dry foods. This is due to the mechanical effect of the dry food and the increased salivary flow.

Local irritants such as occlusal trauma, bruxism, and foreign bodies also have an effect on the development of periodontal disease (13,54). Trauma to the gingival tissues due to malocclusion, crowding, and bruxing (excessive grinding of teeth) are all known to be initiators of periodontal disease. Additionally, hair in the sulcus acts as a typical foreign body, stimulating inflammation, ulceration, and profuse exudation. The hair can be from the animal chewing on itself due to various dermatologic problems or directly from food.

Many animal diets include beef hide as a source of digestible protein. Within the beef hide may be large amounts of hair stubble initially left in the hair follicle, which may be released during palatability treatment.

Indices Commonly Used in Periodontal Disease

While attachment loss and its measurement are the focal aspect of evaluating periodontal disease, there are many other indices that may be used to quantify the extent of inflammation and disease. It is virtually impossible to cover every index available, and some assessments may have numerous evaluation schematics to choose from.

Plaque Index (PI) (92)

0   No plaque
1   Thin film along gingival margin
2   Moderate accumulation, plaque in sulcus
3   Abundant soft material in sulcus

Gingival Index (GI) (93)

0   Normal gingiva
1   Mild inflammation, slight change in color, slight edema, no bleeding on probing
2   Moderate inflammation; redness, edema, and glazing; bleeding on probing
3   Severe inflammation

Sulcus Bleeding Index (SBI) (94)

0   Healthy appearance, no bleeding on sulcus probing
1   Apparently healthy, showing no change in color or swelling, but slight bleeding from sulcus on probing
2   Bleeding on probing, changing of color due to inflammation, no swelling or macroscopic edema
3   Bleeding on probing, change in color, slight edematous swelling
4   Bleeding on probing, change in color, obvious swelling
5   Bleeding on probing, spontaneous bleeding, change in color, marked swelling with or without ulceration

Calculus Index (CI) (95)

0   No calculus
1   Supragingival calculus extending only slightly below the free gingival margin
2   Moderate amount of supragingival and subgingival calculus, or subgingival calculus only
3   Abundance of supragingival or subgingival calculus

Percentage Attachment Loss (PAL) Index (98)

Normal	No attachment loss
Early	≤25% attachment loss
Moderate	<50% attachment loss
Severe	≥50% attachment loss

Radiographic Index (RI) Analysis for Periodontal Disease (PD) (96)

0   Normal
1   Early PD: crestal bone loss around teeth
2   Moderate PD: bone loss <50% around tooth root(s)
3   Advanced PD: bone loss ≥50% around tooth root(s)

The majority of these indices are adapted from human texts and for the most part are applicable to veterinary dentistry. One notable exception is the periodontal disease index, with attachment loss being expressed in millimeter increments. With the wide variability of patient size, particularly when referring to cats, these values are less useful, unless converted into a percentage of attachment loss.

Histologic Changes in Periodontitis

Histologically, there is also a general progression found. Polymorphonuclear granulocytes (PMNs) can be found even in relatively healthy gingiva, and small amounts of gingival fluid can be considered normal. The junctional epithelium will show no changes, in contrast to lateral proliferation in the coronal region as there is progression to an initial and then early gingivitis. This classification is more of a histologic grouping, particularly for mature animals, but more PMNs, some lymph cells, and a few plasma cells may start to accumulate. There will be more vasculitis and exudate and some alteration of fibroblasts with collagen loss.

The time frame for initial gingivitis is 2–4 days once the plaque starts to accumulate and 4–14 days for the early stage. The earliest clinically observable gingivitis is considered to be an established gingivitis, with continued proliferation of the junctional epithelium, more plasma cells, increased exudate, fibroblast injury, and more loss of collagen, at about 1–3 weeks, with a variable length of time for persistence, sometimes years. It is most likely that the accumulation of plaque contributes to the inflammation and even slight sulcus depth, but with no loss of connective tissue attachment and no specific microorganisms involved (1). The migration of PMNs and exudate flow moves parallel to the tooth surface, similar to the movement and sloughing of junctional epithelial cells, providing the host another defense against bacteria.

With the progression to a periodontitis, there are several distinctions, including the virulence of the pathogens (97) and histologic signs of bone resorption, apical proliferation, and ulceration of the junctional epithelium, leading to the continued loss of attachment of the connective tissue. There will be periods of quiescence and exacerbation that can be quite variable from individual to individual, even among individual teeth in the same patient. With the formation of a periodontal pocket and mineralization of calculus on the root surface, the exudate flow changes to a perpendicular direction to the tooth surface, inhibiting the normal cleansing effect of the flow. At this stage, spontaneous healing is no longer possible, and even after root planing, there may be limited healing, although the attachment loss is typically not recovered naturally.

Staging of Periodontal Disease

While this classification helps delineate the characteristics of a disease process, it is still necessary to determine the extent of disease and the clinical degree of severity, or pathomorphologic stage (1). In addition, it is seldom the case that the entire dentition is at the same stage intensity or cycle of the disease, so each tooth should be evaluated separately. As discussed previously, using evaluation guidelines that look at specific pocket depths is not entirely judicious in veterinary medicine due to variation in patient size. Therefore, using percentage attachment loss (PAL) of the total attachment structure provides a viable alternative. Therefore, this veterinary periodontal disease index (PDI) system makes use of a PAL methodology (Table 1).

In *stage 1 (gingivitis) periodontal disease*, gingivitis with no attachment loss is seen (98,99). While some individuals may have significant calculus deposits and minimal gingival inflammation, others may experience profuse inflammation with relatively little plaque and calculus present. Research has shown that in the healthy gingiva of the dog, when plaque is totally controlled, there can be a total absence of a gingival sulcus (8). However, even in a normal healthy gingiva histologically, if the sulcus is a maximum of 0.5 mm, the periodontal probe can still easily penetrate the junctional epithelium, resulting in readings of up to 2.0 mm. For this reason, all probing should be done with an appropriate-size instrument and with minimal pressure.

As gingivitis progresses, there is a lateral proliferation of the junctional epithelium and coronal detachment from the tooth, and the sulcus deepens slightly, allowing bacteria to move into the gingival pocket. With additional inflammation, edema of the gingival tissues increases the height of the gingival margin, resulting in a deeper "pseudopocket," though without attachment loss. Since there is no loss of attachment in these situations, they are not defined as periodontal pockets and, with adequate treatment, are reversible lesions.

The clinical symptoms are evaluated using the indices described earlier, most notably the gingival index (GI) and PDI or sulcus bleeding index (SBI) (1). Healthy gingiva (GI=0; SBI=0) may exhibit a distinct difference between the free gingival margin and attached gingiva with stippling present. Mild gingivitis shows mild redness and edema with minimal bleeding after probing (GI=1; SBI=1), and loss of the stippling may begin. Moderate gingivitis progresses to a more obvious erythema and swelling with notable bleeding on probing (GI=2; SBI=2) with no apparent stippling. Severe gingivitis may exhibit extreme levels of redness and spontaneous hemorrhage with edema significant enough to appear hyperplastic (1) (GI=3; SBI=3–4).

While in many cases gingivitis may persist in an individual with occasional exacerbations of acute disease, it is often possible for the condition to progress to a periodontitis due to the lack of effective preventive treatment or the increased virulence or presence of microorganisms.

In *stage 2 (early) periodontal disease*, the first signs of destructive periodontitis are seen. Probing and radiographic examination may show signs of attachment loss up to

TABLE 1. Veterinary periodontal disease index (PDI)(98, 99)

Stage	Attachment loss (%)	Probing depth (mm)[a]	Dog	Cat
0	Normal	0	<3	<0.5
1	Gingivitis	0	<3	<0.5
2	Early	<25	<5	<1.0
3	Moderate	<50	<7	<2.0
4	Severe	>50	>7	>2.0

From refs. 98, 99.

[a]Probing depth is highly variable according to animal size; percentage of attachment loss is a more accurate measurement.

25% (98,99). In the human PDI system, 30% attachment loss is commonly used in this first stage. However, due to the shorter distance to the furcation in most carnivores (100–101), a reduced percentage for this early stage was selected for the veterinary PDI counterpart. The alveolar crests in the coronal portion tend to be more narrow; therefore, bone loss occurs more easily in a horizontal fashion. However, further bone loss has a tendency to follow blood vessel distribution, and vertical bone loss is also common.

In *stage 3 (moderate) periodontal disease*, the probing and radiographic signs of attachment loss are between 25% and 50% of the root length (98,99). Probing depths may be more pronounced due to the start of vertical defects and infrabony pockets. However, if gingival recession occurs at the same time, there may be little increase in the probing depths (1).

In *stage 4 (severe) periodontal disease*, the attachment loss is greater than 50% (98,99). Often significant infrabony pockets may be localized to a single area, such as the deep palatal pockets seen in maxillary canine teeth. Typically, there is more of a vertical lesion, particularly in teeth that are not closely adjacent to neighboring teeth. With the radius of bone destruction from plaque metabolites averaging 1.5–2.5 mm, broader interdental spaces (septa) allow for greater probability that extensive attachment loss will occur in a more vertical fashion as there is apical extension of bacterial invasion. In more generalized cases, horizontal bone loss is more common. With teeth that are closer together with similar bacterial loads, the bone loss can extend from the region of each tooth, encompassing the entire septa and leading to the more horizontal pattern of bone loss (1).

PATHOBIOLOGIC CLASSIFICATION OF PERIODONTITIS

Many forms of periodontitis exist, each progressing to cause attachment loss at variable rates (13,14). While it is possible to quantitate the degree of periodontal involvement using indices such as the PDI or maximal attachment loss (MAL), classification is sometimes enhanced on the basis of dynamic pathobiology, as is used internationally in human dentistry (8,12). Such a system does not just describe various increments of clinical findings at a finite point in time, but instead elaborates on a typical picture of a distinct disease process. While this particular system was designed for humans, there are specific veterinary entities that correlate with the descriptions provided. The current common international pathobiologic classification of periodontitis includes the following (14):

1. Adult periodontitis (AP)
2. Rapidly progressive periodontitis (RPP)
3. Localized juvenile periodontitis (LJP)
4. Prepubertal periodontitis (PP)
5. Refractory rapidly progressive periodontitis (RRPP)

Adult periodontitis is a slow-progressing form more commonly seen in adults, but it may have had its beginning when the animal was relatively young. It is the most common form of periodontal disease seen, typically experienced as a slow, chronic, gradual development with an irregular distribution. Although it can be generalized, there may be some areas more predisposed than others to more extensive forms of the disease (1). In mild to moderate cases, the bacterial plaque is often formed of gram-positive cocci and rods, though in acute exacerbations more virulent strains may be present. Initially, treatment is typically professional prophylaxis and good home care. It is seen in all breeds and species.

RPP is a rapidly progressive form seen mostly in young adults; it is commonly generalized. In primates, it has been described as occurring more frequently in young adult females (1). In some cases, cyclic episodes of acute infections of gram-negative anaer-obes may be followed by quiet periods. Attachment loss can be quite variable but can be minimized with appropriate therapy of cleaning with supportive antibiotics. There are some individuals with RPP that may have experienced an PP or LJP form of periodonti-tis at an earlier age. This form is seen not uncommonly in the Lhasa apso, Shih Tzu, York-shire terrier, Maltese, and greyhound, and in the Abyssinian and Somali cats.

LJP is a rapidly progressive localized periodontitis most commonly found in young animals. The gingiva will often be normal-looking, but with areas of bone resorption apparent as crater-like lesions radiographically. Aggressive professional prophylaxis, debridement, antibiotics, and home care will help control attachment destruction. In some controlled cases, bone lesions may regenerate with time (1). Uncontrolled cases will usually have continued attachment loss and progress into RPP or RRPP. This condi-tion is seen most commonly in the incisor teeth of the miniature schnauzer and in the pre-molar–molar area of greyhounds.

PP can be a localized or generalized form of periodontitis seen in association with the deciduous teeth. This form can be rapidly progressing with severe gingivitis, gingival recession, and even attachment loss. In the localized form, individual teeth show gin-givitis with little plaque and can usually be treated with mechanical therapy and antibi-otics, in contrast to the generalized form that is more refractory to therapy (1). This form of periodontitis is seen most commonly in Abyssinian and Somali cats.

RRPP is a therapy-resistant periodontitis that may be a subform of RPP (7–14,102). It can be localized or generalized, and is more commonly seen in older animals. In the cat, it is seen more frequently in Abyssinians, Somalis, and any cat with lymphocytic plasmocytic stomatitis (LPS). In the dog, it is most routinely observed in the greyhound, Maltese, minia-ture schnauzer, and any dog with chronic ulcerative paradental stomatitis (CUPS).

Oral Syndromes

There are many conditions and diseases that can affect the periodontal tissues. A more complete listing of periodontal related diseases can be found in the oral pathology chap-ter (see Chapter 5).

A more severe form of gingivitis sometimes seen in the dog is necrotizing ulcerative gingivitis that can be accompanied by pain, halitosis, and even fever. There may be pre-disposing stress factors associated with poor oral hygiene, and spirochetes in the plaque may be elevated (103). Histopathologically, there will be large numbers of polymor-phonuclear granulocytes in the oral epithelium and into the papillae, signifying an acute inflammatory response. The papillary area may become ulcerated and necrotic, flatten-ing out and even becoming concave, eroding away beyond the level of the gingival mar-gin adjacent to the tooth. Careful cleaning of the teeth, debridement of the lesions, antibi-otics, and improved home care are essential (60,104). The use of metronidazole has resulted in a decrease in spirochetes and a concurrent improvement in the disease (105). In the acute stages, no attachment loss is generally noted.

Gingival inflammation can also be elicited by hormonal changes, different drug admin-istration (diphenytoin, cyclosporine), and sensitivities (106). Specific gingival growths or tumors may initially present with an inflammatory or hyperplastic appearance, but they should be biopsied. Autoimmunologic disease such as pemphigus vulgaris and bullous pemphigoid can be severe in appearance, but the lesional destruction involves the epithe-lial layers and does not typically affect the underlying connective tissue, unless secondary infections occur. At the other end of the spectrum, individuals with immunodeficient syndromes may exhibit a host of opportunistic gingival infections by bacteria, viruses, and fungi, often progressing into more severe periodontitis and stomatitis.

Abnormalities in an animal's immune system can have varying effects on the periodontal tissues. Infection, stress, or drugs may lead to alterations in the immune response that may predispose an individual to opportunistic infections. This may be a decrease in response or at times an exaggerated response to relatively normal stimuli. An exaggerated response may be seen in the increase in immunoglobulin G and immune complex deposition in a syndrome of ulcerative stomatitis in Maltese dogs (107). In *"kissing lesions"* of CUPS, there may be a marked ulceration of buccal mucosa that contacts a tooth/calculus surface (48). This condition appears to develop as a result of plaque intolerance with the consequence of an excessive immune response to any deposition. Initially, the condition is primarily localized to areas adjacent to the canine and carnassial teeth, but it may rapidly progress to a more generalized stage. Plaque control appears to be the key; however, due to the pain associated with these lesions, most patients will not allow oral manipulations while awake. In addition, many clients find the fowl odor an obstacle to performing most home oral care. The use of antibiotics, including metronidazole, is helpful only temporarily. Use of topical preparations such as Orabase, Orabase with Benzocaine, or Oralone™ (an preparation with a cortisone) (Thomas Pharmacal, Ronkonkoma, New York) provides a coating effect to temporarily reduce the pain from the ulceration. If effective plaque control cannot be maintained, extractions are often necessary, as anti-inflammatory agents also provide only transitory relief. Additionally, selective extractions customarily only provide temporary relief, as the condition has a tendency to recur at new sites.

Attachment Loss

Attachment loss is the end product of inflammation, involving the supportive tissues, both soft tissue and bone. The direct effect of bacterial byproducts is certainly involved, particularly with increased bacterial presence in periodontal pockets, but the host's defense system can contribute significantly. Destruction of collagen fibers affect many of the supportive tissues, and granulocytes breaking open within the inflamed tissue can release elastase, collagenase, and acid hydrolases. Macrophages can also release hydrolases, proteases, and lysozymes. The destruction of bone is less well defined, because it is difficult to experimentally demonstrate mediators other than cytokines and prostaglandins (PGE_2). These substances stimulate osteoclast differentiation and increase their resorptive capacities; they may also interfere with bone regeneration (1).

In cats, any grossly visible signs of periodontal disease indicate that a significant change has already occurred (7). Because the gingiva is so thin and tightly adherent to the tooth surface, it is difficult to insert even a probe into a healthy sulcus. Attachment loss of 0.5–1.0 mm can result in a substantial decrease in support, particularly in the incisors. There also tends to be a great variability in the relationship of calculus/plaque accumulation and inflammatory response.

In addition to the primary, or *obligate* (1), symptoms of periodontal disease including inflammation, true pocket formation, and bone resorption, a variety of other problems may be present. Gingival swelling, or even hyperplasia, can occur beyond normal levels of gingivitis, often with the accompanying increase in gingival height that can increase pocket depth without concurrent attachment loss.

While the actual, or absolute, pocket depth is important to assess in relation to the amount of attachment lost, the extent and frequency of active periods of periodontitis are essential to determining what process exists and what treatment should be started. A larger portion of quiescent periods with mild-to-moderate signs of active inflammation (bleeding, exudate) will warrant less aggressive attention than a more rapid presentation.

After resolution, either spontaneous or due to therapy, of an active phase of periodontitis, particularly with some of the more slowly progressive forms, the acute inflammation in the gingiva will resolve, and gingival shrinkage may occur. Shrinkage should be differentiated from true gingival recession, which occurs without pocket formation and sometimes in the absence of clinical inflammation (1). Generalized recession does occur, but more commonly only one to several teeth are often involved. Frenulum tension, improper tooth brushing, orthodontic therapy, and even overall aggressive scaling can contribute to the recession. The facial bone plate, very thin to begin with, can be compromised, have fenestration, or even be lost completely (dehiscence). These lesions are sometimes not easily demonstrated radiographically, since the facial bone loss can be "camouflaged." At times, the recession can start by the formation of a small groove, or *Stillman cleft* (1). A fibrotic, noninflammatory response can result in a thickening of the remaining attached gingiva, rolling into a lesion known as *McCall's festoons*. Inflammation can become part of the picture if inadequate hygiene is provided or if the recession extends below the mucogingival line. Shrinkage after periodontitis may be more apparent in papillary regions, while recession is typically found on the facial surface. Gingival shrinkage may result in "smaller" pockets depths, even with significant attachment loss. For the most accurate evaluation, the percentage attachment loss (PAL) should be measured from the cementoenamel junction (CEJ), the initial site of attachment in most teeth, to the depth of the periodontal pocket. Also note that even in healthy tissue, the probing depth can actually be as much as 2 mm more that the sulcus depth itself, as the probe penetrates the histologic bottom of the sulcus. In diseased tissues (gingivitis or periodontitis), the probe may extend through vascular connective tissue, stopping at resistance of intact collagen (1). The final evaluation, then, should be to determine the extent of healthy attachment left, not just probing depth, by assessing the area of the root that is still viable for collagen attachment.

It is extremely helpful in evaluating attachment levels to use radiographs in addition to probing. While extraoral films can provide a general screening capability, it is wise to use intraoral films to isolate specific areas for evaluation. With these views, several items may be assessed, including the area affected (local, generalized), type of bone loss (crestal, horizontal, vertical), extent of the problem and remaining attachment, and sometimes the cause of a specific problem (subgingival calculus). While the films are still only two-dimensional, varying the angulation (horizontal and vertical planes) can help localize specific areas of bone loss and make quantifying easier. In addition, newer methods of computer-assisted evaluations will be used to compare regions pre- and postsurgically. It is important to note is that radiographs will only show bone loss that has already occurred. They will provide no information on the current status of the disease and little data on soft tissue condition.

Types of Recession or Attachment Loss

Attachment loss expresses itself as some form of tissue recession. This recession generally shows as either root exposure, suprabony pockets, infrabony (intrabony) pockets, or a combination of root exposure and pocket formation (8). Sulcus or pocket depth is measured from the gingival margin to the epithelial base of the sulcus or pocket. A sulcus is considered a physiologically normal depth of the crevicular groove. A pocket is considered a pathologic or abnormal depth of the crevicular groove.

Root exposure recession is measured as areas of exposed root between the gingival margin and the CEJ. This can be seen in either horizontal or vertical bone loss in association with gingival margin recession. The combination of loss of the two results in areas of exposed root. A *suprabony pocket* has its base, or bottom of the pocket, coronal to the alveolar crestal bone. It is usually associated with early pocket formation, gingival hyperplasia, or an underlying horizontal bone loss pattern. An *infrabony (intrabony) pocket* has its base apical to the alveolar crest. This means that the pocket, at its depth, is between the tooth and bone (108). It is normally associated with a vertical bone loss pattern. In the dog, this is most commonly seen interproximally between the mandibular 1st and 2nd molars and lingually to the maxillary canine tooth.

Infrabony-Pocket Wall Classification

When infrabony pockets are present, bone loss can contribute to the formation of specific configurations of pocket morphology (109) (Fig. 3). Infrabony pockets are gener-

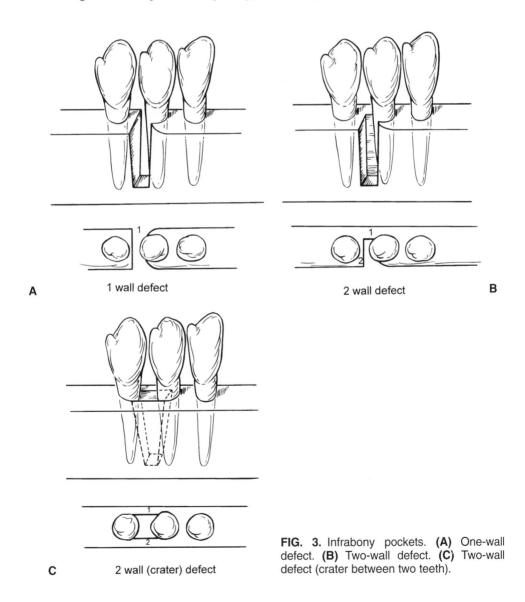

A   1 wall defect   2 wall defect   B

C   2 wall (crater) defect

FIG. 3. Infrabony pockets. **(A)** One-wall defect. **(B)** Two-wall defect. **(C)** Two-wall defect (crater between two teeth).

ally classified by the number of infrabony-pocket walls surrounding the tooth. In an early lesion that extends from and involves one root, the defect is formed by the root as one wall and three osseous surfaces, making it a *three-wall bony pocket*. When this extends interdentally to communicate with the root of an adjacent tooth, the two tooth surfaces make up two walls, and the other two walls are formed by bone on the facial and lingual surfaces, or a *two-wall bony defect*. Apically, if the infrabony defect extends further down the root surface of one or both of the teeth with some preservation of the septal bone, a three-wall defect may be more descriptive of the specific area. A *one-wall bony pockets* extends the lesion just described to include destruction of either osseous surface and its replacement by soft tissue, leaving one bony surface. A defect surrounding the tooth is termed a *cup, moat, circumferential*, or *four-wall defect* (1,108). Combination defects are those with several levels or floors within the defect, resulting in combinations of the above types of defects at the same site (eg, a combined one- and two-wall defect). The degree of bone loss and morphology of the pocket will play a distinct role in determining the mode of treatment that would be most efficacious. Occasionally, combination defects will be seen.

Furcation Exposure

Furcational involvement deals with exposure of areas between roots (110). In addition, the extent of bone loss will often involve the furcation region of multirooted teeth. Extensive problems can occur with attachment loss in these areas, including increasing food and plaque retention, rapid attachment loss, and even erosive or carious lesions (111). Pathologic invasion of a furcation is best determined by careful probing with a curved explorer, although once it is diagnosed, radiographs can aid in determining extent (74). There are various methods of classification of attachment loss involving furcations; the following is a common system used in veterinary dentistry:

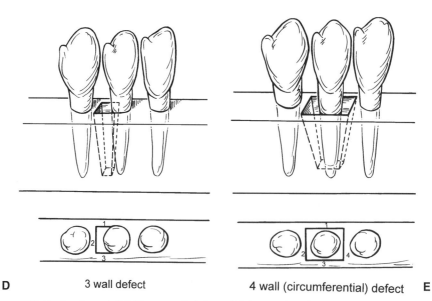

D   3 wall defect   4 wall (circumferential) defect   E

FIG. 3. *Continued.* **(D)** Three-wall defect. **(E)** four-wall defect (circumferential).

Furcation Exposure (FE) (9)

F0   No furcational involvement
F1*   Soft tissue lesion extending to the furcation level with minimal osseous destruction
F2*   Soft tissue lesion combined with bone loss that permits a probe to enter the furcation from one aspect, but not to pass completely through the furcation.
F3   Lesions with extensive osseous destruction that permits through and through passage of the probe, with or without soft tissue obscuring the communication.

*These two classifications are subdivided as F, L, M, D (facial, lingual, mesial, distal) to be used to denote furcation position; example: F2-F = furcation exposure and undermined on facial surface of tooth. The amount of vertical bone loss can further be categorized as to the amount of attachment loss in subclasses (113). Subclass A includes those lesions with 1–3 mm of vertical loss; subclass B, 4–6 mm; and subclass C, >7 mm.

The presence of furcational involvement does result in a poor, but not hopeless, prognosis. The major problems involves access for professional curettage and scaling, and home care. If these problems can be reasonably resolved, the prognosis is no worse than that of a single-rooted tooth with similar attachment loss. Generally, the most difficult cases to treat are the subclasses A and B. With these, food-debris collection and home care are more of a problem. In subclass C, there will often be an associated horizontal bone loss that results in a more open furcation that is easier to keep clean and self-cleans more proficiently. It is not unusual to see subclass C conditions that are stable and have a great deal less of a periodontitis problem than subclasses A or B.

Mobility

Mobility of teeth is a critical diagnostic and prognostic tool. As mobility increases, so do the proportional chances of tooth loss. Some degree of tooth movement is considered normal and is termed *physiologic movement*. The physiologic movement of a tooth is limited to the width of the periodontal ligament and the elasticity of the alveolar support. *Pathologic mobility* is defined as the displacement of a tooth, either vertically or horizontally, beyond its physiologic movement (114). However, a tooth that is loose does not necessarily denote the presence of periodontal disease. Hypermobility can be present in a clinically normal periodontium as the result of previously applied stress, such as orthodontics, or due to a fibrous alveolus, as is seen in mandibular central incisors in a fibrous parasymphysis. In addition, some transient mobility may occur following traumatic injuries, endodontic treatment, and periodontal therapy (74). The following is a classification of mobility in common use in veterinary dentistry:

Tooth Mobility Index (MI)(105)

0   None   Normal
1   Slight   Represents the first distinguishable sign of movement greater than normal
2   Moderate Movement of approximately 1 mm
3   Severe   Movement >1 mm in any direction and/or is depressible.

While mobility of a tooth is primarily influenced by the degree of bone loss associated with periodontal disease (114), occlusal forces can also contribute to progressive mobility (115). Parafunctional occlusal habits such as bruxing, clenching, and cage biting can result in mobility problems (74). In addition, occlusal prematurities, as seen in open bites and base-narrow conditions, may also affect tooth laxity (74). Even the mobility itself can be detrimental to optimal healing in such therapy (116). When this is the case, temporary splinting may be required in addition to other treatments to control the condition. Any condition, injury, or disease that results in alveolar bone loss or weakening can affect tooth movement or mobility (74). Severe mobility nearly always results in tooth loss, which can be considered the final "symptom" of periodontal disease (1). The elimination or even control of pathologic tooth mobility can only be gained by interference with the causative pathology. In the majority of cases, once the tooth is actually lost, the inflammation around the region lessens or even resolves, as the plaque retentive surface is no longer present. In some refractory stomatitis cases, inflammation may persist after extraction or exfoliation.

Periodontal Abscess

If necrotic tissue or debris gets trapped within the confines of the sulcus and is not removed, expelled, or resorbed, a pocket or furcation abscess may result. Penetrating foreign bodies or less-than-thorough subgingival scaling can also result in such a lesion, which can be painful if not draining out the sulcus or fistulated, and may require drainage. In some cases, a submucosal abscess, or parulis, may develop (1).

Generally, periodontal abscesses can be divided into three categories: acute, chronic, and chronic/acute (108). *Acute periodontal abscesses* may be accompanied by pain, swelling, tenderness of the gingiva, tooth sensitivity on percussion, and possibly systemic signs such as malaise, fever, and leukocytosis. These early lesions may present without notable clinical lesions or radiographic changes. Acute lesions, when improperly treated or untreated, may eventually subside but persist in a chronic state. *Chronic periodontal abscesses* are usually asymptomatic. However, a dull pain may sometimes develop that may stimulate grinding of the teeth or a bruxing-like syndrome. Chronic lesions may develop without having ever experienced an acute state, but a chronic state may flare up periodically into an acute condition. *Chronic/acute periodontal abscesses* are acute exacerbations of chronic lesions.

If there is fistulation, the opening will often be seen coronal to the mucogingival line. Because of the complex nature of abscess formation, abscess pockets and sinus opening may not necessarily be located over the same root surface as the actual disease site. Using a periodontal probe or contrast medium with radiographs can help localize the area of abscessation. For those fistula orifices near the mucogingival junction, radiographs are essential to evaluate the possibility of a periapical lesion. The typical appearance of a periodontal abscess is as a discrete area of radiolucency along the lateral root border (108). Abscesses on the lingual or facial surfaces are commonly obscured by the radiopacity of the root. Mobility may be seen, as extensive bone destruction may occur, compromising the dental support structures (27).

Endodontic–Periodontic Relationship

Infection from periodontal disease may have adverse effects on the pulp (108). Generally, pulp involvement occurs from the spread of infection along the root surface, gaining entrance to the endodontic system through lateral or accessory canals or through the apical delta. The endodontic–periodontic relation is discussed in greater detail in the basic endodontics chapter (see Chapter 11).

PERIODONTAL EVALUATION

A systematic and methodical examination is necessary to assess all of the oral structures (see Chapter 4 for a more detailed protocol involving the oral examination).

The examination includes the initial external exam of the facial area, extending to a preliminary check of the labial surfaces of the teeth, the gums, and even a open-mouth view of the alert patient. While this may alert the practitioner to some specific problems, a periodontal examination can never be complete without full probing of all pockets, and normally this can only be accomplished in a sedated or anesthetized animal. All information gathered from the owner during the history gathering should be coupled with any physical clues.

The most important diagnostic tool in periodontal therapy is the explorer/probe. The probe end, marked in millimeters, is gently inserted into the sulcus to measure its depth. Pocket depth, gingival recession, and root exposure should be assessed and combined to determine the total percentage of attachment loss (PAL). Dental radiographs can be aid in this determination, as well as providing other information. These data can then be converted into the staging of periodontal disease (see Table 1).

The explorer is the sharp-pointed end of the explorer/probe, which may be hooked, angled, or straight. It can be gently drawn close to the tooth in the sulcus (with care to avoid soft tissue damage) to help detect hidden calculus, resorptive lesions, or cavities in the subgingival area. The explorer can also be used to aid in detecting open canals due to fractures or cavities.

During oral examination under anesthesia, it is the visual as well as the tactile signs that indicate conditions that may warrant therapy. Evaluations of the gingival index (GI), calculus index (CI), sulcus bleeding index (SBI), furcation exposures (FE), and tooth mobility run index (MI), in association with the periodontal disease index (PDI), can help determine not only the extent of disease but also whether periodontal disease is active or in a period of quiescence. It must be noted that there can be different stages of periodontal disease present in the same oral cavity and even different levels of involvement of different areas of the same tooth. All abnormalities should be properly recorded.

CHARTING

A knowledge of the dental formula of the permanent teeth will help in recognition of abnormalities such as missing teeth, supernumerary (extra) teeth, and even retained deciduous teeth (which should be extracted). Identifying the tooth type is essential for proper charting: *I*, incisor; *C*, canine; *P*, premolar; *M*, molar.

Dog (permanent). $2 \times$ (I 3/3, C 1/1, P 4/4, M 2/3) = 42
Cat (permanent): $2 \times$ (I 3/3, C 1/1, P 3/2, M 1/1) = 30
(**Note:** In a cat, the premolars missing are actually the ones in front; that is, the upper premolars should be numbered from 2 to 4, and the lower premolars should be numbered 3 and 4).

Many methods for charting are available, but consistency is the key. A simple system is to abbreviate the tooth type and then indicate the tooth's number and position by the use of super- and subscripts:

^{1}C Upper left canine
P$_2$ Lower right second premolar

The use of dental charts on the permanent record, either as a stamped impression, sticker, or separate sheet, is one of the easiest methods of simplifying charting. One chart can be used for recording the examination, assessment, and pathology, with a second to denote the specific treatment; otherwise, a single diagram may be used for both. When using charts the following notations are commonly used:

O = Missing tooth	GI = Gingivitis index
X = Extracted tooth	CI = Calculus index
FE = Furcation exposure	PI = Plaque index
RE = Root exposure	SBI = Sulcus bleeding index
CA = Cavity	PDI = Periodontal disease index
CLL = Cervical line lesion	PP = Periodontal pocket
FX = Tooth fracture	M = Mobility
ONF = Oronasal fistula	PRO = Professional prophylaxis

(See Appendix for a more complete set of abbreviations.)

THERAPY

Since the primary cause of periodontal disease is microorganisms, the primary goal of periodontal disease therapy is to control the microorganisms. However, failure to control secondary causes can result in failure to attain the primary goal. Therefore, it is important to address all known possible contributing factors. Therapy is divided into five basic categories:

1. Professional prophylaxis (teeth cleaning)
2. Antimicrobial therapies
3 Periodontal surgeries
4. Dental surgeries
5. Home prophylaxis (home dental hygiene care)

Professional Prophylaxis (Teeth Cleaning)

The benefits of performing a complete and proper prophylaxis to aid in control of early periodontal disease or to help salvage more advanced cases cannot be overemphasized. Gross removal of supragingival plaque and calculus may improve the appearance of the teeth, but full attention needs to be paid to the subgingival tissues, where a majority of the disease process is occurring.

Supragingival calculus scaling can be done in many fashions with many different instruments. Gross removal of supragingival calculus and plaque is accomplished initially by removing larger pieces manually with calculus forceps or a hoe scaler, with care not to injure the soft tissue. This is followed by scaling with either hand or powered scalers. (See Chapter 1 for more information on scalers and curettes.) Hand scaling, although slow, can be gentle to the tooth yet very effective. However, hand scalers should be kept sharp to prevent crushing of calculus and burnishing plaque into the tooth surface. Most hand scalers are made for use only above the gum line and with a pull stroke away from the soft tissues. This is due to the fact that many have a pointed tip, which, if used below the gum line, may lacerate the epithelial attachment and allow bacteria to enter the periodontal tissues more freely. The ultrasonic scaler should always be used on the lowest effective power setting, with a very light touch of the side of the scaler, with adequate water flow to control heat, and for a maximum of 12–15 seconds per tooth, in order to avoid iatrogenic injuries. The heat generated by these instruments may result in hyperthermic pulpitis, which may be reversible or irreversible, necessitating eventual endodontic therapy. Rotary scaling burs are used on high-speed handpieces with a water flow. These burs can be highly effective but can also be highly aggressive to the dental tissues. They should be used with a light touch for no more than 12–15 seconds per tooth. Due to the damage that can be caused to the tooth by these burs, they should be used cautiously.

Various products to facilitate scaling have been introduced on the market, such as Sof-scale™ Calculus Scaling Gel (Ash/Dentsply, York, Pennsylvania). These products have chelating and detoxification agents to ease the removal of calculus. Animal studies have shown that these products facilitate scaling but generally do not provide much of a time savings (117).

Subgingival calculus scaling can be done with ultrasonic or sonic instruments, when proper tips and irrigation are used. Nevertheless, this is still typically performed with the gentler hand instruments or curettes. Subgingival deposits of plaque and calculus (up to 4-mm pocket depth) can often be removed using a curette gently below the gum line. Curettes have a rounded toe that can reduce damage to the epithelial attachment in the bottom of the sulcus, in comparison with hand scalers when used below the gum line. Curette selection must harmonize with the root anatomy to be effective (see Chapter 1 for more information on curettes).

In cases where the root surface is still firm and reasonably smooth, simple subgingival debridement with a periodontal tip on an appropriate ultrasonic instrument may suffice for treatment, as may light use of a curette. However, as the root surface becomes more diseased and the cementum pitted, a process called *root planing* should be utilized to clean and smooth the surface. Pitted and rough root surface areas will only further irritate the gingiva and allow for easy reaccumulation of plaque and calculus. The curette is drawn across the root in several different directions to completely remove all debris and smooth the surface.

Subgingival curettage may also be employed to gently scrape disease tissue and bacteria from the inside layer of the gingival pocket or sulcus. However, in most cases, this procedure is performed inadvertently during subgingival debridement and root planing. Subgingival curettage is seldom an essential part of treatment.

Any type of scaling causes defects in the enamel surface, so *polishing* is necessary to smooth the surface and slow readherence of plaque and calculus. Polishing has been under some scrutiny in human dentistry for its gradual abrasive reduction of the enamel over a 30–60-year period of annual or semiannual treatment, although this has not shown itself to be a problem with pets at this point. However, excessive polishing should be avoided to prevent enamel loss and hyperthermia of the pulp. Most polishing is performed with a slow speed handpiece, a prophylaxis angle (pop-on or screw-on type), an appropriate prophylaxis cup, and a fine-textured polishing paste. The use of light circular strokes for up to 5 seconds per tooth with a fine or extrafine pumice, adequate slurry, and care not to exceed 1–3000 rpm will help avoid hyperthermia. To reach tooth surfaces under the gum line, the foot of the prophylaxis cup can be splayed with light force.

Polishing, as well as minor cleaning, of the teeth can also be performed with an *air/powder prophylaxis unit* (Plaque-Sweep™, Ash/Dentsply). Such units use an air power source to spray a water and abrasive powder across the teeth to polish them. The abrasive is usually a finely ground sodium bicarbonate powder. They create a sandblasting effect that can clean areas in developmental grooves and interproximally, where a standard polishing device often cannot reach. However, the sodium load created by the abrasive may be contraindicated in some cases. Additionally, a few cases of barotrauma have been reported (118). This is the result of the air's blowing open the salivary duct orifice and allowing air, abrasive, and debris to enter. Generally, facial swelling, pain, and possible fever may occur. In many cases, the pneumosialitis literally inflates the gland making it not only painful but easily palpated. Crepitus of the area may also occur if the integrity of the acini is insulted. Most cases are of a mild nature that resolve within 4–5 days with simple treatment. Anti-inflammatory drugs are used to reduce swelling and discomfort, while prophylaxis antibiotics are used because of the chance of contamination of the gland by oral debris.

Polishing is followed by *sulcus irrigation* or *lavage* using water, saline, a chlorhexidine solution of 0.12% or less, or an appropriately diluted fluoride solution. This is done to flush all remaining pumice and debris out of the sulcus to prevent foreign body irritations that might lead to periodontal inflammation or abscess formation. A blunt-tipped irrigation needle and syringe or a periodontal irrigating device can be used.

Application of sodium or stannous *fluoride* in a gel, foam, or varnish to the tooth surfaces may be of some value. The fluoride gels are generally left in place for 3–5 minutes and then blown or gently wiped from the teeth; they are not rinsed off as this will generally deactivate the material. Charting of lesions is necessary for future reference and evaluation.

Professional Prophylaxis and Periodontal Treatment

If the auxiliary steps given in the following outline are required, the treatment is no longer a prophylaxis, but a periodontal therapy.

1. Gross removal of calculus and plaque (supragingival)
   - power or hand (carefully)
2. Subgingival scaling
   - curette
   - remove all deposits

The auxiliary steps constituting periodontal therapy are the following:

3. Polishing
   - light, circular strokes, 15–20 seconds, avoid hyperthermia
   - smooth surface (any scaling causes ridges)
   - "splay" the prophylaxis cup to polish subgingivally
   - aids in slowing readherence of plaque and calculus
4. Sulcus irrigation
   - removes debris that might irritate sulcus or cause abscess
   - can be done with water
   - medicament solutions may be used, such as 0.2% chlorhexidine or 0.4–0.8% stannous fluoride
5. Perio-probing and charting

Depending on the type of pathology, the following auxiliary steps may be required for periodontal therapy:

6. Gingival surgeries
   - gingivoplasty
   - reverse bevel incisions
   - flap surgeries

7. Subgingival debridement or root planing (before polishing)
   - with exposed roots or in pockets (flap needed if >4 mm)
   - curette in several angles to create smooth surface; overlapping strokes in horizontal, vertical, and oblique directions
8. Subgingival curettage (before polishing)
   - remove debris from subgingival gingivae in pockets–microflora and diseased tissue
9. Medicament treatments
   Fluoride treatment (at end)
   - desensitize teeth
   - temporary bacterial resistance
   - air-dry teeth, apply gel or varnish
   Chlorhexidine treatment
   - reduction of oral microflora load
10. Radiology
    - evaluate bone loss, endodontic disease, cavities, resorptive lesions, etc.
11. Chart treatments
12. Home treatments
13. Recheck of professional and home treatment
    - 2 weeks after professional treatment
14. Maintenance through home dental hygiene care
15. Recalls and reevaluations
    - as required according to the PDI, GI, and SBI.

Antimicrobial Therapies

Antimicrobial therapy is based on the theory that bacteria are the underlying cause of most periodontal disease. It is commonly used as an adjunct to teeth cleanings and other treatments, but it should not be used as a substitute for them. There are two basic forms of antimicrobial treatment: local and systemic.

Routine use of local or topical antimicrobials such as chlorhexidine certainly has its place both prophylactically and therapeutically (119). It has been shown to be effective in helping control plaque, gingivitis, and periodontal disease in the dog (120,121). Chlorhexidine may increase staining of the tooth surface and the rate of calcification of calculus. Extended oral contact or a high concentration (>2.0%) can occasionally cause painful ulceration from desquamation (119). Chlorhexidine is typically applied following teeth cleaning as a gel or solution. As a home care product, it is available as a diluted solution (0.12%), a gel, or a bioahesive tablet, such as Stomadhex™ (ImmunoVet, Tampa, Florida) (122). Absorbable antibiotics placed in the sulcus, such as Atridox® (Atrix Labs, Fort Collins, Colorado), a polylactic acid gel with doxycycline, can be injected into the sulcus where it hardens and then proceeds to release antibiotic as the polylactic acid is being absorbed for 3–10 days.

The systemic use of antibiotics has many indications (55). They may be used as a preventive prophylaxis in patients with conditions that might predispose them to infection. For animals with heart conditions, the use of a penicillin-type antibiotic beginning at least 1 hour before professional prophylaxis and lasting for a least 1 hour after the procedure would generally be recommended, based on the short duration of stimulated bacteremia (123). In heavy infection states, antibiotics can also be used to lessen the bacterial load and help prevent systemic migration of the infection to primary organs. They can improve the success in most periodontal treatments. Additionally, they may be used as the treatment in salvage cases in which more appropriate treatments cannot be performed due to the animal's health or client restrictions. However, the oral cavity is naturally a haven for bacteria, and its total sterility is not a logical pursuit. Additionally, the misuse of systemic antibiotics can possibly cause side effects and the development of resistant strains of bacteria. Therefore, judicial but aggressive use of antibiotics is an intricate part of the therapy.

The antibiotics most commonly used in veterinary periodontal conditions are amoxicillin, amoxicillin/clavulanate, clindamycin, doxycycline, and metronidazole (55). The selection is generally based on personal experience, patient sensitivities, and failed responses, rather than oral cultures and sensitivities, which are typically unreliable.

Periodontal Surgeries

The goals of periodontal therapy involve removing calculus or diseased tissue and minimizing pocket depth while preserving at least 2 mm of attached gingiva to protect alveolar bone and mucosa from eroding. If root surfaces are exposed or if the pocket depth is less than 5 mm, closed root planing and subgingival curettage may be performed. When pocket depth exceeds 5 mm or other pathology exists, more invasive procedures are warranted. If any attempts at regeneration or preservation of periodontal ligament cells or at reattachment to any root structure are planned, direct perioperative application of even very dilute concentrations of chlorhexidine is contraindicated (see Guided Tissue Regeneration below).

Gingivoplasty and gingivectomy are similar treatments that are used in different situations. A *gingivoplasty* is a periodontal surgery used to correct gingival deformities of contour not associated with pocketing. This is typically done in cases of minor focal areas of gingival hyperplasia, in which pseudo- or true pockets have not been formed. A *gingivectomy* is the excision of excess gingival tissues to create a new gingival margin level and to adjust contour. This is performed in true cases of gingival hyperplasia, where pocketing has become a problem, and in forms of suprabony pocketing. There will be some cases of gingival hyperplasia with underlying proliferative connective tissue that can get quite large and even ossified, requiring additional effort. Both gingivoplasty and gingivectomy are contraindicated in most cases of infrabony pocketing and in all cases in which the procedure would extend beyond the mucogingival margin or leave an inadequate level of attached gingiva (2 mm).

Gingivectomy and gingivoplasty can be performed with cold steel (blade and scissors), diamond or fluted burs (on a high-speed handpiece), or electrosurgery. Electrosurgery is probably the most controversial of the three, as thermal injuries to the pulp, cementum, alveolar bone, and periodontal ligament are possible. However, the newer units available can, with proper technique, be used safely, efficiently, and with greatly reduced hemorrhage. Cold steel is efficient, but it associated with the most hemorrhage. The contact of the blades with enamel will quickly dull their cutting edge, requiring frequent replacement or sharpening. Diamond and fluted burs permit good contouring, are fairly efficient, and produce less hemorrhage than cold steel. The fluted burs, in comparison with diamonds, will result in less rapid accidental injuries to the tooth surface. Most gingivectomies are performed with a combination of two or more of the above instruments.

In order to reduce pocket depth, an accurate assessment of its dimensions must be obtained. An outline of the pocket depth can be obtained by inserting a probe into the pocket to the base and noting the depth. The probe is then placed externally against the gingiva to the same depth, and the end of the probe is used to puncture the gingiva at that level to produce a bleeding point. This procedure can be repeated around the tooth until a complete outline is obtained. The blade, bur, or cutting tip is then used at an obtuse angle to the tooth to remove the excess tissue while creating a fine, feathered gingival margin edge. Pressure, hemostatic solutions, and electrocautery are frequently used to aid in control of hemorrhage problems. Once the procedure is completed, several layers of Tincture of Myrrh and Benzoin (Sultan Chemicals, Englewood, New Jersey) can be applied to protect the surface and reduce discomfort.

The *reverse bevel gingivectomy* is used for reducing pocket depth in areas where limited attached gingiva is available and infrabony pockets are present; it is also used for releasing flaps. This technique reduces the depth of the pocket, while removing the diseased inner layer of the sulcus. Using the scalpel handle and No.11 blade, a reverse bevel incision is made in the gingiva surrounding the tooth or teeth desired. The incision should extend through the marginal gingiva at an angle back toward the tooth and down into the base of the gingival sulcus. The incision should leave a layer of at least 2 mm of attached gingiva still surrounding each tooth. The loose collar of excised marginal gingiva may slip off the tooth or need to be removed with a sharp curette. This procedure may be used in association with closed or open curettage and citric acid treatment of the root in the hope of reducing the pocket depth by attaining a long junctional epithelium. Long junctional epithelia are not highly stable, unless good oral hygiene is pursued.

Releasing flaps are used to allow additional tooth root exposure for open curettage in areas where closed curettage is ineffective (deep or complex pockets). *Open curettage* enables the operator to have direct visualization to perform quality subgingival debridement by the removal of subgingival calculus, plaque, necrotic cementum, and pocket epithelium. Additionally, this procedure provides the needed exposure for osteoplasty of alveolar bone and facilitates exodontia (extractions). The flaps generally must be full thickness in order to expose bone and root tissues for treatment. The procedure is contraindicated for areas where more conservative treatments (gingivectomy or reverse bevel gingivectomy) would possibly be effective .

The *horizontal releasing incision* is made, with a No.11 blade, by a reverse bevel incision through the marginal gingiva into the base of the pocket. The incision should follow the gingival margin contour. From this point, two approaches can be taken. The first is to extend the marginal releasing incision as far as needed to allow the gingiva to be reflected with a periosteal elevator in an *envelope flap*.

If greater access is required, *vertical releasing incisions* may be made for a *full releasing flap*. The vertical releasing incisions should generally be made at the external proximofacial or proximolingual line angles of the adjacent teeth. External *line angles* represent the theoretical intersection of two of the tooth's external walls (Fig.4). The apical extent of the vertical releasing incisions is determined by the depth of treatment required. For most infrabony pockets, the incision is made only to the mucogingival line. For deeper vertical attachment losses, the incision may be extended well into the alveolar mucosa. Once the releasing incisions are made and the excised gingival collar of tissue removed, the flap is loosened with a periosteal or surgical elevator, such as a No.2, No.4, or No.9 Molt (Fig. 5).

Once the flap is retracted, subgingival debridement and osteoplasty or ostectomy can be completed. *Osteoplasty* is the shaping of bone to restore physiologic contour, without the elimination of walls of a pocket. The *ostectomy* is directed at the removal of osseous defects and infrabony pockets by the removal of bony pocket walls. Either can be performed with a slow-speed handpiece, fluted burs, and sterile saline applied by syringe to

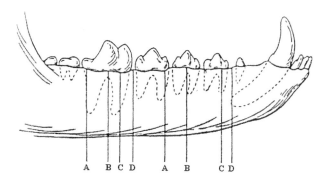

FIG. 4. Line angles. Line angle incision **(A)** and interradicular incision **(B)** are considered appropriate for releasing incisions, while radicular midfacial incision **(C)** and interproximal incision **(D)** are not considered appropriate.

prevent bone damage due to heat generation. Infrabony pockets can be removed in this fashion, as well as bulbous bony margins and bone spicules.

Once subgingival debridement and any required osteoplasty are completed, the flap will need replacement. The flap can be replaced coronally, at the same level, or apically. If the flap is to be repositioned to a new level, the periosteum attached to the flap may have to be severed to allow the flap to have greater movement. This is done by running a blade across the periosteum of the inside of the flap. *Repositioned flaps* are when the gingival attachment is placed back at the approximate original level. *Coronally repositioned flaps* are usually performed in association with guided tissue regeneration procedures (see Guided Tissue Regeneration below). *Apically repositioned flaps* allow the reduction of pocket depth, as successful home care for root exposure is simpler than that for deep pockets. For a flap to be successfully repositioned, the underlying support tissues may need to be reduced by an osteoplasty. The flaps are closed with an interrupted suture pattern through the interdental spaces or with the assistance of sling sutures. All bony tissue should be well covered by the flap. We have found that most absorbable sutures work well for these procedures.

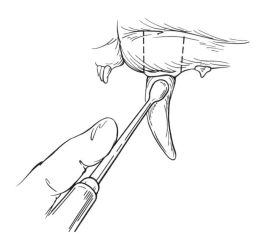

FIG. 5. Mucoperiosteal flap loosened with a periosteal elevator.

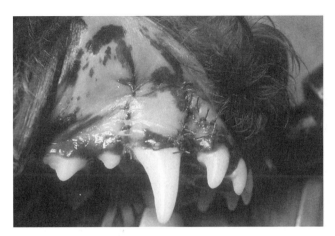

FIG. 6. Sutured sliding (pedicle) flap from mesial aspect of gingival defect associated with maxillary canine. The patient's soft tissue loss was secondary to radiation therapy in the region.

Sliding (pedicle) flaps are used to cover root surfaces denuded of gingiva that have adjacent areas with adequate gingiva for movement. The recipient site is prepared by making a roughly rectangular incision around the site, freshening the edges. The incision should be to the depth of the periosteum and to a 2–3-mm border of bone mesially, distally, and apically. This will provide the needed support for the flap. The resected soft tissue should be removed, with care to leave the periosteum in place and undisturbed.

The periodontium at the donor site should be healthy and have a satisfactory width of attached gingiva. All inflammation and infection at the recipient site should be controlled prior to attempting surgery. A full-thickness or a partial-thickness flap can be used. The partial-thickness flap permits more rapid healing at the donor site. The flap should be made sufficiently wide to more than cover the recipient site—up to 1.5 times as wide. The flap is then sutured in place with simple interrupted sutures of a resorbable material (Fig. 6).

Free Gingival Graft

In areas of loss of attached gingiva, where there is no adjacent tissue to attempt a pedicle flap, tissue may be harvested from another area in the oral cavity with sufficient attached gingiva, such as the upper or lower canine area. The recipient bed is prepared by freeing the periosteum of all submucosal tissue, and a template of aluminum foil is made to fit precisely into the area. The foil is placed at the preselected donor site, 2–3 mm from the gingival margin. A scalpel is used to incise around the pattern to a depth of 1 mm, and the graft is freed from the underlying tissue. Persistent hemorrhage at the donor site is typically controlled by pressure applied with a gauze sponge. The graft tissue is placed on a glass or wood slab and trimmed to correspond to the pattern size. After the graft is held in place with firm digital pressure on the periosteum for 2–3 minutes using a moist gauze, it can be sutured with 5-0 absorbable suture. Shrinkage of up to 20% can be anticipated, with reasonable healing by 1 month.

Follow-up Recommendations

1. Soft diet for 7–10 days.
2. Oral antibiotics for 10–14 days.
3. Home care during the healing stages involves twice daily rinsing with a chlorhexidine solution; additional rinsing with a zinc ascorbate–type product would also be helpful.
4. Home care after healing involves selection of home care product best suited for the pathology originally being treated and prevention of plaque accumulation. Frequency would vary from twice daily to twice weekly.
5. Routine rechecks would be advisable, beginning within 14 days after surgery.

Dental Surgeries

Dental surgeries to aid in healing of periodontal disease are sometimes required. These include placement of needed restorations, readjustment of restorations, odontoplasty, cervical bulge reestablishment, and splinting. Dental lesions close to the gingival margin can act as local irritant to cause inflammation and should be appropriately treated. Additionally, preexisting restorations should be inspected for overhangs and ledging below the gum line, and if these are found, the restoration should be readjusted to correct the problem.

Odontoplasty is the adjustment of the tooth contours, usually along the cervical bulge. The cervical bulge helps to deflect food and debris away from the sulcus of the tooth. However, once gingival recession occurs, the bulge may actually support the retention of debris near the gingival margin. The removal of the bulge may allow for a better physiologic cleansing effect for an area, once gingival recession occurs. It is done with a fluted bur or a white-stone abrasive point. The area should be polished smooth, and if dentin is uncovered, a dentinal sealer should be used to reduce discomfort and seal the tubules. This procedure is considered controversial and should be used only after careful consideration.

At times, teeth that are closely adjacent, such as the upper 4th premolar and 1st molar, accumulate debris apical to their contact points. As attachment loss at the site progresses, the triangular space is even further predisposed to the collection of debris and plaque. The distal surface of the 4th premolar and the mesial surface of the 1st molar can be reduced to open the space and allow more efficient cleansing of the area.

Cervical bulge reestablishment is a procedure to move the cervical bulge apically as recession occurs. This is typically done with composite resin restoratives and bonding agents. The theory is good, but the procedure is very operator-sensitive. The margins of the new cervical bulge restoration will generally be below the gum line. The restoration must be well finished, as any overhangs or irregularities will actually only further irritate the gingiva to cause additional problems.

A *splint* is an appliance used to stabilize mobile teeth. Various permanent and temporary splints are made use of in veterinary dentistry. They are used to assist in the healing of periodontal tissues surrounding mobile teeth following treatment. Splints are used for retention following orthodontic treatment and stabilization of teeth loosened by external traumatic force; they are also used while teeth mobile due to periodontal disease undergo treatment. However, splints compromise plaque control and can assist the spread of periodontal disease throughout the splinted area, if good oral hygiene is not maintained. The teeth can be stabilized by application of acrylics, bonding of composites, and interdental wiring.

Bonding is a quick, effective, and esthetic way of stabilizing teeth. It can be done with or without the removal of dental tissue. One word of caution concerns preexisting restorative work. The application of acrylics and composite bonded across a preexisting composite or glass ionomer restoration may result in their fusion. In addition, they normally bond poorly to glass ceramics, porcelain, and amalgam. The use of reinforcing materials can greatly enhance the durability of the splint. Wire and metal can be used and are easily available at most clinics, but the woven plastic fiber materials, such as Ribbond® (Ribbond, Seattle, Washington), have shown interesting versatility.

Splinting with the woven plastic fiber materials requires a systematic approach to placement (124). The teeth are held in their desired position, and a strip of metal foil is laid on the teeth to be splinted, usually on the lingual surface. The foil is then molded to the contours of the tooth at the level desired. This template is then used to cut the correct length and size of woven fiber material for the reinforcement. Many of these new woven materials must not be handled by hand, until coated with resins. The area to be splinted is then cleaned with a scaler. For a permanent splint, the enamel on the area to be splinted is very lightly roughened with a white-stone or diamond bur, although this is not done for temporary splints. The teeth are then prepared by polishing with pumice and acid-etched, and a thin layer of bonding material is applied and cured. A thin layer of a filled composite resin is then placed across the area. The woven material is coated with unfilled resin, with the excess blotted off. The woven material is then compressed into the composite layer until it makes contact with the tooth. Using a plastic filling instrument, the material should be molded to the tooth contours and tucked it into the interproximal areas. Once the material and teeth are in place, excess composite should be removed and the material cured. An additional layer of a moderately filled composite resin or an unfilled resin is then applied and cured.

Interdental wiring can also be used for splinting (125). However, if not kept high on the teeth, it commonly causes gingival irritation and accumulation of debris. It is best used in teeth that are mobile due to trauma, but it can be used in periodontal disease cases as well. Stout's multiple loop and Essig's wiring techniques are probably the most useful for these procedures (see Chapter 10 for additional information on interdental wiring).

Home Prophylaxis (Home Dental Hygiene Care)

Home care and client education are the keys to success in the control of periodontal disease. Start pets out slowly with home care, and allow the gingiva time to heal following professional prophylaxis or other periodontal treatments. Client education is one area in which the entire staff can play an extremely important role. Client education concerning the products and methods for dental hygiene is crucial to success. Staff members should be well versed in available home care products and their use, so that they are comfortable with them and can demonstrate them to the pet owners. More than just showing a step by step process, the staff should understand the basic concepts and be able to elaborate on their benefits, while instilling confidence and enthusiasm in client.

Client education should start at an early stage by introducing new puppy and kitten owners to the concepts of dental home care as part of normal care and feeding. Most older animals quickly respond to the same calm approach to home dental home care. However, each animal must be assessed individually on the type of home care most appropriate for it, as some pets may be difficult to treat and the risk of injury to the owner or family should not be taken lightly (see the Chapter 21 for more detailed information on home training).

As in any training method, it is best to start out slowly and easily, trying to make it a fun and rewarding experience for all participants. The first step is getting the pet accustomed to being gently handled around the face by rubbing the sides of the cheeks, petting under the chin, etc. Next, the owner should start carefully lifting the lips, while holding the mouth closed with the other hand, and even lightly touching the buccal surfaces of the teeth. Give the pet rewards as the procedures are done, as a positive reinforcement. Once the pet gets used to this type of action, one can progress to using a moist cloth or gauze pad, even with some garlic powder, beef bouillon, or tuna water to provide a pleasant flavor. Any abrasive action is beneficial in removing soft plaque and massaging the gums, but progressing to specific toothbrushes and dentifrices designed for the pet will be more beneficial.

Selection of toothpastes is usually guided by two points: taste and degree of disease. For routine home care in preventing or treating minor disease, a good tasting product that is easy to use is typically selected. The flavored enzymatic tooth pastes, such as C.E.T™. (VRx Products, Harbor City, California), and mild gels, such as Maxigard Gel™ (Addison Biological Laboratory, Fayette, Missouri), appear to fill these requirement extremely well. In the treatment of active or advanced periodontal disease, these same products may be used, but the chlorhexidine oral solutions and gels, such as CHX-Guard LA® (VRx Products), may be used more advanced diseases. Chlorhexidine oral products have all been shown to be among the most effective topicals that can be used in the mouth, although taste has always been a problem.

Toothbrushes should:

- Be easy to clean or disposable.
- Have proper anatomic grip design for the owner.
- Have proper anatomic head and bristle design for the pet.
- Have nonporous bristles or be disposable.

When being used, toothbrushes should:

- Be held at a 45° angle to the tooth.
- Stroke from bottom to top in the anterior teeth.
- Use a circular motion in the posterior teeth.
- Complete their work in under 60 seconds.

For toothpastes:

- Use products designed for the pet.
- Do NOT use human toothpastes; the swallowed detergents and fluoride may cause problems.
- Use salt or baking soda (sodium bicarbonate) only in animals that can tolerate the sodium load.

Even though hard, crunchy chew objects and toys provide chewing exercise that may help reduce tartar buildup, care should be taken in recommending products, as some may cause problems. Many of these chew products can cause damage to the tooth; for example, rawhide bones, cow hooves, and hard plastic bones may result in fractured teeth. Real bones can not only result in tooth fractures and impactions but also, when fed raw (eg, chicken/salmonella), provide a source of infection to the pet, which can be indirectly spread to the owner and family. Many times ice is given to pets as part of training or in the water during hot months, but this should be avoided, as it is common to fracture teeth as well. Crushed ice may be used instead.

The flatter strips of rawhide, such as ChewEzee™ (Friskies Petcare, Glendale, California) and C.E.T.Chews™ (VRx Products), appear to be effective in aiding tartar control without serious risk of fractured teeth. However, a few clients have had problems with their pets' gagging on them at times or causing stomach upsets. The soft, pliable plastic bones, such as Gummy Bones™ (Nylabone Products, Neptune New Jersey), also appear to aid in tartar control without undue risk of tooth fracture, although swallowed sections may occasionally cause concern. The compressed meal bones, such as Milkbone™ (Nabisco, East Hanover, New Jersey), appear to be very safe, while having some tartar control effects. The newer specialty dental diets, such as T/D (Hill's Pet Nutrition, Topeka, Kansas), have been shown to be effective in aiding plaque and tartar control and potentially reducing the risk of gingivitis. Additionally, the products appear to be safe, as no tooth fractures or other significant problems have been encountered. Diet as an aid in the control of periodontal disease appears to be a simple way for most clients to provide some degree of home dental care for their pets. Overall, these products seem to be reasonably effective as an aid in tartar control and are safe for most pets.

Frequency and Type of Routine Home Dental Care

Routine home care must be customized for the client and patient. The frequency of home care depends to a great extent on the degree of disease, while the products used must fit within the client comfort zone and patient acceptance. Table 2 gives some general recommendations by stage for the use and frequency of use of various types of home dental care products.

TABLE 2. General recommendations for the use of various types of home dental care products

Product	Frequency
Stages 0 and 1*	
Special dental diets	Daily as total diet or as treats after meals
Chew biscuits	After meals
Brushing	Once daily to once weekly
Gels, sprays, and solutions	Once daily to once weekly
Acceptable chew treats and toys	Once daily to once weekly
Stage 2*	
Special dental diets	Daily as total diet or as treats after meals
Chew biscuits	After meals
Brushing	Once daily to twice weekly
Gels, sprays, and solutions	Once daily to twice weekly
Acceptable chew treats and toys	Once daily to twice weekly
Stage 3*	
Special dental diets	Daily as total diet or as treats after meals
Chew biscuits	After meals
Brushing	Once daily to three times weekly
Gels, sprays, and solutions	Once daily to three times weekly
Acceptable chew treats and toys	Once daily to three times weekly
Stage 4*	
Special dental diets	Daily as total diet or as treats after meals
Chew biscuits	After meals
Brushing	Once to twice daily
Gels, sprays and solutions	Once to twice daily
Acceptable chew treats and toys	Once to twice daily

*(Stages of veterinary periodontal disease.)

TREATMENT PLAN

After the examination, evaluation, prognosis, and client consultation, the treatment plan is determined. The treatment plan is the strategy for case management. This includes the phases of treatment. In human dentistry, the *phases of therapy* represent six stages of periodontal treatment: evaluation phase, preliminary phase, phase I (etiotropic phase), phase II (surgical phase), phase III (restorative phase), and phase IV (maintenance phase) (108). In veterinary dentistry, due to the need for anesthesia, time considerations, and patient access restrictions, many phases must frequently be combined.

The *evaluation phase* is the examination and history-taking portion of treatment. The *preliminary phase* is the treatment of emergencies, such as acute ulcerations and abscesses. This may include emergency periodontal treatment, lancing of abscesses, or a required immediate extraction. *Phase I therapy* deals with professional prophylaxis, closed root planing, adjustments of restorations, caries or resorptive lesion treatment, occlusal adjustments, splinting, home hygiene care, dietary adjustments, and initial rechecks. *Phase II* encompasses periodontal surgeries and endodontic treatments, as well as reevaluations of their effects. In *phase III*, final restorations and prosthetic devices are placed, together with reevaluations of their effects. In *phase IV*, maintenance of the treatments in all other phases is carried out, as well as treatment of any other pathologies.

Treatment Plan for Stages of Periodontal Disease (Table 3)

In the early phase, or *stage I periodontal disease*, only gingivitis is present, and it is reversible with proper treatment such as a prophylaxis and home care. Sulcus depth should be less than 3 mm in the dog and less than 0.5 mm in the cat. Some pocket depth may be attributed to an increase in gingival height due to edema, not to attachment loss. The patient should be rechecked in 6 months. The prognosis is very good.

In *stage II periodontal disease*, attachment loss of up to 25% has occurred, with some apparent attachment loss. Additional therapy including root debridement and possibly planing to thoroughly clean the root surfaces is essential, in addition to a complete professional prophylaxis. If suprabony pocket formation has occurred and ample gingiva is available, a gingivectomy may be performed. If infrabony pockets or suprabony lesions with limited gingivae are present, reverse bevel flaps to debride the pocket and reduce pocket depth may be selected. Routine home care is required to maintain control. Rechecks at 2 weeks and 4 months will help monitor the patient's condition. The prognosis is good to fair.

TABLE 3. Treatment guide and prognosis for the stages of periodontal disease

Stage	Treatment	Prognosis	Reevaluation
1	Clean, polish, home care	Very good	6 months
2	Clean, debride roots, possible surgery; polish, home care	Good to fair	2 weeks to 4 months
3	Clean, debride roots, possible surgery; polish, home care	Guarded, possible extraction	2 weeks to 3 months
4	Clean, debride roots, possible surgery; polish, home care	Poor, probable extraction	2 weeks to 2 months

In *stage III periodontal disease*, more severe attachment loss of up to 50% may have occurred. If deep pockets are present instead of gingival recession, gingival flaps may be required to attain proper access for subgingival debridement. Therapy involving root debridement and possible planing to thoroughly clean the root surfaces is essential, in addition to a complete professional prophylaxis. If suprabony pocket formation has occurred and ample gingiva is available, a gingivectomy may be performed. If infrabony pockets or suprabony defects with limited gingivae are present, reverse bevel flaps to debride the pocket and reduce pocket depth may be selected. Routine home care is required to maintain control. Guided tissue regeneration or extraction may also be alternatives. Reevaluations should occur at 2 weeks and 3 months. The prognosis is considered guarded.

In *stage IV periodontal disease*, there is more than 50% attachment loss. This means that either very deep pockets, excessive gingival recession, or a combination of both has occurred. Therapy involving root debridement and possible planing to thoroughly clean the root surfaces is essential, in addition to a complete professional prophylaxis. If suprabony pocket formation has occurred and ample gingiva is available, a gingivectomy may be performed. If infrabony pockets or suprabony defects with limited gingivae are present, reverse bevel flaps to debride the pocket and reduce pocket depth may be selected. Routine home care is required to maintain disease control. Although guided tissue regeneration may be considered, extraction is frequently the treatment of choice, but some patient/client situations may warrant intensive therapy. Rechecks at 2 weeks and 2 months are recommended for assessment of treatment and determination of alternatives. The prognosis is considered to be poor.

GUIDED TISSUE REGENERATION

As advances in veterinary dentistry occur, new techniques and materials are being utilized to offer treatment for teeth with advancing periodontal lesions that previously would have been extracted (126,127). Periodontal disease progresses in an cyclic manner of alternating periods of active destruction and dormancy, rather than being linearly continuous (128–130). Many forms of periodontitis exist, each progressing to cause attachment loss at variable rates (13,14). The actual cause of attachment loss is generally considered to include interactions of bacteria, their byproducts, and the various components of the host immune system in response (131–133). Periodontal pockets on the palatal aspect of the maxillary cuspids (upper canine teeth) are easily overlooked, yet they are not an uncommon finding in the dog and, when encountered, have a strong probability for eventual oronasal fistula (ONF) development (134,135). While tooth extraction with appropriate flap closure addresses the problem, preservation of the tooth structure and resolution of the defect using regenerative therapeutic means represent a possible positive alternative (134).

Discussion

With deep palatal pockets (≥5 mm), the depth of the lesions customarily necessitates periodontal flap surgery to adequately expose the lesions for evaluation and treatment (126,127,136). Typically, an increased vascularity of soft tissue and bone in the area occurs, which can be beneficial in the healing process (126). These lesions are not readily demonstrated on radiographs, since they are located medially to the tooth (126). If endodontic involvement or an ONF is demonstrated, the prognosis for guided tissue regeneration is poor, and extraction may be the best alternative. Standard periodontal therapy involving open flaps to facilitate conscientious root debridement and subgingival curettage (126,127,134–137) may be combined with root-surface conditioning using citric acid, along with oral antibiotics, subgingivally placed antibiotics, and oral anti-inflammatory drugs (127,134–137). The oral antibiotic selected should have a good effect on both oral aerobes and anaerobes (138,139). For the passive application of the antibiotic within the pocket, half-inch sections of an absorbable suture material can be soaked in a diluted solution of the antibiotic and then packed into the infected sulcus to protect it from debris invasion. The ultimate goal of periodontal treatment is control of the disease, both the bacteria and host response (140).

Ultimately, regeneration of the supporting tissues to attain a more normal and healthy anatomic and physiologic state may help in maintaining disease control (141). Guided tissue regeneration (GTR) in veterinary dentistry principally deals with the regeneration of periodontal tissues lost due to disease or injury. Tissue regeneration has been demonstrated with alveolar bone, cementum, and the periodontal ligament in specific therapies, locations, and type of materials (142).

Research supports the theory that the category of periodontal reaction and attachment depends on the type of tissue that first repopulates the root surface (143–145). Based on this, there are basically four tissues that can repopulate the root surface, each resulting in various periodontal effects (142). These tissues are the following: gingival epithelium, gingival connective tissue, alveolar bone, and periodontal ligament. In this theory, each cellular type mentioned results in a different attachment consequence. Gingival epithelial cells that migrate along the gingival connective tissues down to the root surface result in a long junctional epithelial attachment that typically, in the long term, breaks down, allowing reestablishment of the disease state. If gingival connective tissue is first to repopulate the root surface, then root resorption usually occurs. Should the cells to repopulate originate from bone, then one of two repercussions occurs: either root resorption or ankylosis. However, when periodontal cells are the first to repopulate the root surface, new attachment results. The periodontal cells have the ability to redevelop cementum on the root surface, and a healthy attachment may be generated (142).

The different forms of response the the bone will exhibit depend on the properties of the substance used in therapy. An *osseoconductive* product is one that will aid in the regeneration of new bone in an osseous site; this applies to almost all of the GTR products. A product is *osseoinductive* if it will aid in the generation of new bone in any site, whether it be muscle tissue, brain tissue, etc. From a practical standpoint, only autogenous bone grafts and bone morphogenic protein (BMP) can do this currently. Freeze-dried bone products and irradiated bone are not osseoinductive because the cells that could have made them so have been killed by treatment of the product. The term *osseopromotive* covers both types of products, describing those that stimulate the growth of new bone osseoconductively or osseoinductively. The term *osseoproductive* is currently considered improper and ill-defined. It has been used incorrectly as a synonym for osseopromotive.

The scientific basis for the principles of GTR are simple, yet they can be difficult to properly attain. The fundamentals are to place a physical barrier between the instrumented root surface and the gingival flap (127,142). The barrier acts as a deterrent to exclude the gingival epithelium or gingival connective tissue from colonizing the root structure. This barrier then provides an area for the progenitor cells of the periodontal ligament and/or alveolar bone to have free access for migration. Since bone development is slower than the development of soft tissues of the periodontal ligament, it is hoped that the latter would develop prior to bony incursion. It is generally believed that periodontal cells have the greatest potential to promote new attachment but that bone also plays a significant role. Studies have suggested that GTR barriers should be in place and intact for a minimum of 28–42 days for the desired effect (142). It must be understood that GTR may not always be as successful as desired, which may be due to material selection, technique, poor client compliance, or other complicating factors.

Site Selection

Current clinical indications for GTR include class II furcations, two- or three-walled vertical interproximal defects, three-walled palatal defects of single-rooted teeth, and circumferential (cup) intrabony osseous defects (142–145). Areas with abundant gingival attachment are generally preferred to facilitate proper flap technique, as well as good defect and barrier coverage. Many other types of defects have been successfully treated, so the indications grow with time and advancement in technique and materials; however, defects of a lesser nature are still best treated by conventional periodontal therapy. Only patients whose periodontal disease is under control and whose maintenance of plaque control is good should be selected for GTR (142). If good home care cannot be provided, the outlook for good results is poor.

Barrier Selection

Selection of barrier materials represents a significant decision-making process for the veterinarian not only because of the wide variation of materials available but also in relation to cost, effectiveness, and client acceptance (134,137). The major decision is between membranes or substance matter barriers. The membranes are thin sheets of pliable material, and substance matter barriers are of a bulkier, more space-filling type of material that acts as a bone matrix superstructure.

Membrane Barriers

Membranes are barriers made from either nonabsorbable or absorbable materials. Millipore filters (Millipore® SA, Molsheim, France) were among the first barriers used in research that demonstrated that GTR membranes might have some beneficial effects (142). Gore-Tex™ (W.L. Gore & Associates, Flagstaff, Arizona) is a nonabsorbable expanded polytetrafluoroethylene (e-PTFE) product that was one of the first to be predictably effective and commercially available specifically for GTR; it does require a second surgery for removal of the material (146). Recently, a new product has been developed, Gore-Tex TR™, a titanium-reinforced barrier that has improved shapeability for easier adaptation. Additionally, there is Resolut™, a bioabsorbable membrane, made from essentially pure lactide and glycolide polymers; it has not yet been introduced in the United States. Vicryl® Periodontal Mesh (Ethicon, Somerville, New Jersey) is woven from polyglactin 910, a synthetic absorbable copolymer of glycolide and lactide derived from glycolic and lactic acids (147), while Guidor® (John O. Butler Company, Chicago, Illinois) is a blend of bioresorbable polylactic acid and a citric acid ester. Both of these products are the newer resorbable-type barriers that do not require a second surgery for removal. Guidor® makes use of a complex multilayer arrangement that may enhance tissue guidance while reducing membrane migration problems. Atrisorb® (Atrix Labs) is a polylactic acid absorbable membrane of a size that allows greater customization, which may be beneficial for some animal procedures. Collagen membranes for GTR represent one of the latest developments in biodegradable barrier technology, although not yet commercially available. The collagen is typically of bovine origin using cross-linking of the fibers to control the time interval of degradation (148). These have additional interesting possibilities for acting as a timed-release delivery system by being impregnated with chemicals, such as chemically altered tetracyclines, growth factors, and other medications, that might improve GTR effects.

Bulk Material or Osseous Replacement Barriers

Bulk osseous replacement packing materials generally come in small natural particulate, granular, or spherical shapes available in nonabsorbable and absorbable substances. Particle size varies with the intended use (GTR, filling empty tooth sockets, or gross bone replacement). HTR® (Bioplant, Norwalk, Connecticut) is a nonresorbable synthetic bone copolymer polymethylmethacrylic (PMMA) polyhydroxylethylmethacrylic (PHEMA), with a small amount of barium sulfate, that is then coated with calcium hydroxide/carbonate. Osteogen® (Stryker Dental Implants, Kalamazoo, Michigan) is a resorbable hydroxyapatite, a form of calcium phosphate. Bon-Apatite™ (Bio-Interfaces, San Diego, California), Calcitite® (Calcitek, Carlsbad, California), and Periograf® and Alveolgraf® (Sterling Winthrop, New York, New York) are additional particulate forms of hydroxyapatite. Perio-Glass™ and ERMI® are forms of Bioglass® (US Biomaterials, Baltimore, Maryland), which is a bioactive glass coated with a hydroxylcarbonate apatite. Another form of Bioglass® available in the veterinary market is Consil™ (Nutramax Labs, Baltimore, Maryland). ADD™ (THM Biomedical, Duluth, Minnesota) is a biodegradable expanded polylactic acid dental surgical dressing that has been used for GTR. Barrier packing materials have been made from or used a myriad of substances and combinations such as sea coral, ceramics, coated acrylic beads, tetracycline, plaster of Paris, hydroxyapatite and bone, among others.

Bone grafting in various forms also has its limitations in availability, convenience, potential cost (126,149), and other compounds such as polylactic acid granules and hydroxyapatite have been used with some success (126,135–137,150). These implants are placed to be incorporated as a matrix for the initial blood clot that is later replaced by supportive tissue, either bone or periodontal ligament; at the same time, they discourage the ingrowth of epithelium or gingival connective tissue (137). Tricalcium phosphate, available in a generic form or as Peri-OSS™ (Miter, Warsaw, Indiana), is yet another compound to be used as a graft (138,151,152).

Whether by themselves or incorporated with graft materials, tetracycline compounds, including doxycycline, are used frequently in oral surgery due to many factors. The most obvious benefit is that that they are antimicrobial, particularly against many oral pathogens (138,139,153), with a gingival crevicular fluid concentration up to ten times greater than in serum (154). In addition, tetracycline compounds have the ability to inhibit collagenase enzymes (152,155), stimulate fibroblast activity (including attachment) (152–155), approximate the demineralizing effect for which citric acid conditioning is used (138,154,156), and bind to dentin and bone (155); they also tend to elicit minimal inflammation when used in low concentrations (152). Doxycycline in particular is less susceptible to chelation than most other tetracycline compounds (152–156) and longer-acting (152). It also keeps its antimicrobial activity when combined with calcium sulfate and tends to improve the effects of tetracycline compounds and other implants synergistically (eg, increased regeneration and decreased crestal resorption, fewer long junctional epithelial attachments, etc.) (151,152). Systemic tetracycline compounds have been shown to be beneficial in refractory periodontal disease cases as well (155).

Calcium sulfate has been used both orthopedically and orally to enhance bone healing (157–160), though some studies have disputed its benefits (160). When used with grafts, such as the tetracycline compound/doxycycline combination, its role as a binder to keep the material together is complemented by its biocompatability, rapid resorption, ability to provide available calcium without elevating serum levels, and porosity to allow fluid exchange while being dense enough to exclude epithelial and gingival connective tissue migration (150,152). In other defects, the calcium sulfate can be molded and trimmed to proper configurations. It is more difficult to introduce material into these deep palatal pockets, so the addition of calcium alginate (Curasorb™, Kendall Company, Mansfield, Massachusetts) was initiated to provide a substrate to carry the other elements into the defect. This wound dressing forms a soft colloidal gel that also aids in mechanical hemostasis, enhances healing, and has been used to aid in postextraction hemorrhage (161). There has been a gradual trend toward substitution for calcium alginate with absorbable collagens, such as Instat™ (Johnson & Johnson, Arlington, Texas) or Collamend™ (Veterinary Products Labs, Phoenix, Arizona).

Objectives

Material placement is aimed at subgingival placement following full-thickness flap exposure, and then closure (127,137,142). Every attempt should be made not to compromise the blood supply of the flap. Local infiltration of lidocaine is acceptable, but the epinephrine concentration should not exceed 1:100,000. The area to be treated is prepared according to need by root debridement and subgingival curettage to remove all epithelial, connective, and granulation tissue from the root surface (142–145). Osteoplasty is sometimes performed to a degree in the curettage or for the removal of spicules that might interfere with the barrier or flap. To possibly enhance reattachment, the root can further be prepared with a dilute tetracycline solution (139) or Citric-Etch™ (Ellman International, Hewlett, New York), a citric acid preparation (12,134,150). Contamination, salivary or otherwise, should be minimized during the surgical placement stage. The oral cavity can have general disinfection with a dilute solution of chlorhexidine not greater than 0.12% (164). It must be kept in mind that stronger solutions are contraindicated in certain circumstances and that root and periodontal ligament exposure to the solution prior to surgery should be kept to an absolute minimum. This is due to the fact that chlorhexidine has two effects on these tissues. First, at strengths greater than 0.12%, it adversely affects the attachment of periodontal cells to the root surface. Second, at strengths as low as 0.0025%, it adversely affects the growth of periodontal cells (164). Due to this dose-dependent inhibition and toxicity to periodontal cells, it is advisable to use caution in its use directly on tissues being grafted or in repeated subgingival applications. There is no indication that postsurgical use of chlorhexidine solution, gel, or bioadhesive tablets has any adverse effects.

Some forms of GTR particulate materials are mixed with saline or blood (141), while others are placed dry and then gently packed into the defect (157–159). The gingival flap is replaced and sutured over the material and defect. With most particulate materials, a slight overfill for a "super clot" is generally preferable (162). This is done with the knowledge that some settling of the material may occur, as well as resorption of some additional support bone due to trauma. However, no material should be left exposed, with the flap fitting securely opposing the tooth surface to prevent particulate material from percolating out or oral contaminates from migrating in (142).

If a membrane is used, it is placed over the affected root area and associated alveolar bone to act as a barrier between them and the soft tissues of the flap closure (142). The membrane barrier should be custom-fitted or seated to the specific defect area by trimming with sterile scissors. All sharp corners, wrinkles, folds, and overlapping of material should be avoided in order to provide appropriate flap apposition. Membranes may need to have the facial and lingual surfaces tucked under the periosteum or the sutures placed through the material to aid in its stabilization. Many have two or more suture leads with attached needles for quick and easy placement and prevention of migration due to pressure or motion. Nonresorbable membranes are generally left in place for 1–9 months to allow for healing and are then removed (142,163).

General Procedure

In healthy animals, local anesthetic with epinephrine can be used in limited amounts to aid in reducing hemorrhage and postsurgical discomfort. However, these are to be use with reasonable caution in association with halothane inhalant anesthesia and in patients with heart or endocrine disease. The general oral cavity can be disinfected with a dilute solution of chlorhexidine not greater than 0.12% (164). Chlorhexidine solutions are contraindicated for treatment of the root and periodontal ligament prior to surgery. A pedicle flap is created using the No.15C blade by making an incision 5 mm medial to a line 3 mm distal to the cuspid in a rostrolateral arc to a point half way between the cuspid and corner incisor. Next, the incision is extended distal to the mesial cuspid sulcus (134). The same procedure is used on the mandibular cuspid, but the flap direction is reversed to incorporate the distal interdental space (134). With the use of a periosteal elevator, a full thickness flap is gently raised. Root debridement is next, utilizing a periodontal or periosteal curette to meticulously remove all granulation and soft tissue between the root and alveolus. The width and depth of the pocket should be measured with a periodontal probe and recorded. Placement of a small amount of citric acid gel into the defect to enhance reattachment can be performed at this time. If used, it should be rinsed after 30 seconds with sterile saline to flush the sulcus clean of the acid and debris. If particles requiring blood or liquid are used, a tuberculin syringe with a 25 gauge needle attached can be used to vacuum some of the blood from the sulcus for mixing. If no free blood is available, saline can be used or the bone within the pocket can be shallowly penetrated with the needle to produce healthy marrow bleeding. The saline or blood can be added to the GTR particles in a Dappen dish or within a carrier syringe. The material can be syringed directly into the defect, or if a Dappen dish is used, a W3 plastic filling instrument can be useful to pickup a small amount of the GTR particles and carry them to the defect. Once in the defect, the particles are gently packed. A slight overfill is acceptable. The flap is then replaced and sutured closed. A sling suture or simple interrupted sutures using large bites of tissue can be used for closure. When it is properly placed, the flap should fit snugly against the tooth. Any open defect from the donor site for the sliding pedicle flap can be protected with a thin covering of a tissue glue.

Postoperative Care

Postoperatively, a soft diet is recommended for 72 hours to prevent undue pressures on the flaps. A vigorous routine home care for plaque control is essential, using dental irrigant solutions (chlorhexidine gluconate or diacetate 0.12%) twice daily until a brushing program can be established at about 2 weeks postoperatively. Antibiotics are generally recommended for a least 3 weeks following the procedure. Doxycycline is considered a good choice in human medicine because of its antibacterial and anticollagenolytic effects, thus aiding in stabilizing collagen locally. Nonabsorbable membranes are normally removed 1–9 months following surgery.

REFERENCES

1. Rateitschak KH. *Periodontology*. 2nd ed. New York: Thieme Medical Publishers; 1989.
2. Harty FJ. *Concise Illustrated Dental Dictionary*. 2nd ed. Oxford: Wright Publishing, Jordan Hill; 1995:180.
3. Goodson JM, Tanner AC, Haffajee AD, Sornberger GC, Socransky SS. Patterns of progression and regression of advanced destructive periodontal disease. *J Clin Periodontol* 1982;9:472.
4. Socransky SS, Haffajee AD, Goodson JM, Lindhe J. New concepts of destructive periodontal disease. *J Clin Periodontol* 1984;11:21.
5. Becker W, Berg L, Becker BE. Untreated periodontal disease: A longitudinal study. *J Clin Periodontol* 1984;11:21.
6. Loe H, Theilade E, Jensen S. Experimental gingivitis in man. *J Periodontol* 1965;36:177.
7. Page RC, Schroeder HE. Pathogenesis of inflammatory periodontal disease. A summary of current work. *Lab Invest* 1976;33:235.
8. Page RC, Schroeder HE. *Periodontitis in Man and Other Animals: A Comparative Review*. Basel: Karger; 1982:58.
9. American Academy of Periodontology. *Glossary of Periodontic Terms. J Periodontol* Nov. 1986;(suppl).
10. *Current Procedural Terminology for Periodontics and Insurance Reporting Manual*. 5th ed. American Academy of Periodontology; Chicago: 1986:26.
11. Deutsche Gesellschaft fur Parodontologie: Neue PAR-Nomenklatur. *DGP-Nachrichten* 1987;1:1.
12. Schroeder HE. Klinik und Pathologie verschiedender Formen von Parodontitis. *Dtsch zahnarztl Z* 1987;42:417.
13. Reddy MS, Jeffcoat MK. Periodontal disease progression. *Curr Op Periodontol* 1993.
14. Ranney RR. Classification of periodontal diseases. *Periodontology 2000* 1993;2:13.
15. Page RC. Gingivitis. *J Clin Periodontol* 1986;13:345.
16. Is periodontal disease a measurement of a pet's general health? *Vet Forum* 1995:66.
17. Loesche WJ. Periodontal disease as a risk factor for heart disease. *Compend Cont Educ Dent* 1994;15:976.
18. Mattila KJ, Nieminen MS, Valtonen VV, et al. Association between dental health and acute myocardial infarction. *Br Med J* 1989;298:779.
19. Syrjanen J, Peltola J, Valtonen V, et al. Dental infections in association with cerebral infarction in young and middle-aged men. *J Intern Med* 1989;225:179.
20. DeStefano F, Andra RF, Kahn HS, et al. Dental disease and risk of coronary heart disease and mortality. *Br Med J* 1993;306:688.
21. DeBowes L. Systemic effects of oral disease. AVDC/AVD Proceedings. 1992:65.
22. Wiggs RB, Lobprise HB, Holmstrom SE, Eisner ER. Periodontal disease and periodontitis incidence rates in the dog and cat. Submitted for publication.
23. National Companion Animal Study, University of Minnesota Center for Companion Animal Health. *Uplinks* Feb 1996:3.
24. Cleland P. Dental splinting using Ribbond®. Veterinary Dentistry. 1993 Proceedings. Auburn University, AL, Sept. 30–Oct. 3, 1993:159.
25. DuPont G. Tooth splinting for severly mobile mandibular incisor teeth in a dog. *J Vet Dent* 1995;12(3):93.
26. Goldman HM, Schuler S, Fox L, Cohen DW. *Periodontal Therapy*. 3rd ed. St Louis, MO: CV Mosby Co; 1964:29.
27. Hurt WC. *Periodontics in General Practice*. Springfield, IL: Charles C Thomas; 1976:7.
28. McHugh WD. The interdental gingivae. *J Periodontal Res* 1971;6:227.
29. Lange NP, Loe H. The relationship between the width of keratinized gingiva and gingival health. *J Periodontol* 1972;3:623.
30. King JD. Gingival disease in Dundee. *J Dent Res* 1945;65:9.
31. Orban B. Clinical and histological study of surface characteristics of the gingiva. *Oral Surg* 1948;1:827.
32. Greene AH. Study of the characteristics of stippling and its relation to gingival health. *J Periodontol* 1962;33:176.

33. Wiggs RB. Canine anatomy and oral physiology. *Compend Cont Educ Dent* 1989;11:1475.
34. Stone S, Kalis PJ. *Periodontics: Biological Basis and Clinical Application.* Baltimore: Waverly Press; 1975
35. Feneis H. Gefuge und Funktion des normalen Zahnfleischgewebes. *Dtsch zahnarztl Z* 1952;7:467.
36. Zwarych PD, Quigley MB. The intermediate plexus of the periodontal ligament: History and further observations. *J Dent Res* 1965;44:383.
37. Genco RJ, Goldman HM, Conen DW. *Contemporary Periodontes.* St. Louis, CU Mosby. 1990:3.
38. Schroeder HE, Listgarten MA. *Fine Structure of the Developing Epithelial Attachment of Human Teeth.* 2nd ed. Basel: Karger; 1977.
39. Listgarten MA. Electron microscopic study of the gingivodental junction in man. *Am J Anat* 1966;199:147.
40. Skougaard MR. Turnover of the gingival epithelium in marmosets. *Acta Odontol Scand* 1965;23:623.
41. Skougaard MR. Cell renewal, with special reference to the gingival epithelium. In: Staple PH, ed. *Advances in Oral Biology*, vol 4. New York: Academic Press; 1970:261.
42. Toto PD, Sicher HJ. Mucopolysaccharides in the epithelial attachment. *J Dent Res* 1965;44:451.
43. Lange DE, Schroeder HE. Cytochemistry and ultrastructure of gingival sulcus cells. *Helv Odontol Acta* 1971;15:65.
44. Wiggs RB. Periodontal disease and its multifactorial cause. Presented at the meeting of the Japanese Dental Society; Osaka, Japan; June 24, 1995.
45. Wiggs RB. Periodontal disease and host factors. Presented at the meeting of the Japanese Dental Society; Oska, Japan; June 25, 1995.
46. Rosenberg HM, Rehfeld CE, Emmering TE. A method for epidemiologic assessment of periodontal health-disease state in a beagle hound colony. *J Periodontol* 1966;37:208.
47. Saxe SR, Bohannon HM, Greene J, Vermillion JR. Oral debris, calculus, and periodontal disease in the beagle dog. *Periodontics* 1967;5:217.
48. Lindhe J, Hamp SE, Loe H. Experimental periodontitis in the beagle dog. *J Periodontal Res* 1973;3:1.
49. Lindhe J, Hamp SE, Loe H. Plaque induced periodontal disease in beagle dogs: A four year study. *J Periodontal Res* 1975;10:243.
50. Egelberg J. Local effect of diet on plaque formation and development of gingivitis in dogs, III: Effect of frequency of meals and tube feeding. *Odontol Revy* 1965;16:50.
51. Hennet P. Periodontal disease and oral microbiology. In: Crossley DA, Penman S, eds. *Manual of Small Animal Dentistry.* 2nd ed. Gloucestershire, UK: Britsh Small Animal Association; 1995:105.
52. Listgarten MA, Mayo HE, Tremblay R. Development of dental plaque on epoxy resin crowns in man. A light and electron microscopic study. *J Periodontol* 1975;46:10.
53. Listgarten MA. Structure of the microbial flora associated with periodontal health and disease in man. A light and electron microscopic study. *J Periodontol* 1976;47:1.
54. Hennet PR, Harvey CE. Aerobes in periodontal disease in the dog: A review. *J Vet Dent* 1991;8(1):9.
55. Hennet PR, Harvey CE. Anaerobes in periodontal disease in the dog: A review. *J Vet Dent* 1991;8(2):18.
56. Hennet PR, Harvey CE. Spirochetes in periodontal disease in the dog: A review. *J Vet Dent* 1991;8(3):16.
57. Boyce EN, Ching RJW, Logan EI, et al. Occurrence of Gram-negative black-pigmented anaerobes in subgingival plaque during development of canine periodontal disease. *Clin Infect Dis* 1995;(suppl):.
58. Ericsson I, Lindle J, Rylander H, Okamoto H. Experimental periodontal breakdown in the dog. *Scand J Dent Res* 1975;83:189.
59. Theilade E. The non-specific theory in microbial etiology of inflammatory periodontal disease. *J Clin Periodontol* 1986;13:905.
60. Loesche WJ, Syed SA, Laughon BE, Stoll J. The bacteriology of acute necrotizing ulcerative gingivitis. *J Periodontol* 1982;53:223.
61. Falkler WA, Martin SA, Vincent JW, Tall BD, Nauman RK, Suzuki JB. A clinical, demographic and microbiologic study of ANUG patients in an urban dental school. *J Clin Periodontol* 1987;14:307.
62. Saxe SR, Bohannon HM, Greene J, Vermillion JR. Oral debris, calculus, and periodontal disease in the beagle dog. *Periodontics* 1967;5:217.
63. Mandel ID. Calculus update: Prevalence, pathogenicity, and prevention. *JADA* 1995;126:573.
64. Harvey CE, Sofer FS, Laster L. Association of age and body weight with periodontal disease in North American dogs. *J Vet Dent* 1994;11(3):94.
65. *Periodontal Syllabus.* Bethesda, MD: US Navy Dental Corps, Naval Graduate Dental School; 1975. NAVMED P-5110:21.
66. Gorrel C. The role of a "Dental Hygiene Chew" in maintaining periodontal health in dogs. *J Vet Dent* 1996; 13(1):31.
67. Watson ADJ. Diet and periodontal disease in dogs and cats. *Aust Vet J* 1994;71:313.
68. Tromp JA, van Rijn LJ, Jansen J. Experimental gingivitis and frequency of tooth-brushing in the beagle dog model: Clinical findings. *J Clin Periodontol* 1986;13:190.
69. Sanges GA. A pilot study on the effect of tooth brushing on the gingiva of a beagle dog. *Scand J Dent Res* 1976; 84:106.
70. Stooky GK, Warrick JM, Miller LL, Katz BP. Hexametaphosphate-coated snack biscuits significantly reduce calculus formation in dogs. *J Vet Dent* 1996;13(1):27.
71. Duke A. How a chewing device affects calculus buildup in dogs. *Vet Med* 1989;84:1110.

72. Jensen L, Logan E, Finney O, et al. Reduction in accumulation of plaque, stain, and calculus in dogs by dietary means. *J Vet Dent* 1995;12:161.
73. Goldstein G, Czarnecki-Maulden GL, Venner ML. Beefhide strips in the maintenance of dental health. World Veterinary Dental Congress Proceedings. Philadelphia, PA; Sept. 30–Oct. 2, 1994:81.
74. Emily P. Tarter control tactics: Dental rinses for home dental care. *Pet Vet* Nov-Dec 1989:35.
75. Berglundh T, Lindhe J. Gingivitis in young and old dogs. *J Clin Periodontol* 1993;20:179.
76. Rosenberg HM. The progression of periodontal disease in the aging beagle hound. 1967. USAEC Argonne National Laboratory Report, ANL-7809.
77. Egelberg J. Local effect of diet on plaque formation and development of gingivitis in dogs, I. Effects of hard and soft diets. *Odontol Revy* 1965;16:31.
78. Studer E, Stapley RB. The role of dry food in maintaining healthy teeth and gums in the cat. *Vet Med Small Anim Clin* 1973;10:1024.
79. Eccles JD, Jenkins WG. Dental erosion and diet. *J Dent* 1974;2:153.
80. Davis WB, Winter PJ. Dietary erosion of adult dentine and enamel. *Br Dent J* 1977;143:116.
81. Harrison JL, Roeder LB. Dental erosion caused by beverages. *Gen Dent* 1991;39:23.
82. Hennet P. Dental anatomy and physiology of small carnivores. In: Crossley DA, Penman S, eds. *Manual of Small Animal Dentistry*. 2nd ed. Gloucestershire, UK: Britsh Small Animal Association; 1995:93.
83. Silness J, Loe H. Periodontal disease in pregnancy. II. Correlation between oral hygiene and periodontal conditions. *Acta Odontol Scand* 1964;22:121.
84. Loe H, Silness J. Periodontal disease in pregnancy. I. Prevalence and severity. *Acta Odontol Scand* 1963;21:533.
85. Muhlemann HR, Son S. Gingival sulcus bleedingóa leading symptom in initial gingivitis. *Helv Odontol Acta* 1971;15:107.
86. Ramfjord SP. The Periodontal disease index (PDI). *J Periodontol* 1967;38:602.
87. Frommer HH. *Radiology for Dental Auxiliaries*. 3rd ed. St.Louis, MO: CV Mosby Co; 1983:290.
88. Van Palenstein-Helderman WH. Microbial etiology of periodontal disease. *J Clin Periodontol* 1981;8:261.
89. *Veterinary Dental Abbreviations*. American Veterinary Dental College, Residency Tracking Committee, suppl; 1994.
90. Wiggs RB, Lobprise HB. Oral disease. In: Norsworthy GD, ed. *Feline Practice*. Philadelphia: JB Lippincott Co; 1993:438.
91. Smith MM, Moon ML, Callan M, Rozum M. Furcation entrance anatomy of the fourth maxillary premolar in dogs. *Am J Vet Res* 1990;51:2050.
92. Smith MM, Massoudi LM, Nunes JD, McCain WC. Furcation anatomy of the first molar in dogs. *Am J Vet Res* 1992;53:242.
93. Loe H, Theilade E, Jensen S. Experimental gingivitis in man. *J Periodontol* 1965;36:177.
94. Mikx FHM, VanCampen GJ, et al. Microscopic evaluation of the microflora in relation to necrotizing ulcerative gingivitis in the beagle dog. *J Periodontol Res* 1982;17:576.
95. Listgarten MA, Lindhe J, Parodi R. The effect of systemic antimicrobial therapy on plaque and gingivitis in the dog. *J Periodontal Res* 1979;14:65.
96. Heijl L, Lindhe J. The effect of metronidazole on the development of plaque and gingivitis in the beagle dog. *J Clin Periodontol* 1979;6:197.
97. Lindhe J, Attstrom R, Bjorn AL. Influence of sex hormones on gingival exudate in dogs with chronic gingivitis. *J Periodontal Res* 1968;3:279.
98. Joffe DJ, Allen AL. Ulcerative eosinophilic stomatitis in three Cavalier King Charles Spaniels. *JAAHA* 1995;31:34.
99. Carranza FA, Perry DA. *Clinical Periodontology for the Dental Hygienist*. Philadelphia: WB Saunders Co; 1986:56.
100. Goldman HM, Cohen DW. *Periodontal Therapy*. 6th ed. St.Louis, MO: CV Mosby Co; 1980:508.
101. Herr Y, Matsuura M, Lin W, Genco RJ, Cho M. The origin of fibroblasts and their role in the early stages of horizontal furcation defect healing in the beagle dog. *J Periodontol* 1995;66:716.
102. Klinge B, Nilveus R, Egelberg J. Bone regeneration pattern and ankylosis in experimental furcation defects in dogs. *J Clin Periodontol* 1985;12:456.
103. Diagnosis, prognosis and treatment planning. In: *Periodontic Syllabus*. Naval Graduate Dental School, Bureau of Medicine and Surgery; Washington DC: 1975:35.
104. Tarnow D, Fletcher P. Classification of the vertical component of furcation involvement. *J Periodontol* 1984;55:283.
105. Greenstein G, Polson A. Understanding tooth mobility. *Compend Cont Educ Dent* 1988;9:470.
106. Svanberg G. Influence of trauma from occlusion on the periodontium of dogs with normal or inflamed gingivae. *Odontol Revy* 1974;25:165.
107. Nyman S, et al. The effect of progressive tooth mobility on destructive periodontitis in the dog. *J Clin Periodontol* 1978;5:213.
108. Wiggs RB, Lobprise HB. Clinical evaluation of Sofscale™ Calculus Scaling Gel in dogs and cats. *J Vet Dent* 1994;11(1):9.
109. Brown FH, Ogletree RC, Houston GD. Pneumoparotitis associated with the use of an air-powder prophylaxis unit. *J Periodontol* 1992;63:642.

110. Robinson JGA. Chlorhexidine gluconate: The solution for dental problems. *J Vet Dent* 1995;12(1):29.
111. Lindhe SE, et al. Influence of topical chlorhexidine on chronic gingivitis and gingival wound healing in the dog. *Scand J Dent Res* 1970;78:471.
112. Tepe JH, et al. The long-term effect of chlorhexidine on plaque, gingivitis, sulcus depth, gingival recession, and loss of attachment in beagle dogs. *J Periodontal Res* 1983;18:452.
113. Gruet P, et al. Use of an oral antiseptic bioadhesive tablet in dogs. *J Vet Dent* 1995;12(3):87.
114. Silver JG, Martin L, McBride BC. Recovery and clearance rates of oral microorganisms following experimental bacteremias in dogs. *Arch Oral Biol* 1975;20:675.
115. Preus HR. Treatment of rapidly destructive periodontitis in Papillon-Lefevre syndrome. *J Clin Periodontol* 1988;15:639.
116. Preus HR, Olsen I. Possible transmittance of *A. actinomycetemcomitans* from a dog to a child with rapidly destructive periodontitis. *J Periodontal Res* 1988;23:68.
117. Grove TK. Problems associated with the management of periodontal disease in clinical practice. In: Manfra-Marretta S, ed. *Problems in Veterinary Medicine: Dentistry.* Philadelphia: JB Lippincott; 1990;2(1):154.
118. Wiggs RB. Basics of guided tissue regeneration. Vet Dent Society Proceedings. Auburn University, AL. Sept. 30–Oct. 3, 1993:23.
119. Goodson JM, Tanner AC, Haffajee AD, Sornberger GC, Socransky SS. Patterns of progression and regression of advanced destructive periodontal disease. *J Clin Periodontol* 1982;9:472.
120. Socransky SS, Haffajee AD, Goodson JM, Lindhe J. New concepts of destructive periodontal disease. *J Clin Periodontol* 1984;11:21.
121. Becker W, Berg L, Becker BE. Untreated periodontal disease: A longitudinal study. *J Periodontol* 1984;11:21.
122. Genco RJ, Evans RT, Ellison SA. Dental research in microbiology with emphasis on periodontal disease. *JADA* 1969;78:1016.
123. Socransky SS. Relationship of bacteria to the etiology of periodontal disease. *J Dent Res* 1970;49:203.
124. Taichman NS, McArthur WP. Current Concepts in periodontal disease. *Annu Rep Med Chem* 1975;10:228.
125. Wiggs RB, Lobprise HB. The Basics of Guided Tissue Regeneration. World Veterinary Dental Congress Proceedings. 1994:147.
126. Grove TK. Surgery on the palatal defects of canine teeth. *Vet Forum.* May 1987:16.
127. Holmstrom SE, Frost P, Gammon RL. *Dental Prophylaxis: Veterinary Dental Techniques.* Philadelphia: WB Saunders Co; 1992:137.
128. Grove TK. Regenerative periodontal therapy. TNAVC Proceed 1992:94.
129. Waleed AA, Bissada NF, Greenwell H. The effect of local doxycycline with and without tricalcium phosphate on the regenerative healing potential of periodontal osseous defects in dogs. *J Periodontol* 1989;60:582.
130. Genco RJ. Antibiotics in the treatment of human periodontal diseases. *J Periodontol* 1981;52:545.
131. Hurt WC. Basic rationale for periodontal therapy. In: Hurt WC, ed. *Periodontics in General Practice.* Springfield, IL: Charles C Thomas; 1976:157.
132. Ashman A. Applications of HTR® polymer in dentistry. *Compend Cont Educ Dent* 1988;(suppl 10):S330-S336.
133. Caffesse RG, Quinones CR. Guided tissue regeneration: Biologic rationale, surgical technique, and clinical results. *Compend Cont Educ Dent* 1992;8:166.
134. Melcher AH. Repair of wounds in the periodontium of the rat. Influence of periodontal ligament on osteogenesis. *Arch Oral Biol* 1970;15:1183.
135. Line SE, Polson AM, Zander HA. Relationship between periodontal injury, selective cell repopulation and ankylosis. *J Periodontol* 1974;45:725.
136. Nyman S, Karring T, Lindhe J, et al. The regenerative potential of the periodontal ligament. An experimental study in the monkey. *J Periodontol* 1982;9:257.
137. Levine RA. Guided tissue regeneration: Clinical Applications associated with dental implants. *Compend Cont Educ Dent* 1992;8:182.
138. Caton J, Greenstein G, Zappa U. Guided tissue regeneration using Vicryl® Periodontal Mesh. *Compend Cont Educ Dent* 1992;8:202.
139. Blumenthal NM. The use of collagen membranes for guided tissue regeneration. *Compend Cont Educ Dent* 1992;8:214.
140. Eisner E. Treating advanced cases of periodontitis in dogs and cats. *Vet Med* 1990:140.
141. Sottosanti J. Calcium sulfate: A biodegradable and biocompatible barrier for guided tissue regeneration. *Compend Cont Educ Dent* 1992;13:226.
142. Evans GH, Yukna RA, Sepe WW, Mabry TW, Mayer ET. Effect of various graft materials with tetracycline in localized juvenile periodontitis. *J Periodontol* 1989;60:491.
143. Pepelassi EM, Bissada NF, Greenwell H, Farah CH. Doxycycline and tricalcium phosphate composite graft facilitates healing in advanced periodontal furcation defects. *J Periodontol* 1992;62:106.
144. Hars E, Massler M. Effects of fluorides, corticosteroids and tetracycline on extraction wound healing in rats. *Acta Odontol Scand* 1972;30:511.
145. Baker P, Evans R, Coburn R, Genco R. Tetracycline and its derivatives strongly bind to and are released from the tooth surface in active form. *J Periodontol* 1983;54:580.
146. Moskow BS, Tannenbaum P. Enhanced repair and regeneration of periodontal lesions in tetracycline-treated patients: Case reports. *J Periodontol* 1991;62:341.

147. Claffey N, Bogle G, Bjornvatn K, Selvig K, Egelberg J. Topical application of tetracycline in regenerative periodontal surgery in beagles. *Acta Odontol Scand* 1987;45:141.
148. Peltier LF, Orn D. The effect of the addition of plaster of Paris to autogenous and homogeneous bone grafts in dogs. *Surg Forum* 1958;8:571.
149. Calhoun NR, Greene GW, Blackledge GT. Effects of plaster of Paris implants on osteogenesis in the mandibles of dogs. *J Dent Res* 1963;42:1244.
150. Radentz WH, Collins CK. The implantation of plaster of Paris in the alveolar process of the dog. *J Periodontol* 1965;36:357.
151. Shaffer D, App GR. The use of plaster of Paris in treating infrabony periodontal defects in humans. *J Periodontol* 1971;42:685.
152. Allen LJ. Oral use of absorbable alginate derivatives to arrest and prevent postextraction hemorrhage. *Oral Surg Oral Med Oral Pathol* 1953;6:444.
153. Miller PD. The concept of the "super clot" in osseous grafting. *Compend Cont Educ Dent* 1992;8:236.
154. Lerner SA. Bone-fill in guided tissue regeneration of periodontal defects. 1991;8:248.
155. Cline NV, Layman DL. The effects of chlorhexidine on the attachment and growth of cultured human periodontal cells. *J Periodontol* 1992;63:598.

9

Oral Surgery

Robert B. Wiggs and Heidi B. Lobprise

Although dentistry for the most part is thought of as a dental operative field, the need often arises for certain surgical procedures for the other oral tissues, both soft and hard. While certain surgical rules and skills necessary for other body systems are applicable for the oral cavity, certain modifications must also be kept in mind. Attempts at maintaining complete sterility are next to impossible in the moist environment and normal status of an oral flora; however, the necessity remains for oral health and function to continue post-operatively in most cases. In fact, the primary goal of any oral surgical procedure is to maintain the overall health and function of the oral cavity, including the teeth.

BASIC SURGICAL PRINCIPLES

In striving to maintain oral function, certain criteria must be addressed. The oral cavity's excellent blood supply can prove to be both a benefit and a hindrance to surgery, and while hemostasis must be provided for proper visualization, preservation of major vessels is essential. The most significant vessels and nerves typically encountered are the infraorbital and palatine structures of the maxilla and the mandibular canal components in the mandible. Short of cases where radical excision will mean some of the vessels must be sacrificed, identifying and retracting the structures may be possible, and certainly ligation is required if they are severed. While the selection of instruments may depend greatly on the operator's preference, typically the smaller scalpel blades allow more refined movement in the oral cavity. Tissue-handling instruments such as forceps and scissors should provide for more delicate handling of the gingiva and mucosa, particularly when they are friable. Preference for suture material may also vary, but typically an absorbable product of 3-0 to 4-0 size with swaged-on needle works best. The type and size of suture can be adjusted according to the size of the patient, condition and thickness of the tissue, and goal of the procedure. For extractions, chromic catgut or other absorbable material may be used, but a product that will stay intact longer (eg, polyglactin 910 or polyglycolic acid) is preferred with oronasal fistula repair and other complicated procedures. In thin, friable tissue, a tapered needle may be preferred, whereas a reverse cutting needle may be needed for thicker mucosa.

Suture technique may also be adjusted according to need, often with a simple interrupted pattern sufficing for most cases and with specialized patterns where indicated. Sutures should incorporate adequate bites of tissue and be secured snugly to resist loosening due to movement of the tongue and lips. They should be placed approximately 0.25 inch apart on average, with care to avoid unnecessary gaping or folds. Interdental sutures should allow good approximation of tissues, as well as keeping the gingiva securely against the tooth. It is best not to have a suture line over a defect, but most important, a suture line should never be placed under tension. Any suture line with tension should be expected to fail. It is also vital to provide a fresh edge or surface for adequate healing. Any chronic area or intact epithelial surface should be debrided or scraped to provide a good healing surface.

Hard tissues must also be dealt with properly during surgical procedures. With high-speed handpieces and burs or electro/radiosurgical units, it is possible to injure or burn bone surfaces, which can later necrose. Often rough bony crests with spicules should be smoothed with alveoloplasty to avoid any further soft tissue damage, but excessive amounts of supportive bone should not be removed. Generally, no area of denuded bone should be left uncovered by soft tissue.

ELECTROSURGERY/RADIOSURGERY

While most surgical procedures are performed with "cold steel," improved methods of electrosurgery make it an option with many procedures. There are four types of units currently available: fully rectified, fully filtered, partially rectified, and fulgurating. *Fully rectified* current provides easy cutting of most oral soft tissue and a good degree of hemostasis. It is useful for gingivectomy, gingivoplasty, palatal soft tissue surgery, frenectomy, and fibrous epulis removal. A *fully filtered* current is the least traumatic of the four types and is used for delicate cutting, but little hemostasis is afforded. Any surgery close to cementum or bone benefits from this type of current, as well as biopsy specimens, gingival grafting, and even widening of the gingival sulcus for crowns. *Partially rectified* current coagulates soft tissues for hemostasis where bleeding is a problem. It can also be used for electrophoresis to stimulate the penetration of solutions into hard tissue, with applications involving bleaching endodontically treated teeth and desensitizing dentin and cementum. The spark-gap technique used at high-power settings to produce the *fulgurating* current is the most destructive of the four. It is used for hemostasis involving osseous surgical sites and destruction of cyst remnants or fistulous tract linings.

While there are disadvantages related to odor, shock hazard, and limitations on use around flammable products, the advantages of hemostasis, improved field visualization, good healing, and speed often outweigh the negatives. A variety of tip shapes can be used for different applications, from a straight wire for most incisions to loops for contouring soft tissues. Ball- and bar-shaped tips are utilized for coagulation without a cutting mode, and the electrophoresis capabilities are best served by the spoon tip.

Tuning the instrument is necessary to provide to adequate cutting, as well as coagulation, with minimal sparking and no drag through the tissue. A new unit can be adjusted by making a series of cuts in a steak, avoiding sparking at too high a setting and dragging or blanching of the meat at too low a setting. As compared to a cutting action, the technique for a lateral heat application includes applying the electrode to any one point for no more than 1–2 seconds, with a 5–10 second interval between applications. Tincture of Myrrh and Benzoin (Sultan Chemical, Englewood, New Jersey) may be placed on the cut edges to reduce discomfort, or a periodontal pack may be applied if extensive surgery has been performed. In veterinary patients, these packs are not always retained for long periods of time.

EXODONTIA

The most commonly performed oral surgery is extraction, or exodontia. While the primary goal of dentistry is certainly to preserve tooth structure, situations may exist in which removing the tooth provides the patient with a better outcome. A number of factors must be included in making the decision to extract a tooth. A complete evaluation of the status of the tooth and the periodontium is combined with the anticipated level of owner/pet compliance with home care and follow-up treatment. As compliance decreases, the probability of exodontia increases.

Indications

Some developmental indications for exodontia may include retained (persistent) deciduous teeth, interceptive orthodontics (extraction of maloccluded deciduous teeth), impacted teeth, maloccluded teeth that are causing trauma to other structures, and supernumerary teeth with associated periodontal disease or malocclusion. Extraction of deciduous teeth is discussed in the pedodontics chapter (see Chapter 7). Severe periodontal disease can often result in highly mobile or diseased teeth that can be candidates for removal, as are extremely damaged teeth or those affected by endodontic complications. As in any dental procedure, the presence of active infection may warrant the use of appropriate antibiotics, particularly in high-risk individuals (eg, poor immune status, valvular disease). Bacteremias have been demonstrated after extraction, and septicemia has been reported as a complication of dental disease in dogs (1,2). The decision for extraction is not always a clear-cut one, and while "toothanasia" should be avoided whenever possible, sometimes exodontia will provide a healthier and more comfortable oral cavity and patient. It must be noted that there is an increasing frequency of complaints from owners in cases in which extractions were performed without the complete knowledge or consent from the owner (3). Even though the treatment may be the optimal one for the patient and possibly cannot be avoided in extremely mobile teeth, communication with the owner must be complete at all times, or potential litigation could result. Even if an owner is informed at the time of initial examination that extractions may be necessary, and approves, it is essential to be able to contact him or her during the procedure should more extensive work need to be done.

At times, the decision for extraction will also be influenced by the relative importance of the tooth to the animal (*strategic teeth*) and to the owner (*esthetic teeth*). The more strategic teeth tend to be the cuspids and the carnassials (upper 4th premolars and lower 1st molars). The esthetic teeth are the maxillary and mandibular incisors. More extensive therapy such as endodontics or periodontal surgery may be considered more practical on these teeth than on *nonstrategic, nonesthetic* teeth. In fact, if periodontal disease is moderate on a nonstrategic tooth that is adjacent to a strategic structure and could potentially endanger its viability, the option to extract the lesser structure may be best.

Technique

Adequate accessibility with use of a mouth gag and good visibility with proper lighting are essential requirements for exodontia. Basic anatomic knowledge of the tooth attachment, crown structure, and root number provides a basic foundation on which to build correct technique. Identification of multiple-rooted teeth will assist the practitioner in deciding to section the teeth into single-rooted segments. Only the maxilla houses three-rooted teeth: the 4th premolars and the 1st and 2nd molars in the dog. Teeth with two roots are the lower premolars and molars: upper 1st–3rd premolars and upper 3rd molars. Occasionally, the 1st premolars (upper and lower) can have just one root. In cats, the only three-rooted teeth are the upper 4th premolars; all other premolars and molars are two-rooted, except the upper 2nd premolars, which have one root like the incisors and cuspids.

These essentials—proper accessibility, visibility, knowledge, and skills—will help make extraction as efficient as possible. Utilizing a systematic approach is the best assurance for reliable results. A radiograph before the procedure can ascertain vital information about ankylosed, fragile, dilacerated, or abnormally shaped roots. Extraoral radiology can be helpful, but intraoral films usually produce a superior image with excellent detail and lack of structural superimposition.

Although veterinary patients are under general anesthesia for extractions and, if managed correctly, should experience no discomfort during the procedure itself, there is a growing awareness of providing pain management for the postoperative period. Topical anesthetic gels can provide temporary relief but are short-lived. Local injectable anesthetics may be administered as an infiltrating injection or deposited in specific areas for individual nerve blocks of defined areas. In recent studies using bupivacaine (average total dose: 2 mg/kg), the following *intraoral regional anesthetic nerve blocks* have been verified (4,5):

A *cranial infraorbital block* is made by injecting at the rostral end of the infraorbital canal to provide analgesia to the incisors, canines, and first two premolars. By insertion of the needle tip caudally into the canal itself and the application of pressure to its cranial opening, the medication can be forced to travel back through the canal, potentially offering a caudal infraorbital anesthesia to encompass the rest of the maxillary dentition. A more specific *caudal infraorbital block* can be placed dorsal to the last maxillary molar at the ventral aspect of the junction of the zygomatic arch. With advancement of the needle tip to the pterygopalatine fossa, the injection is deposited where the infraorbital nerve enters the maxillary foramen at the caudal aspect of the infraorbital canal to anesthetize all maxillary teeth. All mandibular teeth can be covered by a *mandibular alveolar block* with injection at the lingual mandible near the base of the coronoid process. A landmark for starting the injection is the "notch" on the ventral surface of the caudal mandible; the needle tip is advanced dorsally to reach the area. A *mental regional block* placed at the largest mental foramen ventral to the mesial root of the 2nd premolar will provide analgesia to the incisors, canines, and first two premolars. Not only do these blocks provide postoperative pain relief for up to 6–8 hours and smooth the recovery period, but reduction in perioperative pain can allow a lower concentration of general anesthesia to be used.

Pre- and postoperative injections of analgesics such as butorphanol can relieve discomfort and help smooth the recovery period. Oral analgesics dispensed for home care use can continue this level of pain management, which can sometimes deter the patient from mutilating a surgical site due to discomfort.

The first step in extraction is severing the epithelial attachment. A No.11 surgical blade or a small, sharp periosteal or dental elevator can be used for this purpose. The blade is inserted into the gingival sulcus until it meets with the resistance of the alveolar crestal bone. The sulcal incision is extended around the entire tooth, thus releasing the epithelial attachment. The gingiva and even a small amount of the alveolar cortical plate may then be loosened with a No.2 or No.4 Molt surgical periosteal elevator and retracted to provide better visualization of the root structure.

Multirooted teeth must first be divided before any attempts at elevation are made, as there are many anatomic features in an intact tooth that can make extraction difficult. Roots are often divergent to enhance their stability in the oral cavity. Some roots may also have indentations with a corresponding alveolar ridge for additional retentive strength (Fig. 1). On multirooted teeth, once the cortical plate is slightly retracted, a tapered cross-cut bur (eg, a 699L) can be used to resect the tooth by inserting it into the furcation between the roots and passing through the dental hard tissues to the opposite side. This allows each root section to be addressed independently. If this equipment is not available, a Gigli wire passed through the furcation to cut coronally through the tooth, or a tungsten steel hacksaw blade, may be carefully used; however, root splitters should be discouraged as compound tooth fractures are common.

Once the tooth is sectioned into single-rooted portions, or if a single-rooted tooth is being extracted, the periodontal ligament is then severed. Initially, the elevator or luxator is gently pressed into the space between the tooth and alveolar socket occupied by the periodontal ligament, and it is worked circumferentially around the tooth. The elevator is used with a steady, gentle rotational pressure for 10–30 seconds to fatigue the periodontal ligament and cause hemorrhage within its fibers. As the space allows, the elevator is pressed further apically along the tooth, using a slow twisting action on the instrument. Excess force should not be necessary if correct technique is used. Cradling the jaw with the opposite hand and holding the elevator down on the shaft to prevent slippage are important considerations, especially with bone structure of questionable stability (eg, calcium depletion, advanced periodontal disease) that could fracture. A finger should be kept on the shank near the cutting tip to aid in preventing inadvertent forcing of the sharp instrument tip through the alveolus and into other tissues or organs. Injuries to eyes and salivary glands have been reported. Luxators should not be used in a lever action, as their function is to sever the ligament by pressing it apically and sliding it around the root.

With multirooted or even multiple teeth, it often facilitates extraction by using the elevator as a lever between two adjacent sections to put pressure on and fatigue the periodontal ligament. This is done by sliding the dental elevator tip into the interproximal space and then hooking the edge of blade under the cervical bulge. The instrument is then rotated to lift up on the cervical bulge and elevate the tooth. This should be done carefully, as the pressure placed on the adjacent tooth could result in root fractures. If one par-

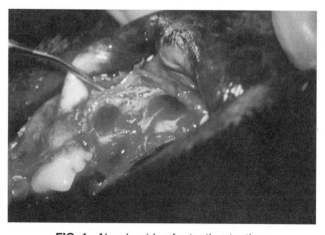

FIG. 1. Alveolar ridge for tooth retention.

ticular tooth or section is a bit more challenging, working on another section and then returning to the original may allow time for the hydraulic pressure from hemorrhage in the periodontal ligament space to help fatigue the ligament and loosen the tooth root.

The size and type of elevator may vary with the shape and size of the tooth, and even the patient size, particularly with feline teeth. The No.2 Molt surgical elevator and the Nos.301s and 301 apical dental elevators work well for most cats, while Nos.301s, 301, and 401 are good general dental elevators for the dog. Once the tooth becomes loose, the elevator can be pressed to the bottom of the alveolus with leverage to remove the tooth. An alternative method would be to use a pair of extracting forceps to grasp the loose tooth. The extraction forceps should never be used forcefully to attempt tooth removal; fracture of the tooth with retention of the root tip is often the consequence. The Nos.27X, 50S, and 3 extraction forceps work well in cats and small dogs, and the Nos.150, 65, and 69 forceps in the larger dogs.

With difficult extractions, a full-thickness gingival flap is sometimes needed to provide good visualization. Once the gingival epithelial attachment is severed (in the sulcus), two vertical releasing flaps are made on the mesial and distal aspects of the tooth. The flap can then be elevated with a No.2, No.4, or No.9 Molt surgical periosteal elevator. At the level of the mucogingival junction, a scalpel blade or small pair of scissors may be used to release the gingival flap more fully by gentle excision of the connective tissue attachment to the periosteum at the base without cutting through the flap. Further facilitation may also be afforded when the buccal alveolar bone plate is removed with a round (No.4), pear-shaped (No.331), or tapered-fissure (No.701) bur on a high-speed handpiece, or rongeurs. Small amounts of bone may be removed, or the bone plate covering the majority of the root may be elevated after a U-shaped outline of the root is cut with a bur. Generally, this removal of cortical plate bone can be performed on the buccal or lingual side, but preferably not to both.

Canines/Cuspids

The combination of gingival flap and buccal bone removal is often necessary in the extraction of canine teeth or cuspids. Frequently, the width of the root nearest the cementoenamel junction is the widest part of the tooth, making simple exodontia very difficult. Once the buccal bone plate is elevated and the majority of the cuspid is exposed, elevators are utilized at its mesial and distal surfaces to loosen the periodontal ligament. Attempt to elevate the maxillary canine teeth lingually may contribute to the formation of an oronasal fistula, especially if marked periodontal disease has affected the region already. There have been studies done comparing removal of the lingual bone plate in mandibular canines (6) to avoid the mental foramina and associated structures, but choice of technique is often due to operator preference. A lingual approach must take into account the soft tissue structures present in the sublingual area and the mandibular symphysis.

Closure of the sites may include alveoloplasty to remove any rough bone edges (7) and to avoid excessive loss of contour, an osteogenic product can be placed to stimulate osseous healing in the region. Various products may aid in bone regeneration in the area, including newer products such as Consil™ (Nutramax Labs, Baltimore, Maryland), a Bioglass® synthetic bone graft particulate product. A tetracycline product (doxycycline) can be placed for both its antibiotic and anticollagenase properties. Care should be taken not to deposit large amounts of tetracycline, as a yellowish staining may occur in adjacent teeth. Extraction of the upper cuspids may alter the facial features slightly because there is no longer any crown structure to support that portion of the upper lip, which is now vulnerable to trauma by the lower cuspid. Additionally, the socket may gradually collapse to some degree, thus further altering the facial features, which some clients may find objectionable. Extraction of the lower cuspids may allow the tongue to protrude from the mouth slightly. More important, the cuspid roots provide over half of the bulk of structure in the rostral mandible. As the sockets collapse after tooth removal, the symphysis and rostral mandible can become thin, fragile, and diminished and thus predisposed to fractures and other complications, so packing the alveolus before suturing would be warranted.

Upper 4th Premolar

The upper 4th premolar is sometimes chosen for extraction because it has been compromised by traumatic fracture and pulp exposure and endodontic therapy has been declined. The same principles of raising a gingival flap and sectioning the tooth with optional buccal bone removal will greatly facilitate the procedure. With a fractured tooth that has been infected, elevation is sometimes quite easy; at other times, however, the roots can be held quite solidly by the periodontal ligament, or even be ankylosed. Extreme care should be used in this region due to the proximity of the suborbital vessels that traverse the space between the mesiobuccal and mesiopalatal roots in the infraorbital canal space. Significant hemorrhage may result from damage to the area, so every attempt should be made to preserve the region (8). Application of pressure and ice packs may facilitate hemostasis if problems occur. Slippage of the elevator when loosening the distal root could also result in damage to nasal sinuses and the orbital contents as well (9–11). Any root tips that have been forced upward should be retrieved carefully. If there is potential damage to the region, the patient should be monitored very closely on recovery, particularly after extubation. If there is any compromise to the nasal passages, a subcutaneous emphysema may result. The animal should be reanesthetized and reintubated at once, and efforts should be made to remove as much of the air as possible, with opening of the extraction site, packing of the region with a solid material such as bone wax, and applying of ice and pressure to the region. If left untreated, the lesion can become quite large and painful and interfere with normal respiration.

Lower 1st Molar

With the proximity of the mandibular canal, the lower 1st molar has its own set of potential problems. Again, slippage or loss of root tips into the canal space should be handled carefully. Extraction criteria for this tooth often include advanced periodontal disease, and with the size of the mesial root specifically, any additional bone loss can make the region extremely weak. This is certainly a site that would benefit from placement of an osseoconductive product to help in osseous healing. In cases where the distal root is severely affected by periodontal disease but the mesial root is still relatively healthy, a tooth or root resection (hemisection) may be performed (see Chapter 12). In this procedure, the diseased distal root is extracted after it is separated from the rest of the tooth, and the mesial root is treated endodontically (12). Elevation and manipulation should be gentle yet precise; otherwise, fracture of the mandible may result, particularly when the large mesial root is involved. Unfortunately, once the region is compromised, any fracture stabilization can be quite challenging due to the periodontal bone loss and the absence of the tooth. Often a combination of transosseous wiring, acrylic splints, and tape muzzles is needed to provide some sort of stabilization.

Embedded Teeth

If a tooth is ever "missing," the area should always be radiographed to insure that the tooth is not present under the gum line. If the tooth is embedded, it is often best to extract it (10,14). An intact tooth under the gingival surface can lead to the formation of a dentigerous cyst originating from the cervical region of the tooth (see Chapter 6) (15,16). If cystic, the embedded tooth can sometimes be found by exploring the defect itself, but radiology is always a helpful tool. Smaller teeth in young animals or those already showing signs of pathology should be removed with a surgical approach involving gingival flaps and buccal bone removal. If a cyst is present, it should be thoroughly curetted and submitted for histopathology. At times, an embedded tooth will be discovered incidentally in an older animal without exhibiting any problems. In such cases, the potential damage that can be caused by the procedure itself, particularly if the tooth is a large one, may outweigh the benefits of continued monitoring. Of course, the owner should be informed of the presence of the tooth, so regular radiographic assessment can be encouraged.

Postextraction radiology should be performed if a procedure was complicated or if there is any concern that tooth material remains, as well as to assess any jaw damage. Any decision to leave a portion of a tooth that is ankylosed should be documented in the record with notification of the owner, and that area should be rechecked on a regular basis.

Once the tooth is removed, the socket is cleaned and curetted of debris or granulation tissue. Bony prominences and spicules are reduced with a bur, curette, or rongeur to simplify closure. Prior to flap closure, empty sockets of the upper and lower cuspids may be best filled with an osteogenic material, such as HTR® (Bioplant, Norwalk, Connecticut) or Consil™, or a tricalcium phosphate product. These materials aid in filling the open sockets with bone and connective tissue rather than allowing them to collapse or granulate in with soft tissue.

A simple gingival sliding flap can be used to cover the extraction site. In some cases, the periosteal attachment may need to be severed on the flap to provide additional slack for closure. This is done by lightly passing a blade across the underside of the flap near its attachment. Simple interrupted suturing using large bites of tissue and absorbable suture material work well in most cases. If needed, 23- or 20-gauge needles can be used to assist passing of the suture material.

Home care can greatly aid in reducing postoperative complications. Medication for pain may be needed in some individuals. A soft diet for a few days is routinely recommended to ease mastication. Antibiotics are recommended if active infections were encountered or anticipated. The patient should be rechecked in approximately 10–14 days to inspect the healing process.

Complications

If all the steps of a correct exodontia are performed, the chances of complications arising will be lessened. Certainly, if the proper radiographs are taken before, during, and after the procedure, the potential problems and their resolution can be assessed and accurately handled. Not every extraction will be a simple one, and the practitioner must know how to deal with the challenges as well.

Fragile teeth, such as those with cervical line lesions (feline) that may have external and/or internal root resorption, often have such debilitated structure that the normal forces used to fatigue the periodontal ligament tend to cause tooth fractures. The periodontal ligament further down the root will be of questionable viability, particularly when external root resorption is extensive. Portions of the root may be ankylosed where bone is growing into the tooth and starting to obliterate the normal root structure. In such cases, total extraction can be extremely difficult. If there is any indication that ongoing infection may be present in the root structure or if any refractory inflammatory process such as stomatitis is present in the oral cavity, it is essential to remove all tooth structure possible. At times, it may be necessary to use a bur on a high-speed handpiece to pulverize the remaining root structure for adequate removal. It is essential to have adequate radiographic capabilities whenever removal of tooth structures in such a fashion is attempted, as extensive damage may occur if this is done blindly. Bone rongeurs or a bur (round, pear-shaped, or tapered-fissure) on a high-speed handpiece with adequate cooling irrigation are used to disintegrate remaining tooth structure and diseased bone that might cause ongoing problems if retained.

A recent study (17), though still considered controversial by some, investigated the results of removing just the crown structure of feline teeth exhibiting erosive lesions and suturing the gingiva over the remaining root structure. Results were generally favorable, with some teeth continuing in their resorption and others maintaining even the periodontal ligament space without adverse signs. Optimally, all root structure should be removed in each case, most importantly in those individuals with stomatitis or evidence of infection in the roots. This technique may be an option in teeth in which attempting to retrieve resorbing or ankylosed roots may cause extreme trauma. If it is used, the owner must be fully informed of the decision, and radiographic follow-up is essential to detect any potential future problems.

More precise visualization can be attained using a gingival flap and buccal bone removal. This technique is also useful with roots that are ankylosed into the socket or have radicular grooves or some degree of dilaceration or cementoid deposition. Any of these conditions greatly interfere with normal elevation and periodontal ligament loosening, necessitating the open method.

In some more complicated cases or those involving excessive force, fractured root tips may be retained in the alveolar socket (Fig. 2). When this occurs, every attempt should be made to remove the remaining structure. Modified elevators with fine working heads, such as root-tip picks, are often helpful in loosening and retrieving these fragments. If the picks

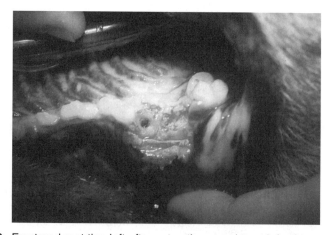

FIG. 2. Fractured root tips left after extraction; persistent infection occurred.

do not provide sufficient assistance in extraction, gingival flap/alveolar bone removal can offer additional access. While as much bone should be preserved as possible, removal of portions of the buccal plate and even some of the interradicular bone is often helpful.

The practitioner must be careful with all instruments, particularly the sharper ones, not letting them slip past the tooth and into the structures beneath, whether soft tissue (sublingual, orbit) or hard tissue (into nasal cavity or mandibular canal). Proper instrument-holding techniques with steadying of the shaft near the working end should limit the possibility of slippage.

A complication described in humans, but not often apparent in veterinary patients, is *localized osteitis* ("dry socket"). While this development is not fully understood, a combination of traumatic procedure, infection, and decreased vascular supply is thought to contribute to this complication (18). If the primary clot becomes dislodged with irrigation and the alveolus is left exposed, severe pain and necrosis can occur. Often it is best to let nature take its course with granulation walling off the necrotic bone and eventual loss of the diseased tissue. Curettage is not recommended, but palliative irrigation and pain control are.

One of the more serious complications that can result from aggressive extraction techniques is an iatrogenic oronasal or oroantral fistula. Formation of a distinct communication between the oral and nasal cavity or sinuses requires a specific correction beyond just poking an instrument through the tissues. Attempts to elevate or rotate an upper canine where the apex is forced medially can cause fistulation.

Oronasal Fistula

If an oronasal fistula is evident either before extraction (due to extensive periodontal disease) or after extraction, it requires closure to prevent a constant influx of food and liquid into the nasal cavity. Though most frequently described in dogs, fistula formation may also occur in cats due to periodontal disease and even resorptive lesions (19). Regardless of the technique used, it is essential to follow the basic guidelines of employing sufficient tissue in the flap, taking large bites, not placing sutures directly over the defect, and allowing absolutely no tension on the suture line.

In minor or acute lesions, a mucogingival flap will often be sufficient. After the fistula margins are debrided to provide a fresh epithelial edge, divergent releasing incisions are made at the mesial and distal aspects of the defect and extended apically into the buccal mucosa. With a periosteal elevator, the gingiva and periosteum are elevated, and the periosteal attachment is released at the depth of the flap to provide enough slack. Simple interrupted sutures of absorbable material should oppose the margins with no tension (Fig. 3).

Larger or chronic fistulas or sites with loss of attached gingiva may require a double-flap technique. The first flap is harvested from the full thickness of the palatal mucosa by joining mesial and distal releasing incisions, sometimes even past the midline, to provide sufficient tissue, while the margin of tissue at the defect itself is preserved. The epithelial surface of the flap is debrided, and the flap is then inverted after elevation, facing the palatal mucosa toward the nasal opening. After this is sutured in place, a second flap may be obtained either by sliding a mucoperiosteal flap as described before or by using a labial buccal pedicle flap (a U-shaped flap) (20). The pedicle flap is a partial-thickness graft from the alveolar mucosa lateral to the defect, with the incision started at the distal aspect of the fistula near the mucogingival line. A second line, approximately one and

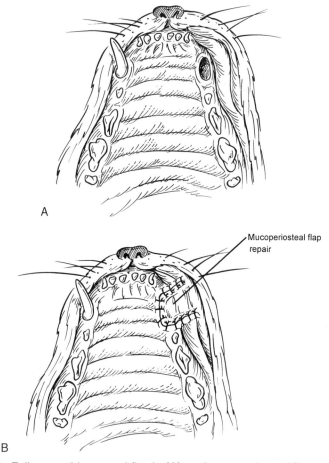

FIG. 3. Feline cuspid oronasal fistula **(A)** and mucoperiosteal flap repair **(B)**.

one-half times the diameter of the fistula away from the first, is made apical and parallel to the initial incision and joined to it mesially by a third incision near the midline of the incisors. After elevation, the flap is rotated and sutured over the palatal flap and its donor site. The donor site edges of the pedicle flap are then closed by undermining the connective tissue, bringing the opposing sides together, and suturing. Gentle cleansing may be helpful postoperatively, but excessive handling of the area should be discouraged. Occasionally, small, recurrent fistulating areas may require additional surgical intervention.

PALATAL DEFECTS

Congenital

Palatal defects can often be found in very young animals and, if left uncorrected, can cause serious complications in the inability to nurse without aspirating liquid into the lungs. These individuals should be tube-fed and nursed until they reach a more reasonable age for the anesthesia and surgery. The type and size of defect will determine what procedure to perform (see later in the chapter), and the practitioner will often have to formulate an individualized approach to each case. Strong owner commitment will be necessary to deal with the additional care and possible multiple surgical procedures necessary to adequately treat the problem. If there is any reason to suspect a potential genetic influence, the animal should not be used for breeding purposes.

Unusually long soft-palatal tissue can sometimes be seen in dogs, particularly the brachycephalic breeds. If the tissue interferes with normal breathing and eating, it can be resected at its edge. To warrant this procedure, the amount of excessive tissue is usually quite significant. The caudal end of the redundant tissue is grasped, and two hemostatic forceps placed from either side. Excessive amounts of mucosa from the nasopharyngeal side should not be removed, so excising one half first, closing that portion, and then continuing with the excision and closure are usually best (21). Clamping the tissue and preplacing mattress sutures are also possible.

Acquired

Acquired palatal lesions are often the result of some type of trauma, most notably being hit by a vehicle or falling from a tall building (high-rise syndrome in cats). Ingestion of caustic chemical or foreign objects or chewing on electrical cords can also cause significant damage to many of the oral tissues, including the palate. At times, the damage may be severe enough to denude the soft tissue down to the palatal bone, or even through the bone itself. Any lesion with communication into the nasal cavity should be corrected, including median separation of the palate that can be experienced after a fall or head trauma. This defect has been known to heal over if left untreated, particularly in animals that were too unstable at the time to withstand the anesthetic required; however, such defects should be closed when possible. Of course, any patient exhibiting traumatic lesions should be thoroughly assessed as to any other areas of damage.

The extent of damage from caustic materials or burns should be thoroughly assessed, even if fistulation has not occurred. Diseased or necrotic tissue should be debrided, but a staged procedure is recommended to avoid removing excessive amounts of tissue at the first round of therapy. In addition, electrical injuries may take several days to demonstrate the full extent of damage. The excellent blood supply of the oral cavity can allow for some significant healing, given a chance.

Though it can be considered a congenital lesion because the initial cause is such, palatal trauma due to malocclusive mandibular canine teeth (base narrow) can be acquired as the teeth erupt further into the palatal tissues (Fig. 4). While many cases will produce only soft tissue trauma and are readily treated by dealing with the cause, occasionally an animal will experience full exposure of the oral cavity, often after chronic trauma from the lower tooth (22). After treatment of the canine (eg, pulp capping, extraction, orthodontic movement), the fistulation must also be repaired (see Oronasal Fistula previously described in this chapter).

Repair Techniques for the Palate

Proper surgical techniques must be adhered to in this region, for surgical sites can be under constant stress from both the effects of respiration and constant movement of the tongue. Absolute absence of tension is essential, and the location of the palatal arteries must always be taken into account to incorporate a blood supply into the flap, if possible.

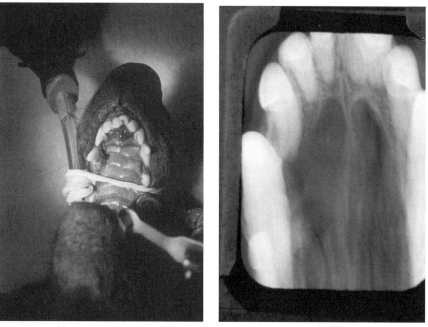

FIG. 4. (A) Palatal trauma induced by maloccluded base-narrow canine tooth. **(B)** Radiograph reveals osseous defect at oronasal fistula site.

All tissue edges should be freshened, and any intact epithelial surface in the surgical field should be scarified. A flap should be at least one and one-half to two times the size or width of the defect to be covered to allow for tissue retraction; sutures should not lie directly over the defect.

Midline Defect Repair

The palatal mucosa is sometimes difficult to work with due to its lack of elasticity (23). The specific technique chosen will depend on the location and severity of the lesion. With significant lesions, an overlapping-flap technique can be incorporated to include the palatine artery on the flap side (Fig. 5). The initial incision is made at the edge of the defect on one side and carried up to 2–3 mm from the dental arch on the other side. This second incision is joined by incisions at its mesial and distal aspects to points near the defect itself. The flap is then elevated carefully to the extent of the defect's edge, with preservation of the flap in one piece. If the harvested flap needs to be large enough to include the region of the palatine artery, the artery can remain with the flap with the use of careful dissection (ligating it at the mesial aspect) to loosen it sufficiently to stretch it as the flap is rotated. The flap is rotated 180° and flipped back over the defect to be inserted into the space created when the initial margin incised was elevated off the palate. An overlapping-suture technique, preplaced, allows the connective tissue surface of each flap to face the other (23).

With smaller (by length or width of defect) lesions, a releasing flap at the lateral aspect by each dental arch can provide enough flexibility to bring the two medial edges together at the midline. The lateral relieving incisions often must be fairly long, incorporating the

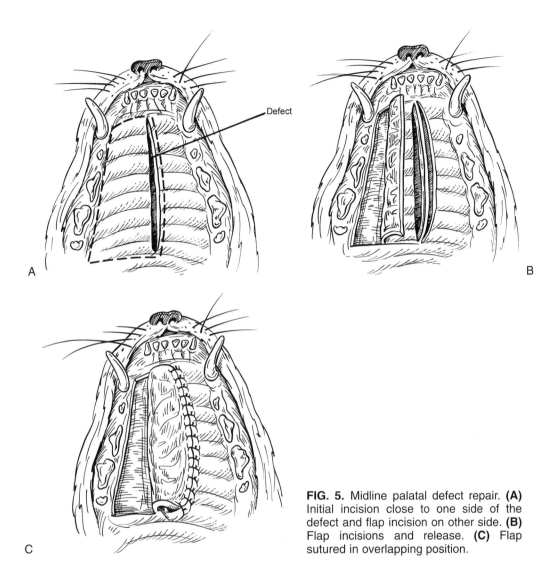

FIG. 5. Midline palatal defect repair. **(A)** Initial incision close to one side of the defect and flap incision on other side. **(B)** Flap incisions and release. **(C)** Flap sutured in overlapping position.

palatine arteries, and the medial edges must be freshened before suturing. Soft palatal defects at the midline can sometimes be closed by a two-layer technique, if sufficient tissue is retained (23).

Asymmetric Defect Repair

Many surgical techniques have been described for palatal defects of varying size and position, illustrating that each case must be evaluated on its own peculiarities. Small circular defects can often be covered by rotation flaps, with care to provide donor tissue of sufficient size (23). Larger defects involving advancement flaps, making use of the flexibility of the soft-palatal tissues, or extraction of premolars to allow future advancement of buccal mucosa often need advance planning (24). Moving large areas of tissue requires consideration of preserving blood supply and ensuring the debridement of any

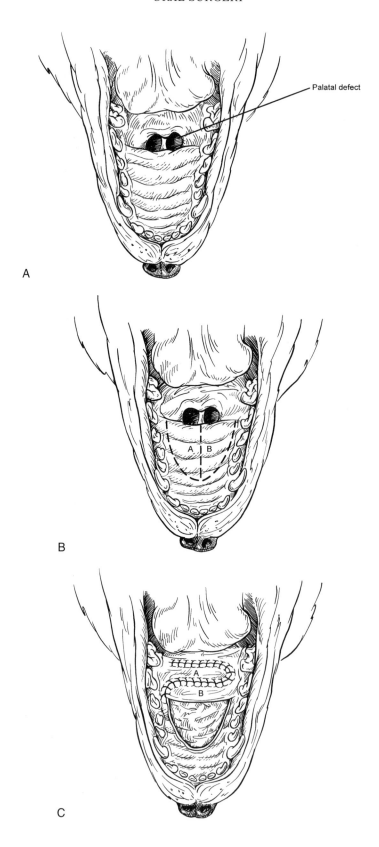

A

Palatal defect

B

C

epithelial surface to be covered. For a larger caudal palatal defect, a split-U flap technique has also been described (25) (Fig. 6). In this technique, a large full-thickness U-shaped flap is created anterior to the defect, extending rostrally to the level of the 1st premolars. The flap is divided at the midline, and the rostral extent of the palatine artery is ligated, with preservation of the rest of the artery for continued blood supply to the flap. The first half of the flap is rotated so the medial border is sutured to the caudal aspect of the defect; then the second flap is rotated and sutured to the now rostral extent of the first flap.

Any attempts at palatal surgery should be accompanied by regular rechecks, as persistent fistulation or communication into the nasal cavity is always possible. If minor defects persist, additional surgical techniques are usually sufficient to provide adequate correction. Small rostral defects may not cause extensive management problems and can at times be monitored. If persistent defects occur, additional surgery may be successful, but multiple procedures often have to rely on tissues that already have some fibrotic areas, so options are limited at times. Obturators, both permanent and removable, can be fashioned to provide closure of the region (26). Such devices generally require owner commitment, as routine hygiene may be required.

For extensive palatal defects and limited tissue to harvest flaps from, the dorsal surface of the tongue can be incised and undermined to use the cut surfaces as flaps, sutured to the palatal defect edges. After 4 weeks of assisted feeding, the tongue is separated from the palate, with enough tissue left to close the defect permanently (27,28).

Another, less serious palatal problem—but one that can contribute to periodontal disease—is deep palatal rugal troughs with embedded hair or foreign objects; this is a particular problem in brachycephalic breeds such as the boxer. If these troughs are left untreated, severe inflammation and infection can develop and extend into surrounding tissues. Cleaning them is helpful, but if their depth is excessive, it may be necessary to obliterate them. Scarifying or removing the epithelial layer with a scalpel blade or 12-fluted bur on a high-speed handpiece and placing sutures to oppose the two walls of the trough often suffice to promote healing to close the lesions (Fig. 7).

LIP AND CHEEK DEFECTS

While some surgery on the lips and cheeks is performed for more esthetic reasons, these structures can be very important in the overall function of the oral cavity, and corrective procedures for problems can significantly improve the patient's health. Surgical techniques may include some consideration of the final visual effect, so modifications are sometimes necessary.

FIG. 6. Split U-flap palatal repair. **(A)** Note the visualization achieved intraoperatively when the patient is placed in dorsal recumbency with the premaxilla taped to the surgical table and the mandible taped caudally in an open position. A large caudal palatal defect is evident. **(B)** The dotted line represents the incision line for creation of the split palatal U-flap. Note that the U-flap is incised along the midline to create flap *A* and flap *B*. **(C)** Following debridement of the edges of the palatal defect, flap *A* is rotated 90° into the palatal defect and sutured in place. Flap *B* is then rotated 90° and sutured to flap *A*. The stippled area represents the donor site devoid of a mucoperiosteal covering. (Reprinted from ref. 25, with permission.)

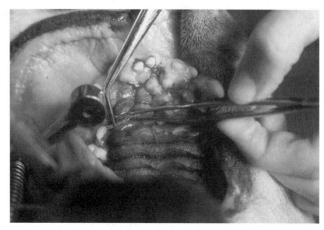

FIG. 7. Removing debris from deep palatal troughs before obliteration of defects.

Congenital/Developmental

While some mild abnormalities can be seen, more serious changes are sometimes present. Any form of cleft lip or sign of tissue-fusion failure should always alert the practitioner to look for other abnormalities. Complete reconstruction of the facial contours can be quite challenging at times, and more advanced procedures beyond two-layer closure of simple defects is beyond the scope of this text. It is important to try to preserve the line of the mucocutaneous junction of the lips and the patency of the nasal passage, if affected.

The Shar-Pei can be affected by tight-lip syndrome, in which the lower lip, due to the lack of proper vestibule development, does not extend to its full length or elasticity and instead folds back over the mandibular incisors and even canines (Fig. 8). The attachment of the vestibule at this point may be very high, contributing to the lifting of the lip up onto the rostral dentition. This mechanical interference can restrict the complete growth potential of the mandible, contributing to a malocclusion in addition to soft tissue trauma

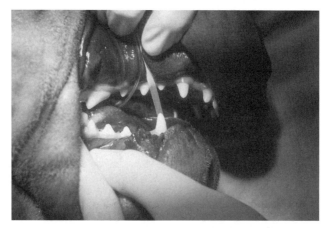

FIG. 8. Chinese Shar-Pei exhibiting tight-lip syndrome. The mandibular lip covers the incisors (and nearly the canines); the mandible is shortened in relation to maxilla.

involving the maxillary teeth on the turned lip. If it is found at an early age, external sutures like those used for entropion are sometimes effective in combination with bilateral mandibular frenectomy (see below); however, there is often enough stricture of fibers to prevent the problem from resolving. In more severe cases, a surgical procedure must be performed to release the tension and provide for a healing period without additional scar formation. Most surgery is based on attempts to reestablish a proper vestibule depth. With the dog positioned in sternal recumbency and the maxilla gently suspended from above to keep the mouth open and give good visibility, the mucosa is incised just below the attached gingiva of the mandibular incisors, and the underlying tissue is released. In extremely tight lips, nearly the entire rostral mandibular tissue needs to be released, approximating a degloving injury. To keep the cut edges from healing back together, a mucosal graft can be placed. This graft can be harvested from buccal alveolar mucosa, but attempting to make the graft initially larger than the site in a oval shape is important. Another option is to cut a piece of Penrose drain lengthwise to open it up and then customize its shape to the desired elliptical defect created. The Penrose template is sutured to the edges of the defect circumferentially, and sutures are used at the depth of the defect to tack down the tubing to the underlying tissue (Fig. 9). Concurrent bilateral mandibular frenectomy may also be performed to release further tension. After the incised edges of the defect have sufficiently epithelialized, the Penrose drain may be removed. Ideally, enough tension on the initial surgery is relieved, because subsequent attempts may not be as successful.

Though not necessarily true congenital defects, other variations in the lips and mandibular frenulum may also be found. In some dogs with tight frenulum, it is thought that this can contribute to periodontal attachment loss due to the tension in the area. Additionally, if the frenulum is tight, trauma from the maxillary canine can cause irritation. Release of the tension is possible by excising the frenulum parallel to the dental arcade and then bringing the mesial and distal cut points together and suturing side to side, perpendicular to the dental arcade. The procedure is generally known as a *frenectomy*; however, the term *frenoplasty* may be more appropriate.

Excessive or redundant lip tissue, normal in some breeds, can be a focal point for saliva and food collection with resulting cheilitis and dermatitis. Particularly in dogs with

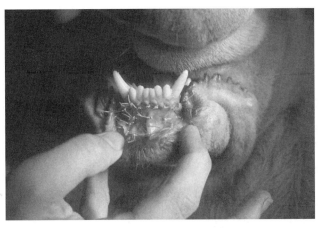

FIG. 9. Surgery for tight lip. Trimmed portion of Penrose drain to cover exposed tissue.

longer hair, collection of debris without regular cleaning can result in active infection. Cheiloplasty can be performed to remove some of the excess tissue, including any pendulous folds that have become infected. A simple resection of the deep lateral furrow will not slow salivation, but it can help in the natural cleansing effect (29). Alternately, a more involved commissuroplasty may be performed to reduce the actual oral opening, allowing the saliva to remain more in the oral cavity. Resection of the tissue should be planned in advance to determine the proper extent of the oral opening and the new position of the commissures. The mucosal margins should be closely approximated to avoid any defects intraorally, with a subcutaneous layer, and the dermal layers should match as well. This procedure can also be used after a mandibulectomy or in cases of nonunion to help provide additional stability to the area and help keep the tongue in the mouth. It should be recognized that any future attempts to clean or treat structures in the caudal portion of the oral cavity will be compromised. Conversely, with fibrotic scarring of the lips due to previous injury, commissuroplasty can be performed to open the stoma further (23).

Acquired

Most of the acquired lesions of the cheeks and lips, other than tumors, are due to trauma of some type. Vehicular injuries can contribute to the nearly complete avulsion of the mandibular soft tissue from the bone and can be quite extensive. Barring any additional injuries to the mandible or other oral structures, repair is typically rewarding if sufficient tissue is present. The area should be thoroughly cleaned and any debris irrigated away. With adequate tissue, the lip can be held in position with sutures from the soft tissue incorporating the canines or incisors. If there is insufficient tissue to cover the mandible completely, a rotation skin flap may be used, with looser skin from the neck to cover the donor site.

Lacerations or cuts of the lips should be sutured back into a normal anatomic position whenever possible, using flaps if necessary. Injury to the tissues due to chemical, thermal, or electrical trauma must be evaluated as to the extent of the injury. If no bone is exposed, debridement of the necrotic areas should be performed with an attempt to preserve as much healthy tissue as possible (30). Again, flaps can be used if bone is exposed or excessive amounts of soft tissue have been damaged.

TONGUE

In other areas of dentistry, there are often similarities between cats and dogs, and variations at times as well. With lingual lesions, the amount of healthy tissue remaining tends to be more critical for cats than for dogs. Canine patients have at times learned to adjust to extensive loss of the tongue, whereas cats typically do not. Their inability to groom themselves properly often leads to severe secondary problems with infections. It has been suggested that a cat that requires surgery involving removal of the tongue may benefit from another cat to help in its grooming habits.

Congenital

While some congenital conditions of the tongue, such as microglossia, obviously have no surgical remedy (31), a report of "tongue-tie" in a dog indicates some benefit from excision of the sublingual frenulum (32). There are few other abnormalities of the tongue to be treated, but individuals with extremely long tongues may benefit from resection of the rostral portion. Excision of the exteriorized portion of the tongue with lateral protrusion in a dog with a neurologic deficit provided sufficient correction (33).

Acquired

Again, most problems associated with the tongue are due to some type of trauma. It is important not to forget to examine the sublingual tissues, for a small laceration or embedded foreign objects can make an individual quite uncomfortable. The dorsal surface of the tongue can also be affected by foreign bodies such as burdock, which may require debridement (34). Lacerations should be sutured where it is feasible. Necrotic tissue as a result of electrical burns should be debrided conservatively, with attempts to preserve as much normal tissue as possible and allow for a staged treatment to remove further tissue if necessary. In one case of nearly complete lingual avulsion, the dog learned to eat and drink quite well after emergency care to stop hemorrhage and close the torn edges (35). The most common tumor of the tongue is squamous cell carcinoma, which can be quite aggressive. Early, rostral lesions often stand a better chance with resection (36–38).

TONSILS

While often overlooked in the oral cavity, the tonsils can be a focal point for severe disease. Surgical resection is warranted in refractory infections, where hyperplasia interferes with swallowing, and certainly when neoplasia is involved. Tonsillar squamous cell carcinoma is extremely aggressive and likely to metastasize. Excision of the tonsil can be performed after infiltration with epinephrine by grasping the tonsil and retracting it forward. The tissue can then be cut away from the tonsillar crypt with curved Metzenbaum scissors (21). The tonsils may also be clamped with forceps, but tonsil snares are less useful due to the fusiform shape of the tissue.

SALIVARY GLANDS

While some congenital problems, such as a branchial cyst, are possible in the salivary glands, they are typically rare (39,40). Obstruction can occur due to sialoliths or foreign objects, with initial pain and swelling followed by eventual atrophy of the gland if uncorrected (41). Surgically opening the duct to remove the obstruction may initiate a full healing process, but if problems continue, the gland should be removed.

Due to the structure of salivary glands with ducts that transport saliva to a distant orifice, trauma can injure and interfere with normal function. Swelling in the neck region may indicate a cervical mucocele, which can get quite large. Draining the accumulation of saliva will temporarily reduce the mucocele, but recurrence is common (41). The term *ranula* describes more specifically a well defined cyst on either side of the tongue that tends to recur if just drained or incised. Marsupialization may be successful in such cases by cutting away the dorsal portion of the cyst and suturing the ventral portions to adjacent mucous membrane to keep the area open permanently. If this is not successful, it is often necessary to remove the mandibular gland and both parts of the sublingual gland on that side.

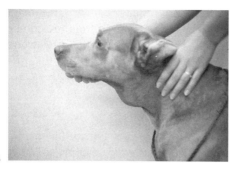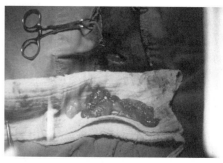

A   B

FIG. 10. Cervical mucocele. **(A)** Swelling is evident externally. **(B)** Resection of mandibular and sublingual salivary glands with cystic structure as well.

Salivary Gland Resection

The parotid salivary gland is best exposed by starting a 6–8-cm incision 2 cm ventral to the ear canal with rostral and caudal incisions of 3–4 cm from the dorsal aspect of the first incision (41). The maxillary vein and facial nerve must be preserved, and it is sometimes easier to remove a portion of the gland first, before the remainder of the gland dissected free.

Using the bifurcation of the jugular nerve near the angular process of the mandible as the starting point, a 6–8-cm incision can be made to expose the mandibular salivary gland. This gland is often removed in conjunction with the sublingual glands, with blunt dissection along the mandibular and caudal sublingual glands to loosen and retract the remaining tissue (41). The cystic structure is often encountered during this process and should be removed and treated as well (Fig. 10).

There are several approaches to the zygomatic salivary gland, as it lies protected below its arch. In the ventral method, a T-shaped incision is started 2 cm below the orbit, with avoidance of the facial nerve as the zygomatic arch is exposed. The masseter muscle should be bluntly dissected from the arch to allow the ventral portion of the bone to be removed (41). This should allow sufficient access to remove the gland itself.

MASS RESECTION

In addition to the basic principles of oral surgery, attaining adequate surgical margins is extremely important when oral masses and tumors are excised, particularly since the majority of tumors encountered in the oral cavity are relatively aggressive in nature. Often the only chance for a reasonable survival rate is early detection and radical excision. Adequate evaluation of the tumor using the tumor-nodes-metastasis (TNM) staging method (World Health Organization tumor classification) to assess local and extended disease can help a practitioner decide on which method to use to treat the case (42). It should also be recognized that if an area is suspicious, biopsy is required to evaluate the lesion fully, especially when it is a recurrent problem, even if previously diagnosed as a benign lesion. In addition, if a tooth has been lost or has been extracted due to mobility without a specific definitive cause such as periodontal disease, the region should be monitored closely in the future for any further changes, including nonhealing extraction sites. At times, this can be the earliest indication that a tumor is forming (43). Regular assessment of pathologic areas such as previously healed fracture sites is warranted. Both cases in the authors' experience—one involving a cat with squamous cell carcinoma appearing in both mandibular bodies 2–3 years after fracture repair and the other a dog with osteosarcoma at a previous fracture site (44), should validate the need for routine examinations. Certainly, areas where masses have been excised should always be closely monitored, for many oral neoplasms are known to recur locally (45).

Some of the surgical procedures described below can also be used for excision of tissue affected by disease other than malignancies. Trauma that contributes to chronic problems may best be resolved by physically removing the affected tissue. One case involving maxillary trauma due to a combination of malocclusion and severe myoclonic episodes was treated with a rostral maxillectomy and mandibular cuspid crown amputation to provide a more comfortable situation for the patient (22). Extensive damage to the mandible, even after attempted, but failed grafting of rib tissue, was managed finally with bilateral mandibulectomy (46).

Conservative Removal

There are only a handful of oral masses that can be treated conservatively; primarily these are benign lesions with slow local invasion and little to no chance of metastasis. Areas of gingival hyperplasia, papillomas, and some epulides fit into this category, but every suspicious lesion should be biopsied and submitted for histopathology. Incisional biopsies are possible as a first step, but it is often more expedient to use an excisional technique and plan additional surgery if the diagnosis is less than favorable. With the benign forms of epulides, full excision with extraction to remove the periodontal ligaments is generally sufficient, but more aggressive surgery is needed for lesions such as the acanthomatous epulis or malignant tumors.

Wide excision with at least a 1-cm normal border, as assessed radiographically, is sometimes difficult to attain without significant removal of alveolar and cortical bone. Due to the aggressive local nature of most oral neoplasms, it is certainly better to err on the wide side.

MANDIBULECTOMY

Rostral Mandibulectomy

Tumors in the rostral mandible that involve both sides can be treated by rostral mandibulectomy up to the level of the 2nd and 3rd premolars (47,48). With very small lesions, preservation of the distal portion of the symphysis will keep both mandibular sides in proper position, but this factor should not preclude complete resection just for cosmetic goals. In fact, with most patients, significant portions of the mandible can be removed with relatively esthetically pleasing results, as well as with the animal's retaining the ability to eat, drink, and groom itself.

Once the initial gingival incisions are made to release the soft tissue, attention should be paid to significant vasculature encountered during resection, including the mental vessels and certainly the mandibular artery once the osteotomy is complete. This latter artery can be grasped with a pair of fine forceps to gently retract it for ligation. The bone edge should be smoothed, and any remaining sections of root past the resection line should be extracted. Generally, there will be no major problems if the two hemimandibles are not stabilized to each other (47–49). In fact, attempting to fix the two sections together in the midline brings teeth medially to hit the palate, potentially affecting the temporo-mandibular joints. Any metallic implant or stabilization should never be placed where roots can be injured, and even if an autogenous rib graft is used to the align the sides, complications may result (23). Closure can be a challenge, but a triangular-wedge resection of excessive tissue on each side or a V-shaped incision at the rostral aspect can provide favorable results (50). Forming a "lip" of rostral gingiva can aid in the retention of saliva (51).

Rostral Hemimandibulectomy

When a lesion is present on one side of the rostral mandible from the incisors to the 1st premolar and does not cross the symphysis, a unilateral rostral mandibulectomy can often be performed. Once the soft tissue is excised, the symphyseal separation or cranial osteotomy should be performed first to provide better access for the caudal osteotomy (50). If the lesions is adjacent to the symphysis without radiographic evidence of its crossing over, an eccentric osteotomy can be performed to incorporate a wider border, including one or two incisors of the contralateral side. Care must be taken with this incision to leave adequate medial cortex around the contralateral cuspid root to maintain its stability (50). With resections back to the 2nd premolar, often no instability results (51). If resection beyond that point is necessary, some instability may occur, but it typically does not require any further stabilization. All other tenets of surgery should be followed, such as hemostasis, root removal, and even commissuroplasty if needed for additional stabilization.

Segmental Hemimandibulectomy (Central, Caudal)

For lesions confined to just a portion of the mandible, a central or even caudal segmental hemimandibulectomy can be performed. Identification of the affected region by radiographs should guide the practitioner to plan wide excisional margins. The mandible can be cut using an osteotome or oscillating saw, or initial resection lines can be made with a dental bur, nearly reaching the mandibular canal. With leverage, the segment can be cracked off the mandible, but it cannot be removed until the mandibular artery is identified and ligated both mesially and distally (23). Cheiloplasty is often helpful to catch saliva and keep the tongue from protruding to that side. In benign lesions, it is possible to perform a central resection involving removal of the dorsal section of the mandible to the extent of exposing the mandibular canal (23).

Caudal hemimandibulectomy is sometimes indicated for a lesion situated in the caudal portion of the body or extending into the ramus of the mandible. The caudal osteotomy may be made ventral to the temporomandibular joint, or a decision may be made to incorporate the joint itself by disarticulation with complete removal of the coronoid process (48). Incising the commissure is often necessary to provide adequate visualization for the procedure (50), followed by closure with cheiloplasty as described previously. More muscle resection is necessary to remove the caudal portions of the mandible, including the masseter muscle on the lateral side and the digastric on the medial side. Careful assistance with retraction of the soft tissues and ligation of the mandibular artery at the appropriate level are issues to be dealt with. With either of the above described segmental hemimandibulectomies, if the lesion is aggressive or malignant, sometimes total removal of the mandible should be considered.

The coronoid process itself can also be resected, if a lesion is present, with access through the zygomatic arch and masseter muscle. Large amounts of the coronoid process can be removed after a portion is dissected free from the temporal and pterygoid muscles. A combination of dorsal coronoid process resection with ventral zygomatic arch resection can be used to relieve "locking" of the coronoid process lateral to the zygomatic arch in cases with temporomandibular joint dysplasia (open-mouth locking) (52).

Total Hemimandibulectomy

With any lesion involving extensive portions of a mandible, complete removal is often the optimal procedure. Initial separation of the symphysis provides the rostral portion of the mandible as a "handle" to facilitate the procedure. Soft tissue incisions should be made to provide a good margin of normal tissue around the lesion itself, and attachments including the lingual tissues should be separated by soft dissection. Elevation of the muscles of mastication is included, with ligation of the mandibular artery as it enters the body of the mandible on its medial surface. Dissection should be careful in this area to avoid excessive damage to the vessel or nerves in the region. If the mandibular artery retracts into the pharyngeal tissues and hemorrhage continues, the carotid artery on that side can be ligated. The temporomandibular ligaments can be exposed by rotating the mandible and then excised, with the muscular attachments bluntly dissected free. Since the contralateral mandible will be deviated medially, the canine on that side can be shortened without exposing the pulp, undergo a crown amputation with vital pulpotomy/pulp capping, or be extracted. Cheiloplasty or commissuroplasty will certainly help keep the tongue from extruding. With any significant length of commissuroplasty, a tape muzzle must be left on initially to prevent the patient from opening the mouth too widely (23).

MAXILLECTOMY

Procedures involving the maxilla have certain considerations unique to the area. Generally, there will be some exposure of the nasal cavity, and most vasculature other than the infraorbital and palatal vessels cannot be specifically ligated, so control of hemorrhage must rely on applied pressure or even carotid artery ligation (23).

Premaxillectomy (Rostral Maxillectomy)

For lesions involving one or both sides of the incisive bone (premaxilla), resection may be confined to the incisive bone itself or may have to incorporate portions of the maxilla and palatine bones along with it. Soft tissue excisions at a reasonable distance from the lesion expose the area of bone that needs to be resected. Unless the lesion extends into the external lip, skin, or nares, these structures can be preserved for optimal esthetic effect. Particularly with a bilateral procedure, some portion of the nasal turbinates will be cut, generally at the same level as the palatal osteotomy, as far back as the canine or 1st premolar (53). Buccomucosal advancements or rotation flaps for closure can be fashioned unilaterally or bilaterally as the need dictates (51). Any trauma to the area caused by the mandibular canines should be considered and treated accordingly.

Partial Maxillectomy

For unilateral lesions in the central or caudal portions of the maxilla, partial maxillectomy can provide sufficient removal. In lesions located in caudal portions, additional consideration must be given concerning the infraorbital vessels (preservation or ligation) and the zygoma or orbit, part of which can be resected without significant problems occurring, if done with care (50). Incision and reflection of the soft tissue expose the regions of bone to be cut in an en-bloc resection. The incision is best done in a rounded, not rectangular, shape, to allow a more tapered area of excision that may be less likely to dehisce (23). If the lesion involves the area around the 4th premolar, it is often best to resect the molars as well to get a more favorable closure. To also maximize the potential gingival healing, electrocautery should not be used on the gingival margins themselves (23,50), and simple interrupted sutures may be reinforced with vertical mattress sutures to minimize tension at the suture line. When suturing involves the palate, small holes can even be predrilled into the bone to assist in retention of sutures (51).

TEMPOROMANDIBULAR JOINT SURGERY

For specific fractures involving the caudal portions of the mandible and the temporomandibular joint (TMJ), see the chapter on oral fracture repair (see Chapter 10). Other problems can exist in the region of the TMJ, particularly with dysplastic or degenerative processes. Luxation due to trauma, generally in a rostrodorsal direction, can often be replaced using a dowel in the mouth while closing the mouth and putting pressure on the mandible to return to a more caudal position (54). If it is luxated caudally, then rostral pressure is used to reduce the luxation.

The syndrome of dysplastic TMJs involving lateral deviation of the coronoid process as it is displaced lateral to the zygomatic arch, as well as its repair, has previously been discussed (55,56). Severe cases of dysplasia or degeneration, including ankylosis, can be treated with a condylectomy with reasonable success (57–59). These cases will often present with the inability to open the mouth, but this can also be seen in cases of false ankylosis, in which extracapsular pathology can limit TMJ movement, as was reported in one case involving squamous cell carcinoma of the ear canal that extended to the TMJ area (60). True ankylosis is due to the bony union across the joint surface (61,62), which is an intracapsular process.

With access through the masseter muscle at the caudoventral aspect of the zygomatic arch (23,63), the lateral ligament of the TMJ is identified and opened. Then the articular condyle is resected and removed, with optional removal of the articular disk. This will allow a more normal range of motion, although arthritic changes can later cause additional problems.

Fractures of the mandibular condyle can also be treated by excision of the fractured portion, as surgical reduction and stabilization are often difficult and can lead to eventual ankylosis. One conservative option in fractures with minimal displacement of the fracture fragments can be afforded by providing a limit in the range of motion during the healing process. With placement of a wire hook or bracket on teeth such as the upper canines and lower 3rd or 4th premolars bilaterally and attachment of elastic orthodontic chains, oral movements can be limited while proper occlusion is maintained; one cat responded favorably to this technique (64).

REFERENCES

1. Withrow SJ. Dental extraction as a probable cause of septicemia in the dog. *JAAHA* 1979;15:345.
2. Black AP, Crichlow AM, Saunders JR. Bacteremia during ultrasonic teeth cleaning and extraction in the dog. *JAAHA* 1980;16:611.
3. Small Animal Update: Dental Consent Forms Should Include Extraction Information. *American Veterinary Medical Association–Professional Liability Insurance Trust*; Vol. 15 (2):2.
4. Tholen MA, Hartsfield SM. Dental anesthesia. In: Tholen MA, ed. *Concepts in Veterinary Dentistry*. Edwardsville, KS: Veterinary Medical Publishing; 1983:23.
5. Anthony JMG. Intraoral regional anesthesia nerve blocks. *World Veterinary Dental Congress Proceedings*. Philadelphia, PA. Sept. 30–Oct. 2, 1994:56.
6. Smith MM. Lingual approach for surgical extraction of the mandibular canine tooth. *World Veterinary Dental Congress Proceedings*. Philadelphia, PA. Sept. 30–Oct. 2, 1994:54.
7. Southerland RM. Post extraction alveoloplasty of an abscessed upper fourth premolar. *J Vet Dent* 1989;6(4):16.
8. West-Hyde L. Applied clinical anatomy: Blood supply to the maxilla. *J Vet Dent* 1990;7(2):8.
9. Swan RH, Rapley JW, Schindler WG, Mathey WS. Hemisection of a molar tooth in a dog: An alternative to total extraction. *J Vet Dent* 1991;8(3):12.
10. Eisner E. Surgical extraction in two cases of impacted, abnormally developed teeth. *J Vet Dent* 1989;6(1):17.
11. Ramsey DT, Manfra Marretta S, Hamor RE, et al. Ophthalmic manifestations and complications of dental disease in dogs and cats. *JAAHA* 1996;32:215.
12. Manfra Marretta S. The common and uncommon clincial presentation and treatment of periodontal disease in the dog and cat. *Semin Vet Med Surg (Small Anim)* 1987;2:230.
13. Kapatkin AS, Manfra Marretta S, Schloss AJ. Problems associated with basic oral surgical procedures. *Probl Vet Med* 1990:85.
14. Hooley JR. Extraction of teeth. In: Levine, Norman, ed. *Current Treatment in Dental Practice*. Philadelphia: WB Saunders Co; 1986:312.
15. Lobprise HB, Wiggs RB. Dentigerous cyst in a dog. *J Vet Dent* 1992;9(1):13.
16. Field EA, Speechley JA, Jones DE. The removal of an impacted maxillary canine and associated dentigerous cyst in a chow. *J Small Anim Pract* 1982;23:159.
17. DuPont G. Crown amputation with intentional root retention for advanced feline resorptive lesions: A clinical study. *J Vet Dent* 1995;12(1):9.
18. Calhoun NR. Dry socket and other postoperative complications. *Dent Clin North Am* 1971;15:337.
19. Manfra Marretta S. The diagnosis and treatment of oronasal fistulas in three cats. *J Vet Dent* 1988;5(1):4.
20. Aller S. Techniques for the repair of oronasal fistulas. *Veterinary Dental Forum Proceedings*. Las Vegas, NV. Nov. 13–15, 1992:95.
21. Leighton RL. Neck and salivary glands: Soft tissue, tonsils, pharyn, larynx and trachea. In: Archibald J, ed. *Canine Surgery*. 2nd ed. Santa Barbara, CA: American Veterinary Publishers; 1974:329.
22. Fiorito DA. Multiple oral procedures performed on a dog with distemper myoclonus. *J Vet Dent* St. Louis, MO; Mosby:1993;10(2):312.
23. Harvey CE, Emily PP. Oral Surgery. In: *Small Animal Dentistry*. St.Louis, MO: Mosby-Year Book; 1993.
24. Howard DR, Davis DG, Merkley DF, et al. Mucoperiosteal flap technique for cleft palate repair in dogs. *JAVMA* 1974;165:352.
25. Manfra Marretta S, Grove TK, Grillo JF. Split-U palatal flap: A new technique for repair of caudal hard palate defect. *J Vet Dent* 1991;8(1):5.
26. Smith MM. Prosthodontic appliance for oronasal fistula in a cat. *World Veterinary Dental Congress Proceedings*. Philadelphia, PA. Sept. 30–Oct. 2, 1994:122.
27. Harvey CE. Palate defects in dogs and cats. *Compend Cont Educ* 1987;9:403.
28. Robertson JJ, Dean PW. Repair of a traumatically induced oronasal fistula in a cat with rostral tongue flap. *Vet Surg* 1987;16(2):164.
29. Clifford DH, Clark JJ. Mouth and teeth. In: Archibald J, ed. *Canine Surgery*. 2nd ed. Santa Barbara, CA: American Veterinary Publishers; 1974:291.
30. Legendre LFJ. Management and long-term effects of electrocution in a cat's mouth. *J Vet Dent* 1993;10(3):6.
31. Wiggs RB, Lobprise HB, de LaHunta A. Microglossia in three littermate puppies. *J Vet Dent* 1994;11(4):129.
32. Wolff A. Tongue tie in a dog? *Canine Pract* 1990;7(2):6.
33. Dent RStC. Operation for correction of lateral protrusion of the tongue in a dog. *Vet Rec* 1952;64:276.
34. Thivierge G. Granular stomatitis in dogs due to burdock. *Can Vet J* 1973;14(4):96.
35. Head KW. Tumors of the alimentary tract. In: Moulton JE, ed. *Tumors in Domestic Animals*. 3rd ed. Berkeley, CA: University of California Press; 1990:347.
36. Withrow SJ. Tumors of the gastrointestinal system: The oral cavity. In: Withrow SJ, MacEwen EG, eds. *Clinical Veterinary Oncology*. Philadelphia: JB Lippincott Co; 1989:177.
37. Hoyt RF, Withrow SJ. Oral malignancy in the dog. *JAAHA* 1984;20:83.
38. King GK. Common oral tumors: Their radiographic signs and treatment options. *Veterinary Dentistry Proceedings*. New Orleans, LA. Dec. 7–10, 1989:45.
39. Karbe E. Lateral neck cysts in the dog. *Am J Vet Res* 1965;26:717.

40. Karbe E, Nielsen SW. Branchial cyst in a dog. *JAVMA* 1965;147:637.
41. Spruell JSA, Archibald J. Neck and salivary glands: Glands of the head and neck. In: Archibald J, ed. *Canine Surgery*. 2nd ed. Santa Barbara, CA: American Veterinary Publishers; 1974:360.
42. Verstraete FJM. Surgical oncology for the veterinary dentist. *Vet Dent Proc* 1993:51.
43. Frankel M. Surgical removal of an odontoma in a dog. *J Vet Dent* 1988;5(4):21.
44. Levin J. Osteosarcoma of the rostral mandible in a geriatric beagle. *Am Vet Dent Proc* 1994:113.
45. Stokes G. Maxillectomy in a nine-year old cat. *J Vet Dent* 1988;5(3):14.
46. Harvey CE, Brown D, Cabell L. Attempted bilateral mandibular body replacement in a dog. *World Vet Dent Congress Proc.* 1994:108.
47. Bradley RL, MacEwen EG, Loar AS. Mandibular resection for removal of oral tumors in 30 dogs and 6 cats. *JAVMA* 1984;184:460.
48. Withrow SJ, Holmberg EL. Mandibulectomy in the treatment of oral cancer. *JAAHA* 1983;19:273.
49. Salisbury AK, Lantz GC. Long-term results of partial mandibulectomy for treatment of oral tumors in 30 dogs. *JAAHA* 1988;24:285.
50. Matthiesen DT, Manfra Marretta S. Results and complications associated with partial mandibulectomy and maxillectomy techniques. *Probl Vet Med Dent* 1990;2(1):248.
51. Manfra Marretta S, Matthiesen DT, Matus R, Patnaik A. Surgical management of oral neoplasia. In: Bojrab MJ, Tholen M, eds. *Small Animal Oral Medicine and Surgery*. Philadelphia: Lea & Febiger; 1990:96.
52. Lobprise HB, Wiggs RB. Modified surgical treatment of intermittent open-mouth mandibular locking in a cat. *J Vet Dent* 1992;9(1):8.
53. Withrow SJ, Nelson AW, Manley PA, Biggs DR. Premaxillectomy in the dog. *JAAHA* 1985;21:49.
54. Nelson DA, Green GW. Rack-and-pinion method of closed reduction of TMJ luxation in the dog. *Tex Vet Med J* August 1991:19.
55. Robins G, Grandage J. Temporomandibular joint dysplasia—open-mouth locking in the dog. *JAVMA* 1977;171:1072.
56. Lantz GC. Surgical correction of unusual temporomandibular joint conditions. *Compend Cont Educ Pract Vet* 1991;13:1570.
57. Lantz GC. Temporomandibular joint ankylosis: Surgical correction of three cases. *JAAHA* 1985;21:173.
58. Brady FA, Sanders B. Traumatic ankylosis of the temporomandibular joint. *Clin Otolaryngol* 1978;3:127.
59. Hatzifoliadis D. Surgical treatment of temporomandibular joint ankylosis. *Int Dent J* 1979;29:269.
60. Anderson MA, Orsini PG, Harvey CE. Temporomandibular ankylosis: Treatment by unilateral condylectomy in two dogs and two cats. *J Vet Dent* 1996;13(1):23.
61. Rowe NL. Ankylosis of the temporomandibular joint. *J R Coll Surg Edinb* 1982;27:67.
62. Miller GA, Page L, Griffith CR. Temporomandibular joint ankylosis: Review of the literature and report of two cases of bilateral involvement. *J Oral Surg* 1975;33:792.
63. Eisner ER. Bilateral mandibular condylectomy in a cat. *J Vet Dent* 1995;12(1):23.
64. Taylor EM. Repair of temporomandibular joint fractures in the cat. *World Vet Dent Cong Proc* 1995:131.

10

Oral Fracture Repair

Robert B. Wiggs and Heidi B. Lobprise

Orthopedic surgery of the oral cavity has many similarities to that of bones in the remainder of the body, but a substantial number of dissimilarities as well. Specific considerations in the area include occasional difficulties in access, lack of complete sterility, variations in fixation possibilities, retention of proper occlusion, and the need for immediate return to a functional state. Often other situations coexist with fractured jaws, whether they be concurrent periodontal disease, metabolic diseases, or other traumatic injuries both in the oral cavity and the rest of the patient. All factors of extent of injury, viability of the bone structure, periodontal status, and overall body condition should guide the practitioner in selecting the appropriate treatment plan.

ASSESSMENT

While some injuries may be readily apparent due to the animal's discomfort and the degree of observable swelling, complete evaluation is generally not possible until some degree of sedation or anesthesia can be safely utilized. Certainly, the patient must be stable enough to withstand whatever level of anesthesia is needed; therefore, any extensive oral examination or therapy may need to be strategically postponed.

The location and extent of the fracture should be determined, from simple and nondisplaced to comminuted or compound. Once the primary lesion is evaluated, the rest of the oral cavity should be thoroughly assessed to detect any additional fractures, broken teeth, soft tissue injury, or hemorrhage. Minor injuries may initially be overlooked, but slightly displaced teeth or torn mucosal surfaces may alert the practitioner to a potential problem. Mandibular symphyseal or temporomandibular joint injuries may often be present but are less obvious. Radiographs are essential for complete diagnosis, particularly in caudal lesions. While intraoral films can provide excellent views of most of the areas associated with dentition, the temporomandibular joint regions are sometimes more challenging to isolate. Ventrodorsal or oblique lateral extraoral films typically provide the best information (1,2).

Fractures of the mandible are more common than those of the maxilla and generally will be more obvious due to the greater mobility. A mandibular fracture may result in a dropped-jaw appearance or result in a malocclusion. Maxillary fractures may be indicated by swelling, epistaxis, and pain, but they are less likely to have the degree of deviation observed in many fractures of the lower jaw, except for some rostral fractures.

Exposure for some dental orthopedic work can at times be challenging, particularly in the caudal oral cavity. Since proper occlusion must be maintained during reduction of the fracture, careful consideration to potential tooth alignment must be made. A pharyngostomy tube may be placed, exiting at the level of the caudal pharynx (3,4).

While there may be differing opinions as to which teeth to salvage when they are associated with a mandibular fracture line, recent reviews of the literature help delineate treatment options (5,6) (Fig. 1). Previous recommendations to extract all teeth in the line of mandibular fractures were due in part to the incidence of osteomyelitis before the introduction of antibiotics (7). A tooth that is relatively stable despite the effects of the fracture can itself contribute to the ultimate stability of the fracture (8,9), as well as facilitating alignment in correct occlusion (10). If a tooth was compromised before the fracture, such as with periodontal or endodontal disease, then extraction would be indicated in most cases, particularly if less than 20% of bone support remains (4). If a particular tooth has just one root that is extensively affected by periodontal disease, tooth or root resection can be performed to salvage the healthy portion of the tooth (11) (see Chapter 12).

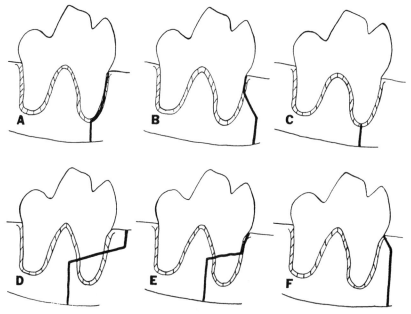

FIG. 1. Recommendations for teeth in the line of mandibular fractures. **(A)** The fracture line creates a communication between the apical area and the oral cavity. Treatment is hemisection or extraction. **(B)** The fracture line involves the coronal one-third of the root. Treatment is to retain tooth and reevaluate in 6 months for periodontal problems. **(C)** The fracture line damages the vascular supply to the root. Treatment is to retain tooth and reevaluate in 6 months for endodontic problems. **(D)** The fracture line is through the bone surrounding the root but not through the root itself. This damages the periapical circulation to the root. Treatment is to retain tooth and reevaluate in 6 months for endodontic problems. **(E)** The fracture line is through the bone surrounding the root but not through the root itself. This fracture damages the peripheral circulation to the root and the coronal portion of the periodontal ligament. Treatment is to retain tooth and reevaluate in 6 months for endodontic and periodontic problems. **(F)** The fracture line does not damage the circulation to the root. Treatment is to retain tooth. (Reproduced from ref. 5, with permission.)

Those teeth having no other problems other than being in the line of the fracture can often be retained, with subsequent therapy for any complications the fracture may cause. If the line of fracture involves any damage to the periapical circulation, the tooth should be reevaluated in 6 months to see whether endodontic therapy is required. The same applies with any fracture lines that may infringe on the periodontal ligament's integrity. In a human study, the type of fracture that most frequently contributed to tooth morbidity involved a fracture line that followed the root surface from the gingival margin to the apical region, affecting both periodontal and endodontic integrity (8).

Another oral injury that involves the bony alveolus but has a more profound effect on the tooth itself is avulsion (see Chapter 12). Key factors in the success of reimplanting avulsed teeth include minimizing the amount of time the tooth is out of the oral cavity, proper handling (it can be stored in cool fresh milk until surgery), and adequate treatment of the endodontic compromise at around 2 weeks after reimplantation.

Depending on the extent of the injury with avulsion, complete soft tissue suturing can occasionally provide enough stabilization, particularly if most of the alveolus is intact and the tooth can be well implanted. With other fractures in the oral cavity with minimal displacement and minimal stability problems, soft tissue suturing will at times be sufficient.

TREATMENT PLANNING

In this chapter, the different types of fractures that may be encountered will be addressed, with brief discussions of recommended treatments. The specific treatments themselves will be covered later in the chapter. A classification of mandibular body fractures has been developed, based on the location of the lesion (12) (Table 1).

Rostral Mandibular Fractures—Region A

The most common rostral mandibular fracture typically involves the symphyseal region, where the most common oral fracture in the cat may be seen. The symphysis in the dog and cat differs from that of humans in that the two sides of the mandible in humans physically fuse together, whereas in the dog and cat the symphysis remains a fibrous union. This union can at times be very slightly mobile yet normal, but any significant laxity or associated deviation in this region necessitates its stabilization. The degree of trauma in this region will determine the extent of treatment necessary (12) (Table 2). In type I injuries, there will be separation with no break in the soft tissues, while type II injuries have soft tissue disruption. A type III lesion will also have com-

TABLE 1. *Mandibular body fractures classification*

Region	Area of mandible affected
A	Symphysis to canine teeth
B	From canine to 2nd premolar
C	From 2nd premolar to 1st molar
D	From 1st molar to the angle of the manible
E	Angle of the mandible
F	Coronoid process
G	Condylar process

(Reproduced from ref. 12.)

TABLE 2. *Classification of mandibular symphyseal injury*

Type	Injury
I	Separation with no break in soft tissues
II	Separation with break in soft tissues
III	Separation with break in soft tissues and comminution of bone; broken teeth not unusual

(Reproduced from ref. 12.)

minution of the bone fragments, often together with broken teeth. If there are no other areas of instability in the oral cavity, this problem has generally been treated with a simple circummandibular or encircling wire to keep the two mandibular halves together, which usually allows healing but not always good reestablishment of the occlusal alignment. Interdental wiring, as with Stout's or Essig's technique, can ordinarily provide both stabilization and proper realignment of the teeth. With severely comminuted fractures of the region, the mouth can be held in proper occlusion yet slightly open with a composite bridge bonded between the upper and lower canines on each side (13). If the patient is not able to lap up liquid food with this device, a feeding tube must be placed. Once sufficient healing has taken place, the splint can be removed.

Mandibular Body Fracture—Regions B,C, and D

Fractures of the body of the mandible are the most frequent oral fractures seen in the dog (13). A unilateral fracture may cause the jaw to be deviated toward the side of the injury, as with a caudoventral luxation of the temporomandibular joint, while rostroventral luxation of the temporomandibular joint will cause deviation away from the injured side (10). With minimal displacement, particularly with a unilateral defect and intact symphysis, a conservative approach with a gauze or tape muzzle may be sufficient. One way to determine the feasibility of using a muzzle would be to see whether the mouth closes easily, while maintaining proper occlusion (13). With the mandible, however, there are a few factors that determine which treatment is best, particularly consideration of the biomechanical effects that the muscles of mastication have on the mandible and any fracture segments. The bulk of the muscles—the masseter, temporal, and pterygoid—works to swing the mandible dorsally, as in closing the mouth, with their insertion on the caudal end of the body of the mandible (13). This movement can lift the caudal mandible in a rostrodorsal direction (14). The digastric muscle works in opposition to these muscles, tending to pull the rostral portion of the mandible caudoventrally, as in opening the mouth.

Fracture biomechanics indicate that the tension side of the mandible is the dorsal or alveolar border of the mandible, where the teeth are (15). Stabilization on this border will provide a natural compressive force on the ventral surface. This can be provided with methods such as interdental wires and splints. Although placement of a plate and screw apparatus has been used, extreme care to avoid important structures is required and difficult.

A unique situation, sometimes seen in cats that have fallen and landed on their chins, is the impacted fracture of the mandible rostral to the 2nd premolar, which is often bilateral (10). Pinning each rostral segment to its caudal counterpart can be accomplished, but great care must be taken not to injure any vital structures.

Favorable/Unfavorable

Biomechanical muscular forces have a particular influence on the type of stabilization needed for fractures in the region. If the fracture line is perpendicular to the long axis of the mandible, some dorsal distraction may occur (14). With a fracture line that runs caudodorsally, the forces tend to keep the segments compressed together, allowing it to be classified as a *favorable fracture* (Fig. 2A). While some favorable fractures can be adequately treated with conservative methods such as a tape muzzle, a single interosseous wire placed perpendicular to the fracture line often provides sufficient reduction and resistance to displacement forces. This is often true when the fracture is unilateral, there is no symphyseal mobility, and the intact opposite mandible provides a good basis for both reduction and stability (10).

When the fracture line runs in a caudoventral direction, however, the larger muscles of mastication exert force upward on the distal segment, and the digastric muscle tends to pull the rostral segment down and caudally, with subsequent displacement; this is classi-

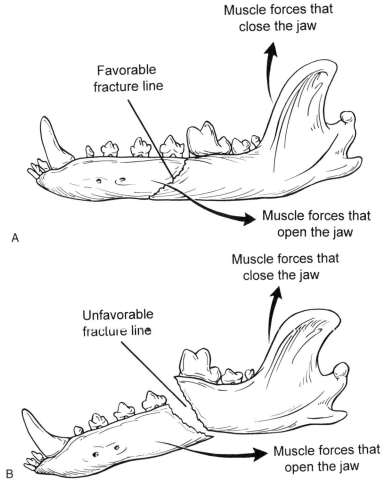

FIG. 2. **(A)** Favorable mandibular fracture. **(B)** Unfavorable mandibular fracture.

fied as an *unfavorable fracture* (see Fig. 2B). Two intraosseous wires can be placed, one dorsally and one ventrally, or just one ventrally with acrylic splint stabilization to compensate for any dorsal gap should be sufficient (13). Alternately, two wires may be placed with a common placement site in the rostral segment and two sites in the distal segment to approximate a perpendicular relationship of the two wires. This triangular method helps to provide additional stabilization against the muscular forces.

Acrylic splints may be used alone or in combination with wire placement, either as additional stabilization for the acrylic incorporated into the material or with acrylic added to an interdental-wiring technique. Interarcade wiring or splinting, involving immobilization of the mouth in partial occlusion to prevent excessive movement while still allowing some ability to drink and eat, is another less invasive method of fracture repair. Incorporating wires into acrylic in edentulous areas can be one means of fixation of pathologic fractures due to periodontal disease at the lower 1st molars.

In more severe fractures, such as comminuted fractures, that have gaps or nonviable tissues, more complicated means of fixation are often necessary. While some axial skeletal fixation means, such as intramedullary pinning, plating, and screws, do not translate well to the oral cavity, some forms of external fixation have been successfully employed (14,16). The combination of using Kirschner wires or Steinmann pins on either side of the fracture site, and even bilaterally, with an acrylic-filled tube to engage the pin ends can provide immediate stabilization. Areas of substantial bone loss due either to fragmentation or necrosis can be held in position with this method to allow the defect to eventually fill in, though this can be a long-term solution, lasting several months if the defect is more than 4–6 cm. Alternately, grafts of cancellous bone chips or even ribs can be used to facilitate bone regrowth (13). If the area is grossly contaminated, the optimum method may be to delay implantation until the epithelial surfaces have healed and then place the material through a sterile, ventral approach (10).

In areas that experience nonunion, the situation may be manageable as a fibrous union if the fracture was unilateral with a stable opposite mandible. Bilateral lesions, particularly those instigated by severe periodontal disease, are often nearly impossible to manage, and while long-term mouth-closure methods (eg, muzzle, interarcade fixation) may eventually provide a functional bite, the management and possible complications are often challenging (14).

Fractures of the Vertical Ramus—Regions E and F

Vertical ramus fractures are less common than fractures of the mandibular body or symphysis (17). In the far caudal region of the mandibular body and even up in the ramus, internal fixation may not be needed if displacement is minimal due to the supportive effect of the surrounding musculature (14). Unilateral fractures dorsal to the condylar process may respond well to a tape muzzle over a 2–3-week period, but fractures below that level may take additional time, up to 4–5 weeks. If the fracture is unstable, the flatter bones, without associated teeth, make it somewhat amenable to plate fixation, but this also has the disadvantage of needing to deal with the substantial muscle masses. Future problems may occur with larger callus formation, if there is any interference with normal oral movements (9). If there is significant malocclusion associated with such a fracture, the temporomandibular joints should be closely examined for any signs of concurrent fracture or fracture/luxation (13).

Fractures of the Temporomandibular Joint—Region F

As with other portion of the vertical ramus, fractures in this region are uncommon (18). If any structures of the temporomandibular joint are affected, complete evaluation with radiographs is necessary to assist in treatment planning. Often these lesions are accompanied by fractures elsewhere in the mandible (19). Luxations of the region can often be reduced (see Chapter 9), while fractures, particularly of the condylar process may require attention. With simple, nondisplaced fractures, conservative therapy with reduction in motion may suffice, particularly if additional fracture sites are reduced and stabilized (19). In addition to tape muzzles and rigid interarcade fixation, another method for limiting movement has been described, involving an orthodontic device (wire hook or bracket) and elastic power-chain installation (20). Any injuries in the area should be monitored carefully in the future, because degenerative or arthritic changes in the joint area can be very painful and can eventually limit effective use (13). In such cases, a condylectomy may have to be performed to relieve the discomfort and provide mobility for the joint (see Chapter 9).

Fractures of the Maxilla

Maxillary fractures are less common than mandibular lesions and may be more difficult to detect and evaluate fully. Epistaxis, swelling, discomfort, and malocclusion may be indications of damage, but displacement can at times be minimal. If such is the case and the occlusion is still correct, little may need to be done. Occasionally, the simple act of suturing any soft tissue defects after digital realignment provides sufficient stabilization (10,13), although some cases benefit from other conservative methods such as tape muzzles or acrylic splints with or without interdental wiring. In more severe cases of comminuted fractures, stabilization may be provided by using Stout's multiple loop interdental wiring technique on both the maxillary and mandibular incisors and then securing the upper and lower loops together to wire the mouth shut (21). Feeding by pharyngostomy tube will be required until a stable callus is formed at around 3 weeks after surgery.

TREATMENT MODALITIES

Tape Muzzle

The conservative use of a tape muzzle has many applications in oral fracture repair (22,23). It is helpful as a first aid treatment with any oral fracture that results in significant displacement to help protect the segments and avoid any further damage (24). In unilateral mandibular fractures or maxillary fractures with minimal displacement, it is often the only modality needed to provide sufficient stabilization (18,25). The oral cavity, with its rich blood supply, does not need complete rigid fixation for adequate healing (16), although the callus formation will be larger in areas that are not totally immobilized. Due to the muscular support afforded in fractures of the mandibular ramus, a tape muzzle may provide additional support for sufficient healing (25); this is also the case in minimally displaced condylar process fractures. Muzzles may also be used as an adjunctive treatment (25).

In addition to fractures with minimal damage, a tape muzzle may be used when other methods of fixation are not possible, as in bilateral pathologic fracture of the mandibles due to severe periodontal disease. Complete union is often not likely, even with attempted osseous regeneration, but if sufficient stability can be afforded initially, a fibrous union may result.

The tape muzzle should be placed with the canines in correct occlusion with allowance of a gap of 0.5–1.0 cm (up to 1.5 cm) in the incisors to permit lapping of water and soft food. The first layer of tape is placed around the muzzle with the adhesive side out, and a second layer around it, with the two adhesive sides touching each other. The head strap is fashioned in a similar fashion, extending from the tape around the nose, back behind the ears, and to the other side to keep the muzzle held comfortably in place. Some contraindications for a muzzle include a brachycephalic head (23) and any problems with vomiting, where the material can be retained in the mouth and aspirated. A patient with respiratory distress would not be a good candidate for a muzzle, which also does not allow for panting if the animal gets overheated (14). Long-term use of a tape muzzle can also cause a significant dermatitis problem (25).

There are other means of limiting oral movements while maintaining occlusion, such as *interarcade wiring* (12,26,27). While this method involving placing circumferential wires around both the maxilla and mandible, or transosseous placement of wires or screws with stabilization between the two arcades (26), is invasive, other means are possible. With the mouth held in proper occlusion and a slight space between the incisors, the canines can be joined together with a composite bridge, with or without pin placement in each tooth. As with the tape muzzle, the same factors apply concerning respiratory distress or vomiting.

Wiring Techniques

Wire has the advantage of being a simple, inexpensive, and versatile tool for repair of osseous fractures in the oral cavity. Wire is useful not only in reducing fractures but also, when used properly, in attaining an excellent realignment of the dentition. Wiring is used in four basic techniques: *osseous*, *interdental*, *adjunct*, and *interarcade*.

Osseous Wiring

Osseous wiring places wire in direct contact with bone to provide direct reduction and support to portions of a bony fracture. This technique can be performed using open or closed surgical approaches, but the visualization attained by open techniques permits a more accurate assessment and realignment of the fractured segments. An open approach also permits the possible visualization of potential complications from hidden foreign bodies and loose bone fragments. The primary function of osseous wiring is to reduce fractures and prevent their displacement by the passive function of the masticatory muscles. However, by itself, osseous wiring cannot be relied on to provide stable fixation if the jaw is to be functional—nonimmobilized—during the initial healing period. If this is the case, the osseous wiring should be augmented by interdental wiring or some additional form of splinting. The first rule of osseous wiring is to do no harm and try to avoid injury to other organs within the jaws such as the mandibular canal, the roots, and the periodontal ligament. The second rule is to always endeavor to reestablish normal functional occlusion. In the osseous category, there are three fundamental forms of wiring: circumferential, transosseous (interfragmentary), and transcircumferential.

In *circumferential wiring*, the wire is typically placed by using a suitable shape and size of suture needle or a large-gauge injection needle to guide its placement. There are many variations of needle placement and direction of wire movement according to the location used: symphysis or mandibular body. Described here is a procedure for treatment of a region A symphyseal fracture.

With use of a large-bore needle, the wire can initially be placed through the skin from the midline under the symphysis into the buccal vestibule behind the canine tooth. It is then passed through the needle bore into the oral cavity (Fig. 3A), and the needle is retracted back through the soft tissue. The needle is then placed in the same way into the opposite buccal vestibule behind the canine tooth, and the lead wire in the oral cavity is passed behind the canine teeth and placed into the needle bore (see Fig. 3B). The needle

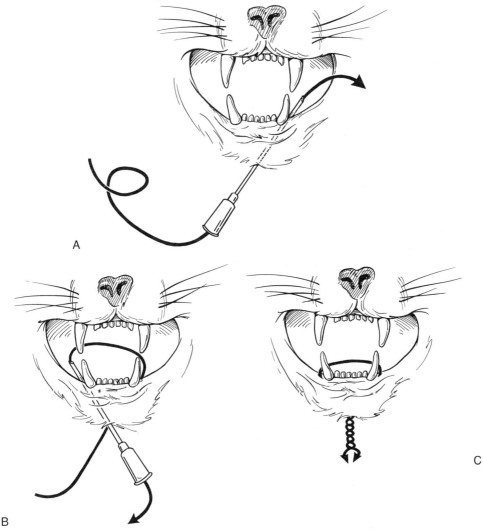

FIG. 3. Circumferential wiring to stabilize symphyseal separation. **(A)** Initial passage of wire through the needle. **(B)** Exit of wire through the needle. **(C)** Tightening of wires.

and wire are then retracted through the soft tissue and out under the mandible. The needle is removed, and the opposite ends of the wire twisted together and tightened to appose the two halves of the mandible (Fig. 3C). In cases involving excessive force or more extensive osseous damage, the mandibular canines can deviate medially, contributing to a malocclusion when the mouth is closed. If such is the case, an additional wire can be used, passed around the canine teeth and under the mandible subcutaneously in a figure-8 interdental configuration, or an acrylic splint may be placed (13).

Circumferential wires can also be used in edentulous areas, where interdental wiring or acrylic splints are not as useful (28). The wire itself can also be incorporated in the acrylic. An alternate method of wire placement involves a lateral incision and use of specific instrumentation, the O'Donoghue Suture Passer® (Richards Manufacturing, Memphis, Tennessee) (29).

In *transosseous (interfragmentary) wiring*, 20–28 gauge stainless steel wire (typically 24-gauge) is used. A large-gauge (14–20 gauge) heavy-duty injection needle and a No.4 to No.6 surgical length ball bur can be used for anchorage-hole placement. During placement of the anchorage holes through the bone, every effort should be made to avoid injury to the roots and periodontal ligament of the teeth and the mandibular canal. When an open technique is used, soft tissue is seldom a problem, but in closed placement, a small cut with a No.11 blade will reduce soft tissue tangling with the bur. In some cases, the large-bore needle can actually be passed through the bone with some twisting manipulations, but the surgical bur is typically faster. However, even the surgical length burs will not always pass entirely thought some mandibles. This is circumvented by placing the guide hole with the bur and then finishing the hole either with the large-bore injection needle or an intramedullary pin of similar size.

For fractures of the body of the mandible, the placement and number of anchorage holes is primarily dependent on the adjacent structures and the type of fracture. Most body fractures are vertically oblique in orientation, resulting in either a favorable or unfavorable type of fracture line. With favorable fractures that reduce well, a single horizontal transosseous wire may provide the needed fixation (Fig. 4). However, with an unfavorable fracture line, additional anchorage is customarily required if transosseous wiring is to be used (Fig. 5). A combination of horizontal and vertical transosseous wires in a triangular configuration with three anchorage holes and two wires may provide the

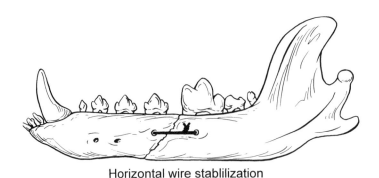

Horizontal wire stablilization
of favorable fracture

FIG. 4. Single horizontal transosseous wire to stabilize a favorable fracture.

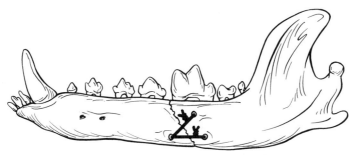

Triangular configuration pattern for
wiring an unfavorable fracture

FIG. 5. Additional anchor with double transosseous wire in a triangular configuration to stabilize an unfavorable fracture.

required stabilization. Two of the holes are placed vertically or at an oblique angle to one another in the caudal segment, and one is placed in the rostral segment. Both wires will make use of the single anchorage hole in the rostral segment. The first wire is placed horizontally and the second obliquely. The wires should be tightened to realign the segment, while the needed retraction is provided to close the fracture line. In some cases, an unfavorable fracture will be stabilized with the combination of a horizontal transosseous wire and interdental wiring.

Transcircumferential wiring is a single-wire technique that involves both a transosseous anchorage and circumferential wiring around the bone (Fig. 6). It is used most commonly for unfavorable body fractures. The transosseous anchorage hole is placed 3–4 mm from the alveolar crest over the fracture site, possibly even between two roots of a tooth. The wire is past through the anchorage hole and then run circumferentially under the mandible with the aid of needles. The lead ends are twisted together and tightened. Interdental wiring performed in combination with transcircumferential wiring provides greater stability for these fractures.

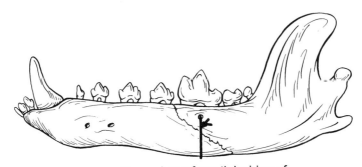

Transcircumferential wiring of
an unfavorable fracture

FIG. 6. Transcircumferential wire technique involving both a transosseous anchorage and circumferential wiring around the mandible.

Interdental Wiring

Interdental wiring is the placement of wires around adjacent teeth to provide reduction and support to a bony fracture that extends between the teeth. Interdental wiring is one technique that can be used for closed fracture repair (30). However, it is used in both closed and open techniques and in adjunct procedures, in which a combination of acrylics, composites, or other devices may be used in association with the wire to provide the needed support once reduction is accomplished. The size of wire used (24–30 gauge) is dictated by the size of the oral cavity and the teeth involved; however, 26-gauge stainless steel orthopedic wire is the most common size used (31). Most wire comes dead soft in rolls. The natural curling of such wire should be corrected by stretching segments of wire to be used with two forceps. Many types of wire handling and twisting instruments are available for use with wire, but needle holders can be used in most cases.

Wires can usually be placed below the cervical bulge of the tooth either with instrument pressure or with the aid of 18–20-gauge needles. A W3 or cord-packing instrument can often assist in holding the wire below the bulge during the tightening phase. Alternatively, a needle can be placed through the gingiva below the bulge to expedite passage of the wire at the proper depth. In most healthy animals, this will cause a transitory inflammation that resolves when the wire is removed. On occasion, notching a tooth with a vertical groove may be required to maintain the wire in either the correct position or at a preferred height above the gingiva. Wire placed at this level will commonly cause gingival irritation. Prevention of infection can generally be accomplished by the routine use of oral hygiene solutions, until the wires are removed, at which time healing is typically rapid and complete. However, if preexisting periodontal disease is present, wire at the gingival level must be inspected routinely, and oral hygiene of the highest caliber must be done. If meticulous care cannot be provided, then other forms of support should be considered. A simple alternative is the placement of the wires higher on the tooth with the assistance of composite bonding, notching of the tooth, or both.

Four basic types of interdental wiring are most commonly used: the Ivy loop, Stout's multiple loop, Essig's, and Risdon's techniques. The Ivy loop and Stout's multiple loop techniques incorporate a single-wire technique, while Essig's and Risdon's techniques require two wires. Placement of these patterns does take some practice, but once the techniques are mastered, they become invaluable in fracture reduction. If the twisted wire ends or any of the loops are irritating to the soft tissues, they can be padded by covering them with a small amount of rubber-base impression material.

The *Ivy loop wiring technique* is most commonly used for reducing simple fractures between two teeth and securing acrylic appliances, as well as for anchorage for other attachments. It involves fastening the two teeth together with a single ligating wire (Fig.7). The wire is folded in half, and an instrument is placed between the two ends at the fold. The wire is then twisted around the instrument to form a loop. The two loose ends are passed through the interdental space between the two teeth to be ligated together to the lingual surface. One end goes around each tooth and back around to the facial side. The distal lead is then passed through the loop and then twisted together with the other lead approximately at the mesiofacial line angle of the mesial tooth. The loop is then lightly tightened over the lead wire that passed through it. The leads and loop are each delicately tightened until the desired tension develops. A slight apical tension on the leads will help keep the wire in place below the cervical bulge. Care must be taken not to overtighten the wire, or it will fatigue and break and the process will have to be repeated. If the Ivy loop is to act as an anchorage for an acrylic appliance on the lingual surface,

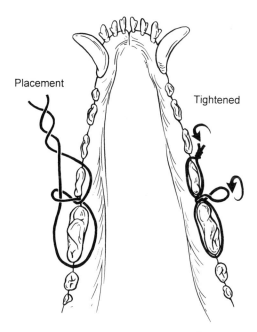

Ivy loop wiring technique

FIG. 7. Ivy loop wiring technique.

loops may need to be created with the leads before they are passed back around to the facial surface. While being tightened, the leads or loops should be grasped as near the tooth or bone as is reasonable to obtain the required reduction of the fracture. The loop and twisted ends can be tucked interdentally if small enough or pressed tightly against the tooth if needed.

Stout's multiple loop wiring technique is another single-wire method, but it incorporates more than just two adjacent teeth. It is in fact a simple continuation of the Ivy loop technique. It is used in the same applications as the Ivy loop but provides greater stability and strength.

The lead ends in Stout's technique are known as the static wire, and the working wire (Fig. 8). The *working wire* is the lead end that is passed back and forth through the interproximal spaces and forms the tightening loops. The *static wire* is the lead that lays against the tooth and is fixed in place by the loops of the working-wire lead. It should be kept in mind that the working lead and static lead are simply opposite ends of the same single piece of wire.

Classically, in Stout's method, the wire loops are placed on the facial surfaces. However, these can be placed on the lingual surface when needed for anchorage or other support. The following description is based on the classic arrangement with loops on the facial surface, but the opposite effect can be obtained by simply reversing the sides on which the leads are used.

The wire is prestretched to remove any kinks or laxity in it. It is taken to the distal surface of the distal most tooth to be included in the wiring. The static lead is brought mesially or rostrally along the facial surface of the teeth near the gingival margin or the desired height. The working lead is brought mesially along the lingual surfaces of the teeth and is passed through the interproximal space between each tooth. The working lead is then passed around the static wire and back through the interproximal space to

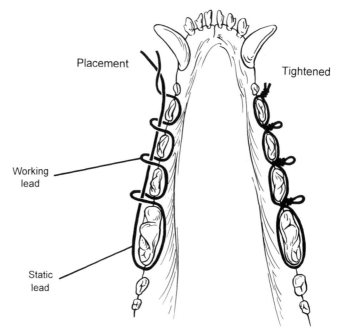

Stout's multiple loop wiring technique

FIG. 8. Stout's multiple loop wiring technique.

the lingual surface. Enough working wire should be left on the facial surface to form the needed tightening loops. The process is continued up the dental arch until all of the desired adjacent teeth have been incorporated, usually at least two teeth on either side of the fracture if possible. The working- and static-lead ends of the wire are then twisted together. The tightening loops should now each be lightly and evenly tightened. Once all have been evenly snugged, the loops and twisted ends can be tightened to the desired reduction point. Care should be taken to avoid overtightening, or the wire may fatigue and break.

Essig's wiring method, sometimes called Esser's (32), is most commonly used to reduce fractures and to stabilize incisor teeth loosened from trauma. It involves a primary wire and multiple secondary wires (Fig. 9). The *primary wire* is the master wire that is passed around all of the teeth to be incorporated in the support, usually the incisors but sometimes the canines as well, and the ends are lightly twisted together. The *secondary wires* are short segments passed interdentally through the interproximal spaces, between each adjacent tooth in the wiring pattern, from the facial surface to the lingual surface and back facially, circling both the lingual and facial strands of the primary wire. Each secondary wire is lightly tightened to hold it in place until all of the secondary wires are placed. The wires are then tightened evenly to the desired tension.

Risdon's wiring technique is used when greater strength of reduction is required, as in some rostral and symphyseal fractures of the mandible. In this technique, there are two sets of primary wires, a left and a right (Fig. 10). In addition, there will be numerous secondary wires. The primary wire is passed distally around the *anchorage tooth* bilaterally, which is typically the mandibular carnassial tooth if healthy. The anchorage tooth should

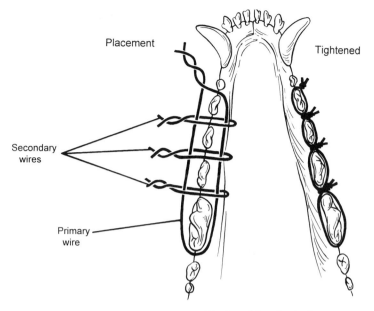

Essig wiring technique

FIG. 9. Essig's wiring technique.

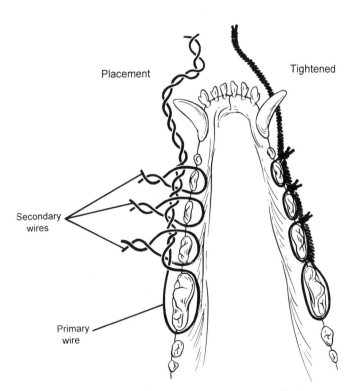

Risdon wiring technique

FIG. 10. Risdon's wiring technique.

be healthy, have a substantial root surface, and be supported in an adequate degree of solid bone. The primary wire is looped around the tooth below the cervical bulge, with the ends meeting at the mesiobuccal-line angle, leaving two long leads of approximately equal length. The two leads are then twisted together in a long braid that reaches past the midpoint of the mandibular symphysis. The secondary wires are looped around the teeth mesial to the anchorage tooth, with one end looped over and one under the primary wire. The ends of the secondary wires should then be twisted together over the primary braided wire. This is repeated on as many teeth as needed to support and stabilize the primary braided wire and to align the incisors properly.

Adjunct Wiring

Adjunct wiring describes a wiring technique used as an adjunct to some other form of stabilization, such as acrylic or composite splints (33), or to some form of orthodontic appliance (34).

Interarcade Wiring or Fixation

The process of interarcade wiring or fixation was briefly discussed under tape muzzle, because the final effect is similar. Options involving composite splinting of the canine teeth or the placing of orthodontic wires or brackets with elastic power chains can provide reasonable stabilization without the invasiveness of wiring. While placement of wires bilaterally with exposure of the furcations of the upper 4th premolars and 1st molars can certainly provide a solid anchor, the potential damage is a distinct disadvantage. A form of circumferential wiring can also be used around both the maxilla and mandible to stabilize the occlusion.

Acrylic Splints

The growing popularity of the use of acrylics in the oral cavity is founded in a variety of reasons, including its being noninvasive, versatile, relatively inexpensive and easy (16). The acrylic can be formed either directly in the oral cavity or on a model in an indirect fashion, and then attached in an appropriate manner. Wires may be used within the acrylic to provide additional strength, or they may be incorporated around other structures such as teeth to enhance retention of the appliance.

Some inherent problems with acrylics include the need for good ventilation, the possibility of soft tissue irritation by rough acrylic edges, and enhanced retention of food particles and debris, which may contribute to a stomatitis (see the discussion of acrylics in Chapter 2). In order to minimize problems, the acrylic edges should be smoothed and well formed to the contours of the oral cavity, the owner should rinse the splint regularly, and any problems should be assessed as they occur. Once the splint is removed, any inflammation usually subsides within a short time.

The fact that an acrylic splint generally incorporates the teeth associated with a fracture, as it is applied to the tension band side, is optimum. With the occlusal forces also in mind, forming the bulk of a mandibular splint on the lingual surface and a maxillary splint on the buccal surface will minimize any occlusal interference by the opposing dentition (16).

Direct Technique 23,28

While many forms of acrylic will generate some heat during the curing phase, excessive thermal damage can be avoided if the acrylic is used in a salt and pepper technique with small amounts of liquid and powder at a time. Use of a cold-curing acrylic or light-cured product will also circumvent this problem. The oral tissues should be prepared prior to acrylic placement by first minimizing any open wound areas. The gingival tissue can be covered by a protective layer of petroleum jelly, and a form using box wax or modeling clay can be made to guide the shape. The teeth to be incorporated into the splint should be cleaned, polished with a flour pumice, and acid-etched. As the fracture is then held in a reduced position, small amounts of powder are placed, followed by small amounts of the liquid, and the sequence is repeated until the desired shape and thickness is attained (15). The thickness of the acrylic should be approximately 1.5–2.0 mm (23,28). A wire may be placed, after the initial layer of acrylic is set, by conforming it to the arcade to be stabilized or by placing a U-shaped piece of wire around teeth incorporated in the splint with the free ends embedded in the acrylic. Any edges of the splint should be rounded and smoothed to avoid excessive soft tissue trauma. The splint can be trimmed with acrylic burs to provide a more accurate fit, with particular attention to the occlusion. Regular examination and client monitoring are essential to flush any debris from the edges.

Indirect Technique

The potential problems of a hyperthermic reaction occurring with a direct application of any acrylic splint can be avoided by making the splint in an indirect method on a stone model (23,28,36). This type of technique does require the additional steps of taking impressions, making a model, forming the splint, and then applying it to the fracture site. Care must be taken to treat the model with a separating agent, such as a foil substitute material (see Chapter 2), to prevent the acrylic from bonding to the model while it is being applied. Many of the same principles are relevant as for direct splints, such as thickness, positioning, maintaining occlusion, and using wires at times to enhance retention. Retaining the indirect splint in the oral cavity may require the placement of wiring (37), for example, around the maxilla or mandible and then inserted through holes in the splint and secured (15). An indirect splint must be secured well, because excessive mobility can interfere with fracture healing.

Internal Fixation

With few exceptions, the use of internal fixators such as intramedullary pins, plates, and screws do not lend themselves to easy application in the oral cavity (38). Although intramedullary pin placement has been attempted, the mandibular canal is not a good site for it due to the canal's curvature and function in protecting the mandibular artery, vein, and nerves. Placement of a pin down the canal can lead to disruption of the reduction, occlusal misalignment, and the loss of important nerves and vessels within it (10,39). An intramedullary pin by itself provides no rotational stability to the fracture site (40). To even approximate a straight-line approach to the mandibular canal for a fracture in the body of the mandible, a rostral approach from the central to intermediate incisor on the ipsilateral side must be used (10). If the fragmented ends are not well aligned, the pin can be placed into the caudal segment and advanced for a retrograde placement. The pin should not extend more than 1–2 cm from the caudal aspect of the mandible before being threaded into the rostral portion as the two fragments are held in place (10). If the mandible is not solid enough . . ."? to maintain such a pin, typically some other method of fracture treatment is preferable.

Screws and plates also are challenging to use correctly in the oral cavity (9,12,40,41). The rigid stability that a plate affords translates into good healing with minimal callus (40), but specialized equipment and skills are needed. The flat surface of the vertical ramus of the mandible may be an area to which a plate can be adapted; however, there is the disadvantage that placing the plate may require removing substantial muscular attachments. Elsewhere in the oral cavity, the biggest detractor to using such devices is the presence of the roots, which occupy up to two-thirds of the mandible. Without careful planning, including radiographs, it is very possible to cause substantial damage to the roots if these devices are placed incorrectly, particularly ventrally (42). While it is optimal to place a plate on the tension side of the mandible, since this is the alveolar ridge, optimal placement is very difficult (38). Use of high-density polyethylene (HDP) plates has been described (43).

External Fixation

Various means of external or *percutaneous skeletal fixation* can be adapted for use in the oral cavity to provide immobilization of fractures with pins or screws placed through the fragments and then connected externally with a metal or acrylic device (16). With good technique that avoids root structures (44) and places the implant on either side of the defect, particularly in comminuted fractures, minimal trauma to the soft tissue will be caused. The size of a Kirschner–Ehmer apparatus makes it too bulky for use in the oral cavity (12,45). A modified form of a biphasic external splint may be useful (12,35,46), but the instrumentation and size of the screws can make use of this process limited. By using Kirschner wires (47) or Steinmann pins in a direct application and not by predrilling the holes with a drill bit (14), even less damage is caused. It is best to put the pins or wires into just one side of the mandible, and not across to the other, to avoid soft tissue damage to sublingual tissues. Transmandibular fixation, even if for a lesion that is unilateral and rostral to the 1st molar (10), can still cause excess damage and is generally not recommended (14). Once the wires or pins are placed, the fracture site is reduced and an acrylic bridge can be formed to incorporate the exposed ends of the pins to stabilize them. A piece of tubing can be connected to each of the pin ends, and acrylic can be injected into it and then allowed to cure. After healing (4–6 weeks), the pins are cut close to the acrylic and removed from the bone.

COMPLICATIONS

Two of the more common complications in attempted fracture repair are nonunion and persistent infection or osteomyelitis (16). With continued signs of infection, culture and sensitivity with appropriate antibiotic usage and curettage of the affected area may be sufficient to allow the oral cavity to continue the healing process. With unresponsive cases, extensive curettage or removal of sequestra may cause a defect or gap in the bone structure. The same may also be true with a nonunion or a pathologic fracture. If such is the case, applying fixation to stabilize both ends stops any movement in the area, and the defect can eventually fill itself in, although the time period may be extensive, up to several months (13). Implantation of osseoconductive or even osseoinductive materials, including cancellous bone chips, may be used in gaps greater than 4–6 cm. A rib autogenous graft can be harvested, with a portion of the rib opened along the long axis to expose the medullary cavity and cancellous bone. The section is positioned to lie in a ventral segment in each fragment and is stabilized with cerclage wires (13). Postoperative care can be difficult, and some degree of failure can be anticipated. In severe cases of infection or nonunion, excision of the affected area with a maxillectomy or mandibulectomy can sometimes resolve continuing problems (48). At times, delaying the grafting procedure until all infection is under control and then approaching the lesion aseptically from a ventral skin incision may be preferable (10). Some patients can eventually adjust to areas of nonunion, and a commissuroplasty may give the area more support (47). *Commissuroplasty* is the alteration of the commissure location of the lips. By removal of the edges of the lips in the commissure area and suturing the opposing edges together, the commissure level can be moved rostrally to provide additional support to the mandible by holding it closer to the maxilla. During the 2-week healing stage, a tape muzzle is required to prevent the commissuroplasty from being separated. It should be kept in mind that this procedure reduces the access to the oral cavity, which may cause difficulties in future dental procedures and intubation.

Placement of an osseoconductive material may also be considered in areas of very thin or weak bone as a *preemptive fracture repair* procedure in an attempt to prevent fractures (49,50). This procedure is frequently done in humans to augment the ridge prior to tooth implant surgery or to build up the bone for adequate bridge placement. After the mucosal epithelium has completely healed, the area should be assessed with radiographs and palpation. Typically, there is a trough or depression in the region (51). A small stab incision can be made at the rostral extent of the lesion, and small hemostats or periosteal elevator can be used to gently dissect the soft tissue off the dorsal surface of the bone. An implant material, such as HTR™ (Bioplant, Norwalk, Connecticut) or Consil® (Nutramax Labs, Baltimore, Maryland), that is supplied in tuberculin syringes or can be placed in a syringe is introduced into the defect and advanced caudally as far as required. The material is then injected into the defect as the syringe is slowly withdrawn; the incision is then closed. The procedure would be beneficial specifically in mandibular regions where severe periodontal disease had compromised osseous health, potentially predisposing the area to a pathologic fracture.

Maintaining correct occlusion during fracture reduction has been emphasized several times already, and certainly major complications may arise when malocclusions result from surgical attempts at fracture repair. This is even more significant in younger, immature animals. Not only can the initial injury itself impair the natural growth of the affected jaw, but rigid fixation may also cause complications involving problems in growth patterns, interference with dental eruptions, injuries to tooth buds, perforations of roots, and damage to the periodontium. In immature animals, staged therapy with more conservative means such as soft tissue suturing and muzzles may provide sufficient stabilization. Often, with minimal assistance, the tremendous healing capability of young animals and of the oral cavity may overcome extensive injuries (52).

REFERENCES

1. Ticer JW, Spencer CP. Injury of the feline temporomandibular joint: Radiographic signs. *J Vet Radiol Soc* 1978; 19:146.
2. Ticer JW. *Radiographic Technique in Veterinary Practice*. 2nd ed. Philadelphia: WB Saunders Co; 1984:231.

3. Verstraete FJM. Surgical repair of mandibular fractures. *Vet Dent Proc* 1993:55.
4. Hartsfield SM, Gendreau CL, Smith CW, et al. Endotracheal intubation by pharyngotomy. JAAHA 1977;13:71.
5. Schloss AJ, Manfra Marretta S. Prognostic factors affecting teeth in the line of mandibular fractures. *J Vet Dent* 1990;7(4):7.
6. Ross DL, Goldstein GS. Oral surgery basic techniques. *Vet Clin North Am Small Anim* 1986;16:967.
7. Neal DC, Wagner WF, Alpert B. Morbidity associated with teeth in the line of mandibular fractures. *J Oral Surg* 1978;36:859.
8. Kahnberg KE, Ridell A. Prognosis of teeth involved in the line of mandibular fractures. *Int Jour Oral Surg*:1979;8:163.
9. Chambers JN. Principles of management of mandibular fractures in the dog and cat. *J Vet Orthop* 1981;2:26.
10. Schrader SC. Dental orthopedics. In: Bojrab MJ, Tholen M, eds. *Small Animal Oral Medicine and Surgery*. Philadelphia: Lea & Febiger; 1990:241.
11. Grove TK. Problems associated with the management of periodontal disease in clinical practice. *Probl Vet Med Surg Dent* 1990;2:110.
12. Weigel JP. Trauma to oral structures. In: Harvey CE, ed. *Veterinary Dentistry*. Philadelphia: WB Saunders Co; 1985:140.
13. Harvey CE, Emily PP. *Small Animal Dentistry*. St.Louis, MO: Mosby-Year Book; 1993:312.
14. Verstraete F. Advanced oral surgery in small carnivores. In: Crossley DA, Penman S, eds. *Manual of Small Animal Dentistry*. Gloucestershire, UK: Britsh Small Animal Association; 1995:193.
15. Smith MM. Oral surgery. *World Vet Dent Cong Proc.* 1995:42.
16. Manfra Marretta S, Schrader SC, Matthiesen DT. Problems associated with the management and treatment of jaw fractures. *Probl Vet Med Surg Dent* 1990;2:220.
17. Alexander JW. *Orthopedic Surgery of the Dog and Cat*. 3rd ed. Philadelphia; WB Saunders Co; 1985.
18. Leighton RL. Treatment of a subcondylar fracture of the mandible in a cat by open reduction and wire fixation. *Feline Pract* 1979;9:30.
19. Salisbury SK, Cantwell HD. Conservative management of fractures of the mandibular condyloid process in three cats and one dog. *JAVMA* 1989;194:85.
20. Taylor EM. Repair of temporomandibular joint fracture in the cat. *World Vet Dent Cong Proc.* 1995:131.
21. Merkley DF, Brinker WO. Facial reconstruction following massive bilateral maxillary fracture in the dog. *JAAHA* 1976;12:831.
22. Manfra Marretta S. The common and uncommon clinical presentations and treatment of periodontal disease in the dog and cat. *Semin Vet Med Surg Small Anim* 1987;2:230.
23. Mulligan TW. Management of mandibular and maxillary fractures. *Amer Anim Hosp Assoc Sci Proc* 1989:149.
24. Zallen RD, Curry JT. A study of antibiotic usage in compound mandibular fractures. *J Oral Surg* 1975;33:431.
25. Withrow SJ. Taping of the mandible in treatment of mandibular fractures. *JAAHA* 1981;17:27.
26. Nibley W. Treatment of caudal mandibular fractures: A preliminary report. *JAAHA* 1981;17:555.
27. Lantz GC. Interarcade wiring as a method of fixation for selected mandibular injuries. *JAAHA* 1981;17:599.
28. Tholen MA. Dental orthopedics. In: Tholen MA, ed. *Concepts in Veterinary Dentistry*. Edwardsville, KS: Veterinary Medical Publishers; 1983:135.
29. Hinko PJ. A method for reduction and fixation of symphyseal fractures of the mandible. *JAAHA*:1976;12:98.
30. Wiggs RB. Jaw fracture management wiring techniques. *Vetadontics Proc* 1988:29C.
31. Wiggs RB. Wire in the oral cavity. *Vetadontics Proc* 1987:74.
32. Shulak FB. Complicated fracture of the mandible repaired with a simple wiring technique. *Friskies Res Digest* 1978;14(2):6.
33. Wiggs RB. Oral surgery: Jaw fractures. *Amer Vet Dent Soc Proc* 1988:25.
34. Wiggs RB. Anterior crossbite corrected using Stout's multiple loop orthodontic wiring technique. *J Vet Dent* 1987;4(3):5.
35. Weigel JP, Dorn AS, Chase DE, Jaffrey B. The use of the biphase external fixation splint for repair of canine mandibular fractures. *JAAHA* 1981;17:547.
36. Ross DL. Anterior mandibular fracture fixation. In: Bojarb MJ, Tholen MA, eds. *Current Techniques in Small Animal Surgery*. Philadelphia: Lea & Febiger; 1975:364.
37. McOwen JS. Intraoral dental splint for mandibular fractures. *J Vet Dent* 1987;4(3):4.
38. Verstraete FJM, Ligthelm AJ. Dental trauma caused by screws in internal fixation of mandibular osteotomies in the dog VCOT. 1992;5:104.
39. Cechner PE. Malocclusion in the dog caused by intramedullary pin fixation of mandibular fractures. *JAAHA* 1980;16:79.
40. Rouh JK, Wilson JW. Healing of mandibular body osteotomies after plate and intramedullary pin fixation. *Vet Surg* 1989;18:190.
41. Brinker WO, Piermattei DL, Flo GL. *Handbook of Small Animal Orthopedics and Fracture Treatment*. Philadelphia: WB Saunders Co; 1983:230.
42. Brinker WO. Types of fractures and their repair. In: Archibald J, ed. *Canine Surgery*. 2nd ed. Santa Barbara, CA: American Veterinary Publishers; 1974:957.
43. Counsell M, McKeown D, Pennock P. Mandibular osteotomy repair using high density polyethylene plates. *JAAHA* 1985;21:685.
44. Sarkiala E. Dental trauma resulting from orthopedic management of jaw fractures. *Vet Dent Proc* 1993:151.

45. Renegar WR, Leeds EB, Olds RB. The use of the Kirscher-Ehmer splint in clinical orthopedics. Part I: Long bone and mandibular fractures. *Compend Cont Educ Pract Vet* 1982;4:318.
46. Greenwood KM, Creagh GB. Bi-phase external skeletal splint fixation of mandibular fractures in dogs. *Vet Surg* 1980;9:128.
47. Manfra Marretta S. A salvage procedure for bilateral pathologic mandibular fractures in the dog. *World Vet Dent Cong Proc* 1995:128.
48. Lantz GC, Salisbury SK. Partial mandibulectomy for treatment of mandibular fractures in dogs: Eight cases (1981-1984). *JAVMA* 1987;191:243.
49. Ashman A. Clinical applications of synthetic bone in dentistry: Part I. General dentistry. *Journal of the Academy of General Dentistry* 1992;40(6):401.
50. Christensen GJ. Ridge preservation: Why not? *JADA* 1996;127:669.
51. Wiggs RB, Lobprise HB. Acute and chronic alveolitis/osteomyelitis "lumpy jaw" in small exotic ruminants. *J Vet Dent* 1994;11(3):16.
52. Schmitz JP, Hollinger JO. The critical size defect as an experimental model for craniomandibulofacial non-unions. *Clin Orthop* 1985;205:299.

11

Basic Endodontic Therapy

Robert B. Wiggs and Heidi B. Lobprise

Endodontics is the branch of dentistry that deals with the diagnosis and treatment of diseases of the pulp and their sequelae in the apical, periapical, radicular, and periradicular tissues. When pulpal tissue is compromised and its vitality threatened or destroyed, some form of endodontic treatment is necessary to preserve teeth that might otherwise be exfoliated or extracted.

Therapy may also serve to resolve dental and peridental infections that can result not only in local but also in systemic complications (1–4). Whichever endodontic procedure is required, a fundamental understanding of basic endodontic anatomy, physiology, pathology, diagnosis, armamentarium, instrumentation, and obturation technique is imperative, as well as an understanding of the post-treatment healing process.

When the pulp is injured and vitality is compromised, the potential for complications, especially infections and abscesses, is substantial. An indifferent attitude of ignoring the problem, particularly if it does not seem to bother the patient, can lead not only to further dental problems and tooth loss but to systemic ramifications as well (1). The option of extracting the affected tooth is preferable to ignoring the problem, but the endodontically aware clinician can offer the client the option of retaining a tooth for both function and esthetics. Most animals can function well with the loss one or more teeth, but many owners are committed to optimum care and even have true esthetic concerns about their pets; for these owners, endodontics may be an unexpected, but appreciated, alternative. Animals trained for special duties (eg, military, police, tracking, retrieving, and protection) often require a sound, functional, complete, or near-complete dentition. For these animals, avoidance of tooth loss can be crucial.

ENDODONTIC ANATOMY

A good working knowledge of the normal tooth, pulp, and pulp cavity morphology and function is essential in assessing abnormalities and making a logical decision concerning endodontic procedures (5). The external shape or anatomy of the tooth is divided into three areas. The first is the *crown*, the portion of the tooth visible above the gingival margin (gum line). The second area is the *neck* or *cervical area*, the junctional point between the crown and the root. The *root*, or third area, is that portion of the tooth apical to the neck and crown, lying under the gingiva and enclosed in the bony socket. The external tooth anatomy gives the practitioner an approximate localization of the internal structure (see Chapter 3). The entire interior tooth vault that the pulp occupies is known as the *pulp cavity*. Some endodontic texts have occasionally referred to the pulp cavity as the *root canal system*. The portion in the crown is referred to as the *pulp chamber*, with its most coronal aspect identified as the *pulp horns*. The part located in the root is defined as the *root canal*. The *apex* of the tooth is the tip of the root. Clinically, as far as standard endodontics is concerned, the most critical area of the pulp cavity or root canal system is that associated with the most apical portion of the root. Humans and nonhuman primates are typically considered to have an *apical foramen*, a single master exit at the apical stricture of the root canal, although in reality many primate teeth have several foraminal openings (6). Dog and cat teeth usually have an *apical delta*, where the main root canal divides into a substantial number of multiple accessory canals opening a few millimeters from the apex. There are typically 6–90 of these small delta openings (5,7) (see Chapter 3). Additionally, lateral or auxiliary canals may provide passage between the pulp cavity and periodontal tissues in locations other than at the apex. While it is impossible to clean and fill all the minute openings of this delta, sealing the canal in the apical one-third generally produces an effective treatment (7).

The soft tissue of this inner cavity, the *pulp*, emerges from the tooth and connects with the periodontal ligament at the apical foramen or delta. The pulp is composed of soft connective vascular and nerve tissue (Fig. 1). It contains odontoblasts, fibroblasts, fibrocytes, collagen fibers, elastic fibers, blood vessels, and nerves. It is this tissue that responds most dramatically to any insult or injury to the dentition.

The bulk of the structure and tissue of a mature tooth is *dentin*, a pale yellow, ivory-like material. It is located in both the root and crown of the tooth, covered by cementum and enamel, respectively. The dentin is covered by the hard substance, enamel, on the crown and by cementum on the root. At the neck of the tooth, the enamel normally meets the cementum of the root. Typically, this *cementoenamel junction* lies just inside the gingival sulcus. In some cases, the cementum may overlap the enamel, but in others it falls short, leaving a gap of exposed dentin underneath.

The pulpal *odontoblasts* produce dentin, which is lower in inorganic composition and somewhat softer than enamel but slightly harder than cementum. Innumerable dentinal

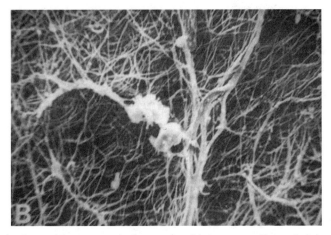

FIG. 1. The pulp tissue is composed of a mass of interwoven fibers (original magnification ×4000). (Reproduced from Baumgartner JC, Mader CL. A scanning electron microscope evaluation of four root canal irrigation regimens. *J Endod* 1987;13:154, with permission.)

tubules perforate the dentin at right angles to the pulp and contain cytoplasmic extensions from the odontoblasts called *Tomes fibers*. The odontoblasts function to produce dentin throughout the vital life of the tooth, resulting in thicker dentinal walls and narrower pulp cavities as the teeth mature. This maturing process is sometimes referred to as *canal calcification*. Dentin can also be reparative, and if attrition is slow enough, or calcium hydroxide is placed on recently exposed pulp, a dentinal bridge may be formed to protect the underlying tissues. Additionally, in some instances reparative dentin may obliterate a portion of the canal. These highly calcified canals can be a problem for endodontic instrumentation (5).

Cementum, covering the external root surface, is produced by the cementoblasts of the periodontal ligament. As enamel is normally thickest at the cusp tip, cementum is thickest at the apex of the tooth. It does have some ability to be regenerated or repaired, as the periodontal ligament continues to produce cementum periodically (5).

Following eruption of a permanent tooth, the apex gradually constricts and calcifies. This is customarily called a *closed apex*, even though in a vital tooth the root never totally closes as foramina or delta openings are always present. The internal root canal apex closes down usually 1–2 mm from the actual external root apex. This internal constriction is generally called the *apical stricture*. Human studies have shown that the apical stricture gradually becomes more distant from the external apex due to additional cementum being laid down at the apex of the root (8). Standard endodontics typically deals with mature permanent teeth with adequate root apex closure. Immature teeth require alternative procedures to deal with their extremely wide canals (blunderbuss) and possibly open apices that may require additional development prior to endodontic therapy (6–9).

In endodontics, it is important to know the normal variation in *root numbers* associated with individual teeth, since all roots of a tooth must be treated. In a normal dog, three-rooted teeth include the maxillary 4th premolars and maxillary 1st and 2nd molars; in cats, only the maxillary 4th premolars have three roots. All incisors and cuspids (canines) are single-rooted teeth, as are generally the maxillary and some mandibular 1st premolars in dogs and the maxillary 2nd premolars (first maxillary cheek tooth distal to

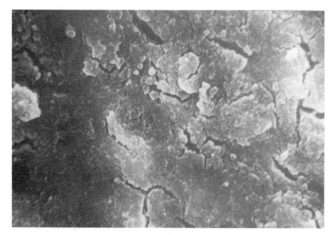

FIG. 2. Typical amorphous smear layer (original magnification ×4080). (Reproduced from Baumgartner JC, Mader CL. A scanning electron microscope evaluation of four root canal irrigation regimens. *J Endod* 1987;13:154, with permission.)

the cuspid or canine tooth) in cats. All other teeth typically have two roots, including the mandibular 1st premolars in some dogs (5,9).

It must be emphasized that a formidable number of variations in dental anatomy exits not only between species but also within species. Even within the same individual, great variations occur in the degree of calcification, dilaceration, and apical status. One of the most reliable guides for the veterinary dentist in most individuals is multiple radiographic views (10).

During endodontic instrumentation, a manufactured or artificial layer is produced within the pulp cavity, known as the *smear layer* (11) (Fig. 2). It consists of a relatively smooth, amorphous layer of microcrystalline debris created by the cutting and/or crushing of the dentinal walls by instruments. Because of its ultrafine composition, it can be superficially forced into the dental tubules, accessory canals, and the apical foramina or delta openings, resulting in a barrier capable of preventing bacteria from entering the dentin (12). However, if excessive organic debris is mixed with the inorganic dentinal debris, bacteria may populate and penetrate the smear layer (13).

ETIOLOGY OF PULPAL AND PERIAPICAL PATHOLOGY

The fact that the tooth is a vital structure makes it important to understand the changes that may occur in response to various stimuli. Inflammation, infective or sterile, of the pulp is termed *pulpitis*, which can be reversible or irreversible (14). *Reversible pulpitis* is generally a symptom of pulpal inflammation caused by some form of irritation such as caries. If the cause can be removed or treated, the pulp can return to a normal state, but if this is not possible, the condition eventual progresses to *irreversible pulpitis*. Treatment is generally of a restorative nature. Irreversible pulpitis is a pronouncement of impending total or partial pulpal death, termed *pulpal necrosis*. Irreversible pulpitis indicates the need for endodontic or exodontic therapy (14).

The tooth can be damaged and the pulp injured by carious lesions, chemical injury during dental procedures, hematogenous infections, feline cervical line lesions (CLL), and trauma, both accidental and iatrogenic. Moderate dental trauma may cause a mild pulpitis or inflamed pulp that is reversible. As the pulp is encased in dentin, any extensive inflammation can cause excessive edema and pressure on this soft tissue can severely compromise it (15). It is the degree of pathologic change that the pulp undergoes as a response to stimuli that determines whether or not endodontic intervention is necessary. In veterinary dentistry, the most common precursor of pulpal disease is traumatic injury typically resulting in tooth fracture, pulpal exposure, inflammation, and bacterial infection—a condition that is the most frequent indication for root canal therapy (9,15). The introduction of bacteria to the pulp tissue may also occur due to deep carious or resorptive lesions (eg, feline CLL) before, during, or after treatment. The *anachoretic effect* (16–18) describes when bacteria reaching the pulp cause a local infectious process. Prior injury of the pulp tissue resulting in inhibition of its defenses is commonly associated with this effect. Bacteria may be carried to the tooth by the bloodstream during transient bacteremias or by the regional gingival lymphatics traveling from the sulcus (16,19). This effect may explain the sudden onset of acute or chronic periapical involvement of teeth that are apparently sound. When the circulation is impaired due to trauma and the pulp becomes nonvital, the necrotic tissue and fluids in the root canal system may result in inflammation of the periapical periodontal ligament, providing a location for opportunistic organisms to populate. Generally, to be in good health, a tooth needs the periodontium with its independent vasculature and nerve supply to maintain a healthy attachment (20). Therefore, extensive periodontal disease can give a tooth a poor prognosis, and then endodontic procedure may be unwise.

While trauma is typically manifested by a broken crown, bruxing forces that are sustained over time (excessive chewing) or are concussive may result in pulpitis in the form of swelling or hemorrhage of the pulp without crown loss (21,22). Blunt trauma may disrupt the apical blood supply to the tooth, while leaving the external tooth structure undamaged. Inflammation may result in edema and swelling that excessively compromise the pulp to the point of irreversible pulpitis (5,15,22). Some of these dental injuries may first present as pink or blue tinging of the tooth. This condition results from a trauma in which vessels supplying the pulp at the apical delta are typically severed. The interrupted blood supply results in blood accumulating within the pulp cavity and the possibility of ischemic death of the pulp and associated odontoblasts. The hemorrhage will only be visibly apparent in the areas where the odontoblasts and their Tomes fibers have died, leaving open dental tubules or dead tracts for the blood to enter. Once the blood or its breakdown components penetrate near the dentinoenamel junction, the hemorrhage becomes visible. If the pulpitis is reversible, the color may eventually diminish and the tooth will return to its normal appearance. If irreversible destruction has occurred, the color changes to a purple–gray as the pulp dies and the blood cell components are degenerated. Initial pain and discomfort during the period when the pulp is acutely inflamed tends to dissipate as the innervation undergoes necrosis (10,23). The necrotic pulp may inflame the periapical periodontal ligament, making it susceptible to the anachoretic effect (16–18) of infection, and eventually the pulp can be expected to exhibit periapical pathologic changes similar to those of an exposed pulp.

Pulpitis may also result from thermal injury to the pulp (24). While this is occasionally accidental (eg, electric cord chewing) (19), most incidents are iatrogenic. Overheating of the teeth due to over-rigorous use of ultrasonic or rotary scalers or polishing units can cause extensive injury. Reasonable care should be taken to prevent thermal damage to the tooth by use of a sufficient water-cooling spray with scalers and rotary burs. With polishing, the use of proper speeds and pressure, an adequate prophylaxis paste, and time restrictions on the use of an instrument on individual teeth will minimize the chance of damage. Iatrogenic pulpal damage with various therapeutic chemicals should also be avoided.

An open pulp cavity allows bacteria to enter the pulpal tissue, resulting in pulpal inflammation and pathology as described earlier. Bacteria extend into the periapical tissues through the apical delta, contributing to abscess formation around the apex and even bone dissolution (5,25). While the infections may sometimes seem subclinical, chronic conditions may affect the patient's general health in subtle ways. More obvious signs occur when abscesses fistulate intraorally (usually apically to the mucogingival junction in permanent teeth and coronally to it in deciduous teeth) or extraorally into the sinuses or through subcutaneous tissues either suborbitally or submandibularly.

Another condition occasionally seen with an exposed canal is *hyperplastic pulpitis* (10). This exhibits itself in one of two forms: hyperplastic granulation and hyperplastic swelling pulpitis. *Granulation* tissue is usually a reddish, rough overgrowth that partially or completely occludes the exposure opening. This results from the pulp's attempt to construct a barrier between itself and the source of inflammation. In primates, it is seen most commonly in carious lesions of the young, whereas with carnivores it is more commonly associated with pulp exposures due to fractures. This hyperplastic activity is an indication of the local immune system's effort to maintain the pulp's vitality. Although removal of the hyperplastic tissue and direct pulp capping can be attempted, a root canal treatment is generally more prudent if the apices are mature. With simple pulpal *swelling*, the tissue will appear reddish to blue and have a smooth tight surface. Pulps in this condition are usually in a terminal change from vital to nonvital, and a standard root canal procedure will generally be best, unless special circumstances are encountered.

PERIAPICAL PATHOLOGY

Once the pulpal tissue becomes infected, organisms will continue to invade, seeking new nutrients. As the apical periodontal ligament is the only directly associated soft tissue in this situation, bacterial involvement will eventually extend to these tissues (26). The periapical tissues have good collateral circulation, which allows the building of a defensive barrier in an attempt to confine the pathogens and their toxins within the root canal system and periapical tissues. In more chronic cases, this barrier generally takes the form of granulation tissue, although it may take purulent or cystic forms at the apex (27,28). However, in acute periapical disease abscess formation is more common (29). Chronic proliferative changes at the apex stimulate dissolution or resorption of periapical bone (30–32). This results in the classic periapical lucency on radiographs (33). Whether an acute or chronic process develops depends on the severity of trauma, pathogenicity of the organism, degree of organism challenge, and host resistance.

Periapical disease generally exhibits itself as one of five conditions: acute apical periodontitis, acute apical abscess, chronic apical periodontitis, phoenix abscess, or chronic periapical osteitis (10). *Acute apical periodontitis* is acute inflammation around the apex (10). Causes can be trauma, bruxing, extension of pulpal disease, and overextension of endodontic instruments. It results in few periapical signs other than tenderness or pain on palpation or percussion. Radiographs generally appear normal, although a slight widening of the periapical ligament space may be seen. It may be associated with either vital or nonvital teeth. In nonvital cases, endodontic therapy is appropriate, while vital teeth require the removal of the cause for correction.

Acute apical abscess implies a painful purulent exudate of sudden onset at the apex (10). The cause is advancement of acute apical periodontitis and a necrotic pulp resulting in extensive suppurative inflammation. Signs are slight-to-severe swelling and pain, with some patients being febrile. Radiographically, as with acute apical periodontitis, no signs may be apparent due to a lack of duration to cause dissolution or resorption of the periapical lamina dura. It can be differentiated from other suppurative abscesses, such as the phoenix abscess, as they typically demonstrate apical bone loss associated with more chronic disease; its differentiation from periodontal abscesses is based on their general association with vital teeth and periodontal pocketing. Exodontic or endodontic therapy along with systemic antibiotics is required. Anti-inflammatory drugs and analgesics may also be necessary.

Chronic apical periodontitis is a long-term inflammation around the apex (10). This can establish itself as a chronic periapical granuloma or cyst, with only histology making the deferential diagnosis in some cases. Abscesses are not seen with chronic apical periodontitis, but rather in acute and phoenix-type disease. Locally, the lesions are generally asymptomatic, although some degree of tenderness can be induced on palpation or percussion in many cases. The equilibrium between the host defense and the extension of the disease constrains the development of clinical symptoms but results in periapical bone loss apparent on radiographs. In some cases, development of a sinus tract allows the escape of toxins and the suppression of symptoms. However, any physical manipulations of the tooth or tissues may induce the release of toxins or bacteria beyond the local host defense systems and into the systemic network to insult or infect other organs (1–4); they may also induce the development of a phoenix abscess (10). Therefore, exodontic or endodontic treatment is necessary.

Phoenix abscesses are simply acute exacerbations of chronic apical periodontitis (10). The symptoms are basically the same as those of acute apical abscess, but they are preceded by the chronic phase. The main diagnostic difference is the presence of radiographic evidence of periapical bone loss, which may be associated with apical root loss. It frequently follows some form of manipulation of the tooth, either occlusal or endodontic. Treatment is exodontic or endodontic, along with systemic antibiotics. Anti-inflammatory drugs and analgesics may also be needed.

Chronic periapical osteitis is the osseous response observed with some low-grade chronic pulpal and periapical inflammations. The three conditions most commonly seen radiographically are osteosclerosis, osteomyelitis, and ankylosis (10). *Periapical osteosclerosis* is the excessive mineralization of the periapical and periradicular alveolar bone. This is relatively asymptomatic in most cases. Low-grade chronic pulpal inflammation of vital teeth, as seen in occlusal stress (eg, bruxing, excessive chewing, etc.), can induce excessive periapical mineralization. Additionally, osteosclerosis is sometimes seen following endodontic treatment. In some chronic pulpitis cases, *radicular ankylosis* eventually occurs. Radiographically, this presents as the loss of the periodontal ligament space, giving the appearance of a tooth root merging with adjacent bone, with the loss of a distinctive root image. *Periradicular osteomyelitis* appears radiographically as an *osteopenia*, with expansion effects involving the alveolus in some cases of chronic pulpal inflammation. This appears most commonly around the cuspids of the cat, involved with cervical, radicular, and apical resorptive activity of the tooth. It is not uncommon in these cases for a degree of osteosclerosis to be present.

ROOT FRACTURES

Fractures of the root structure are seen in domestic animals (34). Flexible, malleable, or padded objects are among the more common causes of root fractures, while sparing the crown of injury (35). The level at which the root is fractured principally determines the degree of mobility in the coronal segment and dictates the need for immobilization. Fractures nearer the cervical area are generally more mobile and have an increased chance of bacterial contamination from the sulcus.

Clinically, root fractures are usually detected only if the coronal segment is displaced, or serious mobility is observed. Radiographically, fractures are not always obvious or detectable. In acute cases, *horizontal fractures* are often obscured by trabecular bone patterns and show no marked radicular change, unless displacement has occurred. Fractures of this type can sometimes be delineated from bone patterns by close observation of whether the pattern extends beyond the bounds of the root-structure image. *Vertical fractures* are seldom detectable on radiographs, except in advanced stages of separation (36).

Most root fractures, if reasonably stable and uncontaminated, heal unaided with the pulp remaining vital (35–39). The alveolus acts as a natural splint, stabilizing and maintaining the segments in close proximity. New cementum or osseous material is laid down on the external root surface, while reparative dentin forms internally to heal the fracture. If mobility is a problem, a temporary acrylic or composite splint is advisable.

Strangulated pulps, periodontal disease, and excessive mobility are problems that can lead to complications in treatment to salvage the tooth (35). Displacement of the coronal segment may result in pulpal strangulation and necrosis. For this reason, displaced segments should be radiographed and suitably aligned as quickly as possible after the injury. If pulpal necrosis does occur, occasionally only the coronal segment is initially involved, allowing for pulpotomy and direct pulp capping in some cases. Should the entire pulp be involved, a standard root canal procedure will be required. Complications of advanced periodontal disease or of fractures transgressing the sulcus can easily influence tooth vitality due to bacterial intrusion and/or mobility from loss of alveolar support. Loss of vitality can be addressed with root canal therapy, but mobility requires realignment and stabilization, which can be a challenge in many animals. Splinting with acrylics can provide a degree of stabilization, but the periodontal disease must also be addressed. When periodontal disease is progressive or extensive, exodontia is most likely the treatment of choice.

ENDODONTIC–PERIODONTIC RELATIONSHIP

The endodontic and periodontic soft tissues are intimately related by various routes. The stable functioning of a tooth is determined by its structural integrity and that of its periodontal attachment and support component (37). Pulpal disease may be primarily endodontic in origin or secondary to periodontal disease (38). Communication between the pulp and periodontal tissues occurs principally through exposed dentinal tubules, lateral or accessory canals, and the apical foramina or delta openings (38,39). Classification of the lesions based on their primary and secondary elements can provide a speculative prognostic guide for treatment.

The relationship can be distinguished as:

Class 0   Primarily endodontic lesion
Class I   Endo-perio lesion: primarily endodontic with secondary periodontal involvement
Class II Perio-endo lesion: primarily periodontal with secondary endodontic involvement
Class III True combined lesion

The classification is based on physical and radiographic findings (40) (Fig. 3). *Class 0* lesions are are primarily endodontic in origin with no signs of true periodontal involvement. They are seen in fairly acute exposures of the coronal endodontic system and in cases in which a sinus tract runs through the periodontal ligament and exits in the sulcus without radiographic signs. The sinus tracts are usually observed visually as materials are evacuated or exposed on probing. These tracts are typically associated with lateral canals and sometimes the apex. A *class I* lesion occurs when a primarily endodontic lesion spreads to the periodontal structures through accessory canals or the apical delta or foramina. *Class II* lesions are primarily periodontal in origin, with the endodontic system involved secondarily through open tubules, accessory canals, lateral canals, or the apical delta. *Class III* lesions occur in teeth that have both primary pulpal and primary periodontal disease, as in a tooth with advanced periodontal disease that becomes fractured. With time, endodontic and periodontic lesions combine and progress to a point where it may become impossible to determine the primary origin. Such lesions are commonly placed in the class III category, although they may not be "true" combined lesions. In addition, with multirooted teeth, radiographs may show class-I type lesions around one root, but class II lesions around another. Such cases are also generally placed in the class III category.

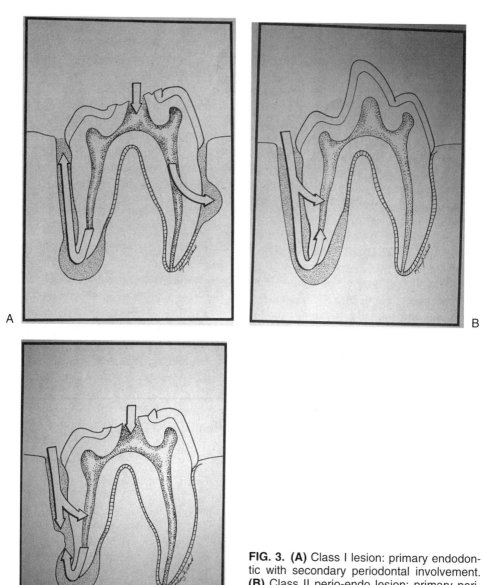

FIG. 3. (A) Class I lesion: primary endodontic with secondary periodontal involvement. **(B)** Class II perio-endo lesion: primary periodontal with secondary endodontic involvement. **(C)** Class III perio-endo lesion: true combination lesion. (Reproduced from ref. 41, with permission.)

Radiographically, class 0 lesions show no periodontal involvement. Class I lesions demonstrate a typical radiolucent halo around root ends and may have a thinner radiolucent area running up the root structure, described as a J-shaped lesion (41). In class II lesions, the radiolucent area running down the root and around the apex is more uniform in thickness, and a degree of attachment loss from periodontal disease is usually present. Class III lesions typical demonstrate a widened periodontal space indicating a deep periodontal pocket, along with a crown pulp exposure and possibly a periapical radiolucent halo.

Each class of lesion carries a different prognosis concerning treatment and therefore may influence practitioners' treatment planning of endodontics or exodontics. With regard to endodontics, when the crown still has good integrity and the roots have not been fractured, prognosis for a class 0 tooth is very good to excellent; for a class I lesion the prognosis is good to very good, and for class II and III lesions fair to poor.

EXAMINATION

The goal of the endodontic examination is to take subjective information and objective data to locate the origin of the problem and obtain an appropriate diagnosis for appropriate treatment planning (36). Subjective information of obscure indications of pain or discomfort are of limited help, although information concerning pain at a specific area can be of help.

Objective information from the owner can be helpful in arriving at an appropriate diagnosis. This type of information typically involves traumatic injuries that cause immediate pain, discomfort, facial swelling, fistula draining, or oral bleeding that the owner readily recognizes. However, many endodontically compromised teeth are not presented with such obvious signs and require an objective examination for specific information. The objective oral examination entails the visual examination, tactile assessment, palpation, percussion, thermal sensitivity testing, transillumination, radiography, and occasionally use of pulp testers (5).

The *visual examination* is the simplest, yet in many cases it can be the most informative for the initial diagnosis. The most obvious finding suggesting that a tooth is endodontically compromised is a fracture of the crown, including cracks and *slab fractures* still attached by the gingiva. If the canal is open, the diagnosis is simple; however, partial crown loss without canal exposure can also lead to irreversible pulpitis. When injuries are recent, the pulp may have conspicuous hemorrhage and be painful. With time, the inflamed pulp becomes necrotic, the tooth generally becomes asymptomatic as far as pain is concerned, and the red or pink exposed pulp site turns dark. Tooth discoloration due to reversible or irreversible pulpitis may display a range of color shades progressing from pink to purple to gray or beige. In the later stages of acute apical abscess, the mucous membranes may swell or discolor, and facial swelling or even fistulation may be discovered, depending on the severity and site involved.

Palpation, percussion, transillumination, and tactile assessment are diagnostic tests that are extensions of the visual examination. Digital palpation of the mucosa above teeth suspected of being compromised may elicit indications of discomfort or reveal a swelling. *Palpation* and *percussion* of the appropriate tooth may induce a suppurative flow from a fistulous tract or disclose tooth mobility or sensitivity. *Transillumination*, also known as diascopy, is the passage of a strong light through body tissues for the purpose of examination. The light penetrating through the tooth may aid in identifying coronal cracks or other defects. Additionally, with time, nonvital teeth may become more opaque to transillumination, due to hemoglobin breakdown, than their adjacent vital counterparts (42,43).

The *tactile assessment* can occasionally be performed on an alert animal, but a proper assessment is best performed with the animal under sedation or general anesthesia. This evaluation is performed using an endodontic pathfinder or explorer to probe for an opening into the endodontic system or pulp cavity (5). Some fine line fractures can be spread to identify and discriminate severity using gentle pressure from probes or rubber-tipped instruments. Periodically, dyes, such as methylene blue, are placed on the tooth to aid in delineating fracture lines.

Thermal testing is used in human dentistry to help identify teeth with pulpitis. It requires a cooperative and alert patient, which is not predictable with animals. It should be noted that a pulpal response can be evoked by various stimuli (eg, cold, heat, electricity, etc.), but pain is the sensation that can be elicited from the patient. In humans, thermal testing is an objective diagnostic tool, as the person verbally responds to the acute onset of sensitivity to stimulus. However, in veterinary dentistry it becomes more of a subjective test because the clinician must interpret the animal's response. For cold testing, a tuberculin syringe with the tip cut off and with water frozen in it can be used. Cold is used in an attempt to determine if the associated nerves are normal, hyper-responsive (acute pulpitis), or not responsive at all (nonvital), as compared with adjacent teeth (5,22). When cold temporally relieves pain, it can be an indication of irreversible pulpitis from pulpal or periapical abscess. Heat testing is a more complex assessment, as all teeth respond to heat; however, those with pulpitis have a more prolonged effect, and those with acute pulpitis respond severely and can be calmed quickly with cold (35,36). Most thermal tests, especially heat, are too subjective or difficult to perform on alert animals to be of serious value.

Radiology is the most important diagnostic, prognostic, and therapeutic evaluation tool in endodontics (5). Diagnostically, radiographs can confirm pulp canal exposure, radicular and alveolar fractures, and periapical disease. Prognostically, they determine the extent of the structural damage due to root fractures, internal or external resorption, and endoliths (pulp stones) and other potential canal blockages, as well as the degree of supportive structure loss due to periodontal disease. Teeth with no clinically tangible signs of endodontic disease may display significant periapical lucency, an indication of probable loss of pulpal vitality (43).

With the exception of obvious visual or radiographic findings, no one single method of diagnosis should totally be depended on. Two or more of the diagnostic tools or methods should be used to aid in confirming the final diagnosis. The subjective and objective examinations provide information for the basis of the prognosis, as well as indicating the courses of action that can then be offered.

ENDODONTIC INSTRUMENTS

Endodontic instruments are those used on the pulp or within the pulp cavity. Understanding the armamentarium of endodontic instrumentation is essential in the selection and proper use of these instruments. The proper selection and use of instruments, in combination with the conscientious application of the endodontic triad, can increase the probability of success in endodontic procedures. The *endodontic triad* is canal preparation, sterilization, and obturation (44). The objective of the endodontic triad is to prepare the canal to accept obturation with a positive seal.

Instrumentation History

Early instruments used for endodontics were developed by individual dental practitioners. Small flat blades, broaches, hickory pegs, and annealed piano wire were used (45). The lack of uniformity of instruments produced numerous instrumentation problems. Ingle in 1961 (46) observed that the Washington Study indicated that improper instrumentation was the second most common reason for endodontic failure, following insufficient obturation.

Ingle was primarily involved with the advocating for standardization of endodontic instrumentation as early as 1955 (47,48). At the annual session of the American Association of Endodontists in 1962, the association's research committee instituted meetings with manufacturers and suppliers of endodontic instruments and began dialogues for standardization. From these conferences, a working committee was formed under the endorsement of the North American Section of the International Association of Dental Research. The American Dental Association (ADA), the National Institute of Dental Research, and the National Bureau of Standards consolidated efforts with the North American Section group in 1964. Later, the American National Standards Institute (ANSI) and its committee Z-156 (Dentistry) were given the worldwide responsibility for standards development. The ANSI Committee Z-156 was later designated Committee MD-156 (Medical Devices). The Council on Dental Materials, Instrumentation, and Equipment of the ADA acts as secretariat for the United States (49).

Under the joint guidance of the Federation Dentaire Internationale (FDI) and International Standards Organization (ISO), the development of worldwide standards for endodontic instruments is governed by Technical Committee 106, Joint Working Group 1 (TC-106, JWG-1). It continues to advance the development of international standards for endodontic instruments in the areas of terminology, dimensions and measuring systems, physical properties, and quality control (50).

In 1976, the American National Standard (Specification No.28) was adopted. In this standard, the shape, dimensions, and diameter of endodontic instruments are defined. In addition, terminology and a color-code identification system are covered (51) (Table 1). Specification No.28 covered only K-type (Kerr) reamers and files. In 1981, the ADA and ANSI Council on Dental Materials, Instruments, and Equipment adopted Specification

TABLE 1. *Terminology, diameter, and color coding of standardized endodontic instruments*

Size	Diameter of instrument (mm)		Color (abbreviation)
	Immediately behind tip at initiation of flutes	$D_{16}{}^a$	
10	0.10	0.42	Purple (pur)
15	0.15	0.47	White (wh)
20	0.20	0.52	Yellow (yel)
25	0.25	0.57	Red (red)
30	0.30	0.62	Blue (blu)
35	0.35	0.67	Green (grn)
40	0.40	0.72	Black (blk)
45	0.45	0.77	White (wh)
50	0.50	0.82	Yellow (yel)
55	0.55	0.87	Red (red)
60	0.60	0.92	Blue (blu)
70	0.70	1.02	Green (grn)
80	0.80	1.12	Black (blk)
90	0.90	1.22	White (wh)
100	1.00	1.32	Yellow (yel)
110	1.10	1.42	Red (red)
120	1.20	1.52	Blue (blu)
130	1.30	1.62	Green (grn)
140	1.40	1.72	Black (blk)
150	1.50	1.82	White (wh)

(From ADA Specification No.28.)
[a] The diameter of the instrument 16 mm from the tip and the end of the operative head in standardized instruments.

No.58 for H-type (Hedstrom) instruments (51). Specifications No.28 and No.58 had revisions approved by the ANSI and ADA in 1988. These became effective on June 30, 1989, and February 28, 1989, respectively. Specification No.63 describes the standards for barbed broaches and instruments of this type. Specification No.57 deals with gutta-percha points or cones. These new guidelines are referred to as the *standard specifications*, whereas the old guidelines are known as the *conventional specifications*.

Instrument Classification

Through the Joint Working Group of the ISO and the FDI, instruments used in endodontics have been grouped according to use (52):

Group I: These endodontic instruments are for hand use only. Included in this group are K-type reamers and files, H-type files, R-type rasps, barbed broaches, probes, applicators, filling pluggers or condensers, filling spreaders, and K-type pathfinders.

Group II: Endodontic instruments in this group are engine-driven, involving a two-part shaft and operative head. These are instruments designed for use only in straight, contra-angle, or specially designed endodontic contra-angle handpieces. The operative heads can be identical with those in group I or specially designed instruments. These include K-type reamers and files, H-type files, R-type rasps, B-2 reamers, quarter-turn reamers, and paste carriers (lentulas).

Group III: Instruments in this group are also engine-driven but have a one-part shaft and operative head. In addition to root facers, this group includes a variety of reamers: B-1, G-type (Gates-Glidden), P-type (Peeso), A-type, D-type, O-type, Ko-type, T-type, and M-type.

Group IV: This group involves endodontic points or cones and includes all types of filling points or cones, as well as absorbent paper points.

Group I

Broaches

Broaches, rasps, probes, and applicators are historically some of the oldest forms of endodontic instruments, dating to before the 19th century (53). Smooth broaches or probes are used to determine whether a canal is present and whether it can be negotiated. They are usually made of a smooth, slender, and fairly flexible round wire that may be tapered and have a point. Probes or smooth broaches are not popular, as most operators use other instruments, such as the Kerr pathfinder (the smallest-size K-type file with a noncutting tip), to perform the functions of probes and broaches. The Kerr pathfinder is not in the broach family.

The *barbed broach* (Fig. 4) in endodontics has only one primary function: removal of the soft pulp tissue from the pulp cavity (52). It is the only instrument in this category that is still in popular use. It is slowly inserted into the canal until light contact is made with the debris or dentinal wall. It is then rotated 180° to entangle the tissue in its extended barbs and drawn back to extract the entangled debris. This debris may be pulp tissue, cotton pellets, medicaments, or loosely seated points.

Barbed broaches are fragile instruments and should be used with caution. They are produced by making small angular incisions into the metal shank of a smooth broach, and

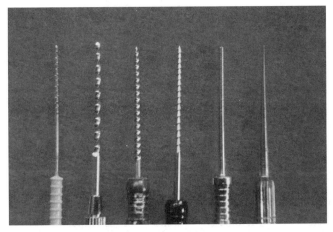

FIG. 4. Group I Endodontic instruments. *(Left to right)* Barbed broach, K-type reamer, K-type file, H-type file, condenser/plugger, spreader.

these are forced open to form barbs. The incisions into the shank of the metal result in areas of weakness in the instrument. If forced down into the canal, the barbs can be compressed. With attempts to remove the instrument, the barbs may spread, digging into the dentinal wall and locking the instrument in place. Any twisting action at this point will usually fracture the delicate instrument at one of the incision points. A surgical endodontic procedure may then become necessary at this disastrous juncture.

A keen tactile sense is required when the barbed broach is being used. Always keep in mind the weakness of the instrument, when selecting the proper size to use within the canal. The size of broach selected should be slightly smaller than the canal, so that little or no contact is made between the barbed tips and the dentinal walls of the canal. This determination of size is extrapolated from critical examination of the scout or diagnostic radiographs of the dentition. In small or finely curved canals, a file will effectively remove pulp material in most cases, without the inherent danger of using a barbed broach. In a young animal with a very large canal, a pair of broaches twisted together and used simultaneously may be necessary to remove the pulpal tissue cleanly.

K-Type Files and Reamers

K-type endodontic instruments are manufactured from prestressed steel wires cut into straight rods and machined into three- or four-sided tapered pyramidal blanks. In cross-section, the three-sided blank is an equilateral triangle and the four-sided blank is either a square or rhomboid. The tapered terminal end of the blank is then twisted to produce the series of spirals that are the operating head of the instrument. The number of twists introduced to the instrument determine whether the blank becomes a file or a reamer. Blanks with 0.1 to <0.25 spiral per millimeter of length produce an instrument with 0.28–0.80 cutting flutes per millimeter of operating head, and are designated *reamers*. Blanks with 0.25 to >0.5 spiral per millimeter of length produce instruments with 0.88–1.97 cutting flutes per millimeter of operating head, and are designated *files*. Reamers have a smaller helical angle of the edge of the flute as compared with files. This results in reamers' having a little better cutting efficiency but a poorer carrying ability than a file. Most operators believe they have a better tactile sense inside the canal with files as compared with reamers, because the greater number of spirals produces more dentinal-wall contact surface with the instrument. Reamers are used in a clockwise-turning fashion. Files are used with a push–pull filing action or with a quarter turn and pull mode (53) (see Fig. 4).

Of clinical importance is the shape of the shaft. One-third rotation of a triangular instrument completes a cutting circle of the root canal. With a square shaft, a quarter turn is necessary to complete a cutting circle, and a rhomboid shaft requires a half turn. Triangular blanks are more flexible than the square, but not as strong. K-type reamers are more flexible than K-type files, but again not as strong. K-type reamers and files are stiffer and stronger than most comparable instrument types, size for size (54). Many manufacturers alter steel, the number of twists, or the shape of the instrument blank in an effort to deliver an endodontic instrument that is more flexible while providing good cutting qualities. Many change their files and reamers from a square to a triangular blank in the larger sizes to improve flexibility. With the change in shape, a subsequent loss of strength occurs. The operator who is not aware of this is likely to experience an increase in instrument breakage at the point of the substitution (55).

Once an instrument is separated or broken off (*disarticulated*) in the canal, it can be difficult if not impossible to remove. Many methods for removing these have been reported in the literature (56). Among them are wrapping cotton on barbed broaches in the hope of entangling a loose fragment to be removed, isolating the fragment with burs and removing it with forceps, working files along side to attempt loosening the fragment, and using trepan burs, ultrasonic vibration, irrigant flushing, or the Massermann extractor (57). No method is totally reliable or without hazards. In many cases, a fragment can be incorporated into the canal filling and bypassed. In other cases, if the fragment is lodged in the apical foramen or delta, the sealer may be forced around the fragment to obtain an apical seal. Teeth with instrument fragments occluding the apical foramen have proven in many cases to be as clinically successful as routine endodontic procedures (58). Prognosis varies with the location of the fragment and chronicity of the lesion being treated. If fragments cannot be incorporated into the filling and do not permit a good apical seal, then a surgical procedure with apicoectomy and retrograde closure should be considered.

H-Type Files

The H-type file, better known as the *Hedstrom file*, is one of the commonly used endodontic instruments in veterinary endodontics. To produce this design of file, a round metal blank is taken and machined down to produce a spiral groove on a tapered, pointed instrument (see Fig. 4). In human endodontic procedures, the H-type file appears to be most commonly used to flare the canal from the apical region to the cervical third of the canal system (56). It is designed in such a fashion that the bulk of the metal in the working blade supporting the cutting surface does not extend out to the edges of the instrument but exists as a central unmachined core. The bulk and size of this type file can be deceptive in its strength. An instrument is only as strong as its central core. Size for size, the H-type files have a smaller central core than K-type files. The large helical angle (≤90°) contributes to the file's effectiveness when it is used in a push–pull filing action. However, it is not designed for rotary motion, and if used for such, it is significantly prone to fracture. Its flutes provide a good carrying effect for the removal of debris from the canal.

Variations and Innovations in Endodontic Files

Originally, most endodontic files were manufactured from carbon steel. These instruments provided an excellent edge on the file flutes for superior cutting effect. In addition, when a file separated and could not be retrieved, the canal could be flooded with normal saline and a temporary filling placed. The carbon steel would then corrode to a weak iron oxide over the next few weeks, which could be easily instrumented from the canal at a later date. Most instruments these days are made from stainless steel, which does not readily corrode. However, it is a great deal more resistant to fracturing and separation and is more flexible. Nickel titanium, memory metal, is the newest metal being used in some files, such as the Hyflex® X-File™ (Hygenic Corporation, Akron, Ohio), ProFile® Series 29™ (Tulsa Dental Products, Tulsa, Oklahoma), and Onyx™ files (Union Broach, Philadelphia, Pennsylvania). These are more flexible than stainless steel files and have a higher stress tolerance, making them more resistant to fracture. Furthermore, this metal has, to a degree, the ability to return to its original shape when heated and cooled. Metals of this nature are the direction of the future in endodontic armamentariums, but cost and instrument life still need improvement.

The popularity of Hedstrom files in veterinary endodontics has arisen primarily because of their availability in extended shaft lengths of 55 mm and 60 mm. This additional length is necessary in many procedures involving the canine, cuspid, or fang teeth because of their long root structure. The 55-mm H-type files have a standardized D_{16}. The D_{16} is the diameter of the instrument 16 mm from the tip and the end of the operative head in standardized instruments. The 60-mm H-type files currently available have an extended operative head, with the classic D_{16} location being approximately 30 mm from the cutting tip, representing a D_{30} for the end of the operative head. With the continued widening of the diameter to support this longer operative head, the 60-mm instrument has a shaft almost twice the diameter of the 55-mm instrument in the same size. Therefore, these 55-mm and 60-mm H-files are not interchangeable during a procedure. The extended length of operative head has superior effect in the long canine cuspid endodontic canals of some young to adult individuals, but in older animals with their narrow canals, this additional instrument width can sometimes be a problem. The extended operative head instrument (60-mm Hedstrom) has improved carrying capacity, provides a greater tapered preparation, and has had fewer reports of instrument separation or fracture. These variations from the standard are helpful for certain veterinary endodontic cases.

Additionally, there are many innovative developments in human endodontic files that no longer fully correspond to the standards of file size. There are two new types of hand files with novel size changes, other than the 0.05- or 0.10-mm steps of standard files. The first of these new types are half-size files: 12.5, 17.5, 22.5, 27.5, and 32.5 (eg, the Hyflex® X-File™); when used in coordination with standard files, these provide increases in file sizes of no greater than 25% at a step. The other type of hand file is the ProFile® Series 29, which provides a uniform 29% increase between each file size. It is presumed that these variations can provide more gradual and uniform enlargement in the instrumentation procedure of the canal. Another innovation in the ProFile® series is the .04 Taper™ (Tulsa Dental Products), a file that provides a 0.04-mm taper per millimeter of operating head as compared with the 0.02 mm of standard files. At the end of the operating head of a standard file, the shaft diameter is 0.32 mm plus the instrument size (ie, a No.20 file would be 0.52 mm), while a 0.04-mm file has twice the base increase, or 0.64 mm, plus the instrument size. Additionally, there is a .06 Taper™ ProFile® Series 29™, with the possibility of a 0.08-mm file in the future. The ProFile® series are available as both hand and rotary instruments. As time moves on, so do the refinements of endodontic instruments, and the need for changes in the endodontic standards.

Use of H-type and K-type Instruments

Within the canal, K-type files produce a clean smooth surface. In comparison, H-type files, though producing a clean preparation, do not result in as smooth a surface (59). Rotary motion used with files produces a fairly round apical preparation, where push–pull rasping actions are less likely to produce the conical preparation that is generally desired. For this reason, K-type files are usually best used for the cylindrical apical retention preparation, and the H-type files for shaping of the occlusal or incisal flare (60). When files are used in a push–pull action, it is normally best to gently prebend them for use in noticeably curved canals. Acute bends or angles should be avoided, as these stress and fatigue the metal and predispose instruments to premature failure.

There is a great deal of variance in resistance to fracture of root canal files, resulting from design and metal type used. The K-type files have their greatest strength, by design, in a clockwise rotational use. They are more prone to fracture when torsional force is applied in a counterclockwise movement (61). In a counterclockwise rotation of 180°, most K-type files and reamers, with their cutting tip firmly bound, will fail suddenly and in a clean, brittle fashion (62). This differs from the clockwise fractures that show a slow, tearing effect. From this, one might suspect that most file fractures occur when files are used in a counterclockwise manner. This is not the case, however. Clinically, most file failures occur during clockwise usage (63). This is simply because counterclockwise use normally relieves the load effect by unscrewing the flutes from the dentinal walls, whereas clockwise use increases load. H-type files fracture both in rotation and in pulling, when used with excessive force. In most cases, when a file becomes bound in the canal, counterclockwise rotation is the best hope of relieving load and removing the instrument intact.

Condensers and Spreaders

Most condensers and spreaders belong to group I endodontic instruments, with the exception of instruments like the McSpadden Condenser™ and Thermal Lateral Compactor™ (Brasseler Company, Savannah, Georgia), which belong to group II. Hand-held spreaders and condensers of this endodontic group have handles that rest in the entire hand. Finger spreaders and condensers are short instruments, similar in size to the files and reamers of group I, that are held in two or more fingers when used (53) (see Fig. 4).

Condensers, also known as *pluggers*, are flat-ended metal instruments with smooth, round, and very slightly tapered sides. They are used to condense or press filling materials vertically or apically into the root canal. *Spreaders* are round, smooth, tapered metal instruments with a point. They are used for laterally condensing the filling material by spreading or pushing it against the walls of the canal (53).

Groups II and III

Engine-Driven Root Canal Instruments

Due to the hazards of instrument fracture and root perforation or fracture, engine-driven instruments have not been widely advocated in the United States (53). However, with new developments in this area, there has been rekindled interest.

Group II endodontic instruments are two-part shaft and operative head, engine-driven instruments (53). Currently, in veterinary endodontics, the only two instruments of this group in common use are the paste fillers (lentula and G-spring) and the McSpadden Compactors™ (Fig. 5). The *paste filler* is used to mechanically pump and distribute cements and fillers down into the root canal and chamber. The *McSpadden Compactor*™ is used to thermoplasticize gutta-percha, while condensing it apically and laterally. Care should be observed in proper use of these instruments. If engaged in reverse and placed into the canal, they act like a corkscrew and either fracture or penetrate the apex. If an instrument enters the apex, it can physically spread the root tip, resulting in vertical fracture of the root structure, an extremely difficult problem to overcome.

Group III endodontic instruments are engine-driven, with a one-part shaft and operative head (53) (see Fig. 5). Of these, only two are currently being used to any extent in veterinary services, the *G-reamer* (*Gates-Glidden*) and the *P-reamer* (*Peeso*). They are

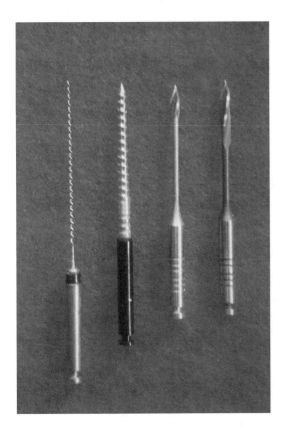

FIG. 5. Group II endodontic instruments. *(Left to right)* Lentula spiral filler, McSpadden compactor, Gates-Glidden drill, Peeso reamer.

primarily used in the enlargement of the canal in its coronal third. On occasion, the G-type reamer is used to aid in removal of gutta-percha from the coronal part of the canal in restorative procedures. The delicate shaft size of these instruments lends to swift fracture and failure, should the tip become bound when mechanically engaged.

Group IV

Absorbent Paper Points

Absorbent points are cones of porous paper (Fig. 6), used to dry the canal after instrumentation (53). They may also be used to apply medicaments or small amounts of irrigants. This is done by dipping the point in the solution and then placing it within the canal. A hemostat or other instrument can then be used to squeeze the exposed end to aid in evacuating the material within the canal. In some cases, these points may be temporarily sealed within the canal.

Silver Points

Silver points are cones of silver metal (53) (see Fig. 6). Metals were used for endodontic filling as early as 1757, when gold and lead were employed.

In addition to its physical properties, silver has a bactericidal effect, referred to as its oligodynamic property. This also refers to its toxic effect on living cells. It is generally accepted that it is the silver salts that are toxic to tissues. These salts form during corrosion. Silver chloride and silver carbonate or silver oxide are the primary salts of corrosion. Most sealers are noncorrosive to silver and even help to protect the cones. Silver points within the canal have little problem, but if they extend through the apex into the periapical tissues, corrosion is common. Toxicity of tissues by silver-point corrosion products has been reported (64). This deterioration of the metal results in alteration to a softer black form that fails to provide good core support to the sealer cements.

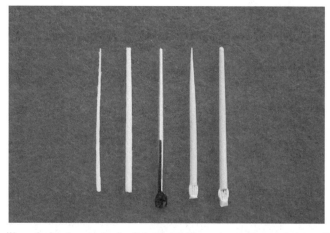

FIG. 6. Group III endodontic point. *(Left to right)* Type 1 paper point, type 2 (standardized) paper point, silver point; type 1 gutta-percha point, type 2 (standardized) gutta-percha point.

The use of silver points in endodontics led to the manufacture of tapered cones designed to match the shaping of the canal. They are available in sizes approximating file sizes. Their use has declined in popularity over the last 20 years, in comparison with use of gutta-percha points.

Gutta-Percha Points

Gutta-percha, an exudate of mazer trees and sometimes called mazer wood, is collected, treated, and mixed to form cones manufactured to approximate the prepared endodontic canals (see Fig. 6). Use of these products is regulated by ADA Specification No.78, and they are available in two basic types of cones: standard (type I) and conventional (type II). *Type I (standard) points* correspond to the sizes of standard endodontic instruments and are used as primary or master points. *Type II (conventional) points* have a taper similar to that of endodontic spreaders and are used as accessory points in lateral compaction. Conventional points have been reported in use as a root canal filling material as early as 1865 (56). Most gutta-percha points have 15–22% gutta-percha and 56–79% zinc oxide, with the remainder being a combination of heavy metal sulfates, waxes, and resins. The viscoelastic state of gutta-percha allows better conformation to natural variations in root canal topography than that of ridged silver point.

Chloroform, eucalyptol, and xylol are common solvents for gutta-percha. Solvent techniques, used to soften gutta-percha, have demonstrated their ability to closely replicate the canal and its intricacies. However, as much of the solvent is lost by percolation within a few weeks, the dimensional stability of the gutta-percha may be lost as shrinkage occurs (65). Therefore, the less solvent used, the less shrinkage would be expected to occur, and the less chance of dimensional deviation. Gutta-percha has a very low cytotoxicity, and once solvents have dissipated, it is the least toxic to tissues of all endodontic materials currently in use (66,67).

As gutta-percha points or cones age, they can become brittle and useless due to alteration in crystalline formations (68) accelerated by light and heat (69,70). This is thought to be a tendency of the actual gutta-percha to change back toward a more natural, brittle alpha state from the softer beta form. No apparent difference in the mechanical properties of the alpha and beta forms are generally observed. However, there are thermal flow, volumetric, and handling differences between the two (71). Storage of cones in dark, dry, cool environments and good management of stocks can reduce cone problems; nevertheless, occasions may arise when aged points may need to be used. Rejuvenation of brittle gutta-percha points to a pliable state can be attempted by immersing the cone in water above 55°C until it begins to soften. It is then plunged into cold water for several seconds (68). Studies have indicated that due to variations in the manufacture of cones, only about 30% are suited for rejuvenation (72).

Instrumentation Aids

Irrigants and Associated Devices

Irrigants are essential in aiding the gross debridement, reduction of microbes, dissolution of necrotic tissue and tissue remnants, and removal of the smear layer. The pulp cavity is an intricate and complicated system that cannot be cleaned in all areas by instruments (Fig. 7). The solutions have been used to aid in debriding the canal for many years

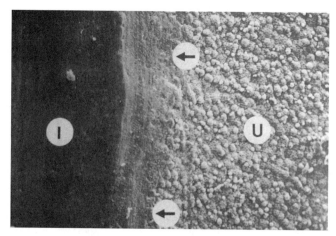

FIG. 7. The junction *(arrows)* between the instrumented *(I)* and uninstrumented *(U)* halves of the canal wall (original magnification ×4080). (Reproduced from Baumgartner JC, Mader CL. A scanning electron microscope evaluation of four root canal irrigation regimens. *J Endod* 1987;13:154, with permission.)

(73). The *law of diffusion* states that "when two or more liquids capable of being mixed are placed together, a spontaneous exchange of molecules takes place in defiance of the Law of Gravity" (74). It is further theorized that it is a *chemomechanical* action that allows these solutions to be effective. This is the chemical cleansing effect combined with instrumentation and the actual mechanical flushing action that loosens and removes materials from the canal. Sodium hypochlorite 5.25% (bleach) aids in dissolving organic debris and destroying bacteria (75). Many practitioners use bleach that is diluted to half strength, or even less for safety reasons. This does reduce both its dissolving effect on organic debris and its antibacterial properties (76). Use of an ethylenediaminetetraacetic acid (EDTA)–urea peroxidase gel (RC-Prep™, ESPE-Premier Corporation, Norristown, Pennsylvania) complements this action, with the urea aiding in bacterial destruction and the EDTA helping dissolve inorganic debris by chelation (77–79). This combination of action helps clean out the smear layer of debris found in the dentinal tubules of an instrumented canal. The alternate use of both solutions appears to produce the most debris-free and cleanest dentinal surface (80–81) (Fig. 8). Copious amounts of a normal sterile saline solution also greatly assist in irrigation.

There are three major considerations with endodontic irrigation. The first is supplying sufficient volumes of irrigant to the working area of the canal. Second is the removal of the expended fluid and debris from the root canal. And third is preventing extrusion of irrigant and other materials beyond the apex into the periapical tissues.

The use of irrigation needles and syringes is important for properly carrying irrigants into the canal and aiding in removal of dentinal chips and debris that can accumulate during instrumentation. Use of endodontic irrigation needles reduces the risk of irrigants and other materials being forced through the apex. This is particularly important when full- or half-strength sodium hypochlorite (bleach) is used as an irrigant, because apical extrusion of this solution can cause severe pain (79,82). There are two basic types of irrigation needles currently in use in veterinary endodontics. The first type has a blunted tip with one side of the tip removed 4–5 mm back toward the hub. The second type of irrigation needle has a blunt, sealed tip with a side window perforation into the lumen of the nee-

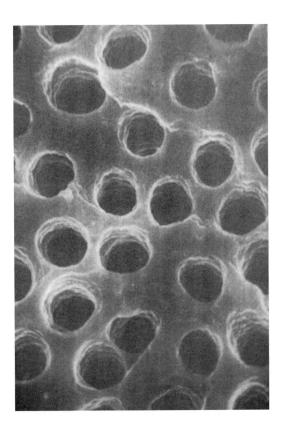

FIG. 8. Sodium hypochlorite and EDTA used alternately regimen. The instrumented half of the canal wall. Note the clean, smoothly planed appearance of the canal wall and the sharply defined orifices of the dentinal tubules (original magnification ×4080). (Reproduced from Baumgartner JC, Mader CL. A scanning electron microscope evaluation of four root canal irrigation regimens. *J Endod* 1987;13:154, with permission.)

dle. These are both designed to allow escape of the irrigating fluids and debris from the apical region by flowing laterally around the needle and out the access site. This type of engineering helps prevent the forceful extrusion of material through the tooth apex.

The inadvertent extrusion of irrigant solutions beyond the apex into the apical tissues during endodontic procedures has resulted in severe injuries (82,83). The degree of reaction is highly dependent on the toxicity of the irrigant, the volume injected, and the location in relationship to nerves, vessels, and osseous canals. Generally, the irrigation needle should be immediately replaced into the canal with syringe attached, and the canal should be aspirated to remove any remaining irrigant. Next, the canal should be rinsed and irrigated with copious amounts of normal saline. In cases concerning bleach, serious delayed pain problems can arise. Therefore, postoperative pain medications should be made available in case of need.

Irrigation needles are sometimes used to aid in drying the canal following irrigation. They should be used to aspirate fluids and never to blow them from the canal. Fatal consequences have been reported from the blowing of compressed air into the open root canals of human (84) and animal (56,85) teeth, resulting in air embolisms. The proximity of the dental site of initiation of the air emboli to the brain appears to be one of the major contributors to the possibility more serious consequences. Should air accidentally be injected in a patient, the head should be immediately lowered and the feet elevated, as air bubbles tend to rise in a fluid and the objective is to keep the emboli as far away as possible from major organs. The frequency of this complication in veterinary endodontics is low. One reason for this may be the combination of the more solid canal apex of a delta in animals as compared to the human foramina and the fact that most veterinary patients are in lateral or dorsal recumbency with their head lowered.

Sonics and Ultrasonics

Endodontic ultrasonic and sonic handpieces have had mixed acceptance since their introduction in 1957 (86,87). They greatly enhance canal cleaning with irrigation solutions (88) but have demonstrated poor canal-shaping efficiency (11). Enhancement of cleaning is due to heating of the solutions and a resonant vibration effect known as acoustic streaming, which was previously considered a cavitation phenomenon (89). Some specialized ultrasonic units have successfully been used for apical resectioning procedures (86).

Automated Mechanical Endodontic Handpieces

Automatic endodontic handpieces are low-speed contra-angles that make use of attached broaches or files to power-mechanically instrument the canal (90). With the Giromatic™ (Micro-Mega, Prodonta SA, Geneva, Switzerland), the files reciprocate back and forth at approximately quarter turns or 90° rotations at about 1,800 rpm (91). It was originally designed to reduce operator fatigue and accelerate instrumentation. The loss of tactile sense, seen with most power instruments, leads to additional risks of instrument breakage, overinstrumentation, and perforation of the apex (92). These instruments should be used clinically only after proper training.

Aids to Measurement

Accurate measurement of the root canal for instrumentation has always been a problem in endodontics. The ability to measure and know canal working lengths aids in keeping instrumentation within the confines of the root canal. Many devices have been manufactured to help with this problem. Sunada (93) in 1962 proposed a method of measuring root canal length based on iontophoresis studies by Suzuki in 1942 (94). The units have been termed electronic locators or *apex locators*. Reports of clinical accuracy vary from 50% to as high as 89%, with some manufacturers claiming much higher accuracy. Additionally, many experienced dental operators working on humans have demonstrated a digital-tactile sense for accurately detecting the apical constriction, without radiographic aids, 60% of the time (56). However, historically, radiography has been the technique of choice.

Electronic root canal measuring devices (*ERCMs*) were first theorized by Suzuki, based on a theory of electrical resistance difference between two probes (94). The theory is that when one probe is attached to oral soft tissue and the other inserted in the canal, a difference of resistance can be measured until the probe in the canal approaches the apex and the soft tissue of the periapical periodontal tissue. The two probes will have no difference in resistance when both are contacting soft tissue. Although some researchers have agreed with this theory of ERCMs' function (95,96), others believe it is a simple physical contact phenomenon (97).

Although these devices are constantly being upgraded, they still have limitations in that they cannot give accurate reading in the presence of conductive tissues or fluids. This means that pulp tissue, pus, and irrigation fluids in the canal can distort readings.

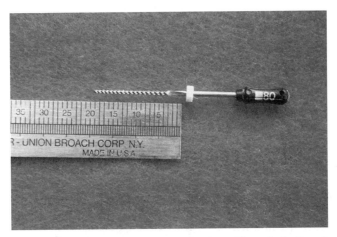

FIG. 9. Endodontic stop on file, measuring with endodontic ruler.

However, at least one study has indicated that calculating the impedance ratio between the two probe frequencies can greatly reduce errors due to fluids in the canal (98). Additional errors with ERCMs can occur when the probe size and apical opening are highly diverse, such as a small file probe and a large or blunderbuss apex (99). In addition, erroneous readings will result if the probe makes contact with the periodontal ligament through perforations or lateral canals or if the exposed probe surface should contact metal restorations. For these reasons, ERCMs should generally not be used as the sole means of length determination, but to reduce the overall number of radiographs needed for a root canal procedure.

In radiographic assessment, a probe is inserted into the canal to the apical constriction as determined by digital-tactile sense. It is then either bent at the occlusal or incisal access as a reference point or a radiopaque endodontic stop is used. A radiograph is then taken. The actual length of the tooth (TA) can then be determined by measuring the radiographic image of the tooth (TR) and the instrument (IR) and then the actual length of the instrument (IA), and using the following mathematical formula:

$$TA = (IA \times TR)/IR$$

Many types of *endodontic stops* are available. Most are color-coded, small circular pieces of rubber or plastic. Directional endodontic stops are fundamentally the same but have a small point on one side. Some operators make their own endodontic stops by using a paper punch, leather punch, or rubber-dam punch on rubber bands of various sizes and colors. The stop is placed on a file or reamer by gently forcing the instrument tip through it. Once the working length of the canal has been determined, the stop can be placed on each file exactly to working length, with help of an endodontic ruler (Fig. 9). This is done to prevent the instrument from passing through the apex and to prevent failure to instrument to full depth.

ENDODONTIC TRIAD

The objectives of endodontic therapy are to address the discomfort and infection from the tooth and periapical tissues by removing the affected canal contents and providing an adequate obliteration of the canal(s) with specific filling materials. This is all accomplished by first understanding and implementing basic endodontic principles and adhering to the *endodontic triad*: preparation, sterilization, and obturation of the pulp cavity (77).

Preparation

The primary goal in preparation is to instrument the canal to create a shape that will allow it to be filled completely (100). Preparation includes accessing and then shaping the canal.

Access deals with the fundamental choice of the site of tooth approach and pulp cavity entry. Its purpose in endodontic therapy is to establish an unrestricted passageway from the crown through the pulp cavity to the apical stricture or the internal commencement of the apical delta (101). An unimpeded pathway to the apex must be customized to facilitate suitable instrumentation and obturation of the root canal in accordance with the specific tooth type and the individuality of the pulp cavity. This should not be misinterpreted to suggest that the most direct route from crown to apex is the proper access. Use of the *access triad* is one way to achieve an unrestricted access to the apex (102). The triad is merely the sequence of chamber access, root canal access, and stricture access—in that order. Each access in the sequence, when properly accomplished, facilitates the pathway to the next, until the apical stricture is reached. The goal of access design is to gain full working length to the stricture for instrumentation, while providing for obturation of the apical third of the canal to be as uncomplicated and complete as possible (102).

Many technical complications confronted in endodontic treatment can be diminished or prevented with appropriate access preparation. One of the cornerstones of proper dentistry has always been the conservation of tooth structure; nevertheless, this should never be allowed to overly influence site selection or design of the access entry (101). This is not to imply that coronal structure should be removed indiscriminately. However, to correctly implement access, it does suggest the necessity for a competent knowledge of the pulp cavity and external root anatomy and the capability to properly analyze radiographic details (36,103). It can be an invitation to unnecessary complications when these basic concepts are not understood and employed.

Unsound tooth or restorative structure that is in the line of access is best removed prior to the initiation of endodontic treatment. In addition to improving visibility, this preemptive action assists in maintaining asepsis and allows a more complete evaluation of restorative requirements prior to root canal therapy (101,102). Failure to remove all diseased structure prior to opening of the access can lead to debris or contaminates falling or being carried into the canal. If restorations are incompletely removed, materials such as composite or amalgam can unintentionally be transported into the root canal. Attempts to use standard instrumentation to remove the material typically leads to the material's being pushed farther into the canal or being packed into the apical third, where, if not removed, it may prevent achieving a proper apical seal. (Techniques for removal of material trapped in the root canal system are discussed in Chapter 12.)

Failure to establish proper access to the pulp chamber and root canals is one of the most common complicating factors in root canal therapy for veterinary practitioners (102). The pulp chamber is generally situated in the central portion of the crown, with the root canals tending to be near the center of the root. However, each pulp cavity is individual in its confines and is dynamic in that it changes during the tooth's vital life. The pulp cavity in vital teeth diminishes in size with age due to secondary dentinal develop-

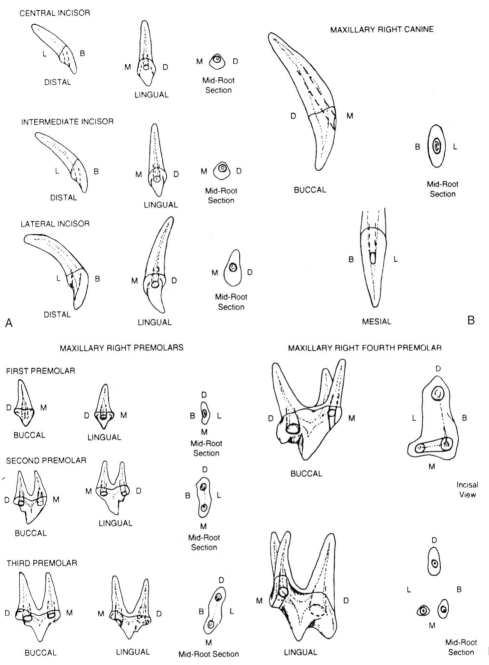

FIG. 10. Endodontic access: **(A)** Maxillary right incisors. **(B)** Maxillary right canine. **(C)** Maxillary right premolars. **(D)** Maxillary right 4th premolar. (For an alternative method to retain more tooth structure, see description of transcoronal approach.) **(E)** Maxillary right molars. **(F)** Mandibular right incisors. **(G)** Mandibular right canine. **(H)** Mandibular right premolars. **(I)** Mandibular right 1st molar. **(J)** Mandibular right molars. (Reproduced from Visser CJ. Coronal access of the canine dentition. *J Vet Dent* 1991;8(4):12, with permission.)

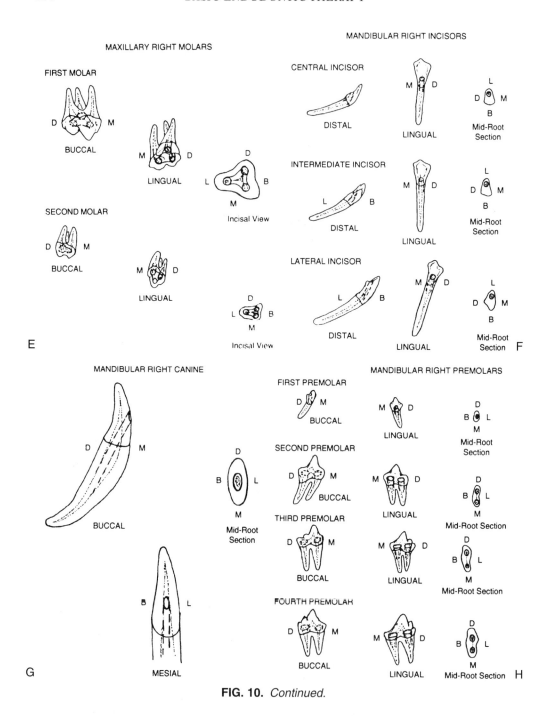

FIG. 10. *Continued.*

ment. Additionally, irritation to the pulp from caries, cervical line lesions, and restorative procedures can lead to dimensional changes at the point of the disturbance due to tertiary or reparative dentin deposition internally. Diagnostic dental radiographs, although only two dimensional, are essential to properly assess the anatomic relationship between crown and root, angle of the root within the arch, and the general condition and position

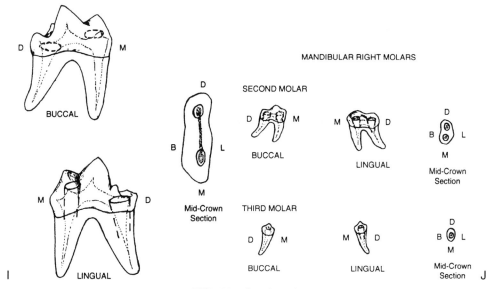

FIG. 10. *Continued.*

of the pulp cavity (104). With abnormalities of the crown or root configuration or with rotation of teeth, radiographs commonly must be angled from mesial or distal aspects to provide the anatomic information required. Use of two-dimensional radiographs for a three-dimensional tooth can occasionally be misleading as to access. Therefore, several views should be taken to reduce the chance of deceptive information.

Even though each tooth must be evaluated as an distinct individual, certain generalities may be drawn as to the characteristic position of approach to the access of teeth in the dog (Fig. 10). One rule of thumb is to avoid making an access opening directly over or through incisal edges, cusp tips, or other developmental ridges or margins, as such openings may predispose to vertical fractures. Typically, the entrance to the incisors is made on the central lingual facet of the crown 1–2 mm above the free gingival margin. However, a labial approach, similarly positioned, can be used, but due to esthetic considerations, it is not in common use. The cuspid or canine teeth can be accessed 1–2 mm from the free gingival margin on the mesial aspect, which allows a more direct line of access to the apex. Individual canals of premolars with two roots may have the access openings made on the buccal or facial surface over the center of each root near the cusp's margin, as confirmed by palpation of the alveolar juga and radiographs. Access to the mandibular 1st molars is basically the same, except that the approach is most commonly made from the lingual aspect. The two-rooted molars have access achieved on the occlusal surface directly over the roots to be entered, with care to avoid cusp tips. The novice will find that the maxillary 4th premolar provides a slight challenge in the access to the mesial roots, especially the palatal. Whereas the distal root access is fundamentally the same as with other premolars, a *transcoronal approach* is the easiest for the mesial roots (105) (Fig. 11). Access to these roots is determined, through a mental extrapolation, by palpation of the mesiobuccal root juga and comparison of the actual location of the mesiopalatal root's cusp tip. The actual opening is generally made between these two determined points and approximately 2–4 mm above the gingival margin on the buccal aspect of the tooth (102). The maxillary molars are three-rooted and may be accessed

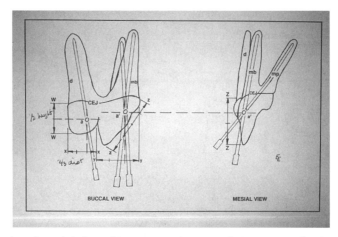

FIG. 11. Buccal and mesial view of transcoronal approach to access of pulp cavity of maxillary 4th premolar. (Reproduced from ref. 105, with permission.)

with a Y- or V-shaped opening on the occlusal surface that exposes each individual canal system (102). The first access point is usually made directly over the lingual or palatal root, with extension of the access with a high-speed bur and following the chamber to expose the two buccal root canals. Straight-line access of the buccal roots must be done cautiously as periodically perforation of the floor of the chamber occurs due to root angulation. In addition, the V- or Y-shaped access aids in the early detection of ribbon canals associated with fused distal and palatal roots, which are not uncommon in the maxillary 1st and 2nd molars (Fig. 12).

If the *pulp cavity is calcified* or reduced in size and poorly visible on radiographs, access approach may be directed to the largest compartment of the chamber or root canal radiographically detectable (106). In cases of diminished pulp chamber space, there is an old adage: "Go for the horns" (101). It is a reasonable doctrine only if the practitioner

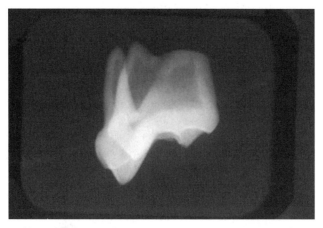

FIG. 12. Radiographic appearance of maxillary 1st molar with fused buccomesial and palatal roots, exhibiting ribbon canal.

understands that the pulp horns represent only a small part of the pulp chamber along its upper and lateral borders. The *pulp horns* are the generally pointed projections of the pulp chamber within the crown and are customarily the most coronal and proximal portions of the system. Once the horn is accessed, it is anticipated that the remainder of the chamber will be evident and access to the root canals can be traced from that location. When these basic guidelines are not satisfactorily followed, problems with failure to locate all canals, excessive structural removal, floor gouging, and perforations of the chamber walls or floor may result (107).

Once access is attained, the type of canal instrumentation must be decided on. There are many types of instrumentation for specific situations, such as *anticurvature filing* for curved canals (see Chapter 12), but two basic styles of root canal instrumentation–shaping procedures are currently in use (108) (Fig. 13). The first is the standard or rigid-core technique, which was developed primarily for silver points but is commonly used with gutta-percha. The second is known as a tapered, flared, serial, telescoping, or funneling technique, which can be instrumented in a step-back or step-down procedure.

In *standard root canal instrumentation*, once cavity access is established, a probe or pathfinder can be used to determine the exact opening location and the general shape and depth of the canal. Next, an appropriate-size barbed broach is inserted. The broach is rotated 180° to entangle the pulp tissue and debris. It is then gently pulled from the canal with the entangled pulp. If the pulp material separates and fails to be removed intact, the

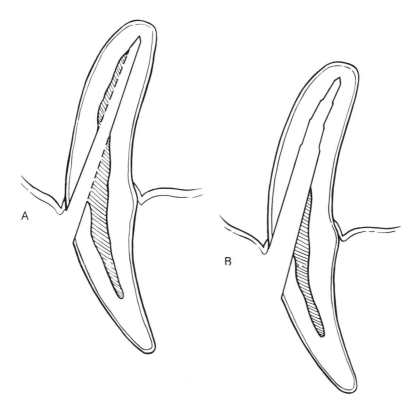

FIG. 13 (A) Standard or rigid-core technique. **(B)** Tapered, flared, serial, telescoping, or funneling technique.

procedure may be repeated. The canal can now be flushed once it is confirmed that the apex is closed, alternately with 4–6% sodium hypochlorite and sterile saline, using an endodontic irrigation needle and syringe. A probe with an endodontic stop is placed in the canal, by digital-tactile sense, to the apical constricture. The stop is slid down the probe or small-size file to make contact with the incisal or occlusal tooth margin for use as a reference point. A radiograph is taken to confirm that the instrument is reaching the apical stricture. *Working length* is then measured from the endodontic stop to the instrument tip using an endodontic ruler.

At this point, working length has been determined by measurement calculations. Most operators will attempt to stay 1–2 mm short of the root apex in apical foramina and level with the apical stricture in apical deltas. According to the length and shape of the canal, the correct type file is then selected for instrumentation. *Endodontic stops* are applied to the files and positioned with the assistance of an endodontic ruler at the appropriate working length. The smallest size file is used first. The file may be coated with a chelating agent (eg, RC-Prep®) that also acts as a lubricant during instrumentation. The file is then inserted into the canal to the working length and is used in a rotation-and-pull or pull-only action, according to the type of file selected. Once that instrument is moving in a smooth, free action, the next size file should be used. Between each file size, the complete irrigation process should be repeated. At the juncture when the file lightly binds at the working tip, the canal should be instrumented to at least three sizes larger. Once this point is reached, a final irrigation should be performed. Next, the canal should be dried using absorbent points. The canal is now ready for obturation. *Obturation* is the final and complete filling and sealing of the root canal system.

Studies indicate that flared, telescoped, or tapered types of preparations possibly permit better debridement and superior obturation and seal (109). In *tapered root canal instrumentation*, the preparation is treated in the same fashion as the standard preparation, except the apical foramen is handled in a more conservative manner. The apical constricture is instrumented to only a size 25 (110). The coronal portion of the canal is then serially widened with Gates-Glidden drills or files in a telescoping style. A No.3 Gates-Glidden drill is inserted into a moist canal at a moderate rate of speed, until light resistance is felt. The drill is then removed, never approaching closer than 5 mm from the apex. The same procedure is repeated with a No.4 Gates-Glidden drill, with care taken to penetrate 1 mm less than the previous drill. The process is repeated with a No.5 Gates-Glidden drill. The canal is then recapitulated to working length with the No.25 file to clean debris. Each file size larger is then placed 1 mm shorter than the last one, as the operator backs out of the canal from the working length (back-stepping). The canal should be recapitulated with the No.25 file to full working length between each size change and back-step. The serial withdrawal should continue to the site of the widening done with the Gates-Glidden drills or to a size 50 file, which ever comes first. The same result can be obtained by working from the crown down in the serial stepping of sizes, once the working length is filed to proper size. This is known as down-stepping, and some reports indicate that it results in less material being forced through the apex (111).

Sterilization

Sterilization of the canal is accomplished during preparation through instrumentation and irrigation. The files cut and remove a portion of the dentinal walls, carrying it free of the canal, while at the same time they remove a large part of the bacterial population inhabiting this space and material. Irrigants, chelators, and lubricants, such as 2% hydrogen peroxide, 2.5–5.25% sodium hypochlorite, urea peroxidase products, and even sterile saline, all actively aid in sterilizing the canal. It has been suggested that the law of diffusion and chemomechanical actions allow these products to reach where instruments cannot to remove debris and bacteria (79).

Sterilization of instruments and obturating materials placed into the canal must also be taken into consideration. Instruments and burs should be autoclaved or sterilized. Bead sterilizers can be used to quickly sterilize the working end of the majority of instruments. Most bead sterilizers attain a temperature of 218-271°C or 424-536°F and sterilize within 5–15 seconds (35). Gutta-percha and silver points are both relatively sterile when removed from packaging, but to assure sterility gutta-percha can be dipped in full-strength bleach (5.25% sodium hypochlorite) for 60 seconds and then rinsed in sterile saline (88). Silver cones can be sterilized in the bead sterilizer. Thermoplasticized gutta-percha is ordinarily well sterilized by the heat used to soften the material.

Packs and sets of instruments can be sterilized by numerous methods. The more common are steam under pressure, dry heat, rapid laminar flow heat, chemical solutions, chemical vapors, and gas, each of which has advantages and disadvantages both to instruments and ability to monitor effectiveness. Some less commonly used are formaldehyde gas, formaldehyde solutions, microwaves, ultraviolet light, gamma rays, x-radiation, laser beam, and electron bombardment. The repeated proper sterilization of good-quality stainless steel endodontic instruments does not result in corrosion, weakness, or an increased rate of fracture from rotation (14).

Obturation

All the efforts of preparation and sterilization are useless without providing a complete sealing and obturation of the canal (112). An apical wall, constricture or apical stop is needed to help obtain a good seal. One study estimated that up to 60% of endodontic failures are the result of incomplete obturation of the canal space (113). A canal must be densely and entirely filled in all its anatomic complexities with a biocompatible hermetic sealing agent to prevent microleakage of microbes in or out of the tooth and to preclude reinfection (78).

The material used to fill the root canal should have certain basic characteristics. The following list is adapted and slightly modified from that by Grossman et al (114):

1. Easily manipulated and placed, and allowing adequate working time prior to setting up.
2. Dimensionally stable: no shrinkage or expansion after compaction.
3. Conformable and adaptable to the various shapes and contours of the canal, while sealing it apically and laterally.
4. Nonirritating to periapical tissues.
5. Nonporous, impervious to moisture.
6. Unaffected and insoluble in tissue fluids; incapable of corroding or oxidizing.
7. Bacteriostatic or nonsupportive of bacterial growth.
8. Radiographically evident dimensions and density irregularities.
9. Nonstaining to dental or peridental structures.
10. Sterile or easily and quickly sterilized for immediate insertion.
11. Removable without difficulty, when necessary.
12. Biologically nonharmful.

An ideal root canal sealer cement should also have certain characteristics. The following characteristics are modified from Nguyen (115):

1. Tacky when mixed and having good adhesion to the canal walls and core material.
2. Having ample setting time for placement and adjustment.
3. Capable of producing a hermetic seal.
4. Having an appropriate particle size for easy mixing with liquid component.
5. Radiographically evident.
6. Capable of maintaining dimensions or slightly expanding on setting, but not shrinking.
7. Bacteriostatic.
8. Biologically compatible; nonirritating to the periapical tissues or dangerous to remote tissues or organs.
9. Insoluble in oral tissue fluids.
10. Nonstaining to tooth or peridental structures and tissues.
11. Soluble in common solvents for removal, if required.
12. Not stimulative of immune responses in or through the periapical tissues.
13. Not mutagenic or carcinogenic.
14. When fresh, acting as a lubricant to aid in placement and seating of the primary and auxiliary cones into the canal.
15. Acting as a filler for discrepancies between cones, as well as between cones and canal.

Gutta-percha in combination with sealer cements is generally accepted as coming closest to fulfilling most of the above criteria, although newer products are being researched and produced (115). The root canal should be obliterated by these products from the apical constricture to the neck of the tooth. The coronal portion of the tooth may be filled with restorative materials, such as composite or glass ionomers, to provide additional structural strength and prevent contamination by the oral fluids.

ADA Specification No.57 provides the basic guidelines for endodontic sealing materials and classifies them as type I and type II endodontic sealers (53). *Type I* materials are sealer cements used with a core material such as gutta-percha. Zinc oxide and eugenol combinations are possibly the most common of this group. Many types of sealer cements are available, from noneugenol products such as Sealapex™ (Kerr Manufacturing, Romulus, Michigan) to those containing calcium hydroxide compounds such as CRCS™ (Hygenic Corporation) (Table 2). Some noneugenol sealers contain epoxy resins (AH-26, L.D. Caulk Company, Milford, Delaware) or polyvinyl resins (Diaket, ESPE-Premier Corporation). Most are very good products, making species, type of procedure, and operator preference the determining choice of products. One compound that may be seen incorporated into sealer cements in the near future is mineral trioxide aggregate (MTA, Tulsa Dental Products), which has shown some promise. *Type II endodontic sealers* are materials that are used without core materials or additional sealer cements. Some endodontic glass ionomers can be used in this fashion.

A simple yet effective type I sealer cement frequently used in veterinary dentistry is zinc oxide–eugenol (ZOE). A small amount of zinc oxide powder [USP] is placed on a mixing slab or paper, followed by a few drops of eugenol liquid [USP]. The liquid is gradually incorporated into the powder with a small flexible cement spatula, until a creamy consistency is obtained. The cement is correctly mixed when a one-inch string can be drawn out between the pad and spatula. The cement may be introduced into the canal on the master (or next size smaller) file as it is spun counterclockwise to coat the apex and lateral walls. A spiral filler on a reduction slow-speed gear may also be used to "pump" the sealer cement into the canal. With larger canals, the material may even be injected,

TABLE 2. *Partial listing of endodontic sealer cements*[a]

Type I
  Zinc oxide–eugenol sealer cements
    CRCS (Calciobiotic) (Hygenic Corporation, Akron, Ohio, 1982)
    Grossman's Sealer Cement (Grossman, 1974)
    Kerr Sealer (Rickert, 1931)
    Proco-Sol Non-Staining (Grossman, 1958)(Star Dental
      Manufacturing Company, Lancaster, Pennsylvania)
    Proco-Sol Silver Cement (Grossman, 1936)
    Rickert's Sealer (Kerr Manufacturing, Romulus, Michigan)
    Super EBA with Alumina (Harry J. Bosworth Company, Skokie,
      Illinois)
    Tubli-Seal (Kerr, 1961)
    Wach's Paste (Wach, 1925)(Sultan Chemicals, Englewood,
      New Jersey)
    ZOE (Zinc Oxide–Eugenol [USP]) Paste
  Noneugenol sealer cements
    AH-26, 1957) (L.D. Caulk Company, Milford, Delaware)
    Chlorapercha (Moyco/Union Broach, Philadelphia, Pennsylvania)
    Diaket (Schmitt, 1951) (ESPE-Premier Corporation, Norristown,
      Pennsylvania)
    Glass ionomers
    Ketac Endo (ESPE-Premier Corporation)
    Kloroperka N-O (Nygaard-Ostby, 1939)
    NOgenol (Coe Laboratories, Chicago, Illinois)
    Polycarboxylate cements
    Sealapex (Kerr Manufacturing)
  Therapeutic sealer cements
    CRCS (Calciobiotic) (Hygenic Corporation)
    Sealapex (Kerr Manufacturing)
Type II
  Therapeutic canal core dressings
    Calasept (J.S. Dental Manufacturing)
    Calcium hydroxide [USP] pastes
    Hypo-Cal (Ellman International, Hewlett, New York)
    Procal (3M Dental Products Company, St. Paul, Minnesota)
    Root-Cal (Ellman International)
    Temp-Canal (Pulpdent Corporation, Watertown, Massachusetts)
    T.E.R.M. (L.D. Caulk Company)
  Canal sealer/core combinations
    Chlorapercha (Moyco/Union Broach)
    Hydron (1978) (NPD Dental Systems)
    Ketac Endo (ESPE-Premier Corporation)
    Kloroperka N-O (Nygaard-Ostby, 1939)
    PCA (variant of Wach's Paste)(Pulpdent Corporation)
    Polycarboxylate sealer cements
    Wach's Paste (Young Dental, Earth City, Missouri)
    ZOE (Zinc Oxide/Eugenol [USP]) Pastes
  Medicated canal sealer/cores
    Endomethasone
    N2 (Sargenti, 1970)
    RC2B
    Riebler's Paste
    Sargenti's Paste
    TCM (Sargenti 1973)

---

[a] Some products may qualify for several categories according to ingredients and the material's usage.

but air bubbles should be avoided. In core or cone techniques it is essential to use a sealer cement, yet minimizing its volume by maximizing the amount of core filling material that approximates the canal shape (78).

Medicated Sealer Cements

In addition to the standard types of endodontic sealers, there is a group that contains various medicaments. These vary from the addition of iodoform to the use of mercury, lead, paraformaldehyde, and other compounds. Proponents of these materials emphasize speed and simplicity. However, due to biocompatability and safety concerns, the materials and techniques for their use have not been advocated by any dental school in the United States, the ADA, or the Food and Drug Administration (116).

Sargenti paste (N-2), endomethasone, and Reibler's paste are a few of the better known of this group of materials, some of which contain paraformaldehyde, a powerful but toxic antiseptic that fixes tissue. The use of corticosteroids as an auxiliary component has been introduced in some of these materials, in the hope of reducing the toxic effects. The addition of lead tetroxide is also common in some of these sealers. Lead greatly increases the sealer's radiopacity and its hardness on setting. This can produce radiographic images that appear well compacted but that can hide large voids. Furthermore, the use of heavy metals carries the additional potential concerns of their dissemination throughout the body to organs remote from the teeth (117).

The potential consequences can be severe if these chemicals are extruded or percolate beyond the confines of the tooth. This should discourage prudent practitioners from their use in standard endodontic procedures, without careful deliberation and client knowledge of potential risks.

Obturation Techniques

There are numerous ways to obturate the canal. Among them are the single-cone method, lateral compaction, vertical compaction, thermomechanical obturation, thermoplastic obturation, chemoplastic obturation, and the paste method. No one method is reliable and recommended for all cases; instead, the clinician should be versatile and proficient in several. No matter how the core material is placed, the primary objective is to completely obturate the canal, especially the apical one-third.

The *single-cone method* is performed in one of two ways: custom-instrumenting the canal to fit a specific size of prefabricated cone or custom-fabricating the cone to fit the canal. The instrumentation of the canal to fit the cone was originally developed for the stiff silver points and was called *rigid-core technique*, but now gutta-percha is more commonly used. The canal is instrumented to the exact size of the type of core used. The sealer cement is used to obtain the apical seal and fill irregularities of the canal. Once the canal is instrumented, a gutta-percha point is inserted for a trial fit and checked for tug-back (115). *Tug-back* is the slight back-pull or resistance to dislodgement of the cone that is felt when it is removed from the canal. If coming from the apical third, this tug-back would be an indication of a good fit. However, irregularities in the upper portions of the system may give a false tug-back sign. For this reason, it is still best to confirm proper fit radiographically. No shrinkage of the core material should be experienced in this method, although eventual loss of sealer cement can occur.

Due to irregularities or size, some canals cannot be instrumented to provide a proper fit for a specific size of prefabricated cone. In some of these cases, *fabrication of a customized single master gutta-percha cone* to fit the canal may be possible (118). Three or more gutta-percha points are heated over a flame and twisted together with all points in the same direction. The warmed points can be placed between two glass slabs held at a slight angle and rolled into a single cone of the required size. Trial fit of the cone while still warm with a light apical pressure can increase the conformation of the fit. If additional cone adaptation is required, the tip can be dipped in chloroform for 1–6 seconds, and the cone can be replaced, with light pumping of it down into the canal. The procedure is repeated until working length and adaptation are suitable. When the cone properly fits the canal, it can be marked at its coronal access with a plugger with a dot at a specific location of the tooth. This will allow the cone to be properly placed both directionally and in depth after the sealer cement is placed. Once the cone is formed, it can be cooled rapidly to make it rigid to prevent distortion during placement by spraying it with ethyl chloride or dipping it in alcohol. Shrinkage of core volume by -1.4% would be expected from loss of solvent within 2 weeks (119). (This is discussed further in the context of the chemoplastic method later in this section.)

Lateral compaction can be accomplished by inserting a spreader alongside the master gutta-percha cone (a type I cone) and using a slight apical pressure and rotational movement to compact the material against the canal wall, making room for additional accessory or type II points (115,120). This procedure is repeated until the canal is filled. The excess material can be seared off with a red-hot endodontic spoon passed across the points in an apical direction. When properly performed, lateral compaction can effectively fill most canal irregularities, but care should be taken not to be overzealous with spreaders, as they can produce vertical root fractures (115). Research has shown no core shrinkage in lateral compaction, but an expansion of +1.13% has been implied by some studies (121). However, this is not true expansion, but merely a rebound memory effect related to points' separating and reconforming to their prefabricated conical state.

Vertical compaction is most commonly used with various heated gutta-percha techniques, although it can be used on cold gutta-percha. A master cone is placed. A red-hot heated instrument is used to remove excess material. If the instrument is not red-hot or if it is allowed to remain in contact with the gutta-percha for more than a brief second, the material will cling to the instrument and possibly be removed or dislodged as it is withdrawn. A nonheated plugger is used to vertically compact the gutta-percha while it is still warm. The plugger can be dipped in zinc oxide powder to reduce its adhesion to the heated mass. Additional segments of gutta-percha can be added, heated, and compacted until the canal is filled. Numerous automated heating devices are available that either heat pluggers or have their own attached heated plugger for vertical compaction. Core volume shrinkage of -0.45% has been reported with warm-compacted gutta-percha 2 weeks following obturation (121).

Thermomechanical compaction involves the use of a compactor instrument on a conventional slow-speed handpiece with a contra-angle at 10,000–12,000 rpm (122). As the compactor is inserted beside the master cone, frictional heat from the dentinal walls is generated that melts the gutta-percha. The blades of the instrument force the softened gutta-percha apically and laterally. Additional points can be fed into the canal as the instrument is being gradually withdrawn, until the canal is filled. The original compactor introduced by McSpadden in 1978 was redesigned and introduced as the Thermal Lateral Compactor™ (Brasseler Company). Technique is important with this method, as instrument fracture, apical overextension, and apical perforation have occasionally been problems with these instruments (115). Mechanical compaction does stimulate heat, which expands the gutta-percha; at 2 weeks postobturation core shrinkage was shown to be –0.62% (121).

Thermoplastic method is the thermal heating of gutta-percha to soften it to improve the quality of the fill. After placement, the gutta-percha can be heated by ultrasonic or heated-plugger devices and vertically compacted. Additionally, it can be heated prior to placement and transported to the canal with a file or endodontic obturator. In most cases, there will be shrinkage or a volume loss due to cooling, similar to that of gutta-percha heated for lateral compaction, as heating will have caused slight expansion (123). For this reason, heated gutta-percha should be compacted as it cools to compensate for the shrinkage.

Currently, there are two types of injection molding devices available commercially: the high-temperature thermoplasticized injection (HTTI) and the low-temperature thermoplasticized injection (LTTI) units (124). HTTI units, such as the Obtura II™ (Texceed Corporation, Costa Mesa, California), heat gutta-percha to 160°C. The device consists of an electronic control unit and an electrical cord attached from it to an injection-syringe pistol that accepts and heats large gutta-percha pellets. The gun has a flexible needle through which the heated gutta-percha is extruded. The needles are available in an extended length for veterinary use. The standard needles are equal in diameter to a No.60 and a No.99 file. Therefore, the access needs to be able to accommodate these sizes. This does not mean that the entire canal to the apex needs to be instrumented to a size 60 or larger. Usually, the preparation is mildly flared, so the needle can reach to within 3–5 mm of an apex instrumented to at least a size 25. Even when this is not possible, if there are no canal obstructions, the heated gutta-percha can be vertically compacted to reasonable depths.

The LTTI units, such as Ultrafil® (Hygenic Corporation), heat gutta-percha to 70°C. The device consists of a portable heater, an unattached injection syringe, and gutta-percha cannulas with an attached needle. The heated cannulas are placed in the injection syringe for use. The cannulas come in three types: a white cannula with a light-bodied, well flowing gutta-percha; a blue cannula with a firm-setting gutta-percha that flows well; and a green cannula, known as Endoset™ (Hygenic Corporation), that does not flow well but sets up quickly. The cannula needles are equal in diameter to about a No.70 file. The gutta-percha used in these cannulas has been prepared, usually with a higher paraffin content, to flow well with the LTTI devices (92).

With the thermoplasticized gutta-percha injection technique, the canal preparation greatly affects successful obturation. The canal should have a slightly flared preparation with a definite apical stop. The flaring allows for easier needle placement and compaction. The apical stop allows vertical compaction with less chance of apical overextension or overfill. The canal should be well dried and a slow-setting ZOE sealer placed. The ZOE will act as a lubricant for the gutta-percha, as well as a sealer of the apex, accessory, and lateral canals. The needle is placed to full depth or 3–5 mm from the apex, and the material is injected. The material should then be vertically compacted and radiographed to examine the apical fill. If the apical fill is good, the rest of the canal can be back-filled and compacted (92).

Thermoplasticized gutta-percha can also be carried into the canal with an obturator or a file carrier. Two of the more commonly used endodontic obturators are Thermafil™ (Tulsa Dental Products) and SuccessFil® (Hygenic Corporation). Thermafil™ obturators are metal or plastic obturators or carriers of sizes corresponding to standard files (sizes 20–140), coated with the alpha phase of gutta-percha. They are placed in a Thermafil™ heater that heats the gutta-percha to the appropriate temperature. The canal is best slightly flared and treated with a slow-setting ZOE sealer. A Thermafil™ obturator the same size as the master file is heated and inserted to full depth. A radiograph is then taken to confirm working length. The file handle is severed with an inverted cone bur 1–2 mm above the level where the root canal opens into the pulp chamber, and the excess discarded. A lubricated plugger is then used to compact the material. If a dowel or post is to be placed in the canal, the file should be notched half-way through the metal carrier at a point that will permit post placement. Once the Thermafil™ obturator is in place, gentle apical pressure can be applied while the file is rotated counterclockwise. This movement will move the gutta-percha apically and cause the unwanted portion of the metal obturator to snap off. Once the device is removed, the remaining gutta-percha is gently compacted vertically.

SuccessFil® is gutta-percha that comes in small tuberculin-like syringes. These are placed in the obturator heater to soften the gutta-percha. The titanium cores provided can be pushed into the open tip of the syringe to the desired depth of coverage. The plunger is then depressed to extrude the core, now covered with the softened gutta-percha. It can now be placed in a similar fashion as the Thermafil™. SuccessFil® also has the ability for the gutta-percha material to be placed without a metal core. This can be highly useful in certain exotic animal endodontic procedures. The apical 2–3 mm of a K-file is coated with the SuccessFil® material. It is then inserted to working length, and the file is rotated counterclockwise. This movement will push the gutta-percha apically and allow it to disengage from the file. It is then vertically compacted, and a radiograph is taken to verify the apical fill. The canal can then be back-filled with additional SuccessFil or Ultrafil product, referred to as the Trifecta Technique.

Chemoplastic method is when a chemical (usually a solvent) is added to the core material (usually gutta-percha) to soften or dissolve it prior to placement in the canal. The chemicals used most commonly are chloroform, eucalyptol and xylol. It is used either as the sole filling material or as a dip technique in conjunction with a well fitting master cone. Studies have demonstrated varying degrees of shrinkage at 2 weeks following placement: –1.40% in core volume for chloroform dip, –4.86% for Kloroperka N-O as the sole filling material, and –12.42% for chloraperka (119). The excessive shrinkage of sole-filler method makes it an unsound procedure, while the dip technique would be considered borderline. An additional concern is more specific to chloroform. Although no malignancy has been directly attributed to endodontic use of chloroform, it is a well known potential carcinogen and should be used judiciously (115).

Chloroform cone-dip technique is a method of placing the master cone in the solvent for varying degrees of time to soften it. It is typically used for oversized canals that need a custom-fit cone. The longer the dipping, the greater the shrinkage. Therefore, the shortest dip time that softens the material sufficiently is the best. One of the more conservative dipping times is 4–6 seconds. A master cone that reaches the apical stricture or approximately 1 mm short of the radiographic apex is marked with a plugger or pliers at its access point into the canal to confirm working length at placement. The cone is held by the base with college pliers, and the apical 4–6 mm of the cone is dipped for 4–6 second in the solvent. It is then reseated into the canal, using the cone markings to assure full depth. Gentle pressure is applied to help diffuse the gutta-percha to conform to the canal. It may be slightly withdrawn and reseated several times with mild pressure to obtain a proper imprint. Radiographs can be taken to confirm the fit. After a few seconds it is removed and inspected. The process is repeated until suitable conformation is accomplished. Once that is accomplished, the cone can be immersed in isopropyl alcohol to firm the cone. The canal should then be reirrigated and dried to remove any excess chloroform. Another similar method is the modified chlorpercha technique. It is basically the same as the chloroform-dip method, except that the master cone is dipped into chlorpercha, a paste formed of gutta-percha dissolved in chloroform. The cone is inserted into the canal, and a plugger is used to apply lateral and vertical pressure to fill accessory canals. Care should be taken, as overfill is common (92,115).

Eucalyptol cone dipping can be used to avoid the carcinogenic possibilities associated with chloroform. However, it is not as strong a solvent, and at room temperature it may take several minutes to achieve any degree of softening of the gutta-percha. For this reason, the eucalyptol may be placed in a glass Dappen dish, and the solution is heated for 20–30 seconds using an alcohol burner to enhance its solvent action. The gutta-percha cone tip is dipped and rotated in the solution for 30–45 seconds before placement and compaction (115).

Paste methods of obturation make use of various soft or semisolid products that eventually harden in the canal. Some of the products that have been used are ZOE, calcium hydroxide, modified Wach's cement, modified methyl methacrylates, N-2 type pastes, silicone, and other assorted sealer cements (115). Methods for their use as the sole filling material have been around for years, with most being pumped or forced into the canal with spiral fillers or pressure-syringe techniques. Problems with overextension, underextension, overfilling, underfilling, and a lack of positive pressure for maintenance of the apical seal have all been problems with paste techniques (115).

Underextension results in a lack of apical seal. Voids allow for percolation of fluids, and if adjacent to accessory canals, lateral canals, or the apex, an incomplete hermetic seal occurs, endangering the success of the endodontic procedure. Because of the liquid nature of most of these products when placed, a positive pressure for sealing is extremely difficult to maintain, as the material can extrude through lateral canals or the apex, negating applied pressure. Overextension can also be a serious problem, as certain components of these products produce varying intensity of toxicity, inflammation, or discomfort when contacting the periapical tissues. The N-2 type materials have paraformaldehyde and heavy metals such as lead and mercury. The potential dangers of these products have been pointed out by scientific studies, and these products are not recommended (125). Silicone resins have received some favorable reports concerning their sealing ability (126), while others indicate they are about the same as other common sealer cements used (127,128). Some reports have indicated that silicone implants are safe (129). However, with public concerns over the use of silicone, implants in the bosom of one's teeth will most likely meet with resistance, until all safety concerns are thoroughly addressed.

Only ZOE and calcium hydroxide pastes have had any degree of professional support, mostly for limited applications (see Chapter 12).

Obturation Complication Terms

Four terms are commonly used with problems of the fill or obturation of the root canal. These are underextension, overextension, underfilling, and overfilling. The differences are subtle but distinct. *Underextension* and *overextension* refer solely to the vertical fill dimension, while *underfilling* and *overfilling* refer to obturation in any dimension (130). A gutta-percha point can be overextended into the periodontal ligament, while the canal still with voids around it is underfilled. Therefore, the obturation was overextended but underfilled. A canal that is fully obturated and has material extruded beyond the apex into the periodontal ligament is overextended, but is more appropriately termed overfilled. A canal that has the apex obturated correctly but has voids is termed underfilled. One that is well obturated except at the apex is termed underextended. A canal with voids around a master cone that also has a void at the apex is both underextended and underfilled.

Basic Lateral Compaction Root Canal Procedure

A diagnostic survey radiograph is taken to fully evaluate the tooth structure and periodontium. In some teeth, pulp cavity exposure at the fracture site provides adequate straight-line access to the canal. However, in most cases, coronal access for proper instrumentation of the canal must be made using a round bur on a high- or low-speed handpiece (9,131). With experience, a practitioner can sense when the bur encounters the canal or chamber, but care must always be exercised to remove the least amount of tooth structure possible, while obtaining an acceptable access (132). A pathfinder or endodontic probe may be used to help locate the canal opening. To remove any remaining pulpal tissue, a barbed broach is carefully introduced into the canal until light contact is made. It is then backed out 1–2 mm and rotated 180° to engage the pulp material, and is then removed (79). This may require repeated efforts to remove the pulp. In extralarge canals, two or more barbed broaches may be twisted together and used. Necrotic pulps can often only be removed with files during instrumentation. A pathfinder or probe is advanced to the fullest depth possible with an endostop in place. A radiograph will help confirm the working length of the canal, which should be recorded and premarked on each subsequent file with an endostop. The coronal portion of the canal can now be flared for improved instrumentation and obturation. This can be done with Gates-Glidden drills, but it is more safely performed with K-type reamers.

The canal is then instrumented, beginning with the smallest file first. Coating the files with a lubricant chelating agent improves handling and cleaning of calcified canals. When K-type files are used in a rotational action, the instrument is turned clockwise 90°, removed, wiped clean with a sterile gauze, and reinserted to repeat the procedure (77,78). Push-and-pull filing (with K- or H-type files) should be performed with a gentle up-and-down stroke (77,78). The files should never be forcibly advanced, as movements that are not passive can create unfavorable results (78,131). In canals with a noticeable curvature, files can be gently prebent to approximate the canal shape (78). When the instrument is moving in a smooth, free action, it is removed and the canal irrigated with 2.5–6 % sodium hypochlorite solution followed by sterile saline. Hydrogen peroxide has been used as an irrigant, but poor effect and complications discourage its use (133). The next file size is used in the same basic technique. As the procedure progresses to larger files, it is best to reuse one of the smaller files to *recapitulate* the canal, loosening any dentinal debris that might be accumulating near the apex (78,134). Copious flushing also aids in debris removal.

Instrumentation is complete when clean, white dentinal shavings are evident on the files, and the canal is properly shaped. One way used to reach this point is the file-binding technique. *File binding* occurs when light, firm contact is made with the canal walls, but the file is not lodged in place. When a light binding of the file at the working tip is noted, instrumentation is generally continued to two or three file sizes larger to provide sufficient debridement, unless excessive binding is encountered (77). At this point, clean, white dentinal shavings should be present on the instruments. If this is not the case or if any hemorrhage persists, additional instrumentation is necessary (see Chapter 12). A radiograph of the largest *(master) file* placed to the full working depth of the canal is taken to verify canal preparation that shows no evidence of perforation or additional canal length beyond the file's tip. A thorough final irrigation, with excessive liquid being aspirated as the needle is withdrawn, is followed by drying of the canal with absorbent paper points that correspond to the size of the master file. At no time should air be blown up into the canal to facilitate drying; this can cause air emboli with potentially serious consequences (84). The canal is then coated with a sealer cement and obturated with gutta-percha. If gutta-percha points are used, they can be dipped in half-strength sodium hypochlorite for 2 minutes or in full-strength for 1 minute to aid in sterilization (88), rinsed, and dried before being placed into the canal. A radiograph should be taken to confirm the master cone fit. If this point will not reach the apex adequately, the next smaller size point may be used. Accessory points can be placed with the aid of spreaders. Once the canal is filled, the excess is seared off with a red-hot endodontic spoon or a beavertail passed across the points in an apical direction so as to not pull them from the canal. While they are still warm, pluggers can be used to vertically condense the gutta-percha and create room for the access closure.

Pulp cavity openings at the fracture site and instrument access are prepared to complete the closure. Undercuts in the dentin, removal of excess gutta-percha and cement, acid-etching the enamel, and preparing the dentin are followed by the placement and finishing of an appropriate restorative. At times, an intermediate restorative is used under the final restorative, as eugenol can inhibit the setting up of most composites. Zinc oxyphosphate cement and glass ionomers are two of the more commonly used to separate ZOE and composites (53).

Antibiotics should be dispensed for postoperative administration. Endodontically treated teeth should be radiographed 9–12 months later and at regular intervals thereafter to monitor for any signs of complications or continuing pathology (135,136). Since a treated tooth can be more brittle than a vital one, placement of a crown for additional strength may be considered.

PERIAPICAL HEALING FOLLOWING ENDODONTIC TREATMENT

Successful endodontic therapy customarily stimulates periapical healing. Under most circumstances, the only clinical criterion to determine healing is radiology. With successful endodontic treatment, the radiolucent periapical signs of disease will dissipate with time. The inflammatory cell infiltrate of the periapical soft tissue (typically granulation tissue), along with excessive vascularity, diminishes as it is supplanted by fibroblastic proliferation. This is followed by osteoblasts evolving from either undifferentiated mesenchymal cells or possibly additional differentiation of fibroblasts (137). Microscopically, small spicules of osteoid are then secreted by the osteoblasts within the fibrous mass. The spicules progressively expand in a loose intersecting pattern, replacing the fibrous aggregate. The organic osteoid matrix gradually undergoes mineralization to form the new periradicular bone. Osteoid is not radiopaque, and newly mineralized trabecular bone contains insufficient calcium salts to be evident radiographically. For this reason, it will frequently be 4–12 months before radiographs may be able to confirm complete healing of a periapical lesion. Rapidity of healing is dependent on the lesion's size, the age and health of patient, and the appropriateness and quality of therapy. Failure of the healing process can be due to incomplete therapy, or persistent periapical cyst. These would be indications for endodontic retreatment or surgical apical treatments (138). Healing following apical surgical therapy works by formation of a blood clot in the void created by treatment. Connective tissue cells and capillaries penetrate the clot, and fibroblasts appear. From this point, healing is fundamentally the same as previously described.

REFERENCES

1. Debowes L. Systemic effects of oral disease. *Veterinary Dental Forum.* 1992:65.
2. Mattila KJ, Nieminen MS, Valtonen VV, et al. Association between dental health and acute myocardial infarction. *Br Med J* 989;298:779.
3. Syrjanen J, Peltola J, Valtonen V, et al. Dental infections in association with cerebral infarction in young and middle aged men. *J Intern Med* 1989;225:179.
4. DeStefano F, Andra RF, Kahn HS, et al. Dental disease and risk of coronary heart disease and mortality. *Br Med J* 1993;306:688.
5. Wiggs RB. Endodontic anatomy, pathology and examination. *NAVC Proc* 1992:106.
6. Hess W, Zurcher E. *The Anatomy of the Root Canals.* New York: William Wood Co; 1925.
7. Hennet P. Apical root canal anatomy in the dog and its significance. *Veterinary Dental Forum.* 1990.
8. Kuttler, Yury. Microscopic investigations of root apices. *JADA* 1955;50:544.
9. Holmstrom SE, Frost P, Gammon RL. Endodontics. In: *Veterinary Dental Techniques.* Philadelphia: WB Saunders Co; 1992:207.
10. Cohen S. Diagnostic procedures. In: Cohen S, Burns RC, eds. *Pathways to the Pulp.* 5th ed. St.Louis, MO: Mosby-Year Book; 1991:20.
11. Pashley DH. Smear layer: Physiology consideration. *Operative Dent* 1984;3:13.
12. Michelich VJ, Schuster GS, Pashley DH. Bacterial penetration of dentin in vivo. *J Dent Res* 1980;59:1398.
13. Brannstrom M. *Dentin and Pulp in Restorative Dentistry.* London: Wolfe Medical Publications; 1982.
14. Iverson GW, von Fraunhofer JA, Herrmann JW. The effects of various sterilization methods on strength of endodontic files. *J Endod* 1985;11:266.
15. Van Hassel HJ. Inflammation. *Am Assoc Endod Proc* 1978.
16. Robinson HBG, Boling LR. The anachoretic effect in pulpitis, I: Bacteriologic studies. *Arch Pathol* 1941;28:268.
17. Boling LR, Robinson HBG. The anachoretic effect in pulpitis, II: Histological studies. *Arch Pathol* 1942;33:477.
18. Grossman LI, et al. Microbiology. In: *Endodontic Practice.* 11th ed. Philadelphia: Lea & Febiger; 1988:234.
19. Eisner E. Endodontics in small animal practice: An alternative to extraction. *Vet Med* May 1992:418.
20. Karzen BH. Endodontic treatment of the adult tooth. In: Levine N, ed. *Current Treatment in Dental Practice.* Philadelphia: WB Saunders Co; 1986:184.
21. Bellows J. Recognizing and treating a dog's broken or discolored tooth. *Vet Pract Staff* 1992;4(1):1.
22. Goldstein GS, Anthony J. Basic veterinary Endodontics. *Compend Cont Educ Dent* 1990;12(2):207.
23. Mulligan TW. Endodontics. In: Kirk RW, ed. *Current Veterinary Therapy X.* Philadelphia: WB Saunders Co; 1989:454.
24. Lisanti VF, Zander HA. Thermal injury to normal dog teeth. *J Dent Res* 1952;31:548.
25. Holmstrom SE. Performing conventional, non-surgical root canal therapy on dogs and cats. *Vet Econ Suppl: Veterinary Dentistry* Feb 1992:14.
26. Wais FT. Significance of findings following biopsy and histopathologic study of 100 periapical lesions. *Oral Surg Oral Med Oral Pathol* 1958;11:650.
27. Hill TJ. Experimental granulomas in Dogs. *JADA* 1932;19:1389.
28. Ross WS. Pulp disease and its prevention. *Br Dent J* 1954;96:108.
29. Mitchell DF. Differential diagnosis of odontalgia. In: Healy HJ, ed. *Endodontics.* St Louis, MO: CV Mosby Co; 1960:15.
30. Thoma KH. A histologic study of the dental granuloma and diseased root apex. *JADA* 1917;4:1075.
31. Towbridge H, Daniels T. Immune response to infection of the dental pulp. *Oral Surg* 1977;43:902.
32. Mortensen H, Winther JE, Birn H. Periapical granulomas and cysts: An investigation of 1600 cases. *Scand J Dent Res* 1971;78:141.
33. Priebe WA, Lazansky JP, Wuehrmann AH. The value of roentgenographic film in differential diagnosis of periapical lesions. *Oral Surg Oral Med Oral Pathol* 1954;7:979.
34. Harvey CE, Emily PP. *Small Animal Dentistry.* St.Louis, MO: Mosby-Year Book; 1993:201.
35. Sommer RF, Ostrander FD, Crowly MC. *Clinical Endodontics.* Philadelphia: WB Saunders Co; 1961:70.
36. Grossman LI. Endodontics. In: Grossman LI, ed. *Handbook of Dental Practice.* 3rd ed. Philadelphia: JB Lippincott Co; 1958:150.
37. Schilder H. The relationship of periodontics to endodontics. In: Grossman LI, ed. *Transactions, Third International Conference on Endodontics.* Philadelphia: University of Pennsylvania Press; 1963.
38. Seltzer S, Bender IB, Ziontz M. The interrelationship of pulp and periodontal disease. *Oral Surg* 1963;16:1474.
39. Seltzer S, et al. Pulpitis-induced interradicular changes in experimental animals. *J Periodontol* 1976;38:124.

40. Simon JHS, De Deus QD. Endodontic-periodontal relations. In: Cohen S, Burns RC, eds. *Pathways to the Pulp*. 5th ed. St.Louis, MO: Mosby-Year Book; 1991:548.
41. Manfra-Marretta S, Schloss AJ, Klippert LS. Classification and prognostic factors of endodontic-periodontic lesions in the dog. *J Vet Dent* 1992;9(2):27.
42. Eisner E. Selecting equipment, instruments, and materials for endodontic procedures. *Vet Med* May 1992:435.
43. Tharaldsen. *Diagnosis by Transillumination*. Chicago: Cameron's Publishing Co; 1927:18.
44. Ingle JI. Root canal obturation. *JADA* 1956;53:47.
45. Sampeck AJ. Instruments of endodontics. *Dent Clin North Am* 1967:579.
46. Ingle JI. A standardized endodontic technique utilizing newly designed instruments and filling materials. *Oral Surg Oral Med Oral Pathol* 1961;14:83.
47. Ingle JI. The need for endodontic instrument standardization. *Oral Surg Oral Med Oral Pathol* 1955;8:1211.
48. Ingle JI, Levine M. The need for uniformity of endodontic instruments, equipment, and filling materials. In: Grossman LI, ed. *Transactions of the Second International Conference on Endodontics*. Philadephia: University of Pennsylvania Press; 1958:123.
49. Council on Dental Materials and Devices. New American Dental Association Specification No.28 for endodontic files and reamers. *JADA* 1976;93:813.
50. American National Standards Institute/American Dental Association. Document No.41. *JADA* 1979;99:697.
51. American National Standards Institute/American Dental Association. Meeting of ISO Committee MD-156; Chicago, 1982.
52. American National Standards Institute/American Dental Association. Meetings of ISO Committee TC-106; (Dentistry). Chicago, 1974.
53. *D.D.R., Materials, Instruments, and Equipment*. 2nd ed. Chicago: American Dental Association; 1983:311.
54. Harty FJ, Stock JR. A comparison of the flexibility of giromatic and hand-operated instruments in endodontics. *Br Endod Soc J* 1983;7:64.
55. Lilly JD, Smith DC. An investigation of the fracture of root canal reamers. *Br Dent J* 1966;120:364.
56. Michael AH, Miserendino LJ. Instruments and materials. In: Cohen S, Burns RC, eds. *Pathways to the Pulp*. 4th ed. Washington, DC: CV Mosby Co; 1987:397.
57. Feldman G, et al. Retrieving broken endodontic instruments. *JADA* 1974;88:588.
58. Crump MC, Natkin E. Relationships of broken root canal instruments to endodontic case prognosis: A clinical investigation. *JADA* 1973;80:1341.
59. Shoji Y. Systematic endodontics. In: *Kie Quentessenz*. Berlin, Chicago: Buchenid Zeitschriften-Verlag; 1973.
60. Fromme HG, Reidel H. Treatment of dental root canals and marginal contact between filling material and tooth, studied by SEM. *Br Endod Soc J* 1972;6:17.
61. Chernick LB, et al. Torsional failure of endodontic files. *J Endod* 1977;3:175.
62. Lautenschlager EP, et al. Brittle and ductile torsional failures of endodontic instruments. *J Endod* 1984;10:349.
63. Roane JB, Sabala C. Clockwise or counterclockwise? *J Endod* 1977;3:175.
64. Seltzer S, Green D, Weiner N, DeRenzis F. A scanning electron microscope examination of silver cones removed from endodontically treated teeth. *Oral Surg* 1972;33:589.
65. Larder TC, Prescott AJ, Brayton SM. Gutta-percha: A comparative study of three methods of obturation. *J Endod* 1976;2:289.
66. Spanberg L, Langeland K. Biological effects of dental materials, 1: Toxicity of root canal filling materials on HeLa cells in vitro. *Oral Surg* 1973;35:402.
67. Rising DW, Goldman M, Brayton SM. Histological appraisal of three experimental root canal filling materials. *J Endod* 1975;1:238.
68. Sorin SM, Oliet S, Pearlstein F. Rejunvenation of aged (brittle) endodontic gutta-percha cones. *J Endod* 1979; 56:1453.
69. Heuer MA. Instruments and materials. In: Cohen S, Burns RC, eds. *Pathways to the Pulp*. 2nd ed. St Louis, MO: CV Mosby Co; 1980.
70. Friedman CE, Sandrik JL, Heuer MA, Rapp GW. Composition and physical properties of gutta-percha endodontic filling materials. *J Endod* 1977;3:304.
71. Goodman A, Schilder H, Aldrich W. The thermomechanical properties of gutta-percha. *Oral Surg* 1974; 37:954.
72. Katz A, Tagger M, Tamse A. Rejuvenation of brittle gutta-percha cones—a universal technique? *J Endod* 1987; 13:65.
73. Callahan JR. Rosin solution for sealing of dentinal tubuli and as an adjuvant in the filling of root canals. *J Allied Dent Soc* 1914;9:53.
74. Johnston HB. A method for filling of the pulp canaliculi by diffusion. *J Dent Res* 1922;4:117.
75. Abou-Ross M, Piccinino MU. The effectiveness of four clinical irrigation methods on the removal of tooth canal debris. *Oral Surg* 54;1982:323.
76. Harrison JW. The effect of dilution and organic matter on the antibacterial property of 5.25% sodium hypochlorite. *J Endod* 1981;7:128.
77. Wiggs RB. Principles of endodontics. *ESVC Proc* Jan 1991:360.
78. Buchanan LS. Cleaning and shaping the root canal system. In: Cohen S, Burns RC, eds. *Pathways to the Pulp*. 5th ed. St.Louis, MO: Mosby-Year Book; 1991:166.
79. Wiggs RB. Endodontic instrumentation. *J Vet Dent* 1991;8(4):4.

80. Senia ES, Marshall FJ, Rosen S. The solvent action of sodium hypochlorite on pulp tissue of extracted teeth. *Oral Surg Oral Med Oral Pathol* 1971;31:96.
81. Barker NA, et al. Scanning electron microscopic study of the efficacy of various irrigation solutions. *J Endod* 1975;1:127.
82. Becker GL, Cohen S, Borer R. The sequelae of accidentally injected sodium hypochlorite beyond the root apex. *Oral Surg Oral Med Oral Pathol* 1974;38:633.
83. Bhat KS. Tissue emphysema caused by hydrogen peroxide. *Oral Surg Oral Med Oral Pathol* 1974;38:304.
84. Rickles NH, Joshi BA. A death from air embolism during root canal therapy. *JADA* 1963;67:397.
85. McCoy DE. Air embolism causing death during an endodontic procedure. Presented at 4th World Veterinary Dentistry Congress. 1995:142.
86. Richman MJ. Use of ultrasonics in root canal therapy and root resection. *J Dent* 1957;1:12.
87. Walton RE. Ultrasonics and sonics: The wave of the future in endodontics? *Ill Dent J* 1988:272.
88. Senia SE, et al. Rapid sterilization of gutta-percha cones with 5.25% sodium hypochlorite. *J Endod* 1975;1:136.
89. Ahmad M, Pitt-Ford TR, Crum LA. Ultrasonic debridement of canals: Acoustic streaming and its possible role. *J Endod* 1987;13:490.
90. Frank AL. An evaluation of the Giromatic endodontic handpiece. *Oral Surg Oral Med Oral Pathol* 1967;24:419.
91. Harty FJ, Stock CJR. The Giromatic system compared with hand instrumenation in endodontics. *Br Dent J* 1974;17:239.
92. Miserendino LJ. Instruments, materials, and devices. In: Cohen S, Burns RC, eds. *Pathways to the Pulp*. 5th ed. St.Louis, MO: Mosby-Year Book; 1991:388.
93. Sunada I. A new method for measuring the length of the root canal. *J Dent Res* 1962;41:375.
94. Suzuki K. Experimental study on iontophoresis. *J Jpn Stomatol Soc* 1942;16:414.
95. Sunada I. New method for measuring the length of the root canal. *J Jpn Stomatol Soc* 1958;25:161.
96. Sunada I. New method for measuring the length of the root canal. *J Jpn Stomatol Soc* 1962;41:375.
97. Huang L. The principle of electronic root canal measurement. *Bull 4th Mil Med Coll* 1959;8:32.
98. Kobayashi, Suda. Ratio method for overcoming false electronic canal measurements. *J Endod* 1994;20:111.
99. Huang L. An experimental study of the principle of electronic root canal measurement. *J Endod* 1987;13:60.
100. Allison CA, Weber CR, Walton RE. The influence of the method of canal preparation on the quality of apical and coronal seal. *J Endod* 1979;5:298.
101. Gutmann JL, Lovdahl PE. Problems encountered in access to the pulp chamber space. In: Gutmann JL, Dumsha TC, Loudahl PE, eds. *Problem Solving in Endodontics*. Chicago: Year Book Medical Publishers; 1988:1.
102. Wiggs RB. Problem solving in veterinary endodontics. *Semin Vet Med Surg (Small Anim)* 1993;8(3):165.
103. Golden AL. New methods for conventional endodontics. *NAVC Proc* Jan 1992:91.
104. Moreinis SA. Avoiding perforation during endodontic access. *JADA* 1979;98:707.
105. Eisner ER. Transcoronal approach for endodontic access to the fourth maxillary premolar in dogs. *J Vet Dent* 1990;7(4):22.
106. Strieff JT, Gerstein H. Access cavity perforations. In: Gerstein H, ed. *Techniques in Clinical Endodontics*. Philadelphia: WB Saunders Co; 1982:1.
107. Gutmann JL. Prevention and management of endodontic procedural errors. *N Z Soc Endod Newslet* 1982;23:15.
108. Christie WH, Peikoff MD. New root canal techniques. *J Can Dent Assoc* 1980;3:183.
109. Allison D, Weber C, Walton R. The influence of the method of canal preparation on the quality of apical and coronal obturation. *J Endod* 1979;5:298.
110. Christie WH, Peikoff MD. New root canal technique. *J Can Dent Assoc* 1980;3:183.
111. Ruiz-Hubard EE, Gutmann JL, Wagner MJ. A quantitative assessment of canal debris forced periapically during root canal instrumentation using two different techniques. *J Endod* 1987;13:554.
112. Dow PR, Ingle JI. Isotope determination of root canal failure. *Oral Surg* 1955;8:1100.
113. Clem WH. Endodontics in the adolescent patient. *Dent Clin North Am* 1969;13:483.
114. Grossman LI, Oliet S, Del Rio C. *Endodontics*. 11th ed. Philadelphia: Lea & Febiger; 1988.
115. Nguyen TN. Obturation of the root canal system. In: Cohen S, Burns RC, eds. *Pathways to the Pulp*. 5th ed. St.Louis, MO: Mosby-Year Book; 1991:193.
116. American Dental Association, Council on Dental Materials, Instruments and Equipment. Council on the use of root canal filling materials containing paraformaldehyde: A status report. *JADA* 1987;114:239.
117. Chong R, Senzer J. Systemic distribution of 210 PbO from root canal fillings. *J Endod* 1976;2:381.
118. Baumgardner KR, Krell KV. Ultrasonic condensation of gutta percha: An in-vitro dye penetration and scanning electron microscopic study. *J Endod* 1990;16:253.
119. Wong M, Peters DD, Lorton L, Bernier WE. Comparison of gutta-percha filling techniques: Three chloroform–gutta-percha filling techniques, part 2. *J Endod* 1982;8:4.
120. Holmstrom SE. Endodontics: A chance to drill, fill and trill. *ESVC Proc* Jan 1991;342.
121. Wong M, Peters DD, Lorton L. Comparison of gutta-percha filling techniques, compaction (mechanical), vertical warm, and lateral condensation techniques, part 1. *J Endod* 1981;7:551.
122. Wiggs RB. Use of the McSpadden compactor for root canal obturation in dogs and Macaques. *J Vet Dent* 1988; 5(3):9.
123. Schilder H, Goodman A, Aldrich W. The thermomechanical properties of gutta-percha. Part V. Volume changes in bulk gutta-percha as a function of temperature and its relationship to molecular phase tranformation. *Oral Surg Oral Med Oral Pathol* 1985;59:285.

124. LaCombe JS, Campbell AD, Hicks ML, Pelleu GB. A comparison of the apical seal produced by two thermo-plasticized injectable gutta-percha techniques. *J Endod* 1988;14:445.

125. Brewer DL. Histology of apical tissue reaction to overfill (Sargenti formula vs. gutta-percha-Grossman). *J Calif Dent Assoc* 1975;3:58.

126. Spradling PM, Senia ES. The relative sealing ability of paste-type filling materials. *J Endod* 1982;8:543.

127. Al Rafei SR, Sayegh FS, Wright G. Sealing ability of a new root canal filling material. *J Endod* 1982;8:152.

128. Lee H, Teigler D. *Review of Biological Safety Testing of Endo-Fill: Research Report RR-82-101*. South El Monte, CA: Lee Pharmaceuticals; 1982.

129. Biggs JT, Kaminiski EJ, Osetek EM. Rat macrophage response to implant sealer cements. *J Endod* 1985;11:30.

130. Schilder H. Filling root canals in three dimensions. *Dent Clin North Am* 1987:723.

131. Anthony J. Endodontics for the nineties. *Am Vet Dent Coll/Acad Vet Dent Proc* Sept 1991.

132. Burns RC, Buchanan LS. Tooth morphology and access openings. In: Cohen S, Burns RC, eds. *Pathways to the Pulp*. 5th ed. St.Louis, MO: Mosby-Year Book; 1991:114.

133. Bhat KS. Tissue emphysema caused by hydrogen peroxide. *Oral Surg Oral Med Oral Pathol* 1971;31:96.

134. Emily P, Tholen M. Endodontic therapy. In Bojrab MJ, Tholen M, eds. *Small Animal Oral Medicine and Surgery*. Philadelphia: Lea & Febiger; 1990:158.

135. Anthony J. Comparative obturation techniques in the canine. *J Vet Dent* 1991;8(4):24.

136. Sicher H. Problems of pain in dentistry. *Oral Surg Oral Med Oral Pathol* 1954;7:149.

137. Saffer WG. Pathology of the periapical area. In: Healy HJ, ed. *Endodontics*. St Louis, MO: CV Mosby Co; 1960:50.

138. Holmstrom SE. Endodontics. *NAVC Proc* Jan 1992:100.

12

Advanced Endodontic Therapies

Robert B. Wiggs and Heidi B. Lobprise

Standard therapeutic endodontics has rapidly progressed from an emerging science to an established part of veterinary dentistry. The excellent results that standard endodontic treatments have provided, founded on scientifically established techniques, have resulted in the professional and public acceptance and expectation of more ambitious treatments for more advanced problems. Anticipation of every possible problem is not feasible; however, the more commonplace can be satisfactorily managed in a proficient manner when correctly identified, in order that appropriate problem-solving steps can be promptly initiated.

DISCUSSION

Many diverse areas of difficulty may be confronted in endodontic treatment (1–3). Some of the more common of these are access to the pulp cavity, attaining and maintaining working length, resolution of periapical pathology, complete obturation, and addressing iatrogenic injury. Perforations of the pulp cavity may result when tissues are diseased, access is complicated, or instrumentation is inappropriate for the situation. When encountered, canal abnormalities and blockages may present an obstacle for adequate access, instrumentation, and filing. In addition, there are pedodontic endodontic considerations such as treatment of deciduous teeth and permanent teeth with immature or poorly developed root structure.

Access

The fundamental purpose in the choice of site of tooth access in standard endodontics is to establish an unrestricted passageway from the crown and through the pulp cavity to the apical stricture or the internal commencement of the delta (1). An unimpeded pathway must be customized to expedite acceptable canal instrumentation and obturation according to specific tooth type and the individuality of the tooth's pulp system. This should not be misinterpreted to imply that the most direct route from crown to apex is the proper access. Following the *access triad* is one of the ways to achieve functional access. This is simply the sequence of *chamber access*, *root canal access*, and *stricture access*—in that order and each in its turn. Each access sequence, when correctly attained, expedites the route to the next, until contact with the apical stricture is achieved. The goal of access design is to gain full working length to the stricture for instrumentation, while providing for obturation of the apical third of the canal to be as complete as possible.

Numerous technical difficulties encountered in many canal therapies can be diminished or eliminated with proper access preparation. A cornerstone of good dentistry has always been the conservation of tooth structure; nevertheless, this should not be allowed to influence the valid selection of site, design, or execution of the actual access opening (1). This is not suggest that an excess of coronal structure should be removed indiscriminately. It does imply the need for a competent awareness of the pulp cavity and external root anatomy and the ability to properly assess radiographic details (2) in order to appropriately implement access and prepare the coronal approach. Failure to follow these basic steps may unnecessarily invite complications.

Tooth or restorative structure that is unsound or unsupported and in the access pathway is better removed before the initiation of endodontic treatment. Such action assists in the maintenance of asepsis and permits a better evaluation of restorative needs before root canal therapy (1), while enhancing visibility. When all diseased structure is not removed before opening of the access, contamination by debris falling or being carried into the canal may result. When restorations are not fully removed, materials such as composite or amalgam can inadvertently be carried into the canal. Undertaking use of standard instrumentation to remove the material frequently results in its being packed into the apical third of the canal; if not removed, this material may interfere with obtaining a suitable apical seal. There are several techniques to remove material trapped in the root canal system, discussed in detail later in this chapter.

Failure to establish proper access to the pulp chamber and root canals is one of the most common complicating factors in root canal therapy for veterinary practitioners (3). The pulp chamber space is typically located in the center of the crown, and root canals are typically located in the center of the root. However, the pulp cavity is a dynamic, changing, cavernous space. With age, the cavity diminishes in size (Fig. 1). In addition, pulp irritation from caries, cervical line lesions, and restorative procedures can result in dimensional changes in the area of the irritation due to deposition of reparative or tertiary dentin internally. Diagnostic dental radiographs, while only two-dimensional, are necessary to properly access the anatomic relationship between crown, root, angle of the root within the arch, and the general condition of the pulp cavity (4). When abnormal crown or root configurations or rotated teeth are present, radiographs often must be angled from mesial and distal aspects to provide the necessary information. Using two-dimensional radiographs as a guide for an access opening in a three-dimensional tooth can sometimes be misleading.

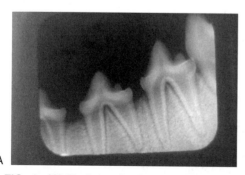
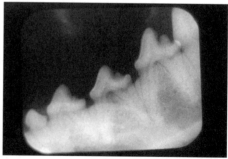

A   B

FIG. 1. (A) Radiograph of mandibular premolars in a young dog showing wide pulp cavity space. **(B)** Radiograph of mandibular premolars in a mature dog showing normal narrowing of the pulp cavity space.

Although each tooth must be assessed individually, certain generalities can be made on the typical location of approach to the more commonly accessed teeth in the dog. The typical entrance to the incisors may be found on the central lingual aspect of the crown 1–2 mm above the free gingival margin. Additionally, a similar labial approach may be used, though commonly not the choice in human dentistry due to esthetics. Cuspids or canine teeth are accessed 1–2 mm from the free gingival margin on the mesial aspect to allow a straighter-line access to the apex. The individual canals of two-rooted premolars may have the access openings made on the buccal aspect over the center of each root near the cusp's margin, as determined by physical palpation of the juga and radiographs. The approach to the lower first molars is similar except that access is most commonly made on the lingual surface. The other two-rooted molars have access achieved on the occlusal surface directly over the roots to be entered. The upper 4th premolar presents a moderate challenge in the access to the mesial roots, especially the palatal. While the distal root access is similar to other premolars, a transcoronal approach has been described using distinct angles (5). This technique is most useful for the novice clinician in gaining an understanding of the basic approach. In most fractured teeth, however, normal anatomy has been destroyed, and determining an adequate exposure by mental extrapolation is required. Palpation of the mesiobuccal root juga and comparison with the actual location of the mesiopalatal root's cusp typically afford sufficient visualization to attain suitable lines of access determination. The actual opening is generally made between these two determined points and approximately 2–4 mm above the gingival margin on the buccal aspect of the tooth. Three-rooted molars may be accessed with a Y- or V-shaped opening on the occlusal surface that exposes each individual canal system. The first access is typically made over the lingual or palatal root, with extension of the access with a high-speed bur and following the chamber to expose the two buccal root canals. Attempted straight-line access of the buccal roots initially will periodically lead to chamber perforation due to the angulation of the roots. Additionally, the V- or Y-shaped access aids in detecting ribbon canals associated with fused distal and palatal roots, which are not uncommon in the upper 1st and 2nd molars.

When the tooth is malaligned or the pulp system calcified or poorly visible on radiographs, access entry may be directed to the largest portion of the chamber visible or to the largest root canal (6). In access opening procedures, there is an old adage, "Go for the horns" (1). In cases of reduced pulp chamber space, it is a reasonable statement, as long as the practitioner realizes that the pulpal horns only represent a small portion of the pulp chamber along some of its borders. The horns are generally pointed projections of the endodontic system within the crown in the pulp chamber and are usually the most coronal and proximal portions of the system. Once in the horn, it is anticipated that the rest of the chamber and root canal openings can be traced from that location. When these basic parameters are not properly followed, problems such as failure to locate all canals, excessive gouging, and even perforations of the chamber walls and floor may occur (7). Generally, *gouging* is the penetration of the floor of the pulp chamber, typically with burs or files during exploration for canals. Root canals can also be "gouged," but this is more appropriately termed *ledging* or *hedging*.

Perforations

Of these errors, the most serious is perforation through the pulp chamber into the oral cavity or the periodontal tissues (1). Should this occur, recognition of the problem as soon as possible can reduce damage to the periradicular tissues from further insult. One of the most common indications of perforation is continued bleeding into the chamber from the injured periradicular tissues. When perforations into the gingival sulcus or above the free gingival margin are present, a simple treatment protocol is best followed. First, control the hemorrhage. This can usually be done with a dry cotton pellet or the large blunt end of a paper point. If the patient is healthy, the use of epinephrine (1:50,000) or another hemostatic agent on the pellet may be considered (1,7). Epinephrine-containing agents should be used cautiously in animals with endocrine imbalances and heart disease, as well as when halothane anesthetic is to be used. This is followed by placement of a gutta-percha or silver point into the root canals to prevent restoratives from entering and sealing them off. Next, place a temporary filling material into the perforation, such as Cavit® (ESPE-Premier Corporation, Norristown, Pennsylvania) or IRM® (L.D. Caulk Company, Milford, Delaware). The root canal procedure should now be completed. A permanent restoration should be placed to seal off the perforation. Additional periodontal treatments, such as gingivectomies or apical repositioning, may prove necessary (8).

When perforations occur at or below the osseous crest or into the furcation, the prognosis is usually very poor (9,10). In attempts to deal with these cases, the following may hold some value in treatment. The perforation should be attended to and sealed as soon as possible. Root canals need to be protected from inadvertent blockage by restorative materials by having a file, gutta-percha cone, or silver point placed into the canals. Hemorrhage must be controlled to obtain a seal in most cases (1). Control can be facilitated with dry cotton pellets or the large blunt end of a paper point. Should bleeding continue, calcium hydroxide powder (11–13) or a fast-setting calcium hydroxide cement, such as DyCal® (L.D. Caulk Company), can be used. Once hemorrhage has been controlled, Cavit® (10,14), zinc oxide–eugenol cements (15), or alloys (16) have all been used to seal perforations. Every precaution should be taken to prevent introducing the restorative material into the periapical tissues (9). Nonsurgical repair of furcation exposures have had reports of clinical successes in humans (12,14), while surgical correction with retrograde fillings has been shown to be almost futile, most often eventually resulting in extraction or hemisection (8,11). When osseous healing is desired, these failures may possibly be due to the drilling out and removal of the cortical plate bone covering the area from which osseous healing of the tooth with osteoid is desired. This is covered in more detail in the section concerning surgical approaches to apexification (see below). However, this could indicate that if a surgical approach is to be perfected with reasonable expectation of success of osseous tooth healing, it will most likely require new creative surgical approaches that maintain the cortical plate in a healthy, intact, replaceable section that totally recovers the exposed area. In single-rooted teeth, a perforation slightly below the osseous crest can sometimes be addressed with orthodontic extrusion. A portion of the crown is sacrificed, and the remainder of the tooth is extruded to bring the perforation above the gum line and out of the soft tissues. A crown preparation is then completed and a new crown placed. This can result in a less favorable crown:root ratio and should be taken into consideration prior to therapy.

Abnormal Canals

In root canal therapy, it is not uncommon to encounter systems that are abnormally configured or dystrophic or have excessive linear calcification (17). Idiosyncrasies such as supernumerary roots and anomalously configured root systems like *ribbon canals* must be detected either by visualization or radiographs. Failure to recognize these quickly can lead to unnecessary delays and problems. *Dystrophic canals* are frequently confronted when standard root canal treatment is attempted on teeth that have previously had direct or indirect pulp capping performed with certain agents. Calcium hydroxide–type products can stimulate an increased layering of tertiary dentin within the pulp cavity, causing dystrophic areas for instrumentation (18,19).

Most cases exhibiting radiographically fine or unidentifiable canals or other calcification blockages are treatable with nonsurgical root canal therapy. Successful identification of calcified orifices requires the use of a knowledge of normal dental anatomy, quality two-dimensional radiographs, and a good three-dimensional imagination. With these, access exploration is initiated using a small-size ball bur directed toward the logical location of the endodontic cavity. Accurate preoperative, as well as frequent operative, radiographs are an absolute necessity for assessment of bur orientation and depth penetration. The search for the canal can be aided with a smooth broach or pathfinder to assist the clinician in identification of the orifice.

Once located, the obstructed canal must be negotiated. At this juncture, the pathfinder can continue to be used, or substitution with a No.8 K-type file is acceptable. The No.6 K-type file is usually too weak to allow appropriate pressure, and the No.10 is typically too large (17). Instrumentation should be performed with a file long enough to reach the apex but not excessive in length, as the longer the instrument is, the more tactile sense is lost (20). If the canal is curved, a slight curve can be placed 1 mm from the apical tip of the instrument to aid in its correct direction of orientation. Endodontic stops should always be used, and if the instrument is curved, a directional stop is mandatory. The directional stop's pointer should be aligned to indicate the direction of the instrument's curvature.

Chelating agents such as ethylenediaminetetraacetic acid (EDTA) can be used to aid in dissolving inorganic calcification within the canal. Products such as RC-Prep® (ESPE-Premier Corporation), a white paste-like substance, combines EDTA, urea peroxidase, and lubricant for use directly on instruments introduced into the canal. Excessive chelation and softening by EDTA preparations is not a problem, as long as the material is not sealed in the canals (21). Frequent copious irrigation with full- or half-strength (3–6%) sodium hypochlorite (bleach) is important to remove debris as the instrument is advanced. Bleach should be used with care in suspected perforation or open apex cases, as it can result in serious complications should it enter the periodontal or periapical tissues. Care should be taken to use true windowed or slotted endodontic irrigation needles in irrigating within fine canals, as injection needles may easily occlude a canal, preventing irrigant from flushing around the needle and thereby forcing it with irrigant and debris through the apex.

When obstruction is met, the file should have gentle force applied and be worked in a very delicate clockwise–counterclockwise rotation. This is sometimes called *stem-winding* or *balance-force* instrumentation. Once appropriate working length is verified radiographically, a filing or up-and-down action should be used until the instrument is functioning in a clean, free movement. Normal standard instruments can commonly be followed from this point, as long as regular recapitulation of the canal with smaller files is employed to loosen any debris or dentin and maintain full length. The use of ultrasonic activated endodontic instruments has been advocated for passive penetration of calcified or blocked canals (22).

In some cases, it is not uncommon to find occlusion of the root canal space from the apex to various levels. If no apical pathology is present or no clinical symptoms are evident, it is clinically acceptable to instrument and fill the canal to the level negotiated, as long as regular monitoring and periodic examinations will be performed (17). The presence of apical pathosis at the time of treatment or at any time during the follow-up observation is an indication to seriously consider reinstrumentation or surgical endodontics with retrograde filling (23).

Procedural Blockage

Procedural canal blockage is the obstruction of a once patent canal preventing full instrument access to the apical stop or stricture. Most blockages result from the packing of dentinal chips, cotton pellets, paper points, or a piece of fractured instrument within the canal (24). Loss of working length due to dentinal chip accumulation at the apical third of the canal can usually be attributed to too rapid an increase in file size, insufficient irrigation technique, inadequate recapitulation, and lack of routine radiographic evaluation (24). Once the condition has occurred, it can be exceptionally difficult to correct. Use of a chelating agent with an EDTA component, such as RC-Prep®, can be of some help. Its action softens inorganic debris such as dentinal chips, and when used in cooperation with reinstrumentation and frequent irrigation with 3–6% sodium hypochlorite, it may facilitate the reestablishment of working length. In other cases, it is a procedural measurement or recording error, and not a true loss of working length. This typically occurs from improper angular placement of the stop on the file, resulting in variations of the measurement to working length according to which side of the file is used to make the measurement.

Cotton pellets and paper points can in most cases be removed with the delicate assistance of a barbed broach or file. Broken instruments in the canal may sometimes be removed by access enlargement and the use of a pair of mosquito forceps to grasp the end. Care must be maintained not to remove excessive amounts of dental tissue to avoid producing unsound tooth structure. The use of a magnetized file, spreader, or plugger can be of assistance with loose instrument pieces. Many spreaders and pluggers with a high ferrous content can typically be magnetized, in the same fashion as screwdrivers, with a strong magnet or magnetizer.

Ultrasonic energy has been demonstrated to be one of the best ways to manage obstruction retrievals in the root canal (25). Ultrasonic instruments and techniques involving them are commonly used to disengage cements and loosen solid objects and material from the frictional hold of the root canal. In some cases, with orientation of the coronal canal access opening in a downward position and then placement of an ultrasonic scaler in contact with the tooth, the fragment may vibrate out of the opening. With those that are more tenacious and in the coronal or upper part of the canal, a different approach can be taken. The access can be slightly enlarged and the scaler placed against the exposed portion of the fragment to loosen it with activation of the ultrasonic device. With deeper instrument fragments, a spreader or plugger may be placed in direct contact with the end of the instrument, and the ultrasonic scaler can be touched to the spreader and activated to vibrate the fragment indirectly with the ultrasonic energy. In other cases when the instrument fragment cannot be loosened, a Gates-Glidden drill can be used to widen the area immediately above the fragment. Canal obturation can be then attempted by leaving the fragment and bypassing it in instrumentation to complete the root canal procedure. Occasionally, when the bypass instrument is in lateral contact with the instrument fragment, it can be energized with an ultrasonic device and loosen the fragment. If the instrument fragment is bound firmly at the apex with no canal distal to the fragment, sealer may be induced around it for an apical seal, and the procedure can be completed.

In these cases, the owner should be advised of the situation, and routine rechecks performed for signs or symptoms of failure. If the fragment is not at the apex and cannot be bypassed, a surgical procedure with a retrograde filling would be advisable.

Cemented posts, silver points, and endodontic instruments can be dislodged more easily when energized with an instrument such as an ultrasonic scaler tip (26). Chemical softening of the cement may be attempted with eugenol, sodium bicarbonate, and oil of orange to ease dislodgement (25). A combination of access and/or canal enlargement with the adjunctive use of chemical softeners may be employed, as well as ultrasonic activation. Removal of gutta-percha seldom represents a serious problem. A Gates-Glidden or gutta-percha extractor (GPX®, Brasseler USA, Savannah, Georgia) drill is customarily effective for gross removal, followed by the use of K-type reamers or K-type files. If necessary, eucalyptol can be used as a chemical softener of the gutta-percha, or heated instruments may be used. In retrieval of any blockage material, the paramount goal is the removal of the obstruction with maintenance of tooth integrity (27). Restorative materials such as amalgam or composite that inadvertently are carried into the canal during access opening can usually be teased out of the canal with a file placed in the canal and energized with an ultrasonic scaler.

Instrumentation Errors

Ledging also causes loss of working length, but it can usually be corrected with use of proper treatment protocol. A *ledge* is a gouge or false canal created during instrumentation with excessive apical pressure; it is primarily associated with curved canals (Fig. 2). Prevention comes from avoidance of excessive apical instrument pressures until the file is working freely in the canal, use of lubricants on the files, and use of prebent

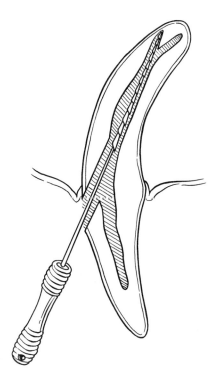

FIG. 2. Ledging or transposition.

files with properly placed directional stops when work involves curved canals. Early recognition of the error is important, and the dilemma is usually obvious if routine radiographs are being taken; however, if missed, it may lead to perforation and a poor prognosis of the endodontic procedure. Even when errors are caught early, the novice will find that attempts at reestablishment of the original canal pathway can be frustrating. This can be overcome in most cases by placing a 45° acute bend 3 mm from the tip of a pathfinder or No.8–15 K-type file. Place the directional stop so that it points to the direction of the angle of the instrument point. The instrument should be well lubricated with Gly-Oxide® (Pfizer USA, New York, New York) or RC-Prep®. The tip of the instrument should be directed away from the ledge. The spring action of the bend of the instrument will normally force the tip to bypass the ledge and compel it to enter the true root canal passageway, thus allowing correct working length to be achieved. Aggressive filing with this instrument will usually result in filling of the ledge with dentinal chips, aiding in its occlusion.

Another procedural error resulting in change of working length is *zipping* or *ellipticatation* (Fig. 3). These terms refer to the transportation or transposition of the apical portion of the canal (28,29). The primary indicted causes of zipping are failure to prebend files, excessive rotation of instruments, and use of too stiff instruments in curved canal systems (24). A stricture known as an *elbow* typically results in this condition (see Fig. 3). Two complications are common with this phenomenon: *apical perforation* and *elbow stricture*. In elbow stricture, the gutta-percha points are commonly seated against the elbow stricture instead of the true stricture or apical stop. This leaves an unfilled apical void or vault in which fluids can accumulate and result in eventual failure of the endodontic procedure. The best approach to treat this problem is an obturation technique that makes use

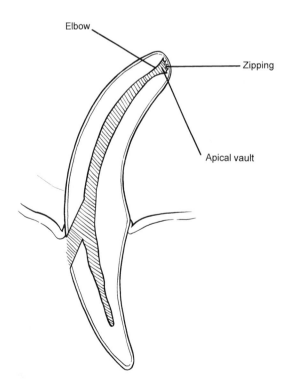

FIG. 3. Elbowing within the apical portion of the root canal contributed to the apical vault and zipping.

of softened gutta-percha that can be compacted past the elbow and into the apical vault. If perforation has occurred, then it is best to use a sealer containing calcium hydroxide instead of the usual zinc oxide–eugenol sealers, which can be more irritating to the periapical tissues. Additionally, the calcium hydroxide products may stimulate formation of a hard tissue barrier when in direct contact with the periodontium (24). Continued signs or symptoms of failure may indicate the advisability of surgical endodontics with an apical retrograde filling.

Stripping is an endodontic complication that results in lateral wall perforation (Fig. 4). This refers to the thinning of a lateral root canal wall, usually in the direction of the root tip curvature. Overzealous instrumentation in the midroot areas is the primary suspected cause, with perforation eventually occurring if not caught early. Judicial use of filing pressure away from the curvature of the root tip and/or toward the more bulky portion of the tooth root (*anticurvature filing*) is normally sufficient to prevent stripping (24). Stripping, when detected early, can be handled by appropriate instrumentation as previously described. Proper radiographs normally provide the differential diagnosis between lateral wall perforation of stripping and apical perforations. Treatment of *lateral wall perforation* is best dealt with in a two-stage nonsurgical endodontic procedure. Nonaffected roots can have standard endodontic treatment completed. The perforated root should be filled with calcium hydroxide powder. A thick paste can be made using calcium hydroxide powder mixed with either sterile saline or a local anesthetic solution. This can be introduced into the canal with a spiral filler, a Thermolateral Compactor (TLC®, Brasseler USA, Savannah, Georgia), or a McSpadden compactor. The use of the McSpadden compactor has been previously described on dogs and macaques (30,31). The material should be gently compacted and a temporary filling placed in the access. The calcium hydroxide normally halts exudate or hemorrhage entering the canal and can stimulate healing

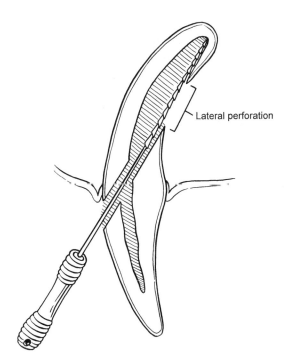

Lateral perforation

FIG. 4. Stripping of the canal wall can result in lateral wall perforation.

with the potential for a calcific barrier formation. The keys to success are rapid identification of the problem, immediate sealing of the perforation to control contamination, and avoidance of forcing sealing material into the periodontium. The calcium hydroxide should be allowed to remain within the root canal system for 4–6 weeks or until all symptoms have subsided. The paste, which by this time will normally be a dry powder, is now removed using anticurvature filing to reduce pressure against the perforation site, as well as copious irrigation. Irrigation should be performed only with normal saline, although 3% hydrogen peroxide is acceptable in most cases. Once the canal has been instrumented and cleaned, it is ready for obturation. Standard treatment is appropriate at this point, although a calcium hydroxide–containing root canal sealer is normally preferred (24). Should symptoms persist, a retrofill surgical approach may be attempted, although chances of success are poor. Hemisection may prove advisable in some refractory cases, and extraction in others.

Apical perforation is the condition when an instrument extends beyond the apical constriction. It is typically associated with one of two scenarios. Loss of the apical constriction (apical stop) customarily occurs due to root resorption from disease or due to excessive instrumentation. This leads to instrumentation damage to the periodontal ligament and alveolar bone and possible inoculation of the area with debris and bacteria. Additionally, in an open apex, overfilling and poor apical seal, as well as patient discomfort, may occur. Continued hemorrhage into the canal is another common sign. Although continued hemorrhage can be an indication of overinstrumentation, it is more commonly an indication of underinstrumentation. Differential diagnosis is often evident with good-quality intraoral radiographs. Prevention comes from appropriate use of instrument stops, quality operative radiographs with periodic verification, and attention to detail during instrumentation. Once apical perforation and loss of apical stop occur, control of hemorrhage is the first step. A new apical stop must then be established within the confines of the root canal system without excessive loss of structural integrity. This is accomplished by establishing a position with the endodontic file tip approximately 1–2 mm from the apex radiographically. With stops in place at this newly established working length, instrumentation should continue to two or three file sizes larger than the first file that shows binding at the tip. This is commonly known as *backup technique* (Fig. 5). A balanced-force, back-and-forth, stem-winding instrumentation should be used when possible. This will aid in forcing dentinal chips into the open apex, forming a chip barrier or plug. Flaring of the coronal third with a Hedstrom file and packing of the dentinal chips can also provide the same results, but caution should be used, as this may also lead to

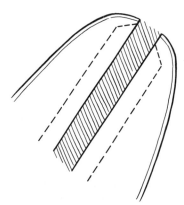

FIG. 5. The backup technique and a tooth without an apical stop. The *dotted lines* indicate the area of instrumentation that allows the reestablishment of the apical ledge or stop for standardized endodontic treatment.

canal blockage. Although clinical success cases support chip packing, it is still considered controversial by some authors (32,33).

Resectioning of Teeth and Roots

The terminology for tooth and/or root resection has been very diverse in the dental literature over the years, such as *radisectomy* (34), *tooth separation* (35), *odontosection* (21), and *tooth sectioning* (36); but *amputation* and *hemisection* are two of the most commonly used terms. Possibly, the more correct term should be tooth or root *resection* (37). *Hemisection* indicates that a tooth is being cut in half, generally through the furcational area. Therefore, the term is accurate only for two-rooted teeth in most cases. The term *sectioning* comes from the Latin word *sectus*, meaning to cut, while *resection* comes from the related Latin word *resectus*, meaning to cut off. Within the parameters being discussed, the structure is being cut off, not just cut. Therefore, *root resection* is the cutting off of a root only (Fig. 6A), while *tooth resection* is the cutting off of a portion of the crown with or without its associated root structure (Fig. 6B).

Resection is performed for many reasons, such as root fracture, root perforation, root resorption, endodontically inoperable tooth or root, periodontal disease, tumors of the jaws, or fractures of the jaws. Root resection involves a horizontal or angular cut to remove the root from the cervix of the tooth. This is most easily accomplished with a high-speed dental handpiece using a carbide steel or a diamond crosscut bur. Generally,

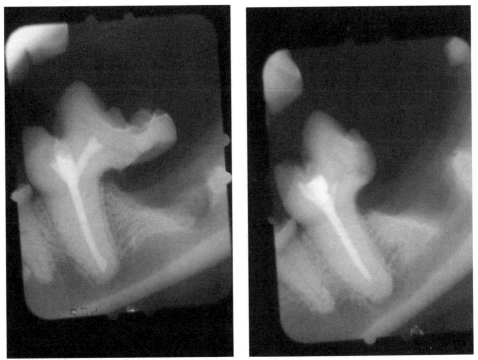

A   B

FIG. 6 (A) Radiograph of mandibular 1st molar exhibiting the root resection technique. **(B)** Radiograph of mandibular 1st molar exhibiting the tooth resection technique.

steel burs are used to cut the tooth in vital resectioning, as they produce less heat to insult the pulp, while diamond points or burs commonly cause bleeding on the pulp amputation. Selection is typically by personal preference. Diamond burs routinely cut faster, but because of their greater contact with the tooth surface, they generate more heat in a shorter period of time. A soft tissue flap and possible buccal bone plate reduction may be necessary in the majority of cases, although in periodontal disease sufficient exposure may already be present. Root resection allows the functional crown structure to remain intact, as compared with tooth resectioning. Currently in veterinary dentistry, both types are performed, but tooth resectioning is the more traditional because of the greater ease and speed of the procedure. The lower 1st molar is the most frequently resectioned tooth in the dog because of periodontal disease involving the distal root. Vital resectioning should be approached with appropriate deliberation because of the risk of loss of pulp vitality as in any pulp amputation or direct pulp-capping procedure (38). For this reason, complete standard endodontics on resectioned teeth deserves serious consideration (39,40).

Immature Deciduous Teeth

Disease and fractures of deciduous teeth occur in young animals. Treatment is determined by the extent of structural damage of the crown and root, the degree of physiologic or pathologic resorption of the root, pulp vitality or lack thereof, and the strategic value of the tooth.

As a rule, due to the short functionality (2–5 months in most dogs and cats) of the deciduous teeth, extraction is the best recourse. On occasion, retention of the tooth may be considered advisable in order to maintain the occlusal spacing and/or interlock. The mandibular cuspids and the maxillary corner incisors can be of strategic importance in maintaining the occlusal pattern in bites that are tight with an inclination toward a class III malocclusion pattern (prognathism). Maintaining these teeth may aid in holding the occlusion in a more normal and functional pattern for the individual. Other teeth may also be of importance in maintaining proper spacing in certain situations. When it is desired to maintain a tooth that still shows indications of pulp vitality, a *pulpotomy* with *direct pulp capping* and a permanent restoration of composite or glass ionomer is advised. If the tooth shows indications of irreversible pulpitis by continued pulp hemorrhage following pulpotomy or other signs, the pulp should be extirpated and the tooth treated as nonvital.

In nonvital teeth, the treatment protocol is greatly influenced by the state of the root structure based on pathologic and/or physiologic resorption. Instrumentation of the canal must be performed carefully not injure the permanent tooth bud by apical perforation of instruments, irrigants, or debris or by bacterial inoculation. Radiographs should be taken to establish working length, which should be 2–3 mm short of the current apex (41). Endodontic stops should be placed at the working length on all instruments to insure safety of the permanent tooth bud. Irrigation should be made with liberal amounts of sterile normal saline, and instruments coated with a chelating disinfectant, such as RC-Prep®. If the apex is intact, the canal can be filled with a thick zinc oxide–eugenol (ZOE) paste (42). The material can be placed by syringe or spiral filler, and a cotton pledget used to gently compact the material. Should air be trapped at the apex, a needle and syringe can be used to remove it. The needle is advanced to the site of the air bubble, and a vacuum is created with the syringe to evacuate it.

If the apex has already begun normal physiologic or abnormal pathologic resorption, the canal may best be filled with a calcium hydroxide paste (43). If the resorption is slight and only a slight overfill will occur, a ZOE paste would still be recommended. The final restoration can be made with an intermediate restorative, glass ionomer, or a composite. With ZOE-paste fills, a composite restoration will require an intermediate separating layer of a zinc oxyphosphate cement or glass ionomer, or the composite may fail to properly set up.

Immature Permanent Teeth

The permanent dentition of the dog has approximately only 50% of its expected root length present at the time of eruption (44). This also means that the apex and apical stop have not formed and the root end is open (Fig. 7). Teeth with undeveloped root apices are not good candidates for standard root canal therapy, as a hermetic seal of the apex is extremely difficult to successfully attain (45). Before the development of procedures to induce apical closure, treatment was typically a surgical approach with retrograde filling. Although this was successful in many cases, mechanical problems were commonly encountered. The thin, fragile dentinal walls proved challenging to attain an apical seal in the less developed apices (41), and removal of weak structure to a more substantial level would at times produce a poor crown:root ratio. For these reasons, two therapies have been developed to treat these teeth to stimulate the eventual closure of the apex (46). In vital teeth, it is termed *apexigenesis*, and in nonvital teeth *apexification* (47).

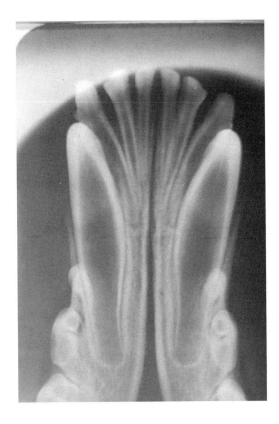

FIG. 7. Radiograph of immature teeth (mandibular cuspids) with open apices.

Apexigenesis is encouraged in immature permanent dentition with open apex and recent coronal pulp exposure, in which the pulp is still vital and salvage of the tooth is desired. The goal of the procedure is to stimulate continued root growth, root-end closure, thickening of the dentinal walls of the root, and dentinal bridge formation at the pulpotomy access site. These are accomplished by maintaining the vitality of Hertwig's epithelial root sheath to encourage continued root growth and closure and by preserving pulp vitality and associated odontoblastic function in laying down additional layers of dentin to thicken the root and bridge the access site (Fig. 8).

The degree of inflammation as determined by the intensity of traumatic insult, the amount of debris and bacterial contamination, and the duration of time from exposure until treatment all play key roles in the likelihood of success in preserving pulp vitality. It can be difficult to determine the true extent of pulp inflammation. However, numerous studies (48–51) have indicated that the depth of inflamed pulp typically does not exceed 2–3 mm from the exposed surface for up to 168 hours, or 7 days, following traumatic exposures. Direct bacterial invasion via pulp tissue does not normally occur, even when left open to saliva, until food and debris contaminated with bacteria are impacted into direct contact with the pulp (48,51).

Pulpotomy and pulp-capping procedures using carbon dioxide laser (52), electrosurgery (53,54), ZOE (55–57), or formocresol (58–60) have been reported with various degrees of success, complications, and failures. However, these treatments should not be

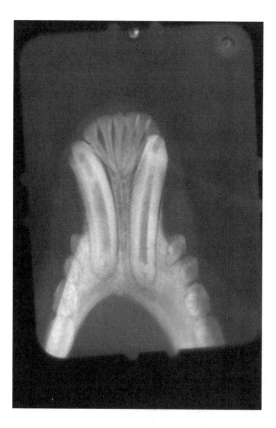

FIG. 8. Radiograph of mandiblar cuspids of a kinkajou showing dentinal bridging within the pulp chamber after crown amputation/pulpotomy/direct pulp capping with calicum hydroxide (6-month recheck).

routinely recommended, until further research has been fully explored and documented. Based on this rationale, only calcium hydroxide application therapy, which has been well documented for this purpose (61–63), will be described.

Once the condition is diagnosed and treatments are decided on, isolation and aseptic conditions should be maintained to prevent further introduction of debris or bacteria. Only exposed pulp deemed inflamed should ordinarily be removed. The instrument of choice is a high-speed dental handpiece with a diamond bur and adequate water flow to remove inflamed tissue, as it has been shown to create the least damage to the underlying pulpal tissues (64). The first few millimeters of inflamed or proliferative tissue should be removed until healthy pulp is encountered (65). In some cases, it may be necessary to remove pulp tissue to a greater depth to reach noninflamed tissue or to provide a suitable depth for restorative requirements. All filaments of the pulp tissue coronal to the selected amputation level should be removed; otherwise, hemorrhage will be difficult to control. Once the pulp is severed, the stump should be thoroughly cleansed with a gentle flow of normal saline or sterile water. Excess moisture can be removed by light syringe vacuum and sterile dry paper points. Blown air should not be used for this purpose, as it can cause desiccation and additional tissue damage. Most hemorrhage can be controlled with cotton pellets dipped in saline and placed against the pulp. Dry cotton pellets or paper points should not be used for this purpose, as they will be incorporated into the clot and, when removed, will dislodge the clot, stimulating additional hemorrhage. Dry paper points or cotton pellets may be placed on top of the wet in order to apply gentle pressure to aid in hemorrhage control. Should the hemorrhage persist, first check for filaments of pulp coronal to the amputation level; if found, they should be removed with an endodontic spoon. Continued bleeding for longer than 5–6 minutes may indicate that not all inflamed hyperplastic tissue has been removed and amputation should be performed more apically. Once amputation enters several millimeters into the root canal and hemorrhage is still insistent, a compromise treatment must be considered. The hemorrhage is then controlled using a hemostatic agent, such as aluminum chloride, applied with a cotton pellet or the blunt end of a paper point (41). Once hemorrhage has been controlled, sterile calcium hydroxide powder is placed against the pulp. An amalgam carrier and the blunt end of a paper point are customarily sufficient to accomplish this treatment. The calcium hydroxide should not be forced into the pulp, as this can result in pressure problems or stimulate excessive calcification within the canal. A calcium hydroxide or ZOE cement is then placed coronal to the powder, and the access is closed accordingly. Composite materials should not be placed directly over ZOE materials because of their tendency to interfere with proper curing and setting up.

The patient should be recalled for radiographic evaluations at 6–9-month intervals for up to 2 years to determine success. Once the apex has closed, the clinician must decide whether to leave the tooth as is or to follow with a complete standard endodontic root canal procedure. The main reason to consider this is periodic reports of calcium hydroxide–treated canals' becoming highly calcified, causing difficulties in endodontic instrumentation if needed at a later date (63,66). However, many other reports indicate that when proper and gentle technique is used, with care not to pack dentinal chips or calcium hydroxide into the underlying pulp tissue, poor negotiability of canals as a sequela of progressive calcification is highly infrequent (58–60).

Apexification is encouraged in the immature adult tooth with an open apex and coronal canal exposure, in which the tooth is pulpless or has a nonvital pulp and tooth salvage is desired. The goal is to stimulate root-end closure, so that eventually a standard endodontic procedure may be carried out. This is accomplished by the removal of all infected or decaying pulp and debris from the canal and by then filling the root canal space with a material to stimulate apical closure with formation of calcified tissue. Numerous materials that successfully promote apexification have been found. The list of compounds includes calcium hydroxide (67), zinc oxide pastes (68), antibiotic pastes (69), Walkoff's paste (70), Diaket (ESPE-Premier, Norristown, Pennsylvania) (71), and tricalcium phosphate (72,73), as well as the stimulation of a granulation bed by manipulating the tissue at the apex to encourage a hemorrhage clot within the canal (74). The use of calcium hydroxide alone or in various combinations has developed into the most commonly accepted protocol for apexification (41,67,75).

Histologic studies indicate that the calcification that occurs at the apical foramen in apexification tends to be *osteoid* (bone-like) or *cementoid* (cementum-like) (72,76–80). These studies have also repeatedly shown an absence of odontoblasts or Hertwig's epithelial root sheath, and thus their lack of involvement in this process. Research has suggested that adjacent cells of connective tissue differentiate in specialized osteoid-producing cells. However, investigators have noted that for apexification to occur, the apex must be entirely encompassed by cortical bone (81); this suggests that migration of these specialized cells from the cortical plate may be more likely than just differentiation occurring alone. Additionally, this means if there is any degree of radiolucency periapically, apexification may be delayed or not occur. Therefore, *radicular curettage and drainage* to simulate bony healing may be required in such cases to improve the prospect of obtaining apexification.

Apexification technique is not complex, but the basic guidelines must be strictly followed for consistent results. The removal of all infected pulp and debris is the first step. In many cases, the pulp will have decayed to a point of fragmentary debris or will have totally dissolved, leaving a pulpless tooth. A file with an endodontic stop applied is advanced until light resistance is met. Radiographs then confirm the location of the tip in relation to the tooth apex or suggest appropriate movement of the file. This is done in order to establish true working length for subsequent instrumentation to minimize periapical instrument trauma, which can affect the eventual outcome of the procedure. The canal should then be instrumented clean using saline as the irrigant of choice. Although sodium hypochlorite greatly improves disinfection and removal of debris, it must be used with extreme caution as it can easily be forced into the periapical tissues with the large open apex, often with dire results. Once all debris has been removed, the canal is dried by syringe aspiration of excess fluid and the employment of sterile dry paper points. The fill material of choice is eight parts calcium hydroxide and one part barium sulfate powder (80,81). The barium sulfate enhances radiopacity for better visualization of appropriate fill technique. The powder combination is then mixed into a creamy mixture using normal saline, Ringer's solution, distilled water, or an injectable local anesthetic solution such as lidocaine. The paste can be placed into the canal with an amalgam carrier, disposable syringe, endodontic pressure syringe, spiral filler, or a McSpadden-type compactor. Large-size pluggers are normally helpful in packing the material to the apex. Success has been reported in underfills or overfills, with overfill being the preferable of the two (75). However, a level or even fill is always best, thereby avoiding introduction of material into periapical tissue yet obtaining a complete fill. Use of some dry powder mix on top of the paste is sometimes helpful in compacting the paste. A cotton pellet can also be useful for this function, but extreme care must be taken not to lose it in the fill paste. Another compound with promise for this procedure, Mineral Trioxide Aggregate (MTA), is in development (Tulsa Dental Products, Tulsa, Oklahoma). Periodic radiographs are necessary to verify appropriate and adequate fill. Composite resin or glass ionomer filling material can be used for access closure.

Apexification normally requires 6–24 months (41). The patient should be recalled at 3-month intervals for physical and radiographic evaluation for symptoms or signs of infection or pathology. If these are found, the canal should be reopened, recleaned, and retreated. Recall is continued until radiographic evidence of a completed apexification is established. The tooth must then be reentered to physically confirm the apexification. Once reopened, the remaining paste mix is removed by gentle instrumentation and frequent saline flushing. A small file is then advanced to the calcified apex, and gentle pressure applied. Should it penetrate through, the canal must again be retreated and sealed to wait for completion of the apexification process. If the file fails to penetrate, then a standard endodontic root canal procedure may be performed at that time. Because of the oversized nature of most of these canals, a custom-formed gutta-percha point or injectable gutta-percha is preferred for obturation.

CLASSICAL SURGICAL ENDODONTICS

Complicating factors in or around the apical third of a tooth may prevent its effective treatment using conservative standard endodontics (82). Surgical endodontic procedures such as *periradicular drainage*, *apical* and *periapical curettage*, *apical resection* or *apicoectomy*, and *retrograde obturation* or *filling* are in many cases the sole alternatives to extraction (83–88). Surgical endodontics, although an advanced procedure, should not be considered radical, but another alternative option (89).

Criteria for Selection

The most common indication for surgical treatment is when standard endodontic therapy is not possible or has been ineffective in resolving periapical problems (90). In such cases, surgical procedures may offer resolution (91). Factors implicated in such problems are numerous but typically can be placed in one of two categories: those with an internal root apex inaccessibility and those with external root end complications.

Inaccessible apices can be present due to a number of reasons. Acute curvature of the canal can occasionally inhibit standard instrumentation, although with newer, highly flexible files, this is not as much of a problem as it once was. Reduced canal dimensions due to secondary or tertiary reparative dentin deposition from age or irritation result in barrier problems in reaching the apex for proper sealing. Decisions of inaccessibility should not be based on radiographs alone. Many canals can be located with pathfinders and instrumented sufficiently for obturation with fine instruments, lubricants, and chelating agents. Broken instruments lodged in the canal may also prevent instrumentation to the apex. Pulp stones (*endoliths*), if unremovable or not bypassable, may preclude apical contact. Malformations of the teeth may provide the same hindrances. Some of these are dentinogenesis imperfecta, dental dysplasia, dens in dente, fusion, dilaceration, and various other root malformations (82,92).

External root end complications can also be reasons for surgical endodontic procedures. Among these is failure of radiographic evidence of resolution of periapical destruction within a reasonable period of time (9–12 months). Cyst formation typically occurs when the rests of Malassez, an epithelial structure caught in a periapical granuloma, rapidly proliferate due to the chronic irritation (85). Failure of a periapical lesion to show indications of healing may indicate periapical cyst formation. Surgical intervention is generally required to address the cystic pathology. Incomplete root development may be cause for surgical endodontics, but apexigenesis and apexification should typically be attempted first. Root fractures in the apical third may prevent complete instrumentation, and in these cases, surgery to remove the fractured root tips may be required. Perforation of the apex by instruments may necessitate surgical procedures, but backup technique to reestablish the apical stop can often alleviate the condition.

Contraindications

There are distinct contraindications for surgical endodontics. These are complex deviations of patient, root, crown, and periodontal health, as well as anatomic location. The patient must be systemically healthy enough to permit the required sedation and anesthesia for the procedure, as well as reasonable healing of the tissues following surgery (90). Excessively weak or damaged roots that require extensive root resection may leave an unfavorable crown:root ratio, permitting easy exfoliation due to trauma or inflammatory disease. If the crown has been damaged beyond reasonable restoration and the root, if saved, serves no useful function, extraction may be best. In cases of advanced periodontal disease, the patient's general health may be best served also by exodontia. Anatomic conditions of the tooth include its location, the value of the bony support that must be removed for access, and the proximity of neural, vascular, sinus, and other important structures (90). Location considerations have to do with the ability to obtain access and visualize structures. In the anterior portion of the mouth, this is not of major concern, but in the posterior region, especially in most herbivores, this can present a problem unless access external to the mouth is utilized.

The value of the bony support tissue to be removed is also important. In the mandible, the posterior buccal cortical plate thickens. Removal of excessive support structure to gain access to root apices can lead to a weakened mandible that may be more prone to fracture in the short term, until complete healing has taken place. If periodontal or other disease has already compromised the mandibular strength, additional bone removal may not be judicious.

The proximity to various structures and organs must also be considered (92). Vessels and nerves exiting from the infraorbital canal of the maxilla just above the mesiobuccal root of the maxillary 4th premolar should be located and isolated if needed to prevent their injury. The same is true in the mandible of those vessels and nerves exiting the mental foramina. The roots of the mandibular premolars and molars generally lie just above the mandibular canal except for the 1st molar roots, which commonly lie just lateral to the canal. Injury to the structures within the canal can lead to nerve loss and other complications. In the maxillary region, other structures to watch for are the palatine arteries, which bleed profusely when cut, and the maxillary sinus above the maxillary 4th premolar. Care should be taken to avoid perforation of the sinus floor. Should this occur, bleeding from the nose may occur during surgery and facial emphysema immediately following it, when the endotracheal tube is removed. This can usually be minimized by proper packing and good flap closure. Additionally, when perforation of the sinus or mandibular canal occurs, caution must be exercised not to allow debris, root tips, infected bone, or filling materials to be pushed into these openings. Reasonable attempts to remove such material should be made if this happens.

Apical and Periapical Surgical Endodontic Procedures

The four major categories of apical surgical interventions are periradicular drainage, periapical curettage, apical resection or apicoectomy, and retrograde obturation or filling (92,93). Each serves a distinct function and is not necessarily linked to another in every case.

Periradicular Drainage

When exudate begins to accumulate due to acute periapical inflammation, the adjacent alveolar bone can be rapidly destroyed (90). This typically leads to pain and swelling. As the condition becomes worse, additional bone is lost and systemic symptoms of fever and malaise may develop (94–97).

Radiographically, periapical lucency develops as the acidic exudate erodes the cortical plate and hormonal response to the inflammation further demineralizes the bone.

Establishment of drainage can relieve much of the pain, swelling, and discomfort (90). Maintenance of drainage can allow periapical healing and the successful use of standard endodontics in many cases. In an emergency situation, antibiotics, anti-inflammatory drugs, and analgesics may give temporary relief. Drainage can be established by two routes. The first is by opening the tooth and extirpating the pulp to allow drainage through the tooth. In dogs, which have apical deltas, this is an unreliable technique for complete relief.

The second drainage technique involves a surgical trephination through the bone (97). The canal is opened and the pulp extirpated. A file with an endodontic stop is then placed and radiographed to establish the appropriate working length and approximate apical location. Selection of the incision site should take into consideration local anatomic consideration such as vessels, nerves, and osseous canal opening. The flap should be patterned for good blood supply and adequate exposure. Injection with a local anesthetic with epinephrine in a healthy patient can aid in hemorrhage control and postoperative discomfort. An elliptical incision is made with a No.15 blade, beginning above an adjacent tooth and 4 mm apical to the point determined as the apical location. The incision is extended in a half-moon shape across the site 4 mm coronal to the apical location and completed to a point 4 mm apically once again, above the opposite adjacent tooth. When possible, the coronal margin should extend into the attached gingiva. This will provide a firm attachment point that prevents the flap from gathering when sutured and resulting in an irregular mucosal pattern or postsurgical lump. A full-thickness mucoperiosteal flap is elevated using a No.2, No.4, or No.9 Molt periosteal elevator. With the bone exposed, a No.4 or No.6 round ball bur on high-speed handpiece—with adequate water flow to prevent thermal injury to the bone—is used to bore a hole through the alveolus and into the diseased pocket. Most hemorrhage problems can be controlled with simple, gentle digital pressure using cotton pellets and gauze, with care taken to remove all material prior to closure. Strands of cotton left embedded in the bone can delay healing and cause inflammatory foreign body problems. Caustics and styptics for hemorrhage control should be avoided, if possible, as they may inhibit proper postsurgical clot formation and result in poor new bone formation (98). Radiographs should be used to pinpoint the trephination site, which is generally 1–2 mm coronal to the root apex. The alveolar juga can be used to aid in locating the apex, as well as needles or gutta-percha points preplaced at intervals for radiographs. Care should be taken in trephination, as an improper approach may result in numerous additional problems. An improper approach may be one above the root tip into other tissues or organs, too lateral and resulting in damage to adjacent vital teeth, or below the desired point and requiring extension of the trephination access. Once the pocket is entered, it can be flushed with saline and a gauze drain of umbilical tape can be placed and sutured in place to keep the incision open to allow healing.

The root canal can be completed at this point. Use of antibiotics is a clinical decision based on the degree of systemic signs and symptoms. The drain is typically removed in 3–6 days, although longer durations may be required in some cases.

Periapical Curettage

Occasionally, apical or periapical curettage is used following apical trephination. At times, this is used to remove apical pathology such as granulomas, but it is more commonly used to eliminate cystic tissue. Once exposure of the root tip is accomplished, a periosteal curette or spoon is employed to peel the lesion free. Periapical lesions can be caused by developmental, metabolic, traumatic, odontogenic, infective, or neoplastic disorders. Therefore, tissue excised from the apical region should be examined, for if removal is justified, so is histologic assessment.

In well circumscribed lesions, once exposed, curettage is quick and simple. However, some periapical tissues are more complicated to remove (98). In some cases, the diseased tissues may be intimately involved with fibrous connective tissue, associated with chronic lesions and fistulas. These typically require extremely sharp curettes or more commonly a scalpel to remove. In cases in which lesional tissue extends into adjacent structures, a more conservative course of action may be prudent to prevent inadvertent injury to adjacent vital teeth, organs, or tissue or the creation of communications with sinus, nasal passage, or osseous canals. In such cases, an incisional biopsy is performed, radicular drainage established, and root canal therapy completed, if possible. If the lesional tissue is granulative, cystic, or infected, prolonged periradicular drainage is generally curative. Should the tissue be neoplastic, a new treatment plan may be required in accordance with histologic findings.

Apical Resection

Apical resection or apicoectomy is performed fundamentally for two reasons: removal of a diseased apex (Fig. 9) and access for retrograde filling. Resection of a necrotic or diseased apex is done in order to stimulate healing, in combination with a standard coronal access obturation. Retrograde filling is accomplished in conditions in which standard access obturation cannot be accomplished due to blockage or it has repeatedly failed. In either case, the most important point is the removal or extraction of the apical tip, once resectioned. If left in place, it will act as a nidus of continued infection, even if a excellent obturation and seal is accomplished.

The procedure is similar to that for trephination, except that a larger flap and bore hole are generally required. Once the root tip is isolated, it is ready for resection. This can be accomplished by burs on standard high-speed or miniature handpieces (Kavo America, Hoffman Estates, Illinois; Union Broach/Moyco, Philadelphia, Pennsylvania; Dyna-Dent, Santa Ana, California). For the veterinarian, the high-speed handpiece will be the most commonly used technique. In resection, for removal of diseased root, it is customarily recommended to remove all pathologic structure (99). This must be done with consider-

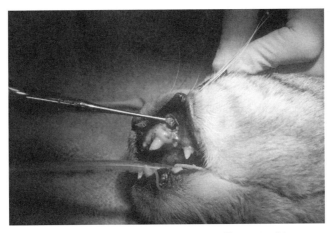

FIG. 9. Apicoectomy of feline maxillary cuspid.

ation that excessive root removal will result in a poor crown:root ratio. If the tooth is to be saved, a conservative approach must be taken with single-rooted teeth demonstrating extensive radicular involvement. A good general rule is to refrain from removing over half the root structure and use periradicular drainage techniques to improve the probability of success. In the dog and the cat, a tapered crosscut bur, such as a 669L, works well in most cases.

An elevator is used to loosen the root tip, and forceps are used for its removal. The exposed socket should be curetted clean. If periradicular drainage is not used, the empty socket area should be packed with an osteogenic product, such as tricalcium phosphate, HTR® (Bioplant, Norwalk, Connecticut), or ADD® (THM Biomedical, Duluth, Minnesota), among others, to control hemorrhage, and the flap should be closed.

Retrograde Obturation or Filling

When a retrograde filling is to be placed, an apicoectomy similar to that previously described is used. The main difference is that only the apical-most 4–6 mm of the apex or root tip is removed. It is resectioned or cut off at a 45° angle in an apical direction. This allows ease of removal of the severed root tip, while providing good visibility of the apical canal anatomy (90).

For cavity preparation for a retrograde filling, generally one of two types is used: a class I cavity preparation or a modified preparation known as the *slot of Matzuri* (87). The class I preparation is customarily preferred, when location allows, as less bone and tooth structure require removal (87).

The class I preparation is made using a small round ball bur (100,101). It is inserted into the apical exposure of the canal to a depth of 3–5 mm. An undercut is then created with the round ball bur or an inverted-cone bur. Because of the restricted space being worked in, the microhead handpiece and microburs may be required (90).

When root location, anatomy, or handpiece size prevents a class I preparation, the slot of Matzuri is customarily used. The root tip is resected as previously described, although additional buccal bone may need to be excavated for extension of the slot. The tip of a tapered-fissure bur is placed in the apical opening of the root canal perpendicular to the long axis of the root. A 3–5-mm long slot is then cut in the root directed coronally. A small round ball bur is placed at the apical canal opening perpendicular to the root, passed down the slot to its most coronal extent, and then pulled through the lateral wall, thus creating an undercut and a preparation appearing like a keyhole.

A clear and dry operative field aids in seeing and placing retrograde-filling materials. Cotton pellets, gauze, Gelfoam® sponges (UpJohn Company, Kalamazoo, Michigan), and bone wax are some of the more commonly used products for clearing the operative site. Gelfoam® dissolves and blends into the area, providing an absorbable barrier. Cotton pellets and gauze can be used with simple pressure or saturated with a hemostatic solution, when necessary. Bone wax is a highly purified beeswax with additives to improve handling. It is gently pressed into the area to form a waterproof barrier between tooth and bone. Bone wax, if used, should be placed prior to apical cavity preparation so that it is not forced inadvertently into the canal, as it may prevent formation of a good apical seal. Bone wax must be removed before closure, just as cotton pellets and gauze must, to avoid healing complications.

Selection of the retrograde-filling material is the next consideration. Amalgam has long been the product of preference, but it has been losing popularity of late to newer products. If amalgam is used, a zinc-free, high copper product is generally preferred, but not required (90). Both zinc and zinc-free amalgam are well tolerated and effective, when placed and compacted in a dry preparation and environment (102–104). If zinc amalgams are placed or worked in even slight moisture, an expansion of 4% and more may occur (105,106), which can result in creep, restorative and root fractures, loss of apical seal, and failure of the procedure. Regardless of the type of amalgam used, a good undercut and use of a cavity varnish in a dry environment greatly improve apical seal and long-term success (107,108). Numerous other products have been studied for retrograde filling, but most have various disadvantages or lack research substantiating effectiveness and safety (94,102,107,109–111). Two zinc oxide–eugenol products that have offered substantial advantages are Super EBA® (Harry J. Bosworth Company, Skokie, Illinois) and IRM® (L.D. Caulk Company (112,113). Another compound with promise for retrograde filling is MTA™ (Tulsa Dental Products).

With amalgam, once the preparation is ready, the cavity varnish is first placed in the cavity preparation, blown thin, and allowed to dry. A small retrograde amalgam carrier is used to pick up the amalgam from the well and carry it to the access site. The tip of the carrier is placed snugly against the preparation and the plugger depressed to force the restorative into the orifice. The carrier is then slid across the bevel to sever any attachment of the amalgam in the preparation and that in the carrier prior to lifting it away. The amalgam is now compacted with retrograde pluggers, and the process is repeated until the cavity preparation is filled. A burnisher can be used to finish the surface, or a carver while an amalgam is setting up.

If Super EBA® or IRM® is used, a different technique can be followed. To begin with, no cavity varnish is used. The product is prepared to a stiff mix, and a microspatula is used to carry a cone-shaped piece of material to the preparation and gently force it into place. The process is repeated until the preparation is filled. As the material begins to stiffen, a plugger can be used to assist in compacting the restorative, and a carver in finishing.

Closure begins with cleaning of the osseous access site. If bone wax, cotton pellets, or gauze were properly placed, their careful withdrawal typically removes all debris. The osseous defect is packed with an osteogenic product, and the flap closure is completed using large tissue bites and a simple interrupted pattern.

Retrograde Root Canal Procedures

A retrograde root canal procedure is totally performed from the apex of the tooth rather than the crown; it has also been called *indirect resection* (98). Ordinarily, this procedure is performed on teeth that were originally vital when they were covered with a restorative or prosthodontic device but have since become nonvital. In some of these cases, the prosthodontic device or restorative cannot be removed without its destruction or that of the underlying tooth structure. Crowns and bridgework can be expensive, and their destruction or that of underlying dental structures removed to obtain a coronal approach may be avoided in some cases with a retrograde root canal procedure.

The procedure is basically a modification of the retrograde-filling protocol. Apical access is made and instrumentation performed customarily with bent files inserted through the apex into the coronal segment. Because of the complex pulp chamber in the coronal section, instruments cannot adequately clean these areas. Nevertheless, certain irrigants' chemomechanical actions can acceptably perform this function. This requires the use of chelating agents with instruments and the frequent irrigation of the canals with suitable amounts of half- or full-strength sodium hypochlorite and the copious use of saline. Once the canals are cleaned and dried, vertical compaction of gutta-percha points—or preferably a technique using heated gutta-percha—is used for obturation, and a standard retrograde apical filling is placed.

Continually Growing and Continually Erupting Teeth

Dental complications have been described, involving species such as rodents and lagomorphs, in which teeth continually erupt (114,115). Traumatic exposure of these open-rooted teeth should be attended to immediately in an attempt to maintain their vitality. A pulpotomy can be performed to remove exposed diseased pulp with a high-speed diamond bur. In a healthy pulp, the bleeding should subside within 2–6 minutes. Next, a direct pulp capping should be performed using calcium hydroxide powder, which is placed over the pulp and gently pushed in place with a paper point. This may be followed with a calcium hydroxide cement, such as DyCal® (L.D. Caulk Company), to provide additional medicament and support. This, hopefully, will lead to the development of a secondary dentinal bridge by odontoblasts and maintenance of the tooth's vitality. The access should be filled with a temporary-type filling material such as IRM®. Failure of vital endodontics typically results in chronic problems with infection, inflammation, occlusion, and/or loss of the tooth. This may inevitably lead to morbid consequences in many rodents and lagomorphs (31,114,115). In certain cases, extractions have alleviated problems, but it must be kept in mind that the opposite occluding tooth may then easily overgrow and produce additional problems that must then be cared for.

REFERENCES

1. Gutmann JL, Lovdahl PE. Problems encountered in access to the pulp chamber space. In: Gutmann JL, Dumsha TC, Lovdahl PE, eds. *Problem Solving in Endodontics*. Chicago: Year Book Medical Publishers; 1988:1.
2. Grossman LI. Endodontics. In: Grossman LI, ed. *Handbook of Dental Practice*. 3rd ed. Philadelphia: JB Lippincott Co; 1958:150.
3. Wiggs RB. Problem solving in veterinary endodontics. *Semin Vet Med Surg (Small Anim)* 1993;8:165.
4. Moreinis SA. Avoiding perforation during endodontic access. *JADA* 1979;98:707.
5. Eisner ER. Transcoronal approach for endodontic access to the fourth maxillary premolar in dogs. *J Vet Dent* 1990;7(4):22.

6. Strieff JT, Gerstein H. Access cavity perforations. In: Gerstein H, ed. *Techniques in Clinical Endodontics*. Philadelphia: WB Saunders Co; 1982:1.
7. Gutmann JL. Prevention and management of endodontic procedural errors. *N Z Soc Endod Newslet* 1982;23:15.
8. Tidmarsh BG. Accidental perforation of the roots of teeth. *J Oral Rehabil* 1979;6:235.
9. Sinai IH. Endodontic perforations: Their prognosis and treatment. *JADA* 1977;95:90.
10. Jew RCK, Weine FS, Keene JJ, et al. A histologic evaluation of periodontal tissues adjacent to root perforation filled with Cavit. *Oral Surg* 1982;54:124.
11. Oswald RJ. Procedural accidents and their repair. *Dent Clin North Am* 1979;23:593.
12. Martin LR, Gilbert B, Dickerson AW. Management of endodontic perforations. *Oral Surg* 1982;54:668.
13. Beavers RA, Bergenholtz G, Cox CF. Periodontal wound healing following intentional root perforations in permanent teeth of *Macaca mulatta*. *Int Endod J* 1986;19:36.
14. Harris WE. A simplified method of treatment for endodontic perforations. *J Endod* 1976;2:126.
15. Nicholls E. Treatment of traumatic perforations of the pulp cavity. *Oral Surg* 1962;15:603.
16. Aguirre R, ElDeeb ME, ElDeeb M. Evaluation of the repair of mechanical furcation perforations using amalgam, gutta percha or indium foil. *J Endod* 1986;12:249.
17. Lovdahl PE, Gutmann JL. Problems in locating and negotiating fine and calcified canals. In: Gutmann JL, Dumsha TC, Lovdahl PE, eds. *Problem Solving in Endodontics*. Chicago: Year Book Medical Publishers; 1988:17.
18. Wiggs RB. Pulpotomy: A case report. *J Vet Dent* 1987;4(2):32.
19. Wiggs RB. Canine oral anatomy and physiology. *Compend Cont Educ Pract Vet* 1989;11:1475.
20. Wiggs RB. Endodontic instrumentation. *J Vet Dent* 1991;8(4):11.
21. Gerstein H. Surgical endodontics. In: Laskin DN, ed. *Oral and Maxillofacial Surgery*. Vol II. St Louis, MO: CV Mosby Co; 1985:143.
22. Stamos DG, Haasch GC, Chenail B, et al. Endodontics: Clinical impressions. *J Endod* 1985;11:181.
23. Taintor JF, Ingle JI, Fahid A. Re-treatment versus further treatment. *Clin Prev Dent* 1983;5(5):8.
24. Glickman GN, Dumsha TC. Problems in canal Cleaning and shaping. In: Gutmann JL, Dumsha TC, Lovdahl PE, eds. *Problem Solving in Endodontics*. Chicago: Year Book Medical Publishers; 1988:18.
25. Goon WWY. Innovative uses of ultrasonic energy for the elimination of problematic root canal obstructions. *Compend Cont Educ Dent* 1992;13:650.
26. Gaffney JL, Lehman JW, Miles MJ. Expanded use of the ultrasonic scaler. *J Endod* 1981;7:228.
27. Goon WWY. Managing the obstructed root canal space: Rationale and technique. *Calif Dent Assoc J* 1991; 19:51.
28. Schilder H. Cleaning and shaping the root canal. *Dent Clin North Am* 1974;18:269.
29. Weine FS, Kelly RF, Lio PJ. The effect of preparation procedures on original canal shape on apical foramen shape. *J Endod* 1975;1:255.
30. Wiggs RB. Use of the McSpadden compactor for root canal obturation in dogs and macaques. *J Vet Dent* 1988; 5(3):9.
31. Wiggs RB. Fractured maxillary incisors in a beaver. *J Vet Dent* 1990;7(2):21.
32. Safavi K, Horsted P, Pascon EA, et al. Biological evaluation of the apical dentin chip plug. *J Endod* 1985;11:18.
33. Brady JE, Hivel VT, Weir JC. Periapical response to an apical plug of dentin filling intentionally placed after root canal overinstrumentation. *J Endod* 1985;11:323.
34. Grossman LI, Oliet S, del Rio CE. *Endodontic Practice*. 11th ed. Philadelphia: Lea & Febiger; 1988:322.
35. Grant DA, Stern IB, Listgarten MA. Periodontics in the tradition of Gottlieb and Orban. St Louis, MO: CV Mosby Co; 1988:921.
36. Goldman HM, Shuman AM, Isenberg GA. *An Atlas of the Surgical Management of Periodontal Disease*. Chicago: Quintessence Publishing Co; 1982:209.
37. Gutmann JL, Harrison JW. *Surgical Endodontics*. Boston: Blackwell Scientific Publishers 1991:420.
38. Kostlin R, Schebitz H. Zur endodontischen Behandlung der Zahnfraktur beim Hund. *Kleintierpraxis* 1980; 25:187.
39. Allen AL, Gutmann JL. Internal root resorption after vital root resection. *J Endod* 1977;3:438.
40. Gerstein K. The role of vital root resection in periodontics. *J Periodontol* 1977;48:478.
41. Camp JH. Pedodontic-endodontic treatment. In: Cohen S, Burns RC, eds. *Pathways to the Pulp*. 5th ed. St Louis, MO: Mosby-Year Book; 1991:692.
42. Bennett CG. Pulpal management of deciduous teeth. *Pract Dent Monogr* May-June 1965:1.
43. Berk H, Krakow AA. A comparison of the management of pulpal pathosis in deciduous and permanent teeth. *Oral Surg* 1972;34:944.
44. Emily P. Problems associated with the diagnosis and treatment of endodontic disease. *Probl Vet Med Dent* 1990; 2(1):152.
45. Camp JH. Pulp therapy for primary and young permanent teeth. *Dent Clin North Am* 1984;28:651.
46. Torneck CD. Endodontic management of partially developed permanent teeth. In: Levine N, ed. *Current Treatment in Dental Practice*. Philadelphia: WB Saunders Co; 1986:171.
47. Webber RT. Apexogenesis versus apexification. *Dent Clin North Am* 1984;28:669.
48. Cvek M, et al. Pulp reactions to exposure after experimental crown fracture or grinding in adult monkey. *J Endod* 1982;8:391.

49. Heide S. Pulp reactions to exposure for 4, 24 and 168 hours. *J Dent Res* 1908;59:1910.
50. Heide S, Kerekes K. Delayed pulpotomy in permanent incisors of monkeys. *Int Endod J* 1986;19:78.
51. Watts A, Paterson RC. Migration of materials and microorganisms in the dental pulp of dogs and rats. *J Endod* 1982;8:53.
52. Shoji S, Nakamura M, Horiuchi H. Histopathological changes in dentinal pulps irradiated by CO_2 laser: A preliminary report on laser pulpotomy. *J Endod* 1985;1:379.
53. Ruemping DR, Morton TH Jr, Anderson MW. Electrosurgical pulpotomy in primates—a comparison with formocresol pulpotomy. *Pediatr Dent* 1983;5:14.
54. Shaw DW, et al. Electrosurgical pulpotomy—a 6-month study in primates. *J Endod* 1987;13:500.
55. Kozlov M, Massler M. Histologic effects of various drugs on amputated pulps of rat molars. *Oral Surg* 1960; 13:455.
56. Masterson JB. The healing of wounds of the dental pulp of man. *Br Dent J* 1966;120:213.
57. Ravn JJ. Follow-up study of permanent incisors with complicated crown fracture after acute trauma. *Scand J Dent Res* 1982;90:363.
58. Fuks AB, Bimstein E, Bruchim A. Radiographic and histologic evaluation of the effect of two concentrations of formocresol on pulpotomized primary and young permanent teeth in monkeys. *Pediatr Dent* 1983;5:9.
59. Peron LC, Burkes DJ, Gregory WB. Vital pulpotomy utilizing variable concentrations of paraformaldehyde in rhesus monkeys. *J Dent Res* 1976;55:B129. Abstract no. 269.
60. Sanchez ZMC. *Effects of Formocresol on Pulp-capped and Pulpotomized Permanent Teeth of Rhesus Monkeys.* Ann Arbor: University of Michigan; 1972. Thesis.
61. Cvek M. Endodontic treatment of traumatized teeth. In: Andreasen JO, ed. *Traumatic Injuries of the Teeth.* 2nd ed. Philadelphia: WB Saunders Co; 1982, 321.
62. McDonald RE, Avery DR. Treatment of deep caries, vital pulp exposure, and pulpless teeth in children. In: McDonald RE, Avery DR, eds. *Dentistry for the Child and Adolescent.* 3rd ed. St Louis, MO: CV Mosby Co; 1978, 149.
63. Seltzer S, Bender IB. Pulp capping and pulpotomy. In: Seltzer S, Bender IB, eds. *The Dental Pulp, Biologic Considerations in Dental Procedures.* 2nd ed. Philadelphia: JB Lippincott Co; 1978, 281.
64. Granath LE, Hagman G. Experimental pulpotomy in human bicuspids with reference to cutting technique. *Acta Odontol Scand* 1971;29:155.
65. Cvek M. A clinical report on partial pulpotomy and capping with calcium hydroxide in permanent incisors with complicated crown fractures. *J Endod* 1978;4:232.
66. Langeland K, et al. Human pulp changes of iatrogenic origin. *Oral Surg* 1971;32:943.
67. Kaiser JH. Management of wide-open canals with calcium hydroxide. Presented at the meeting of the American Association of Endodontics; Washington, DC, April 17, 1964. Cited by Steiner JC, Dow PR, Cathey GM. Inducing root end closure of non-vital permanent teeth. *J Dent Child* 1968;35:47.
68. Cooke C, Rowbotham TC. Root canal therapy in non-vital teeth with open apices. *Br Dent J* 1960;108:147.
69. Ball JS. Apical root formation in a non-vital immature permanent incisor. *Br Dent J* 1964;116:166.
70. Bouchon F. Apex formation following treatment of necrotized immature permanent incisor. *J Dent Child* 1966; 33:378.
71. Friend LA. The root treatment of teeth with open apices. *Proc R Soc Med* 1966;59:1035.
72. Koenigs JF, et al. Induced apical closure of permanent teeth in adult primates using a resorbable form of tricalcium phosphate ceramic. *J Endod* 1975;1:102.
73. Roberts SC Jr, Brilliant JD. Tricalcium phosphate as an adjunct to apical closure in pulpless permanent teeth. *J Endod* 1975;1:263.
74. Nygaard-Otsby B. The role of the blood clot in endodontic therapy: An experimental histologic study. *Acta Odontol Scand* 1961;19:323.
75. Frank AL. Therapy for the divergent pulpless tooth by continued apical formation. *JADA* 1966;72:87.
76. Camp JH. *Continued Apical Development of Pulpless Permanent Teeth Following Endodontic Therapy.* Bloomington: Indiana University School of Dentistry; 1968. Thesis.
77. Ham JW, Patterson SS, Mitchell DF. Induced apical closure of immature pulpless teeth in monkeys. *Oral Surg* 1972;33:438.
78. Nevins AJ, et al. Revitalization of pulpless open apex teeth in rhesus monkeys, using collagen-calcium phosphate gel. *J Endod* 1976;2:159.
79. Steiner JC, Van Hassel HJ. Experimental root apexification in primates. *Oral Surg* 971;31:409.
80. Webber RT. Apexogenesis vs. apexification. *Dent Clin North Am* 1984;28:669.
81. Webber RT, Schwiebert KA, Cathey GM. A technique for placement of calcium hydroxide in the root canal system. *JADA* 1981;103:417.
82. Healy HJ. *Endodontics.* St Louis, MO: CV Mosby Co; 1960:72.
83. Goldsmith JP. Salvaging teeth by molar apicectomy. *N Y J Dent* 1979;49:324.
84. Gutmann JI. Principles of endodontic surgery for the practitioner. *Dent Clin North Am* 1984;28:895.
85. Gutmann JI, Hovland E. A critical reappraisal of the routine use of periradicular surgery in conjunction with endodontics. *JDC Dent Soc* 1978;53:17.
86. Koch C. *History of Dental Surgery.* Vol. 1. Chicago: National Art Publishing Co; 1910:208.
87. Matsura SJ. A simplified root-end filling technique. *J Mich State Dent Soc* 1962;44:40.

88. Uchin RA. Surgical endodontics. *Dent Clin North Am* 1979;23:637.
89. Chivian N. Midsurgery endodontics. In: Arens D, Adams W, Castro R, eds. *Endodontic Surgery*. New York: Harper & Row Publishers; 1983:213.
90. Arens DE. Surgical endodontics, In: Cohen S, Burns RC, eds. *Pathways to the Pulp*. 5th ed. St Louis, MO: Mosby-Year Book; 1991:574.
91. Barnes IE. Surgical endodontics: Introduction, principles, and indications. *Dent Update* 1981;8:89.
92. Healy HJ. Endodontics: Selection of cases and treatment procedures. *JADA* 1956;53:434.
93. Patterson SS. Surgical intervention associated with endodontic therapy. In: Healy HJ, ed. *Endodontics*. St Louis, MO: CV Mosby Co; 1960:244.
94. Bender IB, Seltzer S. Roentgenographic and direct observations of experimental lesions in bone. *JADA* 1961; 62:152.
95. Black CV. *Special Dental Pathology*. 3rd ed. Chicago: Medico-Dental Publishing Co; 1924.
96. LeQuire A, Cunningham C, Pelleu G. Radiographic interpretation of experimentally produced osseous lesions of the mandible. *J Endod* 1977;3:274.
97. Peters D. Evaluation of prophylactic alveolar trephination to avoid pain. *J Endod* 1980;6:518.
98. Sommer RF, Ostrander FD, Crowly MC. *Clinical Endodontics*. Philadelphia: WB Saunders Co; 1961:214.
99. Stabholz A, Friedman S, Tamse A. Endodontic Failures and retreatment. In: Cohen S, Burns RC, eds. *Pathways to the Pulp*. 5th ed. St Louis, MO: Mosby-Year Book; 1991:738.
100. Arens DE, Adams W, DeCastro R. *Endodontic Surgery*. New York: Harper & Row Publishers; 1981.
101. Barry G, Heyman R, Elias A. A comparison of apical sealing methods. *Oral Surg* 1975;39:806.
102. Delivanis P, Tabibi A. A comparative sealability study of different retrofilling materials. *Oral Surg* 1982;45:252.
103. Flande DH, et al. Comparative histopathologic study of zinc-free amalgam and Cavit in connective tissue of the rat. *J Endod* 1975;1:56.
104. Kimura J. A comparative analysis of zinc and non-zinc alloys in retrograde endodontic surgery, 1: Apical seal and tissue reaction. *J Endod* 1982;8:359.
105. Liggett WR, et al. Light microscopy, scanning electron microscopy, and microprobe analysis of bone response to zinc and non-zinc amalgam implants. *Oral Surg* 1980;49:263.
106. Zartner R, James G, Birch B. Bone tissue response to zinc polycarboxylate cement and zinc-free amalgam. *J Endod* 1976;2:203.
107. Abdal AK, Retief HD, Jamison HC. The apical seal via retrosurgical approach, II: An evaluation of retrofilling materials. *Oral Surg* 1982;54:213.
108. Tronstad L, et al. Sealing ability of dental amalgam as retrograde fillings in endodontic therapy. *J Endod* 1983; 9:551.
109. Abdal AK, Retief HD. The apical seal via retrosurgical approach, I: A preliminary study. *Oral Surg* 1982; 53:614.
110. Kos WL, Aulozzi DP, Gerstein H. A comparative bacterial microleakage study of retrofilling materials. *J Endod* 1982;8:355.
111. Stabholz A, et al. Marginal adaptation of retrograde fillings and its correlation with sealability. *J Endod* 1985; 11:218.
112. Coats JM. *Comparison of the Efficiency of Amalgam and IRM as Retrograde Filling Materials*. Detroit: University of Detroit; 1986. Thesis.
113. Oynick J, Oynick T. A study of a new material for retrograde fillings. *J Endod* 1978;4:203.
114. Lobprise HB, Wiggs RB. Dental disease in lagomorphs. *J Vet Dent* 1991;8(2):11.
115. Wiggs RB, Lobprise HB. Dental disease in rodents. *J Vet Dent* 1990;7(3):6.

13

Operative and Restorative Dentistry

Robert B. Wiggs and Heidi B. Lobprise

Today's breeds of dog vary greatly in head type and size, size of oral structures, and type of acceptable dental occlusion. Additionally, most depend to a lesser degree on tooth function than their wild, undomesticated ancestors. However, good oral health, including sound tooth structure, plays a pivotal role in the general overall health of patients, from hard-working police dogs to the spoiled, pampered pet (1). Those individuals using their teeth to perform specialized functions (retrieving, tracking, police work, etc.) frequently run a higher risk of trauma to oral structures, especially the teeth. Furthermore, even everyday pet owners normally wish to maintain their animal's teeth in a reasonable degree of health, function, and esthetic appearance. These client desires have resulted in an increasing demand for all forms of operative restorative procedures.

Operative dentistry is that branch of dentistry that relates to the diagnosis, prognosis, or treatment of teeth with vital or nonvital pulps and to the maintenance or restoration of the functional and physiologic integrity of the teeth as this applies to the adjacent hard and soft tissue structures of the oral cavity (2,3). This relates basically to operations to restore dental tissues as necessitated by resorptive activity, carious action, traumatic injury, impaired function, or the enhancement of esthetic appearance. Restorations may extend beyond the limits normally considered for operative procedures, to such procedures as esthetics procedures for the bleaching teeth. This chapter will focus on chairside restoration; laboratory-assisted restorations (prosthodontics) are handled in Chapter 14.

Restorative Terms

Abutment—a tooth, crown, or portion of an implant used to support, stabilize, or anchor a fixed or removable dental prosthesis, such as a bridge.
Bridge—a dental prosthesis that replaces the crown of one or more missing teeth.
Cap—colloquialism for crown.
Core—a substructure for a crown, which may be part of a post-and-core system.
Crown—a restorative that covers part or all of the clinical crown.
Enamel prisms—basic enamel unit running from the dentinoenamel junction to the surface enamel.
Flashing—a restorative that extends beyond the preparation outline, although, when initially placed, it did not cause an overhang.

Inlay—a restoration made to fit into a tooth.

Onlay—a restoration made to fit over or replace an incisal edge or occlusal cusp either partially or completely.

Overhang—an excess of restoration projecting beyond the parameters of a preparation margin and resulting a projection or shoulder.

Pin—a metal pin or wire cemented or threaded into the dentin at a preparation site to aid in retention of a restoration.

Pontic—the portion of a dental bridge that replaces a missing tooth.

Post—a cylindrical metal rod cemented or threaded into the root canal system as a retentive device for a core or post and crown.

Undercut—a designed feature of a restorative preparation, created by removing a portion of the dentin within the preparation, with the intention of providing retentive qualities to a restoration.

Veneer—a thin restorative covering, generally used to conceal a discoloration, malformation, attritional wear, or other minor injury.

Classification of Cavities and Restorations

For proper treatment, lesions are best classified as to the tooth involved and type and extent of lesion. Individual tooth identification systems can be found in Chapter 4. Carious lesion are classically staged by the G.V. Black classification (Table 1). In addition to location (Fig. 1), tooth pathology can be classified based on type and extent. Some of the more common of these follow:

Elementary Cavity Classification by Location (4)

Simple	Involving only one tooth surface
Compound	Involving two tooth surfaces when prepared
Complex	Involving three or more tooth surfaces when prepared

TABLE 1. *G.V. Black modified cavity preparation classification system*

Class[a]	Tooth type	Location
1	I,PM,M	Beginning in structural defects, such as pit or fissure, commonly found on occlusal surfaces
2	PM,M	Proximal surfaces; when a tooth with a class 2 lesion includes a class 1 lesion, it is still considered class 2
3	I,C	Proximal surfaces; incisal angle not included
4	I,C	Proximal surfaces; incisal angle included
5	I,C,PM,M	Facial or lingual, gingival third; excluding pit or fissure lesions
6	I,C,PM,M	Defect of incisal edge or cusp; not included in Black's original classification

I, incisor; C, canine or cuspid; M, molar; PM, premolar.

[a] Roman numbers (ie, I, II, III, etc.) may also be used. There may be lesions of two different classes on the same tooth (eg, class II and class V) or a combination lesion, where two locations are present and contiguous (eg, class II/V).

(Adapted from ref. 4.)

Class I

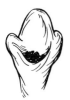

Developmental
groove on the
lingual surface
of an incisor

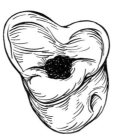

Pits and fissures on
occlusal surfaces of
premolars and molars

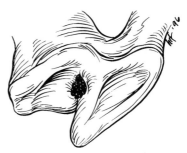

Buccal surface developmental
groove of maxillary fourth premolar

Lesions beginning in pits, fissures or
developmental grooves of teeth

A

Class II

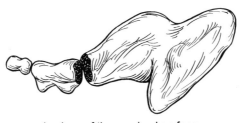

Lesions of the proximal surface
of premolars and molars

B

Class III

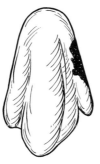

Class IV

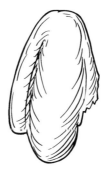

Lesions of the proximal
surface of an incisor
C   or canine tooth

Lesion at proximal surface
of an incisor or canine tooth
that involves an incisal edge   D

FIG. 1. The modified G.V. Black lesion and cavity preparation classification system. The lesions are listed from classifications 1–6. **(A)** Class I: lesions of pits, fissures, or developmental grooves. **(B)** Class II: lesions of the proximal surfaces of premolars or molars. **(C)** Class III: lesions of the proximal surfaces of incisors or canine teeth. **(D)** Class IV: lesions of the proximal surfaces of incisors or canine teeth that involve the incisal edge.

Class V

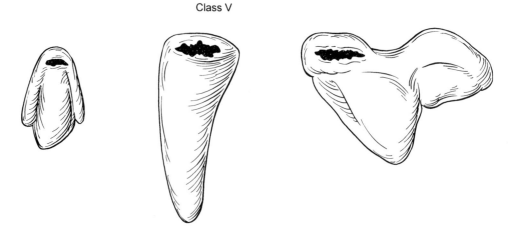

E

Lesions on labial, buccal or lingual surfaces
of an incisor, cuspid, premolar or molar

Class VI

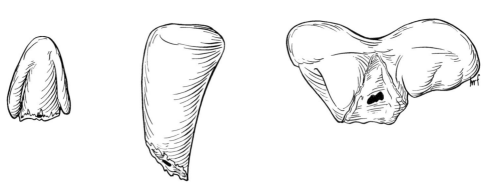

F

Lesions of the incisal edge or cusp tip

FIG. 1. *Continued.* **(E)** Class V: lesions of the labial, buccal, or lingual surfaces of incisors, canines, premolars, or molar teeth. **(F)** Class VI: lesions of the incisal edge or cusp tip of teeth.

Practical Cavity Classification by Location of Restored Surfaces (4)

O = occlusal	DI = distoincisal
MO = mesio-occlusal, or the mesial and occlusal surfaces	MI = mesioincisal
	MID = mesioincisodistal
DO = disto-occlusal	DL = distolingual
MOD = mesio-occlusodistal	ML = mesiolingual
B = buccal	MLD = mesiolinguodistal
L = lingual	MF = mesiofacial
F = facial (labial or buccal)	DF = distofacial
I = incisal	MFD = mesiofaciodistal

Staging of Tooth Injuries

Classifications by extent of pathology generally refer to stages. In combination with G.V. Black's modified classification of tooth lesion locations, the following stages of tooth injuries are commonly accepted (5–7):

Staging of Tooth Injuries

1	Simple fracture of the enamel
2	Fracture extends into the dentin
3	Fracture extends into the pulp chamber; pulp vital
4	Fracture extends into the pulp chamber; pulp nonvital
5	Tooth displaced
6	Tooth avulsed
7	Root fracture; no coronal involvement; tooth stable
8	Root fracture combined with stage 1–2 coronal fracture; tooth stable
9	Root fracture combined with stage 3 coronal fracture; tooth stable
10	Root fracture in combination with stage 1–4; unstable tooth

Feline Dental Resorptive Lesions

Feline dental resorptive (FDR) lesions, also called resorptive lesions (RL), cervical neck lesions (CNL), and cervical line lesions (CLL) (5,8), are generally classified by stage. Stages are used in combination with G.V. Black's modified classification of tooth lesion locations. This staging is a modification of the staging of the tooth injury index:

Staging of FDR Lesions

1	Into enamel only
2	Into dentin
3	Into pulp
4	Extensive structural damage
5	Crown lost, only roots remain

Basrani's Staging of Tooth Injuries

This staging system (9) is based on extent of pathology and is listed as a reference, as some texts make use of it.

Basrani's Staging of Tooth Injuries

A	Crown fractures:
A1	Fracture involving enamel only
A2a	Fracture involving enamel and dentin, but not pulp cavity
A2b	Fracture involving enamel, dentin, and pulp cavity.
B	Root fractures (fractures of root only)
C	Crown and root fractures (involving both crown and root)

Some Common Abbreviations of Dental Restorative Terminolgy (5)

BR = bridge
BP = bridge pontic
BRM = bridge Maryland
BRC = bridge cantilever
C/MOD = cavity, mesio-occlusodistal surface
CA = cavity, fracture, or defect (Classes 1–8)
C1 = occlusal or pit and fissure; molars and premolars; cingulum of incisors (I), premolars (PM), molars (M)
C2 = MOD, mesio-occlusal (MO), OD; M and PM
C3 = mesial or distal; I, no ridge
C4 = mesioincisodistal (MID), mesioincisal (MI), ID; I, with ridge
C5 = lingual or facial; cementoenamel junction; no pit and fissure
C6 = cusp
C7 = root
C8 = root apex
 V = vital (can be added to cavity classification)
  C1V = class 1, pulp exposure, vital
 N = nonvital (can be added to cavity classification)
  C1N = class 1, pulp exposure, nonvital
CR = crown
CM = crown, metal (CMG = gold, CMB = base metal, etc.)
CBU = core buildup
DB = dentinal bonding agent
IL = inlay
OL = onlay
PFM = crown, porcelain fused to metal
P&F = pit and fissure
P&FS = P&F sealer
R = restoration
R/A = restoration, amalgam
R/C = restoration, composite
R/I = restoration, glass ionomer
RL = resorptive lesion (CLL)
 RL1 = into enamel only
 RL2 = into enamel and dentin
 RL3 = into root canal system
 RL4 = into root canal system, with extensive structural damage
 RL5 = crown lost, root tips remain
RR = root resorption
SI = staining, intrinsic (eg, blood, tetracycline, etc.)
SE = staining, extrinsic (eg, metal, etc.)
VBL/NVBL = vital/ nonvital bleaching
VER = veneer

DENTAL DEFENSE MECHANISM

In human dentistry, the dentinal and pulp pain response is considered one of the first diagnostic indicators of pathology—and as an initiator of the dentinal defense mechanism (10). In animal patients, the pain response as a diagnostic and isolatory tool is not as quite as applicable as in humans due to the fact that many animal oral examinations must be done with sedation (see Chapter 4).

The successful dentinal defense mechanism sequence involves the following:

1. Pain (sensible dentin)
2. Pulpitis (reversible)
3. Blockage of tubule with material from dentinal fluid or odontoblast
4. Mineralization of material at exposed dentinal tubule surface and apertures
5. Formation of sclerotic or tertiary (reparative) dentin at the site.

The pain response of dentin in humans has been speculated on for many years, with a fair degree of accuracy (11). The response of a tooth to painful stimuli results in the the tooth's being classified as having sensible or insensible dentin (10). *Sensible dentin* pain can provoke pulp inflammation or pulpitis. Pulpitis can be reversible or irreversible, irreversible pulpitis being the condition of a vital tooth becoming nonvital. Sensible dentin typically implies a tooth that is still vital. However, it does not necessarily indicate whether or not the pulp is in good condition (reversible or irreversible pulpitis). *Insensible dentin* is generally used to suggest a nonvital tooth (12). Nevertheless, there can be areas of dentin in which there are no neural fibers in the tubules to elicit a pain response (10). This can result in an insensible-dentin response in a healthy vital tooth.

A fundamental knowledge of the dentinal tubules and pulp is required to understand the pain response of the tooth and its defense mechanism. There are approximately 30,000–40,000 dentinal tubules per square millimeter of surface dentin (10). In most domestic animals, the odontoblastic process extends from 0.2–1.5 mm into the dentinal tubule. In addition, there may be an afferent nerve fiber extending into the tubule 0.1–0.4 mm from the pulp. These fibers are probably mechanoreceptors, either *A-delta* or *C-delta* types. The A fibers, at the slightest deformation, induce sharp pain; the more slowly reacting C fibers apparently result in dull pain (10). The remainder of the dentinal tubule principally contains dentinal fluid. This means that the dentinal tubule is primarily filled with dentinal fluid, making it a hydrodynamic organ. It is interesting to note that while the afferent nerves endings respond to a variety of stimuli (eg, temperature, pressure, etc.), the perceived sense is one of pain.

The pulp contains free tissue fluid known as *pulp fluid* (10). Capillary permeability and blood pressure in the pulp provide most of the fluid and its drive, resulting in pulp fluid's having a hydrostatic pressure of 20–30 mm Hg. The outwardly directed pressure gradient of the pulp fluid gently drives it into the dentinal tubules and around the odontoblast and nerve fibers to become dentinal fluid. Although the periodontal ligament capillary pressure is 20–30 mm Hg, the hydrostatic pressure in the periodontal ligament space is only about 10 mm Hg (12). A slow, outward flow of water and small molecules occurs through the dentinal tubules even in areas covered with intact enamel or cementum, as these structures are permeable due to the outward pressure gradient. Even if a dentinal tubule's surface is exposed, the normal outward pressure gradient would theoretically result in emptying of the tubule's fluid onto the surface approximately ten times a day, or a flow rate of approximately 1 mm/h (13). This slow normal outward flow would not initiate a pain response (10). However, capillary action is the hydrodynamic factor that can result in a rapid outflow of dentinal fluid at a rate of 2–3 mm/s (13).

Rapid capillary action can be caused by surface dehydration, friction (venturi effect), or fluid contraction, which may be induced by temperature variation on the surface (ice), substances that draw fluid (sugar), or air blown across the surface (friction and dehydration). Due to the composition of dentinal fluid, cold can cause it to contract, while heat may cause dehydration (12). Heat is slow to cause pain and may only effect the C fibers. The rapid movement of fluid from the dentinal tubule can deform the mechanoreceptor nerve fibers in the tubules, stimulating a pain response. In the case of rapid air flow across the surface of an open tubule, a venturi effect may aspirate the odontoblast and nerve fiber into the tubule (10). Water on a tooth can elicit pain in many ways. First, it can cause a temperature change on the surface; second, rapid water movement across the surface may cause a venturi effect or vacuum on the tubule; and third, water flushed directly on an open tubule may cause a negative pressure gradient, forcing fluid back into the tubule. Temperature variations can also cause pain even in areas covered by enamel or restorations by causing the dentinal fluid to expand (heat) or contract (cold). Heat and electricity can also have a direct effect on the pulp to cause pain, while not affecting capillary action in the tubule (14).

Within the pulp are distinct cell zones, each with a specific function in healing. The cell layer closest to the tubules is the *odontoblastic cell layer* or *primary cell layer*. Next, there is a *cell-free zone* followed by a *cell-rich zone* or *secondary cell zone* (10). The odontoblasts of the primary layer are a highly differentiated group of sensitive cells. They can be easily killed by toxins defusing through open tubules or by aspiration during rapid capillary action. The undifferentiated mesenchymal cells in the cell-rich zone are more tolerant of toxins and can traverse the cell-free zone and differentiate into odontoblastic cells. These new differentiated cells can lay down new layers of reparative (tertiary) dentin to block the apertures of the dentinal tubule (15).

Pulp inflammation in association with sensible dentin is the early defense mechanism for the tooth's endodontic system (16). In slight pulpitis, symptoms of clinical pulpitis may not be present. In slight to moderate reactions of the pulp, a positive response occurs to stimulate healing. A more severe form of pulpitis may develop when profuse amounts of toxic products reach the pulp and an excessive immunologic reaction may occur. This may have a negative effect, ultimately leading to pulpal necrosis (10). Additionally, if the inflammatory and immune response is too weak or absent, the infection may result in liquefaction necrosis and pulp death (16). In mature teeth, the pulp cavity may be small with a poor blood supply, and few, if any, undifferentiated mesenchymal cells may be left in a depleted cell-rich zone of the pulp. These can limit the pulp's ability to respond to disease (10).

When tubules are opened on the surface due to injury, disease, abrasion, attrition, scaling, or root planing, material may accumulate at the surface aperture and eventually mineralize (10). This surface mineralization occurs with the assistance of smear layers formed, dentinal fluid flow, salivary substances, fluorides, some lithotropic bacteria, and other substances (10,17). The materials accumulate at the aperture and then mineralize in a fashion similar to that of plaque mineralization into calculus. However, in some cases, continued attrition or abrasion may prevent the tubules from being protectively sealed in this fashion. In these cases, removal of the continued source of wear and some form of dentinal sealer can be used to rectify the problem; more advanced restorative procedures (inlays, onlays, crowns, etc.) may also need to be performed .

Sclerotic dentin is dentin that is more highly mineralized as a result of the tubule's being obliterated as it is filled with additional mineralization (10). This process is similar to the surface mineralization but extends well down into the tubule. For this to occur, the odontoblast must have disappeared, leaving a *dead tract* (unoccupied tubule). *Tertiary (reparative or irregular secondary) dentin* must then form at the tubule access (16). At that point, sclerotic dentin can form. Sclerotic dentin can also form in pulpless nonvital teeth, although it may take more time (10). It is seen in many older patients on exposed root surfaces as a highly translucent root dentin.

Reparative dentin is formed by differentiated mesenchymal cells that migrate from the cell-rich zone (15). It is less permeable and may be atubular. This provides a positive effect to seal the pulp cavity from invasion by toxins and microbes. However, it should also be realized that reparative dentin can also have negative effects (18). First, it can result in insensible dentin that produces no pain response to stimulate pulp inflammation and activate the endodontic immune system in impending disease. Second, it can result in an atypical pulp cavity, which can cause problems in instrumentation during future endodontic procedures.

BASIC CONCEPTS OF RESTORATIVE PROCEDURES

When a defect occurs in the hard tissues of the tooth (enamel, dentin), optimally, it is best to preserve the function and structure of the object by restorative means. It is essential to know basic components of restorative efforts before undertaking therapy, including a knowledge of cavity preparation, from the skills involved to the final preparation that is required. The rules of restoration comprise:

1. Conservation
2. Esthetics
3. Contours and contacts
4. Extension for prevention
5. Cavity preparation
6. Identification and resolution of cause.

Conservation of Natural Tooth Structure

The conservation of natural tooth structure is the first rule of operative dentistry (4). Conservation of tooth structure is essential for protection of the vital pulp. However, not only depth of preparation must be considered, but the size of the area as well. If there are 30,000–40,000 odontoblasts per millimeter of dentinal surface area (10), a 1-cm^2 preparation into the dentin will injure 3–4 million odontoblasts in the pulp cavity by severing their processes or Tomes fibers to some degree. The degree of injury determines whether the individual odontoblast becomes nonvital. Crown preparation for full coverage on a vital tooth will injure and irritate all of the odontoblasts in the crown pulp chamber. The more odontoblasts irritated, the more the pulp will be irritated.

Esthetics

Natural, healthy, unmarred enamel that is supported by healthy dentin, pulp, and periodontium is the most esthetically pleasing. Therefore, the conservation of these healthy tissues is the best esthetics possible. However, when these tissues fail, restorative esthetics come into play. The type of esthetic procedures desired or required then dictate the design of the operative preparation.

Contacts and Contours

A good general knowledge of dental anatomy is required to understand the physiology and function of tooth crown contours (see Chapter 3). *Contact areas, marginal form,* and the buccal and lingual contours must be properly designed to reduce food impaction during mastication. Typically, contact areas should be restored to the condition present when the tooth was young and healthy. Restoration of the axial contours (buccal bulge, etc.) depends heavily on the condition of the periodontium. If the gingival margin is healthy and no recession is present, the tooth should be restored to its original contours. If gingival recession has occurred, the height of the buccal and lingual bulge contour should be moved apically to provide a proper physiologic relationship to the gingival margin.

Extension for Prevention

One of the major goals of operative dentistry is to prevent the recurrence of pathology. This simply means that the preparation outline should be designed to allow for proper oral hygiene to prevent additional disease. Cavity preparation on the occlusal surfaces should include any deep developmental grooves. The lingual and facial proximal cavosurfaces may need to be extended more onto the facial or lingual surfaces to provide margins that can be more properly visualized for completion by the operator—and more easily kept cleaned by the client. The hygienic conditions of the mouth must be taken into consideration, and the preparation outline must be designed accordingly.

Extending the cavity outline below the gingival margin has become slightly controversial. There is compelling evidence for both possibilities, so the operator must design the outline to best suit his or her needs. With placement of the outline above or coronal to the gingival margin, tooth structure is conserved and there is improved visualization of work, easier marginal finishing, less chance of overhangs, and less gingival irritation. However, with full-coverage crowns, placing the preparation outline more apically and below the gingival margin can provide enhanced esthetics and retentive quality. The retentive qualities are improved by providing a greater surface area for cementation, a greater depth of axial crown coverage, and a protected restorative margin. Unprotected or uncovered margins in animals can increase the chance of the crown margin's being caught in prey, food, chew toys, and bite sleeves, thereby providing crown pulling forces to be applied. Cavity outlines at the gingival margin should be avoided or the gingiva recontoured to circumvent this condition, as it typically results in gingival irritation. This makes the marginal finish, whether above or below the gingival margin, one of the most crucial points in restorative placement and finishing.

Identification and Resolution of Cause

If the cause of the disease can be ascertained, steps should be taken to relieve it, if possible. Long-term success of any restoration will be in doubt, if the cause cannot be identified and resolved. In dogs trained in police, military, and protection functions, the source of the trauma can often be identified, but not removed. In the required continuing bite training, the reinforced bite sleeve can sometimes cause damage, as can actual on-duty activity. If the bite sleeve is the cause of an injury, it should be examined to determine if it can be modified or improved to reduce the probability of a recurrence of the injury. In cervical line lesions (CLL) or feline dental resorptive (FDR) lesions, the cause of the disease has not been determined; therefore, restorative attempts have met with limited success (19). If caries is a problem, professional fluoride treatment and home oral hygiene should be implemented. Cage-biter syndrome generally results in wear on the distal surface of the cuspids. When the lesion is due to a behavioral deportment (eg, anxiety from thunderstorms, separation), it must be controlled (see Chapter 21). Dermatologic problems typically result in attrition of the incisor teeth. The skin disease must be controlled, which may require the aid of a dermatologist in order to expect a reasonable result from restorations. Games requiring occlusal gripping (eg, tug of war, Frisbee catching, ball catching) have a tendency to wear down the cusp tips of the canine teeth, with tug of war working primarily on the mandibular cuspids and Frisbees on the maxillary, although this varies with the individual. Tug-of-war games may also result in luxation of teeth. The rougher cloth types of Frisbees appear to cause attrition at a great rate than those constructed of smoother plastic. However, catching the harder plastic type of Frisbee is more likely to cause chipped or fractured cusp tips. Ball catching, like dermatologic problems, most commonly results in attrition of the incisor teeth; balls having a fibrous surface (eg, tennis balls) result in more rapid wear. Hard rubber balls cause less wear but more commonly chip or break teeth. If the games of catch are special to the pet and owner and will be continued, then the owner should be encouraged to use a catch item that is smooth and soft and of sufficient size that swallowing is not probable. In the anterior cheek teeth, attrition or chipping is most commonly the result of carrying (eg, dumb bells) or chewing (eg, bones) hard objects. In the posterior cheek teeth, chewing of objects is the most common cause of wear, chips, and breaks. In our practice, cow hooves, ice, hard plastic bones, rawhide bones, and real bones, in that order, are the most common causes of these lesions. As substitutes for these, the flatter strips of rawhide (Chew-eez®, Friskies Petcare Company, Glendale, California), soft plastic bones (Gummy Bones™, Nylabone Products, Neptune, New Jersey), compressed meal bones (Milkbone®, Nabisco Foods, East Hanover, New Jersey), and specialized dental foods (T/D®, Hill's Pet Nutrition, Topeka, Kansas), as well as Popsicles™ (Good Humor Company, Green Bay, Wisconsin) in place of ice, are less likely to cause such injuries, unless preexisting pathology is present. As each patient's chewing habits differ, the products selected by the practitioner for recommendation should be considered closely for their safety in being swallowed or choked on and for their potential for injuring oral hard or soft tissue.

TREATMENT PLANNING

Treatment planning requires a systematic plan to assess the structures and associated problems that may challenge treatment success. A close study of existing conditions that have lead to the problem is required. It should be determined whether modification in behavior, environment, or a combination of both is required (see Chapter 21). Additionally, the patient's occlusion and periodontal health must be taken into consideration (4). Failure to nullify implicated complicity problems will result in less than optimal chances of operative or restorative success. The tooth structure must be evaluated for the ability to sustain a load, its relative retentive qualities, and esthetic considerations.

Components of Prepared Cavities

Various walls, lines, and angles are created during cavity preparation. The following terms are used to identify the various components of a cavity prepared for restoration.

An enclosing side of a prepared cavity is termed a *wall*. The wall is named in relation to the tooth surface of which it is formed. There are two internal walls possible: the axial and pulpal walls. The *axial wall* is the internal wall formed by the surface of the long axis (axial or vertical plane) of the tooth. The *pulpal wall* is the internal wall in the horizontal plane.

There are numerous noninternal wall surface potentials in a cavity preparation (Fig. 2). Some of these are the following:

Distal wall
Mesial wall
Facial, buccal, or labial wall
Lingual wall
Incisal wall
Occlusal wall
Gingival or apical wall
Facial (buccal or labial) proximal (mesial or distal) wall
Lingual proximal (mesial or distal) wall.

Additionally, there are a few subdivisions of the walls, such as the enamel and dentinal walls. The *enamel wall* is that portion of the preparation wall that consists of enamel. The *dentinal wall* is that portion of the wall that consists of dentin. The *dentinoenamel junction* is that juncture in the wall where the dentinal and enamel walls meet.

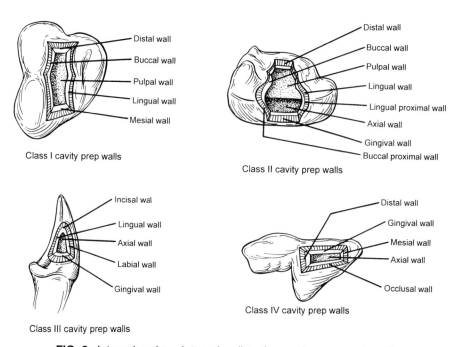

FIG. 2. Internal and noninternal wall surfaces of a prepared cavity.

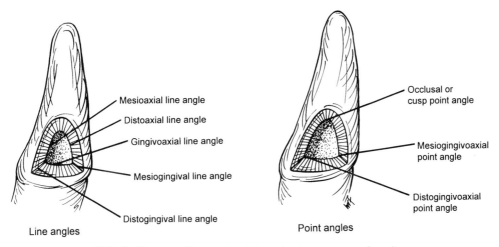

FIG. 3. Common line and point angles in a prepared cavity.

Where two walls meet a *line angle* is formed. At the point where three walls meet, a *point angle* is produced (Fig. 3). The *cavosurface angle* is the line angle formed between a wall of the prepared surface and the unprepared tooth surface. The *cavosurface angle* is also sometimes termed the *preparation margin*, especially once the preparation is restored. The combined peripheral extent of all of the cavosurfaces or preparation margins is termed the *cavity* or *preparation outline*. With regard to restoratives, the *restorative margin* is the restorative surface that abuts the cavosurface angle or preparation margin.

Preparation of Cavosurface Angles or Marginal Finish Lines

Design of the cavosurface angle requires special consideration in its preparation. The preparation marginal restoration greatly affects the retentive qualities of the restoration, resistance to marginal leakage, physiologic contour reactions, gingival health, and resis-

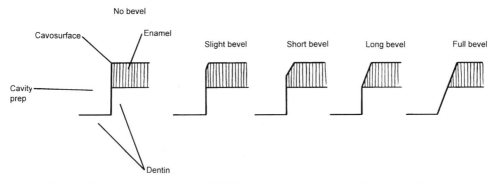

FIG. 4. Basic types of marginal finish lines used on nongingival cavosurfaces.

tance to attrition, abrasion, and fracture of the restoration and restored tooth. Selection of the specific cavosurface angle treatment depends on the type of restoration selected, the restorative materials to be used, the degree of anticipated stress demand on the restoration, and the length and direction of the enamel prisms.

In the consideration of crown preparation for crowns, onlays, and inlays, there are many varieties of marginal finish lines, each with an advantage for use in certain circumstances and specific restorative materials. On the distal, mesial, lingual, facial, occlusal, incisal and proximal cavosurfaces, there are five basic types of marginal finish lines used: slight bevel, short bevel, long bevel, full bevel (chisel), and no bevel (butt) (Fig. 4). On the gingival cavosurface, there are eight more commonly used marginal finish lines: short bevel, long bevel, full bevel (chisel), butt joint (no bevel), shoulder joint, chamfer, deep chamfer, feather (knife edge), and occult (no cavosurface preparation but a feathered restorative margin) (Fig. 5). The beveled finish lines, butt joints, shoulder joints, and chamfers are most commonly used with bonded restorations and inlays and onlays made from composite, metal, porcelains, porcelain-like ceramometals (porcelain fused to metal), and glass ionomers. The knife-edge (feather) and occult finish lines are more typically used with onlays of metals. The use of an occult finish line always results in an oversized restoration, which can be used only in situations where occlusal space allows and esthetics are not of a prime concern.

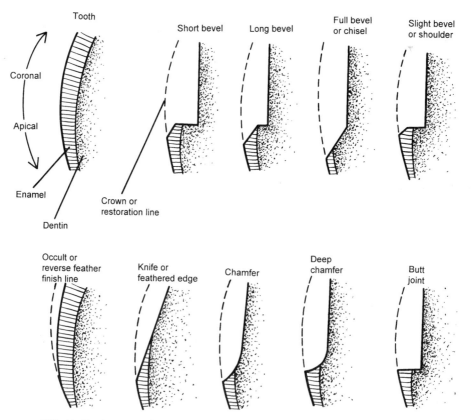

FIG. 5. Basic types of marginal finish lines used on gingival cavosurfaces.

Cavity Preparation

Multiple factors must be taken into consideration prior to the design of the preparation outline being implemented on the tooth:

Location
Extent
Stresses
Tooth condition
Esthetic considerations.

First, classification by location is required using the G.V. Black (see Table 1) or a similar classification. This classification will then direct certain biological mechanical principles being applied. Next, classification by extent is a necessity. This usually does not overtly affect the cavity outline, but rather the depth of the preparation. This in turn determines whether cavity liners, indirect pulp capping, direct pulp capping, or root canal procedures will be required. Third, the occlusal and leverage stresses that must be encountered must be carefully studied. This impacts the types of restorative materials used and whether occlusal height of the crown should be reduced to diminish occlusal and leverage stresses. Fourth, the general condition of the tooth, including other restoratives currently in place or to be placed, must be contemplated. Finally, the esthetic demands by the client will need assessment. The use of porcelain fused to metal for the crown will require greater tooth reduction than the use of a typical metal crown.

STEPS OF CAVITY PREPARATION

Preparation of a tooth to accept any form of restorative material requires specific steps that require forethought as to form, instrumentation skills, and an attention to detail. When these are properly applied, the result is a restoration that is physiologically appropriate and durable in relation to normal functional use. Dr. Black almost a hundred years ago set forth the basic sequence of tooth preparation for restoration (20):

Outline form
Resistance form
Retention form
Convenience form
Pathology removal form
Wall form
Preparation cleansing form.

Outline Form

Outline form consists of the external and internal pattern boundaries of the preparation. This includes consideration of the area of pathology, all undermined enamel, and adjacent pathology, tooth contours, and anomalous anatomy. The preparation margins are placed in areas least susceptible to pathology, where visualization and finishing are suitable for the operator and where access for warranted hygiene by the client is adequate. In addition, the outline form must take into consideration access to the pathology, type restoration, type of restorative material used, functional needs of the patient, and esthetic requirements.

Resistance Form

Resistance form is the shape formulated for the preparation to resist fracture of the tooth and restoration, during both insertion and function. This would encompass the functional needs of the restorative material selected by adequate reduction preparation for the volume of restorative material required, and the correct angulation form of the walls to withstand the functional forces of occlusion.

Retention Form

Retention form is the shaping of the internal aspects of the preparation to assist in preventing the displacement of the restoration. This includes retentive undercuts, groove cuts to prevent rotation, dovetails, pins, posts, and the internal wall angle form.

Convenience Form

Convenience form is the shaping of the preparation in order to provide adequate visualization, suitable accessibility, and reasonable ease in placement of the restoration and its finishing.

Pathology Removal Form

Pathology form is the shaping of the preparation that is necessary to remove or compensate for diseased, injured, or esthetically unpleasing dental tissue. The extent of pathology removal many times determines the need for the use of materials or agents to protect vital pulps. This may also result in the need for specific endodontic procedures.

Wall Form

Wall form is the refinement in the shaping of the preparation. This is typically required to eliminate unsupported enamel rods at the margin or to smooth an irregular or rough outline form.

Preparation Cleansing Form

Cleansing form is typically the final shaping of the preparation, prior to restoration placement. It is generally accomplished with explorers, air, water, spray, cotton pellets, and other agents to remove debris from the preparation.

OPERATING FIELDS

During operative procedures, various isolation schemes are used to enhance visualization and instrumentation, control moisture contamination of instruments, reduce salivary interference, and protect the patient from instrument or chemical injury. The isolation may be either for single teeth or entire arches. There are many methods for isolation, but the type and extent of isolation selected are determined by the type and length of procedure, area anatomy, and operator requirements.

Mouth Mirror and Suction

The mouth mirror in combination with suction can be a highly expedient tool for isolation of an area. The mirror can be used to retract the lip or soft tissue, to aid in indirect visualization, and to redirect light to an area to improve visualization. The suction can provide moisture and debris control for a clear field of view. If the mirror should continue to fog, it can be held up against the tongue surface to warm it. The mirror–suction method for isolation is expedient in that it is easily and quickly removed and replaced when occlusal interference is being checked for.

Cotton Rolls

Cotton rolls are tubes of absorbent material used to help control moisture at a site. They come in an assortment of diameters and lengths (Table 2) and, when in place, may improve or hinder visualization and access. Cotton rolls and hybrid cotton rolls (eg, Parotisroll™, Roeko, Langenau, Germany) can be used be to help isolate teeth, absorb excess moisture, occlude salivary duct openings, and aid in cheek retraction and the application of medicaments. Rolls are used for tooth isolation for restorations and topical treatments, such as fluoride. They are placed in the buccal or lingual vestibule to aid in the control of moisture, and replaced as they become saturated. In the lower arch, cotton rolls and holders are sometimes used to provide retraction for access and improved visualization. The device provides this function by pressing the cotton rolls deeper into the vestibule. Parotisrolls are cotton rolls with a plastic reinforced central core that can be used both for retracting and occluding the parotid and zygomatic salivary gland openings. The Parotisroll can be bent into a U-shape and then inserted with the closed end distal into the buccal vestibule. When released, the reinforced core acts to try to return the roll to its original shape, thus applying a natural retraction within the cheek.

Cheek and Tongue Retractors and Shields

Cheek retractors may be made of metal or plastic and may be single- or double-ended. They are used primarily to displace the cheeks away from the posterior teeth either for dental visualization or shielding of soft tissues in dental procedures or for visualization during photography. Most tongue retractors are made of metal with rubberized tongue

TABLE 2. *Cotton roll sizes*[a]

Lengths available (in.)	Widths available (in.)
Pedo $^3/_4$	—
Short $^1/_2$	Small $^5/_{16}$
Medium 4	Medium $^3/_8$
Long 6	Large $^1/_2$

[a] All sizes and lengths can be combined, but they are not always commerically avaliable.

TABLE 3. *Rubber dam sizes (in.)*

5 × 5
5 × 6

grips, and tongue shields are typically made of plastic or metal. Tongue retractors are used to the move tongue out of the way for procedures, while shields or guards generally partially cover the tongue for its protection.

Rubber Dam

A rubber dam is a thin sheet of rubber or latex used to isolate an operating field in the oral cavity. It can provide an area in which it is easier to maintain asepsis, a dry field, and retraction and protection of soft and hard tissues during oral treatments, as well as preventing debris and instruments from accidentally being swallowed or aspirated. However, as the typical veterinary patient is under anesthesia and intubated, some of these concerns are not warranted. Occasionally, latex gloves with holes punched in them are used as rubber dams in animals, as they can be easily slipped over the muzzle and hold their position more naturally, particularly when cuspids are being worked on. True rubber dams come in various thicknesses and sizes for use according size of oral cavity and teeth (Tables 3 and 4). The heaviest thickness that can be managed for an area is generally best.

Rubber dam templates are generally of no use in veterinary dentistry due to the differences in human and animal anatomy. Quickdam (Vivadent, Tonowanda, New York) is a one-piece type of dam that requires no frame holder. Although such dams have some advantages for veterinary isolation, they are still not ideal for veterinary work. Therefore, the operator must become accustomed to the use of rubber dam material, punches, and hole locations needed for the species of patient being treated (Table 5). The rubber-dam punch also has various sizes of hole punch from which the operator must select.

The rubber dam will generally require some form of stabilization to maintain the isolation. This is done by the use of rubber-dam holders, clamps, ligatures, interproximal devices, and tooth attachments. Dam holders are a frame work that holds the square of rubber stretched out. There are many types of clamps available, none of which is designed for use in animals. Experimentation will generally find the clamp that will work reasonably well for the location desired. However, it should be remembered that clamps should be avoided when possible, as the poor fit in animals commonly results in gingival trauma. Ligatures can be tied around the tooth with dental floss or dental dam cord to help hold the dam down in place. Interproximal devices that can assist in keeping the dam in posi-

TABLE 4. *Rubber dam thickness (in.)*

Thin	0.006
Medium	0.008
Heavy	0.010
Extraheavy	0.012
Special extraheavy	0.014

TABLE 5. *General guide to hole punch sizes*

Punch size	Tooth
1	Cats: cuspids and smaller premolars
	Small dogs: incisors
	Medium to large dogs: central incisors
2	Cats: premolars and molars
	Dogs: incisors, canines, premolars
3	Dogs: premolars and molars
4	Dogs: premolars and molars
5	Dogs: large carnassial teeth

tion are wedges of plastic, wood, floss, or rubber. In addition, tooth attachments can be created with modeling compound or composite applied to the tooth as a ledge to catch the dam under, which is removed following the procedure. The use of beavertail instruments, dental floss, and stretching of the material can facilitate placement. The various stabilizers can then be employed to maintain its position. If the gingiva is traumatized by the apparatus, Tincture of Myrrh and Benzoin (Sultan Chemicals, Englewood, New Jersey) or a periodontal dressing can be applied.

Lesion and Caries Detection

Detection of lesions such as caries and resorptive disease is commonly performed with a sharp explorer, mouth mirror, good lighting, air syringe, and radiographs. Early detection of enamel disease is most reliant on visualization and tactile inspection of the teeth. An incipient carious lesion of enamel may appear rough or chalky white in good light, when air is blown across it. When a sharp explorer is pressed into a carious dental lesion, it will ordinary stick or catch on withdrawal. In moderate to advanced carious lesions of enamel, a brown-to-black appearance may develop in pits, fissures, or developmental grooves, and must be differentiated from staining. In moderate to advanced resorptive and carious lesions, lucent areas may be detected radiographically. Bitewing films are commonly used for this function in humans when carious lesions of the crowns are being searched for.

Dentinal caries (enamel penetration) is sometimes more difficult to distinguish from sound dentin, as healthy exposed dentin often takes on a deep brown–stained appearance. In such cases, a combination of factors is used for diagnosis. Radiographs should be taken to evaluate for lucent areas. The color, texture, and tactile probing can also define a lesion. Decayed dentin commonly has a soft, rough, leathery feel when scraped with a spoon excavator. Additionally, an explorer will often stick in carious dentin or make a dull sound, when drawn across the surface. In contrast, an explorer drawn across the surface of healthy dentin produces a sharp ring.

Once lesions have been detected, the extent of involvement must be ascertained, as well as the relationship to the pulp cavity and pulp vitality. Near-pulpal exposures can typically be detected visually by the pink hue of the dentin. This will usually be an indication for an indirect pulp-capping procedure (see Chapter 11). If the pulp has been exposed but is still vital, a direct pulp capping or possibly a complete root canal procedure may be warranted. If the canal is exposed and the pulp is nonvital or expected to become so, then a complete root canal procedure prior to restoration would be the treatment of choice.

Restorative Materials

Operative chairside restorations generally involve the use of one or more of three basic restorative materials: amalgam, glass ionomers, and composites. These products are held in place by macromechanical retention, micromechanical retention, or chemical crystal formations (see Chapter 2). Macromechanical retention involves undercuts in the dentin and is used with nonbonded amalgams and self- or auto-curing composites. Micromechanical retention is obtained by the use of bonding agents that microscopically interlock in enamel porosities, dentinal tubules, or other microscopic anatomy. This is used primarily with light-cured composites and bonded amalgam restorations. Chemical crystal formations occur with glass ionomers as they form a crystal between the ionomer and the minerals within the enamel and dentin.

Amalgam Restorations

The initial advocation of the use of dental amalgams is credited to M. Traveau in Paris in 1826. It was promoted in the United States by the Crawcour brothers in 1833 as the "Royal Mineral Succedaneum," or the successor of gold. Its less expensive basic combination of mercury and silver made dental restorations more affordable to the general population. However, common problems with expansion resulted in many complications involving broken or split teeth. The subsequent controversies and legal battles over the use of amalgam historically became known as the "Amalgam Wars." It was not until serious research by Dr. G.V. Black and Dr. J. Foster that erratic behavior of amalgam was understood and controlled. The amalgam they developed remained the basic formulation from 1896 until the 1970s. Concerns over mercury toxicity have plagued amalgam in recent years, but no scientific data have yet proven a problem with mercury toxicity related to amalgam fillings. It still remains one of the most easy to use and durable restoratives available to this day. However, toxicity concerns and esthetic image have greatly reduced its use, even in veterinary dentistry.

The concerns over mercury hygiene as related to the patient, dental professionals, and the environment are valid (21). Prudent care when working with amalgam is simply common sense. The following practices regarding amalgam are recommended by some authors (22):

Store in well sealed, break-resistant containers.
Confine spills for easy recovery.
Use spill recovery kits for recovery.
Educate clinic personnel to mercury hazards.
Avoid heating mercury or dental amalgams.
Use protective coats or bonding agents in cavity preparations.
Use in well ventilated areas.
Properly collect, store, and dispose of residual materials.

The clinical properties of amalgam, like all restoratives, are principally controlled by the manufacturer's formulation. However, proper placement can also greatly affect some clinical properties. Clinical properties include setting time, plasticity, setting strength, tensile strength, tarnish and corrosion resistance, dimensional stability, and creep (4). With setting time, the main concern is adequate time to compact the material before it sets; otherwise, strength and marginal adaptation will be compromised (23).

The faster the setting of the alloy selected, the more rapidly and forcefully it must be compacted. Plasticity is the malleability or moldability of freshly mixed amalgam as related to the technique used to compact the material into a prepared cavity site. The higher the plasticity rating of an amalgam, the easier it is to compact it and accomplish acceptable cavity and marginal adaptation. However, to achieve greater plasticity, higher percentages of mercury must typically be incorporated into the amalgam. Setting strength is affected by the quality of compaction and amalgam formula. At about 24 hours after mixing, regular amalgam reaches its highest setting strength, although rapid-setting amalgams may reach that point much earlier (4). Tensile strength relates to the strength of the final restoration and its resistance to cracking and chipping. Mercury can also adversely affect tensile strength, when the content is greater than 52% in the final restoration (24). High percentages of mercury in the final restoration are usually a result of improper mix ratios, poor trituration (mixing or amalgamating), or inadequate compaction. In addition, the finer the lathe cut (ultrafine as compared with fine) of the alloy, the lower the tensile strength typically is (25). Deterioration of the surface and margin by corrosion and tarnishing depends on the alloy combination selected, proper trituration, effective compaction, freedom from moisture during placement, smoothness of final finish, and the oral hygiene levels. However, research has shown that a limited amount of marginal corrosion can benefit the restoration by improving the marginal seal (23,24). Dimensional stability relates to the expansion or contraction of the amalgam on setting. A formulation to provide a very slight expansion is typically used to improve the marginal seal. Nevertheless, excessive expansion, as great as 5%, can be caused by moisture contamination during mixing or placement (4). This can result in postoperative pain, extrusion of the amalgam, cracking of the amalgam, cracking of the tooth, decreased tensile strength, and increased corrosion. Following proper placement and compaction of amalgam, moisture does not affect amalgam's dimensional stability (23). *Creep* is a term used to denote the slow flow or change in shape of amalgams due to chronic pressures. Creep can eventually result in marginal leakage. The American Dental Association's Specification No.6 outlines amalgam alloy standards regarding ingredients, purity, labeling, and packaging (22). (For additional information on amalgam, see Chapter 2).

Amalgam is indicated for restorations that are only small to moderate in size, and it must be supported by sound tooth structure. It is used as restoration in pits and fissures, interproximal lesions, gingival-third restorations, and distal-surface restorations of the canine teeth. It is also used in deciduous teeth in preference to gold, since it will be lost. Amalgam is used as bases, foundations, and cores to help support or retain cast restoration. In endodontics, it is used as root-end fillings and for access closures. The use of amalgam is generally governed by the size of the area to be restored, esthetic demands by the owner, availability of other restorative materials and equipment, and economic restraints. It should not be used in extensive restorations that are subject to excessive stress in occlusion from mastication or bitework.

AMALGAM CAVITY PREPARATIONS

The design of the cavity preparation for amalgam restoration is dictated by certain characteristics of the material's physical properties. The major properties of concern are its low edge and tensile strength, creep or distortion under physical stress, inability to materially bond to dental structure, and high thermal conductivity (4,26). Due to these basic physical characteristics, the following ideals should be contemplated when an amalgam cavity preparation is being designed (4,27):

1. Cavosurface angles should be at a 90° angle to the surface or parallel to the enamel rods.
2. The cavity preparation should be designed so the dentinal tooth structure supports the restoration.
3. Preparation should be complete but conservative in nature.
4. Retention in the form of dentinal undercuts, pin ledges, pins, or posts must be incorporated.
5. In preparations approaching the pulp, a protective insulation layer should be placed between the restoration and pulp.
6. In areas where stress will be a factor (eg, occlusal surfaces), sufficient bulk for strength will be necessary.

Although many possible causes of amalgam restoration failure have been identified, improper cavity preparation is the most common (26,27).

Class I, II, III, and V Restorations

Class I cavities of the pits and fissures are some of the most common carious lesions of humans, nonhuman primates, and dogs. When the pits and fissures, or other anatomy, are of sufficient depth or irregular shape to predispose to the development of caries or other pathology, caries or pathology prophylaxis is generally performed. For caries prophylaxis, a heavy fluoride treatment, prophylactic odontomy, or placement of a pit-and-fissure sealant are the choices from which to select (see Chapter 2 for fluoride treatment). Prophylactic odontomy is the removal of disease-prone dental tissue in the hope of restoring the remaining tissue to normal form and preventing disease. Prophylactic odontomy should be decided on after careful consideration of the possible problems that it may evoke, and it should be done as conservatively as possible. Today prophylactic odontomy is being considered less often in human dentistry, as the use of pit-and-fissure sealants have become more common.

The pit-and-fissure sealants permit a more conservative yet highly effective approach to treatment. The tooth is cleaned meticulously in the pit-and-fissure region. The structure is then polished with flour of pumice and water and rinsed clean. An acid-etching material is applied to the area according to the manufacturer's recommendations, and then rinsed. The tooth is air-dried, and the pit-and-fissure sealant is applied. Most of these sealants are thinly filled composite resins that are commonly fluoride-impregnated. Both chemical-cure and light-cure products are available.

In the cutting of the cavity preparation, the outline form can be established with a high-speed dental handpiece, with adequate water flow, and a straight, tapered (20), or round (4) bur of a size suitable to the dimensions of the tooth. The No.1/2 round p73 and 699L tapered burs work well to start with in most animals. The bur size can be increased according to the tooth and lesion dimensions. When round burs are used to establish outline form, the margins must be checked even more carefully for undermined or unsupported enamel. Once the general outline form is established, a straight or tapered bur can be used to further develop the outline form, with care to avoid undermining the enamel. Wall and angle refinements can also be performed with hand instruments, such as the G.V. Black cavity preparation instruments, Wedelstaedt chisels, etc. Additionally, hand

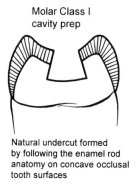

Molar Class I
cavity prep

Natural undercut formed
by following the enamel rod
anatomy on concave occlusal
tooth surfaces

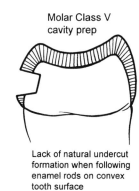

Molar Class V
cavity prep

Lack of natural undercut
formation when following
enamel rods on convex
tooth surface

FIG. 6. Natural angle of undercut following the angle of the enamel rods in cavity preparations of concave tooth surfaces; and the lack of natural undercut in prepared cavities with a convex external surface.

instruments, as well as round, pear-shaped, or inverted-cone burs can be used to create any required undercuts in the dentinal walls. A general tendency toward use of pear-shaped burs has been seen in recent years.

The axial or pulpal walls should be contained to the natural curvature of the tooth surface. If these walls approach or contact vital pulp tissue, then endodontic treatment should be instigated in the form of indirect or direct pulp capping, a root canal procedure, or other appropriate procedures. Due to the lack of tensile strength of amalgam at margins, the cavosurface margins should be structured to result in no unsupported enamel, while providing an approximately 90° cavosurface angle. However, occlusal margins can be modified by beveling to an angle of up to 70°, when required, and if no unsupported enamel rods are created. Greater than 70° modification would predispose the restorative marginal edge to chip and break.

Undercuts are used in the dentinal portion of certain walls to provide the mechanical retention required for amalgam. A natural angle of undercut is often developed in pits, fissures, and occlusal surfaces (classes I and II) by following the angle of the enamel rods; however, the opposite is typically true on walls in the axial plane (classes II–V) and cusp (class VI) (Fig. 6). According to the cavity preparation being performed, undercuts should be placed in the dentin of the gingival and coronal (incisal or occlusal) walls, as well as the distal aspect of the buccal and lingual walls (4). Undercutting all walls is unnecessary and violates the first rule of restoration—conservation of dental structure. Amalgam is not highly advisable in class IV and class VI lesions due to the occlusal stress and pressures. Occasionally, dovetailing the distal and lingual walls is used to improve retention (4).

Class IV and VI Restorations

Class IV, class VI, or extensive lesions are generally best restored with cast or milled restorations. However, amalgam and composite are frequently used for the treatment of these lesions with a reasonable degree of success, when they are skillfully constructed in the correct patient and the cause of the defect has been identified and eliminated. Chairside restoration of these lesions is generally not recommended for working dogs that will be aggressively testing the restoration. Additionally, if the lesion is related to behavioral misconduct, that must be controlled or compensated for; otherwise, long-term success will be in doubt.

When restorations cannot be contained within four walls of sound tooth structure, optimum resistance form cannot be provided. When possible, to compensate for this deficiency, the restoration's bulk may be increased. In lesions in which missing cusps must be replaced by overlay or onlay, the bulk of the restorative must again be increased to prevent occlusal forces from easily fracturing it away from the tooth. This ordinarily means that the overlay area should have a 2.5–3-mm depth of restorative material against the walls that are perpendicular to the lines of occlusal force (pulpal and gingival walls). In addition to undercuts, some cases may require dovetails, pins holes, or pins to provide needed retention or resistance form.

Trituration

Trituration is the amalgamation, or mixing, of the dry dental alloys and mercury into a mass, or amalgam. Hand trituration with a mortar and pestle is past its usefulness, with present new improved alloys. In fact, many older amalgamators or mechanical mixers cannot properly mix the newer alloys. Mechanical trituration with an amalgamator provides a superior mix with uniform consistency of the amalgam.

Most amalgams are provided in a sealed capsule (see Chapter 2). The duration of amalgamation (trituration) depends on the alloy combination, the amount of material to be mixed (single or double spill), the amalgam setting time, and the amalgamator. Most amalgams are mixed for 10–20 seconds, but the manufacturer's recommendations should always be used as a general guideline; and then the time should be refined by experimenting with your individual machine.

Inadequate trituration results in failure to wet the alloy particles with mercury. The mix may still be in a separate powder and liquid form, or simply powdery looking, when spilled into an amalgam well. An *amalgam well* is a holding dish for the amalgam with tapered sides that concentrate the material into the bottom of the well. Undertrituration results in increased expansion, high susceptibility to corrosion and tarnish, a decrease in strength, and a greater failure rate of the restoration (26). Overtrituration results in a contraction of the amalgam, poor flow, and difficulty in complete filling of the preparation.

Cavity Bases and Liners

Amalgam has a high thermal conduction rate. Variations in temperature of a restoration can cause hydraulic movement of dentinal tubular fluid of exposed dentin and the perception of pain. In addition, pulpal and near-pulpal exposures should be capped. The most common and most reliable agents for this purpose are the calcium hydroxide bases and liners. However, calcium hydroxide is eventually absorbed by the body from under restorations, even amalgam (28). This can leave a void under the restoration where fluid can accumulate, causing secondary infection, or it can result in an unsupported restorative that may be more susceptible to fracture. For these reasons, base liners should be used only over the precise areas of need and kept to the minimum depth necessary for the procedure (0.5 mm for indirect and 0.5–2 mm for direct pulp capping).

Cavity Varnishes and Bonding Agents

Under amalgam restorations, cavity varnishes or amalgam bonding agents are used to reduce marginal leakage and sensitivity (29). The varnishes are typically a combination of a volatile solvent and one or more resins from natural gums, synthetic resins, or rosin (see Chapter 2). When the varnish is applied to the wall of a cavity preparation, the solvent quickly evaporates, leaving a thin protective resin film.

Amalgam cements or bonding agents are a newer alternative to the use of cavity varnishes. These are cements that bond to both dentin and amalgam to provide a superior marginal seal and improved retention qualities (30). Most of these cements are designed for the amalgam to be compacted on them while still wet.

Amalgam Insertion and Finishing

The actual placement and finishing of an amalgam restoration involve a fairly straight forward process. The following steps are the general order of treatment:

1. For classes I, V, and VI lesions, go to step 3.
2. For classes II and III lesions, place a matrix band to retain the material within the preparation during placement.
3. Select the amalgam and spill size.
4. Place a cavity base (eg, DyCal®, L.D. Caulk Company, Milford, Delaware), if required.
5. Remove any excess base from the walls of the preparation.
6. Place a calcium hydroxide base or liner, if needed.
7. Place a cavity liner (eg, Copal Cavity Varnish®, Sultan Chemicals, Englewood, New Jersey) or amalgam bonding agent (eg, Amalgambond®, Parkell Products, Farmingdale, New York). Most amalgam bonding agent must still be fresh and moist when amalgam is applied.
8. Triturate amalgam.
9. Empty amalgam into amalgam well.
10. Pick up amalgam from well by loading an amalgam carrier by pressing it into the amalgam ball.
11. Place the tip of the amalgam carrier into the preparation, and press the carrier lever to deliver the amalgam into the cavity.
12. Use a small amalgam plugger to compact the amalgam into all the angles and details of the preparation. Then switch to a larger plugger for heavier compaction.
13. Repeat steps 8–12, until the cavity is slightly overfilled.
14. Use an amalgam burnisher to remove any excess mercury from the restoration. Newer prefilled amalgam capsules are very well proportioned in their alloy:mercury ratio and rarely have excess mercury that can be burnished out.
15. Check the occlusion, using articulation paper if needed. Adjustments can be made with a large discoid carver to remove excess bulk and a cleoid carver to fashion anatomy. It is helpful to partially rest the carver on the tooth surface and carve toward the amalgam.
16. Remove matrix band, if applied.
17. Examine wall covered by matrix band, and use a sanding disk or strip to remove remote proximal excesses.
18. Use the side of an explorer remove excess material from the margins, if needed.

19. Burnish the material lightly to provide some degree of finish or polish. Under normal circumstances, amalgam should be allowed to set for 24 hours before polishing. However, in veterinary dentistry, it is not always possible or prudent to place an animal under anesthesia a second time within 24 hours. But highly finished and polished amalgam margins are more resistant to tarnish and corrosion.
20. When polishing is possible, rubber abrasive points and disks (Greenie® and Super Greenie®, Shofu Dental Corporation, Menlo Park, California) are highly effective on a slow-speed contra-angle.

GLASS IONOMERS

Glass ionomer (polyalkenoic) cements are among the simplest to use dental materials, being less technique-sensitive than most (31) (see Chapter 2). The use of these materials has increased for several reasons, including fluoride release (32) and mild adhesive capabilities to tooth structure (31).

Although relatively easy to work with, there are certain common guidelines for good success. The powder:liquid ratio should be carefully measured, and it is essential to incorporate all the powder into the mix for best results (33). Insufficient powder into the mix substantially reduces the ionomer's strength, results in a slower setting time, and increases its susceptibility to dissolution (34). Most glass ionomers should be mixed in less than 45 seconds in order to assure getting all of the powder incorporated into the mix before placement and commencement of the setting reaction. *Working time* is the time from completion of mixing until the setting reaction begins. With glass ionomers, the working time ends once the surface sheen is gone from the mix. At this point, the setting reaction has begun, and the material becomes spongy and will not adapt or adhere well to the tooth surface. The use of a cool glass slide for mixing will extend the working time (33).

Glass ionomers are also highly sensitive to moisture contamination during working, setting time, and maturation. The dentin should be free of excess moisture but not dried out to the point of desiccation at the time of placement, or adhesion will be greatly reduced. Excess moisture is readily taken into the restorative. Early contamination results in a restorative that easily dissolves and can be washed out of the cavity preparation. Moisture contamination during setting results in cloudy spots at the points of contamination, which is due to crazing or microcracks in the restoration (33). Prevention of these problems can be managed with proper dry-field isolation technique and, if close to the gingiva, with control of gingival crevicular fluid by use of astringents (Hemodent™, ESPE-Premier Corporation, Norristown, Pennsylvania), packing cords (Sil-Trax®, Pascal Company, Bellevue, Washington), or open gingival flap techniques.

Once set, but not hardened, the glass must be prevented from dehydrating during maturation for several hours. If the material is allowed to dehydrate, it will become opaque due to crazing on the surface (35). These microcracks increase leakage and staining and will continue to enlarge due to stress, weakening the restoration toward eventual failure. Dehydration can be controlled by the application of a moisture barrier (36), such as oils, varnishes, or light-cured resins. The ionomer should be coated as soon as the sheen is lost. Light-cured glass ionomers have a resin incorporated within them that is set during curing, which eliminates the separate application of a barrier. The light-cured resins have been shown to be more effective than oils and varnishes (37).

Finishing can be done with simple hand instruments such as a gingival curette. The carving should be done as quickly as possible, and a protective coat should be reapplied to prevent desiccation of the material. Bladed rotary instruments should be used very carefully, as they have a tendency to disrupt the mild bonding effect that the restorative has to the dental structure (38). Once the restorative has set up well, gross reduction and light finishing can be done with an aluminum oxide ("White Arkansas") rotary stone point with a water spray, although some matrix dissolution may occur from the water in chemically cured products (39). Final polishing can be done with a prophylaxis angle, rubber prophylaxis cup, and a composite polish (Glossy Polishing Paste™, Henry Schein Inc., Washington, New York). The polishing should be done at a very slow speed, and in chemical-cure products, it needs to be done quickly to avoid dehydration at this point, when the restorative is stripped of a protective layer. Light-cured glass ionomers need no further treatment, but chemical-cure products should receive an additional protective coating at this point.

Fluoride release varies greatly among products. However, in all glass ionomers, the initial setting reaction creates a reservoir of excess fluoride that is slowly released from the mature restoration by a leaching process (40). It is absorbed more readily by the enamel than the dentin or cementum surfaces and forms a fluorapatite complex (41). The fluoride release aids in preventing carious lesions not only at the immediate site of the restoration but at a moderate distance from it (42).

The mild bond created by glass ionomer cements to the tooth structure is created by a chelation process. The setting reaction of material has an attraction to the calcium of the tooth, as well as that in the silicate of the glass (43). This means that the bond is stronger to enamel than dentin, since it is richer in calcium. However, the bond of glass ionomer to enamel is only about one-third of that of composite resin to enamel (44). Some, but not all, glass ionomer cements make use of a 10-second application of a 10–25% polyacrylic acid or a mild citric acid product to the dentin, which is then rinsed off. This is used to remove the smear layer on the dentin in an attempt to enhance the ionomer's bonding to the dentin (44).

Glass ionomers bond to dentin better than some composite resins with their bonding agents (33). For this reason, glass ionomers are occasionally used as a laminate with composite resins, in what is sometimes referred to as a *sandwich technique* (45,46). The glass ionomer is placed against the dentinal walls. It is then acid-etched for 15–20 seconds with 38% phosphoric acid, rinsed, and dried. A composite resin is then bonded to the glass ionomer and the enamel of the cavity preparation.

Cavity Preparation and Application of a Glass Ionomer Restorative

The cavity preparation for glass is the same as that previously described in the G.V. Black cavity preparation, except that no undercuts are required due to glass ionomers' natural bonding to tooth structure. In domestic cats, due to their diminutive tooth size, it can be difficult to obtain a good cavity preparation without insulting the endodontic system (see Chapter 16). A dry field should be maintained with the use of cotton rolls or pellets and astringents, as previously described. Follow the manufacturer's recommendation as to whether citric acid or polyacrylic acid is to be used for removal of the dentinal smear layer. Dry the cavity preparation lightly, but do not desiccate. Measure out the required powder:liquid ratio on a glass slab. Divide the powder into quarters. Using a W3 plastic instrument, rapidly mix one-quarter of powder into the liquid, and then as quickly as possible add the other three-quarters. The mixing should be completed within 45 seconds to allow for sufficient working time for placement. With the tip of the instrument, pick up a drop of the material and transfer it to the cavity preparation and smooth it into place. The base liner–type materials commonly flow well into preparations. Continue placement of material, until the preparation is filled to the desired level. If using a light-cured material, cure for the amount of time recommended by the manufacture, approximately 45 seconds. If using a chemical-cure product, wait for the sheen to dull and apply a protective coating of an oil, varnish, or light-cured resin. Once the restorative has hardened, check the occlusion. If needed, articulation paper can be used to identify areas that need adjustment. Use a hand curette or rotary Arkansas white-stone point to remove any gross excess of material and obtain a smooth margin. Polish quickly with a composite polishing paste with prophylaxis cup used on a low speed. Light-cured products would be finished at this point, but chemical-cure ionomers will need to have an additional protective coating quickly applied.

Classification of Glass Ionomers

Glass ionomers are classified according to the following types:

I   Luting cements
II   Esthetic restorative
III Bases and liners
IV   Admixtures

Type I luting cements are finely ground ionomers that achieve a film thickness of less than 25 μm. They are commonly used for cementation of orthodontic bands and crowns. Type II glass ionomers are used for restorations when fluorides release is desired but esthetics and strength are not as critical. They are commonly used in the cat for repair of dental resorptive lesions. Type III glass ionomers are base and liner materials. However, this group was originally developed as esthetic restoratives, and many type III products are still used as restoratives, especially in domestic felines. These can be used even in deep cavity preparations due to their enhanced pulp compatibility (47). However, this does not negate the need for proper use of calcium hydroxide liners. Type IV materials are admixtures or have a substantial metallic component. The admixtures are usually gold, silver, or amalgam alloy. They are most commonly used for buildups and cores, but are much weaker than more conventional materials and are contraindicated in stress-bearing areas (33). Composite resins are from three to eight times and amalgam four to ten times more fracture-resistant than glass ionomers (48). Therefore, buildups with composite or amalgam for cores would ordinarily be preferred over glass ionomers.

COMPOSITE RESINS

The potential for the use of acrylic resins for permanent restorations in dentistry first began to be realized in 1955, when Buonocore (49) reported on the use of phosphoric acid on the tooth surface. He found that etching enamel dramatically enhanced the bonding of acrylic to the surface. In 1962, Bowen (50) introduced the new resin today called a *composite*, a reaction product of bisphenol A and a glycidyl methacrylate, commonly abbreviated bis-GMA. The original formula was marketed as a powder–liquid system and a paste–paste form, both of which were self- or chemical-cure products.

Some powder–liquid combinations are still available and used today (Brush Technique Composite®, Darby Dental Supply Company, Rockville Centre, New York). In 1972, the first light-cured composite resins were developed, which used an ultraviolet 365-nm curing light source (33). This resulted in a controlled working and setting time. Most clinically used composites today use the visible light range of 460–480 nm, which provides a more controlled curing in a clinical setting (see Chapter 2). Today's composites can be bonded to enamel, dentin, cementum, metals, porcelain, glass ionomers, and of course to other composites (33).

The composite resins on the market today come as chemical-cure, visible light–cured, and ultraviolet (UV) light–cured. The UV light–cured resins are used mostly for indirect techniques using dental laboratories, while the chemical- and visible light–cured products are used predominately in clinics. The chemically activated resins normally use benzoyl peroxide as an activator. With the light–cured products, most UV systems use benzoin methyl ether, and visible-light systems camphoroquinone (29).

Composite resins are composed of three basic components, often called phases. These are the matrix phase, dispersed phase, and coupling phase. The matrix phase is composed of the various resins. The dispersed phase is composed of the filler particles, such as quartz, lithium aluminum silicate, borosilicate, barium, and other glasses. The coupling phase is the coating on the filler particles that allows the matrix phase to attach or couple with the dispersed phase (33).

Composite resins come in radiopaque and radiolucent forms. In class II and class III lesions and with lesions in proximal surfaces, radiopaque composites help define the extent of the restorative in an area of difficult physical visualization with little interference to radiographic visualization of the remainder of the tooth. However, in class V lesions and veneers, the radiopacity can obscure visualization of the entire tooth radiographically, thereby camouflaging other lesions that may develop.

In addition, composite resins come as macrofilled, intermediate filled or small particle, microfilled, and hybrids. This refers to the size of the filler particles or combination of sizes used in the resin. Microfills polish for excellent esthetics but have a poor resistance to fracture. The intermediate and macrofilled composites have greater strength but, when polished, have only a fair esthetic appearance. Hybrids are a combination of micro- and intermediate-size particles to obtain good levels of esthetics and strength at the same time (29).

Marginal Bevel Considerations for Composite Resins

Beveling of the tooth's cavosurface margins in cavity preparations for composite resins has several positive effects for class III, IV, V, and VI restorations, but it is contraindicated in class I and class II occlusal surfaces (33,51). In classes III–VI, beveled enamel preparations can provide greater retention strength, due to the greater enamel surface area, and improved esthetics, due to the gradual transition from composite to enamel. In a properly beveled cavity preparation, in concert with accurate composite, color matching, and finishing, an almost invisible restoration can be accomplished.

Beveling of the tooth's occlusal cavosurfaces in class I and class II restorations should be avoided; however, beveling of nonocclusal cavosurfaces in these classes is typically recommended (33). Beveling occlusal surfaces is unwise for two reasons. First, this enlarges the surface area of the composite in the occlusion. Composite resins are not as strong as enamel and wear faster, which can result in the need for early restoration replacement. Additionally, the thinned areas of composite along the margins are more prone to fracture from occlusal stress, which results in marginal leakage and deficit areas in the restoration where food and debris can accumulate. These factors can easily result in failure of the restoration. Therefore, occlusal enamel should not be sacrificed for beveling.

In class V and other classes of restoration where the cementoenamel junction is being approached, beveling should not be undertaken if a nonbeveled margin would maintain the enamel margin, while still completing the cavity preparation. The bond strength to enamel and its marginal leakage integrity are greater than those of cementum or dentin (52,53). Therefore, it would be preferred to end the margin in enamel rather than cementum or dentin.

For beveling the cavosurface, the choice of instrument or bur is generally the operator's preference in most cases. When additional bond strength is desired on enamel or dentin, the use of a coarse diamond can dramatically increase the surface area and the potential bonding surface, as well as providing a huge number of miniature interlocking surfaces (51). However, if the bonding procedure is not performed precisely, tiny air bubbles can be trapped between the tooth and bonding material. This can act to prevent the bonding agent from making contact with portions of the dental surface, inhibit resin curing, cause porosities that may lead to discoloration of the resin, and generally lead to a poor retentive bond and marginal leakage (54).

Liners and Bases

Liners and bases with a calcium hydroxide component are the most commonly used products for pulpal or near-pulpal exposures due to their reliable history. However, calcium hydroxide is eventually absorbed even under restoratives (28). This can lead to voids under the restorative that leave areas unsupported and more susceptible to fracture. Additionally, tissue fluids may accumulate in these voids, which may discolor the restoration and be a potential source of infection. This makes it wise to use these liner bases only when needed, in small amounts and directly over the area of need.

Acid-Etching

Acid-etching is used to selectively dissolve some of dental or restorative surfaces. This leaves a surface with more microporosities in which resins can enter to provide a greater micromechanical interlock or bond. In the bonding of a composite resin to a dental cavity preparation, the acid-etching provides greater bonding strength and margins that are a great deal more resistant to leakage.

The most commonly used acid-etchants are nitric and phosphoric acids. The nitric acids require a constant rubbing of the enamel surface to achieve a reasonably etched surface. Phosphoric acids are the most commonly used of the tow agents. A 35–38% gel or solution is used on enamel, and a 10–38% solution on dentin. Dentin requires a shorter application time for etching.

In etching the tooth surface, the first step is to clean the surface to be etched by scaling followed by polishing with flour of pumice and water. Nonfluoride prophylaxis pastes can be used for this purpose only if they are completely water-soluble, which many are not. Fluoride in the paste is contraindicated, as it may counteract the acid to a degree. After etching, fluorinated water can be used for rinsing (55). Moisture contamination can inhibit proper bonding of the resin to the surface. Therefore, adequate dry-field isolation should be used.

Although some feel that dog enamel is more resistant to etching, we have found the manufacturers' recommendations for human use to be fully satisfactory. Generally, etching with a 30–38% phosphoric acid for about 30–40 seconds on enamel and 10–15 seconds on dentin is sufficient. Research has shown the shorter etching periods on enamel to generally be as effective as the longer 60-second etchings in humans (56). Prolonged etching of 120 seconds or longer only creates an insoluble calcium precipitate on the surface, which reduces the strength of the bond (33). The etchant should be applied in a fashion that will not allow the tooth to dry out while being etched. This may mean the reapplication of etchant. Some research has indicated that light agitation of the acid while on the enamel surface can improve the etch pattern and possibly the resin retention effect (57).

Thicker acid gel excesses can be gently removed with a cotton swab. Acid solutions and remaining gel on the tooth should then be rinsed off the surface. Rinsing should last for at least 10 seconds but not exceed 20 seconds (58). Spraying water for more than 60 seconds has shown to damage the etched surface, resulting in a decreased bond strength (59). When the enamel is properly etched and air-dried, the surface will appear to have a lightly chalky appearance. If the surface is still shiny, the etching was unsuccessful. This is usually an indication of a failure either to properly clean the tooth before etching or to prevent moisture contamination. If old resin is still on the tooth surface, it will inhibit etching. It should be scaled off; in some cases, the light use of a diamond bur may be required for its removal.

Enamel Bonding Agents

Enamel bonding agents are liquid unfilled or lightly filled resins. Bonding agents improve restoration retention, while aiding preventing marginal leakage. Marginal leakage is more common along cavosurface margins in cervical enamel than in other parts of the enamel (51). This is due to the fact that the bond between the composite resin and the tooth is weakest with cervical enamel, as a result of its anatomic makeup (52). Gently brushing the bonding resin into a thin coverage rather than using air to blow the layer thin may be better (33). The aggressive use of air may blow air into the resin layer, which can inhibit curing. In addition, the use of three-way air syringes can also cause moisture contamination in the preparation. The use of canned air or electric air dryers can eliminate moisture contamination, and the use of a gentle air stream can avert blowing air into the resin.

Dentinal Bonding

Since the introduction of resin bonding to enamel in 1955, many attempts have been made to achieve a similar quality of bond to dentin (33). This is due to the need for additional retention in some restorations that are under greater stress patterns or have significant amounts of exposed dentin or cavosurfaces of dentin or cementum. There are several reasons for the poorer quality of bond to dentin as compared with enamel in the past. Enamel has approximately a 96% inorganic composition, while dentin has approximately only a 70% inorganic composition, with the remaining 30% being principally water and collagen fibers (see Chapter 3). In addition, during cavity preparation, a smear layer is created on the exposed dentinal surface by the instrumentation, blocking the entrance of the potential bonding surfaces within the tubules.

Dentinal bonding has evolved through what may be classified as four generations. In the late 1950s and early 1960s, the first generation of dentinal bonding agents came on the market, which were cyanoacrylics, polyurethanes, glycerophosphoric acid dimethacrylate, and N-phenyl glycine with glycidylmethacrylate. These had poor clinical success, as they achieved only a 10–20-kg/cm^2 bond strength, with shear-type tests (60).

In the mid 1970s, the second-generation bonding agents were mostly halophosphorous esters of bis-GMA. These undertook to form a phosphate–calcium bond with the inorganic part of the dentin. The bond strength varied widely with the product and skill of the operator, but 30–90 kg/cm^2 was reported (61). However, the oral cavity environment resulted in the bond's being hydrolyzed with time (33). With a bond strength rated only from poor to fair to begin with, and the hydrolization and failure of that with time, resulted in unpredictable and unsatisfactory clinical performance (62,63).

In 1982, the third generation of bonding agents was introduced (64). These were the oxalate systems, which originally had elaborate and time-consuming procedures for mixing and application by the operator, resulting in unpredictable results. In addition, frequently a light-brown marginal discoloration was encountered, which was thought to be due to the acidified ferric oxalate used in the system. However, these systems did demonstrate a bond strength of 100–150 kg/m^2 (64).

A fourth generation of bonding agents has now evolved from the third, with improved handling qualities and bonding strength. There are still some inconsistencies with their application, but they have been reported to have bond strengths of 200–220 kg/cm^2, which approaches the 210–250-kg/cm^2 bond strength of resins to enamel (33). However, standardized testing and research protocols are not used (65), and direct extrapolation of in-vitro tests to the complex environment of the oral cavity has not been possible (66).

With composite resins restorations, dentinal bonding agents are indicated for all exposed dentin surfaces. Additionally, they are indicated for dentin and cementum cavosurfaces. They help control marginal leakage, marginal discoloration, pulp sensitivity, and recurrence of caries. When restoration preparations have little or no enamel for bonding, dentinal bonding should not be used as the sole form of retention, due to a lack of research as to its long-term effectiveness. Dental bonding agents should be used as an adjunct to enamel bonding, dentinal undercuts, dovetails, pin holes, grooves, or pins. In class V lesions, enamel surfaces should be beveled, but if a dentin or cementum cervical cavosurface is present, a light undercut along that surface in the dentin would be recommended. Due to the variety of dentinal bonding agents on the market, their differences in technique of mixing and application, and their sensitivity to variance in technique, the manufacturers' recommendations should be followed closely for each individual product.

Research into dentinal bonding agents will eventually provide the practitioner with agents that have ease of placement, high-quality bonding, marginal security, biocompatibility, and long-term stability in the oral cavity, while being nonirritating or even soothing to the pulp. Dentinal bonding agents are being investigated for their ability to desensitize exposed dentin and root surfaces, as well as to prevent root caries. This may hold some hope for use in the treatment of feline dental resorptive lesions or cervical line lesions.

Composite Polymerization and Shrinkage

Composite resins shrink approximately 3% linearly and 1.5% volumetrically during the curing process (33). This can result in problems with bond strength and marginal leakage. When the shrinkage occurs, some bonding points must suffer. The two weakest points of the bond are at the dentin interface and the cervical enamel cavosurface. This results in the composite resin's pulling away from parts of the dentinal surface, and with the cervical enamel surfaces, either the bond breaks or the enamel rods are pulled out of the tooth. With time, some of the shrinkage is counteracted by expansion of the composite resin due to its absorption of oral moisture. However, areas of bonding may have been permanently disrupted, and some degree of marginal leakage may already have occurred. This problem cannot be solved with stronger bonding agents, as the shrinkage contraction is so strong that either tooth or restoration must give. Only improved composite resins that are not susceptible to volumetric change can solve this problem.

Cavity Preparation and Application of a Composite Resin Restorative

The cavity preparation for composite can be the same as that previously described in the G.V. Black cavity preparations, except marginal beveling in classes III–VI (See Marginal Beveling). Clean the tooth with a scaler and pumice, and rinse it clean. Maintain a dry field by the use of cotton rolls or pellets and astringents, as previously described. Place a liner or base if required. Etch the enamel for 30–40 seconds, and the dentin for 10 seconds with a 33–38% phosphoric acid. Rinse with a clean water spray for 10–20 seconds. Dry with a clean air source to see if the enamel is frosted. If it is not, reclean the surface and repeat the acid-etching (see Acid-Etching above). Follow the manufacturers' recommendation on the dentinal and enamel bonding agents.

The composite can be placed with a composite carrier (eg, Centrix, Centrix Inc., Milford, Connecticut) or plastic instrument such as a W3. If the resin is sticking to the instrument, lightly coat it with some unfilled resin from the bonding kit. The composite should be lightly packed into the cavity to remove any voids and ensure a complete fill.

If a chemical-cure composite resin is being used, the entire cavity can be filled at one time. If a light-cured composite is used, it should not be placed in increments of greater than 2 mm before curing. New composite resin can be applied to preexisting uncontaminated composite within 5 minutes, and the bond between the two will be as strong as if they had been placed simultaneously (67). Cure the composite for the time recommended by the manufacturer, typically 30–70 seconds. Since shrinkage occurs closest to the light source, the margin that you wish to have the best adaptation should have light source applied from that point first, generally buccal or cervical. Continue placement of the material, until the preparation is filled to the desired level.

Check the occlusion, using articulation paper if needed to indicate areas that need adjustment. The restorative can be adjusted and finished with a rotary Arkansas whitestone point or a sanding disk to remove any gross excess of material and obtain a smooth margin. Fluted finishing burs can also be used for this purpose but are highly aggressive and sometimes produce a washboard effect on the surface if not used correctly. Polish with a composite polishing paste with a prophylaxis cup used on a low speed.

With light-cured products, the greatest polymerization and hardness occur at the site closest to the light source. If this was an occlusal surface, much of the hardest composite may have been removed during finishing. Additionally, the surface may have some remaining microporosities not corrected by polishing, and some marginal integrity may have been lost due to shrinkage. To counteract these factors, an additional layer of unfilled resin bonding agent should be applied and cured. All surfaces that were etched should be coated with the bonding agent. Uncoated areas may take as long as 2–3 months to remineralize (54) and, if left unprotected, may stain or discolor and allow a more rapid attachment of plaque and calculus. The restoration is now finished. Repairs of chips or fractures of composite resins are treated with acid-etching, application of a bonding agent, and the placement of the new composite.

Pin Holes and Pin Ledging

Pin holes are holes drilled into the dentin for packing restorative into the dentin to provide retention or resistance for the restorative, or for inserting pins for the same purpose. When a ledge is created on which the pin hole is placed, it is commonly called *pin ledging*.

Restoration Pins

Restorative pins are metal that can be an extension of a cast restorative or an independent entity that extends into both the tooth and the restoration. These should be distinguished from plastic impression pins and metal burn-out pins used in fabrication of cast restoratives. Independent pins will be primarily discussed here, since they are related to normal chairside restoration. Pins are used to provide either resistance form or retentive form. Although they improve retention and resistance to movement of the restoration, the pins actually weaken the tooth and restorative in which it is inserted. It weakens these structures simply by making voids and reducing the structures' bulk. Therefore, if additional retention or resistance to movement is not needed, pins should not be used. Pins should be placed if, in the operators opinion, the risk of restoration failure is increased by not using them. Pins will be used in many cases of core buildup in association with endodontic dowels or posts to provide additional resistance to movement or act as the antagonist of rotational forces.

There are many biological and physiologic factors that must be considered when pins are used:

1. Vitality of the tooth
2. Age of the tooth
3. Pulp cavity location
4. Morphology of the tooth
5. Adequacy of dentin bulk for site of placement
6. Tooth size
7. Bite forces to be countered.

In nonvital teeth the dentin becomes more brittle, losing the elasticity provided by the organic structures and organs that fill the dentin in a vital tooth. Also, teeth lose elasticity as they age, like the rest of the body. Posts and pins that rely on induced stress to provide retention (self-threading and friction-retained posts and pins) may cause crazing in teeth with reduced elasticity (68). Dental *crazing* is the formation of microscopic cracks in the tooth structure induced by stress. Crazing under continued stress may eventually result in cracks and structural failure of portions of the tooth. With threaded posts and pins, even if threads are precut with a guide, crazing may occur during the thread-cutting procedure. Therefore, the use of threaded and friction-retained pins should be carefully contemplated prior to their use in nonvital teeth. Drilled holes and cemented posts or pins are likely to be a more prudent choice. Self-threading and friction-retained pins are best used in vital teeth with their greater elasticity. Pulp location becomes important in pin placement. Vital teeth should not have pins inserted into the pulp cavity to insult the vital structures. In nonvital teeth, the pulp cavity can be used conveniently for endodontic dowels (a pin placed in an endodontic cavity), while reducing the need for the removal of additional tooth structure for a pin-hole site.

Morphology of the crown, root, and endodontic cavity becomes important in determining the structural significance to the remaining tooth and that of the bed in which the pin is placed. This also encompasses the dentinal bulk or depth at the bed site. Insufficient dentinal bulk may preclude the use of a pin at a site. Tooth size becomes a problem in many animals. The majority of the teeth in the domestic cats do not have adequate size for pin placement, except as an endodontic dowel. Additionally, the occlusal stress (compression, shearing, leverage, and rotation) must be taken into consideration. In most carnivores, there are considerable leverage and rotational forces placed on the canine teeth, and compression and shearing forces on the carnassial teeth.

The selection of the type of pin used is also affected by many factors:

1. Pin type or design
2. Pin size
3. Depth of pin holes
4. Pin length into restorative
5. Location of pin holes
6. Pin-hole direction
7. Number of pins.

Most pins are designed as either threaded, cemented, or friction-retained. With cemented pins, a pin hole is drilled and cleaned. Cement is then placed either in the hole or on the pin, and it is inserted into the hole. Friction-retained pins also require a guide hole to be drilled, which will be undersized for the pin. Cement is then placed on the pin or in the hole, and the pin is pressed or malleted into place. Self-threading pins also make use of an undersized guide hole. The pin is then screwed into place with a small driver, or some pins are designed for use with a reduced (1:10 ratio) slow-speed contra-angle (TMS Link®, Whaledent/Coltene, Inc., New York, New York), as they have a latch-attachment base. No cement is used with self-threading pins, unless the hole is oversized in drilling or stripped out by too rapid placement with the slow-speed contra-angle.

The threaded and friction-retained pins can both cause stress resulting in crazing in brittle dentin. Newer designs of threads and placement have reduced but not eliminated the stress. Generally, self-threading and friction-retained pins are best used in young vital teeth (69); however, retentive demands with animals of dictate their use in old and nonvital teeth. Cemented pins can be used in almost any case, young or old, vital or nonvital (68).

Regarding pin size, there are two considerations: the amount of retention required and the amount of structural weakness that is likely to result in the tooth from the pins. The larger the pin used, the more natural tooth structure must be removed for placement, and the greater the weakening of the tooth. Generally, cemented pins have less retentive ability than self-threading pins. A 0.025-inch diameter cemented pin has about 18 lb. of tensile load strength, while a 0.023-inch diameter self-threading pin has closer to 34 lb. In addition, the larger the pin used, the greater is the retention strength, as a 0.031-inch diameter self-threading pin has almost 59 lb. of tensile strength to failure (68). However, the newer resin cements are improving the retentive strength of cemented pins and posts.

Depth of pin placement into the dentin depends on the type of pin used. Self-threading pins achieve their optimum practical retention at 2 mm into the dentin. Cemented pins require a greater number and depth of placement to obtain a comparable effect. The clinically practical depth for cemented pins is usually about 3 mm into the dentin (4).

Pins increase the retention of a restoration. However, they do not reinforce or strengthen the restoration, but actually weaken them (4). Fracture tests have shown that the weak spots in the restoration are around the pins (68). Research indicates the optimum length of pin into the restoration to be approximately 2 mm, as increased length further weakens the restoration without increasing retention (68). The pin can be cut off to the desired length using a No.1/4 round bur; however, many pins are designed with a shear point near the normal desired lengths (TMS® Thread Mate System, Whaledent/Coltene, Inc.).

Location of pin placement primarily depends on tooth morphology and the restorative design. However, certain rules should be followed. Pins should not be placed closer than 0.5 mm to the dentinoenamel junction (DEJ), or crazing of dentin or enamel may occur, as well as pin failure. In vital teeth, all pins should be placed to avoid injury to the pulp. In vital and nonvital teeth, all pins should be placed to circumvent injury to the periodontal ligament. Furcation and fluted root areas should be avoided unless there is sufficient dentinal depth to support a pin, and they should be placed without perforation into the periodontal structures, as this may result in complications that will eventually cause the loss of the tooth. When two or more pins are used, they should be separated as far as morphology will allow for best structural integrity, but typically no closer than 1–2 mm apart (4).

The number of pins used is a clinical decision based on the amount of retention or resistance required and the morphology and size of the tooth. To resist rotation, at least one pin is required. When restoration will overlay cusps, a general rule is one pin for each missing cusp. When retention is the prime requirement, self-threading pins provide greater retentive strength than cemented, and therefore fewer self-threading pins would be required (68).

The direction of pin placement is based on the type of pin and number. For amalgam and resins, greater retention is derived when the pins are not parallel, but divergent to each other. However, in cast restoration, placement of a single pin must be parallel to the line of draw. The *line of draw* is the direction that the restoration must follow to be correctly placed on the tooth without binding. When two or more pins are used for cast restorations, the pin holes need to be parallel to the line of draw and to each other in order to allow placement of the restoration, especially in crown and bridge work (4). Generally, it is safest to place pins 0.5 mm from the DEJ along the lateral line angles of the carnivore cuspid. Due to distal curvature of the crown and root canal, placement distally increases the chance of entering into the canal and fracturing the overlying dentinal surface, or it may easily result in the pin being's exposed to the surface during finishing. Mesial placement in the cuspid should be checked carefully, as the pin may perforate into the periodontal tissues.

In standard pins of normal cavity preparations, the optimum pin placement is customarily in alignment with the long axis of the tooth or parallel to the outside surface (70). However, cleat-type pins (Bondent and Max, Whaledent/Coltene, Inc.) are always placed at a 90° angle to the surface to which they are applied. In slab fractures, this may mean that a cleat-type pin is placed at an angle to the tooth axis.

Endodontic Dowels or Root Canal Posts

The basic information for pin types or design also applies to endodontic posts or dowels (4). Threaded pins and posts make use of friction and wall stress for retention, which increase the possibility of creating internal stress that may eventually result in tooth fracture (69). Many of the threaded pins have a complex superstructure portion for retention of the restorative to the post, known as *Christmas tree*. This superstructure is in alignment with the straight axis of the post. Most carnivore cuspids have a natural distal curvature of the crown. Typically, the post cannot be precurved and screwed into place due to interference of the superstructure or exposed post with the surrounding structures. Once placed, posts should not be bent, as this places severe stress on the root structure, causing crazing and increasing the possibility of splitting the root structure with eventual loss of the tooth.

Standard posts usually require bending to allow them to conform to the gentle curvature of the cuspid root canal. For proper retentive and resistance form, these posts should extend into the canal a distance equal to the height of the eventual restoration. This generally correlates to twice as much post in the canal as is exposed, prior to restoration. Few posts are of a length suitable for this purpose in dog. For this reason, metal intramedullary bone pins are commonly used after being bent and cut to need. In order to improve their retentive qualities for cementation and restorative placement, these customized posts should be scarified on the surface with a bur. Another alternative is the use of Markley Threaded Wire (Almore International, Portland, Oregon), which comes in one foot lengths. The wire can be cut to the desired lengths and cemented in place, without engaging the threads in a screw fashion, only using the threads for cement retention. Additionally, posts do not counteract rotational forces well. For this reason, one or more pins should be strategically placed around the post to resist rotation.

BLEACHING VITAL TEETH

In vital teeth, bleaching (71) is considered an esthetic, conservative treatment modality for teeth discolored as the result of trauma or the systemic effects of injected or ingested substances, such as tetracyclines or fluoride (fluorosis) (72). Ingested tetracycline or excessive fluoride during tooth development can result in significant alterations in enamel color and form. Treatment of these conditions in vital teeth with bleaching has been described in dogs (71).

Discoloration may also occur following traumatization of either permanent or primary dentition (73). Trauma to erupted teeth can result in a pink-to-blue discoloration of the tooth from filling of the pulp chamber and dentinal tubules with blood or blood breakdown products. In addition, staining of the permanent dentition following trauma to the primary teeth is apparently a result of blood breakdown products' seeping from the injured area into the enamel mineralization area during formation.

Vital bleaching of teeth involves the application of heat and a strong hydrogen peroxide solution to the surfaces of discolored teeth. The tooth has been described as acting as a semipermeable membrane (72), the degree of permeability diminishing with age (74). Therefore, younger animals, the ones most commonly presented with lesions of discoloration, have a greater chance of success. Care, however, should be used to avoid hyperthermic damage to the pulp (75) and contact of the hydrogen peroxide with the gingival tissues (76). Prolonged application of a 0.3 mol/L solution of hydrogen peroxide has been reported to produce severe edema of the tongue and frenulum in dogs. Capillary leakage was suspected as the cause of the edema (76,77).

All stained or discolored teeth should be examined and evaluated. A shade guide can be used to establish a baseline color of the teeth. Based on the patient's medical and oral history, the cause of the discoloration should be determined, if possible. Oral radiographs should be taken to determine whether restorations, endodontic treatment, or dental pathology exist. Since bleaching has no effect on the color of most composite materials, restorations that cover facial surfaces may need to be removed and replaced to match the color of the adjacent teeth that are bleached. Discolored teeth that have been treated endodontically should have nonvital tooth bleaching considered (78). Before treatment, a baseline color photograph can be taken to help assess the effectiveness of the treatment.

Adequate isolation of the gingival tissues is imperative before bleaching, because the use of a strong hydrogen peroxide solution can be highly inflammatory. The lingual and buccal gingiva of the area to be treated in dogs should have a thin layer of petroleum jelly applied. A rubber dam should be used with small punch holes to obtain a snug fit around the cervical area of each tooth to be treated. Waxed dental floss ligatures should be placed, where possible, around each tooth and secured with a square knot.

Excessive petroleum jelly and other deposits should be removed from the teeth to be treated with a nonfluoride pumice on rubber prophylaxis cup or rotating brush. Next, use 37% phosphoric acid for 60 seconds to etch the enamel. Although there is no evidence to support the claim, most authors (73,78,79) believe this renders the enamel more porous and therefore more receptive to bleaching. Hydrochloric acid in a 36% solution is sometimes used in heavily stained fluorosis teeth not only to etch the teeth but also to remove the superficial discolored enamel layer (78).

Fill a Dappen dish with 35% hydrogen peroxide (eg, Superoxol®, Moyco/Union Broach Inc., Philadelphia, Pennsylvania). On individual teeth, simple cotton pledgets may be dipped into the prepared solution with hemostatic forceps. Personnel who handle and use strong hydrogen peroxide solutions should always wear protective rubber gloves because of the caustic blanching effect on unprotected skin (80). The saturated pledget can then be placed on the labial surface over the stained area of the tooth to be bleached. For the treatment of multiple adjacent teeth, a single thickness of cotton gauze sponge can be cut to size to fit the facial surface of the teeth to be treated. Once the sponge is placed on the proper surface of the tooth, the hydrogen peroxide solution can be applied to the gauze with a hemostatic forceps and cotton pledgets. In the treatment of fluorosis-discolored teeth, anesthetic-grade ether can be mixed with the hydrogen peroxide. The proportions are five parts 35% hydrogen peroxide to one part ether (81). The ether is believed to be a catalyst that lowers the surface tension of the enamel and therefore increases the bleaching agent's permeability (78). However, extreme care should be maintained when heat is applied to any solution containing ether, and adequate ventilation is imperative.

There are basically two types of heat application units. The first is a bleaching light. This provides high-intensity light and heat necessary to activate bleaching agents. It is designed to concentrate a narrow beam of light. This allows multiple teeth to be treated simultaneously. A rheostat gives the ability to control the intensity of light and heat. A midrange setting, usually 5, gives a good working setting for most animals. The light should be positioned approximately 32–38 cm (13–15 inches) from the teeth. Because of the wide area of heat generated at the site, damp gauze should be placed under the rubber dam to prevent thermal damage to the gingiva and lips. In addition, the animal's eyes should be protected from the high-intensity light. The bleaching light can also result in injury to persons working with or around the light, if proper safety, handling and positioning are not adhered to closely. The second type of heat unit is an individual-tooth bleaching unit. This device is a simple thermal unit that produces heat at the end of a contoured tip. The tip is placed on the hydrogen peroxide–saturated cotton or gauze covering the tooth. It should be applied with a slight pressure, hot enough to create a slight amount of steam when first applied, and should be used on the tooth for 1 second, then off for 3 seconds. This type of unit can also be used to treat multiple teeth. If used for such, it should be applied to each tooth for 3–4 seconds, then moved to the next, and so on.

The recommended temperature for bleaching vital teeth is 46—60°C (115–140°F). Each session should be 20–30 minutes in total bleaching time. Bleaching is different from patient to patient, depending on the severity of the stain, type of stain, number of teeth stained, the age of the patient (reflecting the size of the pulp chamber), and the thickness of the dentin. One to ten treatments are usually necessary for satisfactory results, with the average being three treatments. Each bleaching session should be scheduled 2–4 weeks apart.

After bleaching is completed, remove the gauze using cotton pliers, and rinse the teeth thoroughly with copious amounts of warm water. All dental floss should be removed and then the rubber dam and petroleum jelly, followed by a polish. Sensitivity of the teeth usually disappears within 6–8 hours in humans (72). For the first 24–72 hours, some additional improvement usually occurs in the teeth. But after a few weeks, some slight color reversal may take place. For this reason, slight overbleaching is normally desired. In addition, this may result in the need for some touchups within 1–3 years, which is not uncommon.

Although vital bleaching is not widely practiced, it is effective in improving the color of most discolored teeth. The mechanism of vital bleaching is not known exactly, but photo-oxidation has been suggested as a possible reaction causing the color change (82).

Bleaching Nonvital Teeth

The discoloration of nonvital teeth can be due to causes similar to those in vital teeth, but it is primarily involved with discoloration due to hemorrhage into the pulp chamber (83,84). In trauma-related discoloration, with the color change occurring in the pulp chamber and in the dentinal tubules, it is considered an intrinsic problem. Any serious trauma to a tooth can result in the rupture of a blood vessel within the pulp chamber. Hydraulic pressure may then drive the blood into the dentinal tubules (85, 86). Grossman (87) demonstrated that freed red blood cells in the pulp chamber undergo hemolysis and release hemoglobin. Further degradation of the hemoglobin releases iron. The iron then combines with hydrogen sulfide to form iron sulfide, a black compound. Immediately following a traumatic hemorrhagic injury, the crown will appear slightly pink, but with the progressive breakdown of the red blood cells, the tooth turns orange, then blue, black, or brown. These generally respond well to nonvital bleaching (87).

Pulpal degradation can also occur without hemorrhage (87). This results in various protein-degradation products from the necrotic pulpal tissue. This type of discoloration is not as pronounced as that seen with pulpal hemorrhage, but it does result in a grayish brown discoloration of the crown. By and large, this responds well to nonvital bleaching.

In teeth with pulpal necrosis, the extent of discoloration is directly related to the time duration between pulp death and treatment. The longer the discoloring agents are in the pulp, the deeper will be their penetration into the dentinal tubules, the greater the discoloration, and the greater the difficulty of bleaching the teeth satisfactorily (88).

Iatrogenic discoloration of teeth is considered the negative side effect of some dental procedures (87). These effects are classified as intrinsic because the inner tooth structure is effected. This type of discoloration can result from numerous practices and materials used on or in teeth.

Trauma caused during extirpation of the pulp in the course of an endodontic treatment can result in a diffuse hemorrhage of the pulp. Hemoglobin breakdown may then result in discoloration. Any organic material allowed to remain in the pulp chamber may result in a staining effect (89). To prevent unnecessary discoloration, all blood and other organic materials must be removed thoroughly from the entire pulp chamber during endodontic treatment. This type of staining problem has been known to respond well to nonvital bleaching.

An additional source of iatrogenic discoloration is root canal medicaments. If they reach and enter the dentinal tubules, they may stain the tooth. Other medicaments result in stains on decomposing or combining with another agent or material in the root canal. These may eventually leak and saturate the dentinal tubules. Iodine solutions cause brown, orange, or yellow stains. Silver nitrate results in black or bluish-black discoloration. Chloroazodin, mercuric chloride, and other metallic salts are known to result in staining effects. Volatile oils may create yellowish brown stains (87).

Metal amalgams used as filling materials and root canal sealers containing silver may produce dark-gray or bluish-black to black discoloration (90). Even gold can reflect a discoloration through enamel by mixing with products of decay to enter the tubules and cause a dark-brown stain. Pins can result in blue-grayish stains. Because stains of metallic origin are the most difficult to bleach, alternate forms of restoration may be preferable. Even restorations of acrylics, silicate cements, or composite resins can break down and result in a grayer look to the tooth. These teeth may respond well to bleaching following replacement of the degraded restorations.

Teeth should be carefully evaluated before being selected for bleaching. Teeth restored extensively with acrylics, silicates, or composite resin may not have sufficient tooth enamel surface to respond well to bleaching. Teeth with enamel that is hypocalcified, cracked, or severely undermined is usually best treated with alternate restorative therapy rather than bleaching.

External resorption has been associated with internal bleaching of pulpless endodontically treated teeth on occasion (91). Although this is not proven, it appears that in the young tooth with patent dentinal tubules, the bleaching agents may be able to travel to the cementum and penetrate to the periodontal tissues. In addition, it has been found in humans that in 10% of all teeth, the enamel and cementum do not meet (92). This means that the dentin in the cervical area may be devoid of cementum. Therefore, with the patent tubules of a young tooth, there may be direct communication between the cervical periodontal ligament and coronal portion of the endodontic system. It is possible then that the strong hydrogen peroxide solution placed in the chamber might diffuse through the dentinal tubules to the cervical periodontal ligament to initiate a resorptive inflammatory response. Since cervical external resorption of the tooth appears to be associated with internal bleaching of young teeth, care should be exercised in the selection of a tooth for bleaching to be sure that its internal vitality did not stop at a young stage of development.

Surface bleaching alone in nonvital teeth generally does not yield good results, since the discoloration is usually the result of degradation of materials within the pulp chamber that continue to contribute to the staining mechanism (87). Once the field is ready (see above), the first step is to create an opening of adequate size to allow acceptable access to the complete pulp chamber and orifice of the root canals. This can be done with a round bur. For superior results, the entire pulp chamber and horns need to be fully accessible to the bleaching agents (93). A lingual access opening is preferred for the least noticeable opening.

Removal of the obturating filling material from the pulp chamber and then from the root canal to a depth of 2–3 mm below the gingival margin is the next step. This is commonly done with a Gates-Glidden drill when gutta-percha was used. This type of instrument removal of gutta-percha reduces the chance of disturbing the apical seal of the canal. For additional protection against leakage, a seal of zinc oxyphosphate or polycarboxylate cement is placed over the root canal filling material to a level 1–2 mm coronal to the cementoenamel junction. A slowly rotating bur is then used to remove excess debris along with a minimum surface layer of dentin from the pulp chamber to provide a less restrained penetration of the bleaching solution into the dentinal tubules. This surface layer is often the most highly stained portion of the dentin, so its removal can decrease the amount of bleaching required. The entire prepared chamber and surface of the tooth are cleaned with acetone or chloroform on a cotton pellet to remove the fatty acids, thereby facilitating bleach penetration. The surface and chamber should be dried using alcohol followed by oil-free air.

For in-office bleaching, a cotton pellet should be shaped to loosely fill the pulp chamber. A few strands of cotton or a single layer of cotton gauze should cover the labial surface of the tooth, which is then saturated with 35% hydrogen peroxide from a glass syringe–stainless steel needle combination. The bleaching solution should be delivered slowly to the cotton matrix until it is saturated both on the surface and in the pulp chamber. Excess solution should be carefully removed immediately. The bleach is then activated with an individual bleaching unit at a temperature of 73°C (165°F), as recommended by Caldwell (94) for bleaching nonvital teeth. This has been shown to result in an increase in the bleaching rate by 200 times, when used with 35% hydrogen peroxide. The flap tip of the bleaching instrument is then placed in contact with the cotton matrix on the labial surface of the tooth for a period of 5 minutes, with care to maintain the saturation with the bleaching solution at all times. This procedure is repeated every 5 minutes, with replacement of the cotton matrix, until the desired result is obtained. In most cases, this will take 20–30 minutes of bleaching. Lemieux and Todd (89) outlined a simplified bleaching process using a Woodson No.3 instrument. Its blunt end is heated red-hot with an alcohol burner and applied to the cotton matrix both externally and internally.

When this is completed, remove the cotton matrix and irrigate the chamber and tooth surface thoroughly with saline. Swab the prepared chamber with chloroform. To assure good mechanical bonding, etch the walls of the chamber with 37–45% phosphoric acid for 60 seconds. Flush the acid out with a liberal amount of water and then dry the preparation. Use an unfilled resin in the bleached crown to seal the dentinal tubules. After applying several coats of resin, polymerize with light to prevent recurrence of the coronal stain. The cavity is then filled using a composite resin restorative material. The lightest shade esthetically compatible with the tooth should be used.

The "walking bleach" procedure may be more effective for difficult stains (87), but it does require an observant client who will watch for problems, such as the loss of the seal. After initial preparations, a bleaching paste is made on a glass slide or in a Dappen dish with two or three drops of 35% hydrogen peroxide with enough sodium perborate or sodium peroxyborate (Amoson Powder®, Cooper Labs, Newark, New Jersey) to produce a thick white paste. Because of the bleaching paste's light consistency, a few fibers from a cotton pellet are added to aid in paste placement. Using the impregnated cotton, fill the entire chamber, leaving sufficient space at the access to place a temporary double-seal restoration. The double seal is required because of the continual release of oxygen by the bleaching mixture. The pressure that occurs tends to force open the seal and push material out of the cavity. The inner portion of the double seal is made with a layer of Cavit®

(ESPE-Premier Corporation) and the outer part with a layer of IRM® cement (L.D. Caulk Company).

Reevaluate the tooth every 5–7 days. Repeat the procedure as needed, until the desired effect is reached. Once this point is attained, the same chamber-filling method as previously described for the in-office procedure can be used to complete the protocol. Because of the possible posttreatment cervical resorption problem, periodic examination of the bleached teeth is indicated.

REFERENCES

1. Wiggs RB. Is periodontal disease a measure of a pet's general health? *Vet Forum* Feb 1995;2:66.
2. *Glossary of Operative Dentistry Terms.* 1st ed. Academy of Operative Dentistry.
3. Harty FJ. *Concise Illustrated Dental Dictionary.* 2nd ed. Boston: Wright Publishing; 1995.
4. Howard WW, Moller RC. *Atlas of Operative Dentistry.* 3rd ed. St Louis, MO: CV Mosby Co; 1981:5.
5. Lobprise HB, Wiggs RB. Dental abbreviations. Dallas, TX. *Amer Vet Dent College Prog Training Committee.* 1995:1.
6. Robinowich BZ. The fractured incisor. *Pediatr Clin North Am* 1956;3:979.
7. Torres HO, Ehrlich A. Pedodontics. In: *Modern Dental Assisting.* 2nd ed. Philadelphia: WB Saunders Co; 1980:725.
8. Wiggs RB, Lobprise HB. Dental disease. In: Norsworthy GD, ed. *Feline Practice.* Philadelphia: JB Lippincott Co; 1993:303.
9. Holmstrom SE, Frost P, Gammon RL. *Veterinary Dental Techniques.* Philadelphia: WB Saunders Co; 1992:270.
10. Brannstrom M. *Dentin and Pulp in Restorative Dentistry.* London: Wolfe Medical Publishing; 1982:9.
11. Gysi A. An attempt to explain the sensitivity of dentine. *Br J Dent Sci* 1900;43:868.
12. Brannstrom M. A hydrodynamic mechanism in the transmission of pain-producing stimuli through dentine. In: Anderson DJ, ed. *Sensory Mechanism in Dentine.* Oxford: Pergamon Press; 1963:73.
13. Berggren G, Brannstrom M. The rate of flow in dentinal tubules due to capillary attraction. *J Dent Res* 1965;44:415.
14. Narhi M, et al. Activation of interdentinal nerves by electrical stimulation and heating. *J Dent Res* 1981;60(spec issue A):352. Abstract 167.
15. Sveen OB, Hawes RR. Differentiation of new odontoblasts and dentine bridge formation in rat molar teeth after grinding. *Arch Oral Biol* 1968;13:1412.
16. Symons NBB, ed. *Dentine and Pulp: Their Structure and Reactions: A Symposium.* Edinburgh: E & S Livingstone; 1968.
17. Streckfuss JL, et al. Calcification of selected strains of streptococci. *J Dent Res* 1979;58:1917.
18. Gottlieb B. The formation of secondary dentin and related problems. *J Dent Res* 1946;25:34.
19. Wiggs RB, Lobprise HB. Oral disease. In: Norsworthy GD, ed. *Feline Medicine.* Philadelphia: JB Lippincott Co; 1993.
20. Black GV. *Operative Dentistry.* 4th ed. Chicago: Medico-Dental Publishing Co; 1920.
21. Rupp NW, Paffenburger GC. Significance to health of mercury in dental practice: A review. *JADA* 1971;82:1401.
22. *Guide to Dental Materials and Devices.* 6th ed. Chicago: American Dental Association; 1972.
23. Phillips RW. Research on dental amalgam and its application in practice. *JADA* 1957;54:309.
24. Mahler DB. Physical properties and manipulation of amalgam. *Dent Clin North Am* 1967:228.
25. Mahler DB, Terkla LG, Van Eysden J, Risbeck MH. Marginal fractures vs. mechanical properties of amalgam. *J Dent Res* 1970;49:1452.
26. Healy JH, Phillip RW. A clinical study of amalgam failures. *J Dent Res* 1949;28:439.
27. Nadel R. Amalgam restorations, cavity preparations, condensing and finishing. *JADA* 1962;65:66.
28. Leinfelder KF, et al. Use of Ca(OH)$_2$ for measuring microleakage. *Dent Mater* 1986;2:121.
29. Craig RG. *Restorative Dental Materials.* 7th Ed. St Louis MO: CV Mosby Co; 1985.
30. Arnold TJ. New restorative techniques using phase-transition cementation. *Compend Cont Educ Dent* 1994;16:2.
31. Mount GW. *An Atlas of Glass Ionomer Cements.* Philadelphia: BC Decker Co; 1990.
32. Wilson AD, et al. The release of fluoride and other chemical species from a glass ionomer cement. *Biomaterials* 1986;6:431.
33. Dale BG, Ascheim KW. *Esthetic Dentistry a Clinical Approach to Techniques and Materials.* Philadelphia: Lea & Febiger; 1993.
34. Crisp S, Lewis BG, Wilson AD. Characterization of glass ionomer cements. Effect of the powder:liquid ratio on the physical properties. *J Dent Res* 1976;4:287.
35. Phillips S, et al. An in vitro study of the effect of moisture on glass ionomer cement. *Quint Int* 1985;16:175.
36. Kim KC. The microleakage of a glass cement using two methods of moisture protection. *Quint Int* 1988;18:835.
37. Earl MSA, Hume WR, Mount GJ. Effect of varnishes and other surface treatments on water movement across the glass ionomer surface, II. *Aust Dent J* 1989;34:326.

38. Pearson GJ. Finishing of glass ionomer cements. *Br Dent J* 1983;155:226.
39. Pearson GJ, Knibbs PJ. Finishing an anhydrous glass ionomer cement: An in vitro and vivo study. *Restor Dent* 1987;3:35.
40. Forsten L. Fluoride release from glass ionomer cement. *Scand J Dent Res* 1977;85:503.
41. Retief DH, Bradley EL, Dentin JC, Switzer P. Enamel and cementum fluoride uptake from glass ionomer cement. *Caries Res* 1984;18:250.
42. Hicks MJ, Flaitz CM, Silverstone LM. Secondary caries formation in vitro around glass ionomer restorations. *Quint Int* 1986;17:527.
43. Wilson AD, Prosser HJ. Mechanism of adhesion of poly electrolyte cements to hydroxyapatite. *J Dent Res* 1983; 62:590.
44. Powis DR, Folerars T, Merson SA, Wilson AD. Improved adhesion of a glass ionomer cement to dentin and enamel. *J Dent Res* 1982;61:1416.
45. McClean JW, Powis DR, Prosser HJ, Wilson AD. The use of glass-ionomer cements in bonding composite resins to dentine. *Br Dent J* 1985;158:410.
46. Mount GJ. Clinical requirements for a successful "sandwich" dentine to glass ionomer cement to composite resin. *Aust Dent J* 1989;34:259.
47. Smith DC. Composition and characteristics of glass ionomer cement and its relationship to the setting process. *J Dent Res* 1979;58:1072.
48. Osman E, et al. Fracture toughness of several categories of restorative materials. *J Dent Res* 1986;65:220.
49. Buonocore MG. A simple method of increasing the adhesion of acrylic filling materials to enamel surfaces. *J Dent Res* 1955;34:849.
50. Bowen RL. Dental filling material comprising vinyl silane treated fused silica and a binder consisting of the reaction product of bis-phenol and glycidyl acrylate. US Patent 3,006,112. 1962.
51. Jensen ME, Chan DCN. Polymerization shrinkage and microleakage. In: Vanherle G, Smith DC, eds. *International Symposium on Posterior Composite Resin Dental Restorative Materials*. Netherlands: Peter Szulc Co; 1985:243.
52. Crim GA, Mattingly SL. Microleakage and the class V composite cavosurface. *J Dent Child* 1980;47:333.
53. Davidson CL, Kemp-Scholte CM. Shortcomings of composite resins in class V restorations. *J Esthetic Dent* 1989;1(1):1.
54. Albers HF. *Tooth Colored Restoratives*. 7th ed. Cotati, CA: Alto Books; 1985.
55. Buonocore MG. Retrospection on bonding. *Dent Clin North Am* 1981;24:243.
56. Barkemeier WW, et al. Effects of 15 versus 60 second enamel acid conditioning on adhesion and morphology. *Operative Dent* 1986;11:111.
57. Baharav H, et al. The efficiency of liquid and gel etchants. *J Prosthet Dent* 1988;60:545.
58. Mixson JM, et al. The effects of variable wash times and techniques on enamel composite resin bond strength. *Quint Int* 1988;19:279.
59. Schulein TM, et al. Rinsing times for a gel etchant related to enamel/composite bond strength. *Gen Dent* July-Aug 1986:345.
60. Asmussen E. Clinical relevance of physical, chemical and bonding properties of composite resins. *Operative Dent* 1985;10:61.
61. Fan PL. Dentin bonding systems: An update. *JADA* 1987;114:91.
62. Doering JV, Jensen ME. Clinical evaluation of dentin bonding materials on cervical abrasion lesions. *J Dent Res* 1986;65:173.
63. Dennison JB, Ziemiecki TL, Charbeneau GT. Retention of unprepared cervical restorations utilizing a dentin bonding agent. Two year report. *J Dent Res* 1986;65:173.
64. Bowen RL, Cobb EN, Raapson JE. Adhesive bonding of various materials to hard tooth tissues. Improvement in bond strength to dentin. *J Dent Res* 1982;61:1070.
65. Finger WJ. Dentin bonding agents. Relevance of in vitro investigations. *Am J Dent* 1988;1:184.
66. Retief HD, O'Brien JA, Smith LA, Marchman JL. In vitro investigations and evaluation of dentin bonding agents. *Am J Dent* 1988;1:176.
67. Boyer DB, et al. Buildup and repair of light cured composites: Bond strength. *J Dent Res* 1984;63:1241.
68. Moffa JP, Rozzano MR, Doyle MG. Pins—a comparison of their retentive properties. *JADA* 1969;78:529.
69. Markley MR. Pin retained and reinforced restorations and foundations. *Dent Clin North Am* 1967:229.
70. Dilts WE, Mullaney TP. Relationship of pinhole location and tooth morphology in pin-retained restorations. *JADA* 1968;76:1011.
71. Wiggs RB. Bleaching vital teeth in canines. *J Vet Dent* 1988;5(4):15.
72. Nathanson D, Parra C. Bleaching vital teeth: A review and clinical study. *Compend Cont Educ Dent* 1987;8:490.
73. McEvoy S. Bleaching stains related to trauma or periapical inflammation. *Compend Cont Educ Dent* 1986;7:420.
74. Atkinson HF. An investigation into the permeability of human enamel using osmotic methods. *Br Dent J* 1947; 83:205.
75. Postle HH, Lefkowitz W, McConnell D. Pulp response to heat. *J Dent Res* 1959;38:740.
76. Martin JH, Bishop JG, Guentherman RH, Dorman HL. Cellular response of gingiva to prolonged application of dilute hydrogen peroxide. *J Periodontol* 1968;39:208
77. Dorman HL, Bishop JG. Production of experimental edema in dog tongue with dilute hydrogen peroxide. *Oral Surg* 1970;29:38.

78. Bishop JG, Gage TW, Matthews JL, Dorman HL. In: Squire CA, Meyer J, eds. *Current Concept of the Histology of Oral Mucosa: Proceedings of a Symposium at the University of Illinois College of Dentistry.* Springfield, IL: Charles C Thomas; 1971;15:247.

79. Feinman RA, Goldstein RE, Garber DA. *Bleaching Teeth.* Chicago: Quintessence Books; 1987.

80. Jordan RE, Boksman L. Conservative vital bleaching treatment of discolored dentition. *Compend Cont Educ Dent* 1984;5:803.

81. Goette DK, Odom RB. Skin blanching introduced by hydrogen peroxide. *South Med J* 1977;70:620.

82. Bouscher CF, Dorman HL. Bleaching fluoride stained teeth. *Texas Dent J* 1973:6.

83. Davies AK, et al. Photo-oxidation of tetracycline absorbed on hydroxyapatite in relation to the light-induced staining of teeth. *J Dent Res* 1985;46:936.

84. Wiggs RB. Bleaching of non-vital teeth in the canine species. *J Vet Dent* 1989;6(1):9.

85. White E. Bleaching of pulpless teeth. *S Carolina Dent J* 1974:32.

86. Ingle JI. *Endodontics.* Philadelphia: Lea & Febiger; 1967.

87. Grossman LI. *Endodontic Practice.* Philadelphia: Lea & Febiger; 1970.

88. Nutting E, Poe G. Chemical bleaching of pulpless teeth. *J Dent Child* 1965;32:144.

89. Lemieux JJ, Todd MJ. Simplified bleaching of discolored pulpless teeth. *J Can Dent Assoc* 47:729.

90. Brown G. Factors influencing successful bleaching of the discolored root-filled tooth. *Oral Surg* 1965;20:238.

91. Harrington GW, Natkin E. External resorption associated with bleaching of pulpless teeth. *J Endod* 1979;5:344.

92. Mjor IA, Pindborg JJ. *Histology of the Human Tooth.* Munksgaard: Scandinavian University Books; 1973.

93. Spasser HF. A simple bleaching technique using sodium perborate. *N Y S Dent J* 1961;27:332.

94. Caldwell CB. Heat source for bleaching discolored teeth. *Ariz Dent J* 1967;13:18.

14

Operative Dentistry:
Crowns and Prosthodontics

Robert B. Wiggs and Heidi B. Lobprise

The need often arises to provide additional support to the existing dental structure to enhance oral function, as discussed in Chapter 13 on restorations. Particularly in those pets that require healthy teeth to perform properly, placement of prosthetic devices such as crowns, bridges, and even implants can help restore or maintain function.

Operative dentistry is that branch of dentistry that relates to the diagnosis, prognosis, or treatment of teeth with vital or nonvital pulps and to the maintenance or restoration of the functional and physiologic integrity of the teeth as this applies to the adjacent hard and soft tissue structure of the oral cavity (eg, crowns, inlays, chairside restoration, etc.) (1,2). Dental prosthetics is that branch of dental science dealing with the artificial replacement of one or more natural teeth or associated structures (eg, dentures, bridges, etc.). Prosthodontics is that branch of dentistry concerned with prosthetic dental devices. In many countries, this includes both removable and fixed appliances; however, in some it is considered only to apply to removal prosthetics devices such as dentures (2). This chapter will review restorative devices fabricated principally in laboratories, associated in clinic procedures and surgical procedures.

Restorative Terms

Cap—colloquialism for crown.
Ceramometal crown—see porcelain fused to metal.
Core—a substructure for a crown, which may be part of a post-and-core system.
Crown—a restorative that covers part or all of the clinical crown.
Crown lengthening—a surgical procedure used to lengthen the clinical crown to enhance the retention of an artificial crown.
Dowel crown—crown with a prefabricated post.
Enamel prisms—basic enamel unit running the dentinoenamel junction to the surface enamel.
Extracoronal crown—a crown that covers all or part of the clinical crown (see crown).
Flashing—restorative that extends beyond the preparation outline, but when initially placed does not cause an overhang.
Full crown—restoration that covers the entire clinical crown (eg, full metal crown, full veneer crown, jacket crown).

Full metal crown—a crown made of metal that covers the entire clinical crown (eg, full gold crown), occasionally called a full metal sleeve crown or full metal jacket.

Full veneer crown—see full crown.

Inlay—a restoration made to fit into a tooth.

Jacket crown—a full veneer crown made from porcelain, glass, resin, or metal as a permanent crown, or from acrylics or resins as a temporary crown (see full crown).

Onlay—a restoration made to fit over or replace an incisal edge or occlusal cusp either partially or completely.

Overhang—an excess of restoration projecting beyond the parameters of a preparation margin resulting a projection or shoulder.

Overlay—see onlay.

Partial crown—a restorative crown that covers only a portion of the clinical crown (eg, one-half, three-quarters).

Partial veneer crown—see partial crown.

Pin—a metal pin or wire cemented or threaded into the dentin at a preparation site to aid in retention of a restoration.

Porcelain fused to metal—a cast metal crown to which porcelain is bonded.

Post—a cylindrical metal rod cemented or threaded into the root canal system as a retentive device for a core or a post and crown; it can also be prefabricated as part of a post crown.

Post and core—a substructure for a crown, which is retained by by a post set into the root canal system. It can be a one-piece cast post and core, or a post-and-core buildup made from a prefabricated post surrounded at its exposed part by a core built up of a restorative material (eg, amalgam, glass ionomer, composite, etc.).

Post crown—a crown retained with a metal post (see dowel crown).

Three-quarter crown—see partial veneer crown.

Undercut—a designed feature of a restorative preparation created by removing a portion of the dentin within the preparation for the purpose of providing retentive qualities to a restoration.

Veneer—a thin restorative covering, generally used to conceal or repair discoloration, malformation, attritional wear, or dental injury. It is typically made from acrylic, resin, glass, or porcelain, although it may be made from metal as either a restoration in itself or as an abutment for a bridge.

Classification of Lesions and Restorations

To properly treat lesions, they are best classified as to the tooth involved and type and extent. Individual tooth identification systems can be found in the chapter on oral examination (see Chapter 4). Various classification systems pertaining to carious lesions, cavity preparations, erosive lesions, and staging of injuries can be found in Chapter 13. The G.V. Black modified cavity preparation classification system (see Chapter 13, Table 1) is one of the most universally used systems and the one primarily used in this chapter (3).

Some Common Abbreviations of Dental Restorative Terminology (4)

BR = bridge

BP = bridge pontic

BFF = bridge, fixed-fixed

BFM = bridge, fixed-movable

BRC = bridge, cantilever

BSC = bridge, spring cantilever

BRM = bridge, Maryland

BRR = bridge, Rochette

BCP = bridge, compound
BRT = bridge, temporary
CBU = core buildup
CR = crown
CM = crown, metal (CMG = gold;
   CMB = base metal, etc.)

DB = dentinal bonding agent
IL = inlay
OL = onlay
PFM = crown, porcelain fused to
  metal
VER = veneer

DENTAL DEFENSE MECHANISM

The principles of the dental defense mechanism are as essential in extensive restorative work, such as crowns, as they are in standard cavity preparation. While many teeth requiring such procedures may often be nonvital and have standard endodontic therapy already performed, some vital teeth require attention as well. Overlay and inlay cavity or crown preparation on vital teeth commonly leaves many open tubules, resulting in dental pain and possibly pulpitis. As described in Chapter 13, moderate amounts of injury or wear may expose dentinal tubules, and at times a protective natural defense such as surface mineralization may occur. However, in some cases, continued attrition or abrasion may prevent the tubules from being protectively sealed in this fashion. In these cases, removal of the continued source of wear and some form of dentinal sealer may be used to rectify the problem, or more advanced restorative procedures may need to be performed (eg, inlays, onlays).

Additionally, the amount of dentinal tubules that can be opened or exposed during the crown preparation of a vital structure can play an important role in the eventual health of that pulp. There are approximately 30,000–40,000 dentinal tubules per square millimeter of surface dentin (5). With the hydrodynamics of dentinal tubule fluids, many influences during preparation can cause problems. Rapid capillary action can be caused by surface dehydration, friction (venturi effect), or fluid contraction; these may be induced by temperature variation on the surface (water spray), substances that draw fluid (sugar), or air blown across the surface (friction and dehydration). Whenever a restorative procedure requires exposure of dentin, tubules may be left open. A temporary crown or restorative may be placed to protect the tubules and pulp, but in animals these can sometimes be difficult to maintain on the animal. In these cases, the tubules should at least be sealed with a bonding agent temporarily, until the permanent restoration is fitted. When restoratives are placed on vital teeth, it is prudent to perform followup examinations to reassess and confirm continued tooth vitality.

BASIC CONCEPTS OF RESTORATIVE PROCEDURES

When a defect occurs in the hard tissues of the tooth (enamel, dentin), optimally it is best to preserve the function and structure of the object by restorative means. It is essential to know the basic components of restorative efforts before therapy is undertaken. These include a knowledge of cavity preparation, from the skills involved to the final preparation that is required. The rules of restoration comprise:

1. Conservation
2. Esthetics
3. Contours and contacts

4. Extension for prevention
5. Cavity preparation
6. Identification and resolution of cause.

Conservation of Natural Tooth Structure

The conservation of natural tooth structure is the first rule of operative dentistry (3). Conservation of tooth structure is essential for protection of the vital pulp. However, not only the depth of preparation must be considered, but the size of the area as well. If there are 30,000–40,000 odontoblasts per millimeter of dentinal surface area (5), a 1-cm^2 preparation into the dentin may injure 3–4 million odontoblasts in the pulp cavity by severing their processes to some degree or vacuuming a part of or the entire odontoblast into the tubule. The degree of injury determines whether the individual odontoblasts becomes nonvital. Crown preparation that enters the dentin for full coverage on a vital tooth may injure or irritate the majority of the odontoblasts in the crown pulp chamber. The irritated odontoblasts result in dental pain and possible pulpitis.

Esthetics

Natural, healthy, unmarred enamel that is supported by healthy dentin, pulp, and periodontium is the most ethically pleasing. Therefore, the conservation of these healthy tissues is the best esthetics possible. However, when these tissues fail, restorative esthetics come into play. The type of esthetic procedures desired or required then dictate the design of the operative outline preparation form.

Contacts and Contours

A good general knowledge of dental anatomy is required to understand the physiology and function of tooth crown contours (see Chapter 3). Contact areas, marginal form, and the buccal and lingual contours must be properly designed to reduce food impaction during mastication. Typically, contact areas should be restored to the condition present when the tooth was young and healthy. Restoration of the axial contours (eg, buccal bulge) depends heavily on the condition of the periodontium. If the gingival margin is healthy and no recession is present, the tooth should be restored to its original contours. If gingival recession has occurred, the height of the buccal and lingual bulge contour should be moved apically to provide a proper physiologic relationship to the gingival margin.

Extension for Prevention

One of the major goals of operative dentistry is to prevent the recurrence of pathology. This simply means that the preparation outline should be designed to allow for proper oral hygiene to prevent additional disease. Cavity preparation on the occlusal surfaces should include any deep developmental grooves. The lingual and facial proximal cavosurfaces may need to be extended farther onto the facial or lingual surfaces to provide margins that can be more properly visualized for completion by the operator—and more easily kept cleaned by the client. The hygienic conditions of the mouth must be taken into consideration, and the preparation outline must be designed accordingly.

Extending the cavity outline below the gingival margin has become slightly controversial. There is compelling evidence for both possibilities, so the operator must design the outline to best suit his or her needs. With placement of the outline above or coronal to the gingival margin, tooth structure is conserved, and there is improved visualization of work, easier marginal finishing, less chance of overhangs, and less gingival irritation. However, with full-coverage crowns, placing the preparation outline more apically and below the gingival margin can provide enhanced esthetics and retentive quality. The retentive qualities are improved by providing a greater surface area for cementation, a greater depth of axial crown coverage, and a protected restorative margin. Unprotected or uncovered margins in animals can increase the chance that the crown margins will be caught in prey, food, chew toys, and bite sleeves, thereby allowing crown pulling forces to be applied. Cavity outlines at the gingival margin should be avoided, or the gingiva should be recontoured to circumvent this condition, as it typically results in gingival irritation. This makes the marginal finish, whether above or below the gingival margin, one of the most crucial points in restorative placement and finishing.

Identification and Resolution of Cause

If the cause of the disease can be ascertained, steps should be taken to relieve it, if possible. Long-term success of any restoration will be in doubt if the cause cannot be identified and resolved. In dogs trained in police, military, and protection functions, the source of the trauma can often be identified, but not removed. In the required continuing bite training, the reinforced bite sleeve can sometimes cause damage, as can actual on-duty activity. If the bite sleeve is the cause of an injury, it should be examined to determine whether it can be modified or improved to reduce the probability of a recurrence of the injury. Any predisposing factors such as cage biting, playing tug of war, dermatologic problems, and traumatic chewing behavior should be evaluated as to their potential effect on the restoration.

TREATMENT PLANNING

Treatment planning requires a systematic plan to assess the structures and associated problems that may challenge treatment success. A close study of existing conditions that have lead to the problem is required. It should be determined whether modification in behavior, environment, or a combination of both is required (see Chapter 21). Additionally, the patient's occlusion and periodontal health must be taken into consideration (3). Failure to nullify implicated complicity problems will result in less than optimal chances of operative or restorative success. The tooth structure must be evaluated for the ability to sustain a load, its relative retentive qualities, and esthetic requirements. It must be remembered that a well planned restorative should act not only as a mechanical repair but as a treatment of local dental disease and a prophylaxis against local and systemic disease (6).

Tooth vitality becomes important, as nonvital teeth will first require endodontic treatment. In addition, this means that posts can be placed in the endodontic system, and pulp injury from pin placement will not be a concern. Vital teeth will need a temporary crown or dentinal sealer during the interim between preparation and restorative placement, if laboratory-fabricated.

Tooth mobility should be ascertained in comparison with the adjacent teeth. Any degree of mobility should be checked out carefully, as undue mobility can be not only a contraindication for crown or bridge placement but possibly an indication for extraction.

Components of Prepared Cavities

Various walls, lines, and angles are created during cavity preparation (see Chapter 13). In crown and bridge work the primary walls of concern are the pulpal, axial, and gingival.

Additionally there are a few subdivisions of the walls, such as the enamel and dentinal walls. The *enamel wall* is that portion of the preparation wall that consists of enamel. The *dentinal wall* is that portion of the wall that consists of dentin. The *dentinoenamel junction* is that juncture in the wall where the dentinal and enamel walls meet.

Where two walls meet, a *line angle* is formed. At the point where three walls meet, a *point angle* is produced. The *cavosurface angle* is the line angle formed between a wall of the prepared surface and the unprepared tooth surface. The cavosurface angle is also sometimes termed the *preparation margin*, especially once the preparation is restored. The combined peripheral extent of all of the cavosurfaces or preparation margins is termed the *cavity* or *preparation outline*. With restoratives, the *restorative margin* is the restorative surface that abuts the cavosurface angle or preparation margin.

Preparation of Cavosurface Angles or Marginal Finish Lines

Design of the cavosurface angle requires special consideration in its preparation. The preparation marginal restoration greatly affects retentive qualities of the restoration, resistance to marginal leakage, physiologic contour reactions, gingival health, and resistance to attrition, abrasion, and fracture of the restoration and restored tooth. Selection of the specific cavosurface angle treatment depends on the type of restoration selected, the restorative materials to be used, the degree of anticipated stress demand on the restoration, and the length and direction of the enamel prisms.

In the consideration of crown preparation for crowns, onlays, and inlays, there are many varieties of marginal finish lines, each with an advantage for use in certain circumstances and specific restorative materials. On the distal, mesial, lingual, facial, occlusal, incisal, and proximal cavosurfaces, there are five basic types of marginal finish lines used: slight bevel, short bevel, long bevel, full bevel (chisel), and no bevel (butt).

On the gingival cavosurface, there are eight more commonly used marginal finish lines: short bevel (modified shoulder), long bevel, full bevel (chisel), butt joint (no bevel), shoulder joint, chamfer, deep chamfer, feather (knife edge), and occult (no cavosurface preparation but a feathered restorative margin).

The beveled finish lines, butt joints, shoulder joints, and chamfers are most commonly used with bonded restorations, inlays and onlays made from composite, metal, porcelains, glass, glass ionomers, and ceramometals (porcelain fused to metal). These definitive types of margins provide the laboratory with a distinct finish line and a margin that actually supports weight. With porcelain, glass, and composite materials, these better weight-bearing margins allow support of the restoration margin without spreading the margin when compressed, which could initiate cracks in the restoration. In addition, they allow construction of a restoration that is not oversized.

The knife-edge (feather) and occult finish lines are more typically used with onlays of metals. These preparations are easier to perform, take impressions of, and finish, and they leave a stronger tooth, since less tooth structure is removed. The use of an occult finish line leaves a stronger tooth substructure to support the crown, but it also results in an oversized restoration. The occult finish line is used in cases where additional foundation strength is required (eg, in dogs used by the police, military, etc.). However, it can only be used in situations where occlusal space allows an oversized crown and esthetics are not a principal concern.

Cavity Preparation

Multiple factors must be taken into consideration before the design of the preparation outline can be implemented on the tooth:

Location
Extent
Stresses
Tooth condition
Esthetic considerations.

First, the classification by location by G.V. Black system (see Chapter 13, Table 1) or a similar classification is required. This classification will then direct certain biological mechanical principles to be applied. Next, classification by extent is a necessity. This usually does not overtly affect the cavity outline, but rather the depth of preparation. This in turn determines whether cavity liners, indirect pulp capping, direct pulp capping, or root canal procedures will be required. Third, the occlusal and leverage stresses that must be encountered must be carefully studied. This impacts the types of restorative materials used, and whether the occlusal height of the crown should be reduced to diminish occlusal and leverage stresses. Fourth, the general condition of the tooth, must be contemplated, including other restoratives currently in place or to be placed. The presence of periodontal disease and especially tooth mobility must be considered and controlled. Finally, the esthetic demands by the client will need to be assessed. The use of porcelain fused to metal for the crown will require greater tooth reduction than the use of a typical metal crown.

Operating Field

It is essential for a successful procedure to have adequate access and isolation of the operative field. In addition, protection of other oral tissues from various materials is a consideration (see Chapter 13).

Materials Used in Indirect Forms of Crown and Bridge Work

Indirect inlays, onlays, crowns, and bridges are typically made from metals, glass ceramic, polymer glass, composite, or porcelains. The selection of restorative material has become complicated by the number of restorative materials in current use. However, a knowledge of cavity form, in association with the various restoratives' esthetic, physical, and biochemical properties, can simplify the selection process.

Within indirect form there are two basic techniques: indirect and direct/indirect. In indirect techniques, the cavity preparation is made and impressions are taken and models made; the restorative pattern is then fabricated indirectly on the model, the pattern invested and then burned out, and the restorative cast. With direct/indirect techniques, the cavity preparation is made, a separator medium applied, and the restorative pattern formed directly on the actual cavity; the restorative is then fabricated indirectly by the pattern's being invested and then burned out and the restorative's being cast (7). Porcelain, composites, and polymer glass restorations are fabricated directly on the model, without the need for intermediate patterns, investment, burnout, and casting. These, once patterned on the model, are taken directly to a curing oven (composite, polymer glass) or a baking oven for sintering (porcelain).

Metals

Currently, most dental metal restoratives are custom-fabricated by the lost-wax technique refined by Taggart (8) (Fig. 1). Metals in dentistry are grouped according to degree of nobility and fusing characteristics. *Metal nobility* refers to the degree of noble and precious metals in the alloy, while *fusing* is concerned with the temperature required to melt the metal or alloy (9).

Metals are usually grouped into three classifications regarding their nobility: non-precious (base metals), precious (sometimes called semiprecious), and noble (10). The seven noble metals comprise two groups: gold and platinum. Gold is in a group by itself, and the platinum group includes the remaining six noble metals: platinum, palladium, iridium, osmium, ruthenium, and rhodium.

Basically, metals are classified as noble due to their stability in the oral cavity and fluids and their lack of corrosion with a consequent reduced risk of contact or allergic reaction to the metals. Gold is still an excellent selection in most cases because of its ease of casting, strength, ductility, burnishability, and low allergic-reaction rate (11). The precious or semiprecious metals encompass the seven nobles, plus silver. Silver is not classified as a noble metal due to its tarnishing and corrosion characteristics. The non-precious metals (base metals) are principally nickel- and chrome-based alloys. A group known as *technic metals* also belong to this group. The technic metals are base-metal combinations that usually incorporate copper to provide a gold-tone appearance. Contact

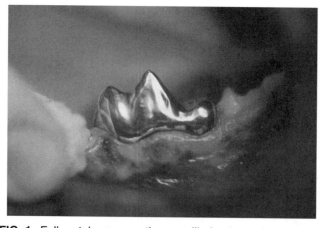

FIG. 1. Full metal crown on the mandibular 1st molar in a dog.

stomatitis, contact dermatitis, allergic reactions, and periodontitis with bone loss due to base metals is more common than in the other two groups (12–14). The more common use of base metals has been due to economic pressures. The proliferation of many new alloy systems has resulted in confusion among practitioners and a greater reliance on laboratory guidance, which unfortunately may also be influenced by economic considerations. However, some of these new alloys often provide very good results more economically than the more costly precious alloys.

Casting alloys are typically classified into two broad groups based on their fusion temperatures. The American Dental Association (ADA) Specification No.5 classifies the properties of casting alloys (15). The *normal-fusing alloys* are formulated for all-metal restoration, while the *high-fusing alloys* are designed for porcelain-fused-to-metal (PFM), or ceramometal, restorations (9). However, high-fusing metals are sometimes used for all-metal restorations. High-fusing metal must be used with PFM restorations so that they do not melt or creep during the repeated heating required to bake on the porcelain layers (16).

The normal-fusing alloys are divided into four types based on increasing hardness. *Type I (soft) alloys* are indicated for dental restorations, primarily inlays, that are not subject to heavy stress (class III and class V restorations). *Type II (medium) alloys* are capable of being used in almost any type of inlay (classes I–V restorations). *Type III (hard) alloys* are suitable for onlays, overlays, and crowns that will be under moderate occlusal stresses (class IV and class V restorations), bridge abutments, and thin partial or three-quarter crowns. *Type IV (extrahard) alloys* are designed for restorations under heavy stresses, fixed bridges, and removable partial dentures (15). Many combinations of alloys can be made to adapt to these specifications, providing the practitioner with a wide selection of materials. When cost is not a concern, the gold alloys are probably one of the best overall selections. However, there are many new precious metal–alloy combinations that provide extremely good results more economically than gold. The base metals, although highly durable and cheap, have many disadvantages that must be taken into consideration (12–14).

The high-fusing metals are generally classified into groups. A common classification comprises seven groups (16):

1 Noble gold
2 White noble
3 Palladium–silver alloys
4 Gold–palladium alloys
5 Nickel/chromium–base metal alloys
6 Cobalt–base metal alloys
7 High-palladium alloys

The noble gold (group 1) is expensive, weaker, and less sag-resistant during the porcelain-firing phases, but it is the easiest to cast and solder, and its light-yellow color aids in color matching light-colored teeth. White noble (group 2) is a combination of gold, palladium, and silver. This combination has improved mechanical properties with better strength and less sag, and is less expensive than group I; however, some porcelain greening or gray coloring sometimes occurs, making color matches for lighter-colored teeth more difficult. Palladium–silver alloys (group 3) have acceptable mechanical properties, but the silver content not uncommonly causes greening of the porcelain, and special porcelains and techniques must often be used. The gold–palladium alloys (group 4) have many good characteristics for PFM use and are considered a good choice by many human clinicians. The nickel–chromium alloys (group 5) are very technique-sensitive in laboratory fabrication and have some degree of allergy problems. The addition of beryllium enhances the porcelain bonding but adds the hazard of beryllium toxicity to laboratory technicians and others, if the alloy is heated (17). The cobalt–base metal alloys (group 6) are harder than the group 5 alloys, but they are even more technique-sensitive and do not have as good a bond strength as group 5. High-palladium alloys (group 7) are a combination of primarily palladium with a moderate amount of base metal and a small amount of gold and silver. They are very hard and compatible with most porcelain systems but are more technique-sensitive and more difficult to cast well (16). Generally, gold–palladium (group 4) is a good all around choice when cost is not a major factor, but you should consult your laboratory, as the metal used is also dictated to a degree by the brand of porcelain used (18).

Indirect Composite Resins Techniques

Indirect composite resin technique describes the fabrication of a composite restoration on a model rather than directly on the tooth. Indirect techniques have some advantages over direct applications.

When cured, composite resins, both direct and indirect have shrinkage in the resin matrix during polymerization. With directly applied composites, this can result in gaps in the marginal seal and possible marginal leakage. With indirect technique, the shrinkage occurs before placement, which is chiefly offset with the luting or bonding agent at the time of placement. This results in less marginal gapping and a decreased risk of marginal leakage (16). In addition, laboratories using composites that are treated with ultraviolet light (direct composites normally use visible light–curing composites), heat, and vacuum can provide a superiorly cured resin restorative (19). This results in a resin that may be harder and have greater tensile strength, thus producing a stronger, longer-lasting restoration (20).

Composite resins have a few advantages even over porcelains. Porcelain is harder than the natural tooth structure, which may cause accelerated wear of the opposing occlusion. Composite resins, being softer than porcelain, do not generally accelerate wear of the opposing natural tooth structure. In addition, once porcelain is bonded into place, areas of adjustments can be difficult to return to the original degree of luster and appearance of vitality. Composite resins on the other hand are easy to repolish following adjustment. These advantages, along with continued improvement in resin technology, may eventually result in resins replacing the use of porcelain in many types of restorations (16).

No undercuts are used in the cavity preparations for indirect techniques. Resins can use a feather margin on veneers with only a 0.25–0.50 mm facial reduction required. However, over incisal, cusp, or occlusal surfaces, a reduction of 1.0–1.5 mm is recommend. With inlays and onlays, margins are usually bevels or butts; shoulders and chamfers can be used at the gingival cavosurface. The gingival cavosurface normally requires at least a 0.5-mm reduction, and incisal, cusp, and occlusal areas require 1.0–1.5 mm of reduction (7).

Once the reduction is completed, impressions are taken and models made for the fabrication of the restorative. When the composite restorative is completed, the inside surface is etched typically with 10% hydrofluoric acid. Once it is received by the practitioner, the first item of business is to have a try-in of the restoration, before intubation and cementation, to check the marginal adaptation, seating, and occlusal articulation.

Adjustments can be made with a white-stone point or fluted bur. If the restorative fits properly, the patient is intubated, and the tooth surface is cleaned, etched with phosphoric acid, and rinsed; a bonding agent is then applied and the restorative is cemented into place. Excess cement can be removed with a hand scaler or white-stone point. The fit should then be rechecked, additional adjustment made if needed, and the restorative polished (16).

The same result can be accomplished by a direct/indirect technique, in which the cavity is treated with a separating medium so that composite will not stick to it. A visible light–curing resin is placed, cured, and finished. The restorative is removed with the tip of an explorer and heat-treated. The cavity preparation is then thoroughly cleaned to remove all separating medium and bonded into place in the same manner as described for the indirect technique.

Cast Glass Ceramic

Cast glass ceramic is one of the restoratives developed as a rival to standard porcelain. It reflects the results of variations of the pyrocerams developed by Corning Glass Works for home cookwear (Corning Wear™). The first adaptation into dental restoration occurred in 1984 as Dicor™ (Dentsply International, York, Pennsylvania).

Dental cast glass ceramic is made with the normal pyroceram materials, but with the addition of various oxides of conventional feldspathic porcelains. Some of the more common oxides used are silicon dioxide, potassium oxide, magnesium oxide, aluminum oxide, and zirconium oxide (16). The newest glass ceramic, Inceram® (Vident, Brea, California) incorporates zirconium oxide (artificial diamond) to enhance the color and strength of the material.

Cast glass ceramic has the same basic fabrication requirements as cast metals. Once the cavity preparation is designed and implemented, quality impressions must be obtained and models made. There are two basic types of cast glass in current use: those cast like metals and those machined from a block of precast material. The machined block is precisely cut by a milling process guided by a computer reading of the model. The blocks of cast glass are colored throughout but come in a limited numbers of colors, which limits esthetic color matching. The conventional casting of a pyroceram restorative, as with metals, requires that a full anatomic wax-up be produced, sprued, and invested. Following burnout of the wax, the glass is cast into the investment (21). Once the cast is removed, the glass must be trimmed and adjusted. The glass from which this is cast may be precolored (Inceram®) or clear (Dicor™). The glass cast at this point does not have full strength. It must now be treated by a process known as *ceramming* to obtain full strength of the restorative by its conversion into a crystalline glass ceramic (pyroceram). The uncolored cast glass pyroceram (Dicor) will now take on a frosted-glass appearance. This cast glass must now have external esthetic color added to give the appearance of a normal vital tooth. This means that the esthetic coloring is a superficial stain on the restorative's surface, and any required adjustments at chairside can remove the color, exposing the frosted glass. This can delay cementation, if the crown must be returned to the dental laboratory for restaining. In the precolored pyrocerams (Inceram®), the color preference was made at the time of casting from a very small, limited color selection, unlike porcelains and stained pyrocerams.

Poor marginal adaptation and rough, porous surfaces may support bacterial colonization, which can result in gingival inflammation (22,23). Cast glass exhibits less surface plaque accumulation than natural tooth surfaces or any restorative material currently being used (24,25). This appears to be the result of the smoothness of the surface, low surface tension, and a form of electrostatic repulsion generated by the cast glass ceramics (22–25).

Porcelain jackets ordinarily have better esthetic qualities than cast glass for anterior restorations. However, formation of Griffith flaws in porcelain results in its being more prone to fracture, crazing, and chipping, making porcelain generally considered too weak for posterior restorations (26,27). Griffith flaws are microscopic defects created during the fabrication of porcelains; they are considered to be responsible for the propagation of cracks in fired porcelains (27). Cast or ceramic glass has a greater compressive strength than porcelains (28,29), and with adequate thickness the vulnerability of cast glass to fracture from lateral and tensile forces can be minimized (29,30). Additionally, porcelains are more abrasive than cast glass, and they can wear opposing natural tooth, metal, porcelain, or other restorative materials (27,30). The wear patterns of cast glass ceramics are more similar than those of other restorative materials to the wear patterns of human enamel (32). This typically makes cast glass a better posterior restorative in comparison with porcelain jackets. Cast glass ceramics are excellent selections for esthetic repairs of dog canine teeth experiencing wear due cage-biter syndrome and other attritional or abrasive forces. However, cast glass ceramics are still vulnerable to the complex shearing forces of animal carnassial teeth, for which metal and ceramometal restorations are generally better suited.

Another form of cast glass ceramic restoration is the porcelain fused to glass (PFG), or Willi's Glass Crown™ (Ivoclar Inc., Tonowanda, New York) (30). This procedure combines the advantages of glass ceramic's strength and porcelain's esthetics (Dicor Plus™, Dentsply International). In the PFG-type crown, the cast ceramic glass is used as a foundation substructure to which porcelain is fused on the surface. This provides superior resistance to the forces of compression as compared with a porcelain jacket, while providing the greater esthetic appearance of porcelain as compared with cast or milled glass ceramics. In addition, slight adjustments can be made at chairside without exposing unstained glass ceramic. PFG restoratives can provide a superior esthetic quality as compared to run PFM and greater fracture resistance as compared with porcelain jackets, although not quite as good as the PFM product.

Polymer Glass

Polymer glass is a new category of restorative for crown and bridge applications (Artglass®, Heraeus Kulzer, Irvine, California). It incorporates a polymer with glass particles of 2 μm and less. The glass particles are fairly spherical but slightly rough. They add strength and esthetics, as they reflect light with little diffusion, helping provide a high-luster appearance with proper finishing. Polymer glass comes in many of the Vita shades, which improves the esthetic color-matching abilities. The material is more impact- and fracture-resistant than standard composites and many ceramics, yet this does not accelerate wear in the opposing occlusion as do many porcelain restoratives (33). It uses a camphoquinone as the initiator of polymerization, which requires a light source in the 470-nm range for activation, as do most indirect composites. However, the polymerization is critical to obtaining the full potential of qualities of the polymer glasses. Therefore, special strobe curing ovens are customarily used for curing. New products, such as the polymer glasses, may provide significant improvements in the quality of dental restorations.

Porcelain

Dental porcelain currently used for restorations is a combination of kaolinite, potash, feldspar, quartz, and glass modifiers (10). The use of vacuum ovens and modifications in the porcelain ingredients have improved the sintering process, resulting in restoratives with improved translucency to better match natural tooth structure and provide a more vital appearance (16). Older techniques result in the porcelain's having a more opaque appearance, and thus the restoration lacks a vital appearance. *Sintering* is the actual fusing of the porcelain powders into a single solid structure (10).

Porcelains are available in low-, medium-, and high-fusing types. The low- and medium-fusing porcelains have the advantage that there is less stress on the metals used in PFM restorations during the fusing of the porcelain to the unit. However, if reheated, these porcelains have a tendency to slump, which is not seen in the high-fusing porcelains. This means that restorations made with low-fusing porcelains cannot be easily repaired by the addition of new porcelain, whereas high-fusing porcelains may be so repaired (10). Other than these two factors, there is little difference between the two fusing types.

When porcelain is used alone with a metal or glass ceramic substructure, it is known as a *porcelain jacket*. The elimination of the metal substructure allows for improved esthetics in limited reduction areas, like those encountered in many anterior restorations. Additionally, it allows the use of high-fusing porcelains, which permit repairs with the addition more fused porcelain. The advantages of an all-porcelain restoration as compared with PFMs are improved esthetics, better biocompatability (no metal allergies or toxins), and no darkening of tooth structure adjacent to the restoration due to metal leaching (16,34). Disadvantages are the low compressive strength, need for substantial remaining tooth structure, and wear to opposing occlusion. These lead to the limitation of all-porcelain use to primarily single-unit anterior restorations, although multiunit bridges have been attempted with limited success (35).

Many techniques have been devised to improve the porcelain jacket's properties. Among these are the alumina-reinforced crown, platinum-bonded alumina crown, and aluminoceramic crown (16). Although each enhances porcelain strength and fracture resistance, together they still have the same basic contraindication: They should not be used with teeth bearing heavy occlusal forces; nor should they be used with short clinical crowns, camouflage techniques, splinting, bridges, tapers greater than 6°, or axial reductions less than 1 mm. However, occasionally, cases with one of these contraindications have been treated successfully. The noncast-metal system can be successfully used with an axial reduction with as little as 0.7 mm, but it is not a true all-porcelain or porcelain-jacket restorative.

Ceramometal or Porcelain-Fused-to-Metal Restorations

Porcelains with a higher coefficient of thermal expansion were developed in the early 1960s (16). They allowed the compatible fusing of porcelains to cast metal dental alloys and the acceptable fabrication of the porcelain-fused-to-metal (PFM) restoration (Fig. 2). Porcelain fuses to the metal by both chemical and mechanical bonding. The chemical bond occurs as the porcelain forms a crystalline attachment to oxides on the surface of the metal alloy. The mechanical interlock occurs both on a gross level from the design and on a micromechanical level from the abrasive treatment of the metal, which forms a

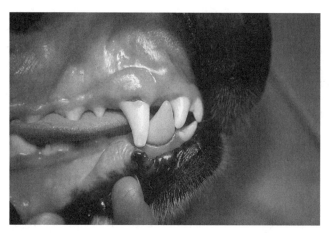

FIG. 2. Porcelain-fused-to-metal crown on the mandibular canine tooth.

surface texture for bonding (10). This combination produces a compressive strength much greater than that of porcelain jackets (10).

The metals for the substructure must be able take repeated firing for the application of the various layers of porcelain without deformation or creep. This means that the substructure metal should be of a high-fusing alloy (see Metals above) (18). The porcelain must be able to resist slumping and devitrification. *Slumping* is the slow deformation of porcelain from repeated heating. *Devitrification* is the crystallization that occurs from the repeated firings, resulting in a clouding of the porcelain and a nonvital appearance to the restoration (10).

Generally, the axial reduction with PFM needs to be in the range of 1.5 mm to allow for a 0.5-mm metal substructure and 1 mm of porcelain needed to cover the metal esthetically. The incisal reduction should be in the 2.0-mm range, and the occlusal in the 1.5-mm range (16). Failure to provide sufficient reduction will result in poor esthetics, a weak restoration, or an oversized restoration (36). In addition, the porcelain layer should generally not exceed 2 mm in thickness, as it is not required for esthetics and the porcelain is the weak link in the restorative. Therefore, the metal substructure should be designed to prevent overlayering of the porcelain (37).

Partial Crowns and Inlays

Partial onlay or *overlay crowns* are restorations that cover a cusp and only a portion of the clinical crown (eg, one-half, three-quarters). *Partial inlay crowns* are restorations that cover a portion of the clinical crown, but not a cusp. Partial crowns, either onlays or inlays, are most commonly used in dogs with cage-biter syndrome. *Cage-biter syndrome* is any condition that initially results in attrition or abrasion that wears the distal surface of a tooth. This is seen most commonly in dogs that grasp wire fence or caging and pull or chew on it, resulting in attrition. This type of wear can be countered in two ways: behavioral training and restoration. Restorations can restore the tooth in most cases, if caught early enough. However, if the underlying behavioral problem is not under control, complications with additional teeth and the restorations may eventually occur (see Chapter 21). The decision whether to restore the wear with an inlay or onlay is usually based

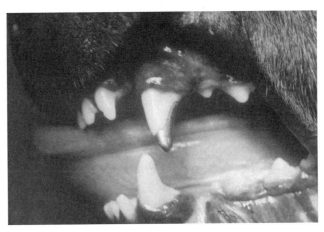

FIG. 3. Partial onlay crown made of metal on the maxillary canine tooth for treatment of cage-biter syndrome.

on the amount and location of wear. Minor wear in the middle and cervical thirds of the distal surface can usually best be handled with the more conservative inlay. More extensive wear or wear to the cusp typically requires an onlay.

The inlay preparation is a class II preparation (see Chapter 13). All undercuts, irregularities, and diseased dental structure at the site should be removed. The cavosurfaces (margins) should be either beveled or chamfered. The lesion can now either be restored with a composite or have impressions made for a laboratory-fabricated restoration. The partial overlay is a class VI preparation (see Chapter 13). The preparation will include the cusp and several millimeters below it on the mesial, lingual, and labial surfaces, while the distal surface will be extended down to a location below the disease or wear. The cavosurfaces can be beveled or chamfered. Impressions are then taken, and a partial crown is made by the laboratory (Fig. 3). These authors have found that both metal and glass ceramic restorations have held up well; however, if the animal continues to chew inappropriately, porcelains are very prone to cracking, chipping, and fractures.

In-Clinic Composite Crown Restorations

Repair of class VI injuries to the crown with in-clinic composites can be esthetically pleasing and less expensive than laboratory-produced devices, and can be fabricated at one setting. However, they are weak in comparison with most laboratory-fabricated restorations and should only be used when the cause of the problem has been eliminated and the animal will not be placing undue shearing stresses on the restoration. The long-term success of such restorations should be considered guarded. (See Chapter 13 for information on composites, bonding, posts, and pins.)

Generally, the fracture is smoothed with a fluted bur or white stone. All unsupported enamel should be removed, and the enamel margins beveled. On nonvital teeth, a post or dowel should be cemented into the root canal system for retention, and one or more pins placed in the dentin to resist rotational forces. A high-quality bonding system should be used on the enamel and dentinal surfaces. The composite can then be applied and cured. The restoration can next be refined and finished using fluted burs or white-stone points.

The final restoration should be etched and have a layer of unfilled resin applied to improve the marginal seal and the wearability of the restoration. Complete curing of the composite is critical. If light-cured materials are used, the composite should be placed in increments and a good-quality light-curing unit should be used. On vital teeth, the same basic process is followed, except that no post is placed and pin placement must not intrude on pulp or periodontal tissues.

Bridges

A *bridge* is a dental prosthesis that replaces the crowns of one or more missing teeth (Fig. 4). In today's dental practice, esthetically minded clients on occasion wish for lost teeth to be replaced, and a dental bridge is one way of accomplishing this. Bridges are a complex restoration and should not be lightly undertaken. Before venturing on fabrication and placement of a bridge, the operator should understand some of the anatomy of a bridge, types of bridges, and retention factors.

The portion of a bridge replacing a missing tooth is termed the *pontic*. An *abutment* is a tooth, crown, or portion of an implant used to support, stabilize, or anchor a fixed or removable dental prosthesis such as a bridge. A *pier* is any abutment other than the terminal abutments. Piers are sometimes called *intermediate abutments*. The portion of the bridge restoration that rebuilds the prepared abutment and pier teeth is known as the *retainer*. With fixed-movable bridges, the retainer on the fixed end is known as the *major retainer*, and the one on the movable end as the *minor retainer*. The *joint* or *connector* is that part of a bridge or prosthetic device that unites the retainer with the pontic. A *dovetail* is a type of connector used as the movable joint for a minor retainer. The portion of the bridge suspended between the abutments is termed the *span*. A *bridge unit* is an individual part of the bridge, such as the pontic or retainer.

Common Bridges Types

There are several common bridge types (2,38):

Fixed-fixed bridge—a one-piece bridge with pontic or pontics attached to the span between retainers at both ends (common bridge) (Fig. 5A).
Fixed-movable bridge—a two-piece bridge with the pontic or pontics integrally attached to the retainer at only one end. The other end of the bridge attaches to the retainer or

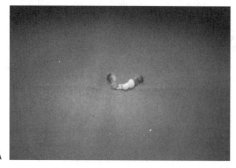
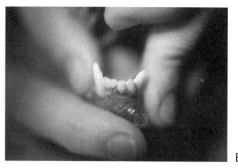

A   B

FIG. 4 (A) Maryland bridge with two porcelain pontics. **(B)** Maryland bridge cemented into place.

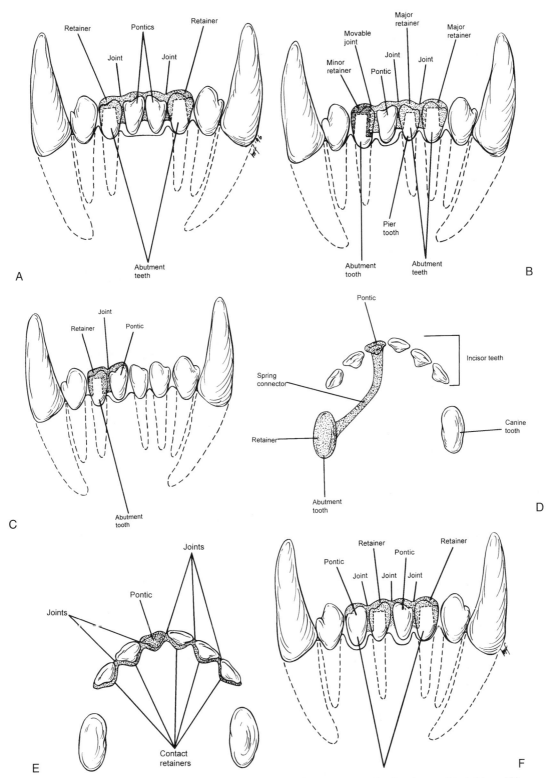

FIG. 5 **(A)** Components of a fixed-fixed bridge. **(B)** Components of a fixed-movable bridge. **(C)** Cantilever bridge. **(D)** Spring cantilever bridge. **(E)** Maryland bridge. **(F)** Compound bridge.

abutment in a fashion that allows some degree of movement. Also sometimes known as a *fixed-free* or *deprecated bridge*, it is most commonly used in the molar/premolar area to allow for occlusal stress patterns (Fig. 5B).

Cantilever bridge—a one-piece bridge with the pontic supported only from one end by a retainer or retainers. The cantilever retainer is generally distal to the pontic to allow a more natural open mesial contact for esthetics (Fig. 5C).

Spring cantilever bridge—a one-piece bridge in which the pontic is remotely attached to the retainer by a spring or bar. This type of bridge is sometimes known simply as a *spring bridge*. This type of arrangement allows for naturally appearing open contacts both mesial and distal to the pontic (Fig. 5D).

Maryland bridge—a bridge in which the retainers are simply acid-etched at the areas that make contact with the tooth to enhance cementation. The retainers do not normally cover a cusp or incisal edge. This is a modified form of Rochette bridge. Maryland-type bridge generally result in the most conservative amount of natural tooth reduction for abutments and piers. At the same time. there is typically a tradeoff in lost retentive qualities (Fig. 5E).

Rochette bridge—a bridge in which the retainers are perforated at the areas that make contact with the tooth to enhance cementation. The retainers do not normally cover a cusp or incisal edge. This type of bridge generally results in the most conservative amount of natural tooth reduction for abutments and piers. At the same time, there is typically a tradeoff in lost retentive qualities.

Compound bridge—a bridge that is a combination of two or more bridge types, such as a fixed-fixed-cantilever, fixed-fixed-movable, or fixed-fixed-spring. Such bridges are used for more complex replacements of multiple teeth that are not all consecutive (Fig. 5F).

Temporary bridge—a bridge constructed and placed on the prepared site for the purpose of protecting the preparation and/or for esthetics, until the permanent bridge can be fabricated and placed.

In deliberation of a bridge placement, the practitioner must consider several factors. First and foremost is whether the owner is willing to maintain a high standard of oral hygiene for the animal. Bridgework commonly results in the entrapment of food particles and conceals plaque accumulation. Daily brushing of the animal's teeth with emphasis on the bridge abutments is extremely important for long-term success, especially if the bridge is replacing teeth lost from periodontal disease (38). Bridges are best used in areas for filling small gaps in the occlusion with an otherwise healthy arch and strong healthy abutment teeth. If the abutment teeth are not in good periodontal health, the additional occlusal stress from the bridge will only lead to complications of mobility. The bridge should be designed to allow natural mastication to assist in hygiene maintenance.

Bridgework must be able to absorb considerable punishment and stress. For this reason, the substructure should generally be made from the more durable high-fusing metals. The greater the masticatory force and the greater the segments of unsupported span are, the greater is the need for strength in the metal framework of the bridge (10,38).

The abutment tooth selection and the type of retainer used greatly affect the retentive qualities of the bridge. Teeth with surface disease (eg, caries, resorptive disease, hypoplasia, hypocalcification, etc.) and nonvital and endodontically treated teeth may have weakened tooth or alveolar structure and should be carefully accessed. These are not necessarily contraindications against their use as abutments, but rather indications for close inspection before use. Tooth mobility, periodontal disease, poor oral hygiene, clinical crowns shorter than 4 mm, splinted teeth, and teeth with bone loss are generally contraindicated for use as abutments. The abutment teeth should provide a total root surface area at least equivalent to that of the teeth to be replaced, but preferably it should be twice that (38) (see the Appendix for approximate root surface areas).

Fixed-fixed, fixed-movable, cantilever, spring cantilever, and compound combinations of these bridge types typically require the abutment teeth have partial- or full-tooth reduction with an appropriate cavosurface margin. Maryland- and Rochette-type bridges generally have a beveled inlay type of preparation for the retainer placement, although some retainers may be designed as various types of ridged bands to provide retention (6).

Tooth reduction for bridges must be carefully considered, as all abutments must eventually have an identical line of draw for the bridge to be seated. In some cases, the bridge can be made to telescope to offset problems with the line of draw. In other cases, telescoping retainers that redirect the line of draw can be used (38).

Tooth Reduction

Reduction of tooth structure should be made with care to remove only to the extent necessary and proper for mechanical and esthetic principles (3). Excessive or unnecessary reduction will only weaken the tooth structure and crown support. In some patients, crowns can be fabricated and seated with little or no reduction of dental structures, but in most cases crown reduction is necessary to achieve function without occlusal interference from the enlargement of tooth dimensions (Table 1). Underpreparation has been reported as a major problem in ceramometal restorations in humans (39). This can result in poor

TABLE 1. *Reduction requirements for restoratives*

Material	Type	Margin at gingival cavosurface	Reduction (mm)	Over area	Reduction (mm)	Taper degrees
Indirect composite resin	Veneers	Feather	0.25	I,C,O	1.00–1.50	6
	Inlay/onlay	Bevel or butt	0.50	I,C,O	1.00–1.50	
Porcelain jacket	Inlay/onlay	Bevel, butt, shoulder, or chamfer	1.2–1.5	I,C,O	1.5–2.0	6
Cast glass ceramic	Inlay/onlay	Anterior teeth: bevel, butt, shoulder, or chamfer	Facially 1.0 Lingually 1.5	I,C	1.5	6
	Inlay/onlay	Posterior teeth: bevel, butt, shoulder, or chamfer	1.2–1.5	O	1.5–2.0	
Porcelain fused to glass	Inlay/onlay	Bevel, butt, shoulder, or chamfer	1.5	I,C O	1.5 2.0	6
Full metal	Veneer/onlay	Occult Feather	0.0 0.3–0.5	I,C,O I,C,O	0.0–0.1 1.0	6
	Inlay/onlay	Bevel, butt, shoulder, or chamfer	0.5	I,C,O	1.0	
Ceramometal or porcelain fused to metal	Inlay/onlay	Bevel, butt, shoulder, or chamfer	1.5	I,C O	2.0 1.5	6

(Compiled from data in refs. 6,7,16.)
I, incisal edge; C, cusp; O, occlusal surface.

TABLE 2. *Common types of finish lines and common uses*

Finish line type	Common use
Occult	Nonreduction areas for MJ
Feather	Slight reduction sites for MJ
Bevels	Cavo- and proximal surfaces for C, PG, MJ, PFM, PJ, PFG
Chamfer	Ideal for most MJ crowns
Deep chamfer	Good for MJ, PJ, PFM, PFG, PG
Shoulder	Good for MJ; ideal for PJ, PFM, PFG, PG

C, composite; MJ, metal jacket; PFG, porcelain fused to glass; PFM, porcelain fused

color matching because the translucency of the porcelain allows the metal matrix shadow to show through, or in overcontouring of the tooth to hide the metal. Theoretically, a full-coverage crown restoration should duplicate the original tooth structure, but it is generally not practical in canine tooth crowns in the dog or the cat. In the cat, the fragility of structure usually does not permit reduction, and in the dog it may be unwise in many canine teeth that will be experiencing substantial occlusal stress. With the limitations of the current restorative materials and the tremendous forces and leverage applied on the cuspid teeth in the dog, certain restrictions on a crown's contour and size are generally prudent. The canine tooth should ordinarily not be restored to original height. Contouring it to just above the height of the fracture is wise, and even in attempts to rebuild height, it is usual not to attempt greater than two-thirds of original height. This reduction takes the tooth slightly out of occlusion and greatly reduces the leverage forces placed on the retentive qualities of the crown. The tip should be contoured to a gently esthetic bluntness. Sharp points increase the potential damage that these restored teeth can inflict. Additionally, sharp pointed teeth will penetrate deeper into bite sleeves and other objects, increasing their anchorage into the object. If substantial jerking or twisting movements are applied while the tooth is deeply embedded, the chances of tooth fracture at the leverage point just below the crown are greatly increased.

Various types of crowns may require not only proportional reduction but a specific type of finish line for either esthetic or support requirements (see Preparation of Cavosurface Angles or Marginal Finish Lines above). The finish line or cavosurface margin is the end point of the apical extent of the crown. Retraction cord should be packed into the sulcus with a cord packer to open the sulcus, if the reduction and finish lines are to come near to or in the sulcus. Several common types of finish lines and their common uses are given in Table 2.

ARMAMENTARIUM

Instruments commonly used—preferably on a high-speed dental handpiece—for crown reduction and finish-line work include:

1. Diamond burs
2. Round ball burs
3. Crosscut burs
4. Fluted burs
5. End-cutting burs
6. Wheel-type disks.

The basic armamentarium divides into two groups of rotary instruments: diamond-coated points and wheels and various steel-type burs. The major differences between the two concern cutting efficiency and heat generation (37). The diamond bur is more aggressive and faster than carbon or carbide steel burs. At the same time, it has greater continuous surface contact, thereby generating greater heat, and this increases the potential of frictionally induced thermal pulpitis in the vital tooth (39). Both steel and diamond devices produce heat, and for this reason, no matter which is used on a vital tooth with a high-speed handpiece, adequate air/water-cooling spray is mandatory. Furthermore, clean, sharp burs are essential for efficient and expeditious structural removal with the least thermal insult.

There is an endless potential variety of shapes, sizes, and coarsenesses that can be manufactured based on demand. A general classification of burs and diamond points can be found in the Chapter 1. Diamond rotary instruments are available in friction-grip, latch-attachment and straight handpiece shanks (40). The diamond grit is applied to the operative in one to three layers, these being electroplated to the bur blanks with either nickel or chromium bonding material. The classification of fineness to coarseness of the bur is determined by the mesh size of the diamond particles, and in the finer sizes, the mesh size is commonly given (eg, 20 μm). Both natural and synthetic diamonds are used, with manufacturers promoting the supposed advantages of each. Instruments with extra-coarse particles are generally used for removal of connective tissues or bone, as in crown-lengthening procedures. Coarse-grit burs are primarily for the bulk removal of tooth structure. The medium grit, sometimes called regular grit, is among the more common types used in routine tooth preparations involving dentin and enamel. The fine-grit instruments are ordinarily utilized for finishing walls and for the marginal preparation. Extrafine, very fine, and superfine rotary diamond instrument were developed for composite finishing and, when used for crown preparation work, frequently do not leave a rough enough finish on the tooth for good cement adherence. A good water flow is recommended to prevent thermal problems with vital teeth and to avoid clogging of the diamond grit bed of the instrument (37).

Metal-cutting rotary burs come in two basic forms: steel (carbon steel) burs and carbide (tungsten) steel burs. Steel burs are initially sharper but also softer than carbide steel burs. This makes the (carbon) steel burs the preferred type for dentinal work, but their soft metal structure is virtually useless on enamel when they are used with high-speed handpieces. When such is applied to enamel, the steel ball disintegrates into a burnt-matchtip appearance almost instantaneously. Only carbide steel holds up well to enamel milling when used with a high-speed handpiece. ADA Specification No.23 standardized the shape, size, and dimensions of both steel and carbide steel burs, as well as their nomenclature, testing, and evaluation (40). Until the development of tungsten carbide burs around 1947, high-speed dental handpieces were not practical.

For enamel-milling work, one of the preferred bur types is the straight-fissure design. This device comes in four basic types: plain end-cutting, plain round end, crosscut end-cutting, and crosscut round end. The operative surfaces of these burs in standard sizes (ie, Nos.57, 557, 1157, 1557) are approximately 4 mm, and in the long operative heads (ie, Nos.57L, 557L, 1157L, 1557L), they are approximately 5.5 mm (49). Additionally, it should be remembered that in each of the four basic types, there are many diameters of burs available; however, the three most commonly used widths are the Nos.56, 57, and 58. This can aid in determining depth of milling during a procedure. The No.556 bur has a 0.9-mm diameter, No.557 a 1.0-mm diameter, and No.558 a 1.2-mm diameter. The four basic types of straight-fissure burs are the following (40):

1. Nos. 56, 57, and 58. These are plain straight-fissure burs with a flat end-cutting tip.
2. Nos. 556, 557, and 558. These are crosscut straight-fissure burs with a flat end-cutting tip.
3. Nos. 1156, 1157, and 1158. These are plain straight-fissure burs with a rounded end.
4. Nos. 1556, 1557, and 1558. These are crosscut straight-fissure burs with a rounded end.

The plain fissure bur cuts a smoother surface than the crosscut burs. Nevertheless, the slightly rougher surface cut of the crosscut fissures allows for a better mechanical retention and a greater surface area for luting (39). However, the rougher-surfaced instruments sometimes cause drag and microscopic tearing of alginate impression materials. The elastic impression materials ordinarily are not effected as much by the rougher surface. The round end burs are most frequently used on the axial surfaces, where a chamfer-type margin is desired.

Round ball burs are sometimes used to cut the margin for chamfers or to cut grooves in the tooth for depth guides in milling the enamel. Although ball burs are made in latch-attachment and straight handpiece shanks only the friction-grip type is normally used for enamel crown preparation work. The standard friction-grip instrument is 19 mm in length, and the surgical-length burs are 25 mm long (40). The surgical-length burs give more reach to work down the sides of some loftier animal teeth, such as the cuspids. The width of the round ball is approximately 0.6 mm for the No.1/2, 0.8 mm for the No.1, 1.2 mm for the No.3, 1.4 mm for the No.4, 1.6 mm for the No.5, 1.8 mm for the No.6, and 2.3 mm for the No.8 bur. Grooves cut into the walls of a tooth by a certain ball size, whether full or partial depth, can then be used as a gauge in reduction of tooth structure to assure proper depth reduction. Once reduction is started, except at the margin, it can sometimes be difficult to know just how much structure has been removed.

Before commencement of the preparation, the operator should visualize the desired design on the tooth to clearly conceive how it will interact with the tooth's current anatomic structure. Milling and tooth reduction are not a continuous grinding of the surface, but are done in stages at a single setting. As work is done, the operator should clear the surface and observe the results periodically during the process.

Reduction should taper 5–7° in toward the tooth's central axial core to allow ease of crown placement while providing good retention (6). The degree of taper can vary with anatomy and directly with the length of clinical crown available. The shorter a tooth is, the greater is the need for more parallelism for retentive purposes (39). Taller teeth can accept a greater taper, while still maintaining good retentive properties (6). The high-speed air turbine turns in only one direction, clockwise, when observed from the turbine to the bur tip. Generally, looking down on the tooth and using a high-speed handpiece, you should endeavor to work counterclockwise around its circumference. Counterclockwise movement around the tooth, in association with the clockwise rotation of the bur, results in the debris' being thrown primarily out behind the preparation path, and an air vortex is created that helps repel the gingival margin (39). When clockwise movement is used, the debris will be thrown into the path of the preparation, diminishing visibility of the working surface. Cut down the tooth uniformly, and strive not to make undercuts or overhangs that will interfere with the seating of the crown. Examine the tooth from above and from the sides, and digitally palpate for irregularities and undercuts. On vital teeth, always use copious amounts of water, and do not keep the bur in contact with the tooth for extended periods of time to prevent frictional heating of the tooth and inflammation of the pulp (33). On vital teeth, always leave at least 0.5 mm of dentin between the reduction and the pulp, as closer proximity may require indirect or direct pulp capping (39). Following reduction, vital teeth should be treated with a dentinal sealer to control sensitivity and reduce the chances of pulpitis until seating of the permanent crown (6). A temporary crown fabricated from acrylic may be advisable in certain patients, although in most animals they can be difficult to retain in place.

PRINCIPLES OF RETENTION

Fabrication and placement of restoratives are pointless if the restoration cannot be kept in place for the long term. Following proper retentive principles is the only way to maximize long-term success (38). The fundamentals of retention comprise:

1. Axial wall taper no greater than 5–7°
2. Maximizing enamel coverage
3. Maximizing tooth coverage (crown lengthening)
4. Retentive grooves
5. Pin holes and pins
6. Core buildup
7. Metal post and core
8. Cross pinning
9. Adhesion system.

Axial Wall Taper

The axial wall taper should be as close to providing parallelism as possible, while still providing a reasonable line of draw for the restoration. This has been generally shown to be in the range of 5° to 7° (6). However, many dog teeth have a natural taper beginning near the neck or at the midcervical third of the tooth out to the cusp. In these teeth, a taper greater than 7° may already exist on some axial walls and cannot be corrected without major structural reduction, which is unwise. In many of these cases, the height of contour will offset the taper discrepancy, or other retentive qualities will need emphasizing.

Maximizing Enamel Coverage

Of the tooth's hard surfaces, enamel provides the bonding surface with the greatest adhesion properties (41). For this reason, reductions should be kept within the enamel layer, when possible, rather than exposing dentin. For the same reason, the margins should be in enamel, when possible, not only for greater adhesion but also for optimal marginal seal against leakage, which can result in bonding fatigue (41–43).

Maximizing Tooth Coverage

The greater the tooth coverage is, the greater is the bonding surface, and, hopefully, the greater the height of contour. Height of contour, or how deeply the crown seats, is one of the primary keys to retentive quality of a crown. At least 3–4 mm of sound exposed tooth structure is the minimum necessary for retention (16). If this is not initially available, there are several techniques for lengthening the clinical crown. However, it should be remembered that a reasonable root:crown ratio must be maintained in these procedures or the tooth's stability will be compromised.

Crown Lengthening

Attempting to increase the amount of crown to be covered may be accomplished in a number of ways. Particularly in teeth with fractures extending subgingivally, some exposure may be necessary anyway.

Certainly, placing the finish margin subgingivally will increase the surface area covered, but this is sometimes difficult to accomplish without gingival flaps to improve access. While subgingival finish lines (at least 1 mm) have been shown to cause no specific problems in some studies where oral hygiene was strictly adhered to (44,45), there are other studies that report increases in gingival inflammation and periodontitis in areas of subgingival restorative materials (46). Direct irritation and plaque accumulation (47), including an increase in gram-negative bacteria (48), seem to contribute to the problems. Therefore, subgingival finish lines should only be considered in specific cases where good oral hygiene will be practiced.

In restorative or crown placement, an understanding and respect for the physiologic principles of biological width are required (16). *Biological width* (49,50) is the distance physiologically maintained by the body's defense mechanisms between the restorative and the base of the sulcus. For the dog, biological width is approximately 2 mm, which represents approximately 1 mm of supracrestal connective tissue and 1 mm of junctional epithelium. This results in a sulcus of 1–2 mm in depth. Restorations that impinge on this can effect a response to rebalance the biological width. The body reacts with an inflammatory response that results in crestal bone resorption and apical migration of the periodontal soft tissues. The inflammatory response will only cease once the biological width has been reestablished, which may take years (16). Occasionally, the crestal bone resorption pattern results in the establishment of infrabony pockets, which may lead to more serious periodontal disease.

Crown lengthening is simply the exposure of more root structure for use as clinical crown for restorative coverage (16). This usually takes the form of one of three procedures:

Type I   Gingivoplasty
Type II   Gingivoplasty and bone recontouring
Type III   Forced eruption.

In individual teeth in which there is sufficient to excessive amounts of attached gingiva, a *type I crown lengthening*, or a simple gingivoplasty, may provide additional length, as long as at least 2–4 mm of attached gingival tissue is maintained (37). This can be done with cold steel, fluted burs, diamond points, or carefully with electrosurgery (Fig. 6).

Type II crown lengthening may be indicated for some teeth if type I crown lengthening failed to provide the needed amount of clinical crown length. To provide optimum retention area without effecting a response to biological-width physiology by placing the restorative margin too close to the alveolar crest, an apically repositioned flap with subsequent alveoloplasty can be performed (16). This type of surgical crown-lengthening procedure can be fairly straight forward in the incisors or premolars, but the conical shape of the canine teeth can make it more challenging.

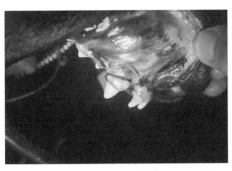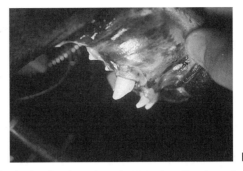

A B

FIG. 6 (A) Incision for removal of part of the gingival collar for a type I crown lengthening of a maxillary canine tooth in a dog. **(B)** Collar removed, demonstrating a substantial increase in clinical crown length.

Simple repositioning with standard mesial and distal releasing incisions on the cuspid teeth is generally not possible, as the gingival soft tissue collar would need to be sutured around a wider portion of the tooth. Therefore, specialized surgical releasing techniques that allow for the expansion of the gingival collar, such as the expanding-collar technique, are required for most type II crown-lengthening procedures involving the dog canine teeth (Fig. 7). The mandibular canine is probably the most difficult for many reasons, including the proximity of the corner or 3rd incisor. At times, extraction of that tooth will permit greater access for apical repositioning and for crown preparation. The procedure is initiated by severing the epithelial attachment around the tooth with a scalpel blade. The specialized pattern of releasing incisions can now be planned. An angled incision is made from a point on the tooth midway between the mesial aspect and buccal surface of

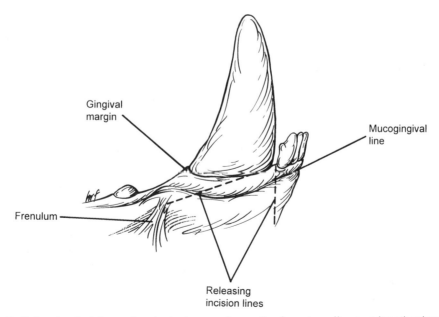

Gingival margin

Mucogingival line

Frenulum

Releasing incision lines

FIG. 7. Releasing incisions of a gingival expanding collar for a type II crown-lengthening procedure on a mandibular canine tooth in a dog.

the tooth, running distally at about a 30° angle to the gingival margin on both the buccal and lingual aspects of the tooth. This will allow for an expanding gingival collar for repositioning at the wider circumference. Additional releasing incisions are made at the mesial aspect, either as a lingual–buccal pair that extends to the mucogingival junction or as a mesial interdental incision to permit exposure and reduction. Often a distal interdental releasing incision is necessary for exposure, and at times excessive gingival folds can be excised before suturing. It is important to ensure that sufficient attached gingival tissue communicates with adjacent attached gingiva to provide a continuous collar around the tooth. A crescent releasing incision on the distal surface, curving around from a buccal starting point to the lingual aspect or vice versa, will also provide more flexibility. Additional releasing incisions may be necessary at the mesial or distal aspects of the tooth to permit adequate soft tissue reflection and alveolar remodeling. Interdental sutures should hold the tissue at an apical position sufficient to provide additional crown height for the preparation.

Type III crown lengthening, or forced eruption, is the extrusion of the tooth orthodontically to increase the clinical crown height. Reach a satisfactory height of contour can be involved and time-consuming (51). Forced eruption must be accompanied by gingival fibrotomy to prevent the coronal movement of periodontal tissue along with the tooth; otherwise, a gingivoplasty may also be required.

Retentive Grooves

In many teeth with irregular contours, the shape of the tooth itself prevents adverse rotational forces from acting on the restoration. However, in the conical-shaped canine teeth, there is little that will prevent rotation of the cast crown around the tooth structure. If a pin is not used specifically for this purpose and the individual tooth will predispose the crown to rotational forces, parallel long-axis grooves may be prepared to provide reasonable stability. As with any crown preparation, the tradeoff exists between the benefits of the procedure and the potential weakening of tooth structure that can occur with additional tooth reduction. Retentive grooves placed in the enamel parallel to the long axis of the tooth and in alignment with the restorative's line of insertion can improve retention by several means. The grooves aid in countering rotational forces on the restoration, for if the crown is even slightly rotated, the bond adhesion can be rapidly broken down. In addition, the grooves increase the potential bonding surface area. When possible, the grooves should be placed in enamel for the best bonding effect (16). These grooves must also be parallel to the line of draw to prevent any inadvertent undercuts that would prevent proper seating of the cast restorative. The groove must also not interfere with the integrity of the marginal finish.

Pin Holes, Pin Ledging, and Pins

Pin holes are holes drilled into the dentin for pins to be inserted to provide retention or resistance for the restorative. The pins are typically one of two forms: pins placed independently for restorative buildup or pins fabricated as a component of the laboratory-constructed restoration. When a ledge is created on which the pin hole is placed, it is commonly called *pin ledging*. The placement and number of pin holes are crucial to successful pinning technique but are affected by many factors, of which tooth vitality status is only one. Pin holes and ledging were discussed in detail in Chapter 13 (6).

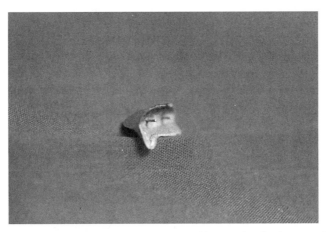

FIG. 8. Gold crown for an upper 4th premolar with two pins for improved retention.

Pin holes can be quite useful in providing additional retention and rotational stability for crown manufacture (37). These benefits should be weighed against the adverse effects of the pins in weakening the tooth structure. In cast restorations, placement of a single pin should be parallel to the line of draw, and if more than one pin is placed, they should be parallel to each other, as well as to the line of draw. With pins that are fabricated as an intricate part of a cast restoration, impression pins must be placed in the prepared pin holes at the time when impressions are made, so that they are incorporated into the impression. This allows the pattern to be duplicated on the model and permits the cast restoration to replicate their position when manufactured properly (Fig. 8). Burnout pins would then be used on the model to be incorporated in the wax pattern used to fabricate the cast restorative (7). Their placement should be snug but not excessively tight, as they are to be cemented into place as part of the crown unit. A try-in of the crown before cementation is necessary to ensure that there has been no deviation of the pin orientation that would prohibit proper seating of the crown.

Core Buildup

At times, there is insufficient tooth structure to provide adequate retention for the restorative desired, or there is a specific need for crown height beyond that which remains. If there is an oblique-type fracture, placement of pins to enhance retention of the core material may be sufficient, if the finished height does not exceed the height of the remaining tooth structure. With tooth injuries of this extent, almost all will be nonvital. This means that endodontic treatment of the tooth is required before dowel placement, since it will be placed to some degree within the endodontic system, usually the root canal space (37).

With fractures perpendicular to the long axis of the tooth, it is usually necessary to provide a superstructure onto which the core material can be built up. A dowel or pin can be placed into the endodontic space of the canal after the appropriate amount of endodontic filler has been removed and the post space is adequately prepared. However, the apical seal (the last 3–4 mm) of endodontic fill must not be compromised, or endodontic failure may occur (38). There are threaded posts and pins available for use as dowels, but as they rely on friction and wall stress for retention, they can result in tooth fracture (52). A Christmas-tree configuration of some posts has a complex superstructure on top of the threaded portion, as well as a straight axis. The only way to fit these posts to an adequate depth in the endodontic space is to drill out a post space to fit the device. This can greatly weaken the tooth. Additionally, in dog canine teeth, the angulation of the root canal system to the crown usually necessitates curving or bending the post, which can only be done after it has been fully seated into the canal. Attempts to redirect the post by bending it after it is placed may result in splitting the remaining root structure with eventual loss of not only the restoration but also the tooth as (see Chapter 13). These human products are not as easily adapted to veterinary dentistry as others.

Standard nonthreaded posts can be bent to conform to the gentle bend of the tooth's natural root canal before placement. Intramedullary pins can provide the length necessary for dog cuspids. While it is best not to be threaded, some form of mechanical retention on the post should be made to improve cementation, such as scoring the surface with a bur at intervals. Markley Threaded Wires™ (Almore International Inc., Portland, Oregon) can also be cut to a desired length and placed without rotational use of the screw threads. Optimally, the post should be placed into the canal system to a depth that will be equal in height to the eventual restoration, which translates to around twice the amount of post in the canal as is exposed before buildup.

With a completely round endodontic canal space, rotational forces can be quite significant, so a different canal shape, such as oval, can reduce some rotation. For specific protection from rotation, one or more pins can be placed or retentive grooves made before core material placement. Once the post and pins are cemented into place, the core material can be placed according to the manufacturer's recommendations for use. Composites, reinforced glass ionomers, and even amalgam can be used for the buildup, which should not extend much beyond the height of the exposed post. However, for most animal and human use, the glass ionomers, even type IV, are generally too weak and prone to fracture for core buildups (16). Once completed, the buildup can then be prepared to specification for the crown type selected. The crown margin should be well within healthy tooth structure, by at least 2 mm, rather than in core buildup material (53).

Cast Dowel Crowns and Post and Core Crowns

Posts or dowels differ from pins only in size and placement. Posts are generally larger than pins and are placed into the endodontic system (endowel) rather than a bed of dentin. A core is a substructure for the seating of the crown. The core is seated above the level of the natural tooth structure and is typically an integral part of a post section that rests in the tooth's endodontic system. Posts can be incorporated into the cast crown restoration itself for additional retention, such as a dowel or post crown (Fig. 9), or they can be a component of a two-piece unit known as a *post/core and crown* (Fig. 10). For a post and core crown, the preparation of the endodontic system is the same as described above for core buildup, and obtaining the impression is basically the same as described above for pins, except that a post-impression pin is used.

If the post is directly incorporated into the crown, it is known as a *dowel crown* (*post crown*). Impression posts are placed into the post preparation, and an impression is obtained. Human dental impression and burnout posts are often not long or wide enough to provide sufficient retention for canine teeth seen in veterinary dentistry. Alternate materials for posts include plastic bristles from combs and hair brushes, particularly those with a wider button on the end to facilitate its incorporation into the impression. Many

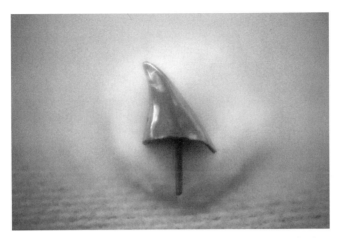

FIG. 9. Post crown. Note that the one-piece unit has a dowel post.

large sizes of brush bristles are available by purchasing inexpensive brushes and plucking the bristles free from the brush. Their sizes can be matched up with the various endodontic reamer sizes. We have found large plastic bristles that match Nos. 60, 90, 120, and 140 reamers. The canal should be prepared with larger-sized (up to No. 140) reamers for the coronal portion of the tooth. The post should reach as deep as is reasonable into the root canal, without dislodging the last 3–4 mm of apical endodontic seal. The post should be well below the cementoenamel junction of the tooth for best retention without increasing the chance of fracturing the tooth just below the apical margin of the restoration. Posts longer than the restoration help distribute the internal shear stresses better during occlusion. Typically, teeth treated in this fashion have significant amounts of tooth structure left and require the post for additional retention and stability. Once prepared, the proper plastic impression post is selected and placed into the canal to full depth. The impression material (elastic type) should lock onto the plastic post once it is fully set. The impression is then removed and sent to a laboratory for restoration fabrication as a post crown.

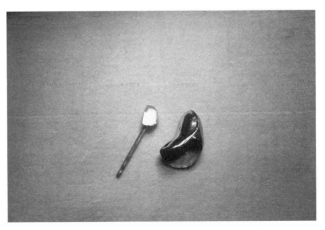

FIG. 10. Post/core and crown. Note the two-piece construction with a separate post-and-core unit.

Another method of fabrication is the direct/indirect method. In this, the casting pattern is made directly on the tooth rather than a model, but it is then indirectly cast into the restoration. This is typically done with either a type I direct inlay wax, such as Kerr® Blue Inlay Wax (Kerr Manufacturing Company, Romulus, Michigan), or an inlay acrylic resin, such AS Duralay® Inlay Resin (Reliance Dental Manufacturing Company, Worth, Illinois) (54). In such, a separating medium is applied to the prepared tooth. A dowel and core can be fabricated by using a plastic burnout post or resin pins and inlay acrylics to form a customized post. With an inlay resin, once the plastic dowel is selected, small amounts of acrylic can be placed on the dowel or into the canal that has been treated with a separator to keep the acrylic from sticking to the walls. As the acrylic begins to set up, a slight rotational movement can keep the post freely moving in the canal. Once fully set, the dowel is kept in the canal while an acrylic resin buildup is made in the general shape required. A standard crown preparation can then be performed on the tooth/acrylic combination, and impressions made for a separate crown manufacture.

Cross-pinning is the placement of a pin through the tooth and crown through the cervical third of the restoration (55). This is typically done by first holding the crown against a block of wood to drill a guide hole through its facial. Many of the harder dental metals will require a cobalt drill bit to cut through them efficiently. The crown is then fully seated on the prepared tooth. The drill bit is then placed in the guide hole, and the guide hole is completed by drilling through the tooth and the opposite side of the crown. The crown and tooth are cleaned of debris, and the crown is cemented into place, cement placed in the guide hole; a firm-fitting pin of the size of the guide hole is then placed through the guide hole, and both ends of the cross pin are cut off with abrasive burs and then polished smooth. This procedure can only be performed on nonvital teeth. Although this procedure provides tremendous retention for the crown, it also makes the tooth more prone to fracture under the crown at the cross-pinning site. We have found this procedure to be unwise in most cases, but especially in animals that will be placing high shrearing stress loads on the crown, such as police and military dogs. Use of the other more practical and safe retentive principles would be advised.

Adhesion systems concern the treatment of the interior surface of the restoration and the type of cementation between the tooth and restoration. Air abrasion is used for the treatment of the interior surface of most restorations; however, tin plating, such as Silicoater® (Heraeus Kulzer), and other systems are used. Air abrading increases the surface area and the microinterlocking capabilities for bonding. Silicoater® is the application of a thin resin coating to the interior surface of the restoration to enhance bonding with resin cements. Panavia™ (J. Morita USA Inc., Tustin, California) does not bond well to gold; therefore, tin plating of the interior surface is commonly performed to enhance the bonding effect. For this reason, the type of restorative and its adhesion treatment play a part in the cementation system selected. Guidance from the dental laboratory can help in making these decisions.

CROWN PREPARATION PROCEDURE

Retraction cord should be packed into the sulcus with a cord packer to open the sulcus, if the reduction and finish line are to come near to or within the sulcus. An astringent solution is used with the packing cord, unless the cord is already impregnated with such. Astringent or hemostatic solutions are basically of three types: epinephrine, epinephrine-combinations, and non-epinephrine (56) (see Chapter 2). Epinephrine constricts the gingival vasculature to shrink tissues and reduce hemorrhage. In retraction cords, racemic epinephrine has been used as high as 8%, that is, 4000 times more concentrated than injectable local anesthetic with the 1:100,000 epinephrine combination. A certain degree of the solution will be absorbed systemically, a condition that can be accelerated greatly in lacerated or injured tissues. Therefore, patients with contraindications to the use of epinephrine (cardiac disease, natural or induced hyperthyroidism, and certain other endocrine disorders) should not be exposed to this type of agent (57). Those wishing to make use of the advantages of epinephrine, but with reduced risk, usually use the combination products. In these, the amount of epinephrine has usually been significantly reduced, and zinc phenolsulfonate, a gentle astringent, has been added to improve the effect. The most common non-epinephrine solution is aluminum chloride. It works by its astringent action to produce shrinkage or contraction of the tissues and reduce sulcal secretions and minor hemorrhage (56–58).

Place a drop or two of the astringent solution in the Dappen dish. Cut two pieces of retraction cord approximately 1.5 times the estimated circumference of the tooth sulcus. Place these cord sections into the Dappen dish with the astringent. Take a piece of the retraction cord, and using a cord packer or a W3 placement instrument, gently force the cord into the gingival sulcus. Scissors can be used to cut away any excess. If the sulcus will accept additional cord material, repeat the procedure with the second piece of packing cord.

Using the high-speed handpiece and bur, begin the milling or crown reduction of the tooth. The type of margin selected guides bur selection. We prefer diamond points or burs to most steel burs (Fig. 11). The level of the apical margin selected for the crown should be either above or below the gingival margin by at least 0.5–1.0 mm for better physiologic cleansing and less irritation to the gingival margin; it should not be at the level of the margin (6). If the margin preparation line is to be below the gingival margin, one or both pieces of the retraction cord may have to be removed to proceed, but the cord should be left in place long enough to spread the sulcus open well to allow good visualization and reduce the chance of rotary instrument injury to the sulcus. The reduction at the apical margin is determined by the type of crown to be placed. The Iwanson calipers can be used to measure the marginal reduction for the appropriate degree of structural reduction.

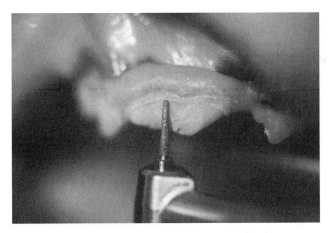

FIG. 11. Use of a high-speed handpiece and diamond point for the crown preparation of an upper 4th premolar.

Failure to remove the appropriate amount of structure can result in the laboratory's having difficulty producing—or being unable to produce—the desired type of crown with a proper contour, color, and fit (38).

Impressions

Good impressions are an absolute necessity for good-fitting crowns (37). Quality impression trays greatly enhance impression stability and the accuracy of the models produced (6). There are several good impression trays on the market, and custom trays can be fabricated. To obtain good sulcal detail, the packed retraction cord should be removed just before the impressions are taken. All impression materials, especially rubber base, should be used with extreme care around loose or mobile teeth, because the teeth may be removed as the impression is removed. (See Chapter 15 for more information on impressions and Chapter 2 for impression materials.)

For the best results, the following impressions are required by the laboratory:

1. Full-mouth impression, upper and lower (alginate)
2. Area-specific impression (tooth to be crowned, etc.)
   A. Elastics (we prefer the properties of the polysiloxane elastic impression materials)
   B. Reversible alginates
3. Bite-registration impression
   A. Wax
   B. Elastics
4. Color registration or matching

Select impression trays for the upper and lower arcade that permit the entire desired area to be encompassed, allowing a minimum of dead space outside the dental structures. Henry Schein Inc. of Port Washington, New York, produces sets of impression trays for both the dog and cat. The Lyman® trays designed for use in the dog can still be found from various distributors from time to time. Mix alginate and take a complete set of *full-mouth* impressions (see Chapter 15 for a more detailed description of taking impressions). The models obtained from these impressions will be used for articulation and occlusal studies for the restoration. Alginate impressions should be kept cool and moist until models are poured, hopefully within 30 minutes and definitely within 2 hours. Wrapping them in a damp paper towel or placing them in a zip-lock plastic bag will usually suffice for the allotted time until the models are poured. The longer the time is between taking the alginate impression and pouring the models, the more distortion may be expected to result. Always pour models with the impressions in the original tray for the least distortion.

Select an *area-specific impression* tray for the individual tooth impression for the actual crown fabrication. Kerr Kwik-Trays™ (Kerr Manufacturing Company) for molars, premolars, incisors, and some canine or cuspid teeth work well; cut-off sections of 12-cc syringe casings will work for most medium- to large-size dog cuspid or canine teeth. Custom trays can be constructed with acrylics, such as Lang's Instant Tray Mix™ (Lang Dental Manufacturing Company, Wheeling, Illinois), or from the newer low-heat moldable plastics, such as Tray Dough™ (Hygenic Corporation, Akron, Ohio).

The following system works best in a four-handed technique (doctor and assistant), but it can be done in a two-handed technique (doctor alone). Inject a light-bodied elastic impression material into the hub of the Kerr Free-Flo™ syringe (Kerr Manufacturing

Company). Pull the packing cord from the sulcus. Using the Kerr syringe filled with a light-bodied material, place the tip at the sulcus and begin injecting to force the elastic impression material down into the depth of the sulcus in front of the syringe; proceed circumferentially around the tooth. Left-over material can be applied to the tooth. To ensure proper infiltration into the sulcus, an air syringe can be used to blow the material into place. While you are using the Kerr syringe, your assistant should be filling the area-specific impression tray with the regular or medium-bodied elastic impression material. Place this tray over the tooth that you have already covered with the light-bodied impression material, firmly pushing it into position; this should result in the merging of the two impression materials types. Keep the tray stable until the material has firmed well; this can be checked with your finger or a small instrument. Once the material has properly set up, the impression can be removed. Elastic impressions should not be poured up for at least 1 hour following setting, as they give off a hydrogen gas that can cause a roughened surface on models.

The final impression taken is the *bite registration* to obtain guidelines for articulating the models. This can be done with a sheet of bite-registration wax or with an elastic impression material. The mouth, with no obstructions, is closed firmly on the wax or elastic impression material to register how it occludes for future reference. Generally, a wax block is the safer of the two to use on an animal under anesthesia, as the wax impression only takes seconds to obtain, while the elastic impression will take 2–5 minutes to set up. With the mouth closed and the tongue pressed back into the mouth for the bite-registration impression, 2–5 minutes of this partial obstruction of airway can lead to problems if the animal's condition and vital signs are not constantly monitored. Bite registrations are of little help to you or the dental laboratory if they are oversized, bulky, block visualization of the model, or prevent it from being put into full occlusion. One way of preventing most of these problems is to make a wax block that can be fitted on the off-side in the premolar portion of the arcade. If the bite registration can be placed on the occluded models in full occlusion and the occlusion can be fully visualized, a satisfactory bite registration has been obtained. Be sure to include instructions to the laboratory on where the bite registration fits to avoid confusion.

Color registration or *matching* is only needed if composite, glass ceramic, polymer glass, or porcelain is to be used in the restoration. There are may types of color-matching systems, so it is best to check with the laboratory you are using and obtain a color guide to match their system, although most laboratories can usually convert your selection from one color system to another with reasonable accuracy.

Models

The dental laboratory, if local, can produce all of your models for you. If you must work by mail or with delays lasting more than a few hours, all alginate impressions should have models poured as soon as possible (10). Keeping the alginate moist and cool will reduce shrinkage problems. The materials used for the pouring of models for prosthodontic devices include:

1. Quality ADA type IV dental stone
2. Rubber mixing bowls
3. Plaster spatula
4. Cement spatula
5. Vibrator

6. Water source
7. Impressions.

   The full-mouth impressions should be poured up with a good-quality ADA type IV dental stone, such as Die Keen (Miles Inc., South Bend, Indiana), or the alginate impressions should be kept cool and moist until they are picked up by the laboratory. (For a more detailed explanation of pouring up models, see Models in Chapter 15; for additional information on dental stone or gypsum, see Chapter 2.) If you pour up your own models, be sure to include the bite registration with the models sent to the dental laboratory or use the bite registration as a guide to mark the lines of articulation with simple arrows drawn on the upper and lower models that point at one another when the bite is properly aligned. If you fail to mark the occlusion pattern or to include the bite registration in the materials to the laboratory, technicians at the laboratory will be forced to make their best guess. Do not worry about the model from the specific-area impression made with the elastic impression material, as it is extremely stable and the dental laboratory can pour it up for you.

   You are now ready to send your models and impressions to the dental laboratory. Before sending them, always talk with your contacts at the laboratory to confirm that you are talking the same language on what you and the client want. Additionally, describe your wishes to the laboratory in writing and, if necessary, with drawings. Place a copy of these with the materials sent to the laboratory, and place a copy with the patient's record in case further discissions with the laboratory are necessary. Many dental laboratories will provide you with a detailed dental laboratory prescription form for this purpose. In most cases, you will wish to have a crown made that closely resembles the original tooth structure. The exception may be with the canine or cuspid teeth. In many of these cases, you will wish to reduce the coronal height to only 65–85% of the original height of contour. Additionally, the cusp tip should be kept slightly rounded and similar to the original shape. Be sure to indicate the type of restoration desired

   Send the laboratory:

1. The full-mouth impressions or models
2. The area-specific impression
3. The bite registration—or mark the articulation on models
4. Color registration
5. Laboratory prescription form filled out in full.

Try-in and Fitting of the Crown

   When the restoration is returned, examine it for quality of workmanship, compliance with the script you ordered, and the fit of the restoration on the models. If all appears well, the client can be called and an appointment arranged for the seating and cementation of the crown.

   The restoration is now ready for the try-in, fitting, cementation, and marginal-finishing process. The try-in of the crown is done to make sure that the restoration fits properly and occludes well with adjacent and opposing teeth. When the animal is sedated the try-in should be done quickly before intubation of the animal in order to check the unimpaired occlusal fit. Place the restoration in position, and then work the teeth together across the crown and observe the interdigitation. Mark areas of occlusal distress with a wax pencil or articulation paper. Minor adjustments in the restoration's contours can be made with abrasive disks or diamonds appropriate for the type of crown material. If major adjustments are required, the restoration should be returned to the laboratory for reworking.

Cementation

Once the crown is fitting well, you are ready for seating and cementation. The actual tooth surface should be cleaned with a flour of pumice and water to remove debris that has accumulated since the preparation. For selection of cement, follow the laboratory's recommendation as to the types of cement that work best with the type of materials used in the restoration. Then follow the recommendations of the cement manufacturer as to application, as many are very technique-sensitive. However, with animals, it is generally best to use the stronger resin cements, such as Panavia (J. Morita USA Inc.). Typically, you will acid-etch the enamel, use a conditioner on the exposed dentin, apply a high-quality dentinal bonding agent, apply the cement according to the manufacturer's recommendations, and allow proper setting of the cement.

Marginal Finish

Once the restoration is cemented, the marginal fit should be checked. Often overlooked, the marginal finishing is a crucial part of a successful restoration. Inspect the marginal adaptation with the side of an explorer/probe. Softer metal restoration, such as gold, can be adapted at the margins by burnishing with a W3 instrument. Harder materials will require white-stone points, abrasive wheels, or diamond bur for reduction. The final adjustment should be smoothed with polishing wheels appropriate for the material.

Wax-Pattern Fabrication

A knowledge of laboratory waxing technique can provide the dental operator with an intimate awareness of prosthetics. This will allow the practitioner to better understand the laboratory's restrictions in production of a restoration. Should a practitioner learn the art of waxing, he or she can produce crowns to own exacting specifications. To do this, the practitioner must be familiar with inlay waxes, basic waxing instruments, and other materials required to treat the models to be waxed. The technique of waxing requires an understanding of basic skills, good eye and hand coordination, and practice to become proficient.

The ADA type I waxes are best used for effective direct waxing techniques, while indirect waxing will utilize ADA type II waxes. Of the waxing instruments, the Roach wax carver and No.7 waxing instrument are used for gross application of wax and some general shaping, while the PKT No.2 waxing instruments are used for delicate application of wax and pressure movement or removal of wax in shaping. The PKT No.4 waxing instrument is a bladed tool used to carve wax in shaping and in creating wax shavings that can be swept off the pattern with a small brush. These instruments can be heated by an alcohol lamp (Buffalo Dental Mfg. Co., Syosset, New York), which can also heat the wax directly. A small section of pantyhose can be used like sandpaper to smooth the waxed preparation.

Preparation of the Model for Waxing

The individual tooth should be isolated by using laboratory or E-type cutters to cut away all of the model except the tooth to be waxed, its margin, and underbase. A round or pear-shaped laboratory cutter on a low-speed bench engine can be used to trim the underbase of the model 1–2 mm immediately below the model margin preparation line. This results in a groove in the base below the margin and is known as *ditching*. This allows the exacting and critical margin work to be done with better detail. A wax pencil (usually red) is then used to outline the preparation margin of the model. This is done to allow better visualization of the margin during waxing and wax trimming. The margin and ditched area are then reinforced, hopefully, to prevent damage to them during waxing. The reinforcing is done by the application of a thin coating of cyanoacrylate cement (Super Glue) applied with a cotton swab.

Next, to make room for the cement between the restoration and tooth, a thin layer of spacer paint is applied to the model. However, the spacer paint should not be applied to the preparation margin or even within 2 mm of it. This is done in order to obtain as tight a margin fit as possible to the tooth to reduce the chances of marginal leakage. The marginal fit and seal can greatly influence the long-term success of a crown. For thin cement, only one thin layer of spacer paint is applied. If a thicker type of cement is to be used for adhesion of the crown, a second layer is normally applied after the first dries. Generally, the spacer paint should be of a different color from that of the inlay wax used to allow easier visualization of the model in areas where the wax is worked very thin. The spacer paint must be allowed to dry before beginning the application of wax.

Procedure

1. Place burning alcohol in alcohol lamp and light the lamp. **WARNING:** Be careful of alcohol spills, as alcohol burns extremely hotly, with a flame that is poorly visible.
2. Apply a thin layer of separator medium to the prepared model. With a three-way syringe, use the air to blow the layer thin.
3. Place the tip of the PKT No.2 wax instrument into the flame until it becomes lightly hot (not red-hot). Overly heated instruments will only burn the wax into vapor.
4. Once the tip is lightly heated, press it into the wax. A small amount should turn to liquid and adhere to the instrument.
5. Transfer this wax to the model. Pay careful attention to the margin fill and work.
6. Apply a thin layer of wax over the entire crown.
7. Once the initial detail work is performed, use the No.7 waxing instrument for the more rapid gross bulking of the wax buildup.
8. Smooth out rough areas by heating the instrument and then gently rubbing it across the areas to reshape the wax.
9. Once sufficient bulking has occurred, use the PKT No.4 to begin the carving process. Do not use the PKT No.4 waxing instrument or any bladed instrument at or near the preparation margin, as it can cut into the model and distort the critical marginal fit. The carving is a bit of an art that can be acquired with time, practice, patience, and a knowledge of tooth anatomy.
10. Perform the marginal finish work using the PKT No.2 waxing instrument once again. Use the blunt curving sides of the instrument to rub and mold the wax to attain a superior marginal adaptation. The instrument can be heated lightly for this work, if necessary.
11. Stretch a small amount of pantyhose between two fingers, and use it like sandpaper to gently file areas and place a smooth finish on the wax.
12. Next, remove the wax pattern from the model and inspect it for defects and thickness. The wax pattern can then be placed on the preparation of the full-mouth model for

articulation. It should be articulated by hand rather than mechanically at this point to prevent damage to the pattern. Check for occlusal movement interference due to mis-shaping or oversizing. Should interference be detected, it is corrected then. Powdered occlusal wax can be applied to the waxed preparation before articulation to aid in discovering interference. Areas that make contact show up as spots with the powdered wax removed.

13. Keep the wax preparation on the preparation model at all times, if possible. This includes when it is sent to the laboratory, in order to reduce the chance of damage or distortion. In addition, do not allow the wax pattern to be exposed to unnecessary heat, or warping and changes may occur. Refrigerate the waxing preparation, if necessary, until it is used or shipped.

DENTAL RESTORATIVE IMPLANTS

Dental restorative implants are a core material that is placed in the alveolar bone of the mandible or maxilla in the hope that it will eventually attach to the bone and then be able to be used as an anchor for an abutment on which a prosthetic device such as a crown or bridge can be placed to replace a missing tooth or teeth. Dental implants for replacement of missing teeth have been used for many years in humans with only a fair degree of success (59). However, experimental studies in the 1980s performed by Branemark in Sweden and Schroeder in Switzerland began the development of new and innovative ways to improve the success rate. Their studies in dogs demonstrated that titanium could be anchored directly to bone. This process involving the metal oxides on the surface of the implant bonding to bone is known as *osseointegration* or *functional ankylosis* (60).

Implant restorations generally consist of three major parts. First is the implant itself, which integrates into the jaw bone. The second part is the abutment, which attaches to the implant with an abutment screw. The third part is the restoration, which typically has a central gold cylinder used as its base. The restoration is formed around this cylinder, which also acts as the interface with the abutment. The restoration is then held in place on the abutment by a prosthetic-retaining screw. There are many types of implants, each varying to some degree in their component parts.

For osseointegration to be successful for the long term, the implant must be biocompatible, it must osseointegrate, and the integration must persist. Pure titanium is used for most implants due to its documented biocompatibility, osseointegration, and long-term success (59–61). The surface of the titanium is often plasma-sprayed to maintain the titanium surface, as well as increasing the total surface area for integration. Surface coatings of hydroxyapatite have been used for osseointegration on implants, but little long-term information is available. In addition, there have been indications that some hydroxyapatite coating may have resorbed from the surface, making long-term success questionable. However, new technologies should soon overcome these problems.

Success of implantation with a reasonable degree of predictability depends on many factors. However, there are three major areas of importance:

1. Surgical technique
2. Implant stability
3. Loading only after osseointegration.

Implant surgery is typically a two-stage procedure (16). The first stage is the placement of the implant, and the second stage its exposure. In stage I, the surgical technique of opening the recipient site must be sterile, precise, low-trauma, and nonheating. The site should prepared as close to the design of the implant as possible. This should be done in a highly sterile fashion, while not traumatizing tissues any more than is necessary. Heat damage to the bone during cutting should be avoided by slow cutting and use of appropriate instrument-cooling systems. The implant must be placed in a stable and protected position in relationship to the bone in order to encourage osseointegration. Typically, to protect the implant, it is submerged by covering the exposed top with a gingival flap. This aids in preventing bacterial migration around the implant, while adding to its stability.

In stage II, the implant should not be uncovered for *loading* (restorative crown attached), until osseointegration of the implant has occurred, usually 3–5 months after implantation. Once osseointegration has occurred, the implant is uncovered and an abutment or temporary abutment placed. A temporary screw is placed in the abutment to protect it and prevent debris from falling inside. Once the tissue surrounding the abutment has healed, the prosthetic appliance can be applied (16).

In the dog, dental implants have been used for the replacement of single teeth and as abutments and piers for bridgework. For the dog, they provide an esthetic alternative to missing incisors and premolars out of occlusion, but they have not held up well as functional bite work or occlusion. In the dog, implants for canine and carnassial teeth are not generally recommended due to the tremendous functional stresses involved. Areas with poor supporting bone are contraindicated for implant placement. Nor should implants be placed for fraudulent purposes of misrepresentation of an animal's occlusal status. In addition, the esthetic results are not always as good as one would wish, due to the restrictions of the restorative implant shape (60). Additionally, unless the owner is committed to good home oral hygiene care of the animal, complications should be expected. Therefore, selection of a dental restorative implant in an animal should be carefully considered and discussed with the owner. The procedure should be considered experimental and the long-term prognosis for success should be considered guarded, until implants are developed that are more considerate of animal anatomy and physiology.

REFERENCES

1. *Glossary of Operative Dentistry Terms.* 1st ed. Academy of Operative Dentistry.
2. Harty FJ. *Concise Illustrated Dental Dictionary.* 2nd ed. Boston: Wright Publishing; 1995:168.
3. Howard WW, Moller RC. *Atlas of Operative Dentistry.* 3rd ed. St Louis, MO: CV Mosby Co; 1981:5.
4. *Veterinary Dental Abbreviations.* American Veterinary Dental College, Residency Tracking Committee, 1994; suppl.
5. Brannstrom M. *Dentin and Pulp in Restorative Dentistry.* London: Wolfe Medical Publishing; 1982:9.
6. Johnston JF, Phillips RW, Dykema RW. *Modern Practice in Crown and Bridge Prosthodontics.* 3rd ed. Philadelphia: WB Saunders Co: 1971:21.
7. Shillingburg HT, Wilson EL, Morrison JT. Guide to Occlusal Waxing. Chicago: Quintessence Publishing Co; 1979:15.
8. Taggart WH. A new and accurate way of making gold inlays. *Dental Cosmos* 1970;49:1117.
9. Bertolotti RL. Casting metals, part I. *Compend Cont Educ Dent* 1990;11:300.
10. Craig RG. *Restorative Dental Materials.* 7th ed. St Louis MO: CV Mosby Co; 1985:354.
11. Bertolotti RL. Selection of alloys for today's crown and fixed partial denture restorations. *JADA* 1984;108:959.
12. Van Loon LAJ, Van Elsas PW, Van Joost T, et al. Contact stomatitis and dermatitis to nickel and palladium. *Contact Dermatitis* 1984;11:294.
13. Magnusson B, Bergman M, Bergman B, et al. Nickel allergy and nickel containing dental alloys. *Scand J Dent Res* 1982;90:163.
14. Bruce GJ, Hall WB. Nickel hypersensitivity-related periodontitis. *Compend Cont Educ Dent* 1995;16:178.
15. American Dental Association. Revised ANSI/ADA Specification No.5 for dental casting alloys. *JADA* 1989; 118:379.

16. Zinner ID, Panno FV, Miller RD, Parker HM, Pines MS. Ceramometal full coverage restorations. In: Dale BG, Ascheim KW. Esthetic Dentistry: *A Clinical Approach to Techniques and Materials*. Philadelphia: Lea and Febiger; 1993:81.

17. Anusavice KJ. *Phillip's Science of Dental Materials, 10th ed.* Philadelphia, PA: WB Saunders Co.; 1996:443.

18. Bertolotti RL. Casting metals, part II. *Compend Cont Educ Dent* 1990;11:370.

19. Berge M. Properties of prosthetic resin-veneer materials processed in commercial laboratories. *Dent Mater* 1989;5:77.

20. Lappalainen R, Yll-Urpo A, Seppa L. Wear of dental restoratives and prosthetic materials in vitro. *Dent Mater* 1989;5:35.

21. Adair PJ, Bell BH, Pameijer CM. Casting techniques of machinable glass ceramics. *J Dent Res* 1980;59:475.

22. Sorenson JA. Rationale for comparison of plaque-retaining properties of crown systems. *J Prosthet Dent* 1989; 62:264.

23. Dragoo MR, Williams GB. Periodontal tissue reactions to restorative procedures. *Int J Periodontal Res Dent* 1981;1:9.

24. Savitt ED, Melament KA. Effects on colonization of oral microbiota by cast glass-ceramic restoration. *Int J Periodontal Res Dent* 1987;7:22.

25. Savitt ED. Clinical applications of oral microbiology in restorative dentistry. In: Perspectives in Dental Ceramics: Proceedings of the Fourth International Symposium on Ceramics. Chicago: Quintessence Publishing Co; 1988:111.

26. Griffith AA. The phenomena of rupture and flow in solids. *Phil Trans R Soc Lond* 1920;A221:63.

27. McLean J. *The Science and Art of Dental Ceramics. Vol II: Bridge Design and Laboratory Procedures in Dental Ceramics.* Chicago: Quintessence Publishing Co; 1980:1.

28. Malament KA. Considerations in posterior glass-ceramic restorations. *Int J Periodontal Res Dent* 1988;8:33.

29. Malament KA. The cast glass-ceramic crown. In: Preston JD, ed. *Perspectives in Dental Ceramics: Proceedings of the Fourth International Symposium on Ceramics.* Chicago: Quintessence Publishing Co; 1988:111.

30. Grossman DG. Cast glass ceramics. *Dent Clin North Am* 1985;29:725.

31. Woda A, Gourdan AM, Faraj M. Occlusal contact and tooth wear. *J Prosthet Dent* 1987;57:85.

32. *International Measurements*. Corning, NY: Physical Properties Department Corning Glass Works; 1987:1.

33. Erdrich AJ. A New Generation of Material for Use in Crown and Bridge Applications. Wehrheim, Germany: Kulzer Co; 1996:2.

34. Eichner K. Einflüsse von Brückenjwishengliedein auf die Gingiva. *Dtsch Zahnarztl Z* 1975;30:639.

35. McLean J. High alumina ceramics for bridge pontic construction. *Br Dent J* 1968;123:571.

36. Staffanov RS. Fixed prosthodontic tooth preparations. In: Eissman HS, Rudd KD, Marrow RM, eds. *Dental Laboratory Procedures in Fixed Partial Dentures, Vol. 2.* St. Louis, MO: CV Mosby Co.; 1990:18.

37. Schillingberg HT, Hobo S, Whitsett LD. *Fundamentals of Fixed Prosthodontics.* 2nd ed. 1981:428.

38. Kantorowicz GF. *Inlays, Crowns, and Bridges: A Clinical Handbook.* Bristol, UK: John Wright & Sons; 1963:117.

39. Freeman SP, Duchan BS. Tooth preparation for full-coverage restorations using the enamel milling technique. *Compend Cont Educ Dent* 1991;12:370.

40. Council on Dental Materials and Devices. Revised ADA Specification No.23 for dental burs. *JADA* 1975; 90:459.

41. Bowen RL, Cobb EN, Raapson JE. Adhesive bonding of various materials to hard tooth tissues. Improvement in bond strength to dentin. *J Dent Res* 1982;61:1070.

42. Finger WJ. Dentin bonding agents. Relevance of in vitro investigations. *Am J Dent* 1988;1:184.

43. Retief HD, O'Brien JA, Smith LA, Marchman JL. In vitro investigations and evaluation of dentin bonding agents. *Am J Dent* 1988;1:176.

44. Silness J. Periodontal conditions in patients treated with dentinal bridge. III. The relationship between the location of the crown margin and the periodontal condition. *J Periodontal Res* 1970;5:225.

45. Koth DL. Full crown restorations and gingival inflammation in a controlled population. *J Prosthet Dent* 1973; 30:156.

46. Larato DC. Effect of cervical margins on gingiva. *J Calif Dent Assoc* 1969;45:19.

47. Loe H. Reactions of marginal periodontal tissues to restorative procedures. *Int Dent J* 1968;18:759.

48. Lang NP, Kiel RA, Anderhalden K. Clinical and microbiological effects of subgingival restorations with overhanging or clinically perfect margins. *J Clin Periodontol* 1983;10:563.

49. Schluger S, Youdelis RA, Page RC. *Periodontal Disease.* Philadelphia: Lea & Febiger; 1977.

50. Gargiulo AW, et al. Dimensions and relationship of the dento-gingival junction in humans. *J Periodontol* 1961; 32:261.

51. Clarke D, Wiggs RB, Lobprise HB. Surgical crown lengthening of the clinical crown in a mandibular canine tooth. Submitted for publication.

52. Markley MR. Pin retained and reinforced restorations and foundations. *Dent Clin North Am* March 1967:229.

53. Phillips S, et al. An in vitro study of the effect of moisture on glass ionomer cement. *Quint Int* 1985;16:175.

54. *Guide to Dental Materials and Devices.* 7th ed. Chicago: American Dental Association; 1974:231.

55. Shipp AD, Fahrenkrug P. *Practitioners' Guide to Veterinary Dentistry.* 1st ed, Beverly Hills, CA: Dr. Shipp's Labs Publishing; 1992:111.

56. *Accepted Dental Therapeutics*. 37th ed. Chicago: American Dental Association; 1977:220.

57. Nicholson RJ, et al. The detection of C_{14} labeled epinephrine in the blood stream of a Rhesus monkey following gingival retraction cord. *ADA Reprinted Abstracts* 1966:317.

58. Woycheshin FF. An evaluation of the drugs used in gingival retraction. *J Prosthod Dent* 1964;14:769.

59. Adell R, Lekholm U, Rockler B., et al. A 15-year study of osseointergrated implants in the treatment of the edentulous jaw. *J Oral Surg* 1981;10:387.

60. Branemark PI, Hanson BO, Adell R, et al. Osseointergrated implants in the treatment of the edentulous jaw: Experience from a 10-year period. *Scand J Plast Reconstr Surg* 1977;11(suppl 15):1.

61. Adell R. Clinical results of osseointegrated implants supporting fixed prosthesis. *J. Prosthet Dent.* 1983;50(2):251.

15

Basics of Orthodontics

Robert B. Wiggs and Heidi B. Lobprise

The term *orthodontics* comes from the Greek *ortho* meaning straight or correct and *odon* meaning tooth (1). Although this term is used to label this area of dentistry, it falls dramatically short of describing what orthodontics has become. In a still oversimplified but more correct definition by the Council on Dental Education of the American Dental Association (ADA), orthodontics is that area of dentistry concerned with the supervision and guidance of the growing dentition and correction of the mature dentofacial structures. It includes those conditions that require movement of teeth and/or correction of disordered relationships of the jaws and teeth and malformations of their related structures (2).

In veterinary dentistry, the enormous number of species and breeds that are encountered makes orthodontics truly a science of infinite variation. Even so, there are major and minor points of similarity in occlusions and malocclusions. Each orthodontic situation is unique according not only to the species, breed, and sex but also to the individual patient presented.

The assessment of the best course of treatment and whether or not to consider treatment or genetic counseling is one of the most critical points in veterinary orthodontics, as the functional dentition and oral support tissues are at risk when the animal's occlusion is abnormal. However, before attempting to assess animal occlusions, a basic understanding of the establishment of norms for species and breeds, as well as the nature of malocclusions, is necessary. There are three basic skull and jaw types that must be dealt with, and they may be either breed- or individual-specific. *Dolichocephalics* are individuals with long, narrow facial profiles, such as collies and greyhounds. The *brachycephalics* have a short, broad facial profile, such as boxers and bulldogs. The *mesocephalics* have a more balanced facial profile that is somewhere between the two other types, such as the beagle and German shepherd. Certain breeds (eg, boxers, bulldogs) have a pronounced class III malocclusion according to dental and medical standards, but according to breed standards, their occlusion is acceptable within a certain range. Therefore, these animals must be classified as having a class 0 normal type 3 occlusion, not a class III malocclusion (see Occlusions below).

A dog's normal occlusion is identified by several factors. The upper (maxillary) incisors should overlap the lower incisors, which rest on or near the cingulum of the uppers in a scissors bite. The lower canine teeth are positioned midway between the upper corner incisors and canines when the mouth is shut. The lower premolar cusps should point to the interproximal spaces of the upper premolars in a pinking-shear fashion, with the cusps of the upper 4th premolars lateral (buccal) to the lower 1st molars (3).

HISTORY OF ORTHODONTICS

Treatment attempts for crooked teeth have been found going back to at least to 1000 BC. Reasonably well designed orthodontic appliances constructed from Greek and Etruscan materials have been unearthed (4). Thoughts concerning crooked teeth can be found throughout recorded history, as in the writings of Hippocrates (460–377 BC) and Aristotle (384–322 BC). Celsus (25 BC–50 AD) was one of the first to record a method of treatment that is still fundamentally correct even today. He stated that "If a second tooth should happen to grow in children before the first has fallen out, that which ought to be shed is to be drawn out and the new one daily pushed toward its place by means of the finger until it arrives at its just proportion" (5). Pierre Fauchard (1678–1761) of France, considered the father of dentistry, wrote what is considered the first comprehensive discussion of what he called "tooth regulation." Another Frenchman, named Le Foulon, in 1839 is thought to be the first person to make use of the term *orthodontia* in dentistry (6). A highly notable text was published in the latter half of the 1800s by Norman Kingsley (7). Responsible for the development of the obturator, he was a pioneer in the treatment of cleft palates and related conditions and was one of the first to use external force in orthodontics. He is closely associated with the development of the concept of "jumping the bite." Immensely influential in dentistry in America, he is considered by some to be the father of modern orthodontics (8–9). His works are considered by some to emphasize tooth alignment and facial proportions rather than occlusion, since the use of extractions was not uncommon (10). The publication of Edward H. Angle's (11) classification of malocclusion and his influence helped develop the concept of natural dental occlusion. His interest in dental occlusions, opposition to extraction, and innovative treatments directly led to the development of orthodontics as a recognized specialty; and for most he is considered the true father of modern orthodontics (10). Those who place Kingsley in that position consider Angle to be the founder of the science of orthodontics (8). However, without a doubt, Angle's work continues to be a substantial influence even in today's orthodontic concepts.

SEQUELAE OF MALOCCLUSION

There are many pathologic possibilities, both short and long range, that may develop from untreated malocclusions (12). The unfavorable consequences vary with the species but include problems with mastication, temporomandibular joint function, caries formation, periodontal disease, dentofacial growth and development, soft tissue trauma, traumatic dental fractures, and dental attrition (13). Each of these is a legitimate reason to initiate orthodontic treatment. Orthodontic treatment should be biologically based for a harmonious occlusion rather than cosmetic orientation of the teeth.

ETHICAL STANDARDS OF ORTHODONTICS

In many cases, it is difficult to ascertain whether an occlusion should simply be classified as a version or variation of *orthoclusion* (normal or correct occlusion) or a malocclusion (an abnormal occlusion). Additionally, in some patients, there will be forms of orthoclusion and malocclusion that are functional yet esthetically unacceptable to the client. In the dog and to a lesser degree in the cat, human intervention has perpetuated some occlusal aberrations. Every animal both deserves and has the medical right to an occlusion as functional and correct as can be reasonably provided by therapy. However, animal club rules, professional association principles, and state and country laws may at times conflict with the an animal's right to proper medical therapy. The American Veterinary Medical Association's (AVMA) *Principles of Veterinary Medical Ethics* (14) states that to perform "surgical" procedures in all species for the purpose of concealing "genetic" defects in animals to be shown, raced, bred, or sold as breeding animals is unethical. In addition, the AVMA recommends that any surgery for the correction of an injury not be grounds for disqualification of a dog from shows and obedience trials, providing that such surgery does not result in improvement in function or cosmetic appearance over preinjury status of the animal; the AVMA does not indicate whether the performance of such procedures would be considered unethical (14). Further, the American Kennel Club's rules of show state that modification of an animal's natural appearance by artificial means, with certain exceptions, is cause not to accept an animal to compete at any show and may result in disqualification (15). The veterinary dentist should adhere to all rightful laws and professional rules of conduct or work for change within the established system. Not every rule or every law is just to humans or animals.

When there are reasonable indications of hereditary involvement, the owner should be informed as to the possibility, and should treatment be considered, the owner or agent should acknowledge his or her responsibilities prior to commencement of treatment (Fig. 1). In many cases, genetic counseling should be advised. Genetic counseling is the action of making recommendations as to the ways to minimize a defect's potential affects on future offspring by either selective breeding or the preclusion of reproduction. No animal is perfect in every way, and just as problems can be bred into an animal, they may be bred out (16). Nevertheless, in many cases, it is impractical to try to breed out defect dilemmas. In these cases, it is generally advisable to counsel the owner that it may be best to remove the animal from the genetic pool either by enforced abstinence or by rendering the animal incapable of reproduction. Of course, termination of reproductive function is wise for any animal with obvious hereditary defects that are inappropriate for the animal or the breed.

One of the major obstacles in advising clients as to dental hereditary involvement is the lack of definitive studies to define hereditary from nonhereditary conditions. It is generally conceded that orofacial skeletal length variations (classes II–IV malocclusions) are hereditary, with the exception of those caused by local oral or systemic influences; and there is reasonable research in the dog to support this (17). However, some hereditary class III malocclusions, actually class 0 type III, are considered within the standard for some breeds. Beyond this point, there are no accepted criteria that have been shown to differentiate between inherited and noninherited oral abnormalities.

ETIOLOGY

In orthodontics, etiology pertains to the science of attempting to identify a specific cause or causes of a malocclusion. When etiology can be determined, the client should be counseled as to preventive measures that may be able to be taken to help control the condition, as well as to the likelihood of the dentofacial deformity's being passed on to offspring.

Dentofacial deformity refers to abnormalities of the teeth in morphology or location and/or of the facial support structures. These deformities typically fall into one or more

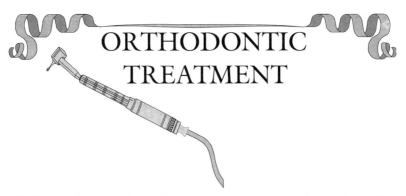

ORTHODONTIC TREATMENT

Unlike most human orthodontic treatments, the correction of malocclusions in pets can have ethical, moral, and legal implications. Any malocclusion may have hereditary involvement, and genetic counseling may be advisable. The American Kennel Club and other related groups have rules against certain animal alterations that may subject an animal to disqualification from showing or other use, and take actions against member owners. Every animal has the medical right to as functional and correct a bite as can be obtained, but without the intent to deceive or mislead. Medical history and treatment information is considered confidential and should not be disclosed by this facility except by owner or legal direction. Therefore, the owner or person directing such treatment must take the responsibility to notify all persons now and in the future that have a need to know about orthodontic or other procedures performed upon an animal under their direction. Signing of this form acknowledges these responsibilities.

Owner or Agent:_____ Pet's Name:_____

Signature:_____Date:_____

FIG. 1. A simple orthodontic treatment release-type form.

of three general categories involving heredity, systemic influences, or local influences. It is not unusual for some influences to fall within several categories or to fall within one yet also exert influence within another.

Heredity is concerned with traits and characteristics that are transmitted from parents or other ancestors to offspring. This can be of great concern in breeding lines and influences the determination of removing an animal from the genetic pool. Teeth and jaws come from different genetic origins (18). Therefore, variations of either or both can be seen in this category. These may include variations in size, number, length, shape, or lack of development of the teeth, jaws, periodontium, or orofacial supporting tissues. Defects in any of these components may affect occlusion.

Numbers of teeth, either too few or too many, can have effects on the occlusal pattern. With the jaws, length, size, and development can all affect occlusion. Almost any alteration may result in some form of orthodontic disturbance; this includes alterations in morphology of the teeth, jaws, or supportive tissues, pattern or chronology of primary tooth exfoliation, lack of primary tooth exfoliation and pattern, and direction or chronology of eruption of primary or permanent teeth.

The tongue, from its size to attachment anomalies, can also play a role in orthodontic problems. *Macroglossia*, a tongue that is too large, may place pressures on the lingual surface of teeth, forcing them facially and out of position. *Microglossia*, a tongue that is too small, may allow the dental arch to collapse lingually. Alterations in attachment of the tongue, such as a short frenulum, may lead to altered tongue posturing, which may release or apply pressures to lingual tooth surfaces.

The muscles and their attachments of the cheeks and lips play a counter role to the pressures of the tongue. This results in a balance or harmony produced between the two opposing forces. The muscles of the orofacial complex exert an influence on positions of the teeth and on growth patterns in the jaw (18). Excessively loose lips may fail to place appropriate pressures on the facial surfaces of the teeth, thereby allowing a facial or even a mesial drift of the teeth (19). On the other hand, *tight-lip syndrome*, a condition involving lip attachment too close to the dentition, can place excessive facial surface pressures on the teeth and jaw, resulting in linguoversion of teeth and even a shortened jaw in the affected arch.

Cleft lips and palates are not uncommonly associated with orthodontic disease. The problems vary greatly according to cleft location and extent, and include alterations of tooth morphology, numbers, impedance, and position of eruption.

Keep in mind that almost all of the problems described here under heredity can be found in the other three categories. Additionally, remember that these conditions can be present without necessarily affecting reasonable occlusal function.

Systemic influences separate out into two general groups: prenatal (congenital) and postnatal (developmental). Prenatal systemic or congenital problems differentiate from hereditary ones in that heredity denotes a genetic origin, whereas congenital involves various influences during pregnancy other than genetic. Postnatal encompasses defects that develop from exposure to a systemic influence after birth. Systemic influences for both groups include nutritional disturbances, infectious diseases, endocrine imbalances, radiational effects, and chemical instigations. Any of these factors may alter development of the teeth or the orofacial complex. These systemic influences may then also result in changes that have local oral influences.

Local influences are those that by their local effects may affect the orofacial complex. An injury that causes loss of teeth is such an influence in that the loss of the teeth allows changes in the orofacial complex to occur. Early loss of any primary or permanent tooth may allow migrational changes. Delayed loss of primary teeth can result in impactions and/or crowding. Periodontal disease, although an infection, is generally considered a local influence, since the systemic disturbances (eg, lungs, heart, liver, kidney) have not been shown to routinely affect the orofacial complex. Only the local influence of periodontal disease reflected in periodontal destruction and tooth loss affect the complex. Cysts, tumors, and other growths can also have dramatic impact on the area (20). Behavioral habits such as cage biting, bruxing, chewing habits, and suckling habits may all likewise alter the complex (21). Whatever the local influence, it must be cured, controlled, or compensated for to expect successful orthodontic treatment (see Chapter 21).

DIVISIONS AND CLASSIFICATIONS OF OCCLUSION
AND MALOCCLUSION

Occlusions must be classified according three general divisions:

Deciduous occlusion—only primary or deciduous teeth
Mixed occlusion—combination of primary and permanent teeth
Permanent occlusion—only primary teeth in the dentition.

The term *deciduous occlusion* is preferred to the terms *primary* or *temporary*, as these confuse the public. When the term *primary* is used, there is a tendency among the public to think of the the problem as not due to some secondary problem; and when the term *temporary* is used, the tendency is to think that the malocclusion is temporary in nature and will go away. Therefore, the use of the term *deciduous occlusion* or *malocclusion* is preferred to the two other terms. The actual classifications within the divisions remain the same, as the terms *deciduous*, *mixed* and *permanent refer* only to the division of the dentitional stages. This means that a puppy with all primary teeth with a simple anterior cross-bite would be classified as a deciduous (division) class I (classification) malocclusion. This division is necessary due not only to the tooth types involved but, more specifically, to the difference in treatment modality for each division.

Dr. Angle's and Dr. Lischen's classifications are the most internationally used formulas of malocclusion (6,11) (Table 1). The following five classifications of veterinary carnivores are modifications of these classifications (Table 2). The first is *class 0 normal*, or *orthoclusion*, which includes true normals and variations of normal. The second is *class I malocclusion*, or *neutroclusion*, in which the teeth are in approximately normal mesiodistal or neutral relation but may have faciolingual disturbances. The third is *class II malocclusion* or *distoclusion*, in which some or all mandibular teeth are distal in relationship to their maxillary counterparts. The fourth is *class III malocclusion* or *mesioclusion*, in which some or all of the mandibular teeth are mesial in their relationship to their maxillary counterparts. The fifth is *class IV special malocclusions*, or *mesiodistoclusion*, which is not typical wry mouth, but a special form in which one of the four jaws is in a mesial relationship to its counterparts, while another is in a distal. By making use of these classifications, veterinary dentists can make better use of the copious amounts of data, research, and publication on humans and animals generated from our human dental counterparts. Being able to speak the same general dental language when discussing cases with our counterparts and human dental laboratory technicians, whom we must make use of, more than makes up for any inconsistencies that must be compensated for in use of this classification.

TABLE 1. *Common human malocclusion classification comparisons*

Dr. Angle's classification		Dr. Lischen's classification
Class 0	Normal occlusion	Normal or orthoclusion
Class I	Malocclusion	Neutroclusion
Class II	Malocclusion	Distoclusion
Class III	Malocclusion	Mesioclusion
Class IV	Special malocclusions	Mesiodistoclusion

(Based on data in refs. 6 and 11.)

TABLE 2. *Basic veterinary carnivore occlusal classification*

Class 0 normal (orthoclusion)
   Types:
   1. True normal
   2. Variant normal
   3. Normal class III occlusion (breed-normal prognathia)
Class I malocclusion (neutroclusion)—both jaws of proper length and
teeth in a normal mesiodistal location
   Categories:
   1. Anterior cross-bite
   2. Posterior cross-bite
   3. Facial cuspids (base-wide canines)
   4. Lingual cuspids (base-narrow canines)
   5. Crowded or rotated teeth
   6. Certain partial level bites
Class II malocclusion (distoclusion)
   Categories:
   1. Short mandible
      Brachygnathism (mandibular)
      Mandibular retrognathism
      Mandibular retrusion
      Unilateral (wry bite)
   2. Long maxilla
      Maxillary protrusion
      Maxillary prognathism
      Unilateral (wry bite)
Class III malocclusion (mesioclusion)
   Categories:
   1. Long mandible
      Prognathism (mandibular)
      Mandibular protrusion
      Level bite
      Unilateral (wry bite)
   2. Short maxilla
      Brachycephalic
      Maxillary retrusion
      Maxillary retraction
      Level bite
      Unilateral (wry bite)
Class IV special malocclusions (mesiodistoclusion)—special classification
of wry bite: one jaw in mesioclusion and the other in distoclusion.

(Adapted from refs. 6 and 11.)

Occlusions

In the discussion of occlusions, there are some terms of which a general understanding may be needed at times:

Occlusion—the contact of the teeth of the maxillary arch with those of the mandibular arch.

Centric occlusion—the position of the arches in relation to each other when the teeth are in maximum occlusal contact.

Static occlusion—the relationship of the teeth when the jaws are closed in centric occlusion. Static occlusion can be studied in the actual patient or on an occluded study cast or model, and it is based on this that most occlusions are classified.

Centric relation—the most functional, unrestrained, anatomically retruded position of the heads of the condyles of the mandible in the glenoid fossae of the temporomandibular joint.

Functional or dynamic occlusion—the active tooth contacts made during mastication and swallowing.

Malocclusions—any deviation from normal occlusion.

Bites

In the discussion of bites, a general understanding of the following terms may be needed:

Scissors bites—the normal relationship of the maxillary incisors overlapping the mandibular incisors, whose incisal edges rest on or near the cingulum on the lingual surfaces of the maxillary incisors.

Anterior cross-bites—a condition in which cusps of one or more anterior teeth (incisors and cuspids) exceed the normal cusp relationship of the teeth in the opposing arch, labially or lingually. Classically thought of as a subclassification of class I malocclusions, they can actually be seen in class I,II,III, or IV.

Posterior cross-bites—a condition in which cusps of one or more posterior teeth (premolars and molars) exceed the normal cusp relationship of the teeth in the opposing arch, buccally or lingually. Classically thought of as a subclassification of class I malocclusions, they can actually be seen in class I,II,III, or IV.

Overbites—the extension of the upper teeth over the lower in a vertical direction, when opposing teeth are in contact and in centric occlusion. Most people incorrectly think that an overbite is a class II occlusion. In addition, what most people consider an overbite is actually an *overjet*, not an overbite. An *overbite* and *vertical overlap* are the same. Overbites can be found in classes I–III malocclusions.

Overjut, overjet, horizontal overlap—the facial projection of the upper anterior or posterior teeth beyond their antagonist in a horizontal direction. These terms all refer to basically the same thing. This can be found in class I and class III malocclusions.

Underbite—a loose term generally applied to certain divisions of class I and class III malocclusions, but most typically to class III malocclusions.

Level bites—when the incisor teeth meet edge on edge (*edge-to-edge bite*) or the premolars or molars occlude cusp to cusp (*end-to-end bite*). This is a traumatic form of bite for the teeth that can cause attritional wearing down of the teeth into a closed bite. This is generally a subdivision of class III malocclusions but can be found occasionally in class I malocclusions.

Open bites—when a part or all of the teeth are prevented from closing to normal occlusal contact. Anterior open bites in the incisal region are the most universal and are commonly seen in association with wry bites. Posterior open bites are most commonly seen in association with traumatic posterior cross-bites. Full open bites are most often seen in traumatic conditions of partially avulsed posterior teeth or posterior cross-bites.

Closed bites—the dental arches close too far when the bite is in static occlusion. This typically is seen when excessive wear of the teeth occurs, allowing excessive closure of the occlusion (see level bite above).

Malpositioning of Teeth

There are terms that will be required to discuss occlusal malpositioning:

Transposition—a condition in which two teeth have exchanged places during the development of the occlusion.

Embrication—irregularly arranged teeth within an arch due to a lack of space (crowding), typically seen in lower incisors. Rotated, tipped, supraerupted (supraclusion), infraerupted (infraclusion), and displaced teeth are not uncommon in embrication.

Shortened tooth—term encompassing infraclusion, infraversion, and variations, such as infralinguoclusion (base narrow and retarded height).

Infraclusion, infraocclusion, or shortened tooth—terms used to describe teeth in which the occlusal surface or incisal edge has not reached the same or appropriate level of other teeth of the same type. This is typically seen in teeth that have failed to fully erupt (partially impacted) or that have been intruded by force or injury.

Supraclusion or supraocclusion—terms used to describe teeth that are above their appropriate occlusal level. It is seen most commonly in teeth that have been extruded due to injury or disease or have overerupted due to a lack of occlusal contact.

Supereruption—term used to describe teeth that have the cementoenamel junction erupted above the normal. The problem may be either supraclusion or supraversion. Additionally, these teeth may be in supraclusion or may not be due to clinical removal or traumatic loss of a portion of the crown.

Rotations, torsiversion, or torsoversion—teeth that are turned or rotated. These can be described by one of two terms: mesiolingual and distolingual. *Mesiolingual rotation* describes a tooth that is rotated on its long axis so that the mesial aspect is moved toward the tongue. *Distolingual rotation* describes a tooth that is rotated on its long axis so that the distal aspect is moved toward the tongue

Tipping, Inclinations, and Versions

Terms describing a tooth in which the crown is tipped or inclined in an abnormal position include:

Mesial inclination, mesial tipping, or mesioversion—condition involving a tooth in which the crown leans in a mesial direction (eg, mesial inclination of a maxillary cuspid in a Shetland sheepdog (sheltie), sometimes incorrectly termed rostroversion).

Distal inclination or tipping, or distoversion—condition involving a tooth in which the crown leans in a distal direction.

Lingual inclination or tipping, or linguoversion—condition involving a tooth tilted so that its crown leans toward the tongue. *Retroclination* is a term sometimes used to describe lingual tilting of the anterior teeth.

Facial or vestibular inclination or tipping, or facioversion—condition in which a tooth is leaning away from the tongue.

Labial inclination or tipping, or labioversion—terms sometimes used to describe facial inclination of the anterior teeth.

Buccal inclination or buccal tipping, or buccoversion—terms sometimes used to describe facial inclination of the posterior teeth.

Displacements

Displacement terminology describes a tooth in which both the crown and root have moved principally in the same direction. These conditions are sometimes described as occlusions (eg, mesial occlusion).

Mesial displacement or occlusion, or mesioclusion—condition in which a tooth is bodily displaced mesially or toward the midline of the arch.

Distal displacement or distoclusion—condition in which a tooth is bodily displaced distally or away from the midline of the arch.

Lingual displacement or linguoclusion—condition in which a tooth is bodily displaced toward the tongue.

Facial displacement or facioclusion—condition in a tooth is bodily displaced away from the tongue.

Labial displacement or labioclusion—terms that can be used to describe this effect in the anterior teeth.

Buccal displacement or buccoclusion—terms that can be used to describe this effect in the posterior teeth.

Versions

Version is a term used to describe malposition of one or more teeth. More specifically, it is used to describe inclinations or tiltings in directions of teeth that are generally in their correct position in the dental arch. These are not bodily moved teeth, such as displaced teeth (see inclinations above).

Labioversion—see labial inclination.

Buccoversion—see buccal inclination.

Linguoversion—see lingual inclination.

Torsoversion or torsiversion—see rotation.

Supraversion—condition involving a tooth that is supererupted and in its proper position in the dental arch, but may have some degree of tilt that allows passage beyond the teeth in the opposing dental arch.

Infraversion or shortened tooth—terms used to describe teeth in which the occlusal surface or incisal edge has not reached the same or appropriate level of other teeth of the same type. This differs from infraclusion in that a degree of crown tilt may be involved.

AIMS OF ORTHODONTIC TREATMENT

The aims of orthodontic treatment are to provide a reasonably functional, esthetic, stable, and harmonious occlusion by altering the position or presence of the natural teeth. To attain these aims in veterinary orthodontics, there are four goals to strive to accomplish:

1. Proper assessment and supervision of the occlusion.
2. Removal of etiologic factors that may disrupt normal growth patterns of the dentofacial complex, when possible, in an interceptive action.
3. Correction, by preventive measures, of conditions that may allow the occlusion to deteriorate.
4. Establishment and maintenance, by corrective acts, of as functional and close to normal an occlusion as is reasonable.

CATEGORIES OF ORTHODONTIC TREATMENTS

Orthodontic treatments, as a rule, can be divided into three general categories: interceptive, preventive, and corrective.

Interceptive orthodontics is generally considered to be the extraction or recontouring (crown reduction) of primary or permanent teeth that are contributing to alignment problems in the permanent dentition. Interceptive measures are not always successful due to time-interval limitations and/or hereditary influences that cannot be overcome. Discovering a discrepancy in jaw-length relationship in immature dogs is not unusual, as each jaw quadrant (two maxillae, two mandibles) grows independently and often in periods of rapid growth. Occasionally, a growth surge of the upper and lower arcade will place the deciduous dentition in an improper interlock, which may interfere with the next growth spurt (22). This is typically seen in a deciduous class III malocclusion, where the upper incisors get caught behind the lowers, or in a deciduous class II situation when the mandibular canines are trapped distally to the maxillary cuspids. In these situations, interceptive orthodontics or selective extraction of the deciduous teeth that are "caught" (usually of the shorter jaw) will help relieve this interlock for unimpeded future growth (23). Selection of teeth to be extracted, as well as the timing of the extractions, is crucial to occlusal outcome. Extraction technique may influence the health and eventual appearance of the unerupted permanent teeth (24). If the hereditary influence involves a specific jaw malocclusion, this procedure will not change the outcome. It will only make a difference in those individuals with genetic potential for a normal occlusion (22–23). (For details of interceptive treatments of deciduous malocclusions, see Chapter 7.)

Preventive orthodontics is the evaluation and elimination of conditions that may lead to irregularities in the developing or mature occlusal complex. Preventive orthodontics basically breaks down into three categories: occlusal assessment and supervision, space control, and behavioral control. *Occlusal assessment and supervision* includes the supervision of timely primary dental exfoliation and permanent dental eruption. Even though exfoliation and eruption supervision is considered preventive, the actual act of assisting exfoliation or eruption is an interceptive orthodontic action. The act of occlusal assessment and supervision is classified as a part of preventive orthodontics; however, the treatment of the assessed problem may fall into interceptive, preventive, or corrective categories. *Space control* includes treatment of traumatic, congenital, or hereditary anomalies, as well as dentally destructive diseases (eg, caries, dental resorption, periodontal disease, etc.), and maintenance of dentally voided spaces. *Behavioral control* deals with treatments to manage deportment, which affect occlusion (see Chapter 21). Behavioral problems typically fall into two categories: habits and anxiety reactions.

Corrective orthodontics has two stages: active treatment and retention. Active treatment refers to the application of devices to restore dental occlusion to a reasonably functional and esthetic state. Before such an action is undertaken, the animal's occlusion should be evaluated, as well as the effects of the various apparatuses that may be selected on the dentofacial complex. Once the *active treatment stage* is completed, it is necessary to have the teeth stabilized in their new position to allow a harmonious state to develop; this is termed the *retention stage*. During active treatment, the alveolar bone has been induced into a state of accelerated resorption and deposition. The retention stage allows this bone to return to a more normal physiologic state, while, hopefully, allowing the bone to eventually provide a sound harmonious tooth support structure. The device that provides the retention is called the *retainer*. Retainers can be either fixed or removable, but in veterinary orthodontics, the fixed retainer is more typical. Occasionally, mild cases of class II or class III malocclusion are treated for cosmetic reasons; this is termed *orthodontic camouflage treatment*.

DIAGNOSTIC AIDS

Diagnosis and treatment planning are principally based on visual assessment accompanied by certain aids (25). These aids help improve the evaluation to reduce the chance of unexpected and possibly disastrous consequences. There are five basic diagnostic tools in veterinary orthodontics: history, physical and oral examination, photographs, dental models and bite registrations, and radiographs.

Written records and history are always important, but in orthodontics they are essential in the determination of progression and response to treatment. History provided by owners can be helpful, but it must be screened carefully due to their lack of understanding of terminology and dental normals. All aspects of previous illnesses and accidents and their treatment are important. Information concerning the line and family can be extremely useful in attempting to classify an anomalous condition as hereditary.

Nothing can take the place of a good physical and oral examination in assessment of occlusion. Only first hand viewing of the true dental articulation can give a reasonable evaluation of the range of motion, potential attritional wear, and interferences to tooth movement. Many temporomandibular joint dysplasias can be felt or heard. Oral soft tissue health is best evaluated by visual and tactile senses.

Photographs provide records of before and after treatment. Additionally, profile and frontal photographs can sometimes aid in treatment planning without the distractions of the patient and owner influences. Color photographs also provide information as to tooth color changes, as well as gingival status.

Dental models and bite registrations of a patient's dental arches and supporting tissues are an excellent source for study of abnormalities and treatment planning. The bite registration allows for a reasonable articulating of the models. With these models, orthodontic appliances can be deliberated, designed, and fabricated.

Radiographs allow analysis of potential complications for treatment and from treatment. Abnormalities and pathologies must be considered prior to treatment. Resorptive lesions, caries, periodontal disease, missing teeth, unerupted teeth, root abnormalities, degree of root maturity, and quality of alveolar bone, among others, must all be taken into consideration, and radiology is the best tool to address many of these.

Cephalometrics and computer treatment simulations are very impressive. However, the lack of cephalometric standards in animals make this tool unreliable. Computerized treatment simulations in animal dentistry at this time are more of a toy than a tool, but they will eventually be an important diagnostic device.

AGE, TIMING, AND TREATMENT

Ideally, orthodontic treatment should be initiated as soon as possible, once favorable conditions exist for assisting orthodontic procedures (1). Young bone is less resistant to tooth movement, young tissues are generally more forgiving, and young animals typically accept placement of oral appliances easier than older. Tooth movement is easier to produce in younger animals due to the fact that their cells are in an active growth phase and readily adapt to changes, whereas there is a more sluggish cellular response in older individuals (1). In addition, with interceptive orthodontic procedures involving deciduous extractions, early institution of treatment is essential for optimal effect. However, the advantages are offset to a degree due to the fact that making an accurate diagnosis becomes more difficult, the younger the animal is. Additionally, treatments in animals with deciduous or mixed dentition may have to be repeated for the permanent dentition, and that too young permanent dentition may require prolonged supervision for retention or retreatment due to drift or recoil.

Regardless of age, it can be a challenge to maintain appliances in many of the smaller terrier breeds. In addition, most interceptive extractions must be delayed until the teeth have erupted or until adjacent teeth will not be injured in the process or interfere. Animals under closer supervision and placement in reasonably confined areas are typically easier to manage during treatment.

The timing of treatment of adjunctive disease is critical in successful orthodontic treatment. A complete treatment plan must include the control of any active dental or oral disease (10). Periodontitis or active periodontal disease must be control prior to orthodontic treatment, as orthodontic tooth movements superimposed on periodontitis can lead to the inevitable destruction of the periodontium (26). Once controlled, the disease should continue to be treated even during orthodontics, as research has shown that regular professional treatment can halt or even reverse attachment destruction (27). Clinical research has shown that orthodontic treatments in both normal and compromised periodontal tissues can be completed without loss of attachment, providing that appropriate treatment had been initiated prior to and during tooth movements (28).

PHYSIOLOGIC AND HISTOLOGIC ASPECTS OF TOOTH MOVEMENT

Unlike most other connective tissues, bone responds to even slight degrees of pressure or tension that deviate from the harmonious occlusal status by changes in form (1). These changes occur due to resorption of existing bone and deposition of new bone. The modifications occur to cortical and cancellous bone alike in quantity and shape that will best withstand the physical demands placed on it with the greatest economy of structure. These are the essentials of *Wolff's law of transformation of bone*:

> The Law of Transformation of Bone is to be understood as that Law under which, as a result of primary alteration in the form and function or of function alone of bone, there follow certain definite changes, determined by mathematical laws, in its inner architecture and as certainly according to the same laws of mathematics, secondary changes in its external form.

This means that the structural form of the bone will be that which is best suited to withstand the forces placed on it, and the quantity of bone tissue will be the minimum needed for its functional requirements. For additional economy of form, part of the structural pressures encountered during mastication are transferred to other parts of the jaws and skull along paths of stress.

Cellular response depends on the degree and duration of applied force (29,30). Changes in capillary pressures stimulate cellular changes in the adjacent tissues. Normal intracapillary pressure in primates falls in the range of 20–30 mm Hg, 20–26 g/cm^2, or 0.65–0.9 oz/cm^2 of tooth root surface (1). The estimation of root surface area is important in determining anchorage and force application. In the dog, some research has been done on root surface areas of the maxillary 4th premolar and mandibular 1st molar (31,32), but there are variations within breeds and from individual to individual. We have attempted to provide some approximations on dog root surface area to act as a general guide (Table 3). Every attempt should be made not to exceed the intracapillary blood pressure. When a light-to-mild force is applied, it acts as a stimulus to initiate cellular activity resorption and deposition of bone, which is termed *physiologic movement*. When these pressures are exceeded with heavy force, there will be necrosis of periodontal tissues on the pressure side and poor to no deposition of bone on the traction side, which is labeled *pathologic movement*.

During orthodontic movements, assuming vital, healthy periodontal tissues, there is a *pressure side* and a *tension* or *traction side* of the tooth. Where pressure is transferred to the bone, there will be resorption, and where there is tension or traction, bone will be deposited.

On the *pressure side* (in the direction of tooth movement), during physiologic movement, the periodontal membrane is compressed to about one-half to one-third its normal thickness. The initial physiologic response is in the periodontal membrane, which is followed by changes in the adjacent bone. This results from an increase in the capillary pressure and blood supply at pressure points, initially the alveolar crest. This results in an increased mobilization of fibroblasts, cementoblasts, osteoblasts, and osteoclasts to the area. These activated cells are responsible for the resorption and remodeling of bone and periodontal tissues. It will take several days for the needed influx of osteoclasts to become established in the bone. The initial bone absorption typically occurs within the tooth socket along the wall near the crest. The osteoblasts will be found in crescent-shaped excavations known as *Howship's lacunae*. Within a few weeks, osteoblasts and osteoclasts will be found within the cancellous bone, where it is being reoriented by absorption and apposition. The trabecular pattern, normally primarily vertically oriented, reorganizes in a more horizontal fashion. The original pattern will gradually be reestablished once tooth movement is terminated.

On the *tension side* (away from the direction of tooth movement), the periodontal ligament is stretched, resulting in a widening of the periodontal membrane space. In response, capillary blood flow and cellular activity increase. This results in the deposition of new bone along the traction areas of the lamina dura.

Most orthodontic movements are simple tipping. This results in the greatest amount of changes occurring near the alveolar crest, lessening as the fulcrum point is approached, and then increasing again as the apex is approached. In correction of infraclusion with

TABLE 3. *Approximate tooth root surfaces (cm²) of the dog*

Tooth root	<10 lbs	<25 lbs	<50 lbs	<90 lbs
Maxillary				
1st incisor	0.7	1.0	1.3	1.7
2nd incisor	0.8	1.2	1.5	1.9
3rd incisor	1.2	1.6	2.25	2.6
Cuspid	3.4	5.4	7.8	9.5
4th premolar	2.5	4.15	5.25	6.75
1st molar	1.5	2.25	3.25	4.25
Mandibular				
1st incisor	0.6	0.9	1.2	1.6
2nd incisor	0.7	1.2	1.5	1.8
3rd incisor	0.9	1.4	1.7	2.0
Cuspid	3.3	5.25	7.65	9.25
4th premolar	1.3	1.9	3.25	3.75
1st molar	2.6	3.8	4.75	6.00

extrusion, deposition of bone normally occurs at the alveolar crest, along the socket walls and at the socket apex. In the treatment of supraclusion with intrusion, resorption of bone along the walls and apex occurs initially. This may be the most potentially hazardous movement in that damage to the periodontal ligament and possible pulpal necrosis may occur due to compression of the apical blood supply. Rotation holds its own risks, especially in movements greater than 45°. If it is performed too quickly, osteoblastic activity will not be able to maintain pace with the osteoclastic activity. This can result in poor support and an unstable position. Rotation movements are best accomplished by light forces for slow transition and by intermittent force application. Teeth should be either overrotated to help compensate for recoil or stabilized securely in position with a retainer for an extended time.

CHANGES IN TISSUES ASSOCIATED WITH TOOTH MOVEMENT

During tooth movement, other various tissues may undergo changes (33). The degree of change and the repair, or lack of it, depend greatly on the intensity and duration of forces applied. The cementum next to the periodontal ligament may undergo some degree of resorption due to clastic cell activity during tooth movement. If light-to-mild pressures are used, the areas will be repaired by cementoblasts once force is relieved to the specific area, even if treatment is still in process.

Dentin on occasion is seen to have resorption following exposure from cemental resorption. These areas are not repaired within dentin, but with cementum, cementoid, or osteoid. The type of reparative replacement varies from individual to individual.

With light force, the pulp typically demonstrates little or no reaction. However, even with mild force, the pulp may develop a slight degree of hyperemia. When heavy forces are applied, hyperemia is common, and partial or even complete pulpal necrosis may occur (34).

Gingival tissues eventually adapt to the tooth's new positioning. However, these changes are commonly less rapid than those of the alveolar bone. In cases in which rapid movement is achieved, this may result in tissue mounding or wrinkling up on the pressure side, as well as its being stretched tight on the tension side until the gingival tissue compensates. This tissue can easily become irritated and inflamed if appliances are allowed to impinge on it. Additionally, the elasticity of the gingival tissue in this condition can act to cause recoil of the tooth back toward its original position, especially in rotation movements (35).

Changes in the temporomandibular joint may also occur during occlusal adjustments from orthodontics (36). Studies have shown that the joint attempts to adapt itself to compensate for changes in the occlusal pattern and pressures (33).

TYPES OF TOOTH MOVEMENTS

Teeth must generally be moved and/or removed to perform orthodontics. There are six basic tooth movements that are utilized or occur in orthodontics: tipping, radicular (root), translation (bodily), rotation (torsion), extrusion, and intrusion. Physiologically, from easiest to hardest, the movements are extrusion, tipping, radicular (root), rotation (torsion), translation (bodily), and intrusion (37–39).

Tipping movements occur when the crown of the tooth carries the primary movement. When compression or tension (traction) is applied to a tooth, the force is transferred through the periodontal ligament to the alveolus, and the alveolar crest usually attempts to act as a pivotal point. However, the true *center of rotation*, or *fulcrum*, created in tipping occurs approximately at the junction of the middle and apical thirds of the root. In tipping, both crown and root typically move, but in opposite directions. The crown and root that is coronal to the fulcrum point move the greater distance as compared with the apex to the tooth. Lighter forces generally provide the best tipping movements, as the lighter the force applied, the more apical will be the fulcrum. This is the most common movement made use of in veterinary orthodontics.

Radicular or *root movements* occur when the apex of the tooth carries the primary or greatest distance of movement in comparison with the crown. Radicular movement is basically tipping from the opposite end of the tooth. Some texts consider root movement as another form of tipping (2); however, almost all other forms of tooth movement involve some degree of tipping. The fulcrum is found approximately at the junction of the middle and cervical thirds of the root. The movement is sometimes used in teeth in which the crown cusp or incisal edge is in the correct position, but the neck of the tooth is not. Typically, the coronal tip of the tooth is held stationary, while compression or tension is applied near the cervical region of the tooth.

Translation or *bodily movement* occurs when the crown and apex both travel in the same direction. Moving a tooth bodily typically requires a fixed attachment to the crown, as a great deal more resistance is encountered from the periodontium than with tipping movements and the movement is therefore more difficult. Lighter forces are initially used for this type of movement, but moderate pressures are typically required to complete the movement in animals within a reasonable time.

Rotation or *torsion movement* occurs when the tooth is rotated on its long axis in one direction or the other. In this movement, all of the periodontal ligament fibers are stretched in the same spiral direction around the tooth. This makes recoil a serious problem in this type of movement. Several things can be done to help counteract recoil from torsion movements. The first is that when teeth are rotated with lighter pressure over a longer time, less recoil occurs. Second, use of alternating periods of movement and stabilization can reduce the recoil effect. Third and most important, the teeth should have some type of retainer applied for several months.

Extrusion is actually movement of the tooth further out of the alveolus, typically in the same direction as normal eruption. If there is no occlusal interference to be dealt with and an appropriate appliance has been designed, extrusion is the easiest movement to accomplish in theory. However, in carnivores, the cuspids or canine teeth with their tremendous root structure and greater occlusal height can sometimes be a challenge. In extrusion, light forces are generally made use of to reduce the chance of accidentally avulsing the tooth.

Intrusion is the movement of the tooth further into the alveolus. The forces required are applied in the same direction as the tremendous forces of occlusion. Therefore, the periodontium is best suited to resist this type of movement, making it the most difficult movement to accomplish. However, once it is attained, coronal recoil is seldom seen. Light forces are best used in order to reduce the chances of apical resorption.

ANCHORAGE

In tooth movements, there must be a stable foundation to which the appliance is attached that acts as the point of resistance. This site of delivery from which force is exerted is known as the *anchorage* (1,38). For every action, there is an opposite and equal reaction. The resistance of the anchorage must be greater than that of the target. The less the anchorage is to move, the greater the anchorage:target ratio of resistance must be (1). For this reason, it is common to make use of multiple teeth in anchorage. These teeth are referred to as the *anchorage unit.*

Resistance to movement is a more complex interaction than one may think (34). Root surface area, quality of root, alveolus surface area, quality of alveolus, leverage of appliance, type of movement, and direction of force all partake in resistance to movement. Appliance leverage is used to help counteract target resistance. By applying the anchorage near the cervical region and the target attachment near the coronal tip of the teeth, a leverage advantage for the anchorage can be obtained. Additionally, the type of movements involved can affect resistance. Bodily movement provides greater resistance than tipping. Direction of movement also plays a role in resistance. There is greater resistance to distal movement in the posterior teeth due to the outward growth patterns of the jaw and the distal inclination of roots (1). For the anterior teeth, there is greater resistance to lingual movement due to tongue pressures, growth patterns of the jaw, and the lingual inclination of the roots.

There are five basic types of orthodontic anchorage: simple, reinforced (planes and stationary), intermaxillary, extraoral, and reciprocal (1).

Simple anchorage occurs when a greater tooth resistance to movement is used in association with an appliance than that of the target of movement in the same dental arch. In view of the factors of resistance, an advantage of at least two to one of anchorage to target teeth is preferred (1). Typically, but incorrectly, this is generally thought of as root surface ratios.

Reinforced anchorage (*planes and stationary*) is used when on occasion the action of an appliance with simple anchorage will be insufficient to resist the reaction of the movement target. In these cases, the anchorage may be augmented for stabilization in one of several ways. These are the use of planes and stationary anchorages. *Planes* are reinforcements to the anchorage that allow a part of the resistance to be transferred from the teeth to paradental tissues, such as the palate. *Stationary reinforcement* is the use of fixed anchorage attachment that is designed so that only bodily movement of the anchorage teeth can occur.

Intermaxillary anchorage is when an appliance anchorage is placed in the opposing jaws or in both the mandible and maxilla. This is a form of reinforcement, but due to its uniqueness it is placed in its own category.

Extraoral anchorage involves seeking anchorage outside of the mouth. This is typically done with various head and neck harnesses (40). Head harnesses are sometimes referred to as occipital traction, and neck harnesses as cervical traction.

Reciprocal anchorage occurs when two teeth or tooth groups are moved to an extent in opposite directions and more or less to an equal extent either away from each other or toward each other. For this to work properly, each group must provide a similar resistance.

APPLICATION OF FORCE

Force may be applied in two ways: intermittently or continuously. *Intermittent force* is when the drive or energy is applied in incremental steps with periods of rest in between. Force application of this type is generally preferred with tooth movements in which recoil is an expected problem. Intermittent force is most commonly applied using orthodontic appliances with screw-type drives and incline planes. With incline planes, the force is self-regulated by the discomfort on the periodontal membranes. With screws, the limiting factor is the adjustment. Most are designed to provide 0.18–0.20 mm of movement per quarter turn (see discussion of expansion screws below). *Continuous force* is when the drive or energy is applied in a constant fashion, until the target tooth is moved to its new target site. This type of force application customarily provides a more rapid movement of the target tooth to the target site than intermittent force. Orthodontic appliances with elastics and springs are most commonly used to provide this type of force application. To maintain continuous force, springs and elastics are readjusted before they become totally relaxed or dead. Springs and elastics can be used in an intermittent-force concept, just as some screws have internal spring devices and can be used in a continuous-force concept. To prevent damage to the periodontium or tooth, the force should be remain below that of capillary blood pressure: 20–26 g/cm^2, 20–30 mm Hg, or 0.5–0.9 oz/cm^2 of tooth root surface.

GENERAL TYPES OF ORTHODONTIC APPLIANCES: REMOVABLE AND FIXED

There are two basic types of orthodontic appliances: removable and fixed. Although both types can be used in most cases, there are certain circumstances in which each is the appliance type of choice. It is necessary to assess and consider treatment of all other oral and dental problems when orthodontics is being considered. Erosions, cavities, and other dental and oral diseases generally need to be treated or controlled before the placement of an appliance. However, when occlusal problems are initiating periodontal disease, orthodontics may be instituted to help in its treatment. Nevertheless, extreme care and supervision is required in such cases, or complications can be expected.

Removable appliances are those designed to be easily and routinely removed and then reinserted. These appliances are preferred in cases in which intensive oral hygiene is required due to oral or dental disease or other dental treatments must be carried on simultaneously. This permits the removal of all food debris, brushing of the teeth, treatment of periodontal infections, cleaning of the appliance, and treatment of other dental problems as necessary. In addition, repairs can be made at leisure or by a technician while the device is removed. In veterinary orthodontics, most of these appliances consist of three parts: a removal base, an active force attached to the base, and a fixed anchorage (41). The base of the appliance, which may be made of acrylic or metal, serves as a platform for the active force. The active force is usually provided by screws, springs, or elastics. The anchorage most often consists of brackets bonded to teeth that allow elastics to attach the base in place for activation. The main disadvantages are that the appliances are frequently bulky, sometimes interfering with normal occlusion, and some astute pets may learn to remove the appliance themselves, presenting the possibility that the appliance may then be swallowed and become an intestinal foreign body (12).

Fixed appliances are typically attached to provide a center for movement force without removal until the tooth attains its target site. Fixed appliances customarily provide greater security of the applied force; they are also less bulky than removable appliances and have improved precision and enhanced gentleness, when properly applied and supervised. The main disadvantage of this type of appliance is the need for greater hygiene care, as food and debris may accumulate beneath its recesses and visual monitoring for disease or trauma may be hampered by the appliance. Additionally, any repairs must generally be be made chairside with a sedated patient. Fixed appliances ordinarily consist of three parts: base plates or bands for anchorage, a framework or bracket for force attachment, and the active force (42). The active force may consist of wires, springs, screws, or elastics (41).

ORTHODONTIC APPLIANCES AND MATERIALS

Orthodontic wire is commonly used in a large variety of orthodontic appliances. There are three basic types of orthodontic wire: round, rectangular, and braided (Table 4). Round wire is the simplest to handle and work with, but when torque is required, specially designed auxiliary parts must be added to achieve a torquing force (2). Rectangular wire, when used with rectangular brackets or tubes, can apply torquing forces with the greatest accuracy (43). Braided wires are made of multiple strands of thinner wires that are twisted or braided together; they provide the most flexibility of the three types (2).

The physical properties and mechanical behavior of wire depends to a great extent on the types of metal employed within them. Stainless steel is the most commonly used metal (2), but many other types and combinations are utilized (44). Nickel–titanium memory-type wire is becoming a more common orthodontic material. ADA Specification No.32 defines all orthodontic wire requirements except those containing precious metals (45).

Bending and forming wires is not beyond the skills of the average practitioner, but it is time-consuming and requires careful consideration, technique, and knowledge. For these reasons, a laboratory is best used by most. However, for simple appliances, bends can be performed with birdbeak, square, Howe, three-prong, or wire-cutter pliers. Bends are basically classified according to the direction of force. There are three basics bends: primary or first-order, secondary or second order, and tertiary or third-order. *First-order bends* are in the horizontal plane and are in-and-out bends. *Second-order bends* are in the vertical plane and are up and down bends. Third-order bends are bends that produce a torque force. There are three types of third-order bends: single-tooth torque, anterior torque, and posterior torque (46).

Springs, *kick*, and *coil* can easily be incorporated into appliances to provide either traction or compression. Open coil springs are used for compression, and closed coil springs for traction. There are many types of kick springs, but the more common are the finger, cantilever, T,W, and Z springs. With fixed appliances, springs can provide bodily movements, but they are normally used for tipping. The longer the wire and the more helical loops applied to the spring, the gentler will be the force and the better the maintenance

TABLE 4. *Orthodontic wire types and uses*

Wire type	Use	Wire-diameter range (in.)
Round	Ligatures	0.007–0.012
	Fixed appliances	0.014–0.022
	Removal appliances	0.160–0.036
	Lingual arches	0.036
	Head gear	
	Inner arch	0.045–0.051
	Facial bow	0.060
Braided	Archwires	0.015–0.020
Rectangular	Edgewise-fixed appliances	0.022–0.028

(Adapted from ref. 2.)

of direction (1). The main disadvantage of the kick spring in tilting movements has been that as the tooth tilts, the spring has a tendency to ride up the lingual surface and possibly over it, disrupting its function. This is best controlled by designing the spring to engage the tooth as close to the cervical area as possible or, in acrylic appliances, by placing the spring into a recessed box cavity. The cantilever, finger, Z, and T springs are usually used for single-tooth movements, unless used in multiple and overlapping patterns. The W spring is most commonly used in veterinary orthodontics with banding for spreading both mandibular cuspids when they are base narrow.

Arch bars, *wires*, and *cast* with their various types and auxiliaries are possibly the most versatile of the orthodontic appliances (2). These can be either labial or lingual to the teeth and be used in the maxilla or mandible. The anchorage attachment is often either bands or brackets. The bands can be matrix or cast. The actual arch wire or bar can also be either prefabricated wire or a cast metal. The cast metal arch bars have the greater strength but are relatively nonflexible. This inflexibility can lead to problems if not compensated for in young or growing animals. Therefore, in young animals, the use of a flexible wire soldered to the anchor bands or in cast bars and the placement of a telescoping central joint alleviate most of these problems. The canine teeth are possibly the most commonly banded teeth for anchorage. These teeth must be carefully examined for paralleling or the lack of it. If the two teeth flare or converge to any degree, a solid cast appliance cannot be placed, unless a joint or flexibility is built into the arch bar.

An *orthodontic band* is a flattened piece of metal constructed as a ring to fit around the clinical crown of a tooth and be cemented in place (2). Bands can be prefabricated on models or formed by an operator with strips of band-metal material for a custom fit. Various brackets are welded or soldered to the brackets to provide the type of force or anchorage required by the design. Custom fits are generally made by the "pinch band technique" in which a roll of band material is fitted around a tooth and the ends pinched together with a pair of Howe pliers. The metal is welded at the pinch, and the loose ends are trimmed, folded over, and welded, thus forming a band.

Base plates are the foundation that provides a surface for direct bonding to the tooth surface. Various brackets and tubes can be attached to the base plate to provide anchorage or movement sites. Base plates typically have a wire mesh or patterned imprint on the side facing the tooth, which allows for greater adherence by the cement. Base plates can be made from plastics, ceramics, or metals. Metals provide the greatest strength, but the plastics and ceramics provide a better cosmetic appearance during treatment.

Orthodontics brackets and *tubes* are devices that are attached to base plates or bands to provide attachment for wires, springs, and elastics (47). Tubes can be round or rectangular according to the needs of the appliance. There is a wide variety of brackets available: slotted, cleats, hooks, and buttons. Buttons are currently the most widely used bracket in veterinary orthodontics.

Many forms of *orthodontic elastics* are available. These are used as sources of force for many appliances. Generally, four forms are in common use: rings, ligatures, tubes, and chains. Elastic rings, which come in various sizes and strengths, can be used as the actual force, but they are also used as the attachment for removable appliances (Table 5). Ligatures are strings of elastic that come in various sizes that affect their strength. Elastic tubes are a form of hollow elastic ligature. The tubes have greater strength than the ligature but a shorter stretch distance, and are more bulky. Chains are flattened elastics with an arrangement of holes to allow their attachment to buttons or similar brackets. The spacing of the holes comes three patterns: long filament, short filament, and continuous filament. The continuous filament is the most practical in veterinary work. "K" modules

TABLE 5. *Elastic rings: size and strength*

Size (in.)[a]	Strength (oz.)
⅛	Light (2)
3/16	Medium (3)
¼	Heavy (4)
5/16	Extra heavy (6)
⅜	

[a]Size is based on approximate relaxed diameter.

are individual filaments with only two attachment sites; they provide a continual gentle force for long periods of time.

Orthodontic acrylics are used to form a framework or base structure from which various inclines, springs, arch wires, or expansion devices can be attached (see Chapter 2). Most are made from heat-cured acrylics in laboratories, but many are made with cold-cure acrylics in the clinic by the operator. Typically, most are made of either clear or pink-shaded resins for cosmetic reasons. When acrylic appliances are formed directly in the mouth, at least two forms of anchorage are usually required due to the occlusal pressures. One weak form of anchorage is acid-etching of the tooth and bonding of the acrylic to the tooth. This is done by acid-etching the lingual enamel surface of the teeth where the acrylic will make contact with a 37% phosphoric acid. Rinsing should be thorough to remove all acid, and the surface is then dried with clean dry air before the acrylic is applied. This will allow the acrylic to lightly bond to the tooth surface. Second, a figure-8 wire placed across the palate and into the acrylic base will provide additional anchorage. Wires based back from the lingual surface of the intermediate incisors can have the leads passed on either side interproximally to the labial surface. The bases of the wires are embedded in the acrylic on the lingual side, and once the acrylic is cured, the lead ends are twisted together labially. Generally, it is best to keep the appliance off the coronal third of the teeth, or it may act as an incline plane, inclining the mandibular incisors further labially, counteracting the labial movement of the maxillary incisors. In addition, the base should not be overbuilt, or the palate and floor space will be overfilled, resulting in an open bite that may allow previously unaffected teeth to drift into malocclusions and even supererupt. It is always important to take into consideration the normal anatomy that may be in the path of the movement bar of the appliance. The incisal papillae of the palate is one structure that must be taken into consideration, and the movement bar should be constructed to prevent its injury. As the movement bar tilts the maxillary incisors labially, it becomes easier for the bar to slip over the top of the incisors. To reduce the chances of this occurring, the expansion bar's contact on the lingual surface of the incisors should be kept as close to the cervical third of the crown as possible, and the expansion of the device should not be hurried. In younger animals, skeletal growth should always be taken into consideration. Appliances should be checked regularly and replaced as needed, or expansion slots or telescoping supports utilized.

Direct construction in-house in the animal's mouth has three draw backs. This type of acrylic does generate a minimal amount of heat, but it is normally insufficient to irritate the oral tissues significantly. It requires a more prolonged initial anesthesia for the animal. The third problem involves the vapors. With the animal under anesthesia and intubated, the vapors are of no serious health hazard to the patient, but they can be to the operator and auxiliaries, unless good ventilation is provided. The advantages of this approach are that it does not require a second anesthesia for installation and treatment can be initiated more quickly.

When an acrylic appliance is indirectly built on a dental model, the model must be coated with a separating medium or the acrylic will bond to it (8). Separating mediums may be metal foils or foil substitutes, such as oils used wet or coating resins applied and allowed to dry. The acrylics should be used in accordance with the manufacturer's recommendations. Actual mixing and application of the acrylic are usually done by brush, salt-and-pepper, or mix-and-pour techniques. However, the most common technique used in-house is the salt-and-pepper technique of applying powdered polymer followed by wetting with the liquid monomer and repeating the process until the desired pattern is achieved. Rope or utility wax can be used on the model as a pattern form to restrict unwanted acrylic flow. The appliance can be trimmed with acrylic burs or white stones. To obtain a smooth surface, an unfilled resin, such as HiSheen™ (Coe Laboratories, Inc., Chicago, Illinois), can be painted on the acrylic, or a rag wheel on a mandrel with a low-speed handpiece may be used with water and flour of pumice to actually polish the acrylic. There are also vapor health hazards with indirect appliance formation, as in the direct method. Good ventilation is always recommended when working with any form of acrylic.

Expansion and contraction screw devices are most commonly used for intermittent movement pressures. They are available in a variety of types designed for single- or multiple-tooth movements. The normal expansion screw operates by the use of a small wire key; when used to turn the central screw properly, the key separates the halves of the unit. With screws, the limiting factor is the adjustment. Most are designed to provide 0.18–0.20 mm of movement per quarter turn (2). Most periodontal membrane spaces are between 0.15 mm and 0.30 mm, with the smaller space seen in smaller breeds and older animals. Typically, younger animals have a larger periodontal ligament space due to eruptive demands. Therefore, application of force should be calculated to no more than 65% of the periodontal ligament space to aid in preventing pathologic injury to the periodontium or tooth. The *piston screw* is used for the movement of a single tooth. One form, the *piston spring screw*, when advanced, has a spring that can maintain a continuous pressure for a movement up to 0.5 mm before requiring readjustment. It is activated with the use of a miniature screw driver. If owners are allowed to adjust the appliance, specific instructions should be given, and, when possible, a directional arrow should be placed on the appliance to indicate the direction of turn to expand the device, as owners have a tendency to become confused and turn the screw in the wrong direction at times.

Incline planes are appliances designed to make contact with the cusps or incisal edges of the teeth of the opposing occlusion to stimulate tooth movement. Inclines have no active movement device but rather rely on the muscles of mastication to provide the movement force (1). When the incline is designed to prevent occlusal closure, it is called a *bite plane*. When the incline covers, a tooth it is known as *incline capping. Half capping* is when the lingual and occlusal surfaces of the tooth are covered, but if the coverage extends over to the facial surface, it is known as *full incline capping*. The plane is classically designed to face apically at an approximate 60° angle (1). Incline planes can be made as removable or fixed appliances and out of acrylics or cast metals. When fixed incline planes are used, one major consideration is to allow for growth. The *Mann incline place* is a cast fixed appliance that is anchored to the upper canine teeth with a telescoping support bar between the two, which allows for skeletal growth. It has one or two spoon-shaped incline planes that engage the lower cuspids to move them labially. The *incisor-capping incline plane* covers a group of incisors, generally the mandibular, to move the opposing incisor teeth.

CONDITIONS TREATABLE BY ORTHODONTICS

Appliances vary greatly, and many different appliances result in the same basic eventual outcome. Appliances should generally not be used on patients with active to advanced periodontal disease, as stability of the movements will be questionable. In some cases, periodontal disease, such as that associated with crowding, improves with appropriate orthodontics, when active disease is first controlled. The success or failure of various appliances rests on the clinician's knowledge of the apparatus' actions, adaptations, and limitations. General treatments will be discussed for torsiversion, infraversion, anterior cross-bites, posterior cross-bites, base narrow or linguoversion of mandibular canine teeth, rostromesial inclination of maxillary canine teeth, distal inclination of maxillary canine teeth, and class II and class III malocclusions.

In the consideration of an appliance, there are certain things that can help guide the clinician. First, select or design the appliance to achieve the desired results in the simplest manner, as complex appliances have complex flaws. The pattern of the appliance should fit the patient with reasonable comfort by ensuring a proper fit. Refrain from overextending the appliance coverage, which may irritate the periodontium. Avoid occlusal interference, except in incline planes where it should be the minimum necessary. Custom-fit brackets and bands for best comfort and adhesion. Always check to make sure brackets and arch wires will be at the level most appropriate for treatment. Select the designs that best accomplish the movements, but always take into consideration hygiene and ease of cleaning for the owner. Do not attempt too many movements simultaneously, but rather stage the treatment. The appliance should be as versatile as possible, so that as many stages can be accomplished as possible with it.

Rotation or *torsion movements* involve rotation of a tooth on its long axis in one direction or the other. They are most commonly encountered in incisors and premolars. The simplest approach to treatment is the use of button brackets and elastic chains. Attach the movement brackets to the facially deviated portion of the facial surface and to the most lingually deviated part of the lingual surface of the tooth. One to two simple anchorage brackets should be placed mesially and distally, as dictated by root surfaces. The anchor bracket should be placed on the facial or lingual surface toward which the mesial or distal surfaces of the tooth are to be rotated, customarily the opposite of the movement bracket. Once the appliance is in place, tighten the elastic chain only one notch to begin. Allow the tooth to move to the point at which the stretch of the elastic is lost. Then tighten one notch again, repeating the process until the tooth has properly rotated. In this type of movement all of the periodontal ligament fibers and the gingival collar are stretched in the same spiral direction around the tooth, making recoil a possible problem (see discussion of rotation or torsion movements in Types of Tooth Movements above).

Teeth with infraversion are those in which their crowns have failed to completely erupt and are frequently either ankylosed or impacted. The first step is to determine the status of the root structure. If the root apex is still vital and open and the impaction cause is relieved, the tooth may erupt on its own (48). If the apex is closed, extrusion orthodontics will most likely be required. When teeth are ankylosed, there is an area of root cementum and alveolar bone that has fused, and this must be relieved before extrusion orthodontics. With impactions, the type of tissue, soft or hard, must be resolved (see Chapter 3). If the impaction is soft tissue, it should be excised. If the impaction is of a bony nature, both soft tissue and bone must be resected. Once the crown tip is exposed, a bracket can be attached for movement, and others can be attached to the adjacent or opposing teeth for sufficient reinforced anchorage. Extrusion typically goes quickly once the impaction cause is relieved, but some precautions should be taken (see discussion of extrusion movements in Types of Tooth Movements above).

Anterior cross-bites are conditions in which one or more incisors are in version to their counterparts in the opposing jaws. Ordinarily, tipping movements will be used to correct the condition (see discussion of tipping movements in Types of Tooth Movements above). Three basic items that must be examined for: crowding, open bite, and whether the incisal version or inclination is in the maxillary or mandibular teeth. If crowding or embrication is a problem, either odontoplasty (stripping) to reduce the tooth size or selective interceptive extractions may be required to make room. When teeth are moved facially, a natural expansion of the arch normally occurs that may correct the spacing problem. Odontoplastic *stripping* is the process of reducing the interproximal contacts using various abrasive strips or thin-fluted burs (10). Stripping reduces the mesiodistal width of the teeth, thus reducing the space required for alignment. It also flattens the interproximal contacts, making that area of the arch more stable. However, as with any procedure that alters the natural contours of the teeth, it should be performed judiciously and not routinely (49). Extractions should not be performed until the owner is consulted. Next, observe the anterior occlusion closely for partial open bites. It is not uncommon to find that the maxillary incisors will not cover the mandibular teeth when the mouth is closed and a small free-way space exists between the uppers and lowers. If there is a partial anterior open bite, then correction will require not only facial or lingual movement but also extrusion to obtain a bite that will not recoil. Lastly, try to determine whether the principal problem is linguoversion of maxillary incisors or labioversion of the mandibular incisors.

According to the findings from the above, one or more of at least six different appliances may be chosen:

1. Elastic ligature ties
2. Lingual maxillary arch bar with kick spring
3. Labial maxillary arch bar with elastics
4. Mandibular or maxillary incline plane
5. Maxillary expansion screw appliance
6. Mandibular brackets and elastic chains.

For mandibular labioversion, the general appliances used to move the mandibular incisors lingually and back into a scissors bite are:

1. Elastic ligature ties
2. Maxillary incisal capping incline planes
3. Mandibular brackets and elastic chains.

For linguoversion of the maxillary incisors, the appliances most commonly used are:

1. Elastic ligature ties
2. Lingual maxillary arch bar with kick springs
3. Mandibular incisal incline plane
4. Maxillary expansion screw appliance
5. Labial maxillary arch bar with elastics.

For partial open bites, the labial maxillary arch bar and elastics and the mandibular brackets and elastic chains are both capable of providing extruding movements in addition to tilting. However, the labial maxillary arch bar is the more reliable of the two for several reasons. First, it can provide a greater degree of extrusion, when properly designed, without moving of the attachments or adding of auxiliaries; and second, the mandibular central incisors in some cases cannot be successfully stabilized when tilted or extruded due to influences of the adjacent fibrous attachment of the mandibular symphysis, which may partially encompass them. In our opinion, the latter two appliances, by themselves or in combination, are the most versatile for most patients.

Elastic ligature ties can be used in either maxillary or mandibular inclinations or versions, but only when there is no crowding. Although ligatures can be used for multiple incisor movements, in the mandible, they are best used for simple single-tooth movements and, in the maxilla, only for single-tooth versions due to the curvature of the arch. Ligature ties, although simple to apply, produce not only lingual or labial movement according to how they are applied but also mesial or distal movement of the adjacent anchor teeth, which can result in embrication. The ligatures must be closely watched to prevent their migration into the soft tissues. For simple single-incisor movement, the ligature is run on the lingual or labial surface near the neck of the tooth, opposite the direction of movement desired. The ligature is brought interdentally on either side of the tooth in the direction of the desired movement across the surface of the adjacent teeth and then interdentally to the opposite surface, and the two ligature leads are brought back to the surface on which the ligature was placed on the movement tooth. The two leads are then tied together with slight tension to the elastic to provide the movement force. Multiple teeth can be moved by expanding the encompassed teeth, but migration below the gum line and slippage above the incisal edge can be additional problems to deal with (Fig. 2).

Lingual maxillary arch bar with kick spring or springs can be fabricated using brackets, arch wires, and attachments or made as a cast unit (Fig. 3). The laboratory-cast units are more durable and thereby provide greater reliability. The cast unit will typically have cast bands to encircle the cervical third of the maxillary cuspids and a lingual arch wire connecting the two bands, with one or more kick springs aligned to press the selected incisors facially. These units should not be heavily cemented in place, as they will typically require periodic removal and reactivation of the spring to continue the movements to completion. Cementation is best performed using a light-cured orthodontic composite cement, as it allows for precise cementation of the nature required. The tooth should be acid-etched on the lingual surface just coronal to the cuspid bands. The cement should be placed only on the lingual surface and slightly under the edge of the band and cured. This

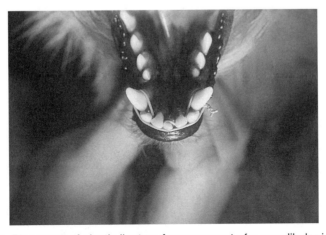

FIG. 2. Placement of elastic ligature for movement of a mandibular incisor.

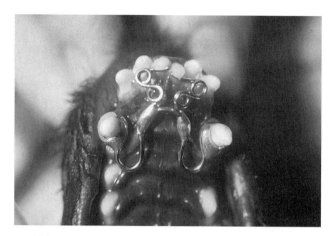

FIG. 3. Lingual maxillary arch bar with kick springs.

allows easy removal of the cement and appliance as needed (see Appliance Removal below). More unruly patients may require a heavier cementation, but this will complicate appliance removal for adjustment. This appliance's main problems are the requirements for removal and readjustments and the ease at which the springs can sometimes be bent out of place by a pet's chewing habits. Additionally, if the animal is young, the arch bar must either be flexible enough to allow for normal continued facial growth or telescope.

Mandibular or *maxillary incisal incline planes* can be constructed from acrylics or cast metals (see discussions of orthodontic acrylics and incline planes in Orthodontic Appliances and Materials above). The cast metals have a greater durability and typically can be cemented in place more reliably. The advantage of these appliances is the lack of moving parts or external activation force. Their primary disadvantage is that they typically block the bite open, until they are removed or movement is complete. This allows occlusal shifts that may further complicate the malocclusion, especially in growing animals. The appliance must be removed carefully to prevent damage to the underlying teeth.

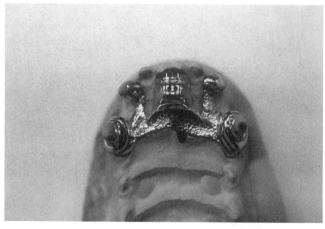

FIG. 4. Maxillary expansion screw appliance on a patient model designed for labial movement of the central incisors.

Maxillary expansion screw appliances are generally of two types: acrylic-base and metal-cast (see discussion of expansion and contraction screw devices in Orthodontic Appliances and Materials above) (Fig. 4). The acrylic appliance's base usually covers much of the palate, unfortunately allowing debris to accumulate and impact against the soft tissues, unless the appliance is a removable type that is detached and cleaned regularly. If it is not, an inflammatory palatitis sometimes occurs and can be quite severe (50). The cast metal appliance is normally less bulky and has less hygiene problems associated with it. The activator is a screw device that, when engaged, places pressure against the maxillary incisors, tilting them facially. Most appliances are adjusted with a small wire key that is inserted into the screw drive and rotated a quarter turn once every 3 days. When an acrylic-base appliance is constructed in-house, several matters must be taken into consideration (see discussion of orthodontic acrylics in Orthodontic Appliances and Materials above).

Labial maxillary arch bar with elastics is one of the most useful of the appliances listed. The arch bar is anchored by bands partially or fully around the cuspids (see discussion of arch bars in Orthodontic Appliances and Materials above). If the occlusion is tight, a partial cast band may be required in a C-shape so that the occlusion of the mandibular cuspids is not blocked. If the animal is young, skeletal growth must be accounted for by using either a flexible or telescoping arch bar (Fig. 5). The bar should come facially far enough to allow the needed movement and have small buttons on it at intervals to allow direction traction by the elastics. In addition, if extrusional movement is required, the bar should be designed to be at the incisal edge to permit coronal traction. Elastic lig-

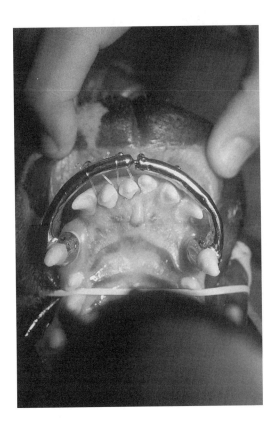

FIG. 5. Labial maxillary arch bar with elastics. Notice the arch bar has a telescoping expansion design near the midline of the animal's arch.

atures or tubes can be used for the activation force. Each tooth to be moved will require an individual ligature from it to the arch bar. Ligatures can easily slip from the incisor teeth due to their anatomic shape, especially in extrusion, unless an mooring-site attachment is placed. The mooring can be either a bracket bonded to the lingual surface of the incisor (51) or something as simple as a small amount of composite bonded as a lip off the lingual surface at the caudal most aspect at the neck of the tooth. The ligature is tied with a square knot around the neck of the tooth with the knot on the facial surface. The leads to the knot are then extended to the arch bar, tightened slightly, and secured to the arch bar with a square knot. As the tooth moves toward the bar, the ligature may require tightening or replacement. Once the teeth have moved into place, the arch bar and either elastics or wires can be used as the retainer device (see discussion of retainers in Categories of Orthodontic Treatments above).

Mandibular brackets and elastic chains are another highly versatile tool (34). Bracket placement and cementation (see Bond and Bracket Placement and Cementation, p. 472) and adjustment of the elastic chains are crucial to successful results. The most commonly used bracket is of the button type, which works well with elastic chains. As well as acting as an active appliance, this type can be used in cooperation with other appliances to act as a retainer for the lower incisors while the uppers are being moved. As the maxillary incisors are being moved labially, their occlusion with the mandibular incisors may act as an incline plane concurrently forcing the lower teeth labially. This can be prevented by the use of brackets and elastic chains on the lower teeth, which act as a retainer.

There are two bracket placement patterns most commonly used in mandibular incisor labioversion and as a retainer. Both patterns use the same basic placement pattern on the incisors but differ in their anchorage locations. In these movements, all of the incisors can be bonded with brackets; however, the central and corner incisors can provide the needed stability, preventing the elastic chain from slipping over the teeth. The brackets on the mandibular incisors should be placed where the least possibility of occlusal trauma from the upper incisors is likely to disrupt their bonding. This means placing the brackets on the cervical third of the crown, which is disadvantageous from a leverage standpoint and must be compensated for in anchorage.

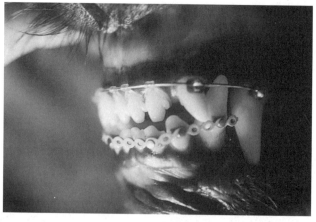

FIG. 6. Mandibular brackets and elastic chains with anterior anchorage to move incisors lingually, used to assist a maxillary arch bar.

In anchorage, there are two patterns most commonly used: anterior anchorage and posterior anchorage. Anterior anchorage makes use of the mandibular cuspid or canine teeth. The brackets are normally bonded in line horizontally with the incisors on the labial aspect of the tooth but free of contact with the maxillary cuspids and corner incisors. The elastic chain can be stretched along the labial surfaces to provide the force to move the incisors lingually (Fig. 6). The disadvantage to this pattern is that the cuspids can also act on one another, causing them to begin to move lingually or base narrow on occasion. Additionally, if the corner incisors need to be moved lingually, this pattern may not provide sufficient movement for them. In this case, the chain may need to be brought interproximally between the corner incisor and the adjacent canine tooth, and attached from the distal direction.

Another approach is to go with posterior anchorage, which can provide a greater degree of anchorage support. The posterior anchorage brackets are placed on the lingual surfaces on the cervical third of the crowns of the mandibular 4th premolar and 1st molar. The developmental groove on the molar can used to advantage to tilt the button brackets slightly caudally, providing superior chain stability. In addition, the longer chain distance from movement tooth to anchorage can provide a traction with either gentler or greater tension than the anterior anchorage pattern, due to the greater volume of chain involved. Direction of the chain labial or lingual to the mandibular cuspids can be used to enhance traction to the incisors when passed lingually or to reduce the traction on the corner incisors when passed labially (Fig. 7).

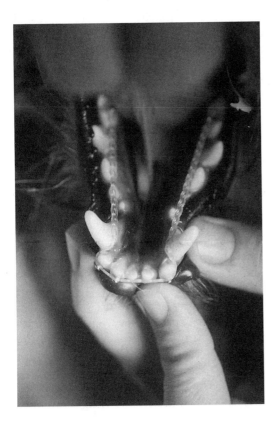

FIG. 7. Mandibular brackets and elastic chains with posterior anchorage for lingual movement of incisors.

Posterior cross-bites in primates are relatively simple in comparison with those in carnivores. Although posterior cross-bites can be seen in almost any breed, the collie appears to be the most commonly affected breed. If it is caught in a deciduous occlusion, interceptive orthodontics should be instigated and the inclined teeth extracted in the hope that the permanent teeth will not follow suit. In most cases presented in permanent occlusion, if the bite is functional, no treatment should be undertaken. In cases of bite interference in which the occlusion is being forced wry, preventive orthodontics should be undertaken with selective extraction of the teeth causing the most disruption. Should corrective orthodontics be undertaken, an incline bite plane will be required to block the bite open to allow the teeth to pass each other during treatment. An expansion screw appliance can be used on the maxillary 4th premolar to force the tooth buccally, while a lingual arch bar with elastics or a similar device will be required to pull the mandibular molar lingually. The bite will be required to be held open for 2–3 weeks during this movement. Corrective treatment should be discouraged, as many problems may arise from treatment, the open bite can allow teeth to drift or supererupt, problems with the temporomandibular joint may arise, and mastication interference may require special dietary care.

Base narrow or linguoversion of mandibular canine teeth can be handled in many ways according to the location of the tooth in relation to the upper teeth. With class I occlusions with anterior cross-bites involving base-narrow teeth, the base of the tooth is in a normal mesiodistal relationship. Those that are involved with mesiodistal discrepancies, especially of the jaw, may be classified as classes II–IV malocclusions, and they are discussed under those categories.

When the condition is caught early in deciduous dentitions, interceptive orthodontics may be performed (see Chapter 7). The degree of lingual inclination can affect the decision-making process on treatment. In very mild cases in which the mandibular cuspid only lightly impales the maxillary diastema gingival margin, preventive orthodontics involving a simple gingivectomy may correct the problem. The gingiva is beveled with a diamond point or fluted bur to a depth that obliterates any gingival impact crater. Tissue hemorrhage can be controlled with a gingival hemostatic solution, and then the tissue can be coated with Tincture of Myrrh and Benzoin (Sultan Chemical, Englewood, New Jersey). This should move the tip of the tooth free of gingival cusp impaction, and the natural incline plane will help to continue the tooth's movement labially.

Corrective orthodontic treatments may involve any one of several types of appliances. Expansion screws, W springs, acrylic incline planes, and cast metal incline planes are among the more commonly used appliances. The expansion screw device is generally used as a fixed cast metal appliance with bands around the lower cuspids and the expansion screw placed between the two bands. The bands and their attachment to the screw should be kept on the cervical third of the crown to reduce mastication and occlusal interference. Most of these appliances lack a flexible attachment to the bands, which results in a bodily movement of the teeth, not a tilting movement. These appliances have on occasion resulted in a spreading of the mandibular symphysis, which is usually evident by a diastemal formation between the central incisors. The bands are cemented into place and the expansion screw adjusted by a quarter-turn expansion every third or fourth day, until the desired movement is attained (see discussion of expansion and contraction screw devices in Orthodontic Appliances and Materials above). The appliance can usually be used as the retainer during the retainer period.

The W spring is a similar fixed appliance using cuspid bands for anchorage, but with a W kick or helix spring between the two as the activator. The flexibility of the spring wire generally results in primarily a tilting movement, although some bodily movement may result. The **W** spring is activated to the desired movement point or slightly further and is then cemented into place. The appliance can normally be used as the retainer during the retainer period.

Acrylic incline planes can be constructed by laboratories but are most typically made in-house. Cold-cure orthodontic acrylics can be used for direct or indirect appliance construction (see discussion of orthodontic acrylics in Orthodontic Appliances and Materials above). Direct construction in-house in the animal's mouth has both advantages and disadvantages, but it is basically used for expediency in beginning therapy. The target locations of incline of the crest are the points at which the mandibular canine teeth make initial contact with the incline. This should be the highest point of the incline, with a sloping angle of approximately 60° toward its target site. If there is uncertainty as to the exact incline crestal target locations, articulation or carbon paper can be placed on the acrylic base, the occlusion closed, and the cuspids tapped against the paper to place marks on the base indicating their position. The incline path can sometimes be enhanced before setting with a plastic filling instrument. Once the acrylic is cured, an acrylic white stone or a laboratory acrylic bur can be used to refine the incline's path. The incline can be smoothed with an unfilled resin or polished with pumice and water.

Cast metal incline planes are more refined, more securely anchored, and have less hygiene concerns. They do require quality impressions and models for the laboratory to fabricate a well fitting and functional appliance. In young animals, the Mann incline appliance accommodates growth with a telescoping central support (52) (Fig. 8).

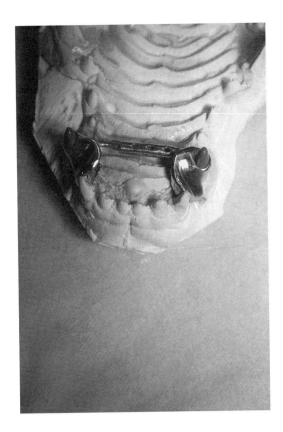

FIG. 8. Cast metal telescoping incline plane (Mann incline) designed on a patient model.

Rostromesial inclination of maxillary canine teeth is most commonly seen in Shetland sheepdogs (shelties). The simplest approach to treatment is with bonded brackets and elastic chains (53). The number and placement of the brackets and the initial tension of the elastic chain are very important for reasonable results with diminished possibility of complications (Fig. 9). Use of button brackets with elastic chains is a sensible combination. The location of the attachment of the movement brackets on the maxillary cuspid should be, if possible, on the labial surface at the middle to coronal thirds of the tooth, with a slight mesial shift to prevent ease of chain loss due to slippage. Occasionally, the cuspid may be wedged against the corner incisor, which prevents placement of the bracket at the desired location. In these cases, either the initial bracket can be placed lingually until the tooth clears the incisor, a slight gingivoplasty can be performed, or a dental wedge can be gently forced between the two teeth to allow space for placement. For good anchorage on cuspid movement, at least a two-to-one advantage would be preferred, which can be approximated by using two or more teeth and making use of a leverage advantage. The maxillary 4th premolar and 1st molar can be used for anchorage, which exceeds the root surface area for the cuspid. By placement of the anchorage brackets near the cervical third, as compared with the middle to coronal thirds for the cuspid, an additional leverage advantage of two or three to one can be obtained. The anchorage brackets should be placed on the buccal surface near the cervical third of the crown. By making use of the tooth's contours, the brackets can be angled slightly distally in many cases to improve their elastic chain–holding ability.

The elastic chain is then applied. For an initial period of 7–10 days, the chain should be tightened only one to two notches to stimulate physiologic movement. As the tooth begins movement, a two-to-three notch tightness can ordinarily be safely used, but excessive traction should not be attempted. Once the tooth reaches the desired position, the elastic chain can be loosened so that it holds the tooth in place during the retention period.

Distal inclination of maxillary canine teeth is more commonly seen in the smaller brachiocephalic breeds. It can be corrected by the use of a maxillary band or sleeve crown with a kick spring. Kick, finger, or Z springs with helices usually work well (Fig. 10). In

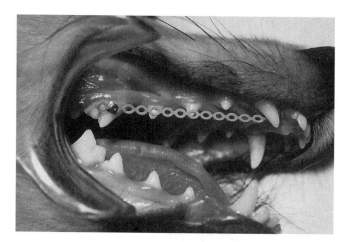

FIG. 9. Button brackets and elastic chain placed for correction of rostromesial inclination or version of the maxillary cuspid. The movement bracket has been placed on the lingual surface of the maxillary cuspid to permit easier movement past the mandibular cuspid. Note the use of only one anchorage bracket on the upper 4th premolar. This can sometimes lead to mesial movement or even partial extrusion of the anchorage tooth.

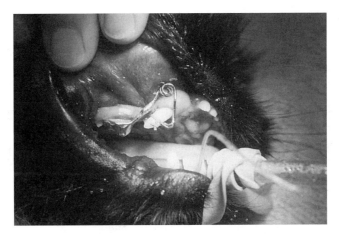

FIG. 10. Band on the upper 4th premolar with kick spring attachment designed for correction of distally inclined maxillary cuspid. Note the use of an elastic ligature to begin movement prior to engaging the kick spring to the distal surface of the cuspid.

some cases, the degree of distal cuspid inclination would result in too heavy a force being placed on the tooth, if the spring is initially brought into direct contact with the cuspid. In these cases, the spring should be allowed to pass the tooth mesially, and an elastic ligature can be tied to the spring, stretched back to the cuspid, tightened, and tied in a square knot. Once mesial movement is sufficient, the kick-spring contact should be placed against the distal surface of the cuspid and allowed to complete the movement. Once the tooth has moved into place, the appliance should be left as a retainer for 4–6 weeks, as these teeth have a strong tendency to recoil toward their original position.

True *class II malocclusions* cannot be corrected completely with orthodontics, since there is an underlying skeletal anomaly. Only orofacial surgery can properly contend with these conditions. In young animals with a deciduous class II malocclusion, interceptive orthodontics may be attempted (see Chapter 7). However, corrective and preventive orthodontics can be performed to make the occlusion functional, or corrective camouflage orthodontics to make the condition less noticeable. In this area, we will discuss only corrective and preventive orthodontics to make the occlusion functional for base narrow class II or linguodistal mandibular cuspid malocclusion. These are cases in which the mandibular canine teeth are not only base narrow or lingually inclined but also moved distally. If the occlusion is functional and causing no dental or oral trauma or predisposition to oral disease (which is unusual), there is no need to consider corrective or preventive orthodontics. There are three basic treatment options: preventive extraction (see Chapter 9), preventive crown amputation and pulp capping (see Chapter 12), or corrective orthodontic incline planes. Extraction of the mandibular cuspids results in a generalized weakening of the rostral mandible and typically should be passed over in favor of crown amputation and pulp capping. Incline planes can be designed in many cases to pass the mandibular cuspids labially, either mesially or distally to the maxillary cuspids, to provide for a functional malocclusion (see discussion of incline planes in Orthodontic Appliances and Materials above).

True *class III malocclusions*, like class II malocclusions, cannot be corrected completely with orthodontics, since there is an underlying skeletal anomaly. In young animals with a deciduous class III malocclusion, interceptive orthodontics may be attempted (see

Chapter 7). However, corrective and preventive orthodontics can be performed to make the occlusion functional, or corrective camouflage orthodontics to make the condition less discernible. In this class, only corrective and preventive orthodontics to make the occlusion functional for base narrow class III or mesiolingual mandibular cuspid malocclusion will be discussed. In these cases, the mandibular canine teeth are not only base narrow or lingually inclined but also moved mesially. If the occlusion is functional and causing no dental or oral trauma or predisposition to oral disease, there is no need to consider corrective or preventive orthodontics. There are three basic treatment options: preventive extraction (see Chapter 9), preventive crown amputation and pulp capping (see Chapter 12), or corrective orthodontic incline planes. Extraction of the mandibular cuspids results in a generalized weakening of the rostral mandible and typically should be passed over in favor of crown amputation and pulp capping, if necessary. On occasion, extraction of the maxillary corner incisors will release mesiolingual entrapped mandibular cuspids, and this is a more logical and medically sound therapy than either extraction or crown amputation and pulp capping of the mandibular cuspids. Incline planes can be designed in some minor cases to move the mandibular cuspids distally and labially into the maxillary diastema to provide for a functional malocclusion (see discussion of incline planes in Orthodontic Appliances and Materials above).

MODELS

Quality dental models and bite registrations of a patient's dental arches and supporting tissues are an excellent source for study of abnormalities and treatment planning (54). The bite registration allows for a reasonable articulating of the models to ensure that appliances fit well and without occlusal interference. Study models permit viewing of the occlusion from all aspects, accurate measurements, assessment of progress to treatment, and collaboration with colleagues and laboratory personnel. With these models, orthodontic appliances can be deliberated, designed, and fabricated. Accurate models come from good impressions, use of appropriate dental gypsum, proper mixing and pouring techniques, and appropriate model trimming. Impressions therefore are many times the foundation of orthodontic appliances.

Impression Trays Preformed and Custom

An impression tray is the apparatus that holds the soft flowable impression material around an area of arch while the material sets or firms in place to hold its negative imprint. Selection of the proper impression tray for the individual provides superior ease of taking the impression and ultimately a more accurate model. The tray should provide complete coverage of the desired area without excessive dead space. It should have a minimum of a quarter-inch clearance in all areas around the facial, lingual, distal, and occlusal surfaces of teeth, while allowing depth for impressions of soft tissues as required (55). The tray should not impinge on the soft tissues so as to distort their true perspectives. However, many trays used in veterinary dentistry are too shallow to achieve required depth. To correct this disparity, utility, box, or rope waxes can be used to extend the tray's dimensions. It is always good to do a try-in of the tray on the patient to be sure it will fit properly before actually attempting to take the impression.

There are several types of preformed impression tray sets available commercially for veterinary use, most which are designed for cats and dogs. Although all of these have deficiencies of one type or another, they are still extremely useful. Due to the wide variety of shapes and sizes encountered in veterinary subjects, no one set of impression trays can cover all situations. For these reasons, custom-made trays may be necessary on occasion.

Custom-made trays can be formed in many fashions, including with the help of a dental laboratory. Dental laboratories most commonly form custom trays from clear plastic sheets by vacuum molding or from acrylic sheets or liquids. These do require a model to begin with to form the tray on. Undercuts on the model are blocked out, and the spacing is created between tray and teeth by the application of a layer of base plate wax. If the tray is to be used for application of medicaments (eg, bleaching chemicals), then the spacer may be left out, and only the undercuts are blocked out. If the model is not totally covered with wax, exposed areas require the application of a separator to prevent bonding of resins or acrylics to the model.

For in-house fabrication, acrylics and molding resins are the most commonly use. In the use of acrylics, generally the same procedure as described previously for laboratories is used in preparation of the model for fabrication of the custom tray. Acrylics for trays come in two types: fast-set (type I) and normal-set (type II). A fast-set acrylic will gel within about 30 seconds, has around a 2.5-minute working time, and sets firm within 4 minutes from the mixing. Type II, normal-set, gels within 2 minutes, has a 4-minute working time, and sets firm within 7 minutes. Lang's Instant Tray Mix™ (Lang Dental Manufacturing Company, Wheeling, Illinois) is a typical acrylic tray mix product. The product comes as a separate powder and a liquid. The two are measured and mixed according to the manufacturer's recommendations and in a volume as needed for the case. (**Warning:** These products should be mixed in a well ventilated area and with an understanding of all of the manufacturer's precautions) (56). Once the mix begins to gel, it will become sticky to the touch and is ready to be removed from the mixing cup. Gently spread the mass over the model, molding it to the desired shape and thickness. While the substance is still in the gel stage, excess can be trimmed off with a blunt instrument and used to form a handle for the tray. Do not remove it from the model until the heat of polymerization has dissipated; otherwise, the tray may distort.

The thermal-softened dental-molding resins are used in a similar fashion as the acrylics in that undercuts must be blocked out and a separator (usually water) applied. One of the more common of these products is TrayDough™ (Hygenic Corporation, Akron, Ohio). Water is heated to 145–185°F, and the TrayDough™ resin pellets are added. Nonplastic containers should be used for the heated water, or the resin may stick to it. Once the beads become translucent, they are ready for use. Remove from the heated water with the use of a nonplastic instrument, and let the water drain off. The mass can now be kneaded into a flat sheet and then molded to the wet gypsum model. Tray resins cannot be applied to plastic models without appropriate separators. The resin will cool within 5–10 minutes, which is evident by its original color's returning, and can then be removed from the model. Most tray resins can be trimmed with scissors or a low-speed handpiece and a plastic cutting bur. Rough edges can be reduced with the use of a light flame, but care should be exercised as plastics can ignite.

Impression and Model Techniques

Orthodontic models or study casts are reproductions of the patient's teeth and arches, typically made from gypsum dental stone. These provide a permanent and lasting record of the condition and permit study and treatment planning of the condition, consultations with colleagues at leisure when the animal is not present, dental laboratory fabrication of an appropriate orthodontic appliance, and articulation of the appliance before insertion to determine any interferences. Impression must first be taken to make study models. Impressions in most animals will be taken under anesthesia. Intubation prevents obstruction of the airway by flowing impression materials, although the bite impression or registration must be taken without intubation.

The following is a basic list of required materials for obtaining impressions:

1. Impressions trays
2. Impression material (alginate type I or type II)
3. Flex bowl or mixing bowl
4. Large laboratory spatula
5. Bite wax or occlusal impression material.

Warning: Precautions must be used with powdered alginate and gypsum dusts, neither of which should not be inhaled. In addition, these products should not be poured down the drain, as they can obstruct the plumbing (56–58). Alginate blockages can usually be removed with standard plumbing techniques; however, gypsum or dental-stone blockages may necessitate replacement of drain pipes. To prevent this occurrence, various types of plaster traps can be installed.

Procedure for Taking the Impression

1. Select an impression tray that allows at least approximately one-quarter inch of space between the teeth and the tray. Excessive tray space can result in more flexibility in the impression and diminished accuracy.
2. Fluff up alginate with the lid closed by gently shaking the container. Allow most of the dust to settle before opening lid.
3. Estimate the approximate number of scoops of alginate that will be required for an impression tray by measuring the amount of dry powder required to fill the tray. After using tray a few times, you can obtain a fairly accurate knowledge of the amount truly required for each individual tray. This should be marked on the tray for future reference. Type I alginate is fast-setting, and type II alginate regular-set (59). Cool water slows setting time, and hot water speeds up setting time. For the neophyte or two-handed work, or when large amounts of impression material need to be mixed, type II regular-set alginate is generally recommended. For most four-handed (two-person) work, type I alginate will reduce the amount of time it takes for taking impressions.
4. Place the powder in the mixing bowl, and add the water. Using a spatula, mix the two together in a figure-8 fashion, until the powder is completely moistened; then spatulate the alginate against the wall of the flex bowl to aid removing air bubbles, until a creamy consistency is obtained. This should take no longer than 60 seconds.
5. With the spatula, transfer the alginate into the preselected impression tray.
6. A small amount of the alginate can be placed with a finger or spatula into small or inaccessible areas, around certain teeth, and in the roof of the mouth against the hard palate, where the alginate may not flow into well. While the alginate is still soft and putty-like, place the tray immediately into the arcade with firm pressure until the teeth and gums are well covered. Try to avoid teeth making contact with the bottom of the tray. When possible, retract the lips from the impression area.
7. Hold the tray as still as possible until the alginate sets up and is firm.

8. Once the alginate is firm, remove the impression and tray from the teeth and mouth in one clean, smooth motion.
9. Rinse the impression, if needed, to remove debris, but do not allow water to stand in the impression, as this additional water may be absorbed, causing it to swell and altering the accuracy of the model. The impressions should be kept moist by wrapping them in a moist towel until the cast or model is poured. Should the impressions dry out to any degree, they will shrink, again causing discrepancies in model accuracy. It is best to pour the model within 30 minutes of taking the impressions to reduce shrinkage of the impression and distortion of the model.
10. With the endotracheal tube removed, place a block of bite wax in the area of the mandibular right 4th premolar and close the mouth firmly to get a bite impression. This will allow the models that are eventually made to be articulated without blocking visual study of the model. Waxes rather than rubber-base materials are generally recommended for veterinary use for bite registration, because rubber-base materials require 2–5 minutes to set up. It must be remembered that your patient will be under anesthesia, with the tongue forced into the back of the throat and the mouth closed. It is not wise to run the risk of impairing proper respiration in an animal under anesthesia for this period of time. Bite wax only takes a few seconds to obtain the registration; however, it can easily be distorted if not properly handled and stored.

Pouring the Cast or Model

The following is a basic list of materials required to produce reasonably accurate models (60,61):

1. Quality impressions
2. Flex bowl or mixing bowl
3. Dental stone
4. Small cement spatula
5. Laboratory spatula
6. Vibrator.

Procedure for Pouring the Cast or Model

1. Measure out the required amount of dental stone (gypsum).
2. Add water to the powder according to the manufacturer's recommendations, and begin mixing with a lab spatula.
3. Once all the powder has been moistened, place the mixing bowl on the vibrator for 10–20 seconds to remove some of the larger air bubbles.
4. Take the impression while still in the original tray, and place it against the vibrator with the anterior portion of the arcade angled down.
5. Take a very small amount of the dental stone mix on the end of a small cement spatula, and apply to the center of the impression. The vibrations should facilitate movement of the stone down the impression and into the tooth depressions. It should fill these voids by gently flowing down the sides and filling from the bottom up. As the teeth are filled, the impression may be tilted back to a level position.
6. Once the teeth and the surface area of the impression have been filled, remove it from the vibrator.
7. Fill the rest of the impression with the stone mix using a regular size lab spatula.

8. Overfill the impression as the stone mix starts to harden to form a base on the impression for added strength, or use boxing wax to form a matrix around the impression for the buildup of stone for the base.
9. Let set for the time recommended by the manufacturer, usually 45 minutes to 1.5 hours, before removing from the impression. The impression material may separate with gentle pressure, or the impression material can be gently and carefully cut free from the cast.

Model Trimming, Identification, Treatment, and Storage

If model trimming is required, it should be done as soon as possible, before the model hardens excessively. If trimming is delayed, soaking thoroughly in water may help. Model nippers can be use to break unwanted small areas off the models, but care should be taken, as careless use can fracture the entire model. Model trimmers, sanders, stone burs, and model saws provide the best contouring.

Always label models and casts as soon as they are dry for permanent identification. Stick on labels can be attached, or a labeling pen may be used to write directly on the models. Models should normally be dated as to the date the impression was taken. Store models in appropriate storage boxes with packing material to assure long-term survival of your models.

If acrylics are to be used or formed on the models, they should be treated with a separator to prevent the acrylic from bonding to the model. Foil substitutes, separators, or petroleum jelly can be used.

If the models are to be used for display, demonstration, or educational purposes, you may wish to treat or coat them. Treatment with model soap or tincture of green soap will produce a light sheen to the model. Models can also be dipped into model resin, such as XXL Model Finish™ (Tlar Company, Pompano Beach, Forida), which leaves a glossy shine on the model surface when dry. Model hardeners, such as Stone Die Hardner™ (George Taub Products and Fusion Company, Jersey City, New Jersey), can also be applied to a dry model. These not only give a shine to the model but also improve the resistance to fracture. Most hardeners are thinned cements that penetrate well into dry gypsum models.

ORTHODONTIC LABORATORIES AND APPLIANCE PRESCRIPTIONS

Initially, it is best to work with dental laboratories that have been working with animal cases. Their knowledge can help guide you to a successful completion of your case. In filling out orthodontic prescription forms, it may be necessary for you to make a rough sketch of the desired appliance, as well as providing a written description. You should make use of the laboratory's expertise by sending your models and written prescription and then calling to discuss the case with your assigned dental technician.

BAND AND BRACKET PLACEMENT AND CEMENTATION

Site Selection

The tooth or combination of teeth used for the anchor must have a greater combined root surface than that of the tooth or teeth to be moved, or have a suitable leverage advantage (see Table 3). Sites selected on the tooth must be located so that the appliance does not obstruct normal occlusion. Additionally, the selection of the site on the tooth, apically or coronally, can provided additional leverage for movement. Generally, for a mechanical leverage advantage, the anchorage tooth site should be near the cervical third of the tooth; on the movement tooth, it should be at the mid- to coronal third of the crown.

Acid-Etching the Tooth

Enamel is smooth and the hardest substance in the body, requiring treatment to enable cementation of bracket base plates directly to the tooth (62,63). A 37% phosphoric acid solution or gel applied to the selected tooth site is customarily used to etch enamel. If dentin requires etching, the 37% phosphoric acid can be used for 10 seconds or a 10% concentration for 15 seconds. Acid-etching lightly roughens the tooth surface, allowing bonding agents, unfilled resins, and other cements to slightly penetrate the enamel or dentin and micromechanically attach.

Selection of Brackets and Custom Fitting

The design of the appliance determines the type of brackets that will be required. Ordinarily, button-type brackets use elastic chains, and slotted brackets use arch bars. The base plates of the various direct-bond brackets differ greatly in size and shape. Selection is based on the available surface space and the tooth contour at the selected site. There are plastic, ceramic, and metal brackets available. The more durable metal brackets are generally preferred for use in animals. The base of the brackets will have a rough imprinted surface or a wire mesh that allows the cement to attach to the bracket. The wire-mesh backs allow better attachment of the cements to the bracket base.

If a bracket does not fit the tooth well, it can often be custom-fitted to match the tooth's size and contours. First, the bracket base plate size can typically be reduced using a diamond point on a high-speed handpiece. Next, the base plate can be adapted to the tooth by bending it. The base plate can be placed into the grip of a three-prong bending plier and lightly squeezed. This will increase its degree of curvature. The bracket is then placed against the site for placement, and using Howe or similar pliers, it is pressed against the tooth, removing unneeded curvature and providing a good customized adaption.

Selection of Bonding Adhesive

For cementing bands on animals, glass ionomers are frequently satisfactory, but the composite resin cements are usually preferred due to their greater retentive qualities. For direct bond–type brackets, the composite resin adhesives are customarily best (64). Glass ionomers and the composite resin cements come in two types: self-curing and visible light–cured. Light-cured products can be used on any type of bracket or band, but they work best with the plastic and ceramic brackets that are clear and allow the light to penetrate well under the bracket. When light-cured adhesives are used on metal brackets or bands, the cement may not be fully cured under the brackets, although proper technique can offset much of this problem. Apply the curing light source at angles that allow it to penetrate under the edges of the band or bracket, and use a good-quality light-curing unit. The light-cured bonding agent's advantages in time and placement easily outweigh the shortcomings.

Application of Direct-Bond Bracket to Tooth

The technique of application is to center the bracket and apply firm gentle pressure until setting is complete. College cotton pliers or direct-bond bracket pliers are routinely used to hold and place the bracket on the tooth. Bracket pliers are spring-loaded to keep a firm hold of the bracket until squeezed to release the bracket. Cotton pliers require gentle pressure to keep a hold on the bracket at all times.

Application of Cement to Bands

Bands can be cemented by two techniques. The first is placement of the cement on the entire inner surface of the band before it is placed. This allows the greatest security for the band. The second technique is to apply the cement after band seating and only to a portion of the tooth just coronal to the band to hold its seating firm.

Cementation Procedure with Orthodontic Resin Cement

1. Select brackets.
2. Custom-fit brackets if required.
3. Using a dental scaler, gently clean the tooth of all gross calculus, plaque, and debris.
4. Using a prophylaxis angle and cup, polish the surface where the bracket is to be applied with flour of pumice and distilled water. Avoid the use of prophylaxis pastes, as most have fluoride, which inhibits the effects of acids, and oils or waxes that prevent the acid from making good contact with the tooth surface.
5. Rinse debris, etc., using water and a three-way syringe.
6. Dry the tooth with a moisture-free and oil-free source (electric dryer or filtered air source).
7. Place a small amount of acid-etchant in a Dappen dish or on a sheet from a paper mixing pad.
8. Using a small application brush, apply a small amount of the acid-etchant to the tooth. Etch only the area where the bracket or band is to be attached.
9. Leave the acid-etchant in contact with the tooth for the recommended time, and then thoroughly rinse the etchant from the tooth by flushing with water for approximately 20 seconds.
10. Dry the tooth with the moisture- and oil-free air.
11. If the site has been properly etched, it should turn a chalky-white color when dried. If this is not apparent, repeat steps 3 through 10.
12. Apply bonding agent according to the manufacturer's recommendations.
13. Carefully remove excess cement, and cure or allow to set.
14. Using the cotton pliers, very gently rock the bracket or band to see if it is well bonded. If it remains attached, proceed to the next bracket or band.
15. Should a bracket fail to attach properly, discard it. With bands, clean it thoroughly by scaling and polishing with flour of pumice. Then repeat the entire procedure from step 1, being sure to remove all of the old cement from the tooth.

HOME CARE INSTRUCTIONS

When orthodontic appliances are placed in an animal's mouth, the owner needs to be aware of the home care and supervision that is required to help in ensuring the best outcome possible. A basic handout outlining owner responsibilities is warranted to reduce confusion. Typical home care instructions for owners to follow include:

1. The patient with corrective orthodontic appliances in its mouth needs special care to help assure safe, speedy, and successful results.
2. The appliance in your pet's mouth should be examined at least two to three times a day to make sure it is in place, working properly, and not causing problems for your pet.
3. Your pet will need to be on a soft diet during treatment and be kept from chewing on materials (eg, chew toys, bone, etc.) that might loosen the appliance or pop brackets off.
4. Try to keep the appliance clean by gently flushing it with a syringe of water at least once daily. Buildup of food and debris under or around the appliance can cause inflammation and infection.
5. Should hair or material become entangled around the appliance or brackets, be careful in attempting to remove it, as you may pop a bracket or elastic free from its functional position.
6. If inflammation, ulceration, or soreness occurs, check with the clinic about the proper care. Soreness may indicate that the appliance is applying too much force and tooth movement may need to be slowed. Ulcerations may indicate that brackets need to have orthodontic wax applied on a regular basis to protect the lips and gums.
7. If something does not look right, call the clinic for instructions.
8. If you cannot contact someone and feel the appliance is causing problems, disconnect or cut any elastics that appear to be causing a problem, and continue to call the clinic.
9. For your pet's appliance to work efficiently, the doctor needs to check your pet on a regular basis. Be sure to schedule appointments for these rechecks. Unsupervised appliances can cause serious damage to your pet's teeth, so keep your scheduled appointments.

RETENTION PERIOD AND RETAINERS

Once active movement has accomplished the desired tooth movements, it is necessary to retain the teeth in their new location (1). The alveolar bone, gingival tissues, and periodontal ligament have been undergoing remodeling and reorganization during tooth movement. For the tooth to stabilize, the bone must transform into firm compact bone, the gingivae must reorganize, and periodontal ligament must tighten. If the teeth are not retained during this transitional period, they may partially recoil or totally return to their original position. Retainers can be fixed or removable. To conserve time, materials, and anesthetics, it is common in veterinary orthodontics to let the primary corrective appliance also act as the retainer. This approach allows for quick response by reactivation of the appliance should recoil commence. In simple movements, a retainer time of 2–6 weeks is required. In more complex movements and those involving torsiversion, 4–12 weeks is recommended. Occasionally, the actual scissors bite or cuspid interlock of the occlusion may act a natural self-retainer. Successful retention depends on correct diagnosis and treatment. Teeth moved to a nonharmonious position typically cannot be stabilized. Histologic studies indicate that alveolar bone is significantly more responsive to pressure for up to 6 months after orthodontic tooth movement (1). Therefore, retention followed by a retention-observation period is highly recommended.

APPLIANCE REMOVAL

Proper removal of an appliance is an intricate component in the successful final results of orthodontic treatment. Crude removal technique can result in enamel fractures and scarification. Failure to remove cements and polish the surface can result in easy plaque accumulation and possible gingivitis. If the surface appears porous, it should be sealed by bonding with an unfilled resin to prevent discoloration from mineral absorption.

Many metal matrix sheet bands can be removed by using an ultrasonic scaler across the surface to loosen the cement and then using the tip of a scaler to hook the cervical line of the band and lift up. Others may require the use of band-removal pliers. The cushioned beak is placed on the cusp, and the other beak positioned under the cervical margin of the band. The handles are then gently squeezed together.

On cast metal bands, a more aggressive approach may be needed. A crown puller may need to be used on the cervical line of the band. If excess cement is present around the band, it can be removed by either using a rotary scaler bur or white-stone point on a high-speed handpiece. Additionally, the bands may need to be cut. A crosscut bur used carefully along the lingual surface of the band to cut it from cervical to coronal margin can be useful. A crown splitter or small screw driver inserted into the slot cut into the band and then rotated slightly will usually separate the band and break loose the cementation. Always make the cut on the lingual surface of the band, in case scarification occurs.

Brackets are usually not difficult to remove. A scaling bur or white stone can be used to remove excess cement. Band-removal pliers used with the cushioned beak placed on the cusp and the other beak under the cervical area of the bracket base plate, and gently squeezed, will remove most. Additionally, needle holders can be used to grasp the bracket and can then be gently rotated back and forth to break the cementation. Always use gentle force, as rapid or uncontrolled movements may fracture the enamel.

Once the appliance is removed, carefully remove all remaining cement with a scaler. Any hard-to-remove material may require the use of a rotary scaling bur or a white-stone point. Inspect the oral cavity for signs of injury to teeth or soft tissues, and treat as required. Polish the tooth with an extrafine prophylaxis paste, and apply a fluoride treatment.

COMPLICATIONS FROM TREATMENT

Deleterious effects from orthodontic force in animals have been recorded (34,65). The four principal areas where effects have been noted are crestal alveolar bone, root structure, periodontal ligament and alveolar attachment, and pulp. Other problems are tooth discoloration, appliance-associated soft tissue trauma, hygiene problems, contact allergy, and elastic slippage.

Remodeling of the *crestal alveolar bone*, as well as the rest of the alveolar bone, occurs during orthodontic movement (10). Orthodontic movements and hygiene problems associated with appliances can contribute to gingival inflammation, which can affect crestal bone loss. However, only the slight loss of height of less than a 0.5 mm is typically seen as a complication of orthodontic treatments, with loss greater than 1.0 mm being rare (6,67). Luckily, alveolar bone will ordinarily "travel" with the tooth, except in certain disease states, such as uncontrolled active periodontal disease. However, even patients with periodontal disease can have orthodontics, if the active disease is under control and sufficient alveolar bone is still present to stabilize the tooth after movement.

When teeth are extruded in a physiologic movement, the alveolar bone will travel with the tooth. This results in the height of the alveolar crest being higher in the arch after treatment but still in approximately the same relationship to the tooth. Conversely, teeth that are intruded have a loss of alveolar height in the arch (68).

Root structure is also affected during orthodontic treatment (69). Tooth movement is only possible due to the periodontal ligament's activity in resorption and apposition of adjacent hard tissues, primarily the alveolar bone (10). However, the remodeling of hard tissues initiated by the periodontal ligament does include some remodeling involving the root structures which are also contiguous with the periodontal ligament. The root cementum repairs itself during periods of quiescence of force (70). Areas of dentinal exposure may also undergo resorption, but repairs are also with cementum, not dentin (10). This means that root remodeling is a constant feature of active corrective orthodontics but that permanent loss of root structure only occurs when cementum is not replaced.

Repair of root cementum is not possible if the cementum becomes separated from the root surface. This can occur in rapid or severe resorptive activity. Such occurrences can take place at any point on the root, but the apex is the most susceptible region due to its anatomic shape. Therefore, root loss primarily occurs at the apex, with some loss in the lateral root walls (10). Some small degree of root loss is probable in almost every orthodontically treated patient, but it is generally minimal and clinically insignificant. However, in some cases, more severe resorption may occur. Resorption may be classified as to degree (71) (Table 6).

In humans, certain teeth have been shown to have a greater probability of having root resorption. These are the maxillary and mandibular incisors and the mandibular 1st molar. Additionally, teeth that have been endodontically treated and have pointed apices, dilacerated roots, a history of trauma, or severe periodontal disease are more susceptible (72,73). Resorption is also more common when excessive or prolonged forces are used. In addition, some individuals are more prone to resorption whether or not orthodontic treatment is performed. However, most of these factors do not play a role in severe or category 3 root resorption. One factor has been shown to be major in the occurrence of severe resorption: root contact with cortical bone (71). This most commonly occurs in cases of orthodontic camouflage treatment of mild class II or class III malocclusion. In these cases, teeth are tilted or rotated to an angle that may force root structure to make contact with the cortical plates.

The *periodontal ligament* is responsible not only for alveolar remodeling but also for its own reorganization during orthodontic treatment (10). The reorganization is necessary for the ligament to detach from the cementum or alveolar bone during movement and

TABLE 6. *Classification of root resorption*

Category	Degree of root loss
0	No loss
1	Slight blunting of apex
2	Moderate resorption: <25% root loss
3	Severe resorption: >25% root loss

(Adapted from ref. 71.)

then to reattach later at more harmonious locations. The periodontal ligament space widens during orthodontic movement due to resorptive activity, which can be seen radiographically in many cases. This, in combination with the reorganization of the periodontal ligament itself, results in a degree of tooth mobility during tooth movements. Excessive mobility is typically an indication of the use of excessive force for movement. When teeth begin to demonstrate signs of excessive mobility, all force should be removed and oral hygiene intensified, until the teeth once again become stable.

The use of heavy force should be avoided, if at all possible, due to the possible complications. Pain during movement with this level of force is common as a result of ischemia of the periodontal ligament and pressures on the apical structures causing a pulpitis (34). The pain often does not occur until several hours after application of the excessive force. Should an owner call concerning a patient with signs of such, instructions to relieve the force should be given, if possible. If the appliance is such that the owner cannot disconnect the force, temporary relief may be obtained by massaging of the affected teeth, which alleviates some of the pressure and allows some blood flow to the ischemic areas.

The use of corticosteroids and nonsteroidal anti-inflammatory drugs (NSAIDs) helps moderate pain and inflammation by interfering with the synthesis of prostaglandins, a major participant in the development of inflammation. Corticosteroids affect this synthesis by helping inhibit the development of the prostaglandin precursor, arachidonic acid. NSAIDs work by blocking some degree of the conversion of arachidonic acid to prostaglandins. However, some degree of inflammation is required for tooth movement (74), and research in animals has shown that many of these drugs slow the rate of orthodontic tooth movement (34,75). This would indicate that if an anti-inflammatory drug or pain medication if used in high enough dosages, could prevent tooth movement.

Ischemic episodes in the periodontal ligament can have other serious consequences. Ischemic areas may undergo necrosis, leaving cementum and alveolar bone in intimate contact. This may result in ankylosis of the root and the inability to move the tooth orthodontically (76). In addition, the ankylosed areas may eventually undergo inflammatory resorption (76).

Under normal circumstances, the *pulp* should have only minimal response to light orthodontic forces. There is a transient reversible pulpitis at the initiation of treatment, probably due to the early response to pressures on the apical vascular and nervous supply (34). This response possibly contributes to the discomfort occasionally seen following activation or reactivation of the appliance; however, it has no long-term significance (10). Loss of tooth vitality can occur under certain conditions. Teeth with a history of past injury are more susceptible to pulpitis, while those with excessive force applied may experience constrained vascular flow and those with misdirected application of force may have the apex moved outside of the alveolus, severing the vascular supply (10). A vital pulp is not required for orthodontic movement; therefore, endodontically treated teeth can be moved as long as a healthy periodontal ligament is present (10,34). However, some studies have indicated that endodontically treated teeth that are moved orthodontically are slightly more prone to root resorption problems, but endodontically treated teeth are generally slightly more prone to root resorption than healthy vital teeth even without orthodontics (69).

Tooth discoloration is typically due to one of two problems: metal impregnation or devitalization. Devitalization generally causes a pink, blue, gray, or beige tooth discoloration. This occurrence requires endodontic assessment (see Chapter 11). Metal impregnation is a result of metal ionization from the base plate or band on the tooth and its penetration into the tooth (77). Ionized metal particles can enter a tooth surface more easily when it is weakened by disease or iatrogenic means. For this reason, all cavity-type lesions should be well cared for. Additionally, in the application of brackets or bands, acid-etching should performed only in the necessary areas, and good oral hygiene for the patient should be encouraged. Some superficial metal discoloration can be removed by polishing, but deeper stains may require a cosmetic restorative camouflage of veneering.

Appliance-associated trauma can occur from many causes. Brackets may cause physical irritation to the lingual and buccal mucosa. This can be controlled by covering them with Hug Caps™ (Orthodontic Supply and Equipment, Gaithersburg, Maryland) or a small amount of a rubber-base impression material. Either lacerations by elastics must be endured, or the elastics must be removed and the appliance readapted to prevent interference.

Hygiene is an owner/patient responsibility. When materials accumulate near the gingiva margins, gingivitis is sure to follow. If materials are allowed to collect under appliance bases covering the plate, a palatitis will result and can sometimes be severe (50). On occasion, actual contact allergies to the materials from which the appliance is constructed may occur. In these cases, either the appliance must be removed and designed with new materials, or anti-inflammatory drugs must be initiated, possibly impeding orthodontic movements.

Elastic slippage is a problem that must be carefully monitored. Simple slippage should be corrected by either movement of the elastic or a new anchorage point designed to prevent it. Should elastics slip under the gingival margin, they can do serious damage to the epithelial attachment. Should the slippage go unnoticed for any period of time, it may cut under the root of the tooth, effectively amputating it. Therefore, elastic placements and progress should be closely observed and recorded until removal.

SUMMARY

Initial involvement with orthodontics should generally be made with a knowledgeable mentor for guidance, as problems or complications are not uncommon for the neophyte. It takes time, knowledge, and experience to properly assess and treat the numerous variations of malocclusions seen in veterinary dentistry.

REFERENCES

1. White TC, Gardiner JH, Leighton BC. *Orthodontics for Dental Students*. 2nd ed. St.Louis, MO: Warren H. Green; 1967:13.
2. *Dentists' Desk Reference*. Chicago: American Dental Association; 1983:182.
3. Ross DA. Orthodontics for the dog: Bite evaluation, basic concepts and equipment. *Vet Clin North Am* 1986; 16:955.
4. Corrucini RS, Pacciani E. Orthodontistry and dental occlusion in Etruscans. *Angle Orthod* 1989;59:61.
5. Weinberger BW. The historical background of modern orthodontics. In: Dewey M, Anderson GM. *Practical Orthodontic*. 6th ed. St. Louis, Mo: CV Mosby Co.; 1942:35.
6. Weinberger BW. *Orthodontics: An Historical Review of Its Origin and Evolution*. St.Louis, MO: CV Mosby Co; 1926:245.
7. Kingsley NW. *Treatise on Oral Deformities as a Branch of Mechanical Surgery*. New York: Appleton; 1880:1.
8. Torres HO, Ehrlich A. *Modern Dental Assisting*. 2nd ed. Philadelphia: WB Saunders Co; 1980:882.
9. Koch C.. *History of Dental Surgery*. Fort Wayne, IN: National Art Publisher; 1910;1:113.
10. Proffit WR, Fields HW. *Contemporary Orthodontics*. 2nd ed. St.Louis, MO: Mosby-Year Book; 1992:2.
11. Angle EH. *The Angle System of Regulation and Retention of the Teeth and Treatment of Fractures of the Maxillae*. 5th ed. Philadelphia: SS White Manufacturing Co; 1899:1.
12. Grove TK. Orthodontic treatment aids in better function. *Pet Talk* Summer 1990:2.
13. Merow WW. Orthodontics. In: Steele PF, ed. *Dental Specialties for the Dental Hygienist*. Philadelphia: Lea & Febiger; 1972:173.

14. Caring for animals. *1995 AVMA Membership Directory and Resource Manual; Principles of Veterinary Medical Ethics.* 44th ed. Schaumburg, IL: American Veterinary Medical Association; 1995.

15. *The Complete Dog Book: An Official Publication of the American Kennel Club.* New York: Howell Book House; 1973:24.

16. Grove TK. Orthodontic techniques can be more effective in treating malocclusion. *DVM Magazine* Apr 1989:1.

17. Stockard CR, Johnson AL. *Genetic and Endocrine Basis for Differences in Form and Behavior.* Philadelphia: Wistar Institute of Anatomy and Biology; 1941:149.

18. Nelson RM. Orthodontics. In: Richardson RE, Barton RE, eds. *The Dental Assistant.* 5th ed. New York: McGraw-Hill Book Co; 1978:527.

19. Moss JP, Picton DCA. Experimental mesial drift in adult monkeys (*Macaca irus*). *Arch Oral Biol* 1967;12:1313.

20. Anderson JG, Harvey CE. Odontogenic cysts. *J Vet Dent* 1993;10(4):5.

21. Lobprise HB, Wiggs RB. Crown amputation and vital pulpotomy to resolve an unusual orthodontic problem in a kinkajou. *J Vet Dent* 1993;10(3):14.

22. Wiggs RB. Basics of orthodontics. *AVDS Proc* 1993:15.

23. Emily P. Adolescent dentistry. *Am Vet Dent Coll/Acad Vet Dent Proc* 1991.

24. Andreasen JO. The influences of traumatic intrusion of primary teeth on the permanent successors: A radiographic and histologic study in monkeys. *Int J Oral Surg* 1976;5:207.

25. Eisner ER. Malocclusions in cats and dogs: Recognizing dental misalignments; selecting the proper therapy. *Vet Med* Oct 1988:1006.

26. Lindhe J, Svanberg G. Influence of trauma from occlusion on progression of experimental periodontitis in the Beagle dog. *J Clin Periodontol* 1984;11:63.

27. Ericsson I, Thilander B, Lindhe J, et al. The effect of orthodontic tilting movements on the periodontal tissues of infected and non-infected dentition in dogs. *J Clin Periodontol* 1991;18:182.

28. Artum J, Urbue KS. The effect of orthodontic treatment on periodontal bone support in patients with advanced loss of marginal periodontium. *Am J Orthod Dentofacial Orthop* 1988;93:143.

29. Graber TM. *Orthodontics: Principles and Practice.* 3rd ed. Philadelphia: WB Saunders Co; 1972.

30. Begg PR, Kessling PC. *Begg Orthodontic Theory and Technique.* 2nd Ed. Philadelphia: WB Saunders Co; 1971.

31. Smith MM, Massoudi LM. Potential attachment area of the fourth maxillary premolar in dogs. *Am J Vet Res* 1991;52:626.

32. Smith MM, Massoudi LM. Potential attachment area of the first mandibular molar in dogs. *Am J Vet Res* 1992; 53:258.

33. Shijo H. An experimental study on effects of the temporomandibular joint in the dog following malocclusion. *J Kyushu Dent Soc* 1990;44:932.

34. Anstendig H, Kronmam J. A histologic study of pulpal reaction to orthodontic tooth movement in dogs. *Angle Orthod* 1972;42:50.

35. Iwai A. Histological study on the changes in the periodontal tissues with labial tipping movement of tooth, in dogs. *J Kyushu Dent Soc* 1990;44:408.

36. Breitner C. Further investigations of bone changes resulting from experimental orthodontic treatment in monkeys. *Year Book of Dentistry.* 1942. Abstract.

37. Weigel JP, Dorn AS. Diseases of the jaws and abnormal occlusion. In: Harvey CE, ed. *Veterinary Dentistry.* Philadelphia: WB Saunders Co; 1985:106.

38. Moyers RE. Biomechanics of tooth movements. In: Moyers RE, ed. *Handbook of Orthodontics.* 3rd ed. Chicago: Yearbook Medical Publishers; 1973.

39. Seiders GW. Orthodontic principles. *Dent Clin North Am* 1972;16:439.

40. Lyons K. *J Vet Dent* 1990;7(3):cover.

41. Schlossberg A. The removable orthodontic appliance. *Dent Clin North Am* 1972;16:487.

42. Way DC. Direct bonding and its application to minor tooth movement. *Dent Clin North Am* 1978;22:757.

43. Thurow RC. *Edgewise Orthodontics.* 3rd ed. St.Louis, MO: CV Mosby Co; 1972.

44. Burstone CJ, Goldberg AJ. Beta titanium, a new orthodontic alloy. *Am J Orthod* 1980;77:121.

45. New American Dental Association Specification No.32 for orthodontic wires not containing precious metals. *JADA* 1977;95:1169.

46. Viazis AD. *Atlas of Orthodontics: Princples and Clinical Applications.* Philadelphia: WB Saunders Co; 1993.

47. Grove TK. Direct bond brackets for orthodontics. *Vet Forum* July 1987:20.

48. Cahill DR. The histology and rate of tooth eruption with and without temporary impaction in the dog. *Anat Rec* 1970;166:238.

49. Gilmore CA, Little RM. Mandibular incisor dimensions and crowding. *Am J Orthod* 1984;86:493.

50. Kertesz P. *A Color Atlas of Veterinary Dentistry and Oral Surgery.* Aylesbury, UK: Wolfe Publishing; 1993:71.

51. Goldstein GS. Basic orthodontics in dogs. *Friskes Vet J* Spring 1992:13.

52. Lyon KF. The straight and base narrow. *Vet Forum* Mar 1990:50.

53. Grove TK. A simple technique for correction of rostrally displaced canine teeth. *Vet Forum* June 1987:10.

54. Chadha JM, Rayson JH. Diagnostic Casts. In: Clark JW, ed. *Clinical Dentistry.* Vol 1. Hagerstown, MD: Harper & Row Publishers; 1981:1.

55. Wilkins ES. *Clinical Practice of the Dental Hygienist.* 5th ed. Philadelphia: Lea & Febiger; 1983:167.

56. Brune D, Beltesbrekke H. Dust and vapors in dental laboratories, part III: Efficiency of ventilation systems and face masks. *J Prosthet Dent* 1980;44:211.

57. Mack PJ. Inhalation of alginate powder during spatulation. *Br Dent J* 1978;146:141.
58. Brune D, Beltesbrekke H. Levels of airborne particles resulting from handling alginate impression materials. *Scand J Dent Res* 1978;86:206.
59. American Dental Association, Council on Dental Materials, Instruments and Equipment. Certification and acceptance programs. *JADA* 1980;101:68.
60. Rigsby BE, Wyss HE. Pouring and trimming casts. In: Peterson S, ed. *The Dentist and the Assistant.* 4th ed. St.Louis, MO: CV Mosby Co; 1977:217.
61. Rudd KD, Morrow RM. A simplified method for mixing stone. *J Prosthet Dent* 1974;32:675.
62. Retief DH, Sadowsky PL. Clinical experience with acid etch techniques in orthodontics. *Am J Orthod* 1975; 68:645.
63. Zachrisson BU. A post-treatment evaluation of direct bonding in orthodontics. *Am J Orthod* 1977;71:173.
64. Retief DH, Dreyer CJ, Gavron G. The direct bonding of orthodontic attachments to teeth by means of an epoxy resin adhesive. *Am J Orthod* 1967:58:21.
65. Goldman HM, Gianelly AA. Histology of tooth movement. *Dent Clin North Am* 1972;16:439.
66. Kennedy DB, Joondeph DR, Osterburg SK, Little RM. The effect of extraction and orthodontic treatment on dentoalveolar support. *Am J Orthod* 1983;84:183.
67. Sharpe W, Reed B, Subtelny JD, Polson A. Orthodontic relapse, apical root resorption and crestal alveolar bone levels. *Am J Orthod Dentofacial Orthop* 1987;91:252.
68. Ingber JS. Forced eruption: Alterations of soft tissue cosmetic deformities. *Int J Periodontal Rest Dent* 1989; 9:417.
69. Wickwire NA, McNeil M, Norton LA, Duell RC, et al. The effects of tooth movement upon endodontically treated teeth. *Angle Orthod* 1974;44:235.
70. Reitan K. Biomedical principles and reactions. In: Graber TM, Swain BF, eds. *Orthodontics: Principles and Technique.* St.Louis, MO: Mosby-Year Book; 1985.
71. Kaley JD, Phillips C. Root resorption. *Angle Orthod* 1991;61:125.
72. Newman WG. Possible etiologic factors in external root resorption. *Am J Orthod* 1975;67:522.
73. Remington DN, Joondeph DR, Artun J, et al. Long-term evaluation of root resorption occurring during orthodontic treatment. *Am J Orthod Dentofacial Orthop* 1989;96:43.
74. Rodan GA, Yeh CK, Thompson DT. Prostaglandins and bone. In: Norton LA, Burstone CJ, eds. *The Biology of Orthodontic Tooth Movement.* Boca Raton, FL: CRC Press; 1989.
75. Davidovitch Z, Shamfield JL. Cyclic nucleotide levels in alveolar bone of orthodontically treated cats. *Arch Oral Biol* 1975;20:567.
76. Guyman CG, Kokich VG, Oswald RJ. Ankylosed teeth as abutments for palatal expansion in the rhesus monkey. *Am J Orthod* 1980;77:486.
77. Maijer R, Lux J, Smith DC. Enamel staining associated with biodegradation of orthodontic bracket bases. *J Dent Res* 1982;61:328. Abstract 1350.

16

Domestic Feline Oral and Dental Disease

Robert B. Wiggs and Heidi B. Lobprise

While there are certainly many similarities in dentistry between cats and dogs, there are also certain considerations that are unique to cats. This chapter will focus on the anatomic variations, disease processes, and treatments that are distinctly feline to complement, but not duplicate, information in previous chapters.

PHYSICAL EXAMINATION

The average feline patient can sometimes be more of a challenge to handle, particularly when it comes to looking at a painful mouth. The initial examination can be quite limited by the temperament of the individual, so full assessment may not be possible until sedation or anesthesia has been administered (see Chapters 4 and 21).

Externally, cellulitis and abscess formation around the facial area may be due to fight wounds, which may mimic dental problems. Swelling of the lips due to eosinophilic granulomas or tumors can also be seen. A general asymmetry of the head can indicate genetic abnormalities or traumatic injuries, such as temporomandibular dislocations or fractures of the mandible or maxilla. Facial asymmetry in Persian cats is not uncommon due to wry mouth, developing secondary to unfavorable deciduous malocclusions of the cuspids.

The oral examination itself should cover all areas, including the sublingual region, to check for linear foreign bodies. In cats, strings or the needles attached to them can be lodged under or around the tongue, with the remainder extending into the intestinal tract. Visualization of the area can be facilitated by pushing a finger up into the intermandibular space to lift the tongue (1). Sublingual oral masses (ranulas), tumors, and foreign bodies can also be examined for in this way. The glossopalatine arches or fauces should also be examined for indications of stomatitis.

ORAL ANATOMY

The dental structures of the dog and cat are anatomically similar, with differences in tooth size, shape, and number. The feline dentition serves a more truly carnivorous function, with few occlusal surfaces.

The dental formula for cats is as follows (2):

Deciduous: (Id 3/3, Cd 1/1, Pd 3/2) × 2 = 26
Permanent: (I 3/3, C 1/1, P 3/2, M 1/1) × 2 = 30

TABLE 1. *Eruption times of deciduous and permanent teeth in the cat*

	Deciduous teeth (wk)	Permanent teeth (mo)
Incisors	2–3	3–4
Cuspids	3–4	4–5
Premolars	3–6	4–6
Molars		4–6

In cats, current scientific thinking is that the premolars that are "missing" from a true phenotypically complete dental formula—(3/3, 1/1, 4/4, 3/3) × 2 = 44)—are actually the most mesial or rostral ones toward the front; that is, the upper premolars should be numbered from 2–4, and the lower premolars should be numbered 3 and 4 (3) (see Chapters 3 and 4).

In addition to a knowledge of the eruption patterns of the deciduous and permanent dentitions in cats (Table 1), it is important to be familiar with number of root tips of the various teeth, particularly in exodontia (extractions) and endodontics (root canal procedure) (2):

One root   All incisors, canines, upper 2nd premolars
Three roots   Upper 4th premolars, upper 1st molar
Two roots   All others

In theory, the upper 1st molar in the domestic cat is a three-rooted tooth. However, clinically, because of its diminutive size in most domestic cats, the classic root structure can be difficult to identify. In addition, close examination of the apical portion of this tooth demonstrates clinical variations. Some of these exhibit no remarkable root structure and appear to almost have a generalized delta across the apical expanse.

ORAL DISEASE

Of oral diseases in cats, periodontal disease is the most commonly encountered. The pathogenesis of bacterial plaque accumulation on the tooth surface to initiate the disease process, including host response, is the same as in many species. In addition to oral bacteria in cats, infectious viral agents have a probable yet indistinct association with the pathogenesis of many forms of oral disease (4). Feline calicivirus (FCV) has been isolated from some cats with moderate-to-severe ulcerative periodontitis, and gingivitis/stomatitis is a frequent finding in cats affected by feline leukemia virus (FeLV) or feline immunodeficiency virus (FIV) (5–8), probably due to their immunosuppressive effects (8). An exact cause-and-effect relationship has not been accurately established for FCV alone, and the role of any two or all three viruses seems to be a synergistic influence on the severity of the disease rather than a absolute increase in prevalence as compared with negative cats (9). Future studies will most likely delineate the viral etiology more completely.

Periodontal Disease

Periodontal disease appears to have its beginnings in young animals as soon as the tooth structure emerges. The early signs of adult periodontitis can be found in immature animals (10,11), including many young cats and kittens (12–14). However, without a doubt, the process leading to periodontal disease begins shortly after eruption, when the tooth is initially exposed to oral microflora. Therefore, the need for appropriate home care in both oral care and diet should be properly emphasized and explained when a kitten is initially examined (see Chapter 21).

Numerous forms of periodontitis occur, each advancing to contribute to attachment loss at variable rates (15–17). Currently, there are five common international pathobiologic classifications of periodontitis for humans. To allow an improved cross-reference of information and use of materials, these same categories have been used in animal classifications (12,13). The categories include adult periodontitis, rapidly progressive periodontitis, localized juvenile periodontitis, prepubertal periodontitis, and refractory rapidly progressive periodontitis (18–23). (These forms of periodontal disease are discussed in more detail in Chapter 8.)

Adult periodontitis (*AP*) is actually instigated shortly after tooth eruption in young animals, but because of its slow progression, it typically does not clinically reveal itself until the animal is an adult and the disease is more advanced (12). Only histology and certain specialized tests have been reasonably reliable in diagnosing AP earlier (24–34). *Rapidly progressive periodontitis* (*RPP*) is a rapidly progressive and generalized form seen mostly in young adult animals, such as in the greyhound, Maltese cat, and Shih Tzu (12). It is typical to see highly inflamed gingival tissue and rapid attachment loss in RPP. *Localized juvenile periodontitis* (*LJP*) is a rapidly progressive localized periodontitis seen to begin development in young animals, as is commonly seen in the mandibular or maxillary incisor region of the miniature schnauzer (13). *Prepubertal periodontitis* (*PP*) is a very rapidly progressing periodontitis found in association with the deciduous dentition. Many cases are simply eruptive gingivitis that has been complicated by rampant oral infection requiring intensive therapy to control. PP may later progress to RPP or even *refractory RPP* (*RRPP*), as some cases may be associated with other diseases or hereditary problems that inhibit normal immune responses. This situation is possibly most commonly seen in young Somali and Abyssinian cats exhibiting lymphocytic plasmocytic stomatitis or FIV involvement (12,35). RRPP, a therapy-resistant periodontitis subform of RPP, may be seen in young or old animals (18–23).

The progression of periodontal disease in cats parallels that in dogs, with differences seen primarily in the extent of the gingival pocket depth, attachment loss as related to tooth size, and bacterial combinations involved. Clinical staging of the grade of periodontal disease in cats, as other species, is done in order to group the type of treatment that is generally appropriate to arrest the disease progression. There are many staging indices, but the following four-stage index is simple for the veterinarian or technician to use, yet clinically highly effective in treatment planning. *Stage I periodontal disease* refers to those conditions of subclinical to more advanced gingivitis with minimal inflammatory changes and minimal to no changes in normal sulcus depth. Any variation is usually attributable to gingival swelling, and not to attachment loss. In stage I disease, the probe can occasionally be introduced 0.5 mm into the crevice, but this depth is usually due to slight inflammation/edema of the gingival margin. Additionally, gingivitis can be indexed into three grades (see Dental and Oral Indices in the Appendix). In *stage II periodontal disease*, inflammation of the periodontal ligament and crestal bone loss are initiated. Pocket depth may increase, but instead of pocket formation, cats may start to develop areas of exposed root structure due to gingival recession and the beginning of attachment loss. As another indication of inflammatory disease, this root exposure uncovers cementum surfaces that are often more sensitive to pain and possibly more susceptible to pathologic changes such as resorptive lesions. The sulcal depth and/or amount of root exposure is still close to the normal range (less than 25% attachment loss or approximately less than 1 mm), and the gingiva is more hyperemic with an increase in sulcal fluid. In *stage III periodontal disease*, inflammation of the periodontal ligament progresses to moderate attachment loss, sulcal pocket depth and/or root exposure increases (up to 2.0 mm), and there is a loss of 25–50% of the bony support, resulting in slight tooth mobility at times. Gingival recession is often more noticeable with advancement of lesions, and radiographs are helpful in monitoring bone loss. *Stage IV periodontal disease* encompasses multiple symptoms of deep pocket/root exposure combinations (theoretically of 2 mm or more, which would be difficult to attain in some teeth of the cat), significant alveolar bone loss (50% or greater), and moderate to great tooth mobility in some teeth. Root exposure can be quite extensive, particularly in cuspids, where over half of the root structure may eventually be uncovered. While not as common in dogs, the chance of an oronasal fistula developing with an infected cuspid may be likely in cats (36). Another sequela may be the formation of reactive bone tissue or even osteomyelitis as a result of chronic periodontal disease (37). Lesions on feline cuspids are more comparable to the situation in humans and dogs, where normal pocket depth is 2–3 mm and a pocket depth of 4–5 mm is substantial. Beyond that depth, the point to which standard periodontal instruments can reach subgingivally, more extensive work with flaps and even regenerative procedures may be attempted (38). With severe lesions, extraction and corrective surgery (alveoloplasty, fistula closure) may be necessary.

Throughout the periodontal examination and treatment, indications of cervical line lesions may be present: hyperplastic gingiva or calculus filling in the defect, involuntary twitching when the sensitive lesion is touched, "hooking" of the pointed explorer end in the concave defect itself. The explorer should be used with great care, so as not to damage any soft tissue, including the epithelial attachment at the depth of the sulcus. This curved, sharp-pointed device is a tactile instrument and can also be used to detect soft carious lesions or subgingival deposits of calculus.

Radiology is another important diagnostic tool, used to discern any alveolar bone loss, tooth or root resorption, and fractures. Intraoral films are extremely useful in the feline mouth and are relatively easy and inexpensive to use (see Chapter 6).

Treatment

It has been estimated that by age 6 years up to 85% of cats have stage 2 or higher periodontal disease that would benefit from some form of treatment (39). Additionally, a study of attachment loss and changes in sulcal enzymes has demonstrated better than a 70% periodontal disease rate in cats approximately 2 years of age (40). To effectively deal with periodontal disease progression in cats, an extensive prophylaxis regimen is required in coordination with regular dental home care (see Chapter 8). Some felines will allow the owner to brush their teeth using a small cat toothbrush. A 45° angle of the bristles into the sulcus and brushing coronally are enhanced with gels and toothpastes, either nonflavored or in a flavor to suit a cat. Daily brushing is ideal, but one to three times weekly is generally recommended. One study indicates that cats that had their teeth brushed one to two times per week showed 95% less calculus than the control group, and those brushed once a week had 76% less (41). The use of oral rinses or gels containing a dilute chlorhexidine or zinc ascorbate compound may be used in conjunction with brushing or alone if brushing is not well tolerated. Weekly stannous fluoride applications would be beneficial to aid in plaque control, but possibly more so in cats with a history of feline dental resorptive lesions. For judicious (small amounts, weekly) use of these products, owners need to be informed of the potential toxicities of excess amounts of ingested fluoride.

While the progression of periodontal disease is the same in cats and dogs, special attention must be given in cats to the smaller, more delicate teeth and diminished sulcal pockets. Even relatively small amounts of attachment loss (1–2 mm) can indicate severe changes in cats warranting more aggressive therapy with gingival flaps and root planing. Loss of attachment only around the distal root of the lower molar might be managed with root resection and removal of that portion, coupled with endodontics of the larger mesial root to preserve it, if still periodontally healthy. Any lesion, particularly sensitive areas or those covered by hyperplastic gingiva, deserves careful examination with an explorer to detect any resorptive lesions. Radiographs may be required to determine root viability or evidence of resorption or ankylosis. With the canine teeth, and the maxillary in particular, a cat's response to periodontal disease can be quite unique. Minor erosive lesions on the surface can mask extreme internal and external resorption evident radiographically, yet with minimal attachment loss or mobility. Sometimes it is a matter of judgment whether to treat conservatively or extract, since these teeth may not appear to be acutely inflamed and the extraction process could cause excessive trauma. The maxillary alveolar bone may have a bulbous appearance, reflecting a chronic osteitis-like condition resulting from constant bacterial exposure. Active, infected areas should be treated appropriately to avoid further progression to potential oronasal fistula. In addition, chronic disease may result in bone changes of osteopenia and the gradual extrusion of the cuspids to the extent that they are no longer covered by the lips (Fig. 1).

Many forms of periodontitis actually begin in the young or juvenile animal (35). In cats with RPP and RRPP and forms of lymphocytic plasmocytic stomatitis, the severe gingivitis/periodontitis may give rise to the secondary development of feline dental resorptive lesions or cervical line lesions due to inflammatory resorption. These forms of periodontitis occur in many young animals without appreciable plaque or calculus accumulation. With these patients, every attempt should be made to keep the oral cavity as free from plaque as possible, with a professional prophylaxis every few months, or as required, and rigorous home care. This is done to minimize attachment loss, in hope that the animal will eventually stabilize or recover from the disease with treatment and maturity. Of course, cats infected with FeLV, FIV, or FCV, among other organisms, tend to

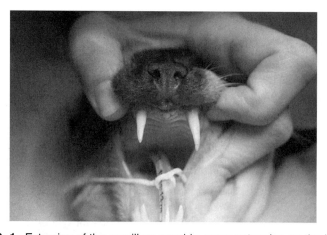

FIG. 1. Extrusion of the maxillary cuspids, more extensive on the left.

have more extensive gingival lesions than the typical patient (35). Young, FeLV- and FIV-negative cats exhibiting a proliferative gingival margin (fibrous papillomatosis) that nearly covers the tooth crowns have responded well to excision in some cases. Rigorous home care and quality dental prophylaxis with appropriate antibiotics and immunomodulators may help decrease the signs.

In view of the serious repercussions that can arise from periodontal disease (12,13), its early control and prevention are extremely important. Since young animals are very impressionable and more readily accept training, it is at this stage of life that it is best to get both the owner and the pet introduced to the concept of good oral health care. By your starting with a strong foundation in the need for oral care and progressing from there to the need for routine oral examination of the pet by the owner, home dental care (including brushing), and regular prophylaxis for the early detection and treatment of problems, the animal can experience the best oral health possible.

Cervical Line Lesions or Feline Dental Resorptive Lesions

During examination of the feline oral cavity or performance of a prophylaxis, it is likely that some lesions on the tooth surface will be encountered. Resorptive lesions of the teeth in cats are currently known under many names. In articles and proceedings, they have been referred to as cervical line lesions (CLL), cervical neck lesions (CNL), cervical line erosions, cervical line resorptions, subgingival resorptive lesions, initiocircocervical desmodentiopathy, osteoclastic resorptive lesions, feline dental resorptive (FDR) lesions, buccal cervical root resorptions, and so on (42,43). These lesions represent currently the most common disease of the tooth structure of the domestic feline (2). The first known report of the disease was in 1955, at which time it was presumed to be root caries (44). The disease was again described in the mid-1960s (45,46) but was not popularly recognized until the mid- to late 1970s, when new descriptions were published and the disease appeared to be increasing in incidence (43,47). Retrospective examination of feline skulls back into the late 1800s revealed a low incidence of the disease (48), and one text by Colyer in 1936 failed to describe any lesions of this nature (42). A reexamination in 1991 of 80 of the skulls originally inspected by Colyer in 1936 did find one skull with a tooth lesion (1.25%) (48). In seven pre-1940 cat skulls examined in Germany and Switzerland, no lesions were found (49). Of 250 pre-1950 museum specimens in the United States, one skull (0.4%) was found to have lesions (50). One of 12 skulls examined in 1960–1969 (8.0%) and 90 of 339 post-1970 skulls (26.5%) examined in Germany and Switzerland demonstrated lesions (49). One problem with the museum skull sample examined is the lack of sex, age, diet, and environmental information to assimilate with surveys. The skulls in museums from earlier times would be expected to be of younger animals, due to shorter life spans. As medicine and diet have improved, animal life expectancies have been enhanced. This would mean that each more recent skull grouping could be of slightly older animals on average as compared with the last. In view of the fact that resorptive lesions are uncommon in young animals and become more common as animals age, there could be some potential disparity in comparing the skulls of these periods. Therefore, a lower rate of disease might be expected from the older-period museum specimens. Thus, the trend toward higher rates in later years is undeniable, and possibly not as remarkable it would appear. Incidences in live animals vary greatly with percentages and population (Table 2). Some studies of stray and feral cat populations have shown a lower rate of lesional formation in the wild population (49,51).

TABLE 2. *Summary of feline resorptive lesion prevalence studies*

Year	Lesion (%)	Patient source[a]	Patients (n)	Country	Reported by/ Reference
1987	65	Dental	465	United States (New York)	Tholen (173)
1987	46	Dental	NR	Austria	Zetner et al (100)
1990	46	Dental	24	Austria	Zetner (50)
1991	43	Dental	306	Netherlands	Remeeus (168)
1991	57	Dental	152	United Kingdom	Crossley (169)
1992	62	Dental	432	Netherlands	van Wessum (51)
1992	67	Dental	78	United States	Harvey (51)
1993	42	Dental	252	United States (Texas)	Wiggs (58)
1987	28	Mixed	NR	Austria	Zetner et al (100)
1990	20	Mixed	NR	United States (California)	Mulligan (172)
1990	52	Mixed	64	Australia (Melbourne)	Coles (167)
1992	26	Mixed	796	United States	Harvey (170)
1992	20	Mixed	50	Germany	Dobbertin (49)
1992	23	Mixed	500	Austria	Zetner and Steurer (174)
1993	37	Mixed	605	United States (Texas)	Wiggs (58)
1982	28.5	Random	200	Switzerland	von Schlup (77)
1984	NR	Random	15	Germany	Reichert et al (55)
1993	28	Random	214	United States (Texas)	Wiggs (58)
1994	29	Random	168	Australia (Melbourne)	Clarke (171)

NR, not reported.

[a] Dental, population from animals examined or treated specifically for oral or dental reasons; mixed, population from animals examined or treated for oral, dental and other reasons; random, population not examined or treated specifically for oral or dental reasons.

Microscopically, two features are sometimes found in clinically normal feline teeth. These are vasodentin and intermediate cementum or osteodentin (52). They have been found in the circumpulpal dentin and root dentin. *Vasodentin* is found to have vascular channels and dentinal tubules traversing through it indiscriminately. Both rounded and flat epithelial-like cells are often found within the channels. It has not been determined whether these channels have peripheral blood circulation or they connect to the periodontal ligament. Dentinal tubules were not found to run through the actual channels. Vasodentin is found in other species, including the dog, and it is typically found in the outer third of the circumpulpal dentin (53). *Osteodentin* is most commonly observed in the root dentin adjacent to the root canal or cellular cementum (53). FDR lesions tend to develop in areas where vasodentin is present. However, vasodentin has been found in teeth with and without FDR lesions in a similar percentage, making any association between the two unlikely.

In early published material, the lesions were thought to be carious and decay-type in nature (44–46). Later, they were described as being progressive subgingival resorptive lesions with osteoclastic involvement (42,47). Histologically, at the cementoenamel junction, these lesions are found to be concave defects lined by odontoclasts (54), with the surrounding dentin appearing normal and no inflammation of the pulp tissue in early-stage lesions (55). Endothelial and epithelial excretion of cytokines can initiate and enhance the odontoclastic activity. Internal resorption of the roots begins when pulpal inflammation eventually stimulates reactions that trigger odontoclast activity (56). Root resorption of teeth can occur with more advanced lesions, and it is not uncommonly found in cats with periodontal disease complications (44,55). Lesions developing more apically or internally may be related to some form of external stimulus of the gingiva. Research has demonstrated dynamic physiologic changes in cat dental pulps, including vasodilation, that can be elicited by many simple noxious stimuli of the gingiva adjacent to a tooth (57). The stimuli causing these effects must pass through the periodontal ligament. This pulpal and periodontal ligament stimulus may very possibly be involved with the development of FDR lesions, especially the more apical and internal lesions.

One European study indicated that Siamese and Persian cats were more susceptible to these lesions (57). However, at least one study in the United States indicated virtually no difference between domestic and Asiatic breeds, except when lymphocytic plasmocytic stomatitis (LPS) was involved, as the Asiatic breeds showed a greater incidence of LPS (58). This study also indicated that there may be more than one form of initial development of resorptive lesions. Gingival crevicular fluid tests demonstrated that levels of aspartate aminotransferase and elastase generally only rose before lesion development in cats showing LPS symptoms but did not rise in most non-LPS lesions after initial lesional development. If these lesions were primarily resorptive (type I FDR) in nature, the enzymes should have risen prior to lesional development. This typically only occurred in cats with LPS, and not with the more common non-LPS (type II FDR) lesional developments. This would indicate that type I FDR lesions are possibly initiated by primary resorption and predisposed by LPS to occur. Type II (non-LPS) FDR lesions are probably secondary resorptive lesions. This means that the type II lesions are most likely not initiated by inflammatory resorption but, once formed, are probably driven by it. This leaves the initiating cause of type II lesions still open to speculation, as well as the predisposing factors.

The theory involving a form of root caries should not be ruled out, especially incipient caries (59,60) with secondary inflammatory resorptive activity (61,62). Predisposing factors of diet have long been speculated on (63,64), but no scientific proof has been forthcoming. Incipient caries is the demineralization of the tooth surface typically due to byproducts of bacteria in plaque (49,60). An incipient carious lesion appears as a white chalky area on the tooth surface. This demineralized area is a weak, porous, brittle zone that is difficult to visually detect, although the use of pointed dental explorers can help (65). In humans, the classic dark-colored caries usually follow incipient caries formation. The incipient caries weakens the tooth structure sufficiently for another form of bacteria to invade the actual tooth structure. This second step seldom occurs in cats, possibly due to differences in their oral microflora as compared to humans.

Periodontal disease and LPS are commonly associated with these lesions (66). Some strains of *Actinomyces* causing periodontal disease in human and animals have been shown also to cause root surface lesions (67,68). Many FeLV-positive patients have periodontal disease and CLL, but the majority of CLL patients are negative for FeLV (4,69). Some have demonstrated increases in immunoglobulins and some have shown immune deficiencies (69). At least one study has demonstrated that a high percentage of patients with CLL are positive for the calicivirus (4), but the significance of this cannot be definitively determined at this time. Human bulimia patients demonstrate a similar form of CLL that results from the chronic exposure of the cementoenamel junction to stomach acids. In view of many cats' periodic episodes of vomiting, some associated with hair, stomach acids may play a part in certain individuals in further exacerbating lesions; in addition, clastic cells work best at a low pH (70). However, it is doubtful that this is a true initiating cause in the majority of cases of feline CLL, since true resorptive lesions of this nature occur on the maxillary palatal surface of the anterior teeth the majority of the time (71,72), yet those in the cat are found on the facial surfaces more than 91% of the time and in the expected location less than 3% of the time (58).

The implications of these studies may reflect the role that inflammation of the periodontal ligament, with fibroelastic activity and cellular differentiation into cementoclasts and odontoclasts, plays in the external resorptive process. If such is the case, then CLL may be an extension of a form of periodontal disease more specific to the feline (73–76), but some feel that the inflammation is secondary to the resorptive lesion (58,70). In pursuit of an alternate theory, some English researchers found that feeding raw liver increased the rate of incidence of lesions (42,46,77). This has lead some to suspect a calcium–phosphorus imbalance as a possible causative agent, but dietary content has not generally been considered a primary factor by many researchers (42,45). On the other hand, the use of calcium-regulating hormones has been suggested to try to control the process of reparative bone–cementum tissue that leads to root ankylosis (54).

Clinical Signs

FDR lesions are common in domestic felines, with recent studies indicating that 28–65% show at least one lesion (78,79) and periodontal disease is commonly found in association with such lesions (66). Lesions are often found to be covered with hyperplastic or hyperemic gingiva and/or plaque or calculus (80). Frequently, the lesions are described as originating at the cervical or cementoenamel junction of the tooth just below the gum line. However, radiographic examination in some individuals has demonstrated lesions further apically on the root structure with no obvious cervical pathology. Most lesions identified in early stages are located at the cervical area with a dental explorer during routine prophylaxis. More advanced lesions may be more conspicuous on simple oral examination. One study found a reduced incidence of the lesions on the lingual and palatal aspects of the teeth, with the vast majority located on the facial and proximal surfaces (58). The lesions are most frequently encountered in the premolars, molars, cuspids, and incisors, in that order (58).

Presenting signs vary greatly according to the stage of lesion development (Fig. 2). Visually, there may be slight to severe gingival inflammation with the gum tissue, which is hypertrophic and hyperemic, and this may progress to gum recession with bone loss

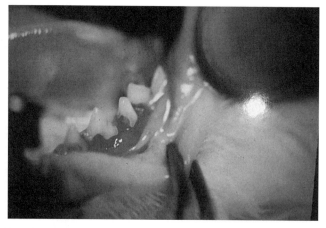

FIG. 2. Feline dental resorptive lesions often progress to involve significant portions of the crown.

and loose teeth. As lesions advance, root resorption and loss of the crown may result as the tooth structure is weakened. A simple gingival lump or swelling where a tooth once existed may indicate a possible root retention below the gum line following crown loss.

A common complaint when owners provide the patient's history is halitosis. Tooth hypersensitivity can be found even in early lesions, but it is more pronounced in deeper lesions with pulpal irritation that causes overt pain. Similar lesions near the cementoenamel junction area in humans are known to be very sensitive (81). In cats, this sensitivity may lead to anorexia, ptyalism, lethargy, dysphagia, and weight loss (70). Head shaking, sneezing, and excessive tongue movement have been observed if the maxillary cuspid is involved.

Diagnosis and Treatment

Most dental resorptive lesions are diagnosed during routine prophylaxis. Even under general anesthesia, a sensitivity response (involuntary twitch) may occur when a dental explorer or probe is drawn across or near a lesion. The explorer/probe should be gently inserted into the gingival sulcus, and the tooth should be probed for any irregularities in the surface (65). If the explorer end is used, care should be taken with the pointed tip to avoid lacerating the epithelial attachment at the bottom of the sulcus.

Generally, teeth should be saved when possible, but exodontia (extraction) is the most common treatment modality for the general practitioner. Some studies have shown that restorative attempts have a poor success rate (54,82). The fact that many lesions have been successfully treated would indicate that restoration is possible (58,83) but not as simple as it may often be presented to be. Probable causes of failure include a range of factors: the small and delicate nature of feline teeth, poor cavity preparation, poor diagnostic classification abilities, questionable restorative materials, poor home care, and inappropriate aftercare. The fact that there may be at least two formative types of lesions, the predisposing causes of which are fully known, further complicates treatment planning.

Should restoration be considered as a viable alternative, careful probing, close visual examination with magnification, and radiographic examination are best performed (81). What appears to be an early stage of the disease by visual and tactile probe examination may prove to be a more advanced lesion radiographically. In addition, we have found that teeth more prone to restorative failure typically have indications of apical external resorption or internal pulp cavity resorption, even when the CLL does not appear to communicate directly with these other lesions.

Type I lesions, primary inflammatory resorptive lesions, require that the inflammatory disease be controlled to have any chance that the actual dental lesions can be treated and controlled. Treatment of LPS is difficult at best, as its cause is seldom ascertained (see Feline Lymphocytic Plasmocytic Stomatitis below). Generally, treatment of both LPS and dental resorptive lesions is attempted simultaneously. The following information on CLL stages can be used in helping determine treatment of the actual lesions. However, unless the inflammatory disease is controlled quickly, most restorative attempts are likely to fail.

Type II lesions have a better prognosis than type I, but restorative attempts should still be undertaken cautiously, as the prognosis for successful restorative treatment is still poor (58). The following classification and staging can aid in determining whether restoration should even be considered.

According to G.V. Black's modified cavity classification (see Chapter 13, Table 1) (84), the lesions, in order of prevalence, will usually be class V (most commonly gingi-

TABLE 3. *Stages of cervical line lesions for feline dental resorptions*

Stage I	Into cementum or enamel only
Stage II	Through the cementum/enamel into the dentin
Stage III	Through the dentin into the pulp cavity
Stage IV	Extensive structural damage, fragile tooth
Stage V	Crown lost, roots still present

(Reproduced from ref. 85, with permission.)

val third of labial or lingual surface), class II (proximal surface of premolars or molars), or class III (proximal surface of cuspids or incisors without involving incisal angle). Many have further broken down the classification into five degrees or stages of pathology to provide specific guidelines in evaluation and treatment (85) (Table 3). Other root caries indices have been proposed (86–88), but these have failed to become popular in veterinary dental classifications.

Stage I

These lesions are shallow with extension only into the cementum or enamel. They are found early in the progression of the disease and should be treated, not extracted, unless radiographs indicate complicating factors. Treatment is simple: after routine prophylaxis, gently burnish the sulcus with a gingival packer or other blunt instrument that has been dipped in a hemostatic solution to control gingival hemorrhage. If additional sulcus exposure is needed, gingival retraction cord should be packed into the sulcus. Do not use an epinephrine-type cord on patients with cardiac or endocrine disease, especially hyperthyroidism. The lesion is then root-planed thoroughly with a dental curette, polished with a prophylaxis paste or flour of pumice, rinsed, and dried. Fluoride varnishes, fluoride-releasing dentinal-bonding agents, or fluoride-releasing pit-and-fissure sealants can then be applied to the dry tooth surface (78,83,89). The varnish products can be applied with microbrushes and dried on the tooth surface with a clean air source. Bonding agents and pit-and-fissure sealants should be applied according to the manufacturer's recommendations. These last two appear to provide superior sensitivity relief.

Stage II

Lesions of this nature have penetrated into the dentin and require treatment evaluation and selection of either restoration or exodontia (extraction). If extraction is chosen, care must be exercised during the process, as these teeth may be fragile from structural loss. Some roots may be ankylosed to the surrounding alveolar bone, making simple extraction impossible. These conditions should be apparent on radiographs taken during initial assessment. (see exodontia).

Restoration of affected teeth in cats is performed differently than in most other species. This is due to the limited dental structures present. The extensive cavity preparations required for amalgam and most composites are not practical for most diminutive feline teeth. Even with the newer bonding agents that improve the retention of amalgam and composite, the additional materials and steps have limited their use. For these reasons, glass ionomer restoratives that can chemically attach to the hard dental tissues (enamel, cementum, and dentin) have been the restorative of choice. Improved bonding agents may enhance the retention of composites with minimal tooth preparation to provide a stronger restoration. Long-term results with a microglass composite in one study showing 10% intact after 2 years (90) are similar to those in other reports. Glass ionomers come in American Dental Association (ADA) type I luting cements and type II base restoratives. The ADA type I glass ionomers have been used for shallow lesions, while type II ionomers have been used for more extensive restorations. Additionally, these are available in auto-cure (self-curing) and visible light–cured varieties. The auto-curing glass ionomers are chemically activated during the mixing of the base and catalyst and self-cure or harden. Light-cured restorative glass ionomers require a visible light (450–500 nm) source (91). This is a blue type of light similar to ultraviolet (320–365 nm), but in a different wavelength range. Certain safety precautions must be observed, as visible light can result in damage to the lens and retina of the patient or administrators, if viewed unprotected for any period of time. Therefore, the patient's eyes should be closed or covered, and administrators should make use of visible-light safety shields or glasses. The use of light-cured restorative materials can noticeably reduce procedure time. Although light-curing has greater initial setup costs than chemical- or auto-curing processes, with the need for special instruments, a light source, and safety equipment, light-cured materials have shown improved initial and long-term success (83).

For restoration, the lesion is initially prepared as in stage I treatment, except that the varnish is omitted. The following describes treatment using a self-curing glass ionomer. The product should be prepared and placed in the lesion according to the individual manufacturer's specifications. The glass ionomer should be covered with Mylar, cocoa butter, or unfilled resin to prevent moisture contamination while setting up. Moisture exposure during the setting stage of the glass may untimely result in deterioration of the glass or failure to properly adhere. Once it is set up, most material irregularities can be corrected by gentle use of a sharp curette. When the finish is acceptable, a coat of waterproof varnish is applied to prevent dehydration of the restorative for a few hours. All restorations should be rechecked for weakening or loss approximately 2 weeks after treatment.

Restorations with light-cured glass ionomers or composites improve restoration adherence by reducing the time involved and the chances of moisture contamination during critical periods of placement and bonding. The glass ionomers reduce time and finishing care. The composite resins, when used with a dentinal agent, may provide affected teeth with superior sensitivity relief, but they do require a more elaborate cavity preparation and application requiring additional steps. However, the more complex cavity preparation may be one of the measures needed to improve the percentage of restoration successes. It would be recommended that the dentinal-bonding agent be one of the newer generation types and preferably one that releases fluoride.

The tooth should be clean prior to application of the restorative. To control sulcal hemorrhage, gently burnish the sulcus with a gingival packer or beavertail instrument, such as a W3 filling instrument, that has been dipped in a hemostatic solution. Several applications may be required in heavily inflamed areas. If additional sulcus exposure is needed, gingival retraction cord should be packed into the sulcus. Do not use epinephrine-type cord in patients with cardiac or endocrine disease, especially hyperthyroidism. Occasionally, a releasing flap may be required for adequate exposure. The lesion is then cleansed thoroughly, and the roughened area smoothed with a dental curette. The cavity preparation should now be polished with a slurry of flour of pumice and distilled water, rinsed, and dried. Standard fluoride prophylaxis pastes should not be used for several reasons. The fluoride mineral may partially occlude some dentinal tubules, reducing restorative bonding ability, as well as reducing the effect of any acid-etching products on the cavity preparation area. Additionally, most prophylaxis pastes use oils or waxes as a binding agent to maintain their paste congregate effect. However, when these agents are polished into the tooth, they may also insulate the tooth against chemical attachments and acid-etching and occlude dentinal tubules, preventing bonding agents from entering. Glass ionomers and composite resins should be prepared and placed in the cavity preparation according to the manufacturer's recommendations.

Stage III

Lesions of this type have pulpal exposure and, according to most practitioners, are generally candidates for exodontia (extraction). If restoration is attempted, a root canal procedure will be required; this is practical only in the cuspids (canine teeth), although other of the larger teeth, such as the upper and lower carnassials, may be treated in some cases. Root canal procedures are performed with a zinc oxide–eugenol sealer and gutta-percha as a core material or with a calcium hydroxide sealer and then filled with a calcium hydroxide paste (see Chapter 11) . These lesion should be evaluated carefully by visual examination, palpation, and radiography before restorative procedures are considered. After endodontic therapy, the restoration should be performed as described previously.

Stage IV

Due to the structural instability of stage IV lesions, they are candidates only for exodontia. In most cases when elevators are applied, the tooth crown will easily fracture. Radiographically, many will show ankylosed roots that defy normal extraction attempts. In some cases, pulverization with a high-speed dental handpiece and a round No.2 bur will be the only practical removal method, with confirmation of complete removal being made radiographically. Recent publications indicate some success with leaving the roots and suturing the gingiva over them, as long as there is no evidence of continuing inflammation or infection (92), which excludes cases of LPS. As a rule, it is best to remove as much of the tooth structure as possible without damaging the surrounding tissues. When excessive force would be needed to remove remaining roots, closing the gingiva may be the best alternative.

Stage V

These are lesions that have progressed to the point that only the roots of teeth are left. In most cases, the gingiva will cover the roots, leaving the appearance of a small bulge in the gingiva. Diagnosis can only be confirmed by radiographs. Many of these roots will be ankylosed. If there is no detectable infection or inflammation in the area, optimally, they can be left alone. If removal is indicated, good light and magnification along with small elevators are necessary tools. At times, pulverization of the root structure and debridement of the alveolus may be necessary, particularly in cases of persistent inflammation.

Professional Aftercare

The animal is placed on appropriate antibiotics and/or anti-inflammatory drugs for 2 weeks. It should then be rechecked for gingival inflammation and/or loss of restoration. If at that time the lesion shows no further indications of problems, it is still best to recheck at 3–12-month intervals according to the stage and treatment. When possible, restorations should be radiographed again at around 12 months after treatment to determine whether lesions are still dormant. Professional prophylaxis to aid in controlling any periodontal disease would be recommended at least yearly. Scaling around the restoration should be done carefully with hand instruments, as ultrasonic and sonic scalers can disrupt small and delicate restorations. The teeth should be cleaned, root-planed, and fluoride-treated. Fluoride in animals may help reduce tooth sensitivity and prevent the deterioration of enamel by certain agents, such as some acids of bacterial byproducts, and possibly even help reduce the bacterial population (92). Topical fluoride gels are applied to the teeth and left in place for 5 minutes and then wiped or blown off the teeth; the gel should not be rinsed from the mouth, and the animal should not be allowed to drink water for 30 minutes after treatment, as this will reduce the effectiveness of sodium-type fluoride products.

Home Care

Home care must be tailored to the individual client and patient in accordance with the degree of the problem and other complicating factors. Based on results of current studies, diet and home dental care are the two primary areas in which the client can help with control of progression of cervical line lesions (CLL) (41). It is evident that high amounts of raw liver and possibly other meats may aggravate the condition (45,77). Therefore, these should be avoided when possible. Chronic vomiting may also play some part in lesion progression (58,70). For this reason, medical investigation and management of such conditions with appropriate medication and dietary changes would be warranted. Although dry food has been shown to reduce the rate of accumulation of plaque on the teeth, felines are discriminating eaters, and owners sometimes have difficulty in grossly changing the textures of their pets' diets. However, a gradual change involving first feeding a semimoist diet before finally changing to a dry diet may reduce a pet's resistance.

Direct dental care by the owner should be approached in a gentle and caring way, if it is to made a stress-free activity for owner and pet (see Chapter 21). Some anxious and distraught animals cannot have home care performed without risk of injury to client and/or patient. Owners should be consulted concerning this matter as to their ability and willingness to perform such tasks in a safe and productive manner. Initially, using only a finger dipped in water saved from a can of tuna fish and gentle rubbing of the facial surfaces of the anterior teeth should be attempted. Once this can be performed in an amiable fashion, a piece of cloth wrapped around the finger is incorporated. From this point, appropriate oral hygiene products can gradually be substituted for the tuna water and a small feline tooth brush for the cloth.

There are many therapeutic oral hygiene products from solutions to gels to pastes on the market. For routine daily to twice weekly use, any of the nonfluoride products may be selected. Frequency of use must be adapted to the degree of oral disease and the ability and commitment of the owner. The use of fluoride gels in the treatment of CLL is common. Stannous fluoride (0.4%) gels, such as Gel Kam® (Gel Kam International, Dallas, Texas) and QyGel™ (Veterinary Products Laboratory, Phoenix, Arizona), and the sodium fluoride gels are among the more popular for such use. The use of fluoride in the mouth should be regulated closely by the practitioner because its effects are seen in other body systems and the effects of long-term ingestion are unknown. Generally, only a very small amount of gel should be applied to the teeth and should be used only once weekly.

Feline Lymphocytic Plasmocytic Stomatitis

Beyond the scope of routine periodontal disease lies a realm of chronic, nonresponsive oral disease usually characterized by a distinct infiltrate of plasma cells and lymphocytes. In the international pathobiologic classification of periodontitis, LPS falls in the categories of rapidly progressive periodontitis (RPP) and refractory RPP (RRPP) according to the interval of disease (12,18–23). The exact etiology of LPS is still unknown, but various factors involving infectious (bacterial, viral) and immunologic capabilities have all been implicated. An unfortunate manifestation of this syndrome is the lack of permanent response to conventional oral hygiene, antibiotics, anti-inflammatory drugs, and immunomodulators (41,94–96). Refractory cases often require eventual extraction of at least the caudal (premolars and molars), if not the entire, dentition.

Pathology

The hallmark of this form of inflammation is evident in its name: Plasma cells, the first line in humoral immunologic response (96), predominate in the lesion in dense sheets (42) with some lymphocytes. This, in conjunction with a polyclonal gammopathy (98–100), lends credence to the supposition that the syndrome has a immunologic basis, possibly that the patient is predisposed to respond excessively to polyclonal B-cell activators in oral bacteria (101). There has been a report of a case of multiple myeloma in a cat initially presented with stomatitis (lymphocytic plasmocytic) that exhibited a monoclonal gammopathy and Bence Jones proteinuria and responded to alkylating agents and corticosteroids (102). The antibodies to specific antigens of plaque bacteria correspond to those seen in other species (eg, dogs, humans) in reaction to *Actinobacillus* and *Bacteroides* species. Though cross-reaction (of A.a.)? to *Pasteurella* species may be one explanation, certain strains of black-pigmented *Bacteroides* have been isolated in affected cats (103–105). The similarities in bacterial types (anaerobic and aerobic) and colony percentage to dogs and humans with similar symptoms may lead to studies to benefit all species (103). However, the severity and prevalence of the disease in cats indicate the possibility of the involvement of cofactors, such as viruses or flagellate bacteria. Viruses have been implicated. One study noted a high feline coronavirus prevalence in affected cats (4,106), but there is no hard evidence for a direct cause–effect relationship. Immunosuppression from infection with FeLV or FIV appears similar and could lead to nonresponsive infections (107–109), but most patients with distinct LPS are negative for these. Those that are positive require special considerations when treatment is determined, especially avoiding corticosteroids.

Although some authors have seen no breed, sex, or age predilection in the classic presentation of LPS (110), some indicate that certain pure breeds (eg, Siamese, Abyssinian, Persian, Himalayan, Burmese) (42,58,111) tend to have more severe disease, which may indicate a possible genetic tendency in those breeds (109,110). These authors have seen a definitively higher incidence in Somali and Abyssinian cats (58). Recently, a somewhat distinct syndrome, *juvenile-onset periodontitis*, has been described. It starts in cats less than 9 months of age (especially Siamese, Maine coon cats, and some domestic short-haired cats) with abundant plaque and calculus resulting in inflammation and causing anatomic changes involving bone loss, gingival resorption, pocket formation, and furcation exposure (109). This is sometimes further differentiated from a hyperplastic response, seen in some young cats, termed *feline juvenile gingivitis* (109). In these particular cats, aggressive early gingivectomy, prophylaxis (even though minimal plaque is usually present), and meticulous home care in the first 2 years may help minimize initial anatomic changes. At that point, these patients often mature into a more normal state (42). This should be differentiated from gingival fibropapillomatosis, a proliferation of the gingival free margin that can cover most of the tooth surfaces in a young cat. This is easily excised and, in our experience, does not recur; nor are any further complications usually encountered.

It has been suggested that the inflammation associated with the plaque bacteria can extend from the gingival margins to other areas by physical contact, leading to pharyngitis and faucitis with acute pain, particularly if untreated (107). There are other stomatitis conditions that seem to be confined strictly to the fauces, with still others that start in that area and extend to the gingiva around the premolars and molars (56).

In general, LPS does not appear to be a distinct disease entity but rather an uninhibited excessive immune inflammatory response (107,109). In light of this, treatment to prevent or control this inflammatory response would appear warranted. Treatments should take into consideration any underlying immune disorders, such as leukemia or acquired immunodeficiency syndrome (feline AIDS).

Clinical Signs

Common presenting complaints of patients with LPS include ptyalism, halitosis, dysphagia, anorexia (notably, reluctance to eat hard foods), and weight loss (108,111). A classic picture of hyperemic, proliferative (though sometimes recessing), ulcerative mucosa with a raspberry or cobblestone appearance is often seen (110,113). This of course represents those cases that have progressed beyond the initial marginal gingivitis as the commissures, glossopharyngeal arches, and palate become increasingly involved (Fig. 3).

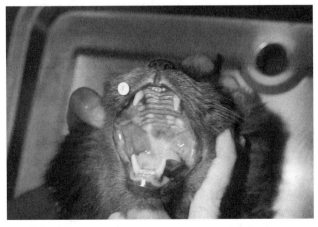

FIG. 3. Stomatitis can progress to involve the commissures of the lips and glossopalatine arches (fauces), as it has in this FeLV-, FIV-positive cat.

Diagnosis

Diagnosis can tentatively be made on the basis of clinical features and the lack of response to conventional oral hygiene techniques; however, biopsy is sometimes necessary to rule out neoplasia (43,113,114) and eosinophilic granulomas to confirm the diagnosis. Histopathology usually reveals an ulcerative mucosa with a dense submucosal infiltrate, consisting primarily of heavy sheets of plasma cells (42,115) but also containing some lymphocytes and neutrophils (108).

Routine laboratory work, including a minimum data base, viral testing, and bacterial culture and sensitivity will help in the patient's overall assessment but will typically fail to reveal any pertinent information, with few exceptions. Autoimmune causes might be suspected in unusual cases with lip ulceration, and hypothyroidism in humans has been implicated in some similar syndromes (116). Bilateral proliferative commissure ulceration may or may not be present in plasma cell pododermatitis, a rare disease of possible immune etiology also represented by an ulcerative granulomatous soft swelling of the foot pads (107,110).

Treatment

Current recommendations for the treatment of feline LPS concentrate on the elimination or control of the excessive inflammatory response described earlier (107). Yet even intense efforts at oral hygiene to control plaque, antibiotics to fight the bacteria, and anti-inflammatory drugs fail to elicit an acceptable response in most cases.

A strong emphasis on frequent professional prophylaxis and additional treatment (eg, root planing, treatment of CLL, resection of proliferative gingiva, and selective extractions) with vigorous home care is the first step. The ideal goal of having no plaque is virtually impossible, however, even in those patients amenable to home care daily or after each meal. The next line of defense in the clinician's arsenal, appropriate antibiotic therapy, is frequently employed, with initial responses that usually decrease in time, even with protracted regimens (43,104).

Since the primary pathogens tend to be anaerobic, metronidazole is frequently prescribed. Published doses vary from 30–60 mg/kg daily or in divided doses twice daily for 5–10 days (42,112,113) up to 250 mg twice daily (43). One regimen suggests, after the initial 5–10 days, administering one-third of the dose every 2–3 days for prolonged periods of time (103). Topical metronidazole solution possibly has a local activity (104). Clindamycin at a dose of 5 mg/kg every 12 hours for up to 3–4 weeks may be an alternate choice (110,114).

If the patient does not respond well to prophylaxis, home care, and antibiotics and is FeLV- and FIV-negative or if the owner is less likely to comply with home care instructions, immunosuppressive doses of anti-inflammatory drugs may be required. Initial doses of prednisolone should be calculated at 2–4 mg/kg one to two times daily; as the patient responds, dosage should be decreased to an every other day schedule (42,43,107,114). If oral administration is difficult, 20 mg of longer-acting methylprednisolone acetate can be given every 2 weeks for three to six treatments and then as needed (110,113). Intralesional injections are also possible in the anesthetized cat, utilizing triamcinolone up to a maximum dose of 10 mg (107). Progesterone, such as megestrol, has both direct and indirect anti-inflammatory effects (104) at a level of 2.5 mg daily for 7 days and then weekly (43), or 5 mg for 3 days, then one-quarter tablet twice weekly (104).

Owners should always be informed about the possible side effects, and this drug should probably be used only when absolutely necessary (107). Other treatments have been attempted with variable results, including gold salts, 1–2 mg weekly for 8 weeks, then monthly (42,43); levamisole 2–5 mg/kg or 30 mg three times weekly (42,43); azathioprine (114); *Lactobacillus*, laser therapy (117); and sodium salicylate, 25 mg/kg once daily for 4 weeks (this does not cause gastric side effects as aspirin does and there is no toxicity if it is given every 3 days long term). Vitamin supplementation, especially vitamins A, C, B complex, and E, and mineral supplementation with zinc may be given to help maintain oral soft tissue health (42,108,112). In our practice, human orthodontic topical anesthetics have shown mixed results in alleviating pain in ulcerative lesions to encourage the patient to eat. Experimental regimens (118) and anecdotal "cures" have been numerous, but no concrete data on a specific therapy have ever been presented.

Throughout the course of treatments, teeth that are unsalvageable should be extracted with meticulous care to remove all root structure and debride reactive bone tissue. In severe or chronic cases, often the only course of action that will help resolve the inflammation is extraction of the caudal teeth (premolars and molars) or the entire dentition in some cases (42,98,108). The discomfort and inflammation frequently subside after extraction, and the partial or complete loss of teeth typically has little negative effect on the animal's ability to eat.

Home Care

In mild-to-moderate cases of LPS, a strong commitment to home care is essential to provide the best chance of saving the teeth. Removing plaque daily, or even after every meal, can be facilitated with the use of chlorhexidine, oral hygiene rinses, fluoride, and other products (see Home Prophylaxis in Chapter 8). Additional care should be taken with more severe cases, as oral discomfort may make oral cleaning and even medication administration more difficult. Often waiting a week or two after a dental cleaning for the inflammation to subside will make things relatively easier.

Acute Necrotizing Ulcerative Gingivitis

Acute necrotizing ulcerative gingivitis (trench mouth, Vincent's stomatitis) is usually seen associated with stress in patients, especially in conjunction with compromised health or immune status (FeLV, FIV). It is caused by fusiform and spirochete bacteria (109). A mass of gray necrotic debris covers the ulcerative lesion that often bleeds and causes discomfort. Dealing with the underlying cause, cleaning, extracting, and antibiotic use are the treatments of choice. In adult cats, this is generally classified as a rapidly progressing periodontitis.

ORAL TRAUMA

Trauma to the oral cavity and associated structures is a prevalent occurrence in domestic felines (119). In the maxillary region, fractures and avulsed teeth are sometimes seen. With the palate, both soft and hard tissue separation can occur. In the mandible, lip avulsions, fractures, symphyseal separations, and temporomandibular joint fractures and luxations are of primary concern. Separation of the mandibular symphysis is currently the most common oral injury in cats (99). In addition, oral burns (electrical or chemical), lacerations, and foreign bodies are seen sporadically.

Clinical Signs

The clinical signs of oral trauma vary with the type, location, and severity of the lesion. The signs of lip avulsion are straightforward in the presenting case, while with fractures and dislocations an open-mouth or dropped-jaw appearance is typical. Characteristic nonspecific symptoms may include halitosis, ptyalism, dysphagia, and pawing at the mouth.

Tooth Fractures

When feline teeth are diseased, as in erosive lesions, dental fractures can occur during occlusal activity. With healthy teeth, this would be unusual, which is unlike the situation in dogs, where chewing on hard objects is not uncommon. External trauma would be a more likely cause of fractured teeth if there is no pathology involved. The most frequently broken teeth are the canine teeth of outside male cats (42).

If there is no canal exposure and the tooth appears healthy, the roughened fracture edges may be smoothed. Nonvital teeth and/or those with pulp exposure should either be extracted or treated endodontically (see Chapter 11). Root canal therapy is usually reserved for salvaging a cuspid, but radiographs must be taken to insure that the root apex is solid (Fig. 4). Often with long-term fractures in cats, there will be internal and/or external resorption of the root, which would be a contraindication for endodontics. In a very recently fractured tooth, a vital pulpotomy would be possible but not easily done on the small feline teeth (see Chapter 12). Again, usually only the canine teeth, though sometimes the first lower molars, will be considered for this procedure. If a tooth is salvaged by endodontics, it will gradually become more brittle in time (103). While not often done in cats, a metal crown may be placed for additional strength, again usually on a cuspid.

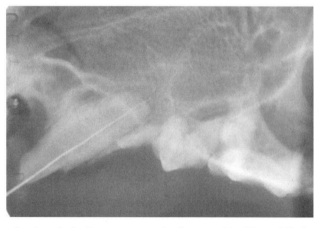

FIG. 4. Radiograph of endodontic assessment of a cuspid with pathfinder in canal. Open apices and internal and/or external resorption may be contraindications for standard endodon-

At least 6 mm of good supragingival tooth structure are needed for adequate retention of a crown. Minimal to no crown reduction or preparation is needed for these teeth.

Extraction typically will be the treatment of choice in the majority of traumatized teeth, and the basic exodontic techniques need few revisions for the feline patient (see Chapter 9). Smaller, more delicate instruments (eg, periosteal elevator, 699L tapered crosscut bur, No.301 elevator, and small extraction forceps) and gentle, patient skills are the keys to excess. Not only can the diminutive tooth size be a challenge, but the incidence of ankylosed roots, particularly in those teeth with erosive lesions, can make the process frustrating. Removal of all tooth structure is ideal, especially in the presence of any infection or inflammation, and sometimes gingival flaps and alveolar bone reduction must be used. Pulverization of root remnants that cannot be fully elevated may need to be done, but very judiciously.

Tooth Avulsion

At times, the force on the tooth will be such that the entire tooth is avulsed from the socket. This most frequently occurs in the maxillary cuspid, and even if other teeth are also avulsed, it is this tooth in which replantation would be considered feasible. Extraction is the treatment of choice for any others. After the injury has occurred, an otherwise healthy tooth should be kept moist in milk or saline (73). Replantation should follow as soon after avulsion as possible, with adequate but not rigid stabilization. Except in rare cases, endodontic therapy is performed either immediately or 3–5 weeks later (see Chapter 12).

Labial Avulsion

In most cases, labial or lip avulsion is seen with mandibular trauma and requires thorough cleansing and debridement as the first step of treatment. The subcutaneous tissue can usually be reattached at the midline to the fascia under the symphysis with absorbable suture material (120). If sufficient soft tissue remains, the lip may be replaced using a mattress suture pattern. In cases in which there is excessive tension, a more extensive suture pattern is required (120). Braided wire placed through the buccal mucosa at the level of and slightly behind the cuspids is passed subcutaneously around through the lip to the canine of the opposite side. The two ends of the wire are then passed through a small-gauge tube immediately behind the canine teeth and tightened until the tissues are brought back to approximately normal position. Once this has been attained, the wire may be tied in a knot, and the tubing slid over the knot. The suture should be left in place until healing is adequate, usually 3 weeks.

Hard Palate Separations

Hard palate separations are common in injuries from falls from high-rise buildings (121) and in head injuries from car accidents. Most soft tissue separation can easily be repaired with a mattress suture pattern using an absorbable suture material. If the separation is extensive with involvement of the palatal midline bones, intra-arcade wiring may be required to reestablish proper occlusion (121). Small holes are placed through the gingiva and interproximal bone mesially and distally to the upper 4th premolars. A wire is placed in a figure-8 configuration around the two upper 4th premolars. Gentle tightening will usually bring the separation back into alignment. In more complicated presentations, where the upper 4th premolars have been damaged or avulsed or are absent due to CLL or periodontal disease, an alternate wiring technique is required. The fracture is compressed with digital pressure. A transverse pin is passed dorsally to the bone of the hard palate at the approximate level of the 3rd or 4th premolars across the fracture line, with both ends extending a short distance from either side of the arcade. A figure-8 wiring technique is then applied, looping over the exposed ends of the pin and across the hard palate and tightening. Acrylic may be applied to the ends of the exposed pin, or orthodontic wax may be dispensed to the client for at-home application, if needed to reduce buccal lip trauma. The soft tissue separation is sutured together in a mattress pattern with absorbable suture material. The wires in a healthy adult can generally be removed in 2–3 weeks. In young, developing animals, interdental wires should be adjusted or loosened every 7–14 days, until removed, to prevent malocclusion. If the wires are left unsupervised by the clinician, occlusal disharmony may ensue, resulting in early contact, open bite, or an anterior cross-bite. In the healthy patient, gingival inflammation due to trauma associated with the wire usually heals rapidly once the wire is removed. Placement of tubing over the wire knot as described previously might also be recommended.

Most other maxillary fractures are treated conservatively, unless compression is a problem. Fractures of the zygomatic arch are treated in a similar fashion. If there is any pressure on the ocular tissues, an incision is made, and the fractured piece can be retracted laterally and stabilized (121). Transverse fractures of the maxillae are very uncommon but can be treated with interdental wiring, figure-8 or Ivy loop, extending from the maxillary canine tooth to the ipsilateral upper 4th premolar.

Oral Burns

Burns involving the oral cavity are usually electrical in nature, being the result of chewing on electrical cords. Lesions are typically distinctive in that they are generally well circumscribed and grayish to tan in color. The commissures of the lips, roof of the mouth, and the tongue are the most frequently affected sites. One report describes the long-term management required in a severe case in which buccal mucosa fused to gingival areas, obliterating the vestibule, as well as causing extensive damage to the palate (122). Damage is the result of heat coagulation of the proteins within tissues. Additionally, the electrophysiologic activity can result in muscle spasms, ventricular fibrillation, unconsciousness, and respiratory distress (123). Pulmonary edema is occasionally seen is some species.

Immediate treatment is symptomatic, using furosemide to treat the potentially dangerous pulmonary edema, but only if needed. Bleeding and other symptoms are customarily treated conservatively (123). Topical application of orthodontic local anesthetics is occasionally used to improve inappetence resulting from oral discomfort.

Severe burns involving the tongue may heal locally, but if any degree of tongue structure is lost, particularly the tip, the animal usually does very poorly (99), not eating well and unable to properly groom itself. Some palatal lesions may require reconstructive surgery, particularly if any defects extend into the nasal cavity.

Oral injury from direct ingestion of chemicals and caustic agents is less likely to occur in cats than in dogs due to their more discriminating eating habits. Cats, however, may get mild to severe ulcerations of the tongue when such agents are contacted through grooming of exposed surfaces of the fur or feet. Symptomatic treatment of the oral cavity is recommended, in addition to washing off any residual chemicals from the fur.

MANDIBULAR TRAUMA

Trauma and fractures of the jaws are common, with 6% of all fractures in the cat involving the mandible (124,125). These injuries range from symphyseal separations, fractures (vertical ramus, horizontal ramus, or condyle), and luxations of the temporomandibular joint (TMJ).

Separation of the mandibular symphysis is the most common oral injury seen in cats due to trauma (99). Midbody fractures of the horizontal ramus are not common, while injuries or luxations of the TMJ are occasionally seen. Fractures resulting from underlying pathology, such as advanced periodontal disease or endocrine disorders, or located distal to the 1st molar on the horizontal ramus can be a challenge to treat.

Clinical Signs

Clinical signs vary to a large degree, based on the location and severity of the pathology involved. Inappetence, ptyalism, dysphagia, dropped-jaw appearance, and malocclusions are some common presenting signs.

Symphyseal Separations/Fractures

Symphyseal separations are normally presented with an anterior malocclusion that may interfere with mastication (Fig. 5). A drop at the midline of the incisors resulting in an uneven or stair-step appearance of these teeth is typical. Should the soft tissues be torn, drooling and bleeding from the mouth may occur. These injuries are often classified according to degree of injury (Table 4).

Treatment

Simple circummandibular wiring may be effective therapy in uncomplicated type I and type II injuries. Inserting a large bore needle through a stab skin incision at the midline ventral mandible and exiting in the mandibular vestibule provide a pathway to guide initial wire placement (126). The 20–22-gauge wire is threaded up through the needle, then directed caudal to the lower canines, and pushed through a preplaced needle (from the ventral midline into the vestibule on the opposite side), exiting ventrally at or near the original wire insertion. The wire is then tightened sufficiently to provide stability and maintain occlusion.

In type III conditions, where mildly comminuted fractures are present, circummandibular wiring aided by a submandibular figure-8 wiring around the canine teeth is generally necessary. The two wire patterns are tightened or adjusted individually until the fracture is stable and occlusion is acceptable. In severely comminuted rostral injuries with the canine teeth intact, Zetner et al (100) have indicated that placing dentinal pins in all four canine teeth and then bonding adjacent cuspids together with composite between the pins can maintain normal occlusion during the 2–4 weeks required to initiate the healing process. This type of treatment results in the animal's inability to open the

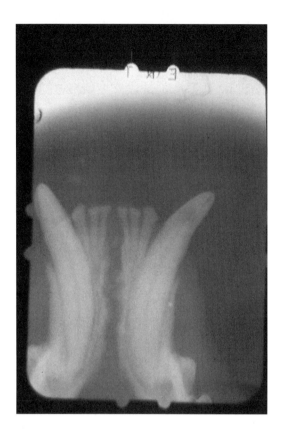

FIG. 5. Radiograph of symphyseal separation. There was no break in the soft tissue in this patient, making this a type I symphyseal injury classification (see Table 4).

mouth, and therefore feeding by gastrostomy or pharyngostomy tubing is typically required (100). Intraoral radiographs to delineate the extent of the pulp cavity and avoidance of the cavity during pin placement are imperative.

Fractures of the Horizontal Ramus

Most fractures of the midbody of the ramus can be treated with an open-front muzzle that fits loosely enough to allow eating and drinking but keeps the canine teeth in proper occlusion interlock at all times for the 2–4-week recovery period. Muzzles may be difficult to maintain in some individuals. For these and more complicated fractures, interarcade wiring of the jaws to keep them closed may facilitate healing. Placement of a wire through the maxilla rostral to the 3rd premolar and either through the mandible rostral to the premolars (using radiographs to avoid the mandibular canal and root structures) or around the mandible can stabilize the fracture site sufficiently. Directing the wire around the mandible

TABLE 4. *Symphyseal injury classification*

Type I	Separation with no break in soft tissue
Type II	Separation with break in soft tissue
Type III	Separation with torn intraoral soft tissues and comminution of bone; broken teeth.

(Reproduced from ref. 125.)

on one side can be helped by using a large bore needle to guide it and a notch placed on the ventral mandible to prevent movement. Others authors have described passing a wire through holes predrilled apically to the furcations of the maxillary 4th premolar and mandibular 1st molar (127). In all cases, the wires are tightened adequately to reduce the fracture while maintaining proper occlusion. Alternatively, TMS® (Thread Mate System, Whale Dent/Coltene, New York, New York) dentinal pins can be placed in the canine teeth, and adjacent canines can be bonded together with composite, as discussed earlier. We have found passing a small wire between the pins to reinforce the composite to be useful in some cases. Others benefit from the bonding of additional teeth further caudal in the arcade. These latter described procedures will necessitate tube feeding. Complicated fractures that are bilateral or severely comminuted with missing teeth or segments of bone may require a more extensive treatment plan. External fixation combining the use of multiple orthopedic pins and an open-end muzzle would be helpful. Pins can be placed transversely across the rostral and caudal segments of the mandible, with care to avoid tooth roots and to slightly alter the transverse angle of each pin. The excess pin lengths are then cut approximately 1 cm from the skin surface. Methyl methacrylate (acrylic) is then injected into an appropriate-size tubing and impaled on the pin segments and allowed to harden, forming an external oral splint (120). A loose-fitting open-end muzzle aids in maintaining occlusion while allowing the animal to eat and drink on its own.

Fractures of the Vertical Ramus

Uncomplicated fractures of the vertical ramus frequently require no specific treatment, as the encompassing muscle mass holds most of the segments in a satisfactory alignment (see below for vertical ramus fractures involving the TMJ).

Temporomandibular Joint Injuries

Details of TMJ injuries, notably fractures, can be difficult to discern clearly on radiographs (128). A ventrodorsal radiograph taken with 20° lateral oblique angulation provides suitable detail in some cases (128).

Acute uncomplicated luxations of the TMJ are relatively easy to replace, and affected animals typically have a dropped-jaw appearance (Fig. 6). A wood or plastic dowel (eg, wooden pencil, plastic toothbrush) should be placed between the upper and lower carnassial teeth of the affected jaw. The nose and rostral mandible are then gently pressed together (120). The mandible can be pulled forward if luxated caudally or pushed back if luxated rostrally, and the jaws are then allowed to close. If the jaws seem unstable, then a loose-fitting open-end muzzle should be applied for approximately 1 week. In cases in which there is difficulty in pressing the jaws together with the dowel pin in place, the affected side should be palpated in the area of the zygomatic arch. If a lateral bulge is felt, the coronoid process of the vertical ramus is flared laterally to the zygomatic arch and locked, thereby preventing the bite from closing. Open the mouth wide, while placing gentle pressure on the area of the bulge, and the mouth will usually close easily at this point, as the ramus returns to a medial position. In these cases, muzzling is highly recommended, because recurrence is more likely. We have frequently found these to have some form of TMJ disease or dysplasia with subsequent laxity, which may eventually require a condylectomy and/or resection of a portion of the ventral zygomatic arch to prevent the locking from occurring repeatedly (129).

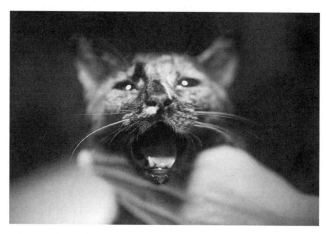

FIG. 6. Open- or dropped-mouth appearance often seen with a temporomandibular joint luxation.

Fractures of the vertical ramus involving the TMJ, fractures of the TMJ, and chronic luxations may result in dysphagia, ankylosis, or pain in the joint. Mandibular condylectomy is frequently the treatment of choice in these cases (130–132). An approach ventrocaudal to the zygomatic arch through the masseter muscle, with care to avoid the facial nerve branches and the parotid duct, provides the best access. After TMJ lateral ligament is severed, the articular condyle and even the articular disc, if injured, are removed with rongeurs. Suturing the masseter aponeurosis, subcutis, and skin completes the procedure, which sometimes results in only minor changes in occlusion.

MALOCCLUSIONS

Malocclusions are not common in most breeds of domestic cats (42). This is probably due in part to the limited variation in skull and jaw types in comparison with the canine species. The classical scissors bite is the correct occlusion of the domestic cat, with the lower incisors fitting slightly behind the uppers and the lower canine teeth fitting between the upper corner incisor and the upper canine teeth. Even the brachiocephalic feline breeds often maintain this proper occlusal pattern. Persians, with their brachycephalic head types, are the breed in which malocclusions most frequently develop (42). The increased rate of malocclusion problems in the brachycephalic breeds may be due in part to the lack of proper dental interlock between the canine and incisor teeth that allows variants to occur during development. A portion of these malocclusions has been attributed to hereditary involvement (42). Malocclusion can also be acquired due to various oral traumas or retained deciduous teeth (133). Ethical considerations should always be taken into consideration, if orthodontic treatment is to be considered.

The prognathism found associated with brachycephalic head types may be seen in the young kitten with deciduous teeth. The proper techniques of interceptive orthodontics as early as 6 weeks of age may be practiced to extract abnormally placed teeth that might otherwise interfere with normal jaw growth.

In a majority of older prognathic animals with the permanent dentition fully erupted, the protruding lower canine teeth hold the lips open or cause trauma to them. Occasionally, tooth-to-tooth trauma is involved, causing attrition, periodontal disease, or dental movements. Treatment usually takes one of three directions. These are exodontia (extraction), orthodontia (tooth movement), and endodontia (crown amputation and pulp capping) (2,42). Exodontia is the straightforward removal of the offending tooth and is the common treatment choice of many clinicians (see Chapter 9). If orthodontics is selected, there is the challenge of keeping small-base, direct-bond brackets on the teeth without causing too much oral discomfort that could make the patient anorectic (see Chapter 15).

Brachygnathic (class II modified Angle's classification) breeds are less common but can be presented with even more severe oral discomfort if the canine teeth are traumatizing the palate. Extraction or crown amputation with pulp capping are typically the only choices in making a more comfortable bite. Orthodontics in such cases, unless extremely mild, can be quite involved.

Other malocclusions, including those with one to two teeth involved, such as base-narrow mandibular cuspids or rostroversion of maxillary cuspids (lance teeth), can sometimes be corrected with orthodontic appliances (eg, palatal acrylic incline plane, buttons and elastics). If these conditions are seen in the deciduous teeth, they should always be extracted. Retained deciduous teeth can even be the cause of such problems as the permanent teeth are deflected into abnormal positions, so retained deciduous teeth should always be extracted as soon as they are noticed.

Wry mouth, where one of the four jaw quadrants is abnormally short or long in relation to the others, is usually unrepairable, but greater comfort can be given to the patient through extraction or crown amputation, if applicable.

CONGENITAL DISORDERS OF TEETH

Congenital abnormalities are seen in the cat, but they are not extremely common (99) (see also Malocclusions above). Variations in the number of teeth are seen rather frequently, as shown by a recent survey (42). With supernumerary teeth, treatment selection has one of two choices. If the additional tooth is causing no pathology, it can be left in place. Should the tooth be evoking a disease process due to crowding, such as periodon-

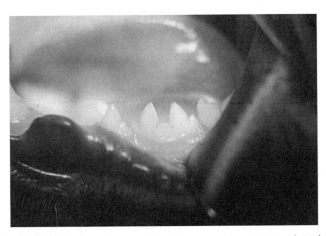

FIG. 7. Gemination lower 4th premolar tooth. In this incomplete attempt by a bud to divide into two teeth, radiographs showed the tooth to have three roots, the central one of which is shared by the two crown structures.

tal disease or malocclusion, extraction should be considered at the earliest possible opportunity (2). Missing teeth seldom cause problems in cats, although occlusion is affected in some cases. The domestic feline copes well without teeth; therefore, missing teeth are of no major consequence, except for esthetics, showing, and breeding purposes. Anodontia, involving the total lack of any teeth, has been reported in a young adult cat (134). Fusion teeth arise from the merging of two tooth buds during development. Teeth of this nature are rarely a problem. Alternatively, gemination teeth are the consequence of a single tooth bud's attempting to divide into two teeth (Fig. 7). These teeth occasionally precipitate crowding in the arch or increased periodontal disease if any irregular surfaces of the tooth contacts the gingival margin, entrapping debris; they periodically require extraction. Fusion and gemination teeth are infrequently observed. Supernumerary roots are sporadically encountered, and sometimes in association with gemination teeth.

PALATAL DEFECTS

Defects in the palates, both soft and hard, have been described in domestic cats (99, 135). They are usually of two general categories: congenital or acquired. Congenital defects may result from hereditary involvement or may be the complication of an insult during fetal development (135). Acquired defects are most notably the consequence of severe chronic infections (stage IV periodontal disease), trauma (eg, electrical cord burns, head trauma), or surgery (eg, aggressive tumor removal) (135). These acquired conditions have been discussed earlier in this chapter.

Clinical Signs

Congenital abnormalities may be manifested as two distinct classifications: a primary palate defect or a secondary (hard and soft) palate defect. A primary palate defect may externally appear as a harelip. The palatal defect itself is located just distal to the upper 3rd incisor and, if communicating with the nasal cavity lingually, can contribute to chronic nasal infections, if left untreated. If the defect is located on the buccal gingival surface alone, minimal side effects occur. Secondary palate lesions affect the midline of the palate and are often found in very young kittens on initial oral examination or when nursing abnormalities (milk coming out of the nose) are suspected. These warrant a more serious prognosis because of the risks of aspiration complications. Additionally, primary and secondary defects may combine to produce a more complicated harelip and midline palatal abnormality. Soft palatal defects may exist with or without concurrent hard palate abnormalities and at either a midline or unilateral position (135). Traumatic palatal injuries have been previously discussed.

Treatment

With uncomplicated cases of primary buccal disorders, corrective surgery of the harelip is generally for esthetic purposes. Simple sliding flaps have poor connective tissue support and are not predictably successful (136). Lingual lesions or deeper buccal lesions that extend into the nasal cavity should be corrected to close the oronasal fistula that can introduce bacteria and food particles constantly into the nasal cavity. Basic rules for gingival/palatal surgery apply here: The flap should be large to minimize tension;

epithelial edges should have fresh surfaces; the suture line should not overlie the defect; tissues should be gently handled; and using large bites in suturing and preserving the blood supply are paramount (135). Using an adequate mucoperiosteal flap and removing any remaining teeth that might interfere with the healing process will increase the chance of success.

Secondary hard palatal defects are often more critical, particularly in young kittens. Tube-feeding the individual to avoid aspiration and to support its growth until 2–4 months of age is often necessary. An overlapping flap is harvested from one side of the defect, with the releasing incision made far enough laterally to provide a generous amount of tissue for the flap, sometimes near the dental arcade. Care must be taken in the area to avoid the palatine arteries. The flap is left intact and hinged at the margin of the defect and then flipped, so the mucosa is facing the nasal cavity. The harvest site must be treated gently, as this tissue is much thinner and more delicate than in the dog. This is sutured (horizontal mattress) to the underside of the opposite-side oral mucosal tissue that has been incised and elevated from the bone along the edge of the defect (135). Alternately, making releasing incisions close to the arcades and elevating the two flaps to bring them together centrally may be done (137), but tension is a potential problem. Extensive defects seen in acquired lesions often require creative corrections, while still relying on the basic principles.

Midline soft palate lesions are managed with a double-flap technique (99). The medial margins on both sides of the edge of the soft palate defect are incised. These are separated by blunt dissection until dorsal and ventral flaps are fabricated. The dorsal flaps are sutured with an absorbable suture material in a simple interrupted pattern to produce an epithelial floor on the nasal side. The ventral flaps are closed similarly to provide an epithelial roof to the oral cavity. The caudal extent of the soft palate should extend just to the level of the caudal extent of the tonsils.

AUTOIMMUNE DISEASES OF THE ORAL CAVITY

Autoimmune disease involving the oral cavity in the feline is not common but should be considered as a differential diagnosis, if lesions resemble chronic ulcerations of the oral mucosa, lips, or philtrum (110). Pemphigus vulgaris is the only form typically seen, and 100% of cases have vesiculobullous involvement and almost 50% have initial sites in the mouth (108).

Diagnosis is made by biopsy with special handling techniques (using Michel's medium). Treatment is aimed at immunosuppression with large doses of corticosteroids (prednisolone 1–3 mg/lb daily) (110), azathioprine (108), cyclophosphamide (138), or gold salts (aurothioglucose 1–2 mg weekly).

NEOPLASIA

The oral cavity is the fourth most common site of neoplasia in cats (139–142), and the great majority of tumors there are malignant (143). Squamous cell carcinoma (SCC) is most frequently seen, followed in rate of occurrence by fibrosarcoma (42) and then melanosarcoma, both of which are relatively rare (142,143). Odontogenic tumors and benign growths are infrequently seen in cats (143–146), and all forms of questionable lesions should be biopsied to accurately differentiate them from other conditions that may be present in the oral cavity (112). Owners are usually alerted to a problem with signs of halitosis, bleeding, dysphagia, anorexia, ulceration, or dental disease (42). For the majority of neoplastic lesions in the oropharyngeal region, simple excision is usually not adequate due to the aggressive local or metabolic actions of the tumors (143).

Squamous Cell Carcinoma

In felines, nontonsillar squamous cell carcinoma (SCC) is the most common neoplasm in the oral cavity, usually in cats older than 10 years without sex predilection (143,145). Initially, the lesion may resemble gingivitis or appear as a white or pink nodule with progressively mobile teeth (110,146). These lesions are seen primarily in the ventrolateral tongue region or frenulum, though sometimes in the gingiva, especially mandibular (145), with occasional ulceration and proliferation (110). Often there will already be radiographic bony changes at the time of presentation, varying from proliferation to lysis or possibly resembling a primary bone tumor or chronic osteomyelitis (147). Metastasis to distant sites is not a significant problem with nontonsillar SCC in cats (145), as aggressive local invasiveness causes the majority of pathologic changes (103,143).

Wide surgical resection, in the form of mandibulectomy or maxillectomy, is effective only in early lesions due to the common event of local recurrence (112,143,148). Typically, lesions are not discovered until they have progressed beyond that point. The use of intraoral radiology before and even during excision is essential to determine the amount of bony involvement in order to accurately remove enough tissue to obtain a 1-cm margin of normal tissue. A poor prognosis is warranted, with only 50% of patients living beyond 1 year (112). Tonsillar SCC carries an even poorer prognosis due to its highly aggressive, extremely early rate of metastasis (147). Excision of lesions under or involving the tongue can also be difficult because, unlike dogs, cats fail to function as well in eating or grooming with part of the tongue excised (99).

Other Oral Tumors

Fibrosarcoma, the second most common oral neoplasm in cats (147), is usually found on the gingiva, palate, or mucosal surfaces (147,149). It is also characterized by highly destructive local invasion, with frequent local recurrence and late metastasis (112). An early lesion, firm, fleshy, red or pink, may be pedunculated at the gingivopalatal margin, even resembling a benign growth (112). But even aggressive resection, as in SCC, is frequently unsuccessful in all but the earliest of lesions, due to eventual recurrence. The poor prognosis reflects the fact that less than 20% of patients live longer than the first year (112).

Malignant melanoma, though very rare in cats (147), tends to act as malignantly as do similar tumors in dogs (112). By the time of detection, no matter how small the initial mass, it can be assumed that distant metastasis has already taken place, as well as significant local destruction (143). Surgical excision is usually only palliative; the total average survival time is 65 days (143).

Tumors of the dental laminar epithelium arising from dental primordium are also rare, with ameloblastoma being the most frequently found (144–147). It is typically seen in middle- to older-aged cats and is a slow-growing, rounded to lobulated, firm, rubbery projection from the gum (146). Radiographically, multiple radiolucent areas may be present with some resorption of tooth roots (146). One other form, in particular, called the inductive fibroameloblastoma is found only in young (less than 18 months) cats, usually at the rostral maxilla (143,145). The term *inductive* refers to the relationship between the ameloblastic epithelial cells and the dental, pulp-like stoma (146,147).

Benign growths, including epulides (145,146), are uncommonly seen in cats (112), but fibromas (141,146–149), odontomas, papillomas (146), and others have been reported. One young cat with extensive gingival overgrowth diagnosed by biopsy as fibropapilloma responded well to excision. Treatment of the benign lesions, including those of odontogenic origin, is usually excision and extraction of any involved teeth.

EOSINOPHILIC GRANULOMA COMPLEX

Often, suspicious oral lesions require biopsy to definitively determine their identity. Sometimes, a suspected neoplasm may be of the granulomatous group, and the converse may also be true. Much has been written about the eosinophilic granuloma complex, a wide variety of syndromes encompassing indolent (rodent) ulcers, eosinophilic plaques, and linear granulomas (150–152). Of the three, indolent ulcers are most frequently found in the oral region on the lips, followed in rate of incidence by linear granulomas, while eosinophilic plaques are rarely seen with oral manifestations (42). Due to probable immune-related causes, treatment generally entails the use of corticosteroids or progesterone compounds (41,109,148,153–157).

Clinical Signs

Indolent ulcers, also referred to as eosinophilic or rodent ulcers, are well circumscribed, ulcerative, red or brown lesions usually found on the upper lip (80%) either bilaterally or unilaterally (157), at the philtrum, or by the maxillary cuspid teeth (153). Females are two to three times more likely than males to have these lesions, and cases with patients aged 9 months to 9 years have been reported, with a higher incidence in the middle- to older-age range (108,112). The exact etiology is unknown but is thought to be inflammatory as a response to irritation (eg, trauma from tooth, excessive grooming) or as a result of allergies (110,155,158). Tissue eosinophilia is an inconsistent finding (159). The possibility that this could be a precancerous lesion (SCC) has been suggested (110,160), so early diagnosis and treatment are essential.

Linear granulomas are the only true granulomas in the grouping, exhibiting degenerative collagen with a granulomatous inflammatory response and tissue eosinophilia (108) initiating in the deeper dermal areas (159). Occasionally, an indolent ulcer will also exhibit these collagen changes, especially if it is present with these intraoral lesions of linear granuloma (159). Typical signs include linear bands on the caudal legs of young cats (159). Oral lesions are smooth or nodular (108,110), sometimes ulcerated (157), frequently found on the tongue, lips, gums, or in the pharynx (159). Peripheral eosinophilia cautions the practitioner to assess a more guarded prognosis, with the possibility of long-term therapy (110,155).

Eosinophilic plaques found on the abdomen and medial thigh are often red and ulcerated, probably due to repeated trauma of licking (155,159). Such plaques are less likely to be found in the oral cavity (110,151), and allergies are also implicated as a possible cause.

Diagnosis of all these lesions often relies on clinical presentation and a positive response to appropriate treatment (157). However, for a definitive diagnosis or in cases refractory to typical therapy, biopsy is recommended (42). In any suspicious oral lesion, it is never too early to obtain a histopathologic evaluation to rule out neoplasia (147).

Treatment

In all three syndromes, the treatment of choice is often an adequate amount of corticosteroids in the early stages (155), since there are likely to be some manifestations of hypersensitivity (159). Some proposed protocols call for immunosuppressive regimens involving prednisolone, 1–2 mg/kg twice daily (42,147) for up to 4–5 weeks (153,158); occasional intralesional administration of triamcinolone, 3 mg weekly (42,147,153); or injections of methylprednisolone, 20 mg every 2 weeks for more than 1 month (106,147). Hormonal therapy may also be used in the form of oral megestrol, 2.5–5 mg every other day (106,161); progesterone, 2–20 mg/kg, or medroxyprogesterone, 50–175 mg/cat every 2 weeks (143); however, the owner should be cautioned about potential side effects (108). Recent responses to antibiotic therapy alone indicate the need to further explore this avenue of treatment (153,158). Radiation treatment, cryotherapy, immunomodulators, hypoallergenic diets, topical erythromycin, aurothioglucose, and even topical cyclosporine have all been suggested as potential remedies (97,153,154,162,163). Frequently, cases are recurrent and require long-term (even lifetime) therapy (110,147). Treatment of insufficient duration with inadequate dosages is particularly prone to failure, and concurrent disease (eg, diabetes mellitus) that contraindicates the use of corticosteroids or progesterones warrants an even poorer prognosis.

SALIVARY GLAND DISEASE

Salivary gland disease is rarely seen in cats, but neoplasia, mucoceles, sialoliths, and even infarctions have been reported (164,165) (Fig. 8). Malignancies are more typically seen in older cats and usually in the mandibular glands, but any gland may be affected. Surgical resection may be sufficient if the lesion is localized to that gland, but local infil-

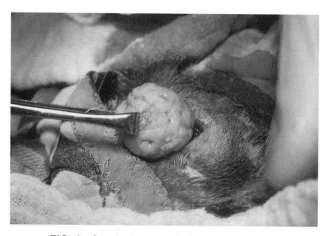

FIG. 8. Surgical removal of a large sialolith.

tration (164) and metastasis to the lymph nodes and lungs are possible (99). Benign growths have also been seen in cats (164).

Salivary mucoceles are most likely the result of some trauma to the gland that caused a salivary leak with accumulation in the tissues (99,165). The sublingual gland and submandibular/mandibular gland complex are most commonly affected, and surgical removal of the gland and defect is usually curative (166). Pharyngeal mucoceles are less common, but rapid salivary accumulation in such lesions can lead to pain and even pharyngeal obstruction (165).

Though not widely reported, salivary gland infarction can occur in cats. The active coagulative necrosis of acinar tissues, usually in the mandibular salivary gland, may result in a firm swelling with associated fever and increased white blood cell count; it usually resolves in 7–10 days (164).

REFERENCES

1. Burrows CF, Harvey CE. Oral examination and diagnostic techniques. In: Harvey CE, ed. *Veterinary Dentistry*. Philadelphia; WB Saunders Co; 1985:23.
2. Frost P, ed. Feline dentistry. *Canine Dentistry*. 3rd ed. Mount Kisco, NY: Day Communications; 1990:60.
3. West L. The enigma of feline dentition. *J Vet Dent* 1990;7(3):167.
4. Thompson RR, Wilcox GE, Clark WT, Jansen KL. Association of calicivirus with chronic gingivitis and pharyngitis. *J Small Anim Pract* 1984;25:207.
5. Loar AS. Feline retrovirus. *Dallas County Vet Med Assoc Proc* Aug 1990.
6. Barr MC, Barlough JE. Feline immunodeficiency Virus. *Cornell Feline Health Center Bulletin* 1989;10:2.
7. Gardner SA. Current concepts of FIV infection. *Vet Med* Mar 1991:300.
8. Sparger EE. Feline T-lymphotrophic lentivirus infection. In: *Feline Medicine IV*. Eastern States Veterinary Conference. Jan 1988:9.
9. Tenorio AP, Fronti CE, Madewell BR, Pedersen NC. The relationships of chronic oral infections of cats to persistent oral carriage of feline calici, immunodeficiency and leukemia viruses. *Veterinary Dental Forum Proceedings* Nov 1990:47.
10. Armitage GC. Periodontal diagnostic aids. *Calif Dent Assoc J* 1993;21:11; Nov: 35.
11. Wiggs RB, Lobprise HB, Capron CM, Bellinger LL. Gingival crevicular fluid aspartate aminotransferase as a marker of naturally occurring active periodontal disease in the cat. 1994; in press.
12. Wiggs RB. Periodontal disease's multifactorial origin. Proceedings of the Japanese Dental Society Meeting; Osaka, Japan. 1995:23.
13. Wiggs RB. Periodontal diseases and oral host factors. Proceedings of the Japanese Dental Study Group Meeting; Tokyo, Japan. 1995:30.
14. American Academy of Periodontology. *Current Procedural Terminology for Periodontics and Insurance Reporting Manual*. 5th ed. 1986.
15. Reddy MS, Jeffcoat MK. Periodontal disease progression. *Curr Op Periodontol* 1993:52.
16. Ranney RR. Classification of periodontal diseases. *Periodontology 2000* 1993;2:13.
17. Page RC. Gingivitis. *J Clin Periodontol* 1986;13:345.
18. Loe H, Theilade E, Jensen S. Experimental gingivitis in man. *J Periodontol* 1965;36:177.
19. Page RC, Schroeder HE. Pathogenesis of inflammatory periodontal disease: A summary of current work. *Lab Invest* 1976;33:235.
20. Page RC, Schroeder HE. *Periodontitis in Man and Other Animals: A Comparative Review*. Basel, Switzerland: Karger; 1982.
21. American Academy of Periodontology. Glossary of periodontic terms. *J Periodontol* 1986 (suppl).
22. Deutsche Gesellschaft fur Parodontologie. Neue PAR-Nomenklatur. *DGP-Nachrichten* 1987;1:1.
23. Schroeder HE. Klinik und Pathologie verschiedener Formen von Parodontitis. *Dtsch Zahnarztl Z* 1987;42:417.
24. Armitage GC. Periodontal diagnostic aids. *Calif Dent Assoc J* 1993;21(11):35.
25. Wiggs RB, Lobprise HB. Assessment of GCF-ALT (SGPT) in fifteen dogs as a marker of active periodontal disease and response to therapy. DDS AC Clinical Study. 1993.
26. Lamster IB, Vogel RJ, Hartley LJ, DeGorge CA, Gordon JM. Lactate dehydrogenase, beta-glucuronidase and arylsulfatase in gingival crevicular fluid associated with experimental gingivitis in man. *J Periodontol* 1985;56:130.
27. Last KS, Stanbury JB, Emberg G. Glycosaminoglycans in human crevicular fluid as indicators of active periodontal disease. *Arch Oral Biol* 1985;30:275.
28. Golub LM, Siegal K, Ramamurthy NS, Mandel ID. Some characteristics of collagenase activity in gingival crevicular fluid and its relationship to gingival diseases in humans. *J Dent Res* 1976;55:1049.

29. Offenbacher S, Odle BM, Van Dyke TE. The use of crevicular fluid prostaglandin E_2 levels as predictor of peri-odontal attachment loss. *J Periodontal Res* 1986;21:101.

30. Palcanis KG, Larjava IK, Wells BR, Suggs KA, Landis JR, Chadwick DE, Jeffcoat MK. Elastase as an indica-tor of periodontal disease progression. *J Periodontol* 1992;63:237.

31. Chambers DA, Crawford JM, Mukherjee S, Cohen RL. Aspartate aminotransferase increases in crevicular fluid during experimental periodontitis in beagle dogs. *J Periodontol* 1984;55:526.

32. Chambers DA, Imrey PB, Cohen RL, Crawford JM, Alves MEAF, McSwiggin TA. A longitudinal study of aspartate aminotransferase in human gingival crevicular fluid. *J Periodontal Res* 1991;26:65.

33. Imrey PB, Crawford JM, Cohen RL, Alves MEAF, McSwiggin TA, Chambers DA. A cross-sectional analysis of aspartate aminotransferase in human crevicular fluid. *J Periodontal Res* 1991;26:75.

34. Wiggs RB, Lobprise HB, Holmstrom SE, Bellinger LL. Clinical gingival crevicular fluid aspartate amino-transferase as a marker of naturally occurring active periodontal disease in the dog. 1994; in press.

35. Williams CA, Aller MS. Feline stomatology. *Vet Dent Forum Proceedings* 1991:101.

36. Manfra-Marretta S. The diagnosis and treatment of oronasal fistulas in three cats. *J Vet Dent* 1988;5(1):4.

37. Eisner E. A case of reactive bone secondary to periodontal disease in a 14-year old cat. *J Vet Dent* 1990;7(1):16.

38. Emily P, Tholen M. Periodontal therapy. In: Bojrab MJ, Tholen M, eds. *Small Animal Oral Medicine and Surgery*. Philadelphia: Lea & Febiger; 1990:121.

39. Tholen M, Hoyt RF. Oral pathology. In: Bojrab MJ, Tholen M, eds. *Small Animal Oral Medicine and Surgery*. Philadelphia: Lea & Febiger; 1990:42.

40. Wiggs RB, Lobprise HB, Holmstrom S. GCF/AST and MAL test results in cats 22–27 months of age, 1994-1996. In press.

41. Richardson R. Dental calculus accumulation in cat. *J Small Anim Pract* 1965;6:475.

42. Frost P, Williams CA. Feline dental disease. *Vet Clin North Am Small Anim Pract* 1986;16:851.

43. Holmstrom SE. Feline dentistry: Small animal dentistry. American Animal Hospital Association Symposium. Apr 1989:12.

44. Builder PL. (Opening paper, untitled) *Vet Rec* 1955;67:386.

45. Joshua JO. *The Clinical Aspects of Some Diseases of Cats*. London: W. Heinemann; 1965:51.

46. Wilkinson GT. *Diseases of the Cat*. Oxford: Pergamon Press; 1966:47.

47. Schenck GW, Osborn JW. Neck lesions in the teeth of cats. *Vet Rec* 1976;99:100.

48. Harvey CE. Dental disease in cat skulls acquired before 1960. *Vet Dent Forum Proceedings* Nov 1990:41.

49. Dobbertin F, Fahrenkrug P. Dental lesions in cats. Unpublished; 1992.

50. Zetner K. Neck lesions bei der Katze, diagnostichatiologische Untersuchungen über Zusammenhänge zwischen Rontenbefund und Futterung. *Waltham Rep* 1990;30:15.

51. Van Wessum R, Harvey CE, Hennet H. Feline dental resorptive lesions. *Vet Clin North Am Small Anim Pract* 1992;22:1405.

52. Okuda A, Harvey CE. Etiopathogenesis of feline dental resorptive lesions. *Vet Clin North Am Small Anim Pract* 1992;22:1385.

53. Okuda A, Harvey CE. Immunohistochemical distribution of interleukeins as possible stimulus of odontoclastic resorption activity in feline dental resorptive lesions. *Proc Vet Dent Forum* 1992;6:41.

54. Okuda A, Harvey CE. Histopathological findings of Features of odontoclastic resorptive lesions in cats' teeth with periodontitis. *Am Vet Dent Coll/Acad Vet Dent Forum* 1991:141.

55. Reichert PA, Durr UM, Triadan H, Vickendey G. Periodontal disease in the domestic cat. *J Periodontal Res* 1984;19:67.

56. Harvey CE. Feline oral pathology, diagnosis and management. In: Crossley DA, Penman S, eds. *Manual of Small Animal Dentistry*. 2nd ed. Gloucestershire, UK: British Small Animal Association; 1995:129.

57. Sasano T, Kuriwada S, Shoji D, Izumi H, Karita K. Axon reflex vasodilation in cat dental pulp elicited by nox-ious stimulation of the gingiva. *J Dent Res* 1994;73:1797.

58. Wiggs RB. Development of feline dental resorptive lesions. *Am Vet Dent Coll/Acad Vet Dent Forum* 1993. Proc?

59. Kikkelsen L, Poulsen S. Microbiological studies on plaque in relation to development of dental caries. *J Caries Res* 1976;10:178.

60. Loesche WJ, Rowan LH, Straffon LH, Loos PJ. Association of *Strepococcus mutans* with human dental decay. *J Infect Immun* 1975;11:1251.

61. Hazen SP, Chilton NW, Mumma RD. The problem of root caries. I. Literature review and clinical description. *JADA* 1973;86:137.

62. Stahl SS. The Nature of healthy and diseased root surfaces. *J Periodontol* 1975;46:156.

63. Keyes PH. Dental caries in the molar teeth of rats. I. Distribution of lesions induced by high-carbohydrate low-fat diets. *J Dent Res* 1958;37:1077.

64. Jordan HV, Sumney DL. Root surface Caries: Review of the literature and significance of the Problem. *J Peri-odontol* 1973;44:158.

65. Newitter DA, Katz RV, Clive JM. Detection of root caries: Sensitivity and specificity of a modified explorer. *Gerodontics* 1985;1:65.

66. Eisner E. Chronic subgingival tooth erosion in cats. *Vet Med* Apr 1989:378.

67. Jordan HV, Keyes PH, Bellack S. Periodontal lesions in hamsters and gnotobiotic rats infected with actino-myces of human origin. *J Periodontol* 1972;7:21.

68. Daly CG, Kieser JB, Corbet EF, Seymourt GJ. Cementum involved in periodontal disease: A review of its features and clinical management. *J Dent* 1979;7:185.
69. Johnesse JS, Hurvitz A. Feline plasma cell gingivitis/pharyngitis. *JAAHA* 1983;19:179.
70. Lyons KF. Feline Dental disease—classification and treatment. *Vet Focus* 1990;2.
71. Hurst PS, Lacey JH, Crisp AH. Teeth, vomiting and diet: A study of the anorexia nervosa patients. *J Postgrad Med* 1977;53:298.
72. Knewitz JL, Drisko CL. Anorexia nervosa and bulimia: A review. *Compend Cont Educ Dent* 1988;9:244.
73. Rossman LE, Garber DA, Harvey CE. Disorders of teeth. In: Harvey CE, ed. *Veterinary Dentistry*. Philadelphia: WB Saunders Co; 1985:84.
74. Seltzer S, Sinai I, August D. Periodontal effects of root perforations before and during endodontic procedures. *J Dent Res* 1970;49:332.
75. Birkendahl-Hansen H. External root resorption caused by luxation of rat molars. *Scand J Dent Res* 1973;81:47.
76. Reichart PA, Althoff J, Eckhardt W. Rippel W. 224Ra and 226Ra experimentally induced dental changes in rats. *J Oral Pathol* 1979;8:157.
77. von Schlup D. Epidemiologische und morphologische Untersuchungen am Kazengebiss I. Mitteilung: Epidemiologische Untersuchungen. *Kleinterpraxis* 1982;27:87.
78. Beard GB, Beard DM. Geriatric dentistry. *Vet Clin North Am Small Anim Pract*. 1989;19:67.
79. Coles S. Prevalence of buccal cervical root resorptions in Australian cats. *J Vet Dent* 1990;7(4):14.
80. Hawkins BJ. Cervical line lesions (neck lesions) in the cat. Acad Vet Dent Nov 1987.
81. Addy M, Dowell P. Dentine hypersensitivity—a review: Clinical and in-vitro evaluation of treatment agents. *J Clin Periodontol* 1983;10:351.
82. Lyon KF. Sublingual odontoclastic resorptive lesions: Classification, treatment, and results in 58 cases. *Vet Clin North Am Small Anim Pract* 1992;22:1417.
83. Emily P. Restoring cervical erosion lesions. *Vet Forum* Oct 1988:22.
84. Emily P, Penman S. *Handbook of Small Animal Dentistry*. Oxford: Pergammon Press 1990:55.
85. *Veterinary Dental Abbreviations*. American Veterinary Dental College, Residency Tracking Committee, 1994; suppl 1..
86. Doff RS, Rosen S, App G. Root surface caries in the molar teeth of rice rats. I. A method for quantitative scoring. *J Dent Res* 1977;56:1013.
87. Katz RV. Assessing root caries in populations: The evolution of the root caries index. *J Public Health Dent* 1980;40:7.
88. Mummia RD. Development of an index for the prevalance of root caries: Discussion of Dr. Katz's presentation. *J Dent Res* 1984;63:818.
89. Hawkins BJ. Desensitization and treatment of feline cervical line lesions in the cat. Proceedings of the World Veterinary Dentistry Congress; 1990:28.
90. Zetner K, Stever I. Long-term results of restoration of feline resorptive lesions with micro-glass composite. *J Vet Dent* 1995;12(1):15.
91. *Dentists' Desk Reference: Materials, Instruments and Equipment*. 2nd ed. Chicago: American Dental Association; 1983.
92. DuPont G. Crown amputation with intentional root retention for advanced feline resorptive lesions: A clinical study. *J Vet Dent* 1995;12(1):9.
93. Furseth R. A study of experimentally exposed and fluoride treated cementum in pigs. *Acta Odontol Scand* 1970:833.
94. Harvey, Shofer, Venner, Haskins. Results following conservative treatment of gingivitis/stomatitis in cats. Philadelphia: Department of Clinical Studies, School of Veterinary Medicine, University of Pennsylvania; 1988.
95. Harvey, Shofer, Venner, Haskins. Clinical features and periodontal indices in cats with chronic gingivitis/stomatitis. Philadelphia: Department of Clinical Studies, School of Veterinary Medicine, University of Pennsylvania; 1988.
96. Lyon K. Spring feline focus: An approach to feline dental disease. 1990;12:493.
97. Joachim F, Barber F, Newman HN, Osborn J. The plasma cell at the advancing front of the lesion in chronic periodontitis. *J Periodontal Res* 1990:25.
98. Pope WT. Plasma cell gingivitis-pharyngitis in a cat. *J Am Assoc Feline Pract* 1988;1:6.
99. Sams DL, Harvey CE. Oral and dental diseases. In: Sherding RG, ed. *The Cat: Diseases and Clinical Management*. New York: Churchill Livingstone; 1989:889.
100. Zetner VK, Kampher P, Lutz H, Harvey CE. Vergleichende immunologische und virologische Untersuchungen von Katzen mit chronischen oralen Erkrankengen. *Wien Tierarztl Monatschr* 1989:303.
101. Smith S, Pick PH, Miller GA, et al. Polyclonal B-cell activation: Severe periodontal disease in young adults. *Clin Immunol Immunopathol* 1980;16:354.
102. Lyon KF. Feline lymphoplasmocytic stomatitis associated with monoclonal gammopathy and Bence-Jones proteinuria. *J Vet Dent* 1994;11(1):25.
103. Sims TJ, Moncla BJ, Page RC. Serum antibody Response to antigens of oral gram-negative bacteria by cats with plasma cell gingivitis-pharyngitis. *J Dent Res* 1990;69:877.
104. Gruffydd-Jones TJ. Gingivitis and stomatitis. In: August JR, ed. *Consultations in Feline Internal Medicine*. Philadelphia: WB Saunders Co; 1991:307.
105. Harvey CE. Bacteriology of oral inflammatory diseases in cats. *Am Vet Dent Coll/Acad Vet Dent Proc* 1990:45.

106. Fiske R. Plasma cell stomatitis. *Texas Vet Med J* Jan-Feb 1985:20.
107. Harvey CE. Stomatitis-gingivitis in the cat. Western States Veterinary Conference. 1991.
108. Burrows CF, Miller WF, Harvey CE. Oral medicine. In: Harvey, CE, ed. *Veterinary Dentistry*. Philadelphia: WB Saunders Co; 1985:34.
109. Williams CA, Aller MS. Feline stomatology. *Am Vet Dent Coll/Acad Vet Dent Proc* 1991:101.
110. Lyons KF. An approach to feline dentistry. *Compend Cont Educ Dent* 1990;12:493.
111. Beard G, Emily P, Mulligan T, Williams C. Cervical line lesions: Gingivitis/stomatitis complex. *CE Semin* 1988:43.
112. Manfra-Marretta S, Matheissen D, Matus R, Patniak A. Surgical management of oral neoplasia. In: Bojrab MJ, Tholen M, eds. *Small Animal Oral Medicine and Surgery*. Philadelphia: Lea & Febiger; 1990:108.
113. Eisenmenger E, Zetner. Veterinary Dentistry. Philadelphia: WB Saunders Co; 1985.
114. Lyon KF. The differential diagnosis and treatment of gingivitis in the cat. *Am Vet Dent Soc Proc* Apr 1991:47. Am Vet Dent Coll/Acad Vet Dent Proc? Also, give volume number?
115. Nisengard R, Newman MG, Sanz M. The host response: Basic concepts. In: Glickman, ed. *Clinical Periodontology*. 7th ed. Philadelphia: WB Saunders Co; 1990.
116. Goldstein G. Some new thoughts on feline stomatitis/gingivitis complex. *J Vet Dent* 1988;5(1):8.
117. Lyons KF. The effect of gallium-arsenide laser application on feline lympho-plasmocytic gingivitis/stomatitis in eight cats. *World Dent* 1990:29.
118. Wiggs RB, Lobprise HB, Matthew JL, Gulliya KS. Effects of pre-activated MC540 in the treatment of lymphoplasmacytic stomatitis in FeLV and FIV positive cats. *J Vet Dent* 1993;10(1):9.
119. Weigel JP, Dorn AS. Diseases of the jaw and abnormal occlusion. In: Harvey CE, ed. *Veterinary Dentistry*. Philadelphia: WB Saunders Co; 1985:106.
120. Todoroff RJ, Pavletic MM. Soft tissue surgery: Oral cavity and pharynx. In: Holzworth J, ed. *Diseases of the Cat*. Philadelphia: WB Saunders Co; 1987:75.
121. Leighton RL, Robinson GW. Orthopedic surgery: Maxilla and mandible. In: Holzworth J, ed. *Diseases of the Cat*. Philadelphia: WB Saunders Co; 1987:133.
122. Legendre LFJ. Management and long term effects of electrocution in a cat's mouth. *J Vet Dent* 1993;10(3):6.
123. Kolata RJ, Burrows CF. The clinical features of injury by chewing electric cords in dogs and cats. *JAAHA* 1981; 17:219.
124. Salisbury SK, Cantwell HD. Conservative management of fractures of mandibular condyloid process in three cats. *JAVMA* 1989;194:85.
125. Weigel JP. Trauma to oral structures. In: Harvey CE, ed. *Veterinary Dentistry*. Philadelphia: WB Saunders Co; 1985:140.
126. Schrader S. Dental orthopedics. In: Bojrab MJ, Tholen M, eds. *Small Animal Oral Medicine and Surgery*. Philadelphia: Lea & Febiger; 1990:254.
127. Umphlet RC. Interarcade wiring: A method for stabilization of caudal mandibular fractures and temporomandibular joint luxations in the cat. *Companion Anim Pract* 1987;1(3):16.
128. Ticer JW, Spencer CP. Injury of the feline temporomandibular joint: Radiographic signs. *Vet Radiol* 1978; 19:146.
129. Lobprise HB, Wiggs RB. Modified surgical treatment of intermittent open-mouth locking in a cat. *J Vet Dent* 1992;9(1):13.
130. Lantz GC. Temporomandibular joint ankylosis: Surgical correction of three cases. *JAAHA* 1985;2:173.
131. Harvey CE. Oral and dental disease in cats. *Am Anim Hosp Assoc Proc* 1986:148.
132. Eisner ER. Bilateral mandibular condylectomy in a cat. *J Vet Dent* 1995;12(1):23.
133. Eisner E. Malocclusions in cats and dogs: Recognizing dental alignments. *Vet Med* Oct 1988:1006.
134. Elzay RP, Hughes RD. Anodontia in a cat. *JAVMA* 1969;154:667.
135. Harvey CE. Oral surgery. In: Harvey CE, ed. *Veterinary Dentistry*. Philadelphia: WB Saunders Co; 1985:167.
136. Howard DR, Merkley DF, Lammerding JJ, Ford RB, Bloomberg MS, Davis DG. Primary cleft palate and closure repair in puppies. *JAAHA* 1976;12:636.
137. Long DA. Surgical repair of cleft palate. *Vet Med Small Anim Clin* 1975;70:434.
138. Withrow SJ, Holmberg DL. Mandibulectomy in the treatment of oral cancer. *JAAHA* 1983;19:273.
139. Dorn CR, Taylor DON, Frye FL, Hibbard HH. Survey of animal neoplasms in Alameda-Costa Counties, California. I. Methodology and description of cases. *J Natl Cancer Inst* 1968;40:295.
140. Dorn CR, Taylor DON, Schneider R, Hibbard HH. Survey of animal neoplasms in Alameda-Costa Counties, California. II. Cancer morbidity in dogs and cats from Alameda County. *J Natl Cancer Inst* 1968;40:307.
141. Dorn CR, Priester WA. Epidemiological analysis of oral and pharyngeal cancer in dogs, cats, horses and cattle. *JAVMA* 1976;169:802.
142. Priester WA, McKay FW. *The Occurrence of Tumors in Domestic Animals*. Bethesda, MD: National Cancer Institute Monographs. NIH Publication No.80-2046.
143. Cotter SM. Oral-pharyngeal neoplasms in the cat. *JAAHA* 1981;17:917.
144. Dubielzig RR, Goldschmidt MH, Brodey RS. The nomenclature of periodontal epulides in dogs. *Vet Pathol* 1979;16:209.
145. Dubielzig RR. Proliferative dental and gingival disease of dogs and cats. *JAAHA* 1982;18:577.
146. Carpenter JL, Andrews JK, Holzworth J, et al. Tumors and tumor-like lesions. In: Holzworth J, ed. *Diseases of the Cat*. Vol 1. Philadelphia: WB Saunders Co; 1987:431.

147. Withrow ST, Norris AM, Dubielzig RR. Oropharyngeal neoplasms. In: Harvey CE, ed. *Veterinary Dentistry*. Philadelphia: WB Saunders Co; 1985:123.
148. Stokes G. Maxillectomy in a 9-year old cat. *J Vet Dent* 1988;5(3):14.
149. Gilmore CE. Tumors of the gastrointestinal tract of cats. In: Kirk, ed. *Current Veterinary Therapy V*. 1974:736.
150. Gorlin RJ, Peterson WC. Oral disease in man and animals. *Arch Dermatol* 1967;96:390.
151. Scott DW. Observations on the eosinophilic granuloma complex in cats. *JAAHA* 1975;1:261.
152. Rosenkratz W. Eosinophilic granuloma confusion. *DVM Spring Skin Seminar* May 1988.
153. Gruffydd-Jones TJ, Evan RJ, Gaskell CJ. The alimentary system. In: Pratt PW, ed. *Feline Medicine*. Santa Barbara, CA: American Veterinary Publishers; 1983:201.
154. Reed JH. The digestive system: Diseases of the mouth. *In: Feline Medicine and Surgery*. 2nd ed. Santa Barbara, CA: American Veterinary Publishers; 1979:154
155. Stover GC. A differential for oral ulcers in cats. *Feline Health Top Cornell* 1987;2(2):1.
156. Freiman HS. Protocol for treating feline indolent ulcers: A lip tip. *Vet Forum* Mar 1991:96.
157. Juliff WR, Helman RG. Linear granuloma involving the tongue of a cat. *Feline Pract* 1984;14:39.
158. Reedy LM. Results of allergy testing and hyposensitization in selected feline skin diseases. *JAAHA* 1982;18:618.
159. Kunkle GA. Update on the feline eosinophilic granuloma complex. *J Am Assoc Feline Pract* 1989;1(2):6.
160. Wiggs RB. Latest practical advances in veterinary dentistry. *Dallas County Vet Med Assoc Proc* Jan 1991:1.
161. Theilen GH, Hills D. Comparative aspects of cancer immunotherapy: Immunologic methods used for treatment of spontaneous cancer in animals. *JAVMA* 1982;181:1134.
162. Hess PW, MacEwen EG. Feline eosinophilic granuloma. In: Kirk R, ed. *Current Veterinary Therapy*. Philadelphia: WB Saunders Co; 1977:534.
163. Willemese A, Lubberink AAMF. Eosinophilic ulcers in cats. *Tijdschr Diergeneeskd* 1978;103:1052.
164. Spangler WL, Culbertson MR. Salivary gland diseases in dogs and cats—254 cases. *JAVMA* 1991;198:465.
165. Feinman JM. Pharyngeal mucocele and respiratory distress in a cat. *JAVMA* 1990;197:1179.
166. Wallace LJ, Guffy MM, Gray AP, Clifford JH. Anterior cervical sialocele (salivary cyst) in a domestic cat. *JAAHA* 1972;8:74.
167. Coles S. The prevalence of buccal cervical root resorptions in Australian cats. *J Vet Dent* 1990;7(4):14.
168. Remeeus PGK. Tandhalsleaesies bij de kat. *Dieren Artz* 1991;7:223.
169. Crossley DA. Survey of feline dental problems encountered in a small practice in NW England. *Br Vet Dent Assoc J* 1991;2:2.
170. Harvey CE. Epidemiology of feline oral diseases. *Proc Vet Dent Forum* 1992.
171. Clarke D. Prevalence of odontoclastic resorptive lesions in cats in Melbourne, Australia: Report to the AVD grant applications committee. July 1994.
172. Mulligan T. Proceeding of Veterinary Dentistry 1990. Las Vegas, NV. (Addendum)
173. Tholen M. Proceedings No.100, University of Sydney Post Graduate Committee in Veterinary Science; 1987:8.
174. Zetner K, Steurer. Pathogenesis and treatment of neck lesions. Proceedings of 1st European Veterinary Dental Congress; 1992.

17

Dental and Oral Disease in Rodents and Lagomorphs

Robert B. Wiggs and Heidi B. Lobprise

With the growing popularity of some of the "pocket pets" and even rabbits, astute practitioners must be aware of the challenges facing them due to the unique characteristics of the rodent and lagomorph oral cavity and dental structures. Being able to recognize normal variations and assess any changes will help in adequately treating many commonly encountered conditions. Between the two groups, there are some similarities and some differences, as there are differences among the various rodents. Where possible, the similarities will be discussed as a whole, while the differences will be pointed out as they are mentioned.

ORAL ASSESSMENT

As with any veterinary patient presented, an accurate history will cover the scope of past medical information and include specific items related to oral and dental disease. Any facts on past and present dental problems, including treatment, dietary information, and chewing or eating habits, can be beneficial. With the owner's assistance, an initial oral assessment can be made in the examination room, but the actual information gathered can vary remarkably depending on the patient's attitude, size, and species. External evidence of swelling, head symmetry, exudate drainage, and anterior malocclusion will

FIG. 1. Dental chart for rabbits. The following routine home dental care is recommended by the British Veterinary Dental Association (Copyright 1993): Rabbits require a tough fibrous diet in order to wear down their continually growing teeth. Dry rabbit pellets, mixed grain and plenty of hay should be provided. Free access to growing grass and provision of other fresh vegetables in moderation is recommended. Avoid sweet fruit and large quantities of cabbage and other brassicas. Rabits seem to enjoy stripping the bark off pieces of non-toxic wood (eg. apple twigs), a practice which helps keep the incisor teeth short and sharp.

Weight loss, inappetence, excessive salivation, lumps around the face, runny eyes, and discharge from the nose are signs of tooth problems. Examine the rabbit's front teeth weekly. If the teeth seem longer or shorter than normal, or if there is any other abnormality, arrange a dental examination by a vet. The examination may require sedation or anesthesia, as it is not often possible to see the back teeth in a conscious rabbit.

Regular health examinations are advised in order to assess dental and general health and to detect and address problems as early as possible. (Adapted from Crossley DA. Dental chart for rabbits. *J Vet Dent* 1993;10(3):13, with permission.)

Rabbit dental chart

Date	Animal's Name	Owner's Name	Reference no. or Address	Age	Breed	Sex

UPPER

RIGHT

LEFT

LOWER

David A. Crossley 1993

Key to Pathology

G   Gingivitis

R   Receding gum margin

P   Periodontal Pocket

X   Extracted tooth

\#   Fractured tooth

●   Missing tooth or cavity

Treatments Performed   Still Required

Scaling/periodontal therapy   { }   { }

Incisor trimming   { }   { }

Occlusal equilibration   { }   { }

Gingival surgery   { }   { }

Extraction   { }   { }

Restoration (filling)   { }   { }

Radiography (x-ray)   { }   { }

Endodontic root treatment   { }   { }

Other, details overleaf   { }   { }

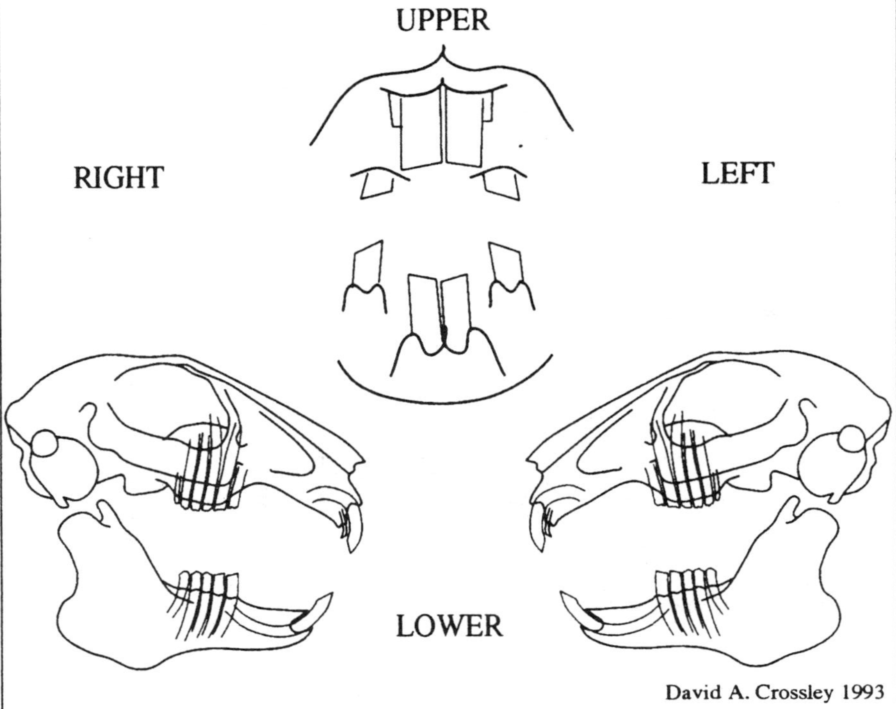

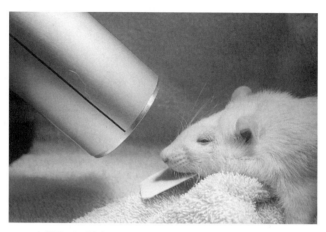

FIG. 2. Using an intraoral dental film in a rat.

be the first signs noted, if present. With gentle lifting of the lips, the gingivae and mucous membranes can be checked for color, hydration, capillary refill, or evidence of swelling, discoloration, hemorrhage, ulceration, or recession. Any changes in the teeth, such as fractures, discoloration, plaque, calculus, caries, erosions, malocclusion, mobility, or developmental defects should be recorded. Although they are sometimes difficult to visualize, the examination should include the palate, floor of the mouth, and all tongue surfaces to check for ulcerations, injuries, tumors, and foreign bodies. Any evidence of epistaxis, halitosis, rhinitis, oral hemorrhage, and masticatory muscle problems should be accurately recorded, along with charting of all oral and dental findings (1) (Fig. 1).

In addition to the information collected during the initial examination and from the history, other oral diagnostics such as biopsies, cultures, transillumination, and radiographs may be utilized. Extraoral radiographic surveys using occlusal No.4 intraoral dental films may sometimes be supplemented by the intraoral use of size 0, 1, or 2 films in sedated patients using the bisecting-angle technique (see Chapter 6) (Fig. 2). Other data such as urine, blood, and fecal assays may not be as helpful as in other species due to the sparseness of significant data to be gathered (2), as well as the difficulty of specimen collection, although urine and feces can sometimes be collected from the table surface following examination.

Complete physical examination of the oral cavity is therefore very important, though at times challenging. Restraint of smaller patients in towels or tubes (3–5)—or by carefully grasping a rabbit by the scruff and supporting the hind legs (3,4,6,7)—can help facilitate the assessment. The oral cavity is typically long and narrow, so the anterior portion is the only part readily accessible in the awake patient. Sedation or anesthesia is often necessary for complete examination (5,7–9), although otoscopes and tongue depressors may be helpful.

ANESTHESIA

In rodents, ketamine hydrochloride is probably the most common injectable anesthetic used, although it requires some special considerations. In lagomorphs and other species, there is usually insufficient relaxation of the oral cavity with ketamine alone, so supplements of additional injectables or inhalant anesthesia may be used. A range of 20 mg/kg

TABLE 1. *Baseline physiologic data for rodents and lagomorphs*

	Life span, mean (yr)	Respiration/ min	Heart rate/min	Body temperature (C°)	PCV (%)	BUN (mg/dL)
Chinchilla	8–10	40–65	40–100	36.1–37.8	27–54	17–45
Gerbil	2–4	70–120	260–600	38.1–38.4	35–45	17–27
Guinea pig	4–5	42–104	230–380	37.2–39.5	35–45	9.0–31.5
Hamster	1.5–3	35–135	250–500	37.0–38.4	45–49.8	12–26
Mouse	1.5–3	94–163	325–780	35.5–38.0	35–40	17–28
Rabbit	5–6	32–60	130–325	38.0–39.6	30–50	17–23.5
Rat	2–4	70–115	250–450	35.9–37.5	35–45	15–21

(Compiled from data in refs. 9,19,25,55,68,74–76.)
BUN, blood urea nitrogen; PCV, packed cell volume.

intramuscular (IM) ketamine (3) (light anesthetic plane) to 30 mg/kg IM (surgical plane) can be used in the chinchilla. In the guinea pig, mouse, and rat, a ketamine dose of 22–44 mg/kg IM produces light sedation to moderate anesthesia but with poor muscle relaxation; 44–100 mg/kg IM will provide the same effect in gerbils and hamsters (3,4,9,10). Anesthetic depth is best monitored by respiration and jaw tension (4,5,11) (Table 1).

Care should be taken using injectable agents alone with rabbits because individual reactions to the drugs may be unusual, especially with barbiturates (2,3), for which there is a very narrow range of safety. Pupil size and corneal or pedal reflexes are too unreliable to be used to monitor the depth of anesthesia, so again jaw tension and respiration should be closely observed (4,5,11). Ketamine can provide a range from sedation to anesthesia at doses of 20–50 mg/kg IM, but with poor muscle relaxation and analgesia (2–5,9,8,11). Combinations of ketamine (25–40 mg/kg) and xylazine (3–5 mg/kg IM with ketamine or 10 minutes before it, for analgesia) (2,4,6,10,12), diazepam (5–10 mg/kg) (9), or acepromazine (0.5–1 mg/kg IM or subcutaneous [SQ]) (2,6,9,11) may help.

While we do not normally recommend it, an intravenous (IV) dose of chlorpromazine (7.5 mg/kg) is better for sedation than the IM route (25–100 mg/kg) due to possible vascular thrombosis or myositis when injected into muscle (2,3). Preanesthetic administration of atropine sulfate (0.2–0.3 mg/kg IM, SQ, or IV) and butorphanol for postsurgical analgesia (0.3–0.8 mg/kg IM, SQ, or IV) can also be given.

In the past, inhalational anesthesia with halothane has been somewhat restrictive in rabbits because they tend to struggle against the mask and cough (11). It can be used at an induction concentration of 3–5% with maintenance at 0.5–2.5% (5,8). Enflurane, ether, and methoxyflurane have been used in rodents and lagomorphs, with proper scavenging units, as in all inhalant anesthesia. Chloroform would not be recommended.

As with most work in the oral cavity, intubation is ideal but, with untrained personnel, can be difficult and even traumatic with the small oral opening and lateral skin folds, and the use of topical anesthetics to control laryngospasms should be restricted (11). Practice and a stiff bendable internal tube guide are helpful for intubation. For very short procedures, where intubation can be avoided, isoflurane, with induction at 3–5% and maintenance at 0.5–3%, can be helpful (based on semi-open anesthetic machine with 2-L/min oxygen flow during induction and 1 L/min during maintenance) (12). For rabbits and larger rodents, a transparent induction chamber can be used, while smaller rodents can be placed into a standard mask held tightly against the table (Fig. 3). Typically, induction is smooth, but rabbits and guinea pigs have been known to initially hold their breath due to an anesthetic sensitivity of the respiration center. This can be followed by their then taking exceptionally deep breaths that could deliver excessive amounts of the anesthetic,

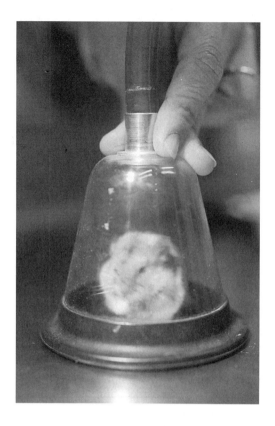

FIG. 3. Isoflurane anesthesia induction in a hamster.

sometimes with even fatal consequences (11). Respiratory assistance can be provided with a straw or eye dropper placed into the back of the mouth and blowing into the trachea. External cardiac massage with rapid, light digital pressure applied to the ribs behind the forelegs can provide some cardiopulmonary resuscitation effects.

DENTAL ANATOMY

Even with excellent techniques of examination and visualization, whether or not the patient is sedated, the practitioner must be familiar with the normal anatomy and physiology to be dealt with. The dentition is a primary reason why rodents and lagomorphs were first placed into a similar classification, and later separated (14).

The Latin verb *rodere* (to gnaw), from which the word *rodent* is derived, reflects a reference primarily to the prominent incisors and the herbivorous nature of many of these animals, although some rat species are omnivorous (15). The Rodentia order is the largest order of mammals, with a wide variety of species including mice, rats, guinea pigs, gophers, beavers, chinchillas, nutria, and many more. The Lagomorpha order consists principally of the Leporidae family with rabbits, hares, cottontails, and pikas. Of all rodents and lagomorphs, domestic rabbits and guinea pigs are most commonly seen by veterinarians, but the occasional "wild" cousin (16) may be in need of dental assistance.

Both rodents and lagomorphs have a *heterodont* dentition, with varying tooth shapes of incisors, premolars, and molars (17). While both groups have generally been considered to be *monophyodonts* (3), there is some debate because of data published by Haber-mehl (18) concerning lagomorphs showing deciduous teeth in rabbits and hares (though probably nonfunctional), which would then classify them as diphyodonts. The rabbit's deciduous teeth start to exfoliate possibly even before birth, with the tips of the maxillary incisors present at that time; total replacement occurs by 3–5 weeks of age (18). Among rodents, there has also been a claim that guinea pigs have deciduous teeth (19) but they may be fetal in nature and nonfunctional (18). The question of the functionality of these teeth and of their fetal or true deciduous nature appears to be pivotal in the decision by anatomists to classify them. Other variations in both rodent and lagomorph dentition indicate the general lack of in-depth research into the area.

The dental formula of rats can vary from $2 \times$ (I 1/1, C 0/0, P 0/0, M 3/3) = 16 in the rats of the Cricetidae family to $2 \times$ (I 1/1, C 0/0, P 1–2/1, M 3/3) = 20 or 22 in squirrels of the family Sciuridae. The presence of four incisors, no cuspids, few to no premolars, 8–12 molars, and a large diastema between the incisors and cheek teeth are the common traits (Table 2).

The primary difference of the lagomorph dentition is the presence of a total of four maxillary incisors as compared with two in rodents, as well as additional premolars (4,20). The most accepted dental formula for rabbits is $2 \times$ (I 2/1, C 0/0, P 3/2, M 3/3) = 28 (3,21–24) (Table 3). At least one author (6) notes a possible variation in the number of maxillary molars (either two or three possible, for a total count of 26–28), which may be due to the fact that the last set of molars is exceptionally small and potentially diffi-cult to visualize.

The standard single row of maxillary incisors in rodents is known as *simplicidentata*, or simple dentition (25). In lagomorphs, the location of the two smaller rudimentary maxillary incisors (peg teeth) (22) directly caudal to the two large grooved incisors is a double-row dentition or *duplicidentata* (Fig. 4). The large incisors of both groups are con-tinuously growing and considered to be aradicular hypsodonts, ie, long-crowned without a true root structure (26). The exposed or clinical crown is the supragingival portion, while the reserved crown is subgingival; combined, they form the *anatomic crown*. The

TABLE 2. *Dental formulas for the order Rodentia*

Hamsters (*Mesocricetidae*)
$\quad 2 \times$ (I 1/1, C 0/0, P 0/0, M 2–3/2–3) = 12–16
Old World rats and mice (*Muridae*)
$\quad 2 \times$ (I 1/1, C 0/0, P 0/0, M 2–3/2–3) = 12–16
Rats and mice (*Cricetidae*)
$\quad 2 \times$ (I 1/1, C 0/0, P 0/0, M 3/3) – 16
Gerbils (*Merionidae*)
$\quad 2 \times$ (I 1/1, C 0/0, P 0/0, M 3/3) = 16
Guinea pigs (*Cavidae*)
Chinchillas (*Chinchillidae*)
Capybaras (*Hydrochoeridae*)
Nutrias (*Capromyidae*)
Old World porcupines (*Hystricidae*)
New World porcupines (*Erethizontidae*)
Beavers (*Castoridae*)
$\quad 2 \times$ (I 1/1, C 0/0, P 1/1, M 3/3) = 20
Squirrels (*Sciuridae*)
$\quad 2 \times$ (I 1/1, C 0/0, P 1–2/1, M 3/3) = 20–22

(Compiled from data in refs. 6,8,17,18,24.)

TABLE 3. *Dental formula for lagomorphs*

Pika
Permanent teeth
2 × (I 2/1, C 0/0, P 3/2, M 2/3) = 26
Rabbits (*Oryctolagidae*)
Deciduous teeth
2 × (i 2/1, c 0/0, p 3/2, m 0/0) = 16
Permanent teeth
2 × (I 2/1, C 0/0, P 3/2, M 2–3/3) = 26–28
Hares (*Lepidae*)
Deciduous teeth
2 × (i 1/0, c 0/0, p 3/2, m 0/0) = 12
Permanent teeth
2 × (I 2/1, C 0/0, P 3/2, M 3/3) = 28

(Compiled from data in refs. 5,6,17,20,21,23.)

"submerged" segment is sometimes called the *clinical root*, but it is not a true root structure, though using the term *open-rooted* is acceptable for these teeth. This can be contrasted with equine teeth, which are radicular hypsodonts, or rooted, long-crowned teeth, with distinct roots that eventually mature into a closed-root structure (17,27). These also have a subgingival reserved crown portion and continue to erupt (not grow) in a coronal direction as the exposed crown is worn away.

All lagomorph cheek teeth and some rodent (eg, chinchilla, guinea pig) molars are also aradicular hypsodonts. Other rodents such as rats, mice, hamsters, and gerbils have molars that are brachyodont (short-crowned, closed roots) that do not continuously grow or erupt. With the aradicular hypsodont incisors, these latter individuals have a *mixed dental crown classification*, as compared with a *mixed dentition* (both deciduous and permanent counterparts present at the same time).

The continuously growing teeth have some interesting characteristics that fit well with their form and function. To begin with, in rodent periodontal ligament (and in developing human teeth), there is an intermediate group of collagen fibers that attach to either the alveolar bone or cementum, not both, with "splicing" in between. This intermediate plexus differs from the traditional view of ligament fibers running the entire

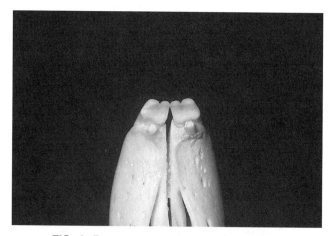

FIG. 4. Peg teeth incisors in rabbit maxillae.

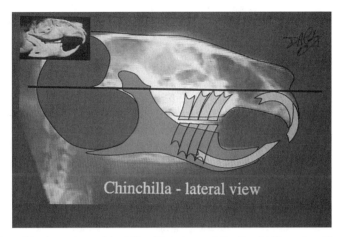

FIG. 5. Position of incisors in a chinchilla. (Courtesy of Dr. David Crossley, Heywood, United Kingdom.)

distance from bone to tooth, and may provide a more suitable mechanism by which continually growing or erupting teeth can have extensive tooth movement using this middle zone (28,29).

Enamel on the incisors of both rodents and lagomorphs is thickest on the facial surfaces, thinning as it extends onto the distal and mesial surfaces; it is nearly nonexistent on the lingual aspect, which is covered with softer dentin and some cementum (30). This configuration of dental hard tissue promotes a wearing pattern that results in a sharp, chisel-like tooth (24). In rabbits, the large maxillary incisors grow at a rate of 2.0 mm/wk, while the mandibular incisors grow 2.4 mm/wk anteromesially. Apparently, there is a faster attrition rate, typically due to dietary influences alone, of the lower incisors to compensate for the difference (22,23,31,32). Incisor teeth of the chinchilla may grow as much as 6–8 cm/yr (21) and are yellow-orange in color, as are most mature rodent incisors.

The position of the most "apical" portion of incisors may vary depending on the animal. Rat maxillary incisors extend for two-thirds of the diastema, while the mandibular

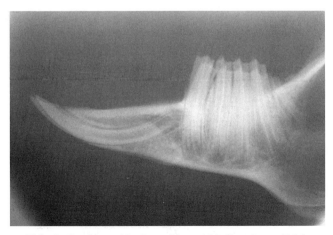

FIG. 6. Position of incisors in a rabbit (hemimandible).

incisors reach distally to the last molar. The maxillary incisors of hamsters reach to one-half to two-thirds of the diastema (mice up to three-quarters), and they are level with or distal to the last molar for the mandibular incisors. Guinea pigs have maxillary incisors that end near the mesial aspect of the first cheek tooth, with their mandibular counterparts traveling lingually and to the level of the second cheek tooth. Chinchilla maxillary incisors reach to one-half the diastema, and the lower incisors to the 1st or 2nd premolars (Fig. 5). Lagomorph maxillary incisors extend for one-third of the diastema, and the mandibulars reach the mesial surface of the 1st premolar (Fig. 6).

In rabbits, mastication is typically performed in a lateral, scissors-like fashion due to a horizontal oral mandibular fossa of the temporomandibular joint. The lower incisor cuts back and forth in between the peg teeth and the larger maxillary incisors (6). The lateral grinding movement is facilitated in the caudal teeth with a flat occlusal surface and deep transverse enamel folds (32,33).

Other structures of interest in the oral cavity of rabbits and guinea pigs is the significant medial folding of skin near the diastema, which limits visualization of the oral cavity (3,7). Golden hamsters have internal cheek pouches, while some other rodents have external, fur-lined cheek pouches found near the oral opening (34).

MALOCCLUSION

With the continually growing nature of lagomorph and rodent incisors (and some molars), it should readily be evident that any disruption in the normal attrition sequence can lead to significant problems with overgrowth (4,11,22). The most common dental problem in rodents (34) and lagomorphs (4,11,22) alike is malocclusion, which is the most common genetic problem in rabbits (9,10,22). Malocclusions are typically classified as atraumatic or traumatic.

Atraumatic

Atraumatic malocclusion results from genetic malpositioning of teeth or dietary causes involving insufficient attrition (9,16,34). Rabbits as young as 3 weeks may exhibit man-

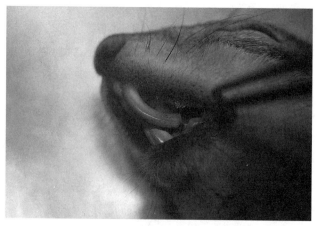

FIG. 7. Incisor overgrowth in a squirrel due to malocclusion.

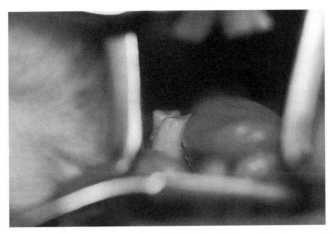

FIG. 8. Overgrowth of mandibular cheek teeth starting to trap the tongue. (Courtesy of Dr. David Crossley, Heywood, United Kingdom.)

dibular incisors that are level with or even extend labially to their maxillary counterparts (3,9,22). An autosomal-recessive gene for a shortened maxillary diastema is the probable cause (2,4,6,7,11,33). The mechanism of abnormal growth of the dorsal and basal skull bones that gives the appearance of a longer mandible (33) may be compared to brachiocephalic conditions in some animals or a class III malocclusion in humans (35).

The teeth continue to grow without proper occlusive wear, with the maxillary incisors starting to curl or twist in the mouth (Fig. 7); they have at times been known to penetrate into the skull if left untreated (3,9). Once the teeth are overgrown, the animal cannot eat properly, may drop its food (quidding), traumatize the tongue, and have excessive salivation (ptyalism or "slobbers") that can lead to *wet dewlap* (moist dermatitis) in rabbits (4, 6,10,11). Excessive overgrowth may cause the maxillary incisors to penetrate into the sinuses or ocular sockets. Malocclusion and overgrowth of the incisors with failure to properly close the mouth can further lead to molar overgrowth and malocclusion in rab-

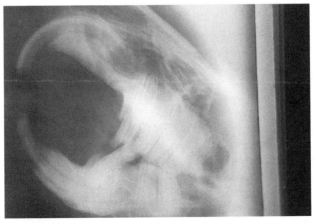

FIG. 9. Advanced problems in a guinea pig with cheek tooth loss and resulting drift and overgrowth of adjacent teeth.

bits and rodents with aradicular hypsodont cheek teeth (3,6). If the condition is left untreated, maxillary molars may flare outward, lacerating the buccal mucosa, while the mandibular molars overgrow lingually, potentially trapping the tongue either ventrally or dorsally (Fig. 8). In the chinchilla, molar overgrowth may be exhibited as an apical displacement or impaction. Primary malocclusion of the cheek teeth, with secondary overgrowth of the incisors as they are prevented from meeting properly, as in guinea pigs, have also been known to develop overgrowth due to excessive selenium intake (3). Whether it is the initial problem or a sequela of other causes, possibly even temporomandibular joint dysplasia, cheek teeth overgrowth is seldom recognized until signs are well advanced, due to the difficulty in routinely examining the teeth, and holds a poor prognosis (Fig. 9).

Traumatic

Traumatic malocclusions are the result of overgrowth of a tooth after the loss or fracture of its opposing counterpart. Loss of proper attrition may lead to many of the same symptoms and problems as in atraumatic malocclusion.

Malocclusion Treatment

The basic rationale behind treatment of malocclusion is adequate crown-height control to approximate the wear that would normally be experienced. Crown trimming or reduction must be done, preferably with a diamond bur or disc (9,16,38), on a regular basis every 3–8 weeks until normal occlusion is reestablished, or in some cases indefinitely (2, 3,7,11,36,37). A tongue depressor held behind the incisors can help protect soft tissue and allow stabilization for more accurate odontoplasty involving shaping the incisor into a chisel configuration that is closer to normal (39). Use of nail trimmers, tooth nippers, bone rongeurs, etc. should be avoided, if possible, due to potential tooth fractures and cracks that could lead to infection (5,8). If a pulp is exposed by crown reduction, it can be treated in the same way as a tooth fractured by trauma after cleansing. A calcium hydroxide paste (eg, DyCal®, L.D. Caulk Company, Milford, Delaware) should be placed to cap the pulp, preferentially stimulating the pulp to form a reparative dentinal bridge. The site should be closed with an intermediate temporary filling material such as IRM® (L.D. Caulk Company) to approximate the wear the tooth should experience (39). Amalgam or composite fillings might disrupt normal attrition, as well as some other temporary filling materials, may not hold up well enough. Crown reduction of the opposing tooth will be necessary, until the damaged crown grows to a correct length, barring the possibility of pulp-capping failure (40–42). Overgrown cheek teeth may also benefit from regular crown reduction, but this procedure is more difficult. A surgical-length diamond bur or more commonly a long-shank diamond bur for the straight handpiece is helpful for premolars and molars, but care should be taken to avoid excess trauma to the tongue, palate, and buccal mucosa (39).

Regardless of whether the incisors and/or the molars were involved, the owner must realize that, with a malocclusion or loss of a tooth causing overgrowth of the opposing tooth, treatment is an on-going, long-term commitment. If a tooth is lost entirely to trauma or has extensive infection that is unresponsive to conservative therapy and antibiotics, extraction of the remaining structure and the opposing tooth may be chosen over the need for regular crown reduction. If the condition is an inherited malocclusion problem, genetic counseling and culling of all affected animals should be considered (3). Patients with poor systemic health (contraindicated for frequent anesthetics), refractory cases, or wild animals that should be released might be candidates for euthanasia as a humane alternative.

In other cases involving abnormalities in the diet, such as hypovitaminosis C in guinea pigs, excess selenium, or inadequate materials for dental exercise, initial treatment with crown reduction will help. If the condition is properly diagnosed, however, rectification of the underlying problem should be sufficient to correct the situation and eliminate the need for frequent occlusal adjustment visits.

There have been some who have advocated tooth mummification, which is the process of applying paraformaldehyde- or formaldehyde-containing materials to the pulp to fix the tissues in hope of stopping the continual growth of the tooth. This is a highly caustic product that works by coagulative necrosis and fixation (43). When the products work properly, the effects should be limited to the immediately adjacent tissues, resulting in a sclerotic zone with preservation of healthy tissue below it (vital pulpotomy). Therefore, simple topical application to the exposed pulp would not be expected to affect Hertwig's epithelial root sheath, and therefore would not affect growth and the enamel organ located on the external apical structure. These compounds have the potential to cause many serious complications because of the numerous toxic compounds they commonly contain (eg, lead tetroxide, phenylmercuric borate, titanium dioxide, paraformaldehyde, etc.) (44). Lead poisoning has been reported in rabbits from various causes (45). Ions from the heavy metals can be disseminated throughout the animal's system to various organs remote from the teeth, posing additional problems (46–49). These products initially fix the tissues from the formaldehyde, but its solubility can result in percolation to adjacent tissues (50), especially in open-rooted teeth. This fixation must reach Hertwig's epithelial root sheath surrounding the apical portion of the reserved crown, which means its influence must make contact with periapical tissues; this has been shown to be very irritating to the periapical tissues in humans (51). This technique can affect not only the periapical soft tissues but also the bone and even the adjacent root structures of other teeth. It should generally not be used in teeth with apical pathology and should be used with extreme care in others, until sound research establishes its efficacy in cessation of tooth growth and safety to the patient's general health.

Another alternative that will also provide a permanent solution and possibly pose fewer serious complications than mummification is extraction. The location of the tooth, type of tooth (hypsodont or brachyodont), and general patient health determine the advisability of extractions. Some individuals are in extremely poor condition at the time of presentation, and antibiotics, anti-inflammatory drugs, fluids, force-feeding, and nursing care may be in order to improve general health prior to anesthetic stress. Location of the tooth becomes important to accessibility. Incisors have good accessibility, while many cheek teeth do not. Occasionally, buccotomies must be performed in some species for visibility and accessibility; however, food impactions, healing problems, and scars may result. Close attention to locations of vascular, neural, and other structures must also be considered.

Closed-rooted cheek teeth (brachyodont), such as those in the rat, can be extracted with some care with an intraoral approach in most cases using bent 18–23-gauge needles as elevators. In the mouse, gerbil, and hamster, the brachyodont cheek teeth are extremely small and difficult to properly remove, unless highly mobile. Broken roots can seldom be addressed without inducing excessive oral trauma in very limited spaces. With extraction, some migration of adjacent teeth and slight supereruption of opposing teeth no longer in satisfactory occlusal contact may occur. These seldom result in serious problems.

Open-rooted cheek teeth (aradicular hypsodont), such as in the guinea pig, chinchilla, and rabbit, have a less favorable outlook for extraction. Since these are continually growing teeth, extraction typically leads to overgrowth of opposing teeth no longer in proper occlusal contact and posterior malocclusions. This results in the need for routine odontoplasty for crown control of the posterior teeth at 3-week to 2-month intervals, or additional extractions. An intraoral approach is usually difficult and time-consuming, while buccotomies have their own associated problems. With the mandible, an extraoral approach through the bone covering the apices is generally best. A simple incision is made over the bony enlargement or abscess site. The specific location is best determined by use of radiographs and a knowledge of the apical anatomy. Guinea pigs commonly have three normal alveolar juga, or bone elevations, that may mimic an abnormality and can be palpated on the ventral surface of the mandible, representing the apical border of the first and last two cheek teeth. The cortical plate can generally be curetted open with a periosteal elevator or a high-speed dental bur. The impacted or infected teeth can often be extracted through this access site. In some cases, teeth will need to be repelled into the mouth from the access with a large endodontic plugger or other devices. If a cystic lesion is encountered, it must be thoroughly curetted. Good closure can be difficult, especially for the intraoral side of the defect. When possible, the attached gingiva should be loosened with a No.2 Molt periosteal elevator on either side of the defect and should be sutured closed with absorbable suture material. The bony defect may be packed with the appropriate osteogenic material. The external access is sutured with absorbable suture material.

The continually growing incisors (aradicular hypsodont) of most rabbits, guinea pigs, and rats are generally not difficult to extract (39,52). The smaller incisors of the mouse and hamster are more of a challenge. If only part of the incisors is extracted, additional overgrowth, migration, and malocclusion in the anterior teeth is not uncommon. Routine odontoplasty may become necessary for these new problems. For this reason, it may be best to extract all of the incisors at the same time. Many of these species have prehensile lips, and only slight, if any, changes in food textures may be required. This is typically not suitable for wild herbivores that are to be placed back into a natural wild habitat because of their great reliance on the incisors in obtaining food (eg, tree bark, etc.), constructing habitats, and defending themselves.

To start, in rabbits, the oral cavity should be cleaned and disinfected with an oral chlorhexidine solution. Complicated or time-consuming extractions should have both pre- and postsurgical radiographs taken. This allows for preoperative knowledge of complicating factors such as reserved crown fractures and weak mandibular support structure (predisposed to fracture). The next step in extraction is the severing of the epithelial attachment. A No.11 surgical blade or a small, sharp periosteal or dental elevator can be used for this purpose. The blade is inserted into the gingival sulcus until it meets with the resistance of the alveolar crestal bone. The sulcal incision is extended around the entire tooth, thus releasing the epithelial attachment. Actual elevation and removal of the tooth can be performed using a No.2 Molt periosteal elevator, a refined No.301 apical elevator, an EX-15 or EX-16 (Cislak Manufacturing, Burbank, Illinois), or an injection needle (18- or 20-gauge) and a small pair of extracting forceps (39). Elevators should be sharpened and shaped on a regular basis specifically for use in small herbivores.

The Molt or the No.301 apical elevator is used to elevate between the tooth and alveolar crest to separate the periodontal ligament. The mesial ligament attachment is typically the most difficult to break down. The instrument is placed against the periodontal

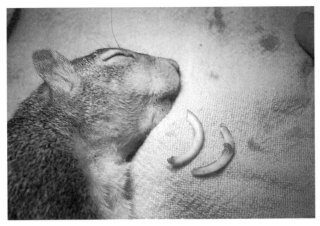

FIG. 10. Extraction of lower incisors in a squirrel after traumatic avulsion of both maxillary incisors.

ligament and used in a sight twisting movement parallel to the reserved crown, while being pressed apically. The angulation of the EX-15 and EX-16 elevators makes them better conform to the tooth's natural curvature, and thus useful on the facial and lingual aspects of the tooth. The process is repeated around the circumference of the tooth, until the reserved crown becomes loose and can easily be removed with small extracting forceps (Fig. 10). The extracting forceps should not be used to attempt forceable extractions, as this can result in fractures of the tooth or supporting bone.

An alternative method is the use of syringe needles in the place of elevators. The needle is inserted beside the tooth and pressed apically with a light twisting force. Extreme care should be observed when the needle is pressed apically, as it can easily penetrate hard and soft tissues and cause serious damage to any structure or organ encountered. In rabbits, 18- and 20-gauge needles work well for most teeth. In rodents, because of the greater size variability, the needle must be selected to fit the incisor, typically 27-, 25-, 23-, or 20-gauge. Owing to tooth curvature, prebending of the needles is possible due to their soft nature but is not ordinarily necessary. The No.2 Molt periosteal elevator and the 18-gauge needle are our most commonly relied on instruments. The smaller rodents such as the mouse are more of a challenge because of the delicacy of teeth and bone. It is very easy, especially in the maxilla, for the needle to penetrate through bone and make contact with underlying structures or organs. For these animals, a 27-gauge 0.5-inch (0.4 mm × 12 mm) needle and gentle manipulation are required.

Once the tooth is removed, the socket is cleaned and curetted of debris or granulation tissue. Bony prominences and spicules are reduced with a bur, curette, or rongeur. If infected, the sockets should be left open for drainage, unless hemorrhage is a problem. In these cases, clean the socket well, flush with saline, fill with tetracycline ophthalmic ointment, and suture closed with absorbable suture material. Antibiotics are recommended if active infection was detected. The patient should be rechecked in approximately 10–14 days to inspect the healing process. Most patients quickly return to eating after surgery in a matter of hours, but occasionally some with sore mouths need encouragement or force-feeding. A liquid diet of fruit or vegetable juice, such as carrot or apple, can be fed with an eye dropper or tuberculin syringe. Blunt-end feeding tubes are available to fit most rodents and lagomorphs, but care should be taken in their use not to injure the animal or inject material into the respiratory system. The owner will need to observe whether the patient has problems with any specific dietary materials and, if necessary, will need either to reduce their size or remove them from the diet, but this is not commonly required.

Should reserved crown tips be broken off in the alveolus, regrowth of the tooth may occur in 4–8 weeks, necessitating a second attempt at extraction at that time. Periodically, the remaining portion may not regrow but become a focus of chronic infection requiring additional attention. Should radiographs at the initial surgery indicate that material is still present, every attempt should be made with a fine elevator or a No.2 Molt to remove this material. The reserved crown of these teeth is hollow with an open apex that has a thin, soft structure. At extraction, soft tissue on the root tip may occasionally be present, representing granulation from infection; on rare occasion the enamel epithelial organ and Hertwig's epithelial root sheath may be present. In chronically infected mandibular retained reserved crown structure that is nonresponsive to normal attempts at extraction, surgical intervention may be required. Radiographs should be used to pinpoint the location, as there is great variation as to the apical location within lagomorphs and rodents (see Dental Anatomy above). An incision is made along the ventral border of the mandible and reflected facially and coronally. Commonly, alterations in normal bone structure will be observed at the pathologic site, indicating appropriate access. If these are not observed, radiographs must be relied on for access selection. In many cases the bony structure will be soft from disease and can be carved away with the sharp No.2 Molt periosteal elevator; otherwise, a No.2 or No.4 round ball bur or a diamond bur can be used to make access. Copious water flow should be used with burs to prevent thermal damage to adjacent hard tissues. Once the reserved crown is exposed, the No.2 Molt ordinarily works well to remove the fragments and to thoroughly curette the lesion. To push reserved crown and debris out, when necessary, an orthodontic wire can be used as a cleaning rod, passed through the apical exposure location and exiting the normal eruption site. Fill the site with tetracycline ophthalmic ointment, and suture it closed using a small-gauge absorbable suture material. In more severe cases, a temporary drain may be placed for a few days.

OTHER DENTAL DISEASE

Besides malocclusion and overgrowth, there are a few other dental problems that lagomorphs and rodents may experience. Minor trauma to or fractures of the teeth that do not involve the pulp may be handled by smoothing the roughened fracture edges and sealing the exposed dentinal surfaces. Occasionally, odontoplasty of the opposing tooth may be needed until the injured tooth grows to a more correct height.

In rats, it is rare to see naturally occurring carious lesions, due to the influences of its normal diet, oral pH, and microflora. Since the shape of molars in rats and hamsters somewhat approximates that of humans (47,53), these teeth are often used in caries research. Rats are most commonly used by feeding high-sucrose diets and decreasing fluoride in pre- and neonatal diets to increase their susceptibility of caries (54). Modifying the amount fed and frequency of meals will promote caries progression, which must often be initiated by introducing particular bacterial strains such as *Streptococcus mutans*. Decreasing salivary flow by surgical removal of glands, inducing diabetes, or radiation exposure of the glands, as well as excising gingival tissue, adding foreign bodies (rat hairs) to the diet, and even placing materials at the gingival line, all may influence their formation.

Since hamsters' mouths can be opened to nearly 180°, regular inspections for caries and plaque research are facilitated. Advantages for using Syrian hamsters include their usual acceptance of cariogenic diet and typical ease in bacterial colonization, but the potential for developing pit-and-fissure caries is relatively low (53,55). Smooth-surface caries is a disadvantage also encountered in gerbils, in addition to their low water consumption that affects oral hydration (56). The continually erupting teeth of guinea pigs and rabbits make them unsuitable for most caries studies.

While caries-like lesions have been described in rabbits (57), these are possibly hypocalcified areas that are most likely sequelae of insults during tooth formation, such as fever, dietary deficiencies, trauma, and infection. If these lesions are minor, treatment is usually unnecessary, as they will eventually be lost as the tooth continues to grow. If extensive or involved, the caries should be removed and a temporary filling material used to restore the teeth, if needed. Any permanent material that may not wear adequately or may produce toxic byproducts if ingested should be avoided.

Brachyodont teeth with carious legions are usually extracted, but standard restoratives may be attempted. Glass ionomers are commonly used in smooth-surface restorations and on occlusal surfaces, and although they lack wearability, they may still be the best alternative (58). Amalgams, with their need for the removal for cavity preparation, would be excessive in these small teeth.

PERIODONTAL DISEASE AND STOMATITIS

Primary periodontal disease is relatively uncommon in rodents and lagomorphs, although it can be induced in laboratory rats with the introduction of *Actinomyces viscosus* (59). A spontaneous form of the disease with plaque and calculus accumulation has been found in gerbils fed a special commercial laboratory diet (60). Periodontal disease can also be reproduced experimentally in rabbits (61), and even hamsters have been used as models for disease transmission (62). However, none of these has been considered very significant clinically, although if periodontal disease is found, it can be treated as it is in other species with a complete prophylaxis, including polishing. Since intubation is usually difficult, hand scaling or use of a sonic scaler without water flow would minimize the chances of patient aspiration of liquids or aerosolized spray. Chlorhexidine solution can also be used to help control plaque accumulation and treat periodontal disease, as has been shown in rats (53).

Most cases of inflammation in the oral cavity are secondary to nonperiodontal causes, as in cheek pouch impaction in the hamster causing a stomatitis (4,42). Removal of the impacted material should be followed by application of an antibiotic ointment or solution in the area.

Hypovitaminosis C, or scurvy, in guinea pigs can cause some serious oral problems, such as gingival hemorrhage, periodontal disease, and loosened teeth that can become maloccluded (9). Treatment with the feeding of vitamin C–rich fruits and vegetables should accompany correction of the diet, including the replacement of outdated foodstuffs. Anorectic animals may require tube-feeding, fluids, antibiotics, and vitamin C supplements.

Overgrown teeth due to malocclusions (21) can also cause irritation to the oral cavity, and crown reduction is usually helpful. Other objects, such as rough edges on water-bottle tubes, feeders, or cages, can lead to abrasions with gingivitis, stomatitis, and excessive salivation. This ptyalism in rabbits may lead to a condition known as *wet dewlap*, a moist dermatitis that often occurs secondary to the causes listed above (3,4). Treating the initial problem usually must be accompanied by clipping the moist area and treating with an antibiotic, as there may be an associated *Pseudomonas* infection (6).

OTHER ORAL DISEASE

Sialoacryoadenitis may affect the salivary glands as a result of a coronavirus infection in rats, causing swellings under the mandible and around the neck (4). Although it is usually self-limiting, it may spread within a colony, and if keratoconjunctivitis is experienced, ophthalmic ointments may be used. The salivary gland virus (cytomegalovirus) in guinea pigs that infects the salivary gland's ductal epithelium seldom causes overt clinical signs (63).

Viral oral papillomatosis in rabbits is usually seen as fixed or pedunculated white growths, usually under the tongue but sometimes on the gingiva (4,10,64–66). Animals with malocclusions that result in abraded epithelial surfaces may be predisposed to the infection (22), which is spread by direct contact; however, it often recedes spontaneously (10). This disease is different from Shope papilloma in the rabbit, which has the potential to transform into malignant squamous cell carcinoma (67–70).

Fusobacterium necrophorum, found in unsanitary conditions, can cause necrobacillosis or Schmorl's disease, with progressive ulceration of the skin and swelling of subcutaneous tissues in the facial, cervical, and oral regions. If abscesses develop at the angle of the mandible, they should be drained and debrided, and the patient should be treated with the appropriate antibiotics (10). Bacteremias and transmission to humans are possible, so these animals should be handled carefully (4).

Other abscesses could be present due to periodontal or endodontic disease and should be treated accordingly. Enlargements associated with the oral cavity other than abscesses may be due to impacted teeth resulting from malocclusion, trauma, or eruption problems. Cysts that are encountered may be treated surgically and thoroughly debrided, while any abnormal mass suspected of being a tumor should always be biopsied.

There are even systemic diseases that will show oral signs, such as lip ulceration in the venereal disease spirochetosis (*Treponema cuniculi*) in rabbits (10). In 6–12-week-old rabbits, tooth grinding may be a common sign of pain associated with the profuse diarrhea of mucoid enteropathy.

No matter what the signs or symptoms, there are many problems pertaining to the oral cavity that the general practitioner can successfully treat in lagomorphs and rodents. Knowing the basic problems that might be encountered and becoming familiar with available treatments can offer patients the best care possible.

ANTIBIOTICS, ANTI-INFLAMMATORY DRUGS, ANALGESICS, AND FLUIDS TREATMENT

Extreme care must be used in the selection of antibiotics and medications, as lagomorphs and rodents have sensitivities and toxicities to many drugs. The most common antibiotics used in rabbit medicine are the penicillins. Penicillin G procaine is commonly used at 20,000–60,000 IU/kg IM twice daily or in the combination of penicillin G benzathine and procaine at 2 cc/10 lb IM or SQ every other day (see caution below). For rabbits or rodents, tetracycline has been used at 30–100 mg/kg orally (PO) in divided doses three times a day or at 400–1000 mg/L in drinking water (4,9,10,36,37). For both rabbits and rodents, 40 mL of sulfamerazine 12.5% solution in a gallon of drinking water for a 0.15% solution has been recommended (9).In rabbits, hamsters, and guinea pigs, almost any antibiotic has the potential to cause a fatal colitis due to potent *Clostridium* toxins, making chloramphenicol the drug of choice in this situation or for other enteropathies because of its effectiveness against *Clostridium* species (71,72). Chloramphenicol succinate in rabbits at 50 mg/kg SQ or IV (10) three times a day and in guinea pigs at 10–30 mg/kg SQ twice a day has been used (3). Chloramphenicol palmitate has been administered orally at the rate of 50 mg/kg three times a day for hamsters and guinea pigs and 200 mg/kg three times a day in mice and rats (9). Lincomycin is contraindicated in rabbits, and ampicillin, erythromycin, and procaine-containing products are to be used with caution (36). Trimethoprim with sulfa drug at a dosage of 30–50 mg/kg SQ or PO once or twice a day is a good general antibiotic for rabbits, gerbils, mice, rats, hamsters, and guinea pigs (9). Enrofloxacin (Baytril®, Miles Inc., Shawnee Mission, Kansas) at the rate of 5 mg/kg PO or 2.5 mg/kg SQ twice a day has been very useful in rabbits for more serious cases.

Although mice, rats, and gerbils typically do not develop the fatal gram-negative enterotoxemias from antibiotics that are seen in hamsters, guinea pigs, and rabbits, they are well known for developing direct toxic effects when certain antibiotics are used. Mice often have antibiotic toxicity problems with streptomycin and procaine, even in low doses (43). Mongolian gerbils are highly sensitive to the streptomycins, with dihydrostreptomycin having a direct toxic effect that results in death within hours (73). Other antimicrobials are of use in rabbits depending on specific pathogens. Several excellent texts on rabbit medicine are available, with extensive drug information (4,10,36,37).

Anti-inflammatory drugs, analgesics, and fluids are required for various procedures. In mice (10) and rats, dexamethasone 1 mg SQ can be used. In rabbits, the dose varies greatly from 0.6 to 6.6 mg/kg SQ or IV according to the severity of the condition being treated (9,74). For analgesia, butorphanol at a rate of 0.05–0.4 mg/kg for both rabbits and small rodents appears to give good pain control (75). Higher dosages published in some texts appear to be unnecessary and unwise. Additionally, fluid therapy of 20 mL/kg SQ twice a day appears to be well tolerated in lagomorphs and rodents (9). With more serious cases in rabbits, a 23–27-gauge indwelling catheter can be placed in the cephalic vein for administration of fluids and medications.

RODENT AND LAGOMORPH COPROPHAGY

In rabbits, one idiosyncrasy associated with the oral cavity that might concern some owners is coprophagy. This is a form of refection that is natural in many lagomorphs and rodents, making them pseudoruminants, as they ingest their own feces for redigestion (36). Rabbits begin this activity around 20 days of age, approximately 3–5 days after they begin eating solid food and maternal feces (11). The cecotrophs, which are about a third of the total fecal output, contain more water, minerals and B vitamins than dry feces produced during the day (11). These animals usually eat these mucus-bound clusters at night and in the early morning hours as part of their natural circadian activity (76).

This behavior can cause a dilemma in evaluation of research data dealing with the teeth and oral cavity. While drugs can be given by gastric intubation or parenteral administration, it must be realized that unabsorbed drugs, their metabolites, modified intestinal bacterial flora, and altered contents of the normal excreta may subject the teeth, oral cavity, and associated structures to covert direct exposure to these components (24). The use of wire-bottom caging aids in reducing this potential complication by allowing some of the cecotrophs to fall through the floor and out of the animal's reach. Unfortunately, many animals ingest them directly from the anus (74). This dilemma should be taken into consideration whenever medications are administered.

REFERENCES

1. Crossley DA. Dental chart for rabbits. *J Vet Dent* 1993;10(3):13.
2. Harkness JE. Rabbit husbandry and medicine. *Vet Clin North Am Small Anim Pract* 1987;17:1091.
3. Williams CSF. *Practical Guide to Laboratory Animals*. St.Louis, MO: CV Mosby Co; 1976:149.
4. Holmes DD. *Clinical Laboratory Animal Medicine: An Introduction*. Ames, IA: Iowa State University Press; 1984:45.
5. Lobprise HB, Wiggs RB. Dental and oral disease in lagomorphs. *J Vet Dent* 1991;8(2):11.
6. Brooks DL. Rabbits, hares and pikas (lagomorpha). In: Fowler, ME, ed. *Zoo and Wild Animal Medicine*. 2nd ed. Philadelphia: WB Saunders Co; 1986:711.
7. Williams CSF. Guinea pigs and rabbits. *Vet Clin North Am Small Anim Pract* 1979:492.
8. Wiggs RB, Lobprise HB. Dental disease in rodents. *J Vet Dent* 1990;7(3):6.
9. Jacobson ER, Kollias GV Jr. *Exotic Animals*. New York: Churchill Livingstone; 1988:179.
10. Russell RJ, et al. *A Guide to Diagnosis, Treatment and Husbandry of Pet Rabbits and Rodents*. Lenexa, KS: Veterinary Medicine Publishing Co; 1981:8.
11. Harkness JE, Wagner JE. *The Biology and Medicine of Rabbits and Rodents*. Philadelphia: Lea & Febiger; 1977:46.
12. Wiggs RB, Lobprise HB. Dental anatomy and physiology of pet rodents and lagomorphs. In: Crossley DD, Penman S, eds. *Manual of Small Animal Dentistry*. Gloucestershire, UK: British Small Animal Association; 1995:68.
13. Zeman WV, Fielder FG. Dental malocclusion and overgrowth in rabbits. *JAVMA* 1969;155:1115.
14. Craigie EH. *Bensley's Practical Anatomy of the Rabbit*. 8th ed. Toronto: University of Toronto Press; 1948.
15. Braithwaite RW. Natural selection in Rattus molars. *J Zool* 1979;189:545.
16. Wiggs RB. Fractured maxillary incisors in a beaver. *J Vet Dent* 1990;7(2):21.
17. Kronfeld R. *Dental Histology and Comparative Dental Anatomy*. Philadelphia: Lea & Febiger; 1937:141.
18. Habermehl KH. *Die Altersbestimmung bei Haus- u. Labortieren*. 2nd ed. Berlin: Verlag Paul Parvey; 1975.
19. Keil A. Über die Frage des naturlichen Vorkommens und der experimentellen Erzeugung echter Zahnkaries bei Tieren. *Dtsch Zahnarztl Z* 1949;4;S:694.
20. Harkness JE, Wagner JE. *The Biology and Medicine of Rabbits and Rodents*. 2nd ed. Philadelphia: Lea & Febiger; 1983:7.
21. Eisenmenger E, Zetner K. *Veterinary Dentistry*. Philadelphia: WB Saunders Co; 1985:25.
22. Weisbroth SH, et al. *The Biology of the Laboratory Rabbit*. New York: Academic Press; 1973:109,357.
23. Craigie EH. *Laboratory Guide to the Anatomy of the Rabbit*. 2nd ed. Toronto: University of Toronto Press; 1973: 26.
24. Navia JM. *Animal Models in Dental Research*. University of Alabama Press; 1977:111,371.
25. Shipp AD, Fahrenkrug P. *Practitioners' Guide to Veterinary Dentistry*. Beverly Hills, CA: Shipp's Labs Publishing Co; 1992:16.
26. Wiggs RB, Lobprise HB. Oral diagnosis in pet rodents and lagomorphs. In: Crossley DD, Penman S, eds. *Manual of Small Animal Dentistry*. Gloucestershire, UK: British Small Animal Association; 1995:74.
27. Kraus BS, et al. *The Study of the Masticatory System Dental Anatomy and Occlusion*. Baltimore: Williams & Wilkins; 1969:274.
28. Allen DL, et al. *Periodontics for the Dental Hygienist*. 2nd ed. Philadelphia: Lea & Febiger; 1974:23.
29. Sicher H, Bhaskar SN. *Orban's Oral Histology and Embryology*. St.Louis, MO: CV Mosby Co; 1972:182.
30. Weisbroth SH. Personal communication between Lindsey JR, Fox RR, and Weisbroth SH.
31. Shadle AR. The attrition and extrusive growth of the four major incisor teeth of domestic rabbits. *J Mammals* 1936;17:15.
32. Weisbroth SH, Ehrman L. Malocclusion in the rabbit: A model for the study of the development, pathology and inheritance of malocclusion. *J Hered* 1967;58:245.
33. Fox RR, Crary DD. Mandibular prognathism in the rabbit: Genetic studies. *J Hered* 1971;62:23.
34. Clark JD, Olfert ED. Rodents (rodentia). In: Fowler ME, ed. *Zoo and Wild Animal Medicine*. 2nd ed. Philadelphia: WB Saunders Co; 1986:727.
35. Neopola SR. The intrinsic and extrinsic factors influencing the growth and development of the jaws: Hereditary and functional matrix. *Am J Orthod* 1969;55:499.
36. Robinson PT. Dentistry in zoo animals. In: Fowler ME, ed. *Zoo and Wild Animal Medicine*. 2nd ed. Philadelphia: WB Saunders Co; 1986:533.
37. Crossley DA. Clinical aspects of lagomorph dental anatomy: The rabbit (Oryctolagus cuniculus). *J Vet Dent* 1995;12(4):137.
38. Wiggs RB. Extraction, pulpectomy, pulpotomy or blunting of macaque canine teeth. *J Vet Dent* 1988;5(1):7.
39. Wiggs RB, Lobprise HB. Prevention and treatment of dental problems in rodents and lagomorphs. In: Crossley DD, Penman S, eds. *Manual of Small Animal Dentistry*. Gloucestershire, UK: British Small Animal Association; 1995:84.

40. Kostlin R, Schebitz H. Zur endodontischen Behandlung der Zahnfractur beim Hund. *Kleinter Prax* 1980;25:187.
41. Burns RB, Hinshaw K. Dentoalveolar Abscess with Sequestra in a Geriatric Porcupine. *J Vet Dent* 1989;6(3):28.
42. Wiggs RB. Pulpotomy failure in a rhesus monkey. *J Vet Dent* 1990;7(1):15.
43. Martin H. Controversies in dentistry. In: Cohen S, Burns RC, eds. *Pathways to the Pulp.* 5th ed. Philadelphia: Mosby-Year Book; 1991:778.
44. Miserendino LJ. Instruments, materials, and devices. In: Cohen S, Burns RC, eds. *Pathways to the Pulp.* 5th ed. Philadelphia: Mosby-Year Book; 1991:388.
45. Hillyer EV. Guinea pigs. *Vet Clin North Am Small Anim Pract* 1994;24:25.
46. Chong R, Senzer J. Systemic distribution of 210 PbO from root canal fillings. *J Endod* 1976;2:381.
47. Goodman L, Gilman A. *The Pharmacological Basis of Theraputics.* 3rd ed. New York: Macmillan Co; 1965.
48. Oswald R, Cohn S. Systemic distribution of lead from root canal fillings. *J Endod* 1975;1:59.
49. Shapiro I, et al. Blood-lead levels in monkeys treated with a lead-containing (N-2) root canal cement. *J Endod* 1975;1:294.
50. Brewer D. Histology of apical tissue reaction to overfill. *J Calif Dent Assoc* 1975;3:58.
51. Brown B, et al. Studies of Sargenti technique of endodontic—reaction to the materials. *J Endod* 1978;4:238.
52. Brown SA. Incisor removal in the rabbit. Tech—North American Veterinary Conference Proceeding 1993;791.
53. Yankell SL. Oral disease in laboratory animals: Animal models of human dental disease. In: Harvey, CE, ed. *Veterinary Dentistry.* Philadelphia: WB Saunders Co; 1985:281.
54. Shrestha BM, et al. Inoculation and pre-weaning conditioning effects on rat caries. In: Hefferren JJ, ed. *Proceedings of the Sixth Conference on Foods, Nutrition and Dental Health.* Chicago: American Dental Association Health Foundation; 1984;5:73.
55. Fitzgerald RL, Keyes PH. Demonstration of the etiologic role of Streptococci in experimental caries in the hamster. *JADA* 1960;61:9.
56. Mundorff SA. Dental decay research in animals. *Lab Anim* 1988;17:19.
57. Hu CK, Greene HSN. A lethal acromegalic mutation in the rabbit. *Science* 1935;81:25.
58. Holmstrom SE, Gammon RL. Glass ionomers. *J Vet Dent* 1988;5(4):34.
59. Baer PN. Use of laboratory animals for calculus studies. *Ann N Y Acad Sci* 1968;153:230.
60. Moskow VS, et al. Spontaneous periodontal disease in the Mongolian gerbil. *J Periodontal Res* 1968;3:59.
61. Horodyski B, Slowik T. Radiograph of periodontal disease in humans and experimental periodontal disease in rabbits. *Czas Stomatol* 1966;19:1191.
62. Jordan HV, Eye PH. Aerobic, gram-positive, filamentory bacteria as etiological agents of experimental periodontal disease in hamsters. *Arch Oral Biol* 1964;9:401.
63. Van Hoosier GL Jr, Robinette LR. Viral and chlamydial diseases. In: JE Wagner, Manning PJ, eds. *The Biology of the Guinea Pig.* New York: Academic Press; 1976:137.
64. Kidd KG, Parsons RJ. Tissue affinity of Shope papilloma virus. *Proc Soc Exp Biol Med* 1936;35:438.
65. Parsons RJ, Kidd JG. A virus causing oral papillomatosis in rabbits. *Proc Soc Exp Biol Med* 1936;35:441.
66. Parsons RJ, Kidd JG. Oral papillomatosis of rabbits: a virus disease. *J Exp Med* 1943;77:233.
67. Shope RE. Infectious papillomatosis of rabbits (with note on histopathology by EW Hurst). *J Exp Med* 1933;58:607.
68. Shope RE. A change in rabbit fibroma virus suggesting mutation. II. Behavior of the variant virus in cottontail rabbits. *J Exp Med* 1936;63:173.
69. Shope RE. Immunization of rabbits to infectious papillomatosis. *J Exp Med* 1937;65:219.
70. Rous P, Beard JW. A virus-induced mammalian growth with the characters of a tumor (the Shope rabbit papilloma). I. Growth on implantation within favorable host. *J Exp Med* 1934;60:701.
71. Manning PT, et al. Biology and disease of guinea pigs. In: Fox FG, Cohen BJ, Loew FM, eds. *Laboratory Animal Medicine.* New York: Academic Press; 1984:149.
72. Gutta GN, et al. Susceptibility of Clostridia from farm animals to twenty-one antimicrobial agents, including some used for growth promotion. *Antimicrob Chemother* 1983;12:347.
73. Wightman SR, et al. Dihydrostreptomycin toxicity in the Mongolian gerbil, *Meriones unguiculatus. Lab Anim Sci* 1980;30:71.
74. Schuekman SM. Individual care and treatment of rabbits, mice, rats, guinea pigs, hamsters and gerbils. In: Kirk RW, ed. *Current Veterinary Therapy VI.* Philadelphia: WB Saunders Co; 1977:126.
75. Short ET. *Principles and Practices of Veterinary Anesthesia.* Philadelphia: WB Saunders Co; 1987:28.
76. Hornicke H, Batsch F. Coecotrophy in rabbits: A circadian function. *J Mammals* 1977;58:240.
77. Collins RG. *Syllabus for the Laboratory Animal Technologist.* Joliet, IL: AALAS.
78. Wallach JD, Boever WJ. *Diseases of Exotic Animals: Medical and Surgical Management.* Philadelphia: WB Saunders Co; 1983:179.
79. Branson PH, et al. Normal hematology and serum chemistry values for the chinchilla. Presented at the AALAS 36th Annual Session; Baltimore, MD; 1985.

18

Exotic Animal Oral Disease and Dentistry

Robert B. Wiggs and Heidi B. Lobprise

Exotic animal dentistry presents many interesting challenges beyond those experienced by the small animal practitioner. However, much can be done to promote good oral health by adapting basic dental skills and knowledge and by gleaning information from previously reported cases.

SPECIAL CONSIDERATIONS

Zoonoses can be of serious or even fatal importance, especially when primates are concerned. Due to the seriousness of some zoonotic diseases that can be easily passed from patient to staff or vice versa, pertinent precautions for each species should be taken (eg, gloves, mask, goggles, gown, etc.). The appropriateness of serum sampling, tuberculosis tests, etc., of patient and staff should be discussed with specialists of the various species. The practitioner must always first address the zoonotic factor before considering diagnosis and treatment.

The lack of close personal contact and of the ability to regularly examine the mouths of most exotic patients can greatly delay the detection of oral problems until they are well advanced. Some general signs might exist, such as a decrease in appetite, weight loss, dropping of food while chewing, external facial swelling or drainage, undigested food in the fecal material, and signs of pain or discomfort such as rubbing the face. Often more subtle indications may be present earlier in the course of the disease, such as a change in attitude, selectiveness of diet (avoidance of hard-to-chew foods), and changes in the method of food prehension. Needless to say, an astute caretaker familiar with the patient and well attuned to any minor changes plays a very important role in early detection of problems. Many problems are first detected during routine yearly physicals performed under chemical restraint. Whenever an exotic is sedated, this is an excellent opportunity to perform an oral examination, dental prophylaxis, and oral treatment.

Once a problem is suspected, the work itself can be quite demanding. A complete oral examination and even very minor procedures quite often necessitate the use of general anesthesia to facilitate the work and protect both the patient and personnel involved. Exotic anesthetic and restraint protocols are beyond the scope of this chapter, and it is highly recommended that persons not familiar with these for a particular type of patient or species enlist the help of a veterinarian who has expertise in the appropriate area. While shortcuts should never be taken that would compromise quality dental care, organization before and during the procedure is necessary to minimize the anesthetic time, especially in exotics. Always keep in mind the patient as a whole.

While basic skills and knowledge can help you address a problem, adjustments must frequently be made to suit a particular species, especially when it comes to instrumentation. Most notably, the biggest shortcomings often concern the use of endodontic instruments in some of the larger patients, such as the big cats. The longer 60-mm veterinary endodontic files can be useful in incisors or smaller species; however, a full-length cuspid on a tiger or lion usually requires custom instrumentation, such as standard endodontic files soldered onto orthodontic wires and the use of threaded Kirschner wires in small canals. In the large canals of young tigers and bears, for example, 3–6-inch long drill bits of various sizes are helpful. Instrument complications, such as decreased efficiency and even breakage at solder joints, are likely, so great care is needed.

Many extractions can be performed with standard instruments, but in oversized and undersized dentitions, adaptation of instruments intended for other uses may be required, such as short-handled sledge hammers, chisels, crowbars, large drill bits, ship augers, and power drills in the elephant. Adjustments in access to the oral cavity are sometimes needed, particularly in the herbivores, so buccotomy approaches may be helpful.

Impressions and models can be facilitated by using various products to make custom trays, but other tools (eg, large feed scoops) may also be used. Instead of the use of custom trays, rubber-base putty impression can be used by mixing and molding it in place in sections around the dental arcade. To improve details, the putty impression can be removed and the dental impressions coated with a wash or light-bodied impression material and quickly replaced in the mouth. Latex gloves or vinyl gloves with powder can easily disrupt the setting of polysiloxane impression materials; therefore, if gloves are to be used, plastic is preferred. With a little imagination (and sometimes desperation), many obstacles can be overcome.

As compared with the situation of small animals, routine postoperative care of larger animals beyond general observation can be minimal. Drug usage may be limited to those drugs that can be added to food or water or administered by dart. Treatment selection should allow the patient to return to normal habits as soon as recovery from anesthesia is complete. Some animals can be worked with postoperatively, but the need for regular handling should be minimized, if at all possible.

All in all, the myriad complications may discourage the practice of good dental care, but the obligation to attempt to provide optimum care must always be recognized. Particularly as related to the oral cavity, a number of iatrogenic problems can occur in captive exotics, primarily as a result of changes made to the diet and surrounding environment. Prepared diets may provide adequate nutrition, but the variety of textures required to provide the physiologic dental and gingival cleaning afforded by chewing roughage for herbivores and rodents or by ingesting prey for predators is lost. Problems of increased periodontal disease, resorptive lesions, lumpy jaw, caries, and dental overgrowth may be related to these dietary alterations. Behavioral problems, such as head or tusk rubbing or abnormal chewing of hard objects and cage bars, can cause significant dental trauma. Trying to provide a diet and environment that approximate what would normally be experienced in the wild would be best for the patient. With good fortune, other problems can be corrected as they occur, thus preserving individuals that might otherwise have perished in their natural habitat.

DENTAL VARIATION

It is nearly impossible to know the distinct dental characteristics and accompanying problems of all the exotic species potentially encountered (1). Nevertheless, as experience in the field grows, our knowledge improves. Starting with elementary dental knowledge and skills and recognizing anatomic differences provide a good starting foundation.

A wide variety of dentitions encountered often closely follow the adaptive pattern of the species in the functions of prehension/incision, mastication, and grooming, as well as social/sexual and defensive capabilities (Fig. 1) (Table 1). Little information is available on deciduous dentition formulas or the eruption times of deciduous or permanent teeth, except for some of the nonhuman primates and a few of the big cats (2,3) (Tables 2 and 3). The distinction between dentition, function, oral access, and temporomandibular joint motion variations among carnivores, omnivores, and herbivores are all important.

True carnivores tend to have teeth adapted for subduing prey and tearing flesh with wide mouth openings and laterally stable temporomandibular joints that allow higher occlusive forces. Although attrition is seen, it is not as extensive as the functional attrition found in herbivores that have constant wear from eating various vegetation, with continually erupting or continually growing teeth. Herbivores also tend to have a much smaller mouth opening with significant lateral temporomandibular joint movement that assists in the grinding of ingesta. The small mouth opening with often a relatively long oral cavity presents unique problems in trying to deal with the caudal portions of the mouth.

Dental structures also reflect adaptive tendencies and function. The carnivore dentition, as well as that of some omnivores and nongrazing herbivores, typically consists of teeth that have specific eruption sequences with maturation and closure of the root apices. The crown length is relatively short in comparison with the root (*brachyodont*) and, once erupted, has less drifting or overeruption due to a more stable periodontal ligament. The crowns are fully covered with enamel, and wear is less of a factor than in herbivores. Omnivorous teeth are similar, though not as specialized, with more occlusal surfaces on caudal teeth and a greater tendency to drift, particularly with adjacent tooth loss (Fig. 2).

Some herbivores (eg, browsing, grazing animals) also have roots with distinctly closing apices but with a relatively long crown (*hypsodont*). While such teeth have a limited

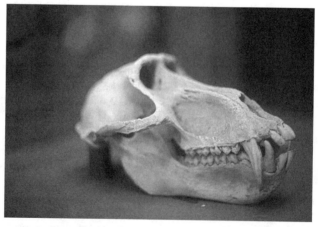

FIG. 1. Skull of a male baboon with large cuspids (as compared with the female sexual dimorphism) for social and defensive functions.

TABLE 1. *Permanent dental formulas*

Taxonomic group	Dental formula				
	Incisors	Cuspids	Premolars	Molars	Total
Insectivora					
Erinaceidae					
Hedgehog (16)	(3/2	1/1	3/2	3/3)	× 2 = 36
or	(3/3	1/1	4/4	3/3)	× 2 = 44
Hedgehog (22)	(2–3/3	1/1	3–4/2–4	3/3)	× 2 = 36–44
Elephantulidae					
Elephant shrew	(1–3/3	1/1	4/4	2–3/3)	× 2 = 36–42
Potamogale					
Water shrew	(3/3	1/1	3/3	3/3)	× 2 = 40
Eremitalpa					
Golden mole	(3/3	1/1	3/3	3/3)	× 2 = 40
Scapanidae					
Moles	(2–3/1–2	1/0–1	3–4/3–4	3/3)	× 2 = 32–42
Chiroptera					
Pteropus					
Fruit bat	(2/2	1/1	3/3	2/3)	× 2 = 34
Rousettus					
Fruit bat	(2/2	1/1	3/3	2/3)	× 2 = 34
Nyctimene					
Fruit bat	(1/0	1/1	3/3	1/2)	× 2 = 24
Paranyctimene					
Fruit bat	(1/0	1/1	3/3	1/2)	× 2 = 24
Desmodus					
Vampire bat	(1/2	1/1	2/3	0/0)	× 2 = 20
Myotis					
Little brown bat	(1–2/2–3	1/1	1–3/2–3	3/3)	× 2 = 28–38
Mystacina					
New Zealand short-tailed bat	(1/1	1/1	2/2	3/3)	× 2 = 28
Edentata					
Myrmecophagidae					
Anteaters	(0/0	0/0	0/0	0/0)	× 2 = 0
Bradypodidae					
Tree sloths	(0/0	0/0	5/4	5/4)	× 2 = 36
Two-toed sloth	(0/0	1/1	4/3	0/0)	× 2 = 18
Dasypodidae					
Nine-banded armadillo	(0/0	0/0	P&Ms	7–9/7–9)	× 2 = 28–36
Tubulidentata					
Orycteropodidae					
Aardvark	(0/0	0/0	2/2	3/3)	× 2 = 20
Lagomorpha					
Ochotonidae					
Pika	(2/1	0/0	3/2	2/3)	× 2 = 26
Leporidae					
Hare	(2/1	0/0	3/2	3/3)	× 2 = 28
Oryctolagidae					
Rabbit	(2/1	0/0	3/2	2 or 3/3)	× 2 = 26 or 28
Rodentia					
Sciuridae					
Squirrels	(1/1	0/0	1 or 2/1	3/3)	× 2 = 20 or 22
Castoridae					
Beaver	(1/1	0/0	1/1	3/3)	× 2 = 20
Cricetidae					
Cricetid mice and rats	(1/1	0/0	0/0	3/3)	× 2 = 16
Muridae					
Old World mice and rats	(1/1	0/0	0/0	2–3/2–3)	× 2 = 12–16

TABLE 1. *Continued*

Taxonomic group	Incisors	Cuspids	Premolars	Molars	Total
Hystricidae					
Old World Porcupines	(1/1	0/0	1/1	3/3)	× 2 = 20
Erethizontidae					
New World porcupines	(1/1	0/0	1/1	3/3)	× 2 = 20
Caviidae					
Guinea pig	(1/1	0/0	1/1	3/3)	× 2 = 20
Hydrochoeridae					
Capybara	(1/1	0/0	1/1	3/3)	× 2 = 20
Chinchillidae					
Chinchilla	(1/1	0/0	1/1	3/3)	× 2 = 20
Capromyiade					
Nutria	(1/1	0/0	1/1	3/3)	× 2 = 20
Monotremata					
Australian duckbill	(0/0	0/0	0/0	0/0)	× 2 = 0
Marsupialia					
Didelphidae					
Virginia, woolly, and mouse opossums	(5/4	1/1	3/3	4/4)	× 2 = 50
or Opossum (61)	(5/5	1/1	3/3	4/4)	× 2 = 52
Vombatidae					
Wombat	(1/1	0/0	1/1	4/4)	× 2 = 24
Macropodidae					
Wallabies and kangaroos	(3/1	0–1/0	2/2	4/4)	× 2 = 32 or 34
Dasyuriade					
Marsupial mice and Tasmanian devil	(4/3	1/1	2–3/2–3	4/4)	× 2 = 42 or 46
Notoryctidae					
Marsupial mole	(3–4/3	1/1	2/2	4/4)	× 2 = 40 or 42
Caenolestidae					
Rat opossums	(4/3–4	1/1	3/3	4/4)	× 2 = 46–48
Phalangeridae					
Bush-tailed opossums, cuscuses, and koalas	(2–3/1–3	1/0	1–3/1–3	3–4/3–4)	× 2 = 22–42
Cetacea (homodont teeth, all similarly shaped)					
Delphinidae					
Common dolphin					160–200
Delphinapteridae					
Beluga dolphin					32–40
Tursiops					
Bottle-nose dolphin					74–102
Phocoenidae					
Harbor porpoise					56–108
Globicephala					
Pilot whale					28–44
Orcinus orca					
Killer whale					40–56
Sirenia					
Trichechidae					
Manatee (16)	(2/2	0/0	0/0	11/11)	× 2 = 52
Manatee (22)	(0/0	0/0	0/0	6/6)	× 2 = 24
Pinnipedia[a]					
Otariidae					
Sea lion and fur seal	(3/2	1/1	4/4	1–3/1)	× 2 = 34–38
Phocidae					
True, hair, and elephant seals (16)	(2–3/1–2	1/1	4/4	1/1)	× 2 = 30–34

TABLE 1. *Continued*

Taxonomic group	Incisors	Cuspids	Premolars	Molars	Total
			Dental formula		
or Elephant seals (22)	(2–3/1–2	1/1	4–6/4–5	0/0)	× 2 = 26–36
Odobenidae					
Walrus (5)	(1–2/0	1/1	3–4/3–4	0/0)	× 2 = 18–26
Carnivora					
Canidae					
Bush dog	(3/3	1/1	4/4	1/2)	× 2 = 38
Asiatic wild dog	(3/3	1/1	4/4	2/2)	× 2 = 40
Domestic dog	(3/3	1/1	4/4	2/3)	× 2 = 42
Fox and wolf	(3/3	1/1	4/4	2–3/2–3)	× 2 = 40–44
Bat-eared fox	(3/3	1/1	4/4	4/4)	× 2 = 48
Ursiade					
Bear	(3/3	1/1	4/4	2/3)	× 2 = 42
Sloth bear (65)	(2/3	1/1	4/4	2/3)	× 2 = 40
Felidae					
Cats, lions, tigers, etc.	(3/3	1/1	3/2	1/1)	× 2 = 30
North American and Canadian bobcats	(3/3	1/1	2/2	1/1)	× 2 = 28
Procyonidae					
Raccoon, kinkajou, and panda	(3/3	1/1	3–4/3–4	2/2–3)	× 2 = 32–42
Mustelidae					
Badger, otter, and skunk	(3/2–3	1/1	2–4/2–4	1/1–2)	× 2 = 26–38
Ferret, mink, polecat and weasel (5)	(3/3	1/1	3/3	1/2)	× 2 = 34
Marten (5)	(3/3	1/1	4/4	1/2)	× 2 = 38
Hyaenidae					
Hyena	(3/3	1/1	4/3	1/1)	× 2 = 34
Viverridae					
Mongoose and genet	(3/3	1/1	3–4/3–4	1–2/1–2)	× 2 = 36–40
Civtes	(3/3	1/1	4/4	2/2)	× 2 = 40
Hyracoidea					
Procaviidae					
Hyrax (16)	(1/2	0/0	4/4	3/3)	× 2 = 34
Hyrax (22)	(1/2	1/1	4/4	3/3)	× 2 = 38
Proboscidea					
Elephantidae					
African elephant	(1/0	0/0	0/0	6/6)	× 2 = 26
or	(1/0	0/0	3/3	3/3)	× 2 = 26
Asian elephant	(0–1/0	0/0	0/0	6/6)	× 2 = 24 or 26
or	(0–1/0	0/0	3/3	3/3)	× 2 = 24 or 26
Perissodactyla					
Equidae					
Horse, ass, and zebra	(3/3	1/1	3–4/3	3/3)	× 2 = 40 or 42
Tapiridae					
Tapirs	(3/3	1/1	4/4	3/3)	× 2 = 44
Rhinocerotidae					
Rhinoceros	(0–1/0–1	0/0–1	4/4	3/3)	× 2 = 28, 32, or 34
Artiodactyla					
Suidae					
Domestic pig	(3/3	1/1	4/4	3/3)	× 2 = 44
Wild swine	(3/3	1/1	4/4	3/3)	× 2 = 44
Babirusa	(2/3	1/1	2/2	3/3)	× 2 = 34
Wart hog	(1/3	1/1	3/2	3/3)	× 2 = 34
Tayassuidae					
Javelina or peccary	(2/3	1/1	3/3	3/3)	× 2 = 36
Hippopotamidae					
Hippopotamus	(2–3/1 or 3	1/1	4/4	3/3)	× 2 = 38–44

TABLE 1. *Continued*

Taxonomic group	Incisors	Cuspids	Premolars	Molars	Total
Camelidae					
Camel, guanaco, llama, vicuna, and alpaca	(1/3	1/1	2–3/2	3/3)	× 2 = 32 or 34
Llama	(1/3	1/0–1	2/2–3	3/3)	× 2 = 30–34
Tragulida					
Chevrotain or mouse deer	(1/3	1/1	2–3/2	3/3)	× 2 = 32 or 34
Ceridae[b]					
True deer	(0/3	0–1/1	3/3	3/3)	× 2 = 32 or 34
Giraffidae[b]					
Giraffe and okapi	(0/3	0/1	3/3	3/3)	× 2 = 32
Antilocapridae[b]					
Pronghorn antelope	(0/3	0/1	3/3	3/3)	× 2 = 32
Bovidae[b]					
Antelope, cattle, goats, and sheep	(0/3	0/1	3/3	3/3)	× 2 = 32
Primates					
Tupaiidae	(2/3	1/1	3/3	3/3)	× 2 = 38
Indridae	(2/2	1/0	2/2	3/3)	× 2 = 30
Daubentoniidae	(1/1	0/0	1/0	3/3)	× 2 = 18
Tarsiidae	(2/1	1/1	3/3	3/3)	× 2 = 34
Lemuridae					
Lemurs	(2/2	1/1	3/3	3/3)	× 2 = 36
Lorisidae					
Lorises	(2/2	1/1	3/3	3/3)	× 2 = 36
Cebidae					
New World monkeys	(2/2	1/1	3/3	3/3)	× 2 = 36
Callithricidae					
Marmosets	(2/2	1/1	3/3	2/2)	× 2 = 32
Cercopithecidae					
Old World monkeys	(2/3	1/1	2/2	3/3)	× 2 = 34
Pongidae					
Great apes	(2/2	1/1	2/2	3/3)	× 2 = 32
Hominidae					
Homo sapiens	(2/2	1/1	2/2	3/3)	× 2 = 32

(Compiled from data in refs. 1,5,16,22,61–64.)

[a]Animals in the order Pinnipedia are closely related to those of the order Carnivora and in many classifications are designated as a suborder of Carnivora (22).

[b]In many of these families, the lower cuspid or canine tooth has migrated mesially and functions similarly to an incisor.

TABLE 2. *Felidae approximate deciduous eruption times (days of age)*

Tooth	Lion	Tiger	Leopard	Puma	Jaguar
1st incisor	22–24	12–20	22–26	14–17	15–17
2nd incisor	25–29	20–24	26–27	17–20	20–25
3rd incisor	33–39	28–29	32–33	23–28	20–32
Cuspid	31–32	31–34	28–30	28–29	29–35
2nd molar	117–152	—	—	—	60–62
3rd molar	60–65	55–59	45–47	40–42	—
4th molar	48–85	52–64	40–69	37–47	—

TABLE 3. *Eruption times of deciduous and permanent teeth in the bobcat*

Teeth	Days
Deciduous	
Eruption begins	11–14
Eruption complete	40–60
Permanent	
Incisor eruption begins	130
Incisor eruption complete	160
Canine eruption complete	190
Maxillary eruptions complete	210
Mandibular eruptions complete	240

(Reproduced from Walker EP. Carnivora (Ursidae). In: *Mammals of the World*. Baltimore: Johns Hopkins University Press; 1964:1169, with permission.)

growth period, they do continually erupt as attrition wears down the anatomic crown height, and the entire tooth structures moves in a coronal direction. Typically, the occlusal surface is rough, covered with varying ridges of enamel, dentin, and cementum that wears away at different rates. These ridges facilitate mastication of fibrous materials. Most of these species have teeth that erupt sequentially in a vertical direction (eg, diphyodont with primary teeth and permanent successors). One exception is the elephant (together with some macropods and manatees), whose molars erupt in a sequential, horizontal direction, moving mesially and breaking off in sections as the next molar erupts behind it. During its lifetime, there are a total of six molars in each quadrant, and the first three are considered to be juvenile. (This will be discussed in further detail in the elephant section below.)

The concept of continual eruption differs greatly from that of continual growth. The latter refers to teeth that have persistently open apices, with growth for the life of the tooth, and no distinct root structure (*aradicular hypsodont*). Typically, these teeth are not completely covered by enamel, if at all, because constant wear is necessary to keep the crown at a reasonable height. Lagomorphs and some rodents (eg, chinchillas, guinea

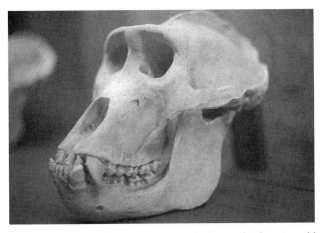

FIG. 2. Skull of a lowland gorilla showing dentition similar to the human with some modifications, particularly cuspids. Premolars and molars have well developed occlusal surfaces.

pigs) have this tooth structure both rostrally and caudally, though in most other rodents only the rostral teeth (incisors) are continuously growing. Needless to say, any disruptions to normal attrition (eg, malocclusion, lack of proper dental exercise) can rapidly lead to tooth overgrowth. In some animals, such as aardvarks (order Tubulidentata), only the caudal teeth continuously erupt.

Other variations in dentition include *homophyodont* teeth, which have a uniform structure throughout the mouth and are brachyodont. Of these, cetaceans are monophyodonts, having just one set of teeth, while sharks and reptiles are polyphyodonts with a potentially endless succession of teeth, either vertically or horizontally replaced. One form of unique development is seen in the alligator and related species, in which the upper jaw rather than the lower is mobile. Most reptilians have limited lateral jaw movement due to the large number of teeth that function primarily for prehension and combat (4).

With this rudimentary overview of various exotic dentitions, the following material will cover problems encountered in different groups of animals. While the treatments listed are typically anecdotal from literature case reports and personal experience, some general knowledge will also be discussed.

DENTAL ABNORMALITIES

Variations in crowns, roots, endodontic systems, and numbers of teeth have all been reported for most species (5). Conditions of heredity, environment, nutrition, dietary textures, and stress may play roles in these abnormalities, with many of these factors being possible causes of the variance between wild and captive individuals.

Enamel hypocalcification and hypoplasia are observed in varying degrees in most species of animals. One study indicates a higher degree of problem in animals raised in zoos than in their wild counterparts (6). Captive chimpanzees, gibbons, baboons, and orangutans are some of the more common nonhuman primates to demonstrate these problems. In brachyodont teeth, treatment is seldom required, unless excessive attrition from the softer teeth results in sensitivity due to dentinal tubule exposure or pulpitis resulting from endodontic exposure. Sensitivities can be controlled with restoratives and pit-and-fissure sealants. Pulpal exposure usually requires endodontic therapy or extraction. Hypsodonts, with their continual eruption and attrition, rarely need any form of therapy, as the diseased structure is eventually worn away. Delayed eruption of teeth can be difficult to timely identify due to problems of examination and a lack of published, obtainable data on eruption times of many species. Eruption problems can be due to endocrine disorders, but mechanical problems of retained deciduous or supernumerary teeth, crowding, tumors, and cysts are more commonly responsible (7). Individual delays can be obvious in the face of eruption of all other teeth, but radiographs are required to determine whether a delay in eruption or a missing tooth is the true problem. However, pathologic bone in the mandrill, bear, and cat have been reported to prevent eruption (5).

Supernumerary teeth can be hereditary or congenital, or the result of disturbances in the odontogenic process through inflammation or excessive pressures (8). Investigations indicate that true supernumeraries are more common in the maxilla than the mandible (5). Polyodontia, or retained deciduous teeth, are not true supernumerary teeth and should normally be treated by exodontia. True supernumerary teeth must be addressed according to the tooth type. Brachyodont teeth, if they are causing no problem, can typically be left alone, but if crowding or periodontal disease occur, extraction would be warranted. Hypsodont teeth are continually growing or erupting. Supernumerary hypsodont teeth

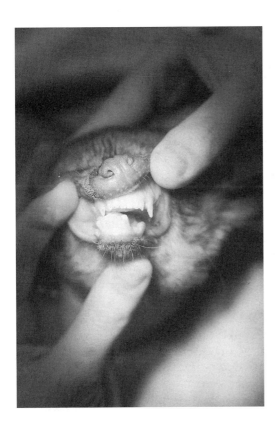

FIG. 3. Kinkajou lateral deviation of mandible caused by "wrist sucking." This individual was orphaned at an early age and developed the habit. Crown amputation with vital pulpotomy and pulp capping were performed to obtain a comfortable bite (postoperative photo).

most often occur in the posterior cheek teeth. Extra teeth in this region customarily result in dental overgrowth due to a lack of contra-attritional surface, and for this reason most require extraction.

Malposition of teeth is also seen in many species (5). Although the same problems are seen in wild and captive groups of animals, the degree of the problem appears to be much higher in captives (7). This may be due to stress, environment, nutrition, dietary textures, trauma, periodontal disease, or abnormal nursing behavior (Fig. 3). With dental drift due to periodontal disease, periodontal therapy and/or exodontia must be initiated along with correction of underlying causes (eg, diet, behavior, etc.). In other conditions, if the malpositioning is not the cause or result of a problem, no treatment is necessary. If trauma or disease results, then extraction or crown amputation and pulp capping should be performed. Attempts at orthodontics in wild species can be complicated; adjustments and maintenance of the appliance are usually difficult.

Carnivores

The most typical lesions found in carnivores, particularly large cats, are fractured, worn, or discolored teeth due to various causes. While the basic tooth/root structure may approximate that of pets seen in a small animal practice, the variation in size can be quite substantial. However, with customized files and pluggers (9), along with softened gutta-percha techniques for fill, most canals can be adequately cleaned and obturated. With small-diameter, deep canals, as in the cuspids of large older African lions (some measuring 0.35 mm × 95 mm), heated gutta-percha carried on the tip of the master file or a size smaller can be vertically compacted by appropriately sized orthodontic wires used for pluggers. In the large canals of some young carnivores, gutta-percha stopping (large sticks of gutta-percha) can be heated on a warm glass slide and rolled to size for a custom fit. In extremely large canals, the stopping can be softened with chloroform and packed into the canal. It is important to not use excessive chloroform, as this technique results in eventual shrinkage of the gutta-percha, which can lead to loss of the apical seal and failure of the procedure. At times, it may be necessary to perform surgical endodontics with apicoectomy in those cases where a standard endodontic technique is not adequate (10,11). As in any endodontic procedure, radiographs are fundamental for good technique, but they are not always available at the sites where the treatment is required to be performed.

Cage-biter syndrome can result in severe dental attrition of the incisal edge of incisors or cuspids and the distal surface of the cuspids. Changes in the physical environment to prevent the chewing or assessment with correction of behavioral stress may correct the bad habit. Teeth with wear may be sensitive and require treatment with pit-and-fissure sealants or placement of a crown. Large crowns fabricated for placement on cuspids can sometimes have problems in being seated due to large amounts of cement being trapped between the cusp tip and the top of the crown. A small vent hole placed at the tip of the crown in fabrication can allow escape of excess cement and ease crown placement.

When damage to the tooth is too extensive, or other conditions exist that would contraindicate endodontics (eg, thin fragile wall, etc.) (11), extraction may be necessary. In deciduous or immature teeth with delicate walls, extraction can be difficult (12), and longitudinal sectioning of the dentinal walls with elevation of each of the segments may prove helpful (10). With large premolars and molars, tooth or root resectioning with accompanying endodontics may preserve a healthy root while removing the diseased one (13).

Crown amputation of cuspids with vital pulpotomy and pulp capping (14,15) may be an alternative to extraction in cases of base-narrow mandibular cuspids (10) or for supposed "disarming" of the animal; however, it must be understood that substantial and serious harm can still be inflicted with blunt cuspids (16).

In animals fed prepared commercial diets, periodontal disease of varying degrees is common (11,17). Standard periodontal treatment protocol (prophylaxis, root planing, polishing, periodontal surgery, etc.) can be followed. In addition, resorptive lesions like

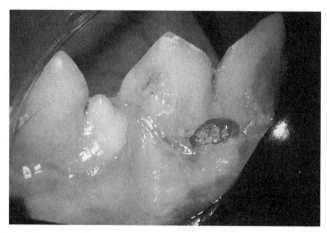

FIG. 4. Buccal erosive lesion on left mandibular 1st molar in a spotted leopard.

those seen in domestic cats have been reported in the larger exotic felines (18,19) (Fig. 4). There has been some concern that lack of texture in prepared diets can play a role in the development of these lesions (20). Treatment can range from restoration of shallow lesions that exhibit no other dental abnormalities (eg, root resorption) to extraction of teeth with more severe lesions.

Other carnivores may experience dental problems; there have been reports of an aged bear that had severe attrition with exposed canals (16), red pandas with periapical and periodontal abscesses (18), and even a polar bear that benefited from multiple endodontic procedures (21). Bears are also subject to tongue problems involving lacerations from worn teeth, penetrating foreign bodies, and neoplasia (22). Basal cell carcinoma in the black bear and melanoma in the Japanese brown bear have been reported (23). One recent case of a 28-year-old sun bear for periodontal problems in one quadrant revealed a squamous cell carcinoma.

In our experience, we have encountered numerous fractured teeth in large cats (lions, leopards, tigers, ocelots, etc.), typically cuspids and incisors. This problem may possible be due in part to these animals' playing with large hard objects and chewing on bars and fencing. Most have responded well to standard endodontic therapy. In addition, metal crowns have been placed both on fractured teeth and on teeth worn from cage biting to prevent fracturing (Fig. 5).

Gingivitis in exotic cats is not an uncommon finding (22). Clinically, signs of halitosis, anorexia, careful food chewing, jaw quivering, and excess salivation can be seen. This problem may associated with periodontal disease, malnutrition, injury or penetrating foreign bodies, viral infection, neoplasia, kidney disease, or teething problems (22). Squamous cell carcinomas have been reported in the Canadian lynx and hemangioma in the cheetah (24).

Omnivores

Parallels can be drawn between dental problems of humans and nonhuman primates (25). Although some have tooth structure and function similar to those of humans, there

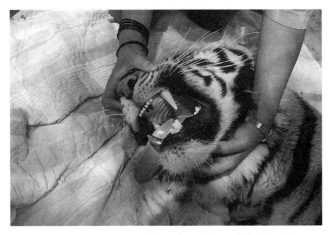

FIG. 5. Steel crown placed on right mandibular cuspid in a Siberian tiger to protect tooth severely worn on its distal aspect (cage-biter syndrome).

are also many differences. Many of the apes have large cuspids and diastemas. The diastema mesial to the maxillary cuspid permits lateral movements of the lower cuspids. In male baboons, the oversized maxillary cuspid passes laterally to the first cheek tooth (3rd premolar). The mesial portion of the 3rd premolar's crown is commonly long and drawn out, providing a specialized shearing action as the jaw closes and the maxillary cuspid moves past it, possibly replacing the carnassial teeth's function in many carnivores. Lemurs typically have the mandibular cuspids and incisors laid out almost horizontally side by side and even, which allows them to function as a comb for grooming. This leads to the lower cuspids' commonly being mistaken for corner incisors. This is further propagated by the fact that the lower 2nd premolar, which is the first cheek tooth, is enlarged and functions as the cuspid would be expected to. Additionally, the upper cuspids of lemurs are elongated mesially to distally, and when trauma exposes the pulp, the canal is typically slot-like in appearance. This requires a modified circumferential instrumentation or a paddling type of instrumentation to suitably clean the canal. New World and Old World monkeys also differ in the number of premolars present (see Table 1). There are also species and individual variations in the absence or presence of the last molar, similar to the wisdom tooth in humans.

Associated problems of periodontal disease and even carious lesions are seen in captive primates, especially when softer prepared diets are fed that may contain refined carbohydrates in contrast to natural fibrous roughage. Treatments will ordinarily follow the basic rules of human dentistry, including infection control.

The progression of periodontal disease starts with the accumulation of plaque and calculus, leading at times to infection and attachment loss and even eventual tooth loss (26). While regular dental care may not be the most practical answer, paying attention to the teeth whenever an individual is under anesthesia for other procedures can help optimize periodontal treatment, while allowing closer examination and earlier detection of dental disease. Most often however, periodontal disease is not found until signs are severe enough to compromise the patient's health (10,16,26–28). Due to large bleeding grooves on the cuspids of some primates, a local periodontitis may be caused by impaction of food and materials in this groove, leading to gingival hyperplasia and periodic periodontal abscesses (15,19) (Fig. 6). This is easily treated by removal of the hyperplastic tissue

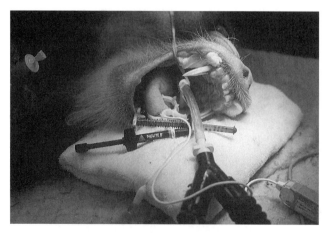

FIG. 6. Hyperplastic gingiva in a male baboon secondary to periodontal disease at the bleeding groove at the mesial aspect of the right maxillary cuspid.

sealing off the sulcus, lancing the abscess, root planing, and packing of antibiotics (eg, doxycycline) into the sulcus.

Gingival tissue may also become hyperplastic or inflamed from vitamin C deficiency (29), causing pseudopockets that would benefit from gingivectomy (10,30). Other oral and gingival swellings should always be closely examined and, if suspicious, should be biopsied for histopathology. While oral neoplasia may be relatively rare in primates, lingual carcinomas and osteogenic sarcomas have been reported in gorillas (28), as has an ameloblastic odontoma in a cynomolgus monkey (3).

Abscess formation may be periodontal or endodontic in origin, due to fractured teeth or deep carious lesions that invade the pulp (32). Whether or not an abscess exists, any exposure or devitalization of the pulp necessitates either endodontics (root canal) or exodontia (extraction). If the lesion spares adequate dental structure, endodontics with the proper restoration would be preferred to minimize drift that can occur after tooth loss (19). Teeth with more extensive damage can be extracted, but that often requires full surgical and sectioning exodontia (10). Facial abscesses and drainage due to fractured maxillary canine teeth are relatively common in captive primates and are referred to as a *malar abscesses.* 22).

Teething problems are sometimes encountered. Teething gingivitis occurs in infant primates, usually with an acute onset of swollen, tender gums, light fever, and occasionally diarrhea (22). Treatment is generally symptomatic with the use of aspirin and antidiarrheal medication. Occasionally, teething abscesses occur due to partially resorbed deciduous teeth with root fractures (Fig. 7). These can be readily diagnosed from radiographs

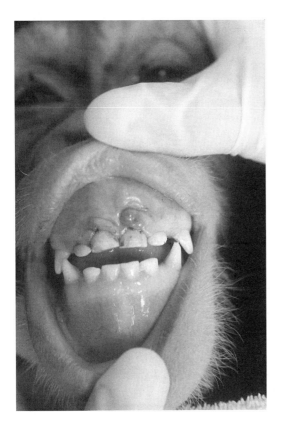

FIG. 7. Abscess of deciduous incisors in an immature chimpanzee; extraction was indicated and performed.

TABLE 4. *Eruption times of deciduous and permanent teeth in the chimpanzee*

	Central incisor	Lateral incisor	Canine	3rd premolar	4th premolar	1st molar	2nd molar	3rd molar
Deciduous teeth (days)								
Maxillary	75–111	87–113	324–354	109–122	282–308	—	—	—
Mandibular	70–96	87–124	349–382	131–149	222–233	—	—	—
Permanent teeth (months)								
Maxillary	66	80–84	110	80–84	83–86	38–40	80–82	136–138
Mandibular	64–71	71–77	106–114	88–90	89	37–40	75–80	125–129

(Compiled from data in Kraus BS, Jordan RE, Abrams L. *Study of Masticatory System Dental Anatomy and Occlusion.* Baltimore: Williams & Wilkins;1969:276; Lombard LS, Witte EJ. Frequency and types of tumors in mammals and birds of the Philadelphia Zoological Garden. *Cancer Res* 1959;19:127; and Effron M, Griner L, Benirsckle K. Nature and rate of neoplasia found in wild captive mammals, birds, and reptiles. *J Natl Cancer Inst* 1977;59:185.)

and by using known eruption pattern information (Table 4). Typically, treatment involves extraction of the deciduous tooth and infected root, with care to prevent iatrogenic damage to the permanent tooth bud.

Carious lesions are not found as commonly in nonhuman primates as in humans; however, changes in diet may increase their incidence, especially in older animals such as gorillas (16). The majority of carious lesions we have encountered have been class I or class II lesions of the premolars and molars. With class II–type lesions, it is common for the proximal surface of the adjacent tooth to have a juxtaposed class II lesion. Shallow lesions that do not involve the pulp generally respond well to standard preparation and restoration techniques with either amalgam or composites (11,19,32). If soft or diseased regions of enamel are found, pit-and-fissure sealants may be used to help discourage future caries formation.

Herbivores

While occasional problems of fractured teeth (10,33) or jaws (33), routine periodontal disease (35), torn or cut lips (36,37), and even infundibular necrosis (38) have been reported in the literature, the most common dental lesion seen in herbivores (especially antelopes and marsupials) is a condition known as *lumpy jaw* (Fig. 8). This acute to chronic alveolitis/osteomyelitis condition is typically manifested by swellings in the facial and mandibular regions, sometimes accompanied by fistulous draining tracts. The pathogenesis seems to be initiation by oral trauma when animals are fed dry, coarse, stemmy hays. The active pathogens are most frequently *Fusobacterium* spp., *Bacteroides* spp., *Peptostreptococcus* spp., Anaerobius spp., Necrobacillosis spp., and *Actinomyces* spp., the majority of which are anaerobes (30,39).

Exodontia is the treatment of choice for most dental abscesses (7,14,16,18,39–42). This can be accomplished by intraoral surgery in many instances. Ease of extraction is determined by the location of the tooth or teeth and the degree of mobility created by disease. The small mouth opening and long, narrow oral cavity make visibility and accessibility a problem. In some cases, a buccotomy may be necessary, although care must be taken with important vasculature and nerves in the area, as well as keeping in mind that some facial scaring may result.

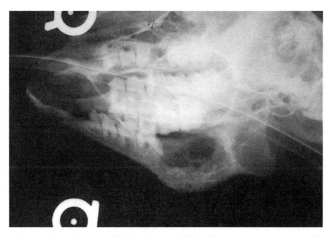

FIG. 8. Radiograph of chronic alveolitis/osteomyelitis (lumpy jaw) of mandibular cheek tooth in a klipspringer.

Routine exodontia principles of severing the epithelial attachment and gradual elevation with gentle force apply here as well. Long, acutely angled extraction forceps can be used to extricate the tooth, once loosened. Tenacious teeth must generally be removed by repelling techniques using radiographs to locate the area (19,43). The socket can then be filled with an osteogenic material, such as tricalcium phosphate, ADD® (Osmed Inc., Costa Mesa, California), or HTR® (Bioplant Inc., New York, New York). The extraoral access is closed with an absorbable suture material. Use of absorbable suture material for the skin sutures is not unusual with exotic animals, as recapture and sedation for removal may pose problems in some cases.

One complication involves empty sockets that epithelialize into the defect, leaving a trough in the mandible between the buccal and lingual cortical plates and leading to food impaction. Mandibular troughing can be prevented after extraction by proper packing and flapping of the sockets. If troughing is already present, a single incision can be made across the mesial proximal border of the defect. A No.2 or No.4 Molt periosteal elevator is then inserted into the incision, and the epithelialized lining is lifted free of the underlying bone, with care to avoid tears, if possible, and curetting the bone surface. Once the lining is properly elevated, a sack-like cavity is produced within the trough. A slender tuberculin syringe of HTR 24 (Bioplant Inc.) (HTR 24 mesh is used for osseous replacement and HTR 40 mesh for periodontal guided tissue regeneration) (44,45) or other osteogenic materials can be used to fill the created cavity; the material is injected as the syringe is withdrawn (46) and the incision closed with one or two absorbable sutures.

While some reports indicate outbreaks with high mortality rates of almost epidemic proportions (39), the results can be favorable if the lesions are recognized early and treated appropriately with extraction, debridement, and antibiotics. Underlying problems such as crowding, sanitation, and coarse feed must be corrected.

Elephants, with their unique dentition characteristics (Table 5; see also Table 1), present an interesting challenge to the practitioner. Problems with tusks are most frequently encountered due to trauma (fractures) (47), self-inflicted injury associated with behavior (rubbing), and even poor development (impaction) (48). The tusk is a modified, continually growing incisor (hypsodont) made of dentin (ivory); it has an excellent ability to remedy injuries with reparative dentin and to fight infections if given a chance (49),

TABLE 5. *Eruption times (years) of deciduous and permanent teeth in the elephant*

Teeth	Eruption	Exfoliation
Deciduous incisors	Birth	
Permanent incisors	1	
Cheek teeth[a] (in order of eruption)		
1st pm/m	Birth	2
2nd pm/m	Birth to 1.5	5
3rd pm/m	2	11
4th PM/M	5	19
5th PM/M	15	60
6th PM/M	26–30	60+

(Reproduced from Walker EP. Carnivora (Ursidae). In: *Mammals of the World.* Baltimore: Johns Hopkins University Press; 1964:1169, with permission.)
[a]There are typically only two sets of cheek teeth fully erupted at any one time. Ordinarily, by age 45–49 years only the sixth set of cheek teeth is still present (pm/m, deciduous premolar/molar; PM/M, permanent premolar/molar).

although some infections can be persistent. When deciduous tusks are present, they are present at birth and are exfoliated and replaced by the permanent tusks by approximately 1 year of age (50). The primary tusks grow from the sulcus, with an initial cap of enamel that is quickly worn away (51). In African elephants, both bulls and cows have tusks, while in the Asian variety, bulls may or may not have tusks, some of which are relatively small. If tusks are present in Asian cows, they typically remain within the sulcus and are barely visible (49). One way to estimate the length of pulp or nerve in the coronal portion of the tusk from the sulcus is to measure the distance from the eye to the tusk sulcus, but this may not hold true with Asian females, as the pulp chambers are customarily located further apically (18). Longer, wider pulp canals are generally found in younger animals, so fractures or attempts at tusk reduction may expose the pulp more quickly than anticipated. Any tusks with fractures, cracks, or cuts that are close to the pulp should be banded with steel rings because splits can occur more readily at that location (49,51). Rings and metal ball caps on the tips may help prevent excessive wear in elephants that habitually rub their tusks (51). One facility now covers all tusks with Ticonium 100™ (Ticonium Co, Albany, New York) (15,52), and others have used Vitallium™ (Howmedica, Inc, Chicago, Illinois) crown halves welded together (47) (post-endo).

If pulp exposure occurs, attempts should be made to prevent or treat infection and to protect the pulp to allow the affected area to grow out. The extent of infection or exposure will dictate the treatment protocol. For minor exposures, removal of the coronal pulp to healthy tissue followed by hemorrhage control and placement of calcium hydroxide to stimulate reparative dentin is usually sufficient with adequate closure. Frequently, the infection goes much deeper, so curettage with copious flushing and application of medicaments (sterile antibiotic) are usually necessary on a regular basis often for long periods of time, until the infected or fistulous area is pushed more coronally with continued tusk growth (54). Keeping the site protected from contamination and continued trauma (rubbing) (55) can be quite frustrating, and many methods have been described (47,52,54–56). Other complications encountered have been refractory bleeding of a large exposed pulp that could only be controlled by inventive cauterization (55) and irregular regrowth of an infected tusk that had previous unsuccessful attempts at extraction (54).

Infected tusks broken into the sulcus or tusk remnants left after attempted extraction will continue to grow, if infection can be controlled. Tusks with longitudinal fractures (57) or with thin walls and refractory infections (18) should be completely extracted, because attempts at surgical or medical management may be fruitless. Tusk extraction has been described (57). It involves cutting off the tusk at the external sulcus with pulp removal to produce a large hollow-core root canal. The dentinal walls are then longitudinally sectioned from the inside out into at least three parts. Each section is elevated using long steel rods with a flattened end and is removed, starting with the smallest section first.

The caudal teeth of an elephant are quite unusual. While some texts identify these teeth as a set of six molars per quadrant that sequentially erupt in a horizontal manner (distally to mesially) (18,49), others have considered them as three premolars and three molars (51) or even the first three teeth as primary teeth because they are present in the juvenile animal (58). The 1st and 2nd molars are present in the newborn and are gradually pushed mesially as more teeth erupt from the back. As a tooth reaches the mesial extent of the jaw, blood supply is lost to that section, and it becomes necrotic and exfoliates (49,58). At any one given moment, there is typically one entire tooth erupted into occlusion with remnants of the one in front and even the initial stages of another distal to it. The ability of the sectional loss is due to the lamellar structure of longitudinal layers of enamel and dentin that become fused with cementum between the ridges (lophodont) (Fig. 9). These teeth are considered to be a type of hypsodont, as well as lophodont (18), with the multiple root structures displaying varying stages of development as the eruption progresses. The molars get progressively larger as they age. The final (sixth) set of molars of the elephant erupts at 26–30 years of age, and by age 45–49 years this is generally the only set of cheek teeth still present in the mouth (59).

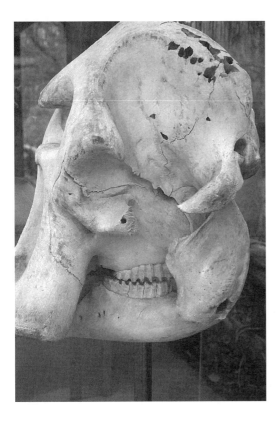

FIG. 9. Large incisor alveoli and ridged (lophodont) cheek teeth in the skull of African elephant.

Abscesses may occur in the molars due to pulp exposure or perforation resulting from trauma (18,60). Treatment strives to address the current problems to minimize complications (eg, infection, etc.), with the understanding that the section will eventually be lost anyway, particularly in younger animals. Debridement of the pulpal space between laminae can be challenging but is often helped by copious irrigation. Previously reported failures were thought to be due to the use of formocresol or extrusion of zinc oxide–eugenol cement (ZOE) beyond the apex (60). A better technique would be to place calcium hydroxide on a surgical patch and pack it into the apex of the dried canal, followed by obturation with a ZOE paste (35) and final closure (60). Malformations or malocclusions can also be treated with conservative crown-length management until exfoliation.

CONCLUSION

While it might seem less trouble to ignore some of the lesions, anecdotes exist of previously intractable, "psychotic" animals showing markedly improved behavior once their dental problem was resolved (18). If, as mentioned earlier, we continue to desire the privilege of having these animals around us, we then carry the responsibility of caring for them to the best of our ability. With information from reported cases—and a little ingenuity—we can provide them optimum dental care.

REFERENCES

1. Colyer JF. *Variations and Diseases of the Teeth of Animals*. London: John Bale, Sons and Danielsson; 1936.
2. Schultz AH. Eruption and decay of the permanent teeth of primates. *Am J Phys Anthropol* 1935;19:489.
3. Schneider KM. The development of the teeth of the lion, with some observations about the teething of several other great cats and the domestic cat. *Der Zoologische Garten* 1959;22:240.
4. Major MA. *Wheeler's Dental Anatomy, Physiology and Occlusion*. 7th ed. Philadephia: WB Saunders Co; 1993:91.
5. Miles AEW, Grigson C (eds). *Colyer's Variations and Disease of the Teeth of Animals*. Rev ed. Cambridge: Cambridge University Press; 1990.
6. Molnar S, Ward SC. Mineral metabolism and microstructural defects in primate teeth. *Am J Phys Anthropol* 1975;43:3.
7. Amand WB, Tinkelman CL. Oral disease in captive wild animals. In: Harvey CE, ed. *Veterinary Dentistry*. Philadelphia: WB Saunders Co; 1985:289.
8. Bernier JL. *The Management of Oral Disease*. St Louis, MO: CV Mosby Co; 1959.
9. Brown WP. Specialized instruments for exotic animal endodontics. Presented at the 1986 Exotic Animal Dentistry Conference; Milwaukee, WI; 1986:29.
10. Kertz P. Exotic animal dentistry in perspective. Presented at the 1989 Exotic Animal Dentistry Conference; Philadephia; 1989:2.
11. Scheels J. Challenging exotic animal cases. Presented at the 1989 Exotic Animal Dentistry Conference; Philadephia; 1989:8.
12. Tinkelman C. Pyogenic granuloma in a young Siberian tiger. Presented at the 1989 Exotic Animal Dentistry Conference; Philadephia; 1989:55.
13. Willis GP. Canine endodontics on large carnivores. Presented at the 1986 Exotic Animal Dentistry Conference; Milwaukee, WI; 1986:18.
14. Hume ID. Nutrition and feeding of monotremes and marsupials. In: Fowler ME, ed. *Zoo and Wild Animal Medicine*. 2nd ed. Philadelphia: WB Saunders Co; 1986:569.
15. Braswell LD. Exotic animal dentistry. *Compend Cont Educ Dent* 1991;13:1229.
16. Robinson PT. Dentistry in zoo animals. In: Fowler ME, ed. *Zoo and Wild Animal Medicine*. 2nd ed. Philadephia: WB Saunders Co; 1986:534.
17. Cook RA, Stoller NH. Periodontal status in snow leopards. *JAVMA* 1986;189:1082.
18. Kertesz P. Dental diseases and their treatment in captive wild animals. In: *A Colour Atlas of Veterinary Dentistry and Oral Surgery*. Aylesbury, UK: Wolfe Publishing; 1993:215.
19. Lobprise HB. Exotic animal dentistry. *Am Vet Dent Coll/Acad Vet Dent Proc* 1993:39.
20. Wiggs RB. Overview of feline resorptive lesions. *Veterinary Dentistry 1993*. Auburn University. Sept 30–Oct 3, 1993. Abstract.

21. Emily P. Root canals restore health to polar bears. *Norden News* Autumn 1987:37.
22. Kraus BS, Jordan RE, Abrams L. *Study of Masticatory System Dental Anatomy and Occlusion*. Baltimore: Williams & Wilkins; 1969:276.
23. Stoller N. Periodontal disease in a population of captive orangutans. Presented at the 1989 Exotic Animal Dentistry Conference; Philadephia; 1989:38.
24. Scheels J. Gorilla dental case reports. Presented at the 1989 Exotic Animal Dentistry Conference; Philadephia; 1989:39.
25. Braswell L. Oral pathology in non-human primates. Presented at the 1989 Exotic Animal Dentistry Conference: Philadephia: 1989:59.
26. Line S, Eisele PH, Markovits JE. Eruption gingivitis associated with scorbutism in macaques. *Lab Anim Sci* 1992;42:96.
27. Emily P. Exotic animal dentistry: The normal, the difficult and the failures. Presented at the 1986 Exotic Animal Dentistry Conference; Milwaukee, WI; 1986:37.
28. Davis JA, Banks RE, Young D. Ameleoblastic odontoma in a *Cynomolgus* monkey (*Macaca fascicularis*). *Lab Anim Sci* 1988;38:312.
29. Fagan DA, Robinson PT. Endodontic surgery for treatment of a fistulated molar abscess in an orangutan. *JAVMA* 1978;173:1141.
30. Meehan TP, Wolff P. Kotz R, Foerner J. Molar extraction in a bactrian camel. Presented at the 1986 Exotic Animal Dentistry Conference; Milwaukee, WI; 1986:88.
31. Howard P. Repair of bilateral fractures in a Bongo. Presented at the 1989 Exotic Animal Dentistry Conference; Philadephia; 1989:77.
32. Phillips L. Dental problems in captive tree kangaroos. Presented at the 1986 Exotic Animal Dentistry Conference; Milwaukee, WI; 1986:63.
33. Reichard T, Heinrichs P. Natural healing of a laceration to the frenulum and associated soft tissue in the lower lip of a nyala. Presented at the 1989 Exotic Animal Dentistry Conference; Philadephia; 1989:86.
34. Huntress S. A technique for lip repair in antelopes. Presented at the 1986 Exotic Animal Dentistry Conference; Milwaukee, WI; 1986:86.
35. Harwell G. Restoration of infundibular necrosis in a Grant's zebra. Presented at the 1986 Exotic Animal Dentistry Conference; Milwaukee, WI; 1986:89.
36. Fraham MW, Emily PP, Cambre RC, Kenny DE. "Lumpy jaw" in herbivores at Denver Zoological Gardens: A retrospective study with thoughts on pathogenesis and treatment. Presented at the 1989 Exotic Animal Dentistry Conference; Philadelphia; 1989:71.
37. Butler R. Bacterial diseases. In: Fowler ME, ed. *Zoo and Wild Animal Medicine*. 2nd ed. Philadelphia: WB Saunders Co; 1986:572.
38. Eisenmenger E, Zetner K. *Veterinary Dentistry*. Philadelphia: Lea & Febiger; 1985:19.
39. Van Foreest AW. Veterinary dentistry in zoo and wild animals. In: Fowler ME, ed. *Zoo and Wild Animal Medicine*. 3rd ed. Philadelphia: WB Saunders Co; 1993:263.
40. Wiggs RB, Lobprise HB. Acute and chronic alveolitis/ osteomyelitis "lumpy jaw" in small exotic ruminants. *J Vet Dent* 1994;11(3):106.
41. Ashman A. Clinical applications of synthetic bone in dentistry—Part I. *Gen Dent* 1992;40:481.
42. Ashman A. Clinical applications of synthetic bone in dentistry—Part II. *Gen Dent* 1993;41:37.
43. Wiggs RB. Basics of guided tissue regeneration. *Am Vet Dent Coll Proc* Mar 1993:23.
44. Reichard T, Heinrichs P, Lentz T. African elephant tusk repair. Presented at the 1986 Exotic Animal Dentistry Conference; Milwaukee, WI; 1986:79.
45. Willis G. Eruption of an impacted elephant tusk. Presented at the 1989 Exotic Animal Dentistry Conference; Philadelphia; 1989:13.
46. Robinson PT, Schmidt M. Dental diseases in elephants and hippos. In: Fowler ME, ed. *Zoo and Wild Animal Medicine*. 2nd ed. Philadelphia: WB Saunders Co; 1986:544.
47. Altevogt R. Elephants. In: Grzimek B, ed. *Grzimek's Animal Life Encyclopedia*. Mammals. Vol 12, No 3. New York: Von Nostrand Reinhold Co; 1975.
48. Schmidt M. Elephants (Proboscidae). In: Fowler ME, ed. *Zoo and Wild Animal Medicine*. 2nd ed. Philadelphia: WB Saunders Co; 1986:885.
49. Braswell L, McManamon R. Tusk fracture in a young African elephant. Presented at the 1989 Exotic Animal Dentistry Conference; Philadelphia; 1989:35.
50. Legendre LFJ. Vital pulpotomy of the broken tusk of an Indian elephant. *J Vet Dent* 1993;10(4):10.
51. Wyatt J. Tusk pulpitis in an African elephant. Presented at the 1986 Exotic Animal Dentistry Conference; Milwaukee, WI; 1986:61.
52. Gardner H, Barr J, Spellmire T. Fractured tusk on a male African forest elephant. Presented at the 1986 Exotic Animal Dentistry Conference; Milwaukee, WI; 1986:56.
53. Heinrichs P, Lantz T. Medical and surgical treatment of tusk. Presented at the 1989 Exotic Animal Dentistry Conference; Philadelphia; 1989:18.
54. Welsch B. Tusk extraction—simplified. Presented at the 1989 Exotic Animal Dentistry Conference; Philadelphia; 1989:22.
55. Kertesz P. Comparative odontology. In: *A Colour Atlas of Veterinary Dentistry and Oral Surgery*. Aylesbury, UK: Wolfe Publishing; 1992:35.

56. Schmidt M. Elephants. In: Fowler ME, ed. *Zoo and Wild Animal Medicine*. Philadelphia: WB Saunders Co; 1978.
57. Welsch B. Dental problems in young African elephants. Presented at the 1986 Exotic Animal Dentistry Conference; Milwaukee, WI; 1986:53.
58. Wallach JD, Boever WJ. Diseases of Exotic Animals: Medical and Surgical Management. Philadelphia: WB Saunders Co; 1983:807.
59. Kronfeld R. *Dental Histology and Comparative Dental Anatomy*. Philadelphia: Lea & Febiger; 1937:141.
60. Nelson B, Cosgrove GE, Gengozian N. Disease of imported primate, *Tamarinus nigricollis. Lab Anim Care* 1966;16:255.
61. Krause MV, Mahan LK. *Food, Nutrition and Diet Therapy*. 6th ed. Philadelphia: WB Saunders Co; 1979:141.
62. St. Louis Zoological Gardens (unpublished data).
63. Crowe DM. Aspects of aging, growth, and reproduction of bobcats from Wyoming. *J Mammals* 1975;56:177.
64. Burton M. Canidae. In: *University Dictionary of Mammals of the World*. New York: Crowell Co; 1962.
65. Crandall LS. Family Canidae. In: *The Management of the Wild Mammals in Captivity*. Chicago: University of Chicago Press; 1964:269.
66. Walker EP. Carnivora (Ursidae). In: *Mammals of the World*. Baltimore: Johns Hopkins University Press; 1964: 1169.
67. Lombard LS, Witte EJ. Frequency and types of tumors in mammals and birds of the Philadelphia Zoological Garden. *Cancer Res* 1959;19:127.
68. Effron M, Griner L, Benirsckle K. Nature and rate of neoplasia found in wild captive mammals, birds, and reptiles. *J Natl Cancer Inst* 1977;59:185.

19

Oral and Dental Disease in Large Animals

Peter Emily, Paul Orsini, Heidi B. Lobprise, and Robert B. Wiggs

EQUINE DENTISTRY

Anatomy

The labia, important in prehension of food, are sensitive structures. They are extremely mobile and well vascularized. The opening of the mouth is small, limiting the examiner's access to the oral cavity. The long narrow oral cavity further limits access to the caudal oral structures. Dental procedures can be accessed via buccotomy approach.

The vestibule is the space between the teeth and the lips and the cheeks. It is continuous with the remainder of the oral cavity at the diastema, which is located in the space between the last incisors and the cheek teeth. The skin of the face is thin and tightly applied to the skull, limiting the capacity of the vestibule. This factor makes examination of the buccal mucosa and the buccal surfaces of the teeth difficult.

The tongue is long, thick, muscular and remarkably strong. Lymphoid tissue aggregates form lingual tonsils at the base of the tongue.

The hard palate, which serves as the roof of the mouth, is composed of the incisive, maxillary, and palatine bones. The lateral boundary is formed by the cheek teeth with the associated alveolar bone. The hard palate is covered by thick, tough, nonmobile mucosa with an extensive underlying venous plexus. The thick mucosa covering the hard palate is thrown into many firm transverse ridges, or rugae. During tooth eruption, the tissue behind the incisors can become swollen from venous distension. *Lampas* was a term used for this condition when it was thought to be a disease process of palatitis (1). The hard palate is continued caudally by the soft palate, which is relatively long compared with that in other species. This junction is located at the level of the 2nd molar. The caudal margin of the soft palate lies ventral to the base of the epiglottis. The ventral (oral) surface of the soft palate is lined with palatine salivary glands.

Dentition

The teeth are well adapted to cope with the abrasive nature of the equine diet. The incisors are specially developed for prehension, but they do contribute to initial mastication. The premolars and molars provide the bulk of mastication. However, dental problems generally occur more frequently in the premolars and the molars than in the incisors.

Dental Formula

The formulas for determining the equine dentition are as follows:

Deciduous teeth: 2 × (Id 3/3, Cd 1/1, Pd 3/3) = 28
Permanent teeth: 2 × (I 3/3, C 1/1, P 3–4/3–4, M 3/3) = 40–44

The inconsistency in the number of premolars is due to the variable presence of the vestigial 1st premolar (wolf tooth). This tooth is much more likely to be present in the upper arcade than in the lower.

The premolar and molar teeth are commonly called cheek teeth and are numbered 1–6 starting with the 2nd premolar. Both the incisors and cheek teeth of the horse has hypsodont or high-crowned teeth (Fig. 1). Since these teeth have a distinct root and continue to erupt as the crowns are worn down, they can be considered *radicular hypsodonts*. The molar form is selenodont, but equine anatomists list it as lophodont. The crown and root are not distinct, so these teeth are considered to consist of body and root only. The body has both free and embedded, or reserve, portions. As the coronal surface continues to wear and the tooth continues to erupt, the reserve crown is decreased in size.

Terminology

The *occlusal surface* is the table or grinding surface of the tooth. This surface contacts the opposing tooth. *Labial* refers to those surfaces of the incisors and canines that face the lips. *Lingual* refers to those surfaces of the mandibular dentition that face the tongue. *Palatal* refers to those surfaces of the maxillary dentition that face the palate. *Mesial* refers to that surface of a tooth that is closest to the midline when the incisors are described, and *rostral* when the other teeth are described. *Distal* refers to that surface of

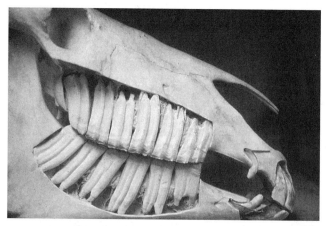

FIG. 1. Equine skull with buccal bone resected to demonstrate the radicular hypsodont cheek teeth (rooted, long-crowned).

a tooth that is away from the midline with reference to the incisors, and *caudal* with reference to the other teeth.

Types of Teeth

Incisors

In normal equine occlusion, the six mandibular incisors and the six maxillary incisors form a nearly level incisal pattern. As these teeth wear, the incisal table broadens. There are various methods of naming the incisors. The most simple method, and the anatomically correct terminology, is to number the incisors from 1–3 from the midline to the right and left. Alternately, the incisors are the central, middle or intermediate, and lateral or corner incisors. The permanent incisors erupt at 2.5, 3.5, and 4.5 years, counting from central to lateral incisors, respectively (see Table 1). The incisal surface of the incisor teeth has a single invagination, also called an *infundibulum* or *cup*.

Due to the continued eruption and wear of the incisors, various parameters may be used to estimate the individual's age. Certain conditions such as abnormal attrition due to malocclusion or rough diet may alter the pattern somewhat. In general, the incisor of a young horse can be twice as wide as it is "thick" (rostral-caudal direction), while an older horse's incisor will be twice as "thick" (Fig. 2). This occurs due to the change in the circumferential shape of the tooth in the apical direction and becomes apparent with normal wear. In a young horse, the incisors will be placed in a semicircular arch that will become

TABLE 1. *Equine eruption/aging sequence*

Tooth	Galvayne(2)			Sisson (9)
	Eruption	Level wear	Cups gone	Eruption
Deciduous Incisors				
1	Birth	—	1 yr	0–7 d
2	14–21 d	2 mo	18 mo	4–6 wk
3	6 mo	8 mo	2 yr	6–9 mo
Premolars				
1	0–14 d	—	—	—
2	0–14 d	—	—	—
3	0–14 d	—	—	—
Permanent Incisors				
1	2.5 yr	3 yr	7 yr	2.5 yr
2	3.5 yr	4 yr	8 yr	3.5 yr
3	4.5 yr	5 yr	9 yr	4.5 yr
Cuspids	—	—	—	4–5 yr
Premolars				
1	—	—	—	5–6 yr
2	2.5 yr	—	—	2.5 yr
3	3 yr	—	—	3 yr
4	4.5 yr	—	—	4 yr
Molars				
1	11 mo	—	—	10–12 mo
2	18 mo	—	—	2 yr
3	3 yr	—	—	3.5–4 yr

(Reproduced from Galvayne S. *Horse Dentition.* 2nd ed. Glasgow, Scotland: Murray & Sons; 1881 and Sisson S, Grossman JD. *The Anatomy of the Domestic Animal.* 4th ed. Philadelphia, Pennsylvania: WB Saunders Co.; 1969:405,451.)

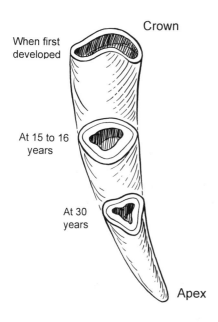

Crown

When first developed

At 15 to 16 years

At 30 years

Apex

FIG. 2. Illustration from Galvayne's *Horse Dentition* showing cross-sectional shape of mandibular incisor as it would appear at different ages. (From Galvayne S. *Horse Dentition*. 2nd ed. Glasgow, Scotland: Murray & Sons; 1881.)

nearly straight in a horse around 21 years of age. The incisors will also change from a nearly perpendicular height to leaning at a 35–40° angle in the older horse.

Galvayne (2) had also described using a "groove" on the upper corner incisor to facilitate the determination of age in a horse. A horse at 10 years of age would just be showing the groove, as it first appears at the apical extent of the exposed crown near the gingival margin. As the tooth continues to erupt, the coronal aspect of the groove should extend to a point halfway down the tooth in a 15–16-year-old and three-fourths of the way down in an 18-year-old. After appearing as a full groove in a 21-year-old, the apical extent of the groove will continue to migrate down the tooth until it is at the incisal edge. It is to be noted that these guidelines are approximate and may vary according to conditions.

Premolars and Molars

The premolars and molars (cheek teeth) are more complex in nature than the incisors. The uppers have two infundibula. The mandibular premolars and molars do not have infundibula and are narrower than the maxillary premolars and molars. The premolars have deciduous precursors. The deciduous premolars erupt in the first 6 months of life. The permanent premolars erupt at 2, 3, and 4.5 years, from mesial to distal, respectively. The molars, which do not have deciduous precursors, become visible at 1, 2 and 3.5 years of age, from mesial to distal, respectively.

The mandible is normally 30% narrower than the upper jaw (exaggerated anisognathism), causing unequal wear of the occlusal surfaces of these teeth. For this reason, as the teeth are worn, sharp edges are formed on the buccal side of the upper arcade and the lingual side of the lower arcade. This is important to remember when routine maintenance of the teeth is being performed. The cheek teeth should have a fairly flat, slightly sloped occlusal profile. Deviation in their formation inhibits the circular grinding motion of the two opposing dental arcades. The premolars and molars are closely associated with neighboring teeth, forming a continuous-table grinding surface that is important for mastica-

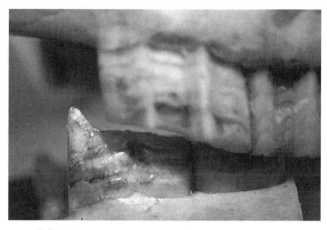

FIG. 3. Hook on distal surface of lower 3rd molar.

tion of fibrous feed. The horse accomplishes this because the temporomandibular joint is far dorsal (superior) to the occlusal line, producing the mechanical or leverage angle to accomplish total occlusal contact at one time. The temporomandibular joint in carnivores is on the same plane as the occlusal line, thereby producing a scissors action to mastication. Normal equine occlusion is slightly mandibular brachygnathic. This results in the formation of sharp points (hooks) on the mesial aspect of the upper 2nd premolars and the distal aspect of the lower 3rd molars (Fig. 3). There is much variability in occlusion between horses, as can be expected. Development of these sharp regions is also variable.

The roots of the upper 4th premolar and all of the molars are located in the floor of the maxillary sinuses. The alveolar bone overlying the roots of these teeth is thin and easily eroded during disease processes. As the cheek teeth continue to wear and erupt, less root is present in the maxillary sinuses and the sinuses become more capacious. Older horses have less root surface in the floor of the maxillary sinuses. Also with age, owing to the curvature of maxillary premolars and molars, the roots move rostrally. In older horses, the roots of the upper 4th premolar are located rostral to the maxillary sinus.

There are certain documented changes seen affecting the endodontic system of equine cheek teeth as they mature (mandibular) (3). At the time of eruption, the apices are still open and dilated, and five to six pulp horns are connected by a common pulp area. The roots and pulp chamber are more distinct 2 years after eruption, with the chamber still communicating with each root canal (two) up to 5 years after eruption. At 6–8 years posteruption, the root canals are distinct and separate cavities—significant information if endodontic procedures are to be performed.

Examination

Examination of the caudal region of the oral cavity is difficult to achieve in the conscious horse. A list of possible diagnoses can be made by considering the history, age, and clinical signs of the patient. The examiner should proceed slowly, when beginning the examination, to avoid apprehension. Appropriate restraint should be provided by an experienced assistant. At times, mild sedation is necessary. Heavy sedation lowers the head excessively, making examination more difficult. Some horses are extremely difficult and dangerous to examine. Possible behavioral problems or painful areas associated with the disease process increase the difficulty even under heavy restraint and sedation. General anesthesia may be required to complete the examination. This can be done in conjunction with radiographic examination.

External Observation

The patient should be allowed to relax and become comfortable before the examination begins. Facial swelling, draining tracts, nasal discharge, foul breath, and facial asymmetry can often be seen with problems. The lips are examined for ulceration, trauma, or neoplasia. The lips are subsequently separated to allow inspection of the incisors for wear, incisal abnormalities, coronal fractures, and retention of deciduous incisor remnants. The teeth should be inspected for periodontal disease and mobility. The patient's age can determined using eruption and wear characteristics of the incisors. The buccal surfaces of the upper 2nd and 3rd premolars are examined for sharp edges by external palpation or palpation with the index finger introduced into the vestibule. The presence of the 1st premolars (wolf teeth) and sharp points on the mesial aspect of the 2nd premolars should be identified.

Examination with Palpation

Intraoral examination is more difficult and can be dangerous. The mouth should be rinsed with warm water before examination. There are traditionally two methods of oral examination with palpation. The first is a two-handed method in which the tongue is held off to one side, placed between the upper and lower dentition, thereby stopping the horse from biting down. A wedge or coil speculum can be used concurrently with this method.

With the one-handed method, the tongue is pushed between the upper and lower dental arcades using the back of the examiner's hand, while the fingers are used to palpate the contralateral arcades. In both methods of palpation, speed is important. Most horses do not readily accept this manipulation. As stated before, those horses that object to palpation and have a history and signs referable to dental disease should be placed under general anesthesia and palpated with the use of a speculum. Various types of specula are available for use, but one should be aware of the dangers with using them. Palpation of the buccal surfaces of the distal teeth is necessary. This should be carried out with care. General anesthesia also allows the examiner to identify dental defects in the infundibulum and periodontal pockets with dental explorers and periodontal probes.

Radiography

Radiographs are essential if dental disease is suspected. Most radiographs can be taken using portable equipment with the animal standing. If necessary, a short-acting anesthetic can be used to facilitate the process. A radiopaque probe is helpful to identify a nidus of infection associated with a draining tract. The probe is inserted to the extent of the fistulous tract before radiographs are taken to identify the direction and origin of infection.

Lateral, oblique, and dorsoventral projections are desirable, although the latter are often difficult to obtain in the conscious patient. For rostral lesions such as fractures, intraoral films are also attainable in the conscious, sedated horse.

The interpretation of skull radiographs can be difficult when the involvement of tooth roots and paranasal sinuses is being evaluated. The oblique views are best for evaluation of tooth roots. Oblique radiographs separate the contralateral arcades. Contrast studies can be performed when a draining tract is present. Radiopaque malleable probes can be used as markers for this purpose. For subtle abnormalities, general anesthesia may be necessary to obtain high-quality radiographs. Intraoral radiographs can be taken for isolated teeth. Size 4 intraoral film (occlusal film) can be used for specific tooth isolation. Occlusal film must be placed far enough apically to capture the apical and periapical pathology. Occlusal film is not long enough to radiograph the entire tooth length. However, the crown is not an important entity as far as apical pathology is concerned.

Endoscopy

Endoscopy can be useful if nasal discharge is present. With chronic discharge, there is often necrosis or granuloma formation at the drainage site, either at the involved root or at the nasomaxillary aperture.

Malocclusions: Definition, Etiology, and Diagnosis

Malocclusion is primarily the result of inherited dentofacial proportions governing the breeding of horses for desired head shapes. It is also seen as a secondary effect of breeding for other desired physical and morphologic features.

Mandibular Brachygnathism

Mandibular brachygnathism (parrot mouth) is the most common malocclusion in horses (Fig. 4). It is believed to be an inheritable trait and is seen consistently in certain Thoroughbred and quarter horse bloodlines. However, the inheritability of this condition has not been ascertained. Mandibular brachygnathism is usually the result of mandibular retrognathism or delayed mandibular growth rather than maxillary overgrowth. The com-

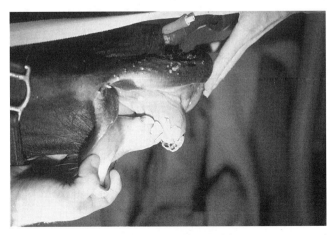

FIG. 4. Malocclusion in a foal: brachygnathism or parrot mouth.

bination overbite and overjet of the maxillary incisors is more noticeable than the corresponding abnormality in the premolars and molars, although in extreme mandibular brachygnathic cases, the upper 2nd premolar and the lower 3rd molar have little occlusal wear and grow unopposed. Anisognathism is more pronounced in mandibular brachygnathism, resulting in excessive overgrowth of the buccal surfaces of the upper premolars and molars, as well as the lingual surfaces of the lower premolars and molars.

Maxillary Brachygnathism

Maxillary brachygnathism (brachycephaly, monkey or sow mouth) is maxillary micrognathism to a greater or lesser degree. It is less common than mandibular brachygnathism and is seen primarily in ponies and dwarf miniature horses. Like mandibular brachygnathism, the maxillary form is believed by most geneticists to be inheritable.

Wry Malocclusion

Wry malocclusion (wry nose) is virtually the same in most mammals. Wry bite is the result of unequal arch development. In severe cases, one side of the head shows overdevelopment, while the opposing side remains normal. Horses may show a total deviation of the muzzle that is severe. However, wry bite can present only as a dental malocclusion without affecting the head. Malalignment can be detected in less severe cases by tracing the midline of the head from the top forward, down the muzzle, and between the teeth. The line between the upper and lower incisors will not match. Wry malocclusion can occur as the result of trauma in the developing foal or in early life; however, it is an inheritable abnormality.

Other Malocclusions

Crowding is rarely seen in standard-sized horses. However, it is often a complication seen in miniature horses. Large teeth generally are dominant over small teeth. Miniature horses with their small mouths are prone to dental crowding. Complications of crowding are many, including soft tissue trauma and periodontal disease. Orthodontic correction is rarely possible due to a lack of room in the mouth to move teeth. Teeth causing soft tissue trauma should be removed.

Cross-bite, either anterior or posterior, is seldom seen in standard-sized horses. However, it can occur in miniature horses as a complication of crowding. Due to the horse's excessive anisognathism, a cross-bite relationship almost always occurs in incisor teeth.

Dental impactions can contribute to malocclusion by allowing adjacent teeth to drift into malalignment. This, however, is not a common dental problem in horses. Anodontia (the total absence of teeth), oligodontia (the congenital absence of many but not all teeth), and hypodontia (the absence of only a few teeth) all can occur in the horse, but like impactions, they can contribute to malocclusion by allowing adjacent teeth to drift.

Treatment

Horses with malocclusion must be examined regularly for development of abnormal dental wear. Prophylactic care is important to prevent aggravation of the malocclusion and advanced disease states. Frequent aggressive filing (floating) of the overgrown premolars, molars, and incisors is often needed to prevent soft tissue trauma.

Orthodontic therapy in the young foal is a consideration. The most correctable malocclusion is mandibular brachygnathism. Initially, a rubber bite plane connected to a harness is placed intraorally and worn by the foal for 7–10 hours per day for 1–3 months. The foals seem to have no problem nursing with the bite plane in place. The bite plane allows the premolars and molars to supererupt, creating an open bite by disoccluding the distal dentition. This clears the mandible and the incisors to advance rostrally before the upper incisors hook over the lower incisors, producing the parrot-mouth effect. This procedure alone may be adequate for correction of less severe mandibular brachygnathic occlusion. Additional correction may be necessary in the more advanced cases to retard maxillary growth. After the bite-plane phase is completed, the upper incisors are ligated together with ligature wire woven in a figure-8 pattern through the interproximal spaces. The upper 2nd premolars are ligated with ligature wire retention braces and retained to the incisors with connecting wires. If active retention is needed, rubber ligatures are placed between the incisors and premolar. The rubber ligatures are retained by wire hook extensions from the ligature wires on the incisor and premolar arcades. Ethical concerns of performing these procedures with knowledge of the potential for propagation of hereditary abnormalities need to be considered carefully.

Abnormalities of Eruption

Ectopic Eruption

Ectopic eruption usually occurs after trauma to the developing tooth bud resulting in occlusal malalignment and soft tissue trauma. Ectopic teeth producing soft tissue trauma should be extracted.

Polyodontia (Supernumerary Teeth)

Supernumerary incisors are more common than supernumerary premolars and molars. There can be a complete duplicate number of incisors or a variable number. Supernumerary teeth can occur both lingually and facially to the normal arcade. Morphologically, supernumerary teeth replicate normal dentition or may present in anomalous forms.

Retention of supernumerary dentition is not common. They may be left in place if no occlusal or soft tissue trauma results. Supernumerary teeth in close proximity or in contract with normal dentition are conducive to food impaction and periodontal disease. Occasionally, extraction of supernumerary incisors can be accomplished in the standing horse under mild sedation and local anesthetic. General anesthesia is commonly required for extraction of supernumerary premolars and molars.

Retained Deciduous Teeth

Retention of deciduous teeth (retained caps) after eruption of the permanent teeth is a common condition. Retained deciduous incisors can deflect the erupting permanent incisors lingually. Detection of retained deciduous teeth at the time of permanent tooth eruption is essential to intercept developmental malocclusions. Timely removal of retained deciduous teeth allows the permanent teeth to erupt into their normal position. A large dental elevator is used to remove retained premolars by elevating the cap from the permanent tooth. The loose cap is extracted with molar forceps. Deciduous tooth removal often can be performed on the standing sedated horse or by means of twitch-restraint.

Tooth Impaction

The 4th premolar is the last tooth to erupt in the horse's mouth. This tooth occasionally becomes impacted between the 3rd premolar and 1st molar. The 4th premolar may oscillate between active and passive states of hyperemia throughout life. Often asymmetric mandibular or maxillary swelling develops. The condition generally resolves spontaneously, but impacted teeth can become endodontically compromised and develop draining tracts (4). The eruption time and stress applied to the 4th premolar is significant in the etiology of dental disease.

First Premolar (Wolf Tooth)

Approximately 20% of erupted 1st premolars are present in horses. They can cause local irritation with pressure from the bit. They are often impacted or erupt into an abnormal position. Mouth sensitivity could be the result of dental projections (hooks) on the mesial surface of the upper 2nd premolar or unerupted premolars in young foals. If the history and clinical signs are suggestive of a problem associated with the 1st premolar, it should be removed. Exposed or impacted 1st premolars can be extracted in the standing horse under sedation and local anesthetic. If the problematic 1st premolar is impacted, it is exposed, elevated, and extracted with dental forceps. Some clinicians prefer a more rapid method using an instrument with a sharp, grooved end placed between the wolf tooth and the 2nd premolar. The tooth is subsequently elevated out of bone. Immediate improvement is usually seen.

Eruption Cyst

During eruption, the vascular forces experienced can cause significant areas of swelling in both the mandible and maxilla (4). Radiographically, these areas can be seen as radiolucent areas at the apices of erupting teeth. In some miniature horses, this swelling can at times be quite significant.

Dentigerous Cyst

While in many species the term *dentigerous cyst* refers to the lesion seen radiographically as a radiolucent halo originating from the neck of an embedded tooth, a variety of the condition is seen in horses. This form of heterotropic polyodontia is a cystic structure arising from the developing tooth substance of a branchial arch remnant (5). The cyst is typically lined with stratified squamous epithelium, and one or more tooth components or even teeth may be contained within it (5). It is often found near the temporal bone in young horses, so the case of a 14-year-old mare with a dentigerous cyst in the ventral conchal sinus was atypical (6).

Dental Abscess

Etiology

The etiology of dental abscesses is controversial and no doubt multifactorial. Severe periodontal disease can progress to alveolar osteitis extending to pulpal involvement. Patent infundibula can become contaminated and later develop pulpal involvement. If the infundibulum of a maxillary cheek tooth is hypoplastic, decay is possible, causing a defect in the surface and allowing food impaction and even fermentation at the site (4). If the situation is managed properly, pulpal contamination can be avoided. Coronal fractures extending into the pulp cavity result in abscess formation. A hematogenous route of infection is probable. Teeth in an active state of hyperemia, such as the 4th premolar that has a more difficult eruption, may pass through an active and passive state of hyperemia. Such teeth are susceptible to blood-borne opportunistic bacterial invasion resulting in anachoretic pulpitis with subsequent abscess formation.

It is rare to find abscesses involving the incisors. The lower 3rd and 4th premolars, followed by the upper 1st molar, are the most common teeth to develop abscesses.

Differential Diagnosis

The clinical presentation can be extremely varied. Vague signs such as weight loss, lethargy, colic, or poor racing performance may be present. Specific clinical signs depend on the tooth involved. Mandibular or maxillary swelling, draining fistulas, foul breath, quidding, and nasal discharge are common clinical signs. The patient may be presented for evaluation of head tilt, behavior abnormalities, or simply not drinking cold water. These varied presentations support the importance of a thorough oral examination in most clinical workups. Physical findings may reveal gingivitis with or without purulent discharge at the gingival margin, mucosal lacerations, fractured teeth, missing teeth, or loose teeth.

Radiographs are essential to differential diagnosis in determination of dental and paranasal sinus involvement. Radiographic interpretation can be challenging in the early stages of the disease process. Endoscopy can be beneficial at times when the upper dentition is suspected or nasal discharge is present. An endoscope may be introduced into the oral cavity of anesthetized horses to closely examine the occlusal as well as the gingival margins of each tooth. This technique is especially valuable in suspected molar tooth involvement. Dental disease may be documented with videoendoscopy.

Treatment

General Guidelines

Endodontic therapy (root canal therapy) has proven to be successful, especially in lower premolar and molar endodontic disease. Dental extraction in the horse is often far from elegant. Equine teeth are extensively embedded in alveolar bone and require great force for removal. The oral cavity and associated structures are well vascularized. Hemorrhage can be extensive. Generally, dental abscesses progress slowly. Often by the time dental disease becomes apparent, the disease process is advanced. It is important to identify the problem as early as possible, so conservative treatment can be attempted. Since tooth removal can have serious complications, it should be performed as a last resort. The importance of dental examination and routine care cannot be overemphasized. The horse owner should be attentive to early signs of dental disease, such as changes in eating habits and the presence of facial swelling. Many horses are presented for tooth abscess of extended duration. The patients often become frustrated, as do owners and veterinarians.

Management

Conservative treatment should be attempted to preserve the tooth. Exceptions include radiographic changes demonstrating advanced dental disease with significant loss of the tooth root or a fracture of the tooth with concurrent signs of infection. Loose teeth are generally a sign of endodontic disease. Tooth extraction is a consideration only if endodontic therapy presents a guarded prognosis or client compliance for endodontic therapy cannot be obtained. Conservative therapy should include a long course of antibiotic therapy. Intramuscular penicillin (22,000 IU/kg twice a day) is the drug of choice. Penicillin has a broad range of activity against anaerobes and other organisms found in the mouth that are most commonly associated with dental abscesses. Regression of signs usually begins within 5–7 days, and therapy should be continued for approximately 1 week after clinical signs have resolved. If there is no initial improvement or if the signs have not resolved in 2–3 weeks of antibiotic administration, further radiographs should be obtained and the therapeutic plan reevaluated. If nasal discharge and radiographic signs of concurrent sinusitis without definitive signs of dental involvement are present, the sinus should be aspirated for culture. Sinus lavage should be repeated daily until signs resolve. The choice of lavage solutions is left to the clinician's discretion. Dilute solutions of povidone-iodine or 0.2% chlorhexidine may be used initially. Balanced electrolyte solutions such as lactated Ringer's are beneficial.

If conservative therapy has been exhausted or if there is recurrence of clinical signs, endodontic therapy or surgical extraction must be considered. Radiographs are repeated to identify the involved tooth or teeth and further progression of the disease. Loose teeth can be removed in standing sedated horses, if extraction has been selected as the therapy of choice rather than endodontic therapy. Short-acting intravenous anesthesia, regional anesthesia, and molar extractors can be used in this procedure.

Endodontic Therapy

Surgical endodontic therapy for mandibular and maxillary abscessed teeth has been successful. Involved roots are treated with retrograde endodontic therapy with Super EBA (Harry J. Bosworth Co., Skokie, Illinois) or IRM (L.D. Caulk Co., Milford, Delaware) cement as the obturating material. Until recently, it was unclear as to whether or not all roots need to be obturated if only one root presents as endodontically involved. Recent studies have shown that there is a communicating canal or chamber between the roots of teeth under 7 years of age. Note that this is a tooth age and not a horse age. Seven-year-old erupted teeth can be seen in a 10-year-old horse. After 7 years of age, the communicating channel calcifies or closes down. Only the infected root needs to be treated endodontically in these older teeth. When in doubt, treat all roots endodontically.

The physiology of continual tooth eruption in equine dentition is rather unclear. Eruption of human and carnivore dentition depends on the presence of a dental follicle. It was thought that endodontic therapy would stop continued eruption. However, continual eruption seems to continue after endodontic therapy. A possible explanation can be the presence of Hertwig's epithelial root sheath fibers, if present in hypsodont dentition. These fibers are found in the periradicular tissues in humans and carnivores. Their function is to aid in root apexogenesis. If present in equine dentition, they could possibly stimulate continued eruption. Hertwig's epithelial root sheath fibers may remain vital irrespective of tooth vitality. Additional research is needed in this area.

Endodontic Procedure

Conventional endodontics as performed in humans via coronal access is not possible. The pulp canal is very difficult to access through the crown in the hypsodont dentition. In addition, intraoral access to premolar and molar dentition is impossible due to the limited oral opening and length of the mandible and maxilla.

Equine endodontic therapy is performed surgically (retrofill endodontics). Success is much better in mandibular premolars and molars due to ready extraoral access and the fact that there are only two roots to obturate, as compared with multiple root apices in maxillary premolars and molars. Maxillary endodontics is possible, though technique-sensitive. The upper 4th premolar in younger horses and all of the upper molar roots lie within the maxillary sinuses. The maxillary extraoral access to the apices is additionally compromised when access is through the sinus. The mandibular procedure will be detailed; however, after access, the retrofill procedures are the same for both mandibular and maxillary dentition.

Under general anesthesia, endodontics always begin with proper radiographic verification of the lesions, because mandibular endodontic disease can be seen without swelling or fistulation directly apical to the involved tooth. The access site is surgically prepared and draped. Access to the involved mandibular apices is directly through the fistula if one is present. The apices are carefully exposed with either an air drill or with a high-speed dental handpiece and sterile surgical-length fissure burs (No.701s). The approach should be as ventral as possible, with adequate exposure so as to establish a clear field of vision. All bone removal must be performed with sterile saline irrigation to prevent heat necrosis. Root exposure is easily accessible because the pathology generally has exposed the root apices. Peripheral bleeding can be controlled with light cautery and bone wax. The endodontic system is entered through the apex of each root along the long axis of the tooth first with 30-mm endodontic Hedstrom files, then longer 30-mm Hedstrom files. The canals are irrigated with a dilute solution of sodium hypochlorite followed by sterile saline throughout the procedure. The entire contents of the canals are extirpated to the 60-mm length, irrigated, and then dried either with extracoarse sterile paper points, cotton swabs, or a small portion of cotton wrapped around the barbs of endodontic files. A rather stiff but tacky mixture of Super EBA cement or IRM cement is condensed into the root canal through the apical access for the entire prepared length. The cement is placed in small increments, allowing intracanal air to be released around the cement during obturation. The cement can be condensed with long dental endodontic pluggers that conform to the prepared canal diameter. Kirschner wires of proper diameter can be utilized for intracanal cement condensation. The obturation with dental cement is carried to the apical extent of each involved root. After all roots are obturated, the surgical site is thoroughly lavaged with a 0.2% chlorhexidine solution. Postoperative radiographs are taken, and the surgical site is closed. Antibiotics are given for 10–14 days postoperatively. Postoperative radiographs are taken at 3 months to check for osseous fill of the surgical site.

Extraction (Exodontia)

Presurgical Examination

Under most circumstances, general anesthesia is necessary. The horse is positioned in lateral recumbency, with the affected side uppermost. Intranasal intubation on the contralateral side should be performed, if possible. Before surgery, additional detailed radiographs should be obtained, and a more thorough oral examination using dental picks and mirrors or an endoscope can be performed. A screw type or other locking type of mouth speculum should be used to keep the mouth open. Caution should always be used with a speculum, because the mandible can be fractured and soft tissue damage can result from the mouth's being left open for long periods of time.

Extraction Techniques

If endodontic therapy is not the treatment of choice or client compliance for endodontic therapy is uncertain, extraction of loose teeth should be attempted using molar extractors. The molar extractors are firmly seated on the exposed crown of the diseased tooth and rocked back and forth, both parallel and perpendicular to the occlusal surface of the teeth. Additional leverage can be obtained by placing a wooden wedge to act as a fulcrum between the shaft of the extractors and the occlusal surface of the mesial tooth. Loose teeth can usually be removed by this method. Caution must be employed with extractors not to fracture the tooth by using excessive force. With extraction of more distal teeth, it may be necessary to cut the tooth with molar cutters for complete removal.

The extracted tooth should be examined to insure that the entire tooth and its roots have been removed. The alveolus should be gently palpated for any tooth root remnants or loose bony spicules. Postoperative intraoral radiographs should always be taken. Trephination may be necessary to remove remnant bone fragments. Draining tracts, if present, can be debrided through curettage, if necessary. This should be followed by lavage using copious amounts of 0.2% chlorhexidine solution.

Aftercare

Rolled gauze coated with a mixture of zinc oxide, iodoform, and petrolatum in equal parts can be securely placed into the alveolus to block feed material from packing in the defect. This is removed in the sedated patient 10–14 days postoperatively. Penicillin is given before and for 3–5 days after surgery. Phenylbutazone is beneficial initially.

Trephination, Sinusotomy, and Tooth Repulsion

If a diseased tooth cannot be removed through an oral approach, tooth repulsion after trephination or sinusotomy or buccotomy with tooth sectioning and extraction must be considered.

Trephination and Tooth Repulsion

This process can be performed on all cheek teeth with roots not located in the maxillary sinuses. It is important to be thoroughly familiar with the regional anatomy of the surgical field, as well as the exact location of the involved tooth root, so that the dental punch can be placed directly over the root. In general, one needs to remember that the mandibular and maxillary 2nd premolars are fairly straight, and the roots are located in line with the occlusal surface. The remaining teeth curve caudally, and one can use the distal (caudal) extent of the occlusal border as the location of the root position. A lateral radiograph should be obtained with a small metallic marker placed over the involved tooth root for proper identification. A stainless steel skin staple can also be used for this purpose.

Surgical Technique

The patient is placed in lateral recumbency under general anesthesia, with the affected side uppermost. A curved or straight incision is made large enough to allow loose placement of a bone trephine. The subcutaneous tissues are retracted and the periosteum incised and elevated. The trephine is placed firmly against the bone. A round section of bone is removed using in a back-and-forth motion. The teeth of the trephine should be cleaned as needed, and the osteotomy site lavaged with saline and 0.2% chlorhexidine solution. An osteotome may be needed to remove the plug of bone.

After exposure of the tooth root, a dental punch is firmly placed against the root apex. Using a mallet, the process of repulsion is initiated. The repulsion is enhanced by having an assistant place one hand on the affected tooth in the mouth, while holding the dental punch in place with the other hand. The punch is tapped with firm but light blows. This is to confirm the correct placement and direction of the dental punch. If the punch is placed correctly, the force of the hammer can be felt directly transmitted through the tooth. A solid sound will also ensure correct placement. More forceful blows are subsequently made until the tooth is freed. Initially, a great amount of force is needed to begin the process of repulsion. The punch may proceed easily at first as it crushes through soft, diseased tooth root. As with oral extraction, the caudal teeth may need to be sectioned and repelled in two or more sections. Caution must be used to ensure that the punch does not move off the tooth, causing bone fracture or, with a maxillary tooth, laceration of the palatine artery.

After extraction, the alveolus and tooth are examined to insure that no remaining pieces of tooth or areas of necrotic bone remain. The surgical tract and alveolus are lavaged, and an oblique radiograph is taken. If remnants remain, they are curetted until all the pieces are removed. Radiographs are repeated as needed.

A dental bridge or plug made of polymethyl methacrylate is placed in the alveolus to form a barrier against feed-material contamination of the deeper aspects of the alveolus. It is important to develop a consistent technique. Placement of the bridge may be the difference between success and failure. The acrylic plug is not packed deeply into the alveolus, but it should fill the defect between adjacent teeth just below the occlusal line and approximately 1.5–2 cm into the alveolus. To obtain a good seal, the material should be flared around the adjacent teeth. The edges of acrylic must be manually smoothed while the material is still soft to avoid any sharp edges. The trephine hole can be packed with rolled gauze. The gauze roll is changed concurrently with incisional cleaning and lavage of the surgical tract every day. Barring any complications, the deficit should heal within 3–4 weeks.

Aftercare

The acrylic plug should stay in place approximately 1 month. If it is lost prematurely, the alveolus can be repacked with a roll of gauze in the sedated horse. Occasionally, the acrylic plug causes oral irritation. The acrylic can be removed with molar extractors in the standing sedated animal. If the plug is packed too deeply and remains in place for an extended period of time, localized irritation may develop and extend into a draining tract. If this occurs, removing the plug usually alleviates the problem.

Sinusotomy

Exploratory sinustomy should be performed if radiographic signs of a dental abnormality associated with the sinus are evident or if conservative therapy is unrewarding. These signs include root lysis, sclerotic bony changes associated with a tooth root, and/or opacities within the region of the sinus. Surgical landmarks for maxillary and frontal sinus exposure should be reviewed by consulting an anatomy text. The maxillary sinusotomy allows exposure to the root of the last four maxillary cheek teeth. The frontal sinus can be used for approaching the caudal maxillary sinus via the frontomaxillary opening. This latter approach is the preferred route for repulsion of the the upper 3rd molar in the young horse because it allows a more direct approach to this tooth root for dental-punch placement.

Surgical Technique

The horse is placed under general anesthesia, with the affected side up. With entrance into the sinus, it is helpful to have suction available so that purulent fluid can be removed without contaminating the adjacent soft tissue. The sinus mucous membranes may be abnormally thickened, and a section may be taken for histopathologic examination, culture, and sensitivity testing. The alveolar bone overlying the involved tooth is often thickened. Occasionally, a defect of the alveolar bone or granulation tissue is encountered, both of which represent signs of infection. This abnormal bone should be removed to allow tooth repulsion using the technique previously described. It is important to avoid damaging the bony plates that separate the diseased tooth from the adjacent teeth. If this occurs, an oral-sinus fistula may develop adjacent to the other tooth, which could necessitate the removal of additional teeth.

Once the diseased tooth is removed and both the alveolus and the tooth are examined to ensure that there are no remaining pieces of tooth or loose fragments of bone, the sinus and alveolar defect are lavaged using copious amounts of fluid. Intraoperative radiographs are obtained at this time to confirm the complete removal of the tooth. The sinus should then be lavaged with a large amount of saline or dilute 0.2% chlorhexidine. The sinus mucous membrane lining should be debrided if it appears grossly necrotic.

Bleeding can be significant at times, and the surgeon should proceed with the procedure as quickly as possible. If bleeding interferes with visibility, it may be necessary to pack the sinus with gauze intermittently. The sinuses should be completely explored to identify any sequestered foreign debris, such as feed or caseous, purulent material. The alveolus is subsequently packed through the mouth with polymethly methacrylate, as previously described. Care must be taken to avoid pressing this material down from the sinus side, which would lock the dorsal aspect of the acrylic plug, making it impossible to remove later.

If the degree of sinusitis is significant at the time of surgery and therefore a considerable amount of postoperative drainage is expected, the nasomaxillary aperture should be enlarged using bone rongeurs. This is often accompanied by a moderate amount of bleeding, and therefore a large piece (5–8 cm) of moistened gauze should be prepared for packing. It is helpful to pass a leader from the sinus through the newly created opening and out the nose. The leader is then tied to the gauze packing and subsequently pulled out the nose. Enough is pulled out to allow adequate packing of the nostril. The remainder of the gauze is firmly packed into the sinus to control the bleeding. It should be folded back and forth on itself to ease removal through the nose.

After adequate hemostasis has been achieved, the bone flap and incision are closed in routine fashion. The nostril is packed with the exteriorized gauze and is sutured closed, incorporating the end of the gauze. An area on the ventral neck should be clipped and cleaned in preparation for an emergency tracheotomy, if needed after surgery.

Aftercare

The packing can be removed 1–2 days postoperatively. If significant bleeding occurs, the removal of the packing should be delayed an additional 12–24 hours.

Buccotomy

Surgical Technique

An alternative for removing premolars and molars in the head is via a buccotomy incision. This exposes the buccal aspect of the involved tooth and its associated alveolar bone. A gingival flap is then elevated and the buccal bone plate removed. The affected tooth is then sectioned using a high-speed and large round bur, and the tooth is removed in pieces. The alveolus is digitally explored for tooth and bone fragments, which should be removed if present. The alveolus is lavaged, and intraoperative radiographs are taken to confirm complete tooth removal. The defect may then be packed with polymethyl methacrylate, or the gingival flap can be closed by primary intention. The buccotomy incision is then closed in 2–3 days.

Soft Tissue Pathology

While the teeth are certainly an area of focus in equine dentistry, the supportive and ancillary structures of the oral cavity may be affected as well. The periodontium plays an important role in dental health of the horse, as it does in other species. It has previously been discussed as to how severe periodontal disease can contribute eventually to endodontic disease, but varying levels of periodontal disease can affect the dentition as well. Since equine teeth work in direct correlation with other teeth, any disruption in the supportive apparatus of the periodontium can cause loosening of teeth and even alveolar disease. Loose teeth can result in drift and then abnormal wear patterns that can escalate to additional pathology.

The soft tissues of the oral cavity may also be a primary site for signs of infectious disease. Intermittent outbreaks of vesicular stomatitis, a reportable viral disease that can impact transport and trade of domestic animals for certain areas. Initial signs of hypersalivation may be accompanied by fever. In the horse, vesicles develop on the surface of the tongue and can progress to significant ulceration, while the signs may vary in other species (7).

RUMINANT DENTISTRY

Extensive dental care is not common in most domestic ruminants, but the very fact that their productivity relies on their ability to ingest feed certainly underscores the importance of the oral cavity. Even without performing specific dental procedures, good husbandry practices of preventing excessive stress, maintaining adequate sanitation, and providing the proper diet can optimize the possibility of supporting good oral health. There may even be the occasional valuable breeding animal that can benefit from specific procedures. Yet another important aspect of veterinary dentistry is the detection of certain infectious diseases that exhibit oral signs to alert an owner or practitioner to the fact that an individual potentially should not be used in food production.

Dentition

Ruminants typically show a rostral ("incisors") and a caudal (cheek teeth) grouping of teeth separated by a diastema. In both the deciduous and permanent dentitions, there are eight mandibular "incisors" and no maxillary rostral teeth; instead, ruminants have a thickened, fibrous dental pad against which the lower teeth grasp food material. This tooth action is more important in the smaller ruminants than in the bovine, in which the tongue is instrumental in prehension of feed (8). The eight "incisors" actually consist of three incisors and one canine tooth on each side, but the teeth are all quite similar and are often grouped closely together. As such, they can be named the central (the largest), medial (first intermediate), lateral (second intermediate), and corner teeth (canines). These teeth have a spatulate shape in cross-section and are hypsodont (radicular). The reserve crown capacity is not as great as in horses, but some continued eruption does occur as they are worn down. Excessive wear can result in attrition of the teeth down to the gingival margin when no further eruption can take place.

The cheek teeth number three in each quadrant in the deciduous dentition and six (three premolars, three molars) in each quadrant in the permanent . The cheek teeth increase in size from rostral to caudal, with the last molar being the largest. These teeth are also hypsodont and have been described as being selenodont, with the cross-sectional

TABLE 2. *Bovine and porcine eruption times (months) of permanent teeth*

Tooth	Bovine (17)	Porcine (21)
Incisors		
1	14–25	12
2	17–36	17
3	22–42	8
Cuspids	32–54	8
Premolars		
1	—	5
2	18–30	12
3	18–30	12
4	18–42	13
Molars		
1	5–9	4
2	12–30	9
3	24–30	17

area in a crescent shape (9,17). There are infundibula present containing cellular cementum, and since this material wears more quickly than enamel, cups develop, facilitating mastication of roughage (10).

The dental formulas for the Bovidae (bovine, caprine, and ovine species) are as follows:

Deciduous teeth: 2 × (Id 0/4, Cd 0/0, Pd 3/3) = 20
   or: 2 × (Id 0/3, Cd 1/1, Pd 3/3) = 20
Permanent teeth: 2 × (I 0/4, C 0/0, P 3/3, M 3/3) = 32
   or: 2 × (I 0/3, C 0/1, P 3/3, M 3/3) = 32

Tooth eruption times in bovine and porcine species are given in Table 2.
Note: all deciduous present within first month

Developmental Abnormalities

There tends to be some degree of prognathism (shorter maxilla in relation to mandible) at birth, but this typically resolves by the time of weaning (10). Abnormal occlusion has been described with both a more exaggerated prognathism and with brachygnathism (parrot mouth) (1,10)

Some calves may also experience a form of achondroplasia, showing a bulging of the frontal sinus region (10,11). Clefts may be present in the palate, lips, and even tongue (10). In some cattle breeds (eg, Holstein, Friesian, Brown Swiss), a genetic defect known as *smooth tongue* may be exhibited. Affected calves tend to be unthrifty and have increased salivation.

Specific dental problems may include hypodontia, or missing teeth, particularly the 1st lower premolar or sometimes incisors. There may also be crowded or rotated teeth, and retained deciduous teeth are also possible (10). Teeth may also exhibit signs of fluorosis, particularly when greater than 100 ppm of fluoride is ingested. They may show mottling and discoloration of the enamel due to a combination of hypoplasia and hypocalcification (12).

Odontogenic tumors are not common in domestic ruminants, but they are biologically similar to those in other species, exhibiting a low-grade malignancy that seldom metastasizes (13). One such case described a rostral growth in a 1-year-old heifer that responded well to rostral mandibulectomy (8). The animal adjusted nicely after the surgery and continued to gain weight. Ancillary therapy such as radiation might be recommended, but it was not necessary in this case. Due to the reliance of smaller ruminants on the lower teeth in prehension, a procedure such as a mandibulectomy may not be always helpful or advisable.

Acquired Diseases

The vast majority of acquired diseases with oral manifestations in cattle and other ruminants are in the infectious (bacterial, viral, etc.) category. However, at times, other problems may exist, such as foreign bodies, trauma, excessive attrition, and even carious lesions. With severe forms of periodontitis, the individual can be quite incapacitated in its eating habits. In cattle, the term *cara inchada*, or swollen face, can be very descriptive of the problems, while *broken mouth* in sheep is also quite accurate (12). Rostral tooth loss in these individuals can lead to weight loss and unthriftiness.

The importance of infectious diseases is apparent not only for the individual but on an epidemiologic basis as well, due to potential spread and even human exposure from food-producing animals. Actinomycosis (*Actinomyces bovis*) often involves the bones of the head, particularly the mandible, and can be a chronic, destructive process (1). Introduction of the bacteria into soft tissues due to rough feed in unsanitary conditions can lead to an extensive osteomyelitis with extensive periosteal reaction (12). This lumpy jaw syndrome can be seen in many ruminants, domestic and exotic as well.

Actinobacillosis (*Actinobacillus lignieresii*) more frequently affects the soft tissue, causing abscesses with thick capsules that appear almost solid (1). Many small, diffuse abscesses in the tongue can cause proliferation of the connective tissue, making it thick and stiff, hence the name *woody tongue* (1,12,14). Excess salivation and decreased ability to eat may be coupled with dysphagia, if any abscesses exist in the pharyngeal region (1).

There are several entities, both viral and bacterial, that can cause stomatitis of various severity, often with ulcerative lesions that can become quite extensive. Primary vesicular-type diseases such as vesicular stomatitis, foot-and-mouth disease, and vesicular exanthema may present somewhat similarly (15). While ruminants are typically more resistant to vesicular stomatitis, lesions can at times be found on the palate and other regions of the oral cavity (7). Foot-and-mouth disease, with its contagious nature, can lead to painful lesions in cattle, while exhibiting a milder form in sheep and pigs (12). Other diseases with ulcerations and other oral signs may include rinderpest, malignant catarrhal fever, contagious pustular stomatitis, and so forth. Blue tongue, transmitted by insects, can cause significant hyperemia and swelling of the oral tissues. The tongue can be quite involved with edema and ulceration of the lateral surfaces (12).

PORCINE DENTISTRY

Pigs have the most complete phenotypical dentition with formulas as follows:

Deciduous teeth: $2 \times$ (Id 3/3, Cd 1/1, Pd 3/3) = 28
Permanent teeth: $2 \times$ (I 3/3, C 1/1, P 4/4, M 3/3) = 44

The first two sets of incisors are larger than and separated from the third set by a diastema. The diastema is closer to the canine teeth, which are modified into a tusk with a triangular crown and enamel on the lateral surface only and are positioned pointing out and forward. The roots appear to remain open in these teeth, permitting continued growth (16). The premolars and molars are bunodont and brachyodont with short crowns and closed roots.

Congenitally, pigs may exhibit signs of a short maxilla, which can at times be confused with the twisted, short jaw that is seen with atrophic rhinitis (16). Mandibular malalignments may also be present with temporomandibular joint changes due to head pressing.

Dental considerations in pigs include the practices of clipping needle teeth on young pigs to keep the sharp teeth from injuring the sow during nursing. The canines and 3rd incisors are generally treated this way. The canines or tusks on boars are sometimes trimmed back every 3–6 months to manage their length. Hypodontia is not uncommon, with the 1st premolars most commonly affected (17). This condition appears to be prevalent in the Vietnamese pot-bellied pig, with one report showing 37% having one or more 1st premolars absent (18). Dentigerous cysts have been reported in the pig (19), as have carious lesions (17).

Acquired diseases can include a variation of vesicular stomatitis and exanthema, which should be differentiated from foot-and-mouth disease, if the latter is possible. Swine vesicular disease can even cause flu-like symptoms in humans at times and includes lameness in some of the porcine patients (16). A widespread staphylococcal infection can affect suckling pigs, with extension of this exudative dermatitis syndrome into the oral area (20).

REFERENCES

1. Frank ER. *Veterinary Surgery*. Minneapolis, MN: Burgess Publishing Co; 1970:128.
2. Galvayne S. *Horse Dentition*. 2nd ed. Glasgow, Scotland: Murray & Sons; 1881:28.
3. Kirkland KD, Baker GJ, Manfra-Marretta S, Eurell JC, Losonsky JM. Effects of aging on the endodontic system, reserve crown, and roots of equine mandibular cheek teeth. *Am J Vet Res* 1996;51(1):31.
4. Baker GJ. Oral anatomy of the horse. In: Harvey CE, ed. *Veterinary Dentistry*. Philadelphia: WB Saunders Co; 1985:203.
5. Baker GJ. Oral examination and diagnosis: Management of oral diseases. In: Harvey CE, ed. *Veterinary Dentistry*. Philadelphia: WB Saunders; 1985:217.
6. McClure SR, Schumacher J, Morris EL. Dentigerous cyst in the ventral conchal sinus of a horse. *Vet Radiol Ultrasound* 1993;34:334.
7. Vesicular stomatitis strikes west. *JAVMA* 1995;207:402.
8. Tetens J, Ross MW, Sweeney RW. Rostral mandibulectomy for treatment of an ameloblastic fibro-odontoma in a cow. *JAVMA* 1995;207:1616.
9. Sisson S, Grossman JD. *The Anatomy of the Domestic Animal*. 4th ed. Philadelphia, PA: WB Saunders Co.; 1969:405,451.
10. Andrews AH. Anatomy of the oral cavity, eruption and developmental anatomy in ruminants. In: Harvey CE, ed. *Veterinary Dentistry*. Philadelphia: WB Saunders Co; 1985:235.
11. Kelly WR. *Veterinary Clinical Diagnosis*. 3rd ed. London: Bailliere Tindall; 1984:99.
12. Andrews AH. Acquired disease of the teeth and mouth in ruminants. In: Harvey CE, ed. *Veterinary Dentistry*. Philadelphia: WB Saunders Co; 1985:256.
13. Walsh KM, Denholm LJ, Cooper BJ. Epithelial odontogenic tumors in domestic animals. *J Comp Pathol* 1987;184:205.
14. Smith HA, Jones TC. *Veterinary Pathology*. 3rd ed. Philadelphia: Lea & Febiger; 1970:500.
15. Blood DC, Henderson JA. *Veterinary Medicine*. 3rd ed. Baltimore: Williams & Wilkins; 1968:468.
16. Harvey CE, Penny RHC. Oral and dental disease in pigs. In: Harvey CE, ed. *Veterinary Dentistry*. Philadelphia: WB Saunders Co; 1985:272.
17. Miles AEW, Grigson C, eds. *Colyer's Variations and Diseases of the Teeth of Animals*. Rev ed. Cambridge: Cambridge University Press; 1990:114,343,344.
18. Otto B, Schumacher GH. Gebissanomalien beim Vietnamesischen Hangebauchschwein. *Z Versuchstierk* 1978;20:122.
19. Gabell DP, James WW, Payne JL. *The Report on Odontomes*. London: British Dental Association; 1914:575.
20. Andrews JJ. Ulcerative glossitis and stomatitis associated with exudative epidermitis of suckling pigs. *Vet Pathol* 1979;16:432.
21. Reiland S. Growth and skeletal development of the pig. *Acta Radiol Suppl* 1978;66:358.

20

Marketing Veterinary Dentistry

Steven E. Holmstrom

Increasing the quality and number of dental procedures performed is a rewarding method of increasing both the quality and income of a veterinary practice. Dentistry is a service that many patients need, and once clients understand what is going on, they are eager to have dental problems in their pets solved. As a reflection of the increased study of dental disease, most practitioners are surprised at the amount of dental disease encountered among their patients. Informing clients about these problems and performing the dental procedures will result in a rise in the esteem of many clients for the practitioner astute enough to spot and solve dental disease in their pets. For this to take place, the practitioner's duty is not only to learn to identify and treat dental problems but also to market these skills in dentistry.

Marketing is defined as a system of activities to identify and satisfy consumer needs and wants. The veterinarian must determine what medical needs the patient has and then inform the clients in such a manner that they will want the services. The first step in effectively marketing a product or service is to determine what the patient's need is. In veterinary medicine, practitioners must first educate themselves and become familiar with all of the aspects relating to the service that is to be delivered. Marketing is more than merely presenting the service to the client. However, this is what many consider to be marketing. In reality, marketing begins by developing your product through education.

GETTING STARTED

Developing Your Product

The veterinarian needs to conceptualize goals and formulate a plan of how to arrive at these goals (1). The plan needs to be reviewed on a periodic basis, and a method of monitoring the achievement needs to be established. The plan should include such items as education and training, equipment acquisition, performance, and the "bottom line."

One way to obtain training is participation in continuing education courses and reading journals and textbooks. As dental theory is learned, the practitioner can start to evaluate how it fits into the practice. For some, learning a little dental theory will persuade them that they want to provide minimal dental services and refer more extensive work to someone else. Others, as they learn more dentistry, will decide they want to become involved in the delivery of even more complex dental services. It is helpful to recognize that there are many subspecialties in dentistry, and a quick glance through this text will leave one with the impression that there is a lot to learn! The reader should plan to start with only those services that he or she is thoroughly familiar with and is able to perform satisfactorily. Other aspects can be added as knowledge and skill levels develop. The necessary skills must be gained before a procedure can be performed, because a substandard job is remembered by the client for a long time.

The dental practitioner has an abundant number of instruments and materials to aid in the treatment of patients. Some of these supplies are mandatory to get the job done. Others ("toys") are optional and may make it easier and/or quicker to perform the procedure. Part of the plan is to establish what is essential for the procedures to be performed and what is not. From there, a budget for equipment and supplies can be determined. While time and time again dentistry has proven itself to be economically viable and a profit center, the expense must be balanced with the income.

As part of the plan, the performance of the dental procedures must be evaluated. A realistic goal should be set as to the number of procedures to be provided over a period of time. This goal may be reevaluated as needed. However, at the time of reevaluation, the practitioner must ask, "Why is the goal being reevaluated?" If the goal was set too low—great! If the goal was set too high, what was the problem? Were expectations unrealistic? Or were there other reasons that the procedure was not performed? Examples of this might include lack of training, lack of equipment, lack of confidence in performing the procedure, or lack of time (eg, the client has been talked into another procedure that takes less time but is not as beneficial for the patient). These factors must be evaluated before setting a new written goal.

Finally, the practitioner must evaluate the "bottom line." Is/was the experience of the education, instruments, and materials worth the time and effort for the practice? The anticipated expenses must be subtracted from the anticipated income. Hopefully, the answer will be in the affirmative.

The best place to start increasing the veterinary dental practice is in the area of the prophylactic or periodontal services. In most cases, practices are already performing dental prophylaxis because periodontal disease is the most common dental disease encountered. The practitioner should reevaluate the dental product provided, improve on it, and introduce other products as needed. Veterinarians are often reluctant to perform a procedure because of lack of experience in doing so. This can be overcome, as there are many situations in the practice that can be used to sharpen skills. For instance, a tooth that is going to be extracted can first be scaled before being extracted. The tooth is subsequently extracted, and a visual check of the work can be performed. The same extracted tooth can be used to perform an endodontic procedure and restorative technique. The tooth can be taken to a colleague or dentist for critique. All of this experience can be gained on just one tooth that was extracted from the patient.

Introducing the Product

As practitioners gain confidence with these skills, the veterinary staff needs to become involved, if they have not already shown an interest. It is best to produce a protocol of how the procedures should be performed. In this way, the entire staff will be better able to assist in the effort. For the most part, the staff can be expected to reflect the positive attitude of the veterinarian toward this new project. The written protocol can be in the form of text alone or text with pictures (Fig. 1).

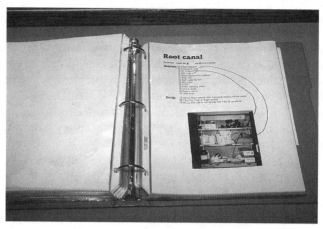

FIG. 1. In this protocol manual, items are listed for procedures, along with where they are stored.

Delivering the Product

After all of this preparation, it is time to go public. Time should be taken to thoroughly examine every patient's mouth. There are many opportunities to use dental skills among patients. Dental disease is rampant in veterinary medicine. Periodontal disease is very widespread, and it is unlikely that it will ever be totally cured in many patients, despite concerted efforts; however, patients will be made more comfortable and their quality of life improved. Evidence of periodontal disease encountered during examination of the patient should be shown to the client, and the importance of preventive care and treatment should be discussed. This can be related to the client's own preventive dental care. The veterinarian and client can start to develop a treatment plan considering the patient's needs, the client's available time, client finance, and the expertise of the practitioner. One of the nice things about dentistry is that it can be delivered one step at a time. Therefore, the patient can be checked for progress, with the treatment plan modified as needed.

Often, when fractured or discolored teeth are discovered, they are ignored. When the indications for treatment are understood and recognized, they should be conveyed to the client. There are only four options for the patient needing endodontic treatment: ignoring the need, extraction, endodontic therapy, or referral. The implications of each approach should be explained to the client. Once educated, most clients want to do something to solve the problem. If the practice charges a fee that is fair to all parties, there will be a mix of both exodontic and endodontic procedures. This also relates to marketing, as options should be presented to clients to let them decide which best suits their needs. If the client is not given the opportunity to accept or reject a treatment by offering the treatment, the treatment will never be performed.

MARKETING TECHNIQUES

Marketing has become a matter of educating the client. Marketing to acquire new clients is known as external marketing. This is marketing outside your practice and has the educational effect of letting potential clients know that you are interested in their pet's health.

Yellow-Page Advertising

A variety of methods have been used in yellow-page advertising. A statement that dental procedures are performed may be useful in promotion of the dental practice and should not be overlooked. You must represent yourself accurately as to your level of expertise.

Direct Mail Advertising

Generally, when you receive direct mail advertising, it is "junk mail." However, when you send it, it becomes advertising. Unfortunately, the response to direct mail is very poor, and in veterinary medicine, this is best left to sending to established clients or newcomers in an area.

Cooperative Direct Advertising (2)

This type of advertising uses numerous special coupon offers from many other local businesses. The cost of mailing is shared by participating companies, resulting in a savings from what a individual mailing would have cost. This type of marketing should be targeted to individuals who are most likely to use the service. A coupon indicating a specific dollar value discount (as opposed to a percentage or a specific fee) should be used for first time clients. This coupon should be as general as possible, in the hope of fitting the needs of as many patients as possible. One problem that can be encountered is a claim of false advertising. Patients who require dental services come in all different sizes, from a small cat to a large Great Dane. They also have different possible dental conditions. For example, if one created a coupon that advertised a set fee for a "teeth cleaning" and the client that responded had a large dog with advanced periodontal disease, the practitioner may be guilty of a bait-and-switch type of offense when it is discovered that the patient needs treatment for advanced disease requiring far more experience. Alternatively, the practitioner is forced to do a hasty, incomplete job that may lead to charges of professional negligence.

Another purpose of direct mail advertising is getting the hospital and/or veterinarian's name out in the public as much as possible. High-quality color photographs and full-color advertising is most likely to achieve the best response (2). This requires consistency and repetition rather than a one-time effort. The first mailing may not build anything but name recognition. Repetitive advertising may pay off. To evaluate the impact of the pay off, the number of responses to the ad campaign should be noted by tracking the number of new clients.

PUBLIC RELATIONS

Public relations can be effectively used to build a veterinary dental practice. It can create a positive image for veterinary dentistry, for the hospital, and for the practitioner. There are several media available to promote veterinary dentistry: Newspapers, magazines, club newsletters, radio, and TV are just a few. One can go out and seek media attention. For example, many dog and cat club newsletter would welcome your information. At other times, the media seek the story. When they come, the practitioner should be prepared. Here are some tips:

Newspaper and Magazines

1. Be willing to change your schedule to accommodate the reporter.
2. Make friends with the reporter, try not to antagonize, and even if you disagree, then disagree politely.
3. Give the obvious answers in your own words. It is usually what the reporter wants to hear from you.
4. Do not respond until you are prepared. Think your answers through, and make sure you are prepared.
5. Double-check quotes and facts with the reporter if you are in doubt that you were understood correctly.
6. Try to turn negative questions into positive answers; keep in mind that newspapers and interviewers have their own styles. Work to understand those styles, rather than becoming defensive. It helps to get a copy of the paper and the reporter's work before the interview to try to anticipate the style.
7. Try to keep a sense of humor.
8. Reporters are people! Tell them when they are doing a good job.
9. Ask when the story will run, and offer to assist in editing.

Radio

1. On the initial telephone call requesting the interview, note the reporter's name and station affiliation. If you are not familiar with the station, listen to it, if possible, to get an indication of the type of questions that may be asked.
2. If possible, discuss the topic and scope of the story before the interview.
3. Find out whether the interview will be taped directly off the telephone. If so, request that the reporter give you a list of questions that may be asked. Or, better yet, offer to fax a list of questions to the reporter (4) (Table 1). If the interview is to be at the studio, get precise directions, including suggestions for parking, entry into the studio, and any other preparations that may be necessary.
5. Avoid personal opinions; answer only with facts.
6. Assume that everything you say will be for the record!
7. Consider ahead of time, and plan your response if possible. Think of the two or three most important messages you want to get across, and then be sure to get them across.
8. Speak sincerely, clearly, and with conviction. Avoid anger and defensive responses.
9. If it is not live, find out when the interview will be played. Ask for an audiotape of the interview.

TABLE 1. *Potential media questions for dentistry*

1. How common is dental disease in pets?
2. How can the pet owner tell if a pet has gum disease?
3. What techniques can be used at home to brush pets' teeth?
4. What products should be used and how often should the teeth be brushed?
5. Are there any other products that help keep the teeth clean?
6. Do pets need to have their teeth professionally cleaned?
7. What can you do if a pet fractures its tooth?
8. Do you have any other tips for dental health care?

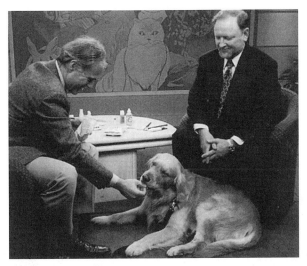

FIG. 2. Dr. Robert Wiggs on television during the 1995 National Pet Dental Health Week. (Courtesy of Harmon Smith Advertising, Inc., Kansas City, Missouri.)

Television (Fig.2)

1. Find out what type of program you will be on and where the interview will be held (eg, at your clinic or hospital or at the studio), and discuss the scope of the interview.
2. Find out if visual aids (eg, videotapes, slides, photographs, enlarged copies of slides) might be helpful.
3. Watch the program beforehand, if possible, to get an idea of the format.
4. Wear appropriate clothing, try to be conservative, and avoid harsh contrasts in colors and patterns. If you are wearing a tie, avoid stripes.
5. Think out in advance the points you would like to get across. Rehearse either orally or mentally to attempt to get these points as concise as possible.
6. During the interview, try to get these points across early. Speak at a normal voice pitch and volume and modulate your voice, avoiding a monotone, "scientific" approach. Avoid wasted words such as "uh," "well," "ah," "you know," and repetitive phrases.
7. Direct your response to the person giving the interview, unless otherwise instructed by the producer or interviewer,
8. Be yourself during the interview; don't be either too stiff or too pushy.
9. Find out when the interview will be played, and ask for a tape.

A final note on public speaking: Consider joining a toastmaster or similar club in your area that would be helpful in honing and improving your public-speaking skills. It is a positive experience to help remove the "ahs," organize your speaking, and learn to speak off the cuff.

SPECIAL EVENTS

Many practices sponsor special events to draw attention to dental health. Increasing awareness through this method can be a way of involving the entire staff. Participation in the National Pet Dental Health Month (currently February) allows the practice to use professional resources for advertising and other materials. In "Pet Dental Checks," veterinarians perform examinations on large numbers of patients, focusing on the oral cavity. A report card can be given to the client (Fig. 3). "The Great Brush Off" is a contest demonstrating the ability to brush teeth combined with dog obedience. A "Dog Walk" can be a community "fun run" or walk. These can be tied into "Pet Dental Checks." Veterinarians and staff can also tie into health fairs that are intended for human health. These

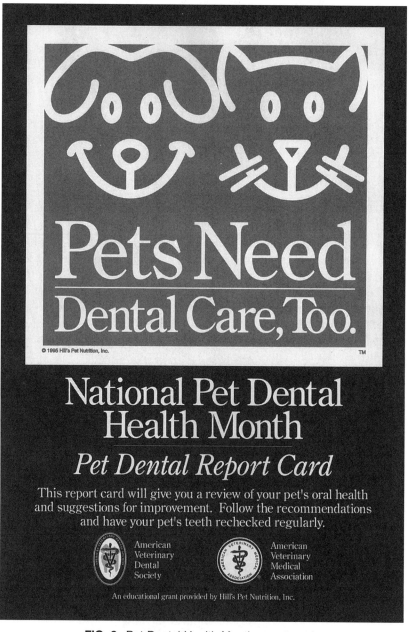

FIG. 3. Pet Dental Health Month report card.

TABLE 2. *Special events timeline*

Three months prior
  Meeting with staff to determine what is to be accomplished, how it will be accomplished, and theme
    (eg, Great Brush Off, Pet Dental...)
  Determine date and time for the event
  Select site for event, considering parking, space needs, and other physical requirements
  Assign tasks: press releases, announcements, visual aids, photography, decorations, invitations,
    prizes, finding photographer
  Design invitations, if any
  Define market (who are you going to invite?)
  Gather information and write articles
  Start computer file/notebook to record information (to use next year)
  Budget
Two months prior
  Progress reports
  Print invitations (if appropriate)
  Alter reminder cards, invoices, etc. to remind clients about event
  Order/design posters
  Decide on refreshments (if appropriate)
  Write press releases/public service announcements
  Order audiovisual equipment (if necessary)
  Plan other entertainment, banners, prizes, flowers (if appropriate)
  Weather considerations
One month prior
  Progress reports
  Address and mail invitations
  Send public service announcements, follow up with telephone call
  Final arrangements for refreshments
  Final arrangements for signs
  Prepare an event kit for guests: free samples, background information, coupons, other take home
    items (as appropriate)
Two weeks prior
  Mail press releases to local media and be sure to follow up with telephone calls
  Make up name tag if names are known, purchase extra name tags, or set up computer to do
  Confirm photographs
  Review assignments with staff
  Confirm all other arrangements
Day of event
  Place banners clearly and securely
  Set up registration table
  Install and inspect audiovisual
  Photographer to take photographs and document event
One week after
  Postevaluation and record keeping: review budget, attendance/response, objectives met—write it
    down!
  Make photo album
  Clip newspaper articles

---

type of opportunities vary from area to area and from practice to practice. Table 2 has been designed to help with planning for a special event.

MARKETING TO EXISTING CLIENTS

For most practices, there is enough untapped dental disease in patients they are already seeing to keep the practitioner busy for a lifetime. For these practitioners, external marketing is not necessary. There are a variety of methods that can be used for client education and *getting to yes*. These aids add credence to the presentation to the client.

Direct Mail Advertising

One effective technique is to prepare and send out a postcard or letter to clients emphasizing the importance of dental examination and care. This advertising can be in association with Pet Dental Health Month or separate from it. Many practitioners may include a discount for their service if performed during a certain time period (which is usually associated with slow periods in a practice). If a discount is offered, it is best written in terms of dollars off rather than a percentage off; this indicates better perceived value. It is recommended that these advertisements be in full color to increase advertisement recall and include photographs. The responses to these efforts should be tracked over a long period of time to make sure that the effort is paying off.

Hospital Brochures

The investment of time, effort, and finances to create a hospital brochure can be very rewarding. The hospital brochure can cover all phases of the hospital, and the dental area should not be left out. The brochure can include information on hospital policies, equipment, and procedures commonly performed and can be a pictorial guide through the hospital.

In-Hospital Displays

Smile Book

A *smile book* is a pictorial essay of procedures performed in the hospital. It can also be before and after photographs of dental procedures. This type of visual aid can be used to educate the client as to expected outcomes. It can also be used to describe procedures or alternative procedures.

Posters

Various posters are available that graphically illustrate dental disease. They can be framed and hung in the reception area or examination room. Other posters can be back-lit on examination room x-ray view boxes (Fig. 4).

Newsletters

A dental section should be included in the practice newsletter. Topics can include causes of periodontal disease, treatment techniques for prevention, treatment of periodontal disease, fractured teeth, dietary considerations in dentistry, veterinary dental orthodontics, cervical line lesions, dental home-care products, and many others. Clip art is available from a number of commercial sources.

Invoices and Statements

Many computer systems allow information to be repetitively printed on invoices and statements. Changed on a regular basis, this can be another source of client education and marketing.

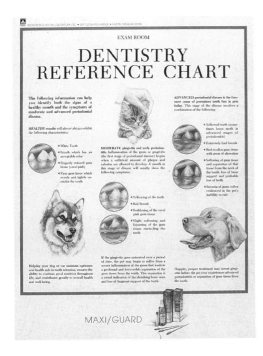

FIG. 4. Dentistry reference chart. (Courtesy of Addison Biological Laboratory Inc., Fayette, Missouri.)

Messages on Hold

Rather than listening to music (or worse yet, a dead line), clients can listen to informative information on veterinary medicine and veterinary dentistry. Messages can be delivered on the need to take care of teeth, home care, periodontal disease, fractured teeth, and other important lesions.

Sign Boards

Some practices have benefited from electronic message boards that list office hours, seasonal reminders, leash reminders, and dental care. Before signing up for any services, be sure that you thoroughly understand all aspects of the contract.

Handouts

Handouts give the client more information on the procedure or procedures that need to be performed. Several pharmaceutical companies have ethical handouts that stay focused on delivering the information, while mentioning a product on the back page. Several commercial companies have produced handouts for purchase. Handouts can also be customized and printed by the practice.

Preoperative

Preoperative handouts inform the client on the need for the procedure. They can be generalized, covering all branches of veterinary dentistry, or specific. Handouts on periodontal disease cover the need for periodontal disease prevention through complete pro-

ROBERT B WIGGS   Number: 0011594 Page: 2

_____ I prefer to be phoned prior to any additional procedures, other than emergencies. However, if I cannot be reached, I authorize unforeseen, non-emergency procedures.

_____ If I cannot be reached, I do not authorize unforeseen, non-emergency procedures.

Discharge Date/time:_____ Doctor talk appointment:_____

I am the owner, responsible agent for, or authorized agent, of this animal. I understand the nature of the procedure(s), that there are risks involved with any surgery or procedure, and that results cannot be guaranteed. I authorize the veterinarians and staff or their designated agents of Companion Animal Hospital to perform all procedures as set forth above, including surgery, treatment, laboratory tests, x-rays, medications, and anesthetics. Further, in case of emergency, I consent to any necessary procedure not set forth on this form, should that procedure be necessary and desirable in the attending veterinarian's professional judgement. I understand that an attendant is not on hospital premises 24 hours per day and that after-hours care is provided as necessary in the judgement of the veterinarian in charge. I consent to the release of medical information.

I agree to pay in full for services performed, including those deemed necessary for medical or surgical complications; or unforeseen circumstances. This is an estimate of services and fees based on the best information currently available. This estimate is not a guarantee of charges or duration of hospitalization. We want to give the best possible care for your special companion. To do so, we sometimes must run tests or do procedures that we did not anticipate when giving you this estimate. We will make an effort to inform you of tests or procedures that cause an increase in this estimate. We want to give your pet the best possible medical and surgical care available at a reasonable cost to both of us. Fees are generally complete when your pet is discharged from the hospital. Some fees from you estimate(s) may not be known at discharge and will be billed at a later date when they are received by us. This estimate is for current recommendations and does not include future diagnostics, procedures, reevaluations, or treatments. These fees are invoiced as the services are provided and are not prorated over the period of hospitalization. Payment is due upon discharge the the hospital or at the time the services are performed. We accept cash, checks, Master Charge, and Visa. We cannot extend the privilege of charging services.

I have read, received a copy of, and understand this authorization and consent.

_____   _____   _____
Signature of owner or responsible agent   Witness   Date signed

FIG. 5. This preoperative estimate includes a release form and information on the treatment of the dental disease.

phylaxis. Handouts on endodontic disease discuss the reasons for performing root canal therapy and the consequences of no treatment. The preoperative handout can be in the form of a dental estimate that discusses fees, expected outcomes, and possible complications (Fig. 5).

Postoperative

Some practices have computer systems that will generate handouts on demand. For example, after a prophylaxis on a patient with stage 1 disease, a handout can be linked to the procedure that describes that stage of the disease, the treatment, and home care. This handout would be different for the patient with stage 4 periodontal disease undergoing periodontal therapy.

Estimate and Consent

While thought of mostly for legal reasons, the estimate and consent form are valuable marketing tools. By using an estimate, a treatment plan may be written up before the procedure. Many veterinarians figure out what to charge the client only after the procedure. Unfortunately, they sit down, think "this costs too much," and start whittling away at their fees. The best method is to write it down before hand, and be fair to the practice and client. Developing a treatment plan and estimate serves as a focus for discussion of the patient's needs and the client's wishes.

Of course, there always can be unexpected procedures that need to be performed. One method to handle this is to give the client three choices on the standard estimate/surgical release/drop-off form. These choices are the following:

1. Do anything the doctor feels necessary.
2. Call first; if I cannot be reached, do what is necessary.
3. Do nothing if you cannot contact me.

These three questions eliminate the game of "give me a call" only to find out the client is not expected in the office for 3 hours (while the patient is under anesthesia!).

Recall System

Recall cards can be a very valuable method of reminding the client to return for repeat visits. Recall reminders should be customized according to the patient's needs. Generally, healthy patients and those with gingivitis should be recalled yearly. Patients with established periodontal disease should be sent a card every 3–6 months, and every 3 months for those with advanced periodontal disease.

Dental Models

One method of presentation is to use plastic dental models. Plastic dental models have become available for the practitioner to use for client education. This education lets the

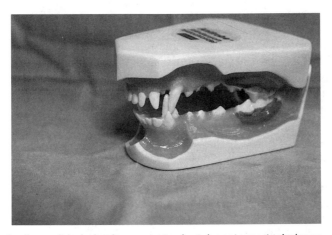

FIG. 6. Plastic tooth models help demonstrate dental anatomy, techniques, and treatment. Antirobe™ Canine Dental Model (Courtesy of UpJohn Co., Kalamazoo, Michigan).

client know the condition that a patient has, as well as what can be done to help the patient. Three companies are currently distributing plastic dental models of the canine and feline oral anatomy and disease conditions. Butler Company (Dublin, Ohio; 800-344-2246) and Henry Schein Inc. (Port Washington, New York; 800-872-4346) make models with excellent representations of dental abnormalities and pathology. Dr. Shipp's Laboratories (Beverly Hills, California; 800-442-0107) has models with plastic teeth embedded in clear plastic. These models are good for demonstrating root structure (Fig. 6). When discussing the patient's dental problem with the client, you should discuss the cause of the condition, the options for treatment, the advantages and disadvantages, the possible complications of each option, your recommended treatment, and the reasonable expectation of the outcome if no treatment is performed. The opportunities for other treatment demonstrations and uses are limitless. Your skills and education must be taken into account when you discuss these procedures with the client.

Canine Models

Retained Primary Maxillary Canine Teeth

This is a violation of the "one tooth of the same type in the same mouth at the same time" rule.

Treatment: Extraction of primary teeth.
Advantage: Will allow space for adult tooth to erupt.
Complications: Retained root fragments may cause infection and disrupt growth of the adult tooth. Fracturing of the root may necessitate the need for a flap procedure and removal of root fragments. Adult tooth may not come in correctly.
No treatment: Permanent displacement of maxillary canine. Periodontal disease may develop due to food impaction and plaque/calculus buildup between primary and adult tooth.

Retained Primary Mandibular Canine Teeth

Treatment: Extraction.
Advantage: Will allow space for adult tooth to erupt.
Complications: Fracturing of root may necessitate a flap procedure and removal of root fragments. There is a slight chance of damaging the adult tooth fragment. Adult tooth may not come in correctly.
No treatment: Permanent displacement of mandibular canine tooth and other teeth. The canine tooth may penetrate into hard palate and cause an oronasal fistula.

Missing Teeth (Oligodontia)

Treatment: Dental radiograph to evaluate for the presence of impacted tooth or retained root fragments. It is often requested by clients in young animals.
Advantages: Diagnostics, preventative dentistry.
Disadvantages: None, other than requirement for general anesthesia and possible need for oral surgery.

No treatment: Possible formation of cyst, infection, or jaw abscess (if tooth is actually present) subgingivally.

Periodontics

Dental models can be used for brushing or wiping instructions. They are preferable to skulls, models made of dental stone, etc.

Stage 1–3 Periodontal Disease
Treatment: Scaling, polishing, fluoride treatment, and home care
Advantage: Preventive dentistry.
Disadvantage: General anesthesia is necessary but is unlikely to be a problem, especially if preanesthesia blood tests are performed to detect problems.
Complications: Improper home care or other causes of disease progression.
No treatment: Continued progression of periodontal disease, tooth loss, systemic disease.

Stage 4 Periodontal Disease
Treatment: Depends on case. Discuss with the client the ability to perform home care, willingness to save teeth, etc. The condition may require periodontal surgery, root planing, splinting, extractions, etc.
Advantage: Improved oral health.
Disadvantage: None.
Complications: Will require general anesthesia and may require extractions. This should be explained to owner before therapy is initiated. There are three things that clients do not like: anesthesia, extractions, and bills. Extracting teeth without permission loses all the way around.
No treatment: Continued shedding of bacteria into body, tooth loss, discomfort.

Oronasal Fistula

Treatment: If tooth present and fistula repair; if tooth is not present, fistula repair.
Advantages: Increased health and comfort as food and other debris will not be packed into oral cavity.
Disadvantages: None, other than expense and anesthesia.
Complications: May require further surgery. Infection may develop.
No treatment: Nasal infection, systemic infection, further loss of maxillary bone.

Maxillary 4th Premolar/1st Molar Crowding

Treatment: Increased professional and home care.
Advantage: Saves teeth
Disadvantage: None
Complications: May require additional therapy.
No treatment: Loss of both teeth.
Optional treatment: Extraction of maxillary 4th premolar.
Advantage: Most of time will allow salvage of maxillary 1st molar.
Disadvantages: Loss of function, extracted tooth, and maxillary 3rd premolar.
Optional treatment: Odontoplasty.
Advantages: Maintains tooth and may allow for natural oral hygiene.

Disadvantage: Potential for undiagnosed complications
Complications: Dental hypersensitivity, tooth death.

Gingival Hyperplasia

Treatment: Gingivectomy and possible biopsy.
Advantages: Removal of excessive gingiva allowing for better natural cleaning as well as home care; diagnostics.
Complications: Oral discomfort. Gingival bleeding is relatively minor problem.
No treatment: Pocket formation allowing progression of periodontal disease, oral discomfort

Gingival Laceration

Treatment: Avoid home care with metal instruments or dental care by untrained, unlicensed individuals.
Advantage: Avoids complication.
No treatment: Further gingival damage.

Slab Fracture of Maxillary 4th Premolar

Treatment: Root canal therapy.
Advantages: Saves tooth as well as function of opposite tooth. Root canal therapy is less traumatic than extraction.
Complications: Previous inflammatory resorption precluding performing endodontics, inability to file canals, inability to completely fill the canal.
No treatment: Dental pain, inflammatory root resorption, fistula formation with discharge below eye, sinus infection.

Fractured Canine Tooth

Treatment: Root canal therapy.
Advantages: Saves function of tooth and prevents upper lip from being pinched between mandibular canine and gums if maxillary canine is extracted. If the mandibular canine is extracted, the tongue may hang out on that side.
Complications: May require surgical root canal, especially if fistula is present.
Optional treatment: Surgical root canal.
Advantages: Seals apex mechanically, removes necrotic tissue from apex, and may establish better drainage.
Disadvantage: Is a more complex procedure, requiring additional anesthesia time.
No treatment: Continued dental disease, loss of tooth, systemic disease.

Acute Fractured Tooth in a Young Patient

Treatment: Vital pulp capping.
Advantages: Preserves a vital tooth, allowing it to continue to lay down dentin to increase wall strength; avoids root canal therapy.

Disadvantage: Need for root canal therapy if procedure fails, thus creating additional expense.

Complications: Failure leading to apical abscess.

No treatment: Death of tooth, abscess, systemic effects.

Orthodontics

The models allow the discussion of proper dental relationships and occlusion, as well as disease states.

Base-Narrow Mandibular Canine Teeth

Treatment: Orthodontics either by incline plane or expansion screw.

Advantages: Will move teeth into proper occlusion, thereby relieving current discomfort. At a young age, when a tooth is hitting another tooth, the periodontal ligament "gives," the tooth moves slightly, and the tooth does not wear. With age, the teeth will wear and saw into each other.

Disadvantage: Will require weekly visits.

Complications: Failure of tooth to move, wear due to appliance, possible staining of teeth due to appliance.

Optional treatment: Amputation and pulp capping.

Advantage: Is a one-step procedure to reduce crown height.

Disadvantages: May kill tooth and require endodontics or extraction at later date.

Complications: Endodontic death of tooth.

Optional treatment: Extraction.

Advantage: Is a one-step procedure.

Disadvantages: Is more traumatic, tooth function lost.

Complications: Biting lip, loss of tooth if a guide.

No treatment: Development of an oronasal fistula, pain, and/or discomfort.

Feline Models

Stage 1–3 Periodontal Disease

Treatment: Scaling, polishing, fluoride treatment.

Advantages: Prevention of disease progression, improved oral health, improved mouth odor.

Disadvantages: None, except general anesthesia.

No treatment: Progression of periodontal disease, possible cause of neck lesions, poor oral and systemic health.

Stage 4 Periodontal Disease

Treatment: Scaling, polishing, fluoride treatment, possibly with dental radiographs and further treatment.

Advantages: Improved oral health, relief of pain and discomfort, improved general health.

Disadvantage: None

Complications: May require other oral treatment such as working up neck lesions, sub-gingival root planing, and curettage; may require extractions.

No treatment: Worsening of condition, tooth loss, decreased appetite, pain and discomfort.

Neck Lesions

Treatment: Dental cleaning, dental radiographs, and possible glass ionomer filling, root canal, or extraction.
Advantages: Relief of pain, improved oral health.
Complications: May require extractions ("toothanasia") to resolve.
No treatment: Continued oral pain (many times cat will not show pain unless under a light anesthesia), oral cavity inflammation, stomatitis. These lesions tend to be very painful with consequent decreased appetite and inability to chew food properly.

Missing Tooth

Treatment: Dental radiographs to check for abscessed root fragments, preventive dental procedures.
Advantages: May prevent further disease, may relieve discomfort.
Disadvantage: Requires general anesthesia.
No treatment: Undetected dental disease, discomfort, worsening of condition.

Canine Tooth, Slab Fracture of Maxillary 4th Premolar

Treatment: Root canal therapy.
Advantages: Saves function of tooth, is less traumatic than extraction.
Disadvantage: None
Complications: Long-standing abscess may be associated with inflammatory root resorption requiring extraction or apical surgery.
No treatment: Chronic systemic bacterial infection, inflammatory root resorption, loss of tooth, pain and discomfort.

SUMMARY

A veterinarian can never start too early in making clients aware of their pets' mouths. New pet examinations should include a thorough inspection of the oral cavity, followed by discussion of routine care. A dental examination should be conducted at age 7–8 months to evaluate the occlusion and to make sure that all primary teeth have exfoliated. At this time, further education may be given to the client. This education may be on the recognition of dental disease, the need to brush and home-care instruction, breed predilection for dental disease, and the need for regular teeth cleanings. If the patient is going under general anesthesia for spaying or neutering, the owner should be offered the option of having the teeth scaled (or even just polished) with fluoride treatment at that time. Dental examinations should be included with the annual physical. The key is to prevent disease, rather than letting it start and then attempting to treat it. Dental examinations in older patients should be performed as appropriate. Some will need dental procedures performed every 3 months, and others yearly. Patients with periodontal disease should be rechecked every 1–2 weeks until the condition is under control. The patient should be recalled every 3 months to make sure oral health is being maintained. Patients with cervical line lesions should be checked in 3 months to make sure the restoration is in place. Patients that have had endodontic procedures (pulp capping or root canal therapy) should be rechecked and radiographed under general anesthesia 6 months after the procedure.

Every patient that comes through the hospital door has a mouth, and in these mouths are many problems that need to be solved. Each problem that needs to be solved can be viewed as a marketing opportunity to provide better service to the patient.

REFERENCES

1. Steinberg T. The business of dentistry: An annual plan. *Dentistry 95* April 1995:12.
2. Bergman LC. Brush up on your marketing. *Dentistry 95* April 1995:4.

21

Behavioral Problems Associated with the Oral Cavity

Janine Charboneau McInnis

Animals use their mouth for many different reasons. Not only do they use their teeth for survival, protection, and grooming, but the individual may also use the oral cavity in ways that are less than desirable. Teeth have been developed for a purpose: to assist animals in their needs. They may also be used to express animals' emotional states. Now that we as a species have worked at domesticating some animals, we have to deal with their instinctual tendencies that often express themselves through use of the mouth. Domestication to some is more an adaptive rather than an inferior trait (1). Behavior with the mouth begins as a way of communication to others. Some behaviors may be a greeting, others may be a sign of being anxious, and still others may be a sign of boredom. From vocal communication to active destructive behavior, pets utilize their ability to use their mouth in many ways.

The study of behavior is becoming an increasing focal point for the veterinarian. It may be of increased concern to the dental veterinarian. Many of the questions asked of veterinarians by clients concern behavioral tendencies that their pet may have. Not only is an animal gotten for a purpose in a person's life, such as protecting a home, but they are also there to keep the people company. Both pleasure and enjoyment are expected when a pet comes into a person's life (2). Behavioral problems can complicate the pleasure that one gets from an animal. Many animals are euthanatized yearly because they have a behavioral problem (3). The practitioner as an animal professional is expected to have a wide education in medicine, including knowledge in dentistry and behavior. Many clients' concerns are for the well-being of the animal and others around them. Their concerns will also be for the surroundings that the pet is kept in. A veterinarian can make many helpful recommendations to improve the situation of clients who come with concerns for their pet and the oral cavity. It's important to educate regarding behavioral problems early and to help encourage a good owner–pet bond (4). Owners will be deeply appreciative of any help that the veterinary staff can give them in a problem situation. A good rapport with clients will help increase the veterinary clientele. Time spent with new clients answering questions can repay itself in a greater amount later on by return business and word-of-mouth referrals to friends and neighbors. Many questions will come when the puppy or kitten is young. This is the opportunity to make a major difference in the eventual outcome concerning the animal's life and the owner's life with the pet. As the practitioner studies the science of behavior, it is important to keep in mind the concerns of his individual clients. In one area of the country, there may be a larger number of apartment animals such as small dogs and cars. In another area, the practitioner may be asked questions of animals kept in a more rural setting. The needs of those animals and their owners will differ. Always keep in mind financial and legal concerns regarding a case, when answering questions. Refer clients to a veterinary behaviorist, a qualified trainer, an attorney, or other important resources when the questions are beyond your realm of knowledge. Be willing to find out information for a client or have one of your staff do so. Some drug therapies may be utilized for behavioral concerns, but caution must be taken as to side effects and the amount of veterinary research on a particular medication (5). The extra effort will be worth the time in return visits by the client and in recommendations to other potential clients. Having an independent knowledge of behavior will help you work with many dental cases that have been presented to the practitioner due to behavioral problems.

The individual pet may exhibit behaviors that are not always desirable to the owner. Each act can be an expression of what the animal thinks it needs or of what it feels. Inappropriate behavior is not desirable according to the standards of the person in the relationship. What some individuals see as acceptable is to others extremely unnecessary and improper in a situation. Often a financial cost as a result of the animal's behavior may result in a client's seeking help to change the behavior. In other situations, the emotional cost to an individual will cause an owner to become frustrated and ask for help. Approximately 25–75% of individuals in animal shelters are there due to behavioral problems (6). Teething, destructive chewing, aggression, and various anxieties are often exhibited by pets, and the owner will turn to the veterinarian for guidance on how to handle these situations. The client may also express concern or already have seen signs of damage to the oral cavity by inappropriate behavior. The doctor can inform the owner on preventive techniques not only for proper dental hygiene but also for avoiding problem situations that can damage a healthy oral cavity. Even if a pet is presented with a dental problem due to inappropriate behavior, working at preventing it from happening again is important.

Encouraging the animal to correctly use its mouth in a way that will not do damage to itself, other individuals, or property is important. Clients need to learn that their efforts can be well spent as an investment in the animal. Owners who get pets, thinking that the only expense is in feeding and basic veterinary care, soon learn otherwise. Without quality time spent initially in training and teaching pets what is allowed in the household, the animals will end up taking the same amount of time—and often more money—in correcting what has been learned incorrectly due to the lack of appropriate time and effort spent in teaching the animal from the start.

Some breeds are more prone to oral tendencies than others. Some animals are hereditarily set to use their mouths for a working capacity. The sporting, herding, and working breeds of dogs have been selected for years to be able to perform out in the field. From bird retrieving, to hunting, to rounding up a herd of sheep, dogs have assisted humans in performing certain tasks of importance. Other animals have been selected for guarding property, other animals, and people. Police and/or military dogs play important roles in drug searches and the pursuit of wanted individuals by the government. They not only assist in important task functions but also decrease the chance of injury for their human partners by being sent into situations before the officers in charge go in. Often, in police work, the mere threat of "sending the dog in" is enough to bring out a potentially harmful individual before someone gets hurt. These dogs have their place in society. Proper health care of the oral cavity is important to insure the ability to do their work. Some individuals have unfortunately been chosen and produced for their aggressive ability with their mouth to hurt or damage other animals for the entertainment purposes of the human species. Although illegal in many areas, animal fighting in some places and in certain parts of our society still involves the status symbol of having an animal that can do great harm to others. Even when organized fighting is not performed, certain individuals take great pride in their animal's having the ability to use its mouth in an aggressive manner. The veterinary staff will be called in to handle these individual animals for both veterinary care and quarantine reasons, if an animal has improperly bitten someone. Even animals whose assertive tendencies make them less preferable can be a liability for owners, as well as for the veterinarian in the clinic. Such animals have to be handled carefully as to when and where they are exposed to others. Caution must be taken in how these individuals are worked with. The staff needs to be highly trained as to how to handle situations with these animals and their owners. The oral cavity is used in many instances both positively and negatively as a working tool for the animal and the owner. Damaged teeth and gum disease decrease their ability to do their job properly. The doctor will be asked questions about the maintenance and care of the animal's oral cavity. Keeping every tooth intact and functional is important in the working animal. The veterinarian needs to use good judgment when advising the client on proper use of the mouth and teeth in the orally active animal.

Good oral hygiene and care are essential for animals' using their mouths for the purposes for which they were meant. In determining the way a client's pet is using its mouth, a veterinarian can explain the best approach to taking proper medical care of the teeth and surrounding areas. In considering whether an animal is using its mouth correctly or incorrectly, the doctor may find a need to refer the case to a veterinary behaviorist or to offer counseling him- or herself. Behavioral education can help clients prevent further abuse of the animal's mouth. Steering owners toward a behavioral program may in the long run decrease the need for extensive dental work. Providing the service of behavioral advice can increase the bond between the veterinarian and the client. Veterinarians should also charge for the time. Monetary compensation should be in line with the degree of effort and knowledge being given. Respect of oneself is important in any profession. Veterinarians need to realize that in offering behavioral advice, they are helping decrease the chances of animals' doing further injury to their oral cavity, to themselves, and to others. Owners and their pets will greatly benefit from the veterinarian's time and knowledge. It is correct to be properly compensated for it. It is suggested that office-call fees be charged per time with a base minimum. Clients should be told this up front when calling to set an appointment. This will help decrease the chances of any misunderstandings. At this initial call, staff can also use this opportunity to stress the importance of proper oral hygiene. If staff members are sincere in their feelings of proper dental care for pets, owners will begin to feel the same way. It is important for a dedicated staff to emphasize the importance of good oral hygiene. They should be knowledgeable enough to assist the veterinarian and clients in achieving this goal. Good oral care along with preventive dentistry is important not only from a medical but also from a behavioral standpoint. Assistance in behavioral problems can help decrease the risk of dental damage.

TEETHING

Puppies and kittens begin teething early in life as their baby teeth erupt through the gum line. Young individual begin to use their mouth for more than just suckling from the mother. The immature teeth become a new source of power for the animals as they learn to use their mouth. When they bite their siblings, they can cause extreme soreness. In behavior, one response may initiate another as puppies or kittens use their mouth. They gain new experiences, both good and bad, from other animals and people. The baby teeth are usually very sharp, so pain is elicited more quickly with pressure than it is in adult teeth. Young puppies' or kittens' teeth are at times like piercing needles when they use their mouth. The mother is often the first to discipline the young if their teeth are causing injury or concern. She will want less and less to be with her babies due to the ability of their teeth to cause her discomfort. This distance will help the bitch's or queen's milk dry up (7), with the decreased stimulus from mouths no longer nursing. Other littermates will also begin to learn to use their mouth to get things that they want because of the positive response that they get. For instance, dominance behavior starts to develop as siblings struggle to get their fare shares at the new food bowl. A dominance hierarchy can begin at this phase. This situation can be the beginning of unacceptable behavior with the individual pet. The animals begin to work in an instinctual manner to defend themselves. The young begin to imprint on the experiences gained at this young age. The longer they are left around other individuals that dominate them, the more problem behaviors they can imprint on at this phase in their life. Once the young have learned they can get a response with their mouth, the smarter individuals especially work at taking advantage of the situation. Critical learning processes start here that will develop into individual behavioral traits later on. When teething begins, the use of the mouth can have major effects on the animals around them.

As puppies begin to get older, behavioral problems begin to develop as the mouth is exercised on new objects besides mom, food, and littermates. Almost all individuals chew on something inappropriate at some time or another in their life (8). Wood, leather, and people's skin are all part of the new field that young pups will try to use their mouth on. Young animals begin to explore with their mouths. By putting things in their mouth, they can test the item for taste, texture, and shape. Teething will often increase when they feel the need to soothe sore gums as their new adult teeth begin to erupt. Then, young individuals begin to learn that the new tools in their mouth called teeth can give them new experiences in life. This is all part of the learning process for pups. Some feel that it is instinctual for dogs to automatically use their teeth on items and individuals. Chewing is a common need in puppies. They have not yet learned what is acceptable to chew on and what is not.

The veterinarian can inform the litter owner what to look for and how to rechannel teething behavior correctly. If the dominant puppy is left in with the rest of the litter, long-term psychological situations can develop for both the assertive individual and the others in the litter. The litter owner must make a judgment call to separate pups or correct the situation. Appropriate chew toys should be provided. Various objects that are all right for dogs to chew on should be left in the area for the pups to play with. They can become bored if not continually given items to occupy them. If chewies and toys are not given, puppies will find other objects to use their mouths with. By keeping them in a closed-in "puppy area" that is void of furniture and valuable property, owners can decrease the chances of having problems with the young teething puppies. Educating clients properly can help avoid problems later on. Owners will often appreciate guidance in how to properly raise the litter and channel them correctly. When clients come to the clinic, a little time spent talking to them about their new venture can pay off in the future with veterinary referrals to the new puppy owners. The doctor can also train a staff member to precede him or her in the examination room to answer questions and help steer clients toward raising the litter correctly. This can save time for the veterinarian up front. A qualified and personable staff person can provide a good service for both doctors and clients. Informing clients on how to guide new puppies into using their mouth correctly can get the animal off to a good start and help provide dog owners with a good puppy education.

PUPPY ORAL TENDENCIES

Young dogs have not learned that there is much difference between new owners and their littermates. They will try to wrestle and play in an instinctual way with both their siblings and their owners. In the litter, pups will wrestle and pull ears and tails in play. They are competitive with one another to feed with the mother dog, along with trying to be the first to the food bowl as they get older. No one is teaching them manners with their littermates. Anything goes when they are together. Their individual personalities start coming to surface as they learn new experiences with each other both for the good and otherwise. They may growl at and learn to be unsure of one another. Remember: The new teeth are very sharp and can do damage along with causing quite a bit of pain. The mother dog's actions also play a part in animals' learning experiences. She may not teach them things that will be beneficial for them later on as a family dog in the household. The young dog have not learned what is acceptable when communicating with people. They only know the actions and reactions from their exposure to siblings, their mom, and any other animals they have come across. When human exposure occurs, the experience with that individual becomes the norm or what is accepted or allowed when dealing with a person. Where owners differ from littermates is in their ability to teach the young animals according to human standards. These standards may vary among individuals. It is important to teach young pets how to use their mouth in an acceptable manner. A common complaint to veterinarians is that the new puppy likes to jump and snap at the hands or feet of the individual. A young dog may learn to get what it wants by using its mouth. Training should be sought early in puppies' lives. Owners who wait to start teaching until dogs are older have unfortunately allowed the animals far too much time to establish inappropriate habits (9). Puppies can soon learn the difference between the expectations of people and the normal interaction with littermates and their mom.

When considering where to train animals, owners may turn to their pet's doctor for advice. Veterinarians should encourage owners to ask a lot of questions when they are hiring a trainer. Communication skills are critical for a good trainer with regard both to animals and to owners (10). It is recommended that clients should observe classes or lessons conducted by an obedience instructor, before entrusting their new pup to certain behavioral techniques. Verbal recommendations by other clients may clue a veterinarian as to who is a good trainer in the area. Training should be encouraged for small breeds just as much as for large breeds. If dogs show early behavioral problems, special help besides basic training should be found. Knowledgeable people in the field of animal behavior (above and beyond basic obedience skills) are necessary for consultation with owners whose pets have special problems. If animals in a regular training class are consistently disruptive or may pose a danger to other animals or people, their owners should seek help from professionals trained in the field of animals behavioral problems, before regular obedience classes are considered. Veterinarians are often asked to guide pet owners in finding such a person. The local veterinary association or other veterinarians may have knowledge of where to find such help. In the decision as to whom the veterinarian should refer clients, credentials are important, as are verbal recommendations. Many basic trainers call themselves behaviorists, but the practitioner must be cautious in recommending someone who may not have the necessary knowledge to handle the case. Special training in behavior and/or psychology is necessary to have the insight to help owners with pets with behavioral problems.

Common concerns with young animals are the use of the mouth in both play and in serious actions. Many individuals will not take a young puppy's oral tendencies seriously because they think this is "normal" for an adolescent. They also feel that if aggression is exhibited during play, it is acceptable because the animal enjoys it. Some encourage such aggression. It is important to be aware at this stage that the animal is exercising the ability to use its mouth on its own terms. It is not being taught to discriminate when to use and not to use its mouth on someone or something else. The puppy phase should be an active phase of teaching, and it should consist of dogs' being taught what is allowable in the household. The first 2 years of a young animal's life should be an intense interaction period between owner and pet. Clients need to understand that they are the guide for teaching their pets proper behavior. Owners should show animals how to respect others when they consider using their mouth in an assertive manner. The angle to teaching is critical. If it is not done correctly, the animal may later show problems due to an inappropriate approach. Both trainers and owners should pick their training approach carefully. Not only is it important when to teach pets appropriate use of their mouth, but it is also critical how it is done.

Many animals reach the age 5–6 years, having never received any training. Many have not learned the word "no." In some cases, owners have allowed pets to get away with multiple behaviors without teaching them what should be allowed. Often, animals start getting away with so much that in time the people living with them cannot handle them. It is then that they ask their veterinarians about their dogs' behavioral problems. In some situations, some owners have tried training but have been given the wrong advice, and the effects of that advice begin to show in the animal's temperament. Training advice, including that given in books and pamphlets, should be reviewed and carefully selected by the person giving it to help guide pet owners. This can make a difference in the end result. Dog owners turn to veterinarians for guidance in raising their dog in the correct manner. A lot of behaviors that animals exhibit when young are not what owners are going to want to live with later on. However, owners do not always realize this at the time. The animal's doctor has the opportunity to practice good medicine, including advising clients on behavior, to help make a difference in both pets' and owners' lives together.

Clients will appreciate the extra effort taken not only in return visits to the doctor but also in talking to friends to whom they may recommend the veterinarian. When working with clients and their dogs, the practitioner may be able to pinpoint trouble spots before the client does. They need to choose how to talk to owners about the subject carefully. Some oral behaviors may surface, and clients will not even admit that these behaviors could become potential problems. Alerting owners to things that could happen later on if the behavior continues could decrease the chances that they will occur if the pet's family takes the situation seriously. Veterinarians should be sincere in talking about problems but also considerate of owners' feelings about their pet. Remember: Sometimes clients are not aware of the potential of animals' behavior with their mouth. Instead of finger-pointing at the particular animal exhibiting problems, it may be advisable to talk about experiences that other clients have had with similar situations and what happened later when owners did not address the issue soon enough. Make sure not to mention any specific names so as not to offend anyone. By your talking about other situations without being personal, owners may be able to utilize the information given to help them guide their own situation in the right way. Identifying problems early and guiding pet owners correctly can clearly avoid problems.

TEETH BRUSHING AND CONDITIONING

Veterinarians need to teach owners to condition their pet to having their teeth brushed. As oral hygiene awareness increases in the veterinary community, practitioners must pass on their knowledge to their clients. Pet owners expect doctors to be well informed on the latest medical procedures and techniques for their animal's welfare. This includes behavioral education along with dental education. More clients want to know how to teach their animal to have its teeth brushed. It may be a new concept for some, but as veterinarians help educate clients, they can get more people open to the idea of decreasing the tartar on their pet's teeth by brushing them. Many people are not aware that with a small amount of effort, brushing done correctly on a daily basis can avoid many problems. There are clients who are skeptical about putting their pet under anesthesia and would like to prevent the need to have a regular dental checkup for as long as possible. They also want to provide good health care that includes minimizing the accumulation of plaque and calculus to help reduce gum disease. Veterinarians have an opportunity to work with clients in brushing their animal's teeth and decreasing problems.

It is important for practitioners to remember that a part of conditioning animals to having their teeth brushed includes teaching them to get used to having their mouth handled. Many people expect pets to sit still while a toothbrush is moved back and forth over their teeth without any prior conditioning for the experience. Remember that it takes time for both animals and clients to get adjusted to it. Many would not consider it a natural instinct for animals to accept teeth brushing. Getting used to the procedure is a learned behavior. In some cases, when animals get fractious or restless during teeth brushing, individuals may not understand why. Some may get angry about it. They may not understand that an animal is mouth-shy to start with. The first step in conditioning is to take small amounts of time, often, to teach an animal to get used to having its teeth worked on. The initial approach should be just to get the animal used to having its mouth touched. Working with the animal to let the owner sit next to it is first on the agenda. Then, while the animal is laying down, the individual should work on handling its muzzle. Some animals may have no opposition to this, but others may be a challenge in accomplishing the task. Some animals are so active that they cannot sit still. Basic obedience is important in getting the animal to lay down and stay for a period of time. This is before the owner can get to the point of handling the animal's mouth. Once this is accomplished and the owner has spent the necessary amount of time to condition the animal to letting the owner hold its muzzle in a gentle fashion, the owner will want to slowly introduce a foreign object near the mouth. A sterile surgical gauze is a good material to start to condition the animal to handling over its teeth. The gauze sponge can be slowly touched to the front of the incisors and then carefully moved over the front of the teeth. Caution should be taken not to force the animal into accepting a lot of oral work all at once. If it is hesitant, move slowly in the amount of both exposure of and pressure on the teeth. Short periods of working with the pet will be time well spent. Owners may choose to give the pet treats as they continue to proceed with conditioning the animal to this new procedure. In addition, toothpaste oriented toward the animal's taste preference can be added to the gauge sponge to increase acceptance of the procedure. Later, the toothpaste can be added to a small toothbrush to increase its acceptability when it is introduced. This special veterinary paste in custom-made flavors can be ordered and offered for purchase by veterinary clients. A good time to mention this is when you educate them in the examination room on teeth-brushing procedure.

Clients should not expect quick changes in a pet's acceptance of the procedure. Patience is important. After continued efforts, clients will start to see a small amount of improvement in the animal's learning to handle having its teeth brushed (Fig. 1). Teachers should be gently firm and encouraging to the animal as they work toward the goal of getting their pet to allow them to brush their teeth. Veterinary practitioners should accom-

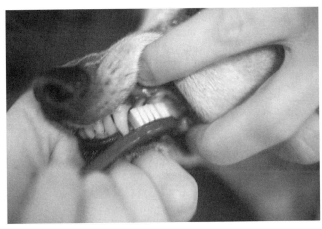

FIG. 1. Conditioning the animal to accepting teeth brushing.

plish the task of teaching an animal proper oral brushing themselves, before instructing pet owners on the subject. Clinicians are important in getting clients to follow through and condition their animal to accept good tooth-brushing techniques. They need to be able to do it themselves first to be better able to teach the technique to their clients. This would be helpful if possible. If there is a clinic dog, kept for blood donation or other purposes, the veterinarian and staff may want to work and practice with this animal, which can be used as a demonstration dog. In addition, the doctor may consider making a short videotape of the procedure that clients can watch while waiting for the doctor to come into the examination room. Again, staff members can assist in teaching the technique to owners and in showing the video. If owners are taught to coach the dog correctly, the animal has an increased chance of learning to sit still and actually enjoy having its teeth brushed.

BEHAVIORAL CONCERNS WITH ANIMALS IN THE CLINIC

Veterinarians and staff are required to handle behavioral concerns with clients' pets in the clinic on a daily basis. Owners are often deeply attached to their animals. Practitioners need to be educated on how to handle these situations. In dealing with behavioral problems in animals, it is very important to put the safety of clients, staff, veterinarians, and pets first. Many problems can be avoided by careful questioning of owners about the nature of the animal before examination. A questionnaire form in the waiting room may be used in this respect to inform the doctor and staff what to expect before a pet gets into the room for examination. Careful observance of the animal's body stance and actions will give insight to what it is feeling and how it may react with handling. Anytime the staff or a doctor handles a new animal, the time necessary should be taken to calmly work with the pet. Some animals become very stressed in new situations or areas. Others are uncomfortable with strangers. Every effort should be taken to make animals and owners comfortable with the situation at hand. A caring staff can take the edge off of a potentially uncomfortable situation. With an animal known for being aggressive, the staff may prefer to schedule the appointment at a time when it is slow in the clinic. If the pet dislikes other animals, the client should be taken into an examination room right after registering at the front desk. Many potential problems can be avoided by a staff sensitive to the needs of pets. Owners will appreciate the special care and concern given their animal's needs. Every care should be taken to relax the animal during the visit. If drug intervention is needed to decrease an animal's anxiety, clients should be asked about the possibility of giving this early, before the examination is done. Some pets will do better with tranquilization before being handled. This type of medication is used in the management of animals on a temporary basis. Drugs are not a cure for a pet's problems (11). Some animals, due to more involved emotional concerns, may need anesthetic intervention to allow the practitioner to do a thorough medical workup and examination, including a dental exam. It is good to talk to clients early about the behavioral needs of the pet as dental work is being considered. This gives the staff and doctor insight as to the pet's needs. Owners will appreciate the care shown toward their pet and themselves in this situation. This helps build client relationships and potentially increase a good client base. In being aware and careful about animals' behavioral needs, the pet professional can increase client rapport and decrease the chance of liability concerns.

Once in a while, although not often, a practitioner may have a behavioral problem with an animal right after surgery. Although to many pets, surgery is a discomfort, most of them go through the procedure uneventfully. There will, on an unusual occasion, be an animal that has a hard time working through the situation. It has been known that an animal may become uncontrollable and unmanageable after a procedure. This individual needs to be handled carefully. Again, it is important to be careful that no one is hurt. If the animal is in a large cage, it risks damaging itself with the extra room. In many cases, the size of the space can increase the chance of injury. In addition, the more the animal can see outside their cage, the more it may become excited. In certain individuals, the stress of being away from home and a change in regular schedule are hard to handle. Then, the challenge of surgery is added on top of things. In a few cases, animals may not be able to handle the situation at hand. Some animals cannot handle the added stress and discomfort even of what we consider a routine spaying or declawing procedure. Although most pets adjust to the change, each case is different. The veterinarian will need to make a judgment call. Some animals can be sent home fairly soon after surgery. Other animals need to be kept and tranquilized to decrease their psychological discomfort while their medical condition is being managed. Most surgeries and medical procedures run smoothly without unusual behavioral concerns. However, there are a few cases that require extra attention, and doctors need to give special attention to these clients. It is important to remember that not only do animals have medical concerns but they also have behavioral needs. We are coming into an age in which pets are very important to their owners. Medical doctors need to start showing increased concern and giving importance to the psychological aspects of veterinary medicine. Many questions will be asked by clients regarding the behavioral needs of their animals. Not only do doctors need to increase their knowledge of the subject, but it is also to their advantage to know the subject well to help decrease the possibility of injury to themselves and their staff. Because some animals have a hard time with hospitalization, caring, compassionate veterinarians are needed to help in this situation. Clients cannot help but appreciate when they see a practitioner sincerely trying to help such animals. This alone can help sell a veterinary clinic to the general public. Word of mouth often spreads fast when clients feel well taken care of. Especially in problem situations, owners pick up on it right away when the veterinarian appears calm and concerned for a pet's feelings. So will the staff members. Their respect for the doctor will increase when a tough situation is handled well. In being aware that some animals will have special behavioral needs from the challenge of surgery, the veterinarian can decrease problems by handling those cases carefully.

One of the goals of veterinarians when examining an animal's mouth is to make it as pleasurable an experience as possible. It is important to be not too forceful or rough when handling the animal. The doctor helps the pet through the examination by handling the animal carefully. Verbal communication with the individual can help calm the animal and reassure clients that they have a caring doctor. Anything that can scare the animal can decrease his willingness to want to return to the vet's office. Remember that the veterinary staff can work at conditioning animals to enjoy being at the doctor's. Even if the veterinarian needs to do uncomfortable procedures, concern for the animal's sensitivity is critical.

FELINE ORAL BEHAVIORAL CONCERNS

Cats have become a very popular household pet as owners' schedules have become increasingly busy and their living space has decreased. Oral tendencies in the pets may develop with time. Owners may notice unusual behavior before other medical clinical signs are exhibited (12). Clients with felines are becoming more educated about their furry companions and want the best for them. Cats also need good dental care. In the past, they used to be more active as they served their purpose of keeping the rodent population under control on the farm and in the house. The animals were actively working with their mouths. Some cats are still utilized for the same purpose, but many more are starting to lead a highly inactive life. Inappropriate behaviors such as aggression or furniture scratching may increase. It is important to direct behavior like clawing furniture to the proper place to do so (13). There are also correct places for cats to use their mouth, as well as incorrect places. Some animals use their mouth in a proper fashion, such as eating, but they may overdo or underdo the behavior. The teeth are important in transforming food taken into the mouth to a more easily digestible matter for the gastrointestinal system. Cats can be finicky about not only the flavor of food but also its size and shape. Cats may decrease their appetite if they are not offered the type of food that they prefer. It is important that the animal is actively eating within a short period of time to decrease the chances of having internal problems. It is also important that owners observe the animal's eating behavior to prevent obesity or, on the opposite end of the scale, an unhealthy, underweight condition.

If cats have dental problems causing pain or irritation in the oral cavity, these problems may lead to cats' decreasing their food intake. Observation of how pets eat their food may help owners understand what is going on with their pet. Visualization of the behavior is important in helping find a diagnosis. If the animal drops its food while chewing, there usually is a reason for this. A good oral physical examination by the veterinarian may reveal abnormalities in the oral region. Observation by the veterinary staff can also yield insight, if the animal is hospitalized and watched carefully during mealtimes. Pain may be the cause of an animal's being unable to chew food properly on the affected side. Some animals may drop their food from their mouth while eating due to an oral problem. Weight loss may be noted. To help in diagnosis, it is important to determine where the pain is coming from. Behavioral abnormalities may be the first sign of dental problems. Listening to the client can give the doctor a better idea of what is going on with the animal. Some cats may prefer to have canned food rather than dry. Other cats want only dry food. They may just prefer a certain consistency of food. Others will desire only a softer type of food as the result of pain with chewing. Teeth can be missing due to age or poor oral hygiene. The pet may need a special consistency to its meal to assist in the eating process. With all consideration, careful history taking, proper observation, a thorough physical examination, and good assessment skills, a correct diagnosis can be reached.

Obesity can be a behavioral problem in some felines. Overeating is a common behavior that doctors have to address with owners in the examination room. Recording the weight of animals every time they come in for a physical examination will help the veterinary staff determine whether or not the animals are gaining weight. Free-choice feeding is becoming increasingly popular in caring for cats due to convenience. In a number of cases, pets do not know their own limits. To many, feeding time is the highlight of the day. With a less active lifestyle and an increased exposure to food, the average feline has a high ability to gain weight. Obesity is no more healthy in cats than it is in other animals. It is important for veterinarians to educate clients on how to keep animals' weight down. Increased activity through play interaction with the owner and other pets in the household helps burn calories. The activity can be a good bonding experience for owners and cats. Various toys are offered for the feline fancier: from play mice on a simulated fishing pole to balls with bells in them. Cat owners should take some time at the local pet shop to browse and find a number of toys that their cat may be interested in. It is important to choose toys that the animals will not destroy or ingest parts of. Again, being familiar with the animal's behavior and particular personality will help owners choose these toys correctly. Next, choosing a proper diet will assist clients in keeping their cat's weight down. Calorie levels and fiber content should be noted in the choice of a food that is best for a particular situation. Once again, veterinary practitioners can guide owners in the selection of a proper diet for their pet. The weight and activity level of the animal should be taken in consideration. Along with the choice of the right diet to help control obesity, the decision must be made whether to leave food in the bowl all day long or to set up special feeding times. Many cats do well without having access to food all day long. By limiting the food, owners can help decrease the amount of time that animals are exposed to their food. Overeating can be controlled by proper attention on the part of owners. Veterinarian can help clients by properly educating them on the subject. Through proper exercise, a good diet, and scheduled feeding times, animals' weight can be kept at a healthy level.

Cats' potential behavior can be developed at an early age. It is important for kittens to be exposed to different people and situations at an early age, so that they get used to variety later in life. Some social behavioral traits may be hereditary, while others may depend more on how well animals have been socialized (14). Holding and petting is very important for young kittens to help decrease the chances later in life of their being afraid of people (15). The goal is to properly socialize pets for their benefit and the owners'. Cats unaccustomed to being around people and objects may be more aggressive later in life. It is important how young cats are raised and to whom they are exposed.

Cats may have increased oral tendencies with others if they are not properly socialized when young. Owners need to ask a lot of questions, when bringing a new cat into the household. Cats should be watched closely for oral behavioral tendencies. If owners observe inappropriate oral tendencies, they should seek help early.

FELINE ORAL EXAMINATION

Examination of the feline oral cavity is a regular part of a normal physical examination. After looking at the animal's overall appearance, many doctors usually begin the physical by looking at the mouth and its anatomic contents. Many cats exhibit a fearful behavior in the veterinary clinic. Cats are often not as sociable as dogs, especially in strange situations and with people that they are not exposed to on a regular basis. If there is increased noise or activity in the building, this may also increase an animal's apprehension. As the patient is handled, it may grow increasingly nervous especially if the approach is not properly done. Veterinarians should take special consideration in dealing with pets of this type. Care must be taken if there is the potential for aggressive behavior by the animal; precautions should be taken to decrease the chance of anyone's being hurt, including the owner. If handled carefully, an oral examination can be successful and well done and can inform the doctor and client of any abnormalities or concerns in the mouth.

It is important to encourage all cat owners to bring their cats in a travel box or carrier to decrease the chance of their losing control of the animal during the visit. Cats like to hide and often feel more secure in a pet carrier. Owners need to condition pets to the travel bag or box long before they are taken to the doctor's. Sometimes animals will not come out of their traveling container once they are at the clinic, preferring the security of their container. Cats should be handled carefully and patiently. Understand that just the car ride alone is a major event for many of these household pets. They are used to being in a home setting. The car ride is not quite what they expected to make their day complete. Talking in a calm, stable voice will help many through a tough situation. It is recommended that animals not be forced to come out of the carrier too quickly. Whether an animal appears to have the potential for aggression should be assessed and established right away. Tranquilization before transport may be needed to help calm some animals, but it has also been noted that they may work very hard to overcome the effects of it. It is important to understand that an antianxiety medication is not necessarily an antibite pill. Caution needs to be used even if the animal has been tranquilized.

With potentially fractious cats, care should be taken to protect the doctor, staff, owner, and the animal. First, the veterinary staff should take note to see if the individual has been declawed. Putting the animal in a cloth-type cat bag or wrapping it in a towel carefully tucked under the rear claws may help decrease injury with the feet. The person assisting the doctor by holding the animal should make sure that his or her face is not too close to the mouth, teeth, or any parts of the animal that can cause damage. The person restraining the animal should assess its behavior at all times to be aware of any potential actions that the cat may make. Once the animal is gotten under control, the doctor can carry on with the oral physical examination. One hand should grasp the head and maxilla to raise the upper lip and jaw, while the other hand will lower the bottom lip and mandible. Starting with assessment of the incisors and canine teeth, the clinician should take special care to check the gum line and the neighboring mucous membrane area. Checking for abrasions, broken or cracked teeth, ulcers, and abnormal coloration of the gums and teeth, the veterinarian should note any abnormalities that exist. The doctor will want to move as calmly and quickly as possible without forfeiting a thorough and professional job. If the animal is getting anxious, the doctor may want to give it a short rest, without letting the restraining hold loose, before he continues with the examination. The procedure should then be continued, covering the premolars, the molars, the tongue, and the rest of the oral cavity. Care should be taken especially in a potentially fractious animal that the clinician's fingers stay out of the animal's mouth as much as possible during the examination. The less they are in the mouth cavity, the fewer the chances are that the animal will clamp down and cause injury. By taking special care and considering the animal's temperament, the clinician can direct attention to proper restraint and techniques for decreasing the chances of injury during the oral examination.

The mouth is a very important tool for animals to survive, when it used for eating and consuming daily meals. It is also used in defensive modes, when animals are uneasy about situations. Cat bites can be very serious if not treated. The wounds are often deeply penetrating and can cause extreme damage. Clinicians and staff members should be extra cautious when handling a potentially fractious cat. Owners should be encouraged to stand back in the examination room if an animal could lash out. Some veterinarians prefer to take animals into a back room for the mouth examination to help decrease the chances of injury to clients in stressful situations. Animals should be taken to an area where there is not a lot of activity and confusion going on. Room should be given for staff persons doing the restraining to be able to move freely around the animal and be able to get out of the way if necessary, if the animal gets extreme. Care should be taken to calm the animal with medication for the safety of all concerned. Permission should be received from owners to use drug therapy. Again, concern for the animal and those involved in handling it is top priority.

Techniques for helping animals stay calm in the clinic can make a difference in the outcome. Many animals will be cooperative in allowing the doctor to perform the mouth examination. Each individual should be assessed as to its ability to be handled and restrained in a veterinary setting. Seeking information from clients early, before the examination, will be helpful for the staff to approach the situation properly. Cats are often stressed in being handled by someone they do not know. Special care and consideration of an animal's feelings will help put it at ease. Owner will appreciate the extra steps taken by the veterinary staff to make their pet comfortable and secure during the examination. The overall environment in the veterinary clinic can affect certain animals' temperament. Some veterinarians have found it helpful to have a separate waiting room for cats to help them feel less stressed during the visit. Quiet music in the area may be calming for both animals and clients. Scheduling the visits of clients with cats during a less busy time of the day or on days that are less active is recommended. Cats do not appear to be as socially active as dogs. They tend not to like to have a lot of other animals around them, especially when they are unsure of what is going on. Staff should take special consideration in approaching cats, moving in a careful, nonthreatening way. Talking to the animals may be helpful for some individuals. Gentle petting to help reassure that everything is all right can be a prerequisite for helping cats adjust to the situation, but it should be recognized that a few cats do not like handling. In taking careful consideration of cats' needs in the veterinary clinic, the staff can decrease the chances of having animals that may be afraid and fractious in the situation.

DENTAL INJURY DUE TO BEHAVIORAL PROBLEMS

Occasionally, animals may be presented to the veterinarian with a dental injury or concerns due to behavioral problems. Traumatic injury to the gums, teeth, tongue, and the surrounding areas could cause permanent damage. Separation anxiety, thunderstorm anxiety, obsessive chewing, licking, and grooming, and aggression are a few of the many behavioral concerns that can cause dental problems. Doctors need to be aware of potential damage to the mouth and its different parts from inappropriate behavior. A thorough examination of the oral cavity, along with a good history from clients, can yield important information about how an animal has damaged its mouth. The breed of animal should be taken into consideration of why the injury is there and how it got there. A pet's individual personality can also predispose it to having mouth problems. Fence and kennel chewing can wear teeth down or break or crack them. There have been cases of extreme injury to the oral cavity when dogs are frustrated about being closed up in an enclosure. This does not mean that animals should not be put in a pen, but it does mean that owners need to seek help in teaching animals that it is "no big deal" to be in one. Animals should learn to be separated from other parts of the household or backyard to decrease the chances of destroying or hurting other objects or individuals. Some animals have an extreme need to chew. It may be necessary to teach them to be in a special enclosure with their toys, so that they learn what is all right to play and interact with. Especially early in life, when individuals are more orally oriented, it is important not to allow pets to get themselves into trouble. Even when animals are channeled to exercising their mouth on a toy or chew article that is all right to use, injury can still occur due to the intensity of the chewing. Again, psychological help may be recommended, but this needs to come from a trained professional who is used to dealing with these types of problems. If an individual of this caliber cannot be found in the area, it is advised that the veterinarian seek as much behavioral training and education as possible through articles, lectures, and books. One goal of good dental work is to help clients prevent problems from occurring again. Proper assessment of the situation at hand when pets are presented can help veterinarians steer clients into preventing further abuse of their pet's oral cavity.

FENCE AND KENNEL BITING

Veterinarians will occasionally get a case involving fence and kennel biting. Injury and/or breakage of teeth may be present. In some cases, a history of blood found in the area is received without owners' knowing where it came from. With a good physical examination, lacerations of the gums and surrounding areas may be found. The type and severity of the mouth trauma should be assessed. A thorough examination of the oral cavity is essential to assist in the diagnosis. Checking the surface of the teeth for any cracks or wearing down of the teeth should be done. In some cases in which the animal is chewing on wire or fencing, portions of affected teeth will exhibit a gray metal–looking coloration and at times increased wear. The gums may or may not be intact. In addition, cuts and/or lacerations to the lips or tongue may be seen. Doctors should ask about visual damage to the pen or area where the animal is kept. Some injuries are more serious than others. Owners have different reasons why they feel they need to keep the pet in a secure area. They will need help in getting the animal to adjust to the situation. This may be an opportunity to work with clients to decrease the chances of the behavior recurring, before severe injury to the oral cavity occurs.

Assessing the situation by asking clients a lot of questions is the starting point for offering behavioral advice. Some animals have not gotten used to being away from their owners for a length of time. Owners more than ever have a busy schedule and have an increased need at times to use a pen for their pet. This at times can result in oral injury. Questions about the situation need to be asked to give practitioners a better picture of what is happening. It is important to know an animal's usual routine before it is put in the pen. The location of the kennel area should also be known. Where the pen is located may lead to increased stimulation of the animal, thus causing it to try to get out. Some animals react to certain stimuli. Changing the location in this situation can make a difference. Exposure to other animals, people, noise, or activity should be avoided. At the same time, the consistency of the kennel should be looked at. Building a sturdier structure or changing the type of material that the pen is made of can decrease the chance of injury.

If possible, it is good to see what area the animal is biting at. Building a barrier that the animal is not interested in using its mouth on should be considered. Are there other things in the area to keep the animal occupied? Is boredom or stress predisposing the animal to feeling the need to exercise its mouth on the pen? Many areas should be looked into to get a good idea of the situation. In reviewing these questions with clients, veterinarians should consider recommending behavioral modification techniques such as desensitizing to the confined area for animals that have damaged or are on the way to injuring the oral cavity. Drug therapy may be a consideration, but behavioral techniques are recommended before turning to medication. Many cases can be worked through without drug intervention. In some extreme cases, however, after an owner has tried everything else, including seeking professional advice, medical therapy is necessary. The type of medication should be based on the past medical history and the present situation of the animal. As low a dose as possible should be used to maintain the situation safely—on a temporary basis, if possible. In some cases, a combination of behavioral modification techniques, drug therapy, and active participation by owners will be needed to help the situation. Through proper questioning, careful assessment, good communication skills, and client involvement, a good behavioral program for the cage-biting animal can be achieved.

DESTRUCTIVE CHEWING

Some animals will be presented with dental problems due to destructive behavior with their mouth. In addition to medical problems associated with injury to the oral cavity, other veterinary problems from ingesting articles may be exhibited due to abnormal behavior. Some behaviors with the mouth are instinctual. Others may reflect emotional causes. Dogs suffering from separation anxiety may chew destructively as a way to get to the individual that they desire to be with (16). These individuals may be neurologically different either chemically or anatomically (17). Larger breeds of dogs have the ability to do more damage than smaller breeds. The animal may go outside in the backyard and chew on a tree limb, and it may not be noticed by the owner as a problem. But when the animal comes into the house and chews on the expensive table leg, it is now in big trouble. In actuality, the behavior exhibited outdoors can be a problem, although not causing a financial problem as far as replacement goes. The animal can still find itself on the examining table being examined for destruction of the oral cavity. Injuries such as broken teeth, lacerated gums, wood splinters wedged between teeth, and ingestion of wood pieces or other items can occur. These can cause vomiting, abdominal pain, and gastrointestinal problems. Owners may notice that the animal is having medical problems right away or may not notice problems for some time. Destructive behavior can be a major concern in animals that exercise their ability to use their mouth on objects that can break, bend, splinter, or peel. Animals do not necessarily know what is or is not good for their health. Not only can the ordeal be expensive for owners, but it can also do irreparable damage to the body if foreign or toxic objects or materials are ingested. This behavior, whether instinctual or psychological, can cause major concerns for animals and owners.

Boredom can be a cause of excessive chewing and destruction. Some animals are highly intelligent and need activities to keep them occupied. As our lifestyles get busier, the household animal often gets pushed to the side or ignored and has to occupy its time by itself. Years ago, animals were next to their master's side, assisting in catching the day's meal by hunting and retrieving. They also helped herd the sheep and the cattle on the farm. They were a more active part of the family, guarding the area and working with family members. Then, later in the evening after a long day's work, they would lay down in front of the fireplace to rest before the next day of activity began. Often, one adult was around to watch what went on and to call for the animal's assistance. The dog was highly counted on to do its part in the family setting. Now, in our mobile society, not only have our fast-paced schedules pushed the animal into the background, but we are also looking for easier and more convenient ways to manage pets without involvement of our time. From free-choice feeding to installed dog doors, animals are to manage themselves throughout the day by themselves. When owners come home exhausted from a long day's work, they want to sit and rest, but it is the highlight of the animal's day having its master home. Often, owners get upset with the animal's overexuberance at this time and shoo the animal away, wanting to be left alone. This is the psychological basis of some destructive chewing behavior.

Frustrated from the lack of attention and activity in their lives, some animals may start to exhibit inappropriate behaviors such as chewing articles in the house when no one is at home. It may be anything from pulling books and magazines around or off shelves to seriously destroying expensive shoes, clothes, and other items in the house. The medical problems associated with this destruction oral behavior range form lacerated gums to broken or fractured teeth. In some cases, owners get highly upset because of the financial aspect of the situation and get down on the animal more for the destructive behavior, frustrating it even further and beginning the cycle again. Owners will present the case to the veterinarian to help correct the medical concerns associated with the problem behavior and will also ask for advice in changing what is going on.

Again, certain breeds may be more prone to destructive chewing than others. The larger the dog, the more damage can be done to a home. Animals can also do damage to outdoor possessions such as patio furniture, air conditioning wires, shrubbery, flower beds, and barbecue covers. Electrical burns in the oral cavity and even death from electric shock can occur if the pet has used its mouth on cords and other electric devices. Portions of the lip, gums, and tongue may be blistered from an electrical charge when animals chew on wires with current running through them. A proper medical workup should be done to assess the extent of damage. If an animal is highly sensitive to having its mouth examined, tranquilization or anesthetic intervention may be necessary. The overall medical condition of the animal should be properly assessed and taken into consideration before any medication is administered. Breed disposition and animal size may help determine whether an animal is a candidate for destructive chewing and can correlate with the amount of damage done.

Not only should good medical care be given to treat the traumatic injury, but owners must be steered toward measures to prevent this type of injury. Depending on the situation at hand, it may be necessary to keep the animal in an area where it is unable to get to its owner's possessions or things that can hurt it, if chewed on. Proper teaching and giving the animal safe toys and chew articles are important. Owners must help an animal learn what is allowable to chew on. Veterinary practitioners can inform clients which toys and chew items are good. They can also channel clients into selecting chew toys that are large enough and strong enough so that the dog will not tear pieces from them and ingest them. Other articles made for dogs to chew on need to be assessed and chosen, or avoided, by the type of dental damage that can be done with them. Some toys or chew articles, if too hard, have been known to break or crack teeth after extensive chewing on them. By giving animals proper articles to chew on, owners can decrease the animals' interest in other items to exercise their mouth on. In this way, owners can prevent pet oral injuries and establish a better relationship with their pet.

PICA AND WOOL SUCKING

Some animals, both dogs and cats, may be presented with the complaint of excessive eating of objects in the house. This behavior can start as simple chewing or sucking on an object, but in time it progresses to ingesting multiple objects or pieces of articles. Pica can be a secondary problem to an initial problem involving the esophagus, pharynx, stomach, or intestines (18). Many behaviors can start as a simple oral tendency to be active with the mouth. Many owners may disregard the actions because they do not appear to be serious or because the owners think that they are just natural behaviors, having seen them since the animal was young. Many do not realize that in time this condition can intensify in frequency. Pica is seen in both dogs and cats and is most noticed in younger animals, although it can be well established in an older individual. Sometimes an animal does it in the presence of the owner, but at other times, owners see only traces of the behavior after they have been out of the animal's presence for a while. Holes may start to appear in sweaters, or torn carpeting is noticed after a pet has been left alone. Others may not recognize that something has been ingested until it is passed through the gastrointestinal system and appears in the stool. Severe internal injury can occur due to the ingestion of plastics, carpeting, pantyhose, towels, and other objects that the animal can get its mouth on. Major surgery may need to be performed to remove the ingested articles from the animal's stomach and intestinal region. So there is both a physical and financial aspect to this problem. Clinical signs include vomiting, diarrhea, anorexia, weight loss, blood in the stool, and pieces of the ingested item in the feces. Excessive eating and ingesting of items can be a psychological disorder in the animal. Special care and concern must be given affected animals to decrease the chances of exposure to these articles. Inquiry into its background may reveal why an animal is exhibiting such unusual behavior.

In cats, "wool sucking" is a common oral misbehavior (19). They tend to chew or suck on items that have wool in them. Later, they may move on to other types of fiber. Knitted sweaters, afghans, carpeting, and upholstery fabric are a few of the items that cats might chew. They seem to seek out clothing or articles made of cloth. Severe damage to the items can cause serious frustration in the owner. The financial aspects of the situation can play a role in clients' seeking help with the situation. Injury to the cats' internal system can cause major problems. Passing the material ingested may be a challenge and can cause severe injury and even death if the behavior is not caught, prevented, or corrected.

Dogs tend to ingest a greater variety of objects. Excessive chewing in puppies can lead in time to a serious pica problem. Toxic or poisonous plants or materials may pose an increased risk to animals ingesting them. Children's toys, pencils, remote control devices, and other household items are often destroyed and ingested by animals with this particular chewing and eating disorder. Some dogs may start by stealing an article and running away from their owners. In time, many things are picked up and transported in a dog's mouth. Out of desperation, not wanting to give the item up, the animal may swallow it. Other items in the house will be picked up and ingested for similar reasons. In time, the dog is now ingesting multiple articles in the house. Especially in families with children in the household, toys, crayons, plastic army soldiers, and plastic building blocks are often left out, and the animal has increased access to them. The more an animal ingests items, the greater the risk the animal has for internal damage to be done. Owners need to be careful about the amount of exposure that they want the animal to have to these articles. They also need to be aware of any abnormal behavior, such as anorexia or lethargy, that may be caused by the ingestion of nonfood objects. Clients who have an animal with this type of problem should be aware of the consistency of its stool at all times. If problems arise or if the possibility of pica exists, the animal should visit the veterinarian for a physical examination to rule out any major medical concerns.

MOUTH SHYNESS

Some animals appear to be mouth-shy, when presented to the veterinarian. They hesitate to allow anyone to touch or examine their mouth or parts therein. As the doctor approaches, a mouth-shy animal's ears may tip backward, and the animal may pull away. Some animals lay peacefully on the examination table, but as soon as the veterinarian starts moving to examine the mouth, they start to appear anxious and will not allow anyone to touch them. If someone forces the issue, the animals may snap or get ornery in some cases. Mouth-shyness is seen in a variety of breeds and in both males and females. It may be apparent in young individuals or may not manifest itself until an older age, when an animal becomes more unsure of someone handling it. Many of these animals have not had anyone touch their mouth on a regular basis, or when they have, it has not been a good experience for them. The veterinary clinic makes matters more difficult because it is a relatively strange place for animals to be in. They will not be as comfortable there as in their own home. Many animals will have no problems with being examined, but the one that is mouth-shy can be very difficult to deal with. How such animals are handled is important. The approach should be carefully chosen to help decrease the problem with the individual animal, while geared to achieve the goal of accomplishing the task once set out (Fig. 2).

Owners will also have problems with some of these pets, while trying to pill them. Medication must be given, but owners may not know how to handle a mouth-shy pet. Some may be bitten if they force the issue. Cats can bite and cause deep puncture wounds that may predispose to serious infection. The veterinary staff needs to teach owners how to pill an animal properly. Taking some time with clients before the problem occurs can make a difference in the outcome. Although owners may know how to properly pill a pet, they may still not be able to do so with some animals. Other modes of medicating may be needed. A liquid medication may help decrease the hesitancy problem in cats, puppies,

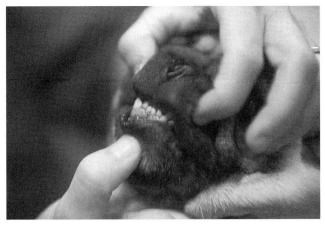

FIG. 2. Conditioning the animal to allow handling of the facial area and opening of the oral cavity.

and difficult animals, but it still must be administered properly. This approach may be more advantageous than pilling. For other pets, owners may crush the pill and put it in a highly palatable canned food. If an animal poses a serious problem in medication administration, the client and the veterinarian may decide that hospitalization and handling by a professionally trained staff may be desirable to help lessen the chance of injury. Injections may be necessary. In these cases, it is important that the animal is medicated. If owners are not able to do so at home, the veterinarian should offer the option of keeping the pet in the hospital to accomplish what medically needs to be done. It is recommended to advise clients of the expense of hospitalization when they are informed of this medication option. Regardless of cost, clients may have to decide to have the veterinary staff deal with the pet's concerns in the clinic as opposed to keeping the animal at home and risking being bitten. Home care recommendations for such individuals should be carefully considered.

When an animal has a behavioral problem such as mouth-shyness, it should be noted in the record. Any problem that the staff should be aware of should be written in a special place in the animal's chart, so the doctor's assistants can be aware at a glance of particular needs of the pet. A different-colored ink or a special code may be used to make the instructions legible and easy to see. If an animal is fractious, it should be noted. It should also be written on the identification card in the kennel that the animal is put in. The staff should make the needs of the animal a priority before it is handled. Keeping the staff informed can prevent problems. Special instructions on how to handle mouth-shy animals will lessen the chance of accidents when staff members work with such individuals.

ORAL EXAMINATION IN THE POTENTIAL SHOW DOG

Veterinarians may be working with clients who show dogs or plan on doing so and are interested in teaching animals to accept examination of the mouth. The animals will need to learn to accept this when it is done not only by the doctor but also by a dog show judge. It is important for veterinarians to remember that when they are working with a puppy on the examination table, this may be the animal's first experience with having its mouth handled. The animal will remember what type of first experience it was, and it is important that it be a good experience, even if it takes more time. Veterinarians need to stress to owners that if the animal is going to be shown, they need to get the dog used to an oral examination. Some dog-show oral examinations may be more extensive than others depending on the breed. The working breeds may need to allow the molars and premolars to be examined and counted. Toy and nonsporting breeds, such as the poodle and the Lhasa apso, need only to have the incisor and canines looked at. The extent of the oral examination is up to the judges and their interpretation of the breed standard. Again, veterinarians may want to refer their clients to an experienced show breeder or handler for lessons or classes on teaching the animal to stand for examination, which should include the oral examination. It is important to remember that many animals' first experiences with the procedure are with their doctor. Veterinarians can be an important part of the animal's learning to accept an oral examination correctly.

COPROPHAGIA

Veterinarians occasionally get complaints concerning coprophagy. Some dogs will ingest their stool after defecation or consume the stool of other animals. The problem is not often see in cats, while dogs are known to be more inclined to it (20). Many clients find this behavior rather repulsive. Especially if they have close contact with the animal's face, the odor of the animal's breath is less than desirable. The animals can be well groomed and healthy in appearance. The doctor will be asked about why the animal is doing such a thing. Some owners get so irritated with the pet that they may abuse the animal, thinking they are disciplining it. Owners may take the situation personally in the fact that they could not consider ever doing anything close to what the animal is doing. They do not understand how their beloved pet could act in such a manner and even perhaps appear to enjoy it. In answering clients' questions, veterinarians can help owners with their frustrations and in time may help lessen the severity with which they handle the animal and its behavior.

Not a lot of animals will exhibit coprophagic behavior, but those that do can cause owners concern. Dogs in the wild often eat food, digest it, and defecate the remains. In establishing an area that animals claim as their territory, they will later consume the stool to help keep the area clean of feces. It is also a way of recycling undigested food stuff that is still in the stool and did not get fully utilized by the body. Some animals will go out, kill their prey, and then bring the food back to their territory. Often, dogs will defecate shortly after ingesting food, so the stool is near his living area. Whether animals' coprophagic behavior is for keeping their territory well kept, utilizing undigested foodstuff in the stool, or decreasing the scent in the area, it is not totally clear why they act the way they do. Some have felt that there might be something in the stool that is needed in the animal's diet. It could be a needed enzyme or type of foodstuff that animals are seeking. The reason for this behavior is really not completely known. Animals have not had formal training on proper etiquette according to human standards. The do's and don'ts may not have been covered enough or in the correct fashion by owners to get the message across to the household dog. The problem needs to be approached with understanding as to why the animal would be doing the behavior. It is not doing it to hurt or make an owner angry. Clients may tell the doctor that the dog "knows better," but they often need to understand the cause underlying the situation. Telling the animal once or twice in an extreme disciplinary form may teach the pet to avoid the owner rather than the stool. Veterinarians can help clients understand the cause and use a more rational approach in dealing with this unwanted behavior.

First, it is important to pursue the possibility of an underlying medical problem. Any medical concern that may increase the desire to eat objects excessively can increase the tendency for coprophagy in an individual (20). A connection with a pancreatic insufficiency problem has been suggested in some cases of coprophagy. A proper medical workup including blood work should be done. Some animals with this behavior are actually craving food as the result of a problem with improper digestion and absorption of the food they are given. Many nutritional elements are still maintained in the stool because they were not utilized by the body the first time around. The animal may be basically hungry. The clinician needs to pursue the medical possibilities that may a basic cause of coprophagy. During the initial physical examination, a proper history needs to be taken. History as to when and how often the dog attempts to ingest the stool should be recorded. Is the animal overanxious when eating his food? Is it eager to go into the backyard where the stools are? Is it adamant about eating the stool? Does it defecate a large amount of stool? What consistency is the stool? Is there a particularly unusual smell to the feces? Is the color different? As the physical continues, the veterinarian should look for signs of pancreatic insufficiency or other digestive problems. Is the animal thin and/or underweight even though it consumes a large amount of food? Does it appear unthrifty? Other possible medical causes should be ruled out, including internal parasites or other conditions that may semidebilitate an animal and keep its system from receiving the necessary nutrients from the foods given it. Is the animal constantly wanting to go outside or having accidents in the house? This again may point to higher stool volume from a medical condition. Are the stools voluminous in size? These are all questions that can be asked of the client during the history-taking process. The answers may lead the clinician to finding the cause of the problem. Inquiry into the animal's medical history is important to reaching a proper diagnosis in cases of coprophagy.

It is important to remember that different causes may predispose an animal to coprophagic tendencies. The cause may be medical, nutritional, or psychological. Once an animal starts the behavior, with time, it may get used to doing the activity, making it harder to stop. Not only is it unpleasant for owners to experience their animal's doing an unacceptable behavior such as coprophagy, but it is also not healthy for the animal to ingest aged stool because of its bacterial and potential fungal content. This can increase the chances of infection. It is important for veterinarians to determine a possible cause and then to help owners develop a plan to help decrease the behavior.

In considering how to approach the problem of coprophagy, pet owners must look at the possible techniques that may be used. One recommendation is aversion conditioning. This involves making the feces adversive to the animal. Adding an ingredient to the stool that is repulsive to the pet will deter the animal from ingesting it. There are commercial products that can be purchased from the veterinary distributor and offered to the client at a retail price. It is important to give clear instructions on how to use the product. Following the manufacturer's recommendations is always suggested. Others have tried to add a natural product such as pumpkin filling or meat tenderizer to the diet. Modifying the pet's meal in this way modifies the end product, and at times this may make the stool undesirable to the animal. Other approaches may entail continued teaching of the pet that eating the stool is unacceptable. The owner must watch the animal closely when it is let outside and, after it defecates, must go out to the dog and constantly stress that it must stay away from the stool after it has been left alone in the yard. It is important in using this technique that the owner not discourage the actual act of defecation. The owner must praise the act but discourage going back to the area where the animal might ingest the fecal material. Careful watch over the situation can increase a positive outcome. The owner needs to assess which approach is best for the particular animal with the problem. There is no product or technique that will work at all times in all cases, but these are some different approaches that have been used to help decrease problems associated with coprophagy.

EXCESSIVE ORAL GROOMING

Some animals may groom themselves excessively. Clinical signs of this include worn-down teeth, gum disease from excess hair between the teeth and gum line, alopecia, secondary dermatitis, and severe skin ablations called "hot spots." A pet may be presented that appears moth-eaten or debilitated and unkept. Damage can depend on the type of bite or dental occlusion (or malocclusion). Some pets with an extreme underbite may collect the hair along the gum line in an extreme manner. The bottom jaw acts as a scoop as the animal licks and bites the skin area. Some of these pets are simply doing regular grooming to keep the coat and skin clean. Others may have a parasitic or dermatologic condition predisposing them to the behavior. Where animals are infested with a severe flea infestation, the chronic irritation keeps them obsessively licking and chewing to decrease the itching sensation caused by the parasite. Other causes of obsessive grooming with the mouth should be asked about and analyzed accordingly. Allergies, bacterial infections, hypothyroidism, and other internal causes may be a prerequisite to this excessive behavior. Veterinarians should be thorough in the history taking to uncover underlying causes of obsessive grooming or dermatologic destruction.

When examining an animal for excessive oral behavior involving the coat and skin, veterinarians will start with the oral cavity. Worn or missing teeth or hair embedded into the gingival sulcus may be present due to the behavior. In older pets who have advanced gum disease, loose teeth may actually fall out or be ingested during the process of grooming. The extent of damage should be assessed. Other abnormalities should be noted during the physical examination. Various clinical signs may help practitioners focus on a hormonal cause that increases the chances of having hot spots or excessive dermatologic damage due to the animal's chewing on the skin. If warranted, blood work should be done according to the clinical signs that the animal exhibits. Proper diagnosis of parasitic infestation is important, and a treatment program must be set accordingly. Certain types of mange can cause extreme pruritic conditions, leading animals to scratch and chew and cause increasing damage. Allergies to food, grasses, chemicals, and other irritants can initiate excessive grooming. In addition to treatment, the causative agent must be removed to increase the benefit of a respectable medical treatment plan. Various causes are the prerequisite to excessive licking and chewing. To decrease the potential for dental damage, the source of the problem needs to be found and diagnosed accordingly.

Excessive grooming in cats is often noted in medium- to long-haired cats. Hairballs can become a major problem in the feline species. There may also be a medical basis for increased grooming. External parasites such as fleas may increase the animal's desire to heavily groom itself. Skin conditions, such as a bacterial infection with pruritus, may also lead to continuous grooming. Abdominal obstruction can occur if the cat excessively grooms itself. Veterinarians should recommend managing a hairball problem with a proper laxative. There are several on the market. It needs to be palatable and given on a regular basis whenever the animal actively grooms itself. Doctors should ask clients about their cat's grooming habits on a regular basis.

Dogs can also have an excessive grooming problem associated with skin or parasitic problems. Hairballs in dogs usually travel the gastrointestinal system and are passed in the stool, but they may also be vomited up. Owners may not know what they are, especially in the long-haired breeds. It is important for clients to work at keeping their pet parasite-free. If skin concerns do arise, owners should seek veterinary care and guidance as soon as possible. This may decrease the animal's desire to groom excessively.

A pet's excessive grooming can cause internal problems. Owners should be aware of their pet's grooming habits. Veterinarians should encourage owners to observe their pet's behavior. Any potential complications should be prevented by early detection and proper treatment for the problem. Vomiting, hair loss, lethargy, loss of appetite, and even shock and death may be clinical signs of potential gastrointestinal blockage due to excessive intake of hair at grooming. The animal should be treated according to the clinical signs. Radiographic confirmation of a possible blockage may be necessary. Hairballs due to heavy grooming can be medically unhealthy in both cats and dogs. It is important to question clients on the behavior to try to prevent problems. Proper veterinary advice can help prevent problems with hairball buildup and help animals function internally better.

Excessive grooming can cause many potential medical complications, including worn-down teeth, gum disease, hair loss, and gastrointestinal problems. By taking a proper history and doing a thorough examination, practitioners can help decrease those problems.

It is important to find the cause of the behavior. By questioning owners and being aware of the possible underlying causes, veterinarians can often decrease this often destructive behavior.

INGESTION OF PLANTS AND GRASSES

Veterinarians are often asked why animals eat plants and grasses. It is well known that many cats enjoy grazing on the catnip plant. Owners later observe the aftereffects of plant ingestion. Dried catnip is contained in some cat toys to increase the interaction between the animals and the toys. Some cats will spend hours on end playing with the toy because of the attraction to the catnip. Some companies encourage owners to grow their own catnip and grass for their cat to ingest. The fresh plant is very attractive to the animal. Catnip is usually an acceptable plant for cats to eat.

Some clients complain that their pets are eating and chewing household plants. First, they are unhappy about the situation because they do not like having indoor plants that have holes chewed in them and look rather moth-eaten. They also have concerns about the toxicity of these plants. Dieffenbachias, poinsettias, and other household plants are known to have potential poisonous effects. Owners need to be cautious about placing the plants in an area that is accessible to the animals. Puppies and some adult dogs will also destroy and eat plants. Not only can the situation cause a mess in the household, but animals also can get ill from ingesting plants. There may also be a financial aspect to the problem involving the loss of the plants, damage to household furnishings, and the veterinary bills for treating the animal that gets sick or needs medical attention because of the potential toxicity of the plant ingested. The question of death as the result of eating toxic plants may arise with clients. If an animal is presented with the concern that it may have eaten plant material, a thorough history should be taken, including the type of plant or a description of it. Owners should also asked whether they saw the animal eat the plant and how much of the plant is missing. If a client calls in to make an appointment out of concern for the potential consequences of household plant ingestion, the receptionist should recommend bringing the plant or a plant leaf in for identification. Owners need to be aware whether the animal has vomited or has had bouts of diarrhea since exposure to the plant. Is the animal showing clinical signs besides those that point to plant toxicity? Medical attention should be given accordingly. It needs to be stressed that plants should be kept away from where the animals can reach them. If the client has a dog, plants should be placed high enough so that the pet cannot get them. For cats, plants should be kept in a side room that is off limits to them. Animals can be taught to avoid the plants if they are continuously supervised and taught to avoid the material. Repetition is critical in teaching pets that plants are off limits to them. Veterinarians should recommend training techniques that allow animals learn to stay away from the plants but to still have a good relationship with the owner. In handling this matter, doctors should educate clients that efforts early in the life of the animal can help prevent this problem from occurring. Clients should also be encouraged to watch young pets for any interest in household plants. They should automatically set the house up to keep plants out of reach of the animal. Preventing plant eating is far superior to having to treat its consequences.

Some dogs eat grass outside and then vomit the material. Owners often ask practitioners why the animal does this. It has been theorized that grass-eating is associated with gastrointestinal irritation or with a certain pH level in the stomach. Owners may observe that once they let the dog into the yard, it will almost frantically start pulling the grass near the base and ingesting the material. Quite a bit of grass may be ingested before the animal vomits the plant material with an amount of stomach fluid. Owners should observe the animal after an episode of this type for other clinical signs of irritation or upset of the gastrointestinal tract. If the animal begins to exhibit behavioral or other signs of a problem, they should seek help from their veterinarian. When a behavioral problem or change is first noted, it can sometimes be the first sign of a medical problem. Practitioners should listen to clients, who know their pet better than anyone. Clients can detect early changes that help catch a medical condition in its elementary phases. This can help decrease the chances of illness if correctly diagnosed and treated. The grass that an animal ingests can be a source of fiber and other nutrients. Often, though, the animal vomits after ingestion. It is not completely known why animals do the behavior, but it is recommended that owners take it as a possible early sign of a problem.

ACRAL LICK GRANULOMA

Acral lick granulomas are caused by an animal's excessive licking and chewing on the skin. They are often seen on legs and over joint areas of the appendages but can be found in other areas. Some animals start by simply licking the coat in one area. After some time, they continue to go to the spot, chewing and excessively mouthing the area until they start to wear it down to an irritated, unhealthy state. Others begin by chewing the area directly, without licking it first. Signs of irritation begin to appear when the first areas of hair loss are noted. Even though the alopecia is seen, owners may not take the behavior as a serious problem at this stage, and the animal continues to mutilate itself in the same area. Redness, heat, and swelling may appear along with bleeding or serous drainage. The animal is continually be drawn to the area. More hair loss can occur, along with deterioration of the dermal region. The animal may begin to self-destruct the area through the dermal and epidermal regions. Severe debilitation can occur in some animals as they totally disregard any other distraction to focus on continuing this destructive behavior in the same location. Veterinary practitioners must inquire into what starts the behavior. They should be aware of the possibility of an underlying medical condition in the area being damaged. If the destruction is over a joint area, practitioners should recommend a radiologic examination to rule out the possibility of a veterinary problem. Arthritis or joint deterioration may be a consideration in such excessive behavior. The pet may have a slow, progressive problem with calcification, minor fractures, or other orthopedic conditions. Other conditions, such as a parasitic infestation, may also be the cause of this inappropriate behavior. The cause should be determined first before a treatment program is prescribed.

DENTAL DAMAGE DUE TO EXCESSIVE CHEWING INTENSITY

In veterinary dentistry, it is not unusual to come across cases in which an animal has broken a tooth or teeth while chewing an article that is commonly recommended as a chew toy or object. In behavior, we work at teaching pets what is acceptable to exercise the mouth on. Some animals, however, chew so intensely that they actually crack or break a tooth or multiple teeth. Some of these animals have very powerful jaws. In the wild state, dogs used their teeth to crush bone, as bone from prey was a source of calcium. Some domesticated dogs still have traits from their wild ancestry. These animals may also exert their frustrations from other sources on the chew bone or other acceptable objects given them to use. Some dogs also enjoy crushing and chewing ice cubes, especially in warm or hot weather. Owners often give them the ice to occupy them. Some will actively play with the cubes for quite a long time and then bite and chew them until they are gone. Damage can be done on the oral cavity even with a natural product such as ice cubes. The intensity of the bite on the object can sometimes split teeth. The problem in this situation is that if owners do not give pets appropriate objects to chew on, the animals may start to chew other things such as patio furniture or expensive items. Still, it has to be a judgment call on the part of veterinarians and clients as to what should be allowed for dogs to chew. If extensive dental damage occurs or can occur, this needs to be taken into consideration. A softer chew toy that will not split teeth can be substituted for a harder toy, as long as there is little chance that the animal can ingest the article. Popsicles can be a replacement for ice cubes if the animal wants to cool off. Remember that owners want to decrease the chances of dental damage. An object to mouth helps satisfy an animal's oral need and can help prevent problems. It is also recommended that owners be active in training their pet to help occupy its interests. Training for dogs helps keep them active in something they can use their mind on. It makes them feel more useful. In some working and sporting breeds, training helps decrease boredom and at times possibly the frustration that animals may feel if they are not as actively interacting with family members as they would like. Animal may channel their frustration into chewing hard toys, hooves, ice cubes, and chew articles. Between the power in their jaws and the intensity of the bite on the article, broken or split teeth can occur. Other oral damage is also possible. Sometimes owners may not recognize the problem when it happens, because dogs do not complain verbally of the discomfort as a person would. However, they may do it in other ways. This may be when clients start to notice a behavioral change in their pet and not know why. Pets may start to show signs that something is wrong, anything from a decreased appetite to increased irritability in attitude. Again, the physical examination, including a good oral examination, is the course of action of choice. Veterinarians need to examine all teeth in the mouth for any signs of cracking, breakage, or loss. In addition, signs of abscesses in the teeth should be sought. A proper medical workup, including dental or head radiographs, may be necessary if problems are suspected. Clinicians should be suspicious of dental involvement if owners report a behavioral change. Proper questioning of owners about an animal's particular temperament is important, including how active the animal is with chew objects. The location of broken teeth in the mouth and the presence or absence of marks on the teeth made by the chewed object will help in assessing what the animal may have broken the teeth on. It needs to be considered whether the animal is a fence chewer. That type of damage should show metal marks on the teeth and may be more anterior than teeth breakage and splitting from chew toys. Animals are able to get a chew toy or article farther back in the oral cavity, so damage is usually in the posterior portion of the oral cavity. Proper assessment of the location of the damage and the type of damage is important to helping clients keep the problem from happening again. Care needs to be taken to decrease the chances of pets' breaking teeth and doing dental damage from intense chewing.

AGGRESSION

Aggression can be a major problem with animals using their mouth in an unacceptable way. There are different types of aggression in animals. Some pets will have conflicts with other animals. Individual animals may have problems with dogs, cats, large animals such as horses, or small animals such as rabbits, squirrels, opossum, and raccoons. Aggressive animals may not like individuals of the same sex as themselves, while others are not choosy. Some may dislike small dogs but may not mind a larger animal that is their type. Others have not been able to accept humans as a nonthreatening source. They return their actions by lashing out and can cause quite a bit of damage by biting. Some will accept older individuals, while not allowing a small child by them. Others may be aggressive with a person of one sex but not with someone of the other sex. The stimulus varies with each individual. Some animals, through fear or rage, may interpret that they may be hurt or are in danger (21). This interpretation may not always be correct. The presence of uniforms, hats, umbrellas, and other objects may make some animals skeptical of a person. In some cases, animals can assert themselves by redirecting the aggression. This involves the animal's directing its aggressive behavior inappropriately—not at the object or person that triggered it but at someone or something else. This can sometimes occur when the initiating object is unavailable to or unreachable by the animal (22,23). This problem is seen in dogs, cats, and other animals kept in a domesticated situation. Cats, for example, may see a cat outside through a window, get upset, and redirect the aggression toward the owner (24). Many clients will turn to veterinarians for help with this problem. Some animals can do great damage with their mouth not only because of the power of their jaws and the sharpness of their teeth but also from the intensity of the attack. Some dogs have teeth conformations similar to those of their wild ancestors. The mouth was used for tearing muscle from prey and can do quite a bit of damage on the individual bitten. Some animals will give a warning before they make their move, whereas others will not. Owners must be careful both in the physical and in the legal aspects of the bite. Secondary injury can occur in some cases, if the person or animal injured or involved has underlying medical problems. A person with cardiac problems is a good example of this. Veterinarians can help their clients by getting them to seek help early, before something adverse occurs. Some people do not realize the potential of the situation, until severe or serious injury has already occurred. In some cases, it is too late. Owners need to be aware that help can be gotten early, if they seek the advice of a qualified person well versed and trained in the field. If a veterinary behaviorist is available, practitioners are advised to be in touch with him or her and to refer clients as early as possible for assistance. Some pet owners are willing to travel several hours and pay decent referral fees for the benefit of their pet (25). Dominance types of aggression, aggression related to fear, and intraspecific aggression are some of the most common types that client will turn to practitioners for help with (26). Be careful if only trainers and not veterinary behaviorists are available to help in individual aggression cases. Make sure that their expertise and personal experience are what is needed for the the case. These professionals need to have more than just a basic obedience program for animals. In these special cases, the approach taken in aggressive situations must be properly set and utilized to get the required results. Aggression is an important issue that needs to be handled carefully.

In speaking to clients with an animal with a potential aggression problem, veterinarians need to take a special approach. They can help emphasize the potential seriousness of the situation to clients without making them overly paranoid or sensitive about the subject. It may be beneficial to talk about similar cases without mentioning specific names. Clinicians may say that in their experience certain actions have happened when the problem was left to solve itself. Some clients will respond that they think the animal will outgrow the behavior. However, this is often not the case. If the behavior is noted in puppies and kittens, it is likely to be intensified as the animals go through puberty; puberty is not likely to calm them down. People do not realize that problems often get worse with age if they do not seek help in handling the situation properly. Some clients think that if they simply neuter the animal, the behavior will cease to exist. This may be the first step in helping decrease the problem, but the animal will often need more help than that. There may be a decrease in aggression in male dogs that have been castrated, but owners need to seek other help if the problem continues after the surgery. In female dogs, spaying is recommended to decrease hormonal swings that may affect them, but the problem may be more than just hormonal. Of course, prevention by early neutering is recommended to help decrease the chances of problems. This is the first step in an overall behavioral program for helping animals and clients. It is important for clients to understand that the approach for helping potentially aggressive animals must combine not only decreasing sex hormones but making other changes as well. Animals may also have other medical conditions that could predispose them to this behavioral change. Internal conditions can affect temperament (27). Talking to clients early and in an appropriate manner can help decrease this behavioral problem. Taking aggression concerns seriously can help decrease the chances that a problem will develop.

In working with potentially aggressive animals, clinicians and staff must be extremely careful. A fractious animal can do great damage if it bites the hands or face, although any bite can do damage. Animals will more commonly bite a stranger rather than their owner (28). Veterinarian must be careful when staff members work with a potentially aggressive animal. At all times they must make sure that the animal is current on its rabies vaccination. Especially in states that have recently had problems with rabies or a rabies quarantine, veterinary staff members risk exposure if an animal's vaccinations are not current. The history and background of the animal will also help in determining the potential for exposure to such serious disease. It is important to emphasize that preventive measures can also help decrease the chances of injury; these include proper gloving and using specialized equipment such as restraint poles or cat bags. A restraint cage is worth its cost if it avoids one bite wound in a staff person. Clinicians should be careful not to let untrained kennel help or other untrained individuals handle potentially fractious animals. Cat bites can be very serious because the feline canine teeth can penetrate deeply and do serious damage, thus increasing the chances of infection and abscess developing. Cats can attack and move very fast, taking a person by surprise. Muzzles, including cat muzzles, of all sizes, styles, and types should be available in the clinic. There are also special muzzles for chow or pug-nosed breeds. A good-fitting muzzle is essential; it should be snug, but not too tight. Some animals are still able to bite through a muzzle. Cages and records should be specially marked to alert staff of potential problem animals. Teaching proper restraint methods by introducing them at staff meetings can avoid problems. Training new individuals as they are hired will be critical to helping decrease bite wounds in the veterinary practice. Practitioners may prefer to pay for continuing education in animal behavior for their technicians and other staff members at veterinary conventions. In handling aggression cases carefully and correctly, the staff can keep a lot of problems from occurring.

Problems can be decreased by placing animal-aggressive animals, when boarding or hospitalized, in an isolated or far away cage or run. Animals of this type may also be placed in a cage or run near the door so that they do not need to walk past others, when entering or exiting the room. In addition, a towel or sheet may be placed over the front of the cage to obstruct animals' vision of others. It is important to make sure that there is proper ventilation when the front of the structure is covered. This practice is acceptable as long as the animals are not able to pull the towel in and chew it up. A thorough history at the start will help establish whether or not an animal is a destructive chewer. It is important to ask owners about the particular animal's temperament before accepting the pet into the hospital. This will help in determining how to properly handle it while it is in the clinic. The receptionist will also want to schedule such animals at an off time, if a clinic works on an appointment basis. If the owner of such an animal is a walk-in, the staff needs to keep attuned to what is going on in the waiting room. If the animal exhibits aggressive tendencies, it should be taken to an examination room as soon as possible. Concern for everyone's safety is the top priority. Even if an animal is aggressive only with other animals, people may get in the way of a potential fight and can get hurt. Owners often do not realize the seriousness of their pet's problem. The veterinary staff should be aware of potential problems. It can make a difference in the outcome. When boarding, an animal-aggressive dog should at least have an empty run between it and other dogs. Another option is to exercise the animals separately from one another in the runs. Even if the bottom portion or base of the fenced runs are solid, such as painted cement blocks, some dog can reach over the top of the fenced area or scrap with or attack another animal through the fence. This can do injury to the pet, especially dental damage. Any decreased vision of other animals when a pet is aggressive toward them will help in managing the individual correctly. In handling dogs and cats according to their needs, practitioners can lessen the chances of problems with them and their owners.

When animals exhibit the ability to be aggressive to people, clinicians and staff should proceed with caution. These animals should be watched cautiously for signs of uneasiness and potential aggressive symptoms. The position of the ears, head, tail, and the hair on the back should be observed carefully. The eyes can also reveal much if the observer is sensitive to the signs. Animals will often bite after being exposed to a certain stimulus that is respected as a sign of danger (21). It may be a certain noise or a hand movement. Some owners will totally deny that their pet has a problem. Veterinarians need to approach the situation carefully with regard not only to the animal's emotional state but also to the feelings and concerns of clients. If the clinician annoys the owner, whether rightly or wrongly, his or her ability to help the animal and the client is compromised in the long run. Even if doctors do not push the issue with clients, they need to work cautiously with the animal and alert the staff to work carefully in the situation. It is better to limit who is handling the particular pet than to have a problem develop. Preventive medicine in all aspects is important. Practitioners want to be careful not to push the issue too much with clients, but stating their position in a careful manner, they can help owners realize that problems can occur. Even if clients at first refuse to believe what may be obvious, it may begin to dawn on them that everyone in the situation wants to help, for the benefit of the animal. Referring clients to professional knowledgeable in these types of cases may be the treatment of choice in the situation. If accredited individual is not available, practitioners may be able to steer clients to appropriate reading material.

Veterinarians should keep on hand in the clinic proper restraint articles. These may include thick leather gloves, restraint poles (both short and long), a squeeze restraint cage, a small fiberglass tank in which to anesthetize unmanageable animals, cat bags, slip leads, nylon muzzles of all sizes and styles, long thin leather strips or leads to double-muzzle if necessary, and other articles that are humane and appropriate for individual behavioral needs. Staff should be appropriately trained in using these articles. It is important for pet care professional, when handling emotional situations, to stay calm and in careful control, thinking of the individual's safety and well-being at all times. It is important not to handle the situation in a rough or inhumane way. It is recommended that when an animal with aggressive tendencies needs to be handled, the proper time be chosen when the doctor and staff are not under pressure to complete the procedure. Time and patience are required in handling these situations correctly. It may also help in doing an appropriate job with such cases if a procedure can be scheduled outside the busy portion of the day. With appropriate equipment and scheduling, dental veterinarians can lessen the chances of complications developing in the clinic, when handling animals with behavioral problems.

BEHAVIORAL SIGNS BEFORE CLINICAL SYMPTOMS

Animals often exhibit behavioral signs before the clinical symptoms of a medical condition appear. An animal may not show common signs and symptoms of disease such as vomiting, diarrhea, coughing, or sneezing, among others, but its owner will present it for crying, or hiding, or acting unusually hyperactive in certain situations. Veterinarians need to be careful about dismissing these complaints too quickly. An animal may be feeling pain or sensing that something is wrong in an early phase of a disease process. Some animals become more aggressive or start urinating on the floor when a system in the body is having problems. Behavioral complaints may be the initial phase of an underlying veterinary medical concern.

The history taking before the physical examination is important and can help increase the ability to properly diagnose a case. The time spent with clients at this point can be well invested in learning about the particular needs of the pet. Correct diagnosis can be reached by connecting all of the signs of medical illness, including the behavioral aspects. Specific questions about changes in behavior should be asked in the history. One thing to watch for is behavior that differs from the norm for a particular animal. That an animal that has been aggressive since puppyhood bites is not as relevant as biting that has started recently and was never noticed before. If a cat is urinating on the floor, other signs will help practitioners determine whether it is of medical or behavioral origin. Is the individual doing it frequently? Does the animal appear to be straining when urinating? Has the pet's appetite changed during the course of the problem? Are there other medical signs? Are there other behavioral signs? Veterinarians have gone too long in ignoring the importance of behavioral signals in illness. They should be at the top of the list when the history is taken. In dental medicine, dogs may show pain by acting ornery or hard-headed when they are really just not feeling well. Animals do not feel like cooperating when all they really want to do is to lay down and not do much, nor do they want to chew a chew toy if they have a broken or fractured tooth. Some animals will stop eating or cry when eating when their mouth hurts. A normally quiet animal may become outgoing, when ill. On the other hand, an active pet may become very low-keyed when it does not feel like interacting because of an underlying medical problem. The key is noting the change in the norm for the animal. The behavioral portion is critical in the history taking to help reach a correct diagnosis. It is important for practitioners to remember that in some animals, the first sign of a medical illness may simply be a behavioral change.

CONCLUSION

In veterinary dentistry, it is important to realize that behavior is an integral part of the situation in some cases. Doctors should be knowledgeable about the behavioral clinical signs that can helpful in diagnosis. Veterinary staff members should be trained in how to handle both clients and animals in matters involving behavioral problems. Educating pet owners on early warning temperament signs can help prevent dental injury. Understanding the normal oral tendencies of young animals will also help pet professionals guide pet owners in teaching their dogs and cats proper use of the mouth. Conditioning pets to accept proper oral care, including teeth brushing, will help decrease dental disease. Animals are as integral in their psychological make up as they are in their physiologic aspects. As practitioners acknowledge this aspect of veterinary medicine, clients will be helped in providing their animals a better and higher-quality life.

REFERENCES

1. Boice R. Domestication. *Psychol Bull* 1973;80: 215.
2. Anderson RK. Make euthanasia the last resort. *Vet Forum* 1990:26.
3. Shaw FP. No more bad dogs. *Focus:* Veterinary Product News 1995:34.
4. Hunthausen W. Behavioral problems find long-term solution instead of a quick fix, part 2. *Vet Econ* May 1996:39.
5. Polsky RH. Guidelines to follow when using drugs in behavioral therapy. *Ani Behav Vet Med* 1995:829.
6. Landsberg GM. The distribution of canine behavioral cases at three behavioral referral practices. *Vet Med* 1991; 86:1011.
7. Vervaeke-Helf SA. *Lhasa Lore*. Loveland, CO: Alpine Publications; 1983.
8. The Monks of New Skete. *How To Be Your Dog's Best Friend: A Training Manual for Dog Owners*. Boston: Little, Brown; 1978.
9. Long C, Strader R. *The Pictorial Encyclopedia of Dogs*. New York: Gallery Books; 1989.
10. Myles S. Trainers and chokers. *Vet Clin North Am Small Anim Pract* 1991;21:239.
11. London P. *Behavior Control*. New York: Harper & Row; 1969.
12. Loxton H. *The Nobel Cat: Aristocrat of the Animal World*. New York: Portland House Publishing; 1990.
13. Beaver B. *Veterinary Aspects of Feline Behavior*. St. Louis, MO: CV Mosby Co; 1980.
14. Landsberg G. Feline behavior and welfare. *JAVMA* 1996;208:502.
15. Bateson P, Martin P. Behavioral development in the cat. In: Turner DC, Bateson P, eds. *The Domestic Cat: The Biology of Its Behavior*. Cambridge: Cambridge University Press; 1988.
16. Hetts S. *The Effects of Differential Separation Periods on Separation Distress in Domestic Dog Puppies*. Ft. Collins, CO: Colorado State University; 1989. Thesis.
17. Overall K. Diagnosing separation anxiety can be difficult for practicing veterinarians. *DVM Newsmagazine* 1996:15S.
18. Strombeck DR. *Small Animal Gastroenterology*. Philadelphia: Stonegate Publishing; 1979:69.
19. Houpt K. Feeding and drinking behavior problems. *Vet Clin North Am Small Anim Pract* 1991;21:281.
20. Tams TR. Gastrointestinal symptoms. In: *Handbook of Small Animal Gastroenterology*. Philadelphia: WB Saunders Co; 1996.
21. Arieti S. The structural and psychodynamic role of cognition in the human psyche. In: *The World Biennial of Psychiatry and Psychotherapy*. Vol 1. New York: Basic Books; 1970.
22. Borstock M, Morris D, Mounihan M. Some comments on conflict and thwarting in animals. *Behavior* 1953;6:66.
23. Overall K. Animal behavior case of the month. *JAVMA* 1995;207:305.
24. Capman BL, Voith VL. Cat aggression redirected to people: 14 cases (1981-1987). *JAVMA* 1990;196:947.
25. Hart BL, Hart LA. *Canine and Feline Behavioral Therapy*. Philadelphia: Lea & Febiger; 1985.
26. Horwitz D. Aggressive behavior in dogs. *Pedigree Breeder Forum Magazine* 1995;4(4):11.
27. Campbell WE. Behavior problems in dogs. In: *Physiology and Behavior. Part II: Diseases, Disorders, and Behavior*. Santa Barbara CA: American Veterinary Publishing; 1985.
28. Wright JC. Canine aggression towards people: Bite scenarios and prevention. *Vet Clin North Am Small Anim Pract* 1991;21:299.

Glossary of Terms

Abfraction   Flexure of the tooth resulting from forces of mastication near the cementoenamel junction causing imperceptible cracks or chips in the cementum or enamel.

Ablations   Taking away, wearing down, erosion of an area.

Abrasion   Mechanical wearing away of teeth by abnormal stresses. This could result from toothbrushing habits or other abnormal stresses on the teeth.

Abrasive points   Rotary instruments that have an abrasive coating on the operative head.

Absorbent points   Cones of porous paper used to dry the root canal after instrumentation.

Abutment   A tooth, crown, or portion of an implant used to support, stabilize, or anchor for a fixed or removable dental prosthesis, such as a bridge.

Acanthomatous ameloblast *See*   acanthomatous epulis

Acanthomatous epulis   A benign but locally aggressive epulis that can even infiltrate into bone; also known as acanthomatous ameloblast, adamantinoma, or basal cell carcinoma.

Access   The fundamental choice of the site of tooth approach and pulp cavity entry.

Access triad   Sequence of proper tooth access in the order of chamber access, root canal access, and stricture access.

Accessional   Permanent teeth that do not replace deciduous teeth but rather become an accession (an addition) to the deciduous or succedaneous teeth or to both types.

Accessory parotid salivary gland   Small lobules to glandular masses with small ducts located above the parotid duct in the dog.

Accessory root canals   Extra openings into the pulp, usually located on the sides of the roots or in the bifurcations.

Acellular cementum   Cementum that has no cells trapped in it.

Acidic fluorides   Fluorides with acids added to enhance greater penetration and remineralization of the tooth with a fluoride-rich superficial zone.

Acquired   Pertaining to something obtained by oneself, not inherited.

Acrodont   Teeth not set in sockets, having no true root structure and ankylosed directly to underlying bone (eg, agomid, turatara).

Acromegaly   Disease resulting from an excess of growth hormone, causing some bones in the body to continue to grow after normal growth has been completed.

Acrylic   Plastics, basically methyl methacrylate, mixed from a powder (polymer) and liquid (monomer). These were once used extensively as restoratives.

Active treatment stage   Stage of corrective orthodontics in which devices are applied to restore dental occlusion to a reasonably functional and esthetic state.

Acute apical abscess   A painful purulent exudate of sudden onset at the apex.

Acute apical periodontitis   Acute inflammation around the apex.

Acute hypersensitivity   Drug reaction that can start as ulceration and hemorrhage.

Acute periodontal abscess   Sudden suppurative periodontal lesion with pain, swelling, and systemic signs.

A-delta fibers   Nerve fibers responsible for sharp pain.

Adamantinoma   *See* acanthomatous epulis

Adhesion systems   Types of bonding or cementation materials used between the tooth and a dental device.

Adjunct wiring   Wiring methods used in combination with other stabilization.

Adult nonodontogenic gingival cyst   Cyst arising from the traumatic implantation of gingival epithelium into the gingival connective tissue.

Adult odontogenic gingival cyst   Cyst arising from remnants of dental lamina, enamel organ, or epithelium associated with the periodontal ligament.

Adult periodontitis (AP)   Slowly progressing form of periodontal disease seen in adults.

Aerobic bacteria   Those that thrive in the presence of oxygen.

Afunctional   Not performing a purpose or action.

Ala (pl. alae)   Latin for *wing*, referring to the sides of the nostrils of the nose.

Alginate   Irreversible hydrocolloid impression material used frequently in veterinary dentistry, especially when partial- or full-mouth models are needed that require decent, yet not excellent detail.

Alignment   Arrangement of teeth in a row.

Allele   An alternative form of a gene.

Alopecia   Loss of hair.

Alveolar bone   Bone forming the sockets for the teeth.

Alveolar bone proper   *See* cribriform plate.

Alveolar crest   Highest part of the alveolar bone closest to the cervical line of the tooth.

Alveolar crest fibers   Alveolodental periodontal ligament fibers running from the cementum to the alveolar crest of bone.

Alveolar eminences   Bulges on the facial surface of the alveolar bone that outline the position of the roots.

Alveolar juga   *See* alveolar eminences.

Alveolar mucosa   Mucosa between the mucobuccal fold and gingiva.

Alveolar process   Part of the bone in the maxillae and mandible that forms the sockets for the teeth. *See* alveolar bone.

Alveolar ridge   Bony ridge formed by the alveolar process of the mandible and maxilla. It may reduce in size when teeth are lost and functional demand for support is reduced.

Alveolar socket   Cavity in the alveolar process in which the tooth root is held in place by the periodontal ligament.

Alveolodental fibers   Periodontal fibers running between the tooth and alveolar bone (alveolar crest, horizontal, oblique, apical and interradicular fibers).

Alveolus (pl. alveoli)   Cavity or socket in the alveolar process in which the root of the tooth is held.

Amalgam   An alloy or combination of finely powdered metals that are mixed, or triturated, with mercury to wet the particles and form a condensable mass.

Amalgamation   The process of combining an alloy with mercury (eg, silver or copper alloy triturated with mercury makes up an amalgam).

Amalgamator   A mechanical device or a ground glass mortar and a glass pestle used to triturate an alloy.

Ameloblast   Enamel-forming cell that arises from oral ectoderm.

Ameloblastoma   The most common tumor of the dental laminar epithelium. It is slow-growing but often shows a multiple cystic structure and can extend into bone.

Amelogenesis imperfecta   Condition of abnormally formed enamel caused by a hereditary reduction in the amount of enamel matrix laid down during its formation.

Anachoresis   Exposure to bacteria through a hematogenous route.

Anatomic crown   That part of the tooth covered by enamel.

Anatomic root   That portion of the tooth covered by cementum.

Anchorage   Site of delivery from which force is exerted in orthodontics.

Anchorage unit   Multiple teeth used in anchorage.

Angle   Juncture of two or more surfaces.

Angle lines   *See* line angle.

Angle of the mandible   Point at the lower border of the body of the mandible where it turns up onto the ramus.

Angstrom units   Radiation wavelength measurement

Angular process   Portion of the vertical ramus of the mandible.

Anisognathism   Condition of having unequal jaw widths in which the mandibular molar occlusal zone is narrower than the maxillary counterpart. It is seen in the feline, canine, bovine, equine, and other species.

Ankyloglossia   *See* Tongue-tie

Ankylosis   Fusion of the cementum of a tooth with alveolar bone.

Anodontia   Condition in which most or all the teeth are congenitally absent.

Anomaly   Any noticeable difference or deviation from that which is ordinary or normal.

Anorexia   Loss of appetite.

Anterior   Situated in front of. This term is commonly used to denote the incisor and canine teeth or the area toward the front of the mouth.

Anterior cross-bite   Condition in which cusps or one or more anterior teeth (incisors and cuspids) exceed the normal cusp relationship of the teeth in the opposing arch labially or lingually. Classically thought of as a subclassification of class I malocclusions, it may actually be seen in classes I–IV malocclusions.

Anticurvature filing   Use of judicial filling pressure away from the curvature of the root tip and/or toward the more bulky portion of the tooth root.

Apex   Terminal end or tip of a root.

Apexification   Physiologic process of the apex's closure with hard tissue by the action of cementoblasts and odontoblasts.

Apexogenesis   Continued maturation and closure of a immature root.

Apex locators   An electronic device for determining when the apex has been reached with an endodontic instrument.

Aphthous ulcers   Painful, necrotic, gray-to-yellow bleeding ulcers of the gingiva and tongue, covered at times with a thin, grayish pseudomembrane. Aphthous means "to set on fire."

Apical   Direction toward the root tip or away from the incisal or occlusal surfaces.

Apical delta   Multiple openings through which vessels, nerves, or other structures pass into the tooth at the apex.

Apical fibers   Alveolodental periodontal ligament fibers running from the apex to the alveolar bone to resist extrusional forces.

Apical foramen   Aperture, or opening, at or near the apex of a tooth root through which the blood and nerve supply of the pulp enters the tooth.

Apical perforation   Extension of an instrument beyond the apical constriction and into the periapical structures.

Apical stricture   Closure of the internal root canal apex.

Apically repositioned flap   Gingival flap attached in a position more apical than its original site. This is often done to reduce pocket depth.

Appliance trauma   Physical irritations or lacerations to the lingual and buccal mucosa caused by use of appliances.

Aradicular hypsodont   A subdivision of hypsodont, long-rooted, describing dentition without true roots (sometimes called open-rooted) that produces additional crown throughout life. As teeth are worn down, new crown emerges from the continually growing teeth, as in lagomorphs and the incisors of rodents.

Arch, dental   *See* dental arch.

Area-specific curettes   Curettes with an offset blade with only one cutting edge.

Articular disc   Fibrous disc between the condyle and the mandibular fossa.

Articular process   Portion of the vertical ramus of the mandible that is part of the temporomandibular joint.

Atraumatic malocclusion   Condition of teeth malpositioning from genetic or dietary causes involving insufficient attrition.

Attached gingiva   Tightly adherent gingiva extending from the free gingiva to the alveolar mucosa.

Attachment apparatus   Consists of the cementum, the periodontal ligament, and the alveolar bone or process.

Attachment epithelium   Cells that attach the gingiva to the tooth. Originally, these are cells of the reduced enamel epithelium.

Attrition   Process of normal wear on the crown, usually due to mastication or chewing.

Auxiliary canals   Additional natural opening into the root canal system. *Also see* lateral canals.

Aversion conditioning   Causing one to dislike something by negative conditioning.

Avulsion   Tearing away of a part, such as a tooth.

Axial   Pertaining to the longitudinal (long) axis of the tooth (eg, labial, buccal, lingual, mesial, and distal surfaces).

Axial root center   An imaginary line passing through the geometric center of a tooth root parallel to its long axis.

Axial wall   Internal wall of a cavity formed by the surface of the long axis (axial or vertical plane) of the tooth.

Backscatter   Radiation originating from x-rays interacting with the patient's tissues that may bounce back through the reverse side of the film.

Balance-force instrumentation   *See* stem-winding instrumentation.

Barbed broach   Endodontic instrument with hooks on the sides that functions to snag and remove the soft pulp tissue from the pulp cavity.

Basal cell carcinoma   *See* acanthomatous epulis

Base material   Provides a physical support for the final restoration when structural loss is being replaced and helps protect the pulp from irritating substances and thermal changes.

Base narrow   Condition in which one or both of the mandibular canines are tipped too far lingually or toward the tongue, resulting in the cusp tip(s) making contact with the palate.

Base plates   Foundation that provides a surface for direct bonding to the tooth surface.

Bell stage   Third stage of enamel organ formation in which the crown form is established.

Benign   Nonmalignant. Such lesions do not destroy the tissue from which they originate or spread to other parts of the body (metastasize).

Bevel   An inclined plane formed by one line joining another at not a right angle; a cut with an angle of more than 90° with a cavity wall.

Bevel gingivectomy   Cutting of the gingiva to approximate a feathered edge of the gingival margin. It may be used, if sufficient attached gingiva is present, in areas to remove excessive gingiva or to minimize pocket depth.

Bicuspid *See* premolars.

Bifid tongue Tongue with developmental splitting at the midline. (fissure tongue).

Bifurcation Division into two parts or branches, as any two roots of a tooth.

Biological width Distance physiologically maintained by the body's defense mechanisms between a dental restoration or device and the base of the sulcus.

Bird tongue *See* microglossia.

Bisecting angle Technique of taking radiographs to minimize linear distortion by aiming the beam perpendicular to the line that bisects the angle formed by the long axis of the tooth and the film.

Bite plane Appliance in which the incline is designed to prevent occlusal closure.

Bite registration wax Used to orient opposing dental models for articulation.

Bitewing film Packet that has a tab or wing across the center of the packet front to allow a human patient to bite on to hold in position.

Biting force The pressure (pounds per square inch) exerted by teeth when engaged by the muscles of mastication.

Bleaching agents Used for in-office bleaching of vital and nonvital teeth; typically hydrogen peroxide or complexes of it such as urea peroxide.

Blue tongue Insect-borne disease that can cause significant hyperemia and swelling of the oral tissues in ruminants. The tongue can be quite involved with edema and ulceration of the lateral surfaces.

Body of the mandible Horizontal portion of the mandible, excluding the alveolar process.

Bolus of food A ball of food that has been chewed and mixed with saliva and is ready to be swallowed.

Bone Hard connective tissue that forms the framework of the body. The hardness is attributable to the hydroxyapatite crystal.

Boxing wax Flat sheets of wax used to form a box around an impression to hold freshly mixed plaster or stone solution in and on the impression when poured.

Brachycephaly Condition in which individuals have short, broad facial profiles, such as boxers and bulldogs.

Brachyodont Teeth with a shorter crown:root ratio (eg, primates, dogs, cats, and carnivores in general).

Branchial arches I and II Developmental sections of the facial region present around day 21 of development.

Bridge Dental prosthesis that replaces the crowns of one or more missing teeth.

Bridge unit An individual part of the bridge, such as the pontic or retainer.

Broken mouth Condition in sheep caused by severe periodontitis that encumber the ability to eat.

Bruxism Abnormal grinding of the teeth.

Bucca Latin for "cheek."

Buccal Pertaining to the cheek; toward the cheek or next to the cheek; also called facial.

Buccal contour Posterior teeth facial contours. *See* facial contours.

Buccal developmental groove Groove separating the buccal cusps on a buccal surface.

Buccal embrasure *See* embrasure.

Buccal inclination (buccal tipping, buccoversion) Terms used to describe facial inclination of the posterior teeth.

Buccal molar salivary gland Several small ducts—in cats, the molar gland—located between the orbicularis oris muscle and the mucous membrane of the lower lip at the angle of the mouth.

Buccal object rule *See* SLOB rule.

Buccal salivary glands Numerous small, serous or mucous ducts in the submucosa of the buccal cavity.

Buccal surface Surface of a posterior tooth positioned immediately adjacent to the cheek.

Buccocclusion Posterior teeth bodily displaced away from the tongue.

Buccopharyngeal membrane A wall separating the stomodeum and foregut. It is located at a level called the oropharynx.

Buccoversion *See* buccal inclination.

Bud stage First stage of development of the enamel organ. It develops from the dental lamina.

Bullous pemphigoid An autoimmune disease in which oral lesions, frequently at the mucocutaneous junction and with some mucous membrane ulceration, are present in about half of affected individuals.

Bundle bone Extra thickness of bone added to the cribriform plate.

Bunodont dentition Having cheek teeth with low, rounded cusps on the occlusal surface of the crown.

Bunolophodont dentition Having cheek teeth with both rounded cusps and transverse ridges on the occlusal surface of the crown.

Bunoselenodont dentition Having cheek teeth with both rounded cusps and crescentic ridges on the occlusal surface of the crown.

Burs Rotary dental instruments with cutting blades as an active part of the operative head.

Cage-biter syndrome Any condition that initially results in attritional wear of the distal surface of a tooth.

Calcification Process by which organic tissue becomes hardened by a deposit of calcium salts within its substance. Literally, the term denotes the deposition of any mineral salts that contribute toward the hardening and maturation of tissue.

Calculus Mineralized dental plaque that adheres to tooth surfaces and prosthetic dental materials.

Canal Long tubular opening through a bone or tooth root.

Canal calcification Maturing process of dentinal walls and pulp cavities that reduces their size and patency.

Cancellous bone Less dense bone situated between surrounding denser cortical plates. *See* spongy bone.

Canines *See* cuspids

Canine eminence Extra bulk of bone on the labial aspect of the maxillae, overlying the roots of the canine teeth.

Canine fossa Depression in the maxillae below the infraorbital foramen.

Cantilever bridge One-piece bridge with the pontic supported only from one end by a retainer or retainers. The cantilever retainer is generally distal to the pontic to allow a more naturally open mesial contact for esthetics.

Cap Colloquialism for crown.

Cap stage Second stage of enamel organ development.

Capsule, joint Fibrous band of tissue surrounding a joint and limiting its motion.

Cara inchada Condition in cattle caused by severe periodontitis that can incapacitate the animal's eating habits. The term describes a swollen face.

Caries Condition of decay, usually applied to teeth.

Carious caries The classic black cavity with a more rapid demineralization of the dentin.

Carnassial teeth   The largest shearing teeth in the upper and lower jaws (upper 4th premolar and lower 1st molar in dogs and cats).

Cartilaginous perisymphysis   Condition in which the ossification of the rostral angle of the mandible is deficient, resulting in a fibrous portion and loose teeth. It may be inherited.

Carving   The manual process of placing anatomic landmarks on the surfaces and margins of a restoration or a wax pattern.

Casting waxes   Used to produce the patterns for the metallic framework of removable partial dentures, some orthodontic frames, and other similar structures.

Caudal infraorbital block   Intraoral regional anesthetic nerve block achieved by injecting the infraorbital nerve at the caudal aspect of the infraorbital canal.

Cavity floor   The enclosing base portion of the cavity preparation. It pertains to the pulpal and gingival walls of the cavity preparation.

Cavity margin   Junction of the cavity wall and the enamel surface of the tooth.

Cavity outline   Combined peripheral extent of all of the cavosurfaces or preparation margins.

Cavity preparation   A surgical operation that removes the caries and excises hard tissue in order to shape the tooth to receive and retain the restoration.

Cavity preparation, principles   Composed of the steps essential to the preparation of a cavity to assure the eradication of the carious lesion and to enable the retention of a restoration.
1. **Outline form**   Curved shape and border of the restoration and the tooth surface.
2. **Resistance form**   Form and thickness given to the tooth and its restoration to prevent displacement or fracture of either structure.
3. **Retention form**   Relationship of the tooth surfaces (walls) to prevent the dislodgement of the restoration.
4. **Convenience form**   Methods used by the operator to gain access to the cavity preparation for the insertion and finishing of the restorative material.
5. **Removal of caries**   Procedure of removing the decayed and decalcified enamel and dentin and possibly the placement of medicated bases or liners in cavity preparations.
6. **Finishing of the enamel wall**   Process of angling, beveling, and smoothing the walls of the cavity preparation (eg, using an enamel chisel or gingival margin trimmer on the enamel margins of the cavity preparation).
7. **Cavity debridement**   Performing the "toilet" or cleansing of the cavity; the removal of all decay and the debris from the preparation to assure a clean, dry surface for the placement of the restoration.

Cavosurface angle   Line angle formed between a wall of the prepared surface and the unprepared tooth surface.

Cavosurface bevel   A bevel found at the cavosurface angle of the cavity preparation.

C-delta fibers   Nerve fibers responsible for dull pain.

Cell-free zone   Cell layer in the pulp between the odontoblastic cell layer and the cell-rich zone.

Cell-rich zone   Cell layer in the pulp consisting of undifferentiated mesenchymal cells.

Cellular cementum   Cementum that has cells trapped within it.

Cement   Used to apply orthodontic brackets, appliances, crowns, or other prosthodontic devices.

Cementoblasts   Cells that form cementum.

Cementoclasts   Cells involved with resorption of cementum.

Cementocytes   Cementoblasts that have become entrapped within cementum.

Cementodentinal junction (CDJ)   Junction where the cementum and dentin contact.

Cementoenamel junction (CEJ)   Junction of enamel of the crown and cementum of the root, ie, cervical line.

Cementoid   Term meaning cementum-like.

Cementoma   Benign proliferation of the connective tissue that produces cementum or cementum-like tissue.

Cementum   Layer of bone-like tissue covering the root of the tooth.

Central developmental groove   A groove crossing the occlusal surface of a tooth from mesial to distal sides, dividing the tooth into buccal and lingual parts.

Central developmental pit   A pit that occurs in the central fossa.

Central fossa   A fossa that occurs in the center of the central groove.

Central groove   *See* central developmental groove.

Centric occlusion (central occlusion)   Relationship of the occlusal surfaces of one arch to those of the other when the jaws are closed and the teeth are in maximum intercuspation.

Centric relation   Arch-to-arch relationship of the maxilla to the mandible when the condyles are in their most upward position, the mandible is in its most posterior position, and the jaw is most braced by its musculature.

Ceramometal crown   *See* porcelain fused to metal.

Cervical (neck, cervix)   That portion of a tooth at the junction of the anatomic crown and anatomic root.

Cervical bulge   Reestablishment procedure for moving the cervical bulge apically as recession occurs.

Cervical embrasure   Embrasure or spillway located cervically to the contact area of the teeth.

Cervical line   Line formed by the junction of enamel and cementum of a tooth, ie, cementoenamel junction.

Cervical loop   Deepest point in the root prior to its complete calcification (the stellate reticulum and stratum intermedium are missing).

Cervical mucocele   *See* mandibular salivary gland mucocele.

Cervical third   That portion of the crown or root at or near the cervical line.

Cervix (neck)   Narrow or constricted portion of a tooth in the region of the junction of crown and root.

Chairside   A light-safe box with a light-selective see-through cover in which to develop films in the operatory.

Chamber   A finish or curve from the axial wall to the cavosurface on the extracoronal cavity preparation.

Chamber floor   Bottom of the pulp chamber.

Chamber horns   Most coronal part of the pulp chamber in which the pulp horns reside.

Cheeks   Lateral boundary of the oral cavity.

Cheilitis   Inflammation of the lips.

Cheiloschisis   *See* cleft lip

Chemical fogging   Darkening of the radiographic film caused by improper mixing or exhausted processing solutions.

Chemoplastic method   Method of endodontic obturation when a chemical is added to the core material to soften or dissolve it prior to placement in the root canal.

Chlorhexidine digluconate   Solution used in the treatment of periodontal disease that has been shown to inhibit the development of plaque and calculus and the onset of gingivitis in humans.

Chronic/active periodontal abscess   Acute exacerbation of a chronic lesion.

Chronic apical periodontitis   Long-term inflammation around the apex.

Chronic periapical osteitis   Osseous response observed with some low-grade chronic pulpal and periapical inflammations.

Chronic periodontal abscess   Slowly progressive lesion that is usually asymptomatic but may stimulate a dull pain.

Chronic ulcerative paradental stomatitis (CUPS)   A marked ulceration of buccal or lingual mucosa that contacts a tooth/calculus surface; sometimes called a "kissing lesion."

Cingulum   A bulbous convexity on the cervical third of the lingual surface of a tooth.

Circular gingival fibers   Gingival periodontal ligament fibers found in the free gingiva running in a circular pattern around the tooth, providing additional support to hold it firmly against the tooth.

Circumferential defect   *See* four-wall defect

Circumferential wiring   Placing wire around the bone (mandible) to assist in reduction.

Clark's rule   *See* SLOB rule.

Class 0 normal   Occlusions that are true normals and variations of normal; also known as **orthoclusion.**

Class I malocclusion   Condition in which teeth are in approximately normal mesiodistal or neutral relation but may have faciolingual disturbances; also known as **neutroclusion.**

Class II malocclusion   Condition in which some or all mandibular teeth are distal in relationship to their maxillary counterparts; also known as **distoclusion.**

Class III malocclusion   Condition in which some or all of the mandibular teeth are mesial in their relationship to their maxillary counterparts; also known as **mesioclusion.**

Class IV special malocclusions   Special forms of wry mouth in which one of the four jaws is in a mesial relationship to its counterparts, while another is in a distal position; also known as **mesiodistoclusion.**

Cleft lip   Defect or gap in the upper lip, occurring during fetal development.

Cleft palate   Lack of joining together of hard or soft palate.

Cleoid   Claw-shaped instrument used to form corners in a cavity preparation.

Clinical crown   That portion of the tooth protruding above the gingiva.

Clinical root   That portion of the tooth below the gingiva.

Closed apex   Natural constrictive closing of the tooth apex.

Closed bites   Condition in which the dental arches close too far when the bite is in a static occlusion.

Closed curettage   Periodontal therapy and root planing of a periodontal pocket shallow enough to allow the apical extent to be reached with hand instruments.

Coalescence   Fusion of lobes during crown formation, resulting in grooves of various depths.

Col   Area of the interdental papilla lying cervical to the interproximal tooth contacts.

Color registration or matching   Process of matching the color of a restoration with that of the tooth.

Combination defect   Infrabony pocket with different levels or floors within the defect, resulting in combinations of the defect types, such as a combined one- and two-walled defect.

Commissure   Junction of the upper and lower lip at the angle of the mouth.

Commissuroplasty   Surgery to recontour the commissure either to close the angle of the mouth further rostrally or to open it up further.

Common bridge   *See* fixed-fixed bridge.

Complex odontoma   Mixed odontogenic tumor composed of both epithelial and mesenchymal cells in a disorganized mass that contains no tooth-like structures. Can have a cystic component.

Composite   Type of restorative typically composed of an organic polymer matrix of high molecular weight, usually a bisphenol A-glycidyl methacrylate (bis-GMA) resin, with or without fillers.

Compound bridge   A bridge that is a combination of two or more bridge types, such as a fixed-fixed cantilever, fixed-fixed movable, or fixed-fixed spring. It is used for more complex replacements of multiple teeth that are not all consecutive.

Compound odontoma   Mixed odontogenic tumor composed of both epithelial and mesenchymal cells and containing small tooth-like structures (denticles) with various levels of differentiation. Can have a cystic component.

Concrescence   A fusion of the cementum and sometimes dentin of two teeth along their roots.

Condensation   Mechanical process of compressing a restorative substance into the cavity preparation.

Condensers   Flat-ended metal instruments used to press filling materials vertically or apically into the root canal; also known as **pluggers.**

Condyloid process   That portion of the vertical ramus of the mandible that is part of the temporomandibular joint.

Congenital   Present at birth.

Conical papillae   Soft, long papillae in the root area, pointing caudally, with a probable mechanical function.

Connector   *See* joint.

Contact allergies   Allergies to the materials from which a dental device is constructed.

Contact area   That region of the mesial or distal surface of a tooth that touches the adjacent tooth in the same arch.

Contact point   Specific point at which a tooth from one arch occludes with another tooth of the opposing arch.

Continuous force   The drive or energy that is applied in a constant fashion until the target tooth is moved to its new target site.

Contour   Shape of the tooth.

Contrast   Relates to the variation in the black and white density on areas of radiographic film.

Conventional points   *See* type II gutta-percha points.

Coprophagy   The act of eating feces.

Core   A substructure for a crown that may be part of a post-and-core system.

Coronal   Direction toward the crown

Coronally repositioned flap   Gingival flap that is attached at a point coronal to its original position.

Coronoid process   Bony projection at the upper anterior portion of the vertical ramus. It is the attachment location for the temporal muscle.

Corrective orthodontics   Consists of two stages: active treatment and retention.

Cortical plate   Dense bone on the outer buccal and lingual surfaces of the alveolar bone.

Cranial infraorbital block   Intraoral regional anesthetic nerve block achieved by injecting at the rostral end of the infraorbital canal to provide analgesia to the incisors, canines, and first two premolars.

Craniomandibular articulation (CMA) *See*   temporomandibular joint

Craniomandibular osteopathy (CMO)   Enlargement of the horizontal ramus, often caudally, due to periosteal proliferation. It is often seen in terrier breeds (eg, West Highland white terrier).

Creep   Used to denote the slow flow or change in shape of amalgams due to chronic pressures.

Crest   As pertains to radiation, the height of the wave.

Cribriform plate   Dense bone that forms the actual wall of the tooth socket.

Cribriform plate of ethmoid   Small perforations of ethmoid bone beside the crista galli that provide passages for olfactory nerves from the nasal to the cranial cavity.

Cross-bite   Condition in which the cusps of a tooth in one arch exceed the normal relationship with cusps of a tooth in the opposing arch facially or lingually. *See also* class I malocclusion, anterior cross-bite, and posterior cross-bite.

Cross-pinning   Placement of a pin through the tooth and crown at the cervical third of the restoration.

Crown   That portion of a tooth covered with enamel that is normally visible in the oral cavity. *See also* anatomic crown and clinical crown.

Crown   A restorative that covers part or all of the clinical crown.

Crown lengthening   Procedure for lengthening the clinical crown in order to enhance the retention of an artificial crown.

Crown lengthening, type I   A simple gingivoplasty.

Crown lengthening, type II   Gingivoplasty and bone recontouring.

Crown lengthening, type III   Forced eruption.

Crypt   Term used to describe the early tooth socket.

Cup defect   *See* four-wall defect

CUPS   *See* chronic ulcerative paradental stomatitis

Curette   Instrument of choice for removing light subgingival calculus, root planning, and gingival and subgingival curettage.

Cusp
   1. A pronounced elevation on the occlusal surface of a tooth terminating in a conical, rounded, or flat surface.
   2. Any crown elevation that begins calcification as an independent center.

Cuspid (canine teeth, fang teeth)   One of four pointed teeth situated one on each side of each jaw, immediately distal to the corner or lateral incisors.

Cyclic neutropenia   *See* gray collie syndrome

Cyst   Sac of fluid lined by epithelial cells; it may grow to varying sizes.

Dead tracts   Empty dentinal tubules resulting from death of odontoblasts and their process that filled that area.

Deciduous (milk, primary, baby) teeth   The first dentition; that which will be shed.

Deep waves   One of the four basic categories of x-radiation wavelengths, used for deep therapy.

Definition evaluation   A localization technique by determining that the structures with better definition are those positioned lingually, closest to the film.

Deglutition   Action of swallowing.

Dens   Tooth.

Dens in dente ("tooth within a tooth")   Formed when the top of the tooth bud folds into itself, producing additional layers of enamel, cementum, dentin, or pulp tissue inside the tooth as it develops.

Dens invaginatus   A developmental anomaly involving an invagination on the lingual or palatal surface of an incisor. *See also* dens in dente

Dental abrasion   Excessive wear from the friction of an externally applied force, such as brushing.

Dental arch   All teeth forming an arch in either the maxillary or mandibular jaw.

Dental attrition   Increased amount of wear or loss of tooth substance due to normal masticatory forces.

Dental crazing   Formation of microscopic cracks in the tooth structure induced by stress factors.

Dental lamina   Embryonic downgrowth of oral epithelium that is the forerunner of the enamel bud. Ectodermal-origin epithelium pushes into mesodermal tissues underneath.

Dental luxator   Instrument with a wider, more delicate blade than an elevator that is used in the periodontal space to sever the periodontal ligament attachment.

Dental papilla   Mesodermal structure partially surrounded by the inner enamel epithelial cells. The dental papilla forms the dentin and pulp.

Dental sac   Several layers of flat mesodermal cells partially surrounding the dental papilla and enamel organ. It forms the cementum, periodontal ligament, and some alveolar bone.

Dentes canini   Canine, cuspid, eye, or fang teeth.

Dentes decidui   Deciduous teeth.

Dentes incisivi   Incisor teeth.

Dentes molares   Molar teeth.

Dentes permanetes   Permanent teeth.

Dentes premolares   Premolar teeth.

Denticles   Small, tooth-like structures.

Dentifrice   Any substance used for cleaning teeth.

Dentigerous cyst   Cystic structure arising from all or a remnant of the developing dental follicle at the neck of the tooth; also know as an **eruption** or **follicular cyst.**

Dentin   Hard calcified tissue (formerly called dentine) forming the inside body and bulk of a tooth, covered by cementum and enamel, and surrounding the pulp tissue.

Dentinal bonding agents   Material to enhance bonding of a restorative material to dentin.

Dentinal fluid   Liquid within the dentinal tubule.

Dentinal tubules   Space or tubes in the dentin occupied by the odontoblastic process.

Dentinal wall   That portion of the wall consisting of dentin.

Dentinocemental junction (DCJ)   *See* CDJ.

Dentinoenamel junction   Juncture within the crown of the tooth where the dentinal and enamel walls meet.

Dentinogenesis imperfecta   A hereditary condition in which dentin is abnormally formed.

Dentition   General character and arrangement of the teeth, taken as a whole, as in carnivorous, herbivorous, and omnivorous dentitions. Primary dentition refers to deciduous teeth; secondary dentition to permanent teeth. Mixed dentition refers to a combination of permanent and deciduous teeth in the same dentition.

Dentofacial deformity   Abnormalities of the teeth in morphology or location with or without abnormalities of the facial support structures.

Dentogingival fibers   Gingival periodontal ligament fibers running from the cementum to either attached or free gingiva, providing a firm support for these tissues.

Deprecated bridge   *See* fixed-movable bridge.

Depression   Lowering of the mandible or opening of the mouth.

Dermal papilla   The interdigitation of the submucosal connective tissue into the epithelium.

Desiccation   Condition of extreme dryness of the tooth substances by chemical or mechanical means. Overdrying (desiccation) of the tooth structures is injurious to the pulp.

Developer   Solution to make the latent image on an exposed x-ray film visible.

Developmental depression   Noticeable concavity on the formed crown or root of a tooth, occurring at the junction of two lobes.

Developmental grooves   Fine depressed lines in the enamel of a tooth that mark the union of two lobes of the crown.

Developmental lines   *See* developmental grooves.

Developmental pit   Small hole formed by the junction of two or more developmental grooves.

Devitrification   The crystallization of porcelain that occurs from repeated firings, resulting in a clouding of the porcelain and a nonvital appearance to the restoration.

Diagnostic waves   One of four basic categories of x-radiation wavelengths. It is used in most dental and standard x-ray units for diagnostic radiographs.

Diastema   Any spacing between adjacent teeth in the same arch.

Digastric muscle   Muscle of mastication arising from the jugular process of the occipital bone and inserting on the ventral border of the mandible to open the jaws.

Digestive tract   In the embryo, the roof of the entodermal yolk sac enfolds into a tubular tract forming the gut. Initially, a blind tract closed at both ends (anal-cloaca and oral-stomodeum).

Dilaceration   Crown or rooted structure that is bent or crooked from developmental causes.

Dimple   Embossed concavity on the back side of the film for orientation during exposure and after development.

Diphyodont   The feature of having two sets of teeth, one designated deciduous or primary and the other permanent. Most domesticated animals (eg, cats, dogs, cows, horses, etc.) and humans are diphyodonts.

Direct acrylic splint   Acrylic splint formed in the oral cavity for fracture stabilization.

Direct/indirect technique   Technique of directly forming a restoration or a model of a restoration on or in a cavity preparation, with the restoration treated or cured indirectly out of the cavity or the model used indirectly make the permanent restoration.

Disarticulated instrument   The separation or breaking off of an instrument, as in the root canal.

Disc derangement   Damage and displacement to the articular disc, as that of the temporomandibular joint.

Disclosing agents   Solutions or wafers that are effective in staining plaque, calculus, and bacterial deposits on the teeth, tongue, and gingiva.

Discoid   Disc-shaped excavator used to cut or dig out diseased dentin in a cavity preparation.

Discoid lupus erythematosus (DLE)   An autoimmune disease with possible oral lesions involving ulceration of the tongue or hypopigmentation of the nasal planum, gums, and lips.

Displacement   Condition of a tooth in which both the crown and root have moved principally in the same direction; sometimes described as an occlusion.

Distal   Farthest away from the median line of the face.

Distal contact area   *See* contact area.

Distal displacement (distocclusion)   Condition of a tooth bodily displaced distally or away from the midline of the arch.

Distal inclination (distal tipping, distoversion) Condition of a tooth in which the crown leans in a distal direction.

Distal proximal surface Proximal surface on the posterior side of a tooth.

Distal surface Surface of a tooth facing away from the median line following the curve of the dental arch.

Distal third Portion of a surface farther from the midline, viewed from the facial or lingual surface.

Distoclusion *See* class II malocclusion.

Distolingual cusp Most distal of the lingual cusps.

Distolingual rotation A tooth that is rotated on its long axis so that the distal aspect is moved toward the tongue.

Ditching Technique involving a round or pear-shaped laboratory cutter to trim the underbase of a dental model 1–2 mm immediately below the model margin preparation line, resulting in a groove in the base below the margin.

Dolichocephaly Condition marked by a long, narrow facial profile, as in collies and greyhounds.

Domestication Adjustment of animals to living with humans; taming.

Dominance behavior Control over another individual; a strong personality that affects others.

Dominance hierarchy Position within a group according to personality traits from strongest to weakest.

Dominant An allele that produces an effect on the phenotype even when present in a single dose.

Dorsum of the tongue Top surface of the tongue.

Dot Embossed button for orientation during exposure and after development of radiographic film, visible on the outside of the film packet.

Dovetail
1. A fan-shaped detail of the cavity preparation designed to increase the retention of the restoration and its resistance from displacement.
2. Type of connector used as the movable joint for a minor retainer.

Dowel crown Crown with a prefabricated post.

Dr. Black's Instrument Numbering Formula Universally accepted three- or four-number formula for identifying cutting instruments.

Duplicidentata Double-row dentition.

Dynamic occlusion *See* functional occlusion.

Dystrophic canals Canals with abnormal configurations.

Ectoderm Outer embryonic germ layer that forms skin, salivary glands, hair, sweat glands, sebaceous glands, nerves, etc.

Edge, incisal *See* incisal edge.

Elbow Stricture near the apex, resulting in an apical vault.

Electromagnetic spectrum Spectrum of wavelengths with both electric and magnetic fields, encompassing x-rays and gamma radiation.

Electronic root canal measuring devices (ERCMs) Based on a theory of electrical resistance difference between two probes. *See* apex locators.

Elevation Raising the mandible, or closing the mouth.

Elevator Instrument used to elevate the tooth or root section out of the alveolus during extraction.

Elliptication *See* zipping.

Elongation Distortion of a radiographic image because of too little vertical angulation.

Embrasure   A "V"-shaped space between the proximal surfaces of two adjoining teeth in contact.

Embrication   Irregularly arranged teeth within an arch due to a lack of space (crowding), typically seen in lower incisors.

Embryonic oral (stratified squamous) epithelium   Begins to thicken on the 25th day of development.

Enamel   Hard calcified tissue covering the dentin of the crown portion of a tooth.

Enamel cuticle (Nasmyth's membrane)   A thin membrane that covers the crown of a tooth at eruption.

Enamel hypocalcification   Condition in which tooth enamel may be soft and poorly mineralized, appearing white to yellow to brown in color, usually due to arrested development. *See also* hypocalcified enamel.

Enamel hypoplasia   Condition in which the enamel layer is thin or reduced. *See also* hypoplastic enamel.

Enamel lamellae   Imperfections or cracks in enamel caused by trauma or imperfect enamel formation.

Enameloma   *See* enamel pearls

Enamel organ   Ectodermal epithelial structure that leads to the formation of tooth enamel.

Enamel pearls   Small enamel growths on the root of the teeth; considered abnormal structures.

Enamel prisms   Basic enamel unit running the dentinoenamel junction to the surface enamel.

Enamel rod   Individual pillars of enamel formed by ameloblasts.

Enamel spindle   Odontoblastic process trapped in enamel at the dentinoenamel junction.

Enamel tuft   Area of hypocalcified enamel at the dentinoenamel junction.

Enamel wall   That portion of the preparation wall that consists of enamel.

Endoderm   Inner germ layer of an embryo that forms the epithelial lining of organs such as the digestive tract, liver, lungs, and pancreas.

Endodontic ruler   Instrument used to measure endodontic instruments from tip to endodontic stop.

Endodontic stops   Small, circular pieces of material placed on endodontic instruments to mark the depth of canal penetration.

Endodontic triad   The steps of canal preparation, sterilization, and obturation.

Endoliths   Calcifications within the endodontic system; sometimes referred to as **pulp stones.**

Envelope flap   Raising of the gingiva from an underlying lesion by using a periosteal elevator at a horizontal releasing incision for exposure.

Eosinophilic granuloma complex   In cats, a group of similar lesions, often with an eosinophilic component, with possible immune ramifications and some oral lesions (eg, indolent/rodent ulcers, collagenolytic granulomas, eosinophilic plaques).

Epiglottis   Mucosal-covered cartilage that helps cover the laryngeal opening.

Epithelial attachment   Substance produced by the reduced enamel epithelium that helps secure the attachment epithelium at the base of the gingival sulcus to the tooth.

Epithelial diaphragm   Deep part of the epithelial root sheath that is turned horizontally.

Epithelial rests   Cells from the epithelial root sheath that remain in the periodontal space and cells that remain at areas of embryonic fusion.

Epithelial rests of Malassez *See* epithelial rests.

Epithelial root sheath Downgrowth of the inner and outer enamel epithelium that outlines the shape and number of the roots.

Epoxy Model material in the form of a paste with an activator added to initiate hardening.

Epulis The most common form of benign growth arising from the periodontal ligament. It may be fibromatous, ossifying, or acanthomatous.

Erosion External loss of tooth hard tissue due to a chemical process without active bacterial involvement.

Eruption Movement of a tooth as it emerges through surrounding tissue so that the clinical crown gradually appears longer.

Eruption cyst A form of dentigerous cyst surrounding the tooth crown during eruption.

Eruption times General times for anticipated eruption of teeth.

Eruptive stage Period of eruption from the completion of crown formation until the teeth come into occlusion. The prefunctional eruptive stage occurs at the beginning, before the teeth move into occlusion.

Essig's interdental wiring technique Multiwire technique with one primary wire passed around all the teeth and secondary wire anchors passed interdentally.

Esthetic teeth Teeth important to the owner, usually the incisors and canine teeth.

Evaluation phase Phase of periodontal therapy in which the examination and history taking occur.

Exfoliation Shedding or loss of a primary tooth.

Exostoses Small extra growths of bone on its surface; usually seen on the buccal cortical plate.

Expansion and contraction screw devices Most commonly used for intermittent movement pressures.

Extension for prevention Extension of the outline form of the cavity preparation beyond the caries-susceptible area in compliance with the anatomy of the tooth surface to prevent the recurrence of decay.

External resorption Loss of outer substance of the roots due to traumatic forces.

Extirpation Complete surgical removal or destruction of a part, such as a pulp.

Extracoronal crown Crown that covers all or part of the clinical crown.

Extract To pull out or remove.

Extraoral anchorage When anchorage is sought outside of mouth.

Extrinsic Originating outside a structure.

Extrinsic muscles of the tongue Innervated by the hypoglossal (twelfth cranial) nerve: *m. styloglossus* draws tongue caudally; *m. hypoglossus* retracts and depresses tongue; and *m. genioglossus* depresses and protrudes the tongue.

Extrusion Movement of the tooth further out of the alveolus, typically in the same direction as normal eruption.

Eye teeth *See* cuspid.

Facial Term used to designate the outer surfaces of the teeth collectively (buccal or labial).

Facial contours Curvature of the facial surface of a tooth.

Facial displacement (linguoclusion) Condition in which a tooth is bodily displaced away from the tongue.

Facial embrasure *See* embrasure.

Facial or vestibular inclination (tipping, facioversion) Condition in which a tooth is leaning away from the tongue.

Facial nerve   Cranial nerve VII, innervating the caudal belly of the digastric muscle.

Facial surfaces   Labial and buccal surfaces collectively.

Facial third   The third of that surface closest to the facial side, from a proximal view.

Facultative anaerobes   Bacteria that can live in either aerobic or anaerobic conditions.

False temporomandibular ankylosis   Condition in which extracapsular pathology limits the movements of the jaw.

Familial   Used to describe conditions that affect a family to an extent that is considered greater than expected by random chance or circumstance.

Fauces   Space between the left and right palatine tonsils.

Favorable fracture   Mandibular fracture in a caudodorsal direction, allowing muscular forces to compress segments together.

FDI system   System for tooth identification promulgated by the Federation Dentaire Internationale (International Dental Federation).

Fibromatous epulis   Fibrous form of epulis that may be single or multiple, pedunculated or sessile.

Fibrosarcoma   Malignant tumor comprised of fibrous connective tissue. The third most common tumor in dogs that is locally invasive with a high recurrence rate but metastasizes late.

File binding   When light firm contact is made with the canal walls.

Filiform papillae   Small pointed projections pointing caudally that heavily cover most of the dorsum of the anterior two-thirds of the tongue.

Film fogging   When part or all of the developed x-ray film is darkened by sources other than the useful primary beam.

Film mount   Plastic or cardboard devices to hold and protect intraoral films.

Finishing   Process of refining the anatomic landmarks, surface, and margins of restorations to provide the ultimate function of the tooth and avoid irritating the soft tissue of the oral cavity.

First-order bends   Bends in orthodontic wire in the horizontal plane.

Fissure   Cleft or crevice in a tooth surface thought to result from the imperfect fusion of the enamel of adjoining cusps or lobes.

Fixed appliances   Devices typically attached to provide a center for movement without removal until the tooth attains its target site.

Fixed-fixed bridge   One-piece bridge with pontic or pontics attached to the span between retainers at both ends; also called a **common bridge.**

Fixed-free bridge   *See* fixed-movable bridge.

Fixed-movable bridge   Two-piece bridge with pontic or pontics integrally attached to the retainer only at one end. The other end of the bridge attaches to the retainer or abutment in a fashion that allows some degree of movement; also called a **fixed-free** or **deprecated bridge.**

Fixer solutions   Used to preserve and enhance the latent image on the radiographic film.

Flashing   Restorative that extends beyond the preparation outline but, when initially placed, does not cause an overhang.

Flour of pumice   Abrasive material used to polish teeth, restoration, and acrylics.

Fluorosis   Disruption in the mineralization of forming teeth due to excess ingestion of fluoride, often seen as chalky white spots or discoloration of the enamel.

Focal–film distance (FFD)   Distance from the focal spot on the tube's target to the film.

Foliate papillae   Poorly developed papillae that appear as small vertical folds in the posterior part of the sides of the tongue, immediately rostral to the palatoglossal fold. They contain the taste buds.

Follicular cyst   Dentigerous cyst or dilation of the follicular space around the crown of a tooth that is unerupted or impacted.

Foramen   Short circular opening through a bone.

Foreshortened   Shortened distortion due to excessive vertical angulation.

Fossa   A rounded or angular depression on the surface of a tooth. There are three common types:

1. **Lingual fossa**   A broad shallow depression on the lingual surface of an incisor or canine.
2. **Central fossa**   A relatively broad, deep angular valley in the central portion of the occlusal surface of a molar.
3. **Triangular fossa**   A comparatively shallow pyramid-shaped depression on the occlusal surfaces of posterior teeth located just within the confines of the mesial and/or distal marginal ridges.

Four-wall defect   An infrabony pocket defect surrounding the tooth.

Fractious   Unpredictable aggressive behavior that has the potential to occur suddenly.

Free gingiva   Gingiva that forms the gingival sulcus; also known as **marginal gingiva.**

Frenectomy   Excision of the frenulum.

Frenoplasty   Excision of part of the frenulum to alter its contours.

Frenulum   Fold of alveolar mucosa forming a noticeable ridge of attachment between the lips and gums. *See also* frenum.

Frenum   Fold of skin or lining tissue that limits the movement of an organ (eg, tissue under the tongue).

Frequency   Number of oscillations per second in a wave.

Frontal prominence   Forehead area of the embryo, occurring in coordination with the stomodeum and mandibular processes.

Fulcrum   Center of rotation of the tooth, usually occurring approximately at the junction of the middle and apical thirds of the root.

Fulgurating current   Destructive form of electric current used in electrosurgery.

Fulguration   Therapeutic destruction of tissue by means of electrical sparking effect.

Full bevel   Bevel involving the entire wall of a cavity preparation.

Full crown   Restoration that covers the entire clinical crown (eg, full metal crown, full veneer crown, jacket crown).

Full incline capping   When a half cap extends over to the facial surface of the tooth.

Full metal crown   Crown made of metal that covers the entire clinical crown (eg, full gold crown); occasionally called a **full metal sleeve** or **full metal jacket.**

Full releasing flap   *See* releasing flaps.

Full veneer crown   *See* full crown.

Fully filtered current   Electric current used in electrosurgery that is the least traumatic of the four common types of current. It is used for delicate cutting but affords little hemostasis.

Fully rectified current   Electric current used in electrosurgery that provides easy cutting of most oral soft tissue and a good degree of hemostasis.

Functional ankylosis   *See* osseointegration.

Functional eruptive stage   Stage when teeth erupt or move into actual occlusion; also known as the **posteruptive stage.**

Functional occlusion   Active tooth contacts during mastication and swallowing; also called **dynamic occlusion.**

Fungiform papillae   Small circular mushroom-shaped papillae scattered throughout the anterior two-thirds of the dorsum of the tongue.

Furcation   Point at which roots diverge.

Fusion tooth   Result of two separate tooth buds joined at the crown by enamel and possibly dentin.

Galvanism   Uninterrupted electric current that may be created by the contact of two dissimilar metals.

Gamma-radiation   Radiation of the same approximate wavelength as x-radiation that is naturally occurring rather than man-made.

Gemination   Disorder in which the developing bud attempts to split but fails to do so completely, resulting in duplication of part of the tooth but not total twinning.

Gene   A unit of information in DNA that codes for a particular disease or trait.

Genetic   Term describing the condition of being hereditary.

Genotype   The genetic makeup of an animal.

"Geographic tongue"   Zones of desquamation of filiform papillae in a well demarcated but irregularly shaped area (in humans).

Giant cell epulis   Lesion appearing similar to acanthomatous epulis that can only be differentiated by histopathology.

Gingiva   Part of the gum tissue that immediately surrounds the teeth and alveolar bone.

Gingival crest   Most occlusal or incisal extent of gingiva.

Gingival crevice (sulcus)   Subgingival space that under normal conditions lies between the gingival crest and the epithelial attachment.

Gingival embrasure   *See* cervical embrasure.

Gingival fibers   Periodontal fibers in the gingiva.

Gingival hyperplasia   Proliferation of the attached gingiva.

Gingival margin   Crest of gingiva around the tooth.

Gingival papillae   That portion of the gingiva found between the teeth in the interproximal spaces gingival to the contact area; also called **interdental papillae.**

Gingival stippling   Small dimples in the gingival tissue caused by the insertion of rete pegs (not a consistent indication of gingival health).

Gingival sulcus   *See* gingival crevice.

Gingivectomy   Excision of excessive gingival tissues to create a new gingival margin.

Gingivitis   Inflammation involving the gingival tissues only.

Gingivoplasty   Periodontal surgery used to correct gingival deformities of contour not associated with pocketing.

Glass ceramic   Restorative developed as a rival to standard porcelain, made with the normal pyroceram materials but with the addition of various oxides of conventional feldspathic porcelains.

Glass ionomers   Compounds that chemically bind to enamel and dentin by ions forming salts that bond to the calcium in the tooth, even if slight moisture is present.

Glossectomy   Surgical removal of part or all of the tongue, or a lesion of the tongue.

Glossitis   Inflammation of the tongue.

Glossolalia   Baby talk.

Glossoplegia   Paralysis of the tongue, either unilateral or bilateral.

Gomphosis   Type of fibrous joint in which a conical object is inserted into a socket and held.

Gouging   Excavations of the floor of the pulp chamber, typically with burs or files during exploration for canals, that may result in perforation.

Granular layers of Tomes   Hypocalcified dentin that occurred during formation, found next to the cementodentinal junction.

Gray collie syndrome A simple autosomal-recessive disease producing a cyclic neutropenia that can exhibit stomatitis and pharyngitis with fever.

G-reamer Endodontic instrument used to enlarge the root canal in its coronal third.

Grenz waves One of the four basic categories of x-radiation, used for superficial therapy.

Groove Shallow linear depression on the surface of a tooth. There are two common types:
1. **Developmental groove** Marks the boundaries between adjacent cusps and other major divisional parts of a tooth.
2. **Supplemental groove** An indistinct linear depression, irregular in extent and direction, that does not demarcate major divisional portions of a tooth.

Ground substance Glue-like substance composed of a substance known as a mucopolysaccharide that serves as the background for connective tissue, including cartilage and bone.

"Gum-chewer's" syndrome Self-trauma to the buccal mucosa and tongue from chewing on the tissues.

Gutta-percha Endodontic filling agent that is about 60% crystalline and slightly viscoelastic.

G.V. Black classification Classification of dental lesions according to location.

Gypsum Naturally occurring chalky porous white mineral, chemically known as calcium sulfate dihydrate.

Hairy tongue Tongue with long filiform papillae that resemble hair and can be darkly stained.

Half-capping Capping involving the lingual and occlusal surface of the tooth.

Halitosis Bad or foul breath.

Handle parallelism Technique that allows the handle of a universal curette to be parallel to the working surface for orientation below the gum line.

Hard palate Bony vault of the oral cavity proper covered with soft tissue.

Hard tissue Calcified or mineralized tooth tissues or bone.

Haversian system System of blood vessels located within the bones to provide nourishment.

Hedging *See* ledging.

Hemangiosarcoma Red, raised, friable lesion with high rate of malignancy and early metastasis.

Hemisection A tooth being cut in half generally through the furcational area.

Hereditary Term describing traits received from past ancestors that produce specific characteristics.

Hertwig's epithelial root sheath *See* epithelial root sheath.

Heterodont The feature of having more than one type (shape, size) of tooth represented in the dentition, such as incisors, cuspids, premolars, and molars. The domestic dogs and cats have heterodont dentition.

High-fusing alloys Alloys designed for porcelain-fused-to-metal or ceramometal restorations.

High-speed handpieces Dental handpieces that provide great speed of operation but lower tactile sense than slow-speed handpieces. High speed handpieces can be used for efficient removal of enamel, dentin, bone, and other hard tissues.

Homodont The feature of having all teeth that are of the same general shape or type, although size may vary, as in fish, reptiles, and sharks.

Horizontal angulation Movement of the position-indicating device in a direction mesial or distal from the center of the object.

Horizontal fibers   Alveolodental periodontal ligament fibers running from the cementum to the alveolar crest to resist horizontal tooth movements.

Horizontal overlap   *See* overlap, horizontal.

Horizontal ramus   That portion of the jaw composed of the body and symphyseal area of the mandible.

Horizontal releasing incision   Made by reverse bevel through the marginal gingiva into the base of a pocket.

Hot light   Bright light available for viewing films displaying marginally excessive density or darkness.

Howship's lacunae   Crescent-shaped excavations in bone.

Hydraulic scalers   Scalers that work as a water and abrasive stream on the tooth to "sandblast" the tooth clean.

Hydrogen peroxide in a 3% solution   Mild oxidizing agent that kills certain anaerobic bacteria.

Hydroxyapatite   Crystal found in hard substances of the body such as bone, cementum, dentin, and enamel; sometimes spelled hydroxylapatite.

Hypercementosis   Increased thickness of cementum, usually seen at the apex of the root.

Hyperemia   Congestion of blood, seen in pulp.

Hypersialism   Excessive salivation or drooling.

Hypocalcifed enamel   Condition in which there is either an insufficient number of enamel crystals or insufficient growth of the crystals. *See also* enamel hypocalcification.

Hypodontia   Condition in which some teeth are missing.

Hypoplastic enamel   Thin enamel, commonly seen in conjunction with enamel hypocalcification. *See also* enamel hypoplasia.

Hypsodont   The feature of having dentition with a submerged longer anatomic or reserved crown and in comparison to short roots.

Imbrication   Visible horizontal striae of Retzius on the exposed surface enamel; also known as **Perikymata lines.** These are not distinctly described in dog or cat teeth.

Impacted   Teeth not completely erupted that are fully or partially covered by bone or soft tissue.

Impression compound   Rigid plastic used in sticks or sheets that softens when heated and becomes rigid again as it cools.

Impression plasters   Plasters similar to dental plasters that have a fine grain and a higher water:mix ratio to allow recording of fine details; also known as **type I gypsum.**

Impression waxes   Combination of low-melting paraffin wax and beeswax, used most frequently for bite registration in combination with other impression materials.

Imprint   To permanently instill on the mind a situation that may affect the individual's actions in life.

Incipient caries   First indication of enamel demineralization seen as a chalky white spot.

Incisal   Coronal portion or direction in incisors.

Incisal bone   The premaxilla, rostral most area of upper jaw that accommodates the maxillary incisors and is formed solely by the medial nasal process; also known as the **primary palate.**

Incisal edge   Edge formed at the labioincisal line angle of an anterior tooth after an incisal ridge has worn down.

Incisal embrasure   *See* embrasure.

Incisal ridge   Rounded ridge form of the incisal portion of an anterior tooth.

Incisal third   That aspect of the surface closest to the incisal edge, from a proximal, lingual, or labial view of an anterior tooth.

Incisive ducts   Ducts communicating with the cavity of the vomeronasal organ through the palatine fissure to the floor of the nasal fossa.

Incisive foramen   Foramen at the midline of the anterior palate region.

Incisive papilla   Small, rounded, oblong mound of tissue directly behind or lingual to the maxillary central incisors and lying over incisive foramen.

Incisivomaxillary suture   Articulation of the incisive bone and the maxillae.

Incisors   Center teeth in either arch that are essential for cutting.

Incisor capping incline plane   Covers a group of incisors, generally the mandibular, to move the opposing incisor teeth.

Inclinations   *See* tipping.

Incline capping   When an incline covers a tooth.

Incline planes   Orthodontic appliances designed to make contact with the cusps or incisal edges of the teeth of the opposing occlusion to stimulate tooth movement directed by the incline.

Incremental lines of von Ebner   Incremental growth pattern lines in dentin, similar to those of the striae of Retzius found in enamel.

Indirect acrylic splint   Splint manufactured on a stone model for eventual placement in the oral cavity.

Inferior border of mandible   Lower edge of the lower jaw.

Infrabony pocket   Periodontal pocket that has its base apical to the alveolar crest; also known as **intrabony pocket**.

Infraclusion   Condition of the teeth in which the occlusal surface or incisal edge has not reached the same or an appropriate level of other teeth of the same type.

Infraversion   Condition of the teeth in which the occlusal surface or incisal edge has not reached the same or an appropriate level of other teeth of the same type, differing from infraclusion in that a degree of crown tilt may be involved.

Inlay   Restoration made to fit into a tooth.

Inlay waxes   Used to make wax patterns for crown, bridges, and some other dental appliances. These waxes are more precise and have better control than other waxes.

Inner enamel epithelium (IEE)   Group of epithelial cells in the enamel organ that eventually form the enamel of the crown.

Inorganic matrix   Hydroxyapatite crystals in the early matrix.

Inorganic matter   Mineral deposits such as calcium or phosphorus.

Insensible dentin   Dentin that does not register pain.

Instinct   An innate ability.

Instinctual   Natural ability to perform certain tasks or actions.

Instrument adaptation   Way in which the instrument contacts the intended surface.

Interalveolar Septa   *See* interdental septum.

Interarcade wiring   Various mean of securing the maxilla and mandible together with wires and other implements to restrict oral movements.

Interceptive orthodontics   Generally considered to be the extraction or recontouring (crown reduction) of primary or permanent teeth that are contributing to alignment problems of the permanent dentition.

Intercuspation   Relationship of the cusps of the premolars and molars of one jaw with those of the opposing jaw during any of the occlusal relationships.

Interdental   Located between the teeth.

Interdental papilla   Projection of gingiva between teeth.

Interdental septum   Bone between the roots of adjacent teeth.

Interdental wiring   Placement of wires around adjacent teeth to provide reduction and support to a bony fracture that extends between the teeth.

Interfragmentary wiring   *See* transosseous wiring

Interglobular dentin   Areas of hypocalcified dentin between normal areas of dentin, found in both crown and root dentin.

Intermaxillary anchorage   When an appliance anchorage is placed in the opposing jaws or in both the mandible and the maxilla.

Intermediate abutment   *See* pier.

Intermittent force   Drive or energy that is applied in incremental steps with periods of rest in between.

Internal fixation   Surgical stabilization of fracture with pins, plates, screws, etc.

Internal resorption   Loss of the dentinal structure internally.

Interproximal   Between the proximal surfaces of adjoining teeth in the same arch.

Interproximal space   Space between adjoining teeth.

Interradicular fibers   Alveolodental periodontal ligament fibers in multirooted teeth that go from the interradicular crestal bone to cementum.

Interradicular septa   Bony partitions between adjacent teeth.

Intertubular dentin   All dentin that is not tubular or peritubular.

Intrabony pocket   *See* infrabony pocket

Intraradicular septum   Bone between the roots of multirooted teeth.

Intraspecific aggression   Aggressive behavior within one special individual; aggression within the same species.

Intrinsic   Lying entirely inside a structure.

Intrinsic muscles of the tongue   Unit of muscles that produces the complicated protrusion and prehensile movement of the tongue. They innervated by the hypoglossal nerve.

Intrusion   Movement of the tooth further into the alveolus.

Inverse square law   In radiology, the ability to reduce the exposure time as a inverse square proportion to the length of the focal–film distance (FFD) (eg, an 8-inch FFD requires only one-quarter the exposure time of a long 16-inch FFD technique).

Ionizing radiation   Radiation produced when an orbiting electron is ejected or ionized from its place in an electrically stable or neutral atom. This includes x-rays, gamma rays, and some particulate radiation.

Irreversible pulpitis   Inflammation of the pulp that cannot be resolved, leading to the death of the vital pulp.

Isognathism   Condition of having equal jaw widths, in which the premolars and molars of opposing jaws align with the occlusal surfaces facing each other, forming an occlusal plane.

Ivy loop interdental wiring   Single-wire technique incorporating two teeth.

Jacket crown   Full veneer crown made from porcelain, glass, resin, or metal as a permanent crown, or from acrylics or resins as a temporary crown. *See also* full crown.

Joint   That part of a bridge or prosthetic device that unites the retainer with the pontic.

Junctional epithelium   Epithelium that acts to hold mucosa in the base of the gingiva sulcus to the tooth.

Keratin   Substance that makes up the surface cells of skin, hair, and nails.

Keratinized cells   Dead cells of the stratum corneum.

Keratinized stratified squamous epithelium   Multilayered epithelium, such as skin, whose upper layers are dead cells similar in the composition to hair.

Keratohyalin granules   Granules in the stratum granulosum that help produce the dead layer of cells on the skin surface.

Kilovoltage selector   Control unit of a radiographic machine that regulates the kilovoltage (kVP)

"Kissing lesion"   *See* Chronic ulcerative paradental stomatitis (CUPS).

Labium (pl. labia)   Latin for "lip."

Labial   Next to or toward the lips.

Labial displacement   Condition of an anterior tooth that is bodily displaced away from the tongue; also known as **labioclusion**.

Labial frenum   Fold of tissue that attaches the lip to the labial mucosa at the midline of the lips.

Labial inclination (labial tipping, labioversion)   Terms used to describe facial inclination of the anterior teeth.

Labial salivary glands   Numerous small, serous or mucous ducts scattered throughout the submucosa of the lips.

Labial surface   Surface of an anterior tooth positioned immediately adjacent to the lip

Labioversion   *See* labial inclination.

Lactoperoxidase and glucose oxidase   Enzymes that are used to augment normal salivary peroxidase production for a mild antiplaque and antibacterial effect.

Lamina dura   Radiographic term denoting the cribriform plate, bundle bone, and the dense alveolar bone surrounding a root.

Lampas   Swelling of the soft tissue behind the incisors from venous distension during tooth eruption.

Lance tooth   Significant mesiorostroversion of a maxillary canine.

Latent image   Image contained on a radiograph after it has been exposed but before it is developed.

Lateral canals   Additional natural root canal openings on the lateral surface of the root. *See also* auxiliary canals.

Lateral compaction   Method of endodontic obturation accomplished by inserting a spreader alongside the gutta-percha cones and compacting them against the canal wall.

Lateral excursion   Movement of the jaws sideways.

Lateral protrusion   Lateral deviation of the tongue, due at times to hypoglossal nerve damage.

Lateral pterygoid muscle   Muscle of mastication arising from the sphenoid bone area and inserting on the mandibular condyle and articular process to act to close the mouth.

Law of diffusion   "When two or more liquids capable of being mixed are placed together, a spontaneous exchange of molecules takes place in defiance of the law of gravity."

Learned behavior   Behavior learned through experience and reaction to it.

Ledge   Gouge or false canal created during instrumentation with excessive apical pressure, primarily associated with curved canals.

Ledging   Gouging of root canals; sometimes called **hedging.**

Leishmania stomatitis   Systemic infection with *Leishmania* that produces proliferative lesions on the mucosa, including the oral cavity.

Lethargy   Lack of energy or reduced activity.

Level bites   When the incisor teeth meet edge on edge or the premolars or molars occlude cusp to cusp.

Ligament   Regularly arranged group of collagen fibers that attach bone to bone.

Light fogging   Fogging of a radiographic film when it is exposed to a light source before or during processing.

Line angle   Formed by two walls or surfaces (eg, mesial and lingual: the junction is called the mesiolingual line angle).

Line angles in cavity preparation   Junction of the two walls of a cavity preparation (tooth surfaces) forming an angle, with the name taken from the two surfaces involved. In the identification of the line angle, the names of the surfaces are combined. The ending of the first word used is changed to *o* (eg, axial pulpal becomes axiopulpal). Additional examples of line angles are as follows: mesiofacial, distopulpal, distogingival, mesiolingual, gingivoaxial, mesio-occlusal, distofacial, linguoaxial disto-occlusal, distolingual, facioaxial, axiogingival, faciolingual, faciogingival, axiomesial, linguopulpal, linguogingival, axio-occlusal, mesiopulpal, mesiogingival, axiodistal.

Line of draw   Direction that the restoration must follow to be correctly placed on the tooth without binding.

Liner   Thin coating of a material in a cavity preparation to protect the pulp and decrease dentinal sensitivity.

Lingual   Next to or toward the tongue.

Lingual arteries   Primary blood supply to the tongue.

Lingual contours   Curvature of the lingual surface of a tooth.

Lingual crest of curvature   Most convex or widest portion of the lingual surface of a tooth.

Lingual displacement   Condition in which a tooth is bodily displaced toward the tongue; also called **linguoclusion**.

Lingual embrasure   *See* embrasure.

Lingual fossa   Slight concavity just above the cingulum on the lingual surface of an incisor.

Lingual frenum   Fold of tissue that attaches the undersurface of the tongue to the floor of the mouth.

Lingual groove   Developmental groove that occurs on the lingual side of the tooth.

Lingual inclination (lingual tipping, linguoversion)   Condition in which a tooth is tilted so that its crown leans toward the tongue. *See also* retroclination.

Lingual molar salivary gland   In cats, small gland with numerous small openings in the membranous molar pad just lingual to lower molar, with mixed salivary secretions (serous and mucous).

Lingual mucosa   Thick rough cornified mucous membrane covering the dorsum of the tongue.

Lingual salivary glands   Numerous small, serous or mucous ducts in the submucosa and muscles of the tongue in the caudal third.

Lingual surface   Surface of a tooth immediately adjacent to the tongue.

Lingula   Small projection of bone just in front of the mandibular foramen, found in primates.

Linguoversion   *See* lingual inclination.

Lining mucosa   Mucosa (nonkeratinized) of the soft palate, lips, cheeks, vestibule, and floor of the mouth.

Lips   Most rostral extent of the oral cavity. The upper and lower lips converge at the angles of the mouth to form the commissures.

Loading   Attachment of the restorative crown to a prepared tooth or implant.

Lobe   Major division of a tooth erroneously believed to be formed during development from a separate center of calcification.

Local influences Influences that may affect the orofacial complex by their local effects.

Localized juvenile periodontitis (LJP) A rapidly progressive localized periodontitis in which gingiva is normal-looking but there are crater-like areas of bone resorption. It is most commonly initiated in young animals.

Localized osteitis Complication caused by a combination of traumatic procedure, infection, and decreased vascular supply; commonly known as a **dry socket.**

Long bevel Bevel involving no more than the external two-thirds of a cavity wall (more than the external one-third of a cavity wall).

Long-cone technique An increase in the focal–film distance in a parallel technique to reduce distortions.

Lophodont The feature of having teeth that have a lamellar structure of longitudinal layers of enamel and dentin that become fused with cementum, with cusps that connect to form ridges, as in the cheek teeth of the rhinoceros and elephant.

Lumpy jaw Condition caused by *Actinomyces bovis* infection in which there may be extensive osteomyelitis with an extensive periosteal reaction in the jaw in herbivores.

Luxation Partial or complete dislocation from a joint, as in the temporomandibular joint or a tooth.

Lymphocytic plasmocytic stomatitis (LPS) Syndrome describing an inflammatory condition of the oral soft tissues with a component of lymphocytes and plasmacytes.

Lymphosarcoma A malignant tumor comprised of lymphoblasts and lymphocytes that may be present in the oral cavity as involvement of the tonsils or as a more diffuse ulcerative or proliferative stomatitis.

Lyssa Fusiform cord composed of fat, muscle, and islands of cartilage surrounded by a fibrous sheath and located in the ventral portion of the tongue along the midline. It may act as a stretch receptor for the rostral portion of the tongue.

Macrodontia Teeth that are disproportionally large.

Macroglossia Oversized or large tongue.

Magnetostrictive Type of ultrasonic scaler that uses a ferromagnetic stack or a ferrite rod to create electromagnetic energy and results in the scaler tip's moving in an ellipsoid pattern.

Major retainer Retainer on the fixed end.

Major sublingual salivary duct Duct that takes saliva from the monostomatic portion of the sublingual salivary gland to the sublingual caruncle.

Malar abscess Facial abscess and drainage due to fractured maxillary canine teeth. It is relatively common in captive primates.

Malignant Term to describe tumors that show an uncontrollable growth and destructive growth pattern of the tissue of origin and that may exhibit metastasis.

Malocclusion Abnormal occlusion of the teeth. *See also* class I, class II, and class III malocclusions.

Mamelon One of three rounded or conical protuberances of the incisal ridge of a newly erupted incisor tooth.

Mandible Lower jaw.

Mandibular Pertaining to the lower jaw.

Mandibular alveolar block Intraoral regional anesthetic nerve block achieved by injecting at the lingual mandible near the base of the coronoid process.

Mandibular arch First pharyngeal arch that forms the area of the mandible and maxillae. It is the lower dental arch.

Mandibular condyle   Rounded top of the mandible that articulates with the mandibular fossa.

Mandibular duct   Duct for the mandibular salivary gland that opens on the small sublingual papilla or caruncle near the rostral attachment of the lingual frenulum.

Mandibular expansion device   Orthodontic appliance placed to move base-narrow canine(s) laterally into position.

Mandibular *foramen*   Opening on the medial surface of the ramus of the mandible for entrance of nerves and blood vessels to the lower teeth.

Mandibular fossa   Depression on the inferior surface of the skull in the temporal bone that articulates with the condyle of the mandible.

Mandibular salivary gland   Ovoid, compact, yellow to buff-colored gland just caudal to the angle of the jaw and easily palpable; the mandibular duct opens at the sublingual papilla or caruncle; with mixed salivary secretions (serous and mucous).

Mandibular salivary gland mucocele   Retention cyst of salivary fluids from the mandibular gland that produces an enlargement under the mandible or near the throat area; also known as a **cervical mucocele**.

Mandibular symphysis   Point at which the mandibular processes merge, forming the mandible.

Mann incline plane   A cast fixed appliance that is anchored to the upper canine teeth with a telescoping support bar between the two to allow for skeletal growth.

Marginal development groove   *See* marginal groove.

Marginal gingiva   *See* free gingiva.

Marginal groove   Groove that crosses a marginal ridge.

Marginal papillae   Small, soft tissue protrusions present at birth along the margins of the rostral half of the tongue. They are mechanical in nature to aid in nursing vacuum.

Marginal ridge   Ridge or elevation of enamel forming the margin of the surface of a tooth, specifically, at the mesial and distal margins of the occlusal surfaces of premolars and molars and at the mesial and distal margins of the lingual surfaces of incisors and canines.

Maryland bridge   Bridge in which the retainers are simply acid-etched at the areas that make contact with the tooth to enhance cementation. The retainers do not normally cover a cusp or incisal edge. It is a modified form of Rochette bridges.

Masseter muscle   Muscle of mastication arising from the zygomatic arch and inserting on the lateral ramus of the mandible. It acts to close the mandible.

Mastication   Act of chewing or grinding.

Masticatory mucosa   Mucosa (parakeratinized or keratinized) of the hard palate and gingiva.

Masticatory muscle myositis   Inflammatory and possibly immune-mediated disease that affects the muscles of mastication innervated by the trigeminal nerve, sometimes with a local or systemic peripheral eosinophilia. It results in the inability to open the mouth.

Matrix   A mechanical device placed near or around the tooth cavity preparation to provide the missing walls of the tooth during condensation of plastic-type restorative material. A cylindrical matrix may supply more than one missing wall of a tooth (eg, mesio-occlusodistal cavity preparation [circumferential]).

Matrix band   Metal or plastic band fitted around a tooth when interproximal fillings are placed, preventing the filling material from squeezing out.

Maturation stage of calcification   When the crystals grow in size, becoming tightly packed together with the enamel rod.

Maxillae   Paired main bones of the upper jaw.

Maxillary   Pertaining to the upper arch.

Maxillary arch   Upper dental arch.

Maxillary sinuses   Paired paranasal sinuses located in the maxillae medially and dorsally to the maxillary 4th premolars.

McSpadden compactor   Instrument used to mechanically thermoplasticize gutta-percha while condensing it apically.

Medial displacement (medial occlusion, mesioclusion)   Condition in which a tooth is bodily displaced mesially or toward the midline of the arch.

Medial nasal processes   Two medial (and lateral) processes forming the upper lip, found on either side of the nasal pits.

Medial pterygoid muscles   Muscles of mastication arising from the sphenoid bone and inserting on the condyle and articular processes of the mandible. They serve to close the mandible.

Median line   Vertical line that divides the body into right and left (eg, the median line of the face).

Median raphe   Midline of the palate dividing the right and left sides.

Median rhomboid glossitis   Inflammation of the dorsal surface of the tongue in a regular-shaped pattern (developmental).

Melanosarcoma   (Malignant melanoma) Malignant neoplasm derived from melanin-producing cells; the most assertive oral tumor with aggressive invasion, recurrence, and a high rate of early metastasis. It may or may not be pigmented.

Mental foramen   Foramen on the lateral side of the mandible, below the premolars.

Mental regional block   Intraoral regional anesthetic nerve block achieved by injection at the largest mental foramen ventral to the mesial root of the 2nd premolar. It provides analgesia to the incisors, canines, and first two premolars.

Mesaticephaly   Condition marked by a head shape of medium proportions.

Mesenchymal cells   Embryonic connective tissue that begins the development stage of the dental papilla and the dental sac.

Mesenchyme   Connective tissue derived from mesoderm.

Mesial   Toward or situated in the middle (eg, toward the midline of the dental arch).

Mesial contact area   *See* contact area.

Mesial drift   Phenomenon in which the permanent molars continue to move mesially after eruption.

Mesial inclination (mesial tipping, mesioversion)   Condition in which in which the crown of a tooth leans in a mesial direction.

Mesial proximal surface   Proximal surface closest to the midline.

Mesial surface   Surface of a tooth facing toward the median line, following the curve of the dental arch.

Mesial third   From a facial or a lingual view, third of the surface closest to the midline.

Mesioclusion   *See* class III malocclusion.

Mesiodistoclusion   *See* class IV special malocclusions.

Mesiolingual cusp   Most mesial of the lingual cusps.

Mesiolingual rotation   Condition in which a tooth is rotated on its long axis so that the mesial aspect is moved toward the tongue.

Mesocephaly   Condition marked by a balanced facial profile, somewhere between dolichocephalic and brachycephalic, as in beagles and German shepherds.

Mesoderm   Middle germ layer of the embryo that forms connective tissue, muscle, bone, cartilage, blood, etc.

Metal nobility   Degree of noble and precious metals in an alloy.

Metastasis Dissemination of tumor cells to other parts of the body.

Microcheilia Condition in which there is a small oral opening or stoma. Literally, the term means "small lips."

Microdontia Teeth that are disproportionally small.

Microglossia A small tongue; also known as **bird tongue.**

Middle third *See* mesial third.

Midline Imaginary line that divides the body into right and left halves.

Midsagittal plane Imaginary plant that divides the body vertically into right and left halves.

Migration Filling of the groove between the medial and lateral nasal processes with connective tissue.

Milliamperage selector Control unit of a radiographic machine to regulate the milliamperes (mA).

Mineralization stage of calcification Stage at which enamel matrix is laid down at the end of the bell stage. All crystals placed within the rods are laid down at this time.

Minor retainer Retainer on the movable end.

Minor sublingual salivary ducts Ducts that carry secretions of the polystomatic sublingual salivary gland to the sublingual area.

Mixed dentition The feature of having primary and permanent teeth in the dental arches at the same time.

Moat defect *See* four-wall defect

Molars Teeth with occlusal surface that can be used to grind food or break it down into smaller pieces.

Monophyodont The feature of having only one set of teeth that erupt and remain functional throughout life. There are no deciduous teeth.

Motion of activation Way in which scalers and curettes are used in the hand to effect proficient work.

Mottled enamel Enamel that is opaque or chalky and may be discolored due to its porous nature. *See also* hypocalcified enamel.

Mouth Entrance to the oral cavity.

Mucobuccal fold Point at which the oral mucosa and the top or bottom of the vestibule turn toward the alveolar ridge.

Mucocele *See* sialocele

Mucogingival junction Point at which the alveolar mucosa becomes gingiva; also known as the **mucogingival line** or **margin.**

Mucolabial fold *See* mucobuccal fold.

Mulling Manipulation of a triturated mass of silver amalgam placed in a sterile square of rubber dam or between two finger cots. In the process, the mass of amalgam is kneaded and rolled briefly in the rubber covering, until it becomes a coherent, homogenized mass.

Multiple root Tooth with multiple roots.

Nasal pits Beginning of the nasal cavities, first revealed by two small depressions found low on the frontal prominence.

Nasal septum Wall between the left and right sides of the nasal cavity, made up of the ethmoid and vomer bones.

Nasmyth's membrane Membrane covering the surface of the tooth crown at the time of eruption.

Neck Where the crown and root meet; also known as **cervix.**

Neoplasia A new growth or tumor.

Nerves of the periodontal ligament Provide additional senses to the tooth (eg, pain, pressure, heat, and cold fibers).

Neutral sodium fluoride Typically a 2% sodium fluoride topical solution or thickened gel that is freely soluble in water with a resultant neutral pH. It is one of the most common topical fluoride preparations.

Neutroclusion *See* class I malocclusion.

Newborn gingival cyst Cyst arising from the remnants of dental lamina in newborn animals.

Noble metals Metals used in dentistry because of their stability in the oral cavity and fluids and their lack of corrosion, with consequent reduced risk of contact or allergic reaction to the metals. The seven noble metals are gold, platinum, palladium, iridium, osmium, ruthenium, and rhodium.

Nonprecious metals Nickel- and chrome-based metal alloys.

Nonscreen films Films that do not use intensifying screens, such as intraoral films.

Nonspecific plaque hypothesis States that there is a superinfection of mixed bacterial population that causes periodontitis.

Nonsuccessional (nonsuccedaneous) teeth Permanent teeth (classically molars) that do not succeed a deciduous counterpart.

Nontonsillar squamous cell carcinoma Malignant tumor of squamous epithelium (not tunsillar) that is locally invasive and slow to metastasize.

Normal-fusing alloys Alloys formulated for an all-metal restoration.

Object–film distance (OFD) Distance between the film and the object during radiography. Minimizing OFD can reduce distortion.

Obturation Complete filling or closure of a space, such as the root canal system.

Oblique fibers Alveolodental periodontal ligament fibers that extend from the cementum in a coronal-oblique pattern to the alveolar bone. They resist occlusal stresses.

Obtundent Substance that causes a dulling of the the patient's sensitivity to a stimulus of pain.

Occluding Contacting opposing teeth.

Occlusal Articulating or biting surface; the coronal surface of some premolars and molars.

Occlusal assessment and supervision Includes the supervision of timely primary dental exfoliation and permanent dental eruption.

Occlusal embrasure *See* embrasure.

Occlusal films Intraoral films typically positioned in the occlusal plane of the patient (size 4 film).

Occlusal plane Side view of the occlusal surfaces.

Occlusal relationship Way in which the maxillary and mandibular teeth touch each other.

Occlusal ridge Ridge of the premolars that does not make contact with opposing teeth.

Occlusal stress Pressures on the occlusal surfaces of teeth.

Occlusal surface Surface of a premolar or molar within the marginal ridges that contacts the corresponding surfaces of antagonists during closure of the posterior teeth.

Occlusal table Area bordered by the cusp tips and marginal ridges, as seen from an occlusal view.

Occlusal third That portion of a surface closest to the occlusal surface, from a proximal, lingual, or buccal view of a posterior tooth.

Occlusal trauma Injury caused by one tooth prematurely hitting another during closure of the jaws.

Occlusion   When the teeth of the mandibular arch come into contact with the teeth of the maxillary arch in any functional relationship; relationship of the mandibular and maxillary teeth when they are closed or when there are excursive movements of the mandible.

Odontoblast   Dentin-forming cell that originates from the dental papilla.

Odontoblastic cell layer   Layer in the pulp that is closest to the tubules.

Odontoblastic process   Cellular extension of the odontoblast, located along the full width of the dentin.

Odontogenic cyst or tumors   Lesions arising from cellular components of the developing tooth structure.

Odontoma   Mixed odontogenic tissue tumor containing both epithelial and mesenchymal cells. It may be either compound (disorganized mass) or complex (with denticles).

Odontoplasty   Adjustment of the tooth contours, usually along the cervical bulge.

Oligodontia   Condition in which some teeth are missing.

One-wall defect   Infrabony defect that involves destruction of one osseous wall (facial or lingual) of a two-wall defect with extension to an adjacent tooth.

Onlay   Restoration made to fit over or replace an incisal edge or occlusal cusp either partially or completely.

Opaque   Not easily able to transmit light.

Open bites   When a part or all of the teeth are prevented from closing to normal occlusal contact.

Open contact   Space between adjacent teeth in the same arch; an interproximal opening instead of a contact area where the teeth touch.

Open curettage   Therapy and root planing of an area that has been exposed by a flap for additional visualization.

Operculectomy   Excision of an operculum to allow further eruption and crown exposure.

Operculum   Persistence of a thick, fibrous gingiva over a partially or even fully erupted tooth.

Oral cavity (cavum oris)   Area extending from the lips to the oral pharynx at the level of the palatine tonsil.

Oral cavity proper   Area extending from the alveolar ridge and teeth to the oral pharynx. It does not include the vestibule.

Oral eosinophilic granuloma in dogs   Raised, firm, yellow-brown to pink lesions, somewhat ulcerated, that appear on the lateral margins and frenulum of the tongue in young Siberian huskies. It is possibly inherited.

Oral epithelium   Lining membrane of the oral cavity consisting of stratified squamous epithelium.

Oral mucosa   Stratified squamous epithelium running from the margins of the lips to the area of the tonsils and lining the oral cavity; also known as **oral mucous membrane**.

Oral mucous membrane   *See* oral mucosa.

Oral-oriented   Used to describe individuals that like to make use of their mouth.

Oral papilloma   Benign tumor, caused by a virus in dogs, consisting of multiple pedunculated masses on the oral mucosa.

Organic matrix   Noncalcified framework in which crystals grow.

Ornery   Irritable and undesirable temperament.

Oropharynx   Section between the tonsils and the base of the tongue.

Orthoclusion   *See* class 0 normal.

Orthodontic acrylics   Materials used to form a framework or base structure from which various inclines, springs, arch wires, or expansion devices can be attached.

Orthodontic band   Flattened piece of metal constructed as a ring to fit around the clinical crown of a tooth and be cemented in place.

Orthodontic brackets and tubes   Devices that are attached to base plates or bands and provide attachment for wires, springs, and elastics.

Orthodontic camouflage treatment   Cosmetic treatment of class II or III malocclusions.

Orthodontic elastics   Items used as force for many appliances.

Orthodontic wire   Special type of wire commonly used in a large variety of orthodontic appliances.

Orthodontics   That area of dentistry concerned with the supervision and guidance of the growing dentition and correction of the mature dentofacial structures. It involves those conditions that require movement of teeth and/or correction of malrelationships of the jaws and teeth and malformations of their related structures.

Oscillating angles   Prophylaxis angles that need no lubrication, reducing the throwing of prophylaxis paste, and do not catch patient hair.

Osseoconductive   Characteristic of a product that aids in regenerating new bone in an osseous site. Almost all guided-tissue regeneration-products are osseoconductive.

Osseoinductive   Characteristic of a product that aids in the generation of new bone in any site, even muscle tissue. Autogenous bone grafts and bone morphogenic protein can do this; however, freeze-dried bone and irradiated bone are not osseoinductive because the necessary cells have been killed by treatment of the product.

Osseointergration   Process in which a material's surface becomes attached or bonded to bone; also known as **functional ankylosis**. In the process, metal oxides on the surface of an implant bond to bone.

Osseoproductive   Currently considered an improper and ill-defined term used incorrectly as a substitute for osseopromotive.

Osseopromotive   Characteristic of a product that stimulates the growth of new bone either by osseoconductivity or osseoinductivity.

Osseous wiring   Placement of wires in direct contact with bone to provide reduction and support to segments of a bony fracture.

Ostectomy   Removal of osseous defects and infrabony pockets by the removal of bony pocket walls.

Osteoblasts   Cells that form bone.

Osteoclasts   Multinucleated cells responsible for destroying bone, as well as cementum and dentin.

Osteocytes   Osteoblasts that have surrounded themselves with bone.

Osteoid   Term meaning bone-like.

Osteoplasty   Shaping of bone to restore physiologic contour, without the elimination of walls of a pocket.

Osteosarcoma   Osseous tumor of the mandible or maxilla that is locally invasive but has less metastatic potential than its counterpart in the appendicular skeletal.

Outer enamel epithelium (OEE)   Outer epithelial layer of the enamel organ. It serves as a protection for the developing enamel.

Overbite   Relationship of the teeth in which the incisal ridges of the maxillary anterior teeth extend below the incisal edges of the mandibular anterior teeth when the teeth are placed in a centric occlusal relationship. *See also* overlap, vertical.

Overextension   Excessive filling of the root canal system in the vertical fill dimension.

Overfilling   Excessive filling of the root canal system in any fill dimension.

Overhang   Excess of restoration projecting beyond the confines of a tooth preparation margin, resulting in a projection or shoulder.

Overjet   *See* overlap, horizontal.

Overjut   *See* overlap, horizontal.

Overlap, horizontal (overjet, overjut)   Facial projection of the upper anterior and/or posterior teeth beyond their antagonists in a horizontal direction.

Overlap, vertical (overbite)   Extension of the upper teeth over the lower teeth in a vertical direction when the opposing teeth are in contact in centric occlusion.

Overlay   *See* onlay.

Overlay crowns   *See* partial onlays.

Palatal   Pertaining to the palate or roof of the mouth.

Palatal surface   Lingual (medial) surface of maxillary teeth.

Palate   Roof of the mouth.

Palatine fissures   Fissures in the maxillae caudal to the incisors to allow passage of the palatine vessels.

Palatine raphe   Ridge of masticatory mucosa extending posteriorly from the incisal papilla along a median path of the palate.

Palatine rugae   *See* rugae.

Palatine salivary gland   Serous or mucous glands in the submucosa of the ventral surface of the soft palate.

Palatoschisis   *See* cleft palate.

Palmer notation system   System of coding the teeth using brackets, numbers, and letters.

Papillary gingiva   Gingiva that forms the interdental papillae.

Papillary squamous cell carcinoma   Nontonsillar malignant tumor involving the papillary gingiva in young animals.

Papilloma   *See* oral papilloma

Parakeratinized layer   Stratum corneum in which some cells are dead and some are still alive.

Parakeratinized stratified squamous epithelium   Multilayered epithelium in which top layers of cells are not completely dead.

Paralleling technique   Method of taking radiographs that supposedly gives the most accurate representation of proper tooth dimensions by keeping the film and the object as parallel as possible.

Parotid duct   Duct formed by two to three tributaries from the parotid salivary gland. It opens at the parotid papilla at the level of the distal root of the maxillary 4th premolar.

Parotid papilla   Location of the opening for the parotid duct.

Parotid salivary gland   "V"-shaped serous gland located beneath the ear and behind the posterior border of the mandible and the temporomandibular joint. It has superficial and deep portions. *See also* parotid duct.

Partial anodontia   Condition in which some but not all of the teeth are missing.

Partial crown   Restorative crown that covers only a portion (eg, one-half, three-quarters) of the clinical crown.

Partial inlay crowns   Restorations that cover a portion of the clinical crown, but not a cusp.

Partially rectified current   Electric current used in electrosurgery when bleeding is a problem to coagulate soft tissues for hemostasis. It is also used for electrophoresis treatments.

Partial onlays   Restorations that cover a cusp and only a portion (eg, one-half, three-quarters) of the clinical crown.

Partial veneer crown   *See* partial crown.

Passive eruption   Condition in which the tooth does not move but the gingival attachment moves farther apically.

Paste filler   Instrument used to mechanically push and distribute cements and fillers down into the root canal.

Paste methods of obturation   Various soft or semisolid products that eventually harden, to obturate the root canal.

Pathologic movement   Orthodontic tooth movement that occurs when a heavy force exerted, resulting in necrosis of periodontal tissues on the pressure side and poor to no deposition of bone on the traction side.

Pedicle flap   *See* sliding (pedicle) flap.

Peg tooth   A small tooth with a cone-shaped crown. *See also* microdontia.

Pellicle   A thin film of salivary proteins found on teeth.

Pemphigus vulgaris   An autoimmune disease in which up to 90% of patients have oral lesions frequently at the mucocutaneous junctions, with some mucous membrane ulceration.

Percutaneous skeletal fixation   Use of pins or wires extending from fracture fragments and secured externally with an additional device (eg, rod, acrylic tubing).

Perforation   Producing a hole through the pulp cavity into the oral cavity or the periodontal tissues.

Periapical   Around the tip of a tooth root.

Periapical abscess   Active infection around the root tip or apex, with suppuration.

Periapical cyst   Cystic reaction around the root tip, often developing from epithelial cells from the rests of Malassez.

Periapical film   Intraoral films used to isolate apical regions (sizes 0, 1, and 2).

Periapical granuloma   Granulomatous reaction around the root tip or apex without demonstrable bacteria.

Periapical osteosclerosis   Excessive mineralization of the periapical and periradicular alveolar bone.

Pericoronitis   Inflammation of the gingiva during eruption.

Perikymata   Transverse wave-like lines found on the outer surface of enamel, thought to be external manifestations of the lines or striae of Retzius.

Periodontal   Surrounding a tooth.

Periodontal disease   Inflammation of the gingiva or periodontium, their active recessive alteration, or their alteration state with or without disease.

Periodontal membrane or ligament   Collagen fibers attached to the teeth roots and alveolar bone, serving as an attachment of the tooth to the bone.

Periodontal packs   Adhesive putties applied over periodontal surgery sites.

Periodontal probes   Flat or round-tipped instruments that have various lengths in millimeters marked on them.

Periodontitis   An active disease state of the periodontium.

Periodontium   Supporting tissues surrounding the teeth.

Periosteum   Fibrous and cellular layer covering bones and containing cells that become osteoblasts.

Peripheral odontogenic fibroma   Term used to describe both fibrous and osseous epulides.

Periradicular osteomyelitis   Radiographic osteopenia and expansion effects of the alveolus seen in some cases of chronic pulpal inflammation.

Peritubular dentin   Dentin immediately surrounding the tubule. It is slightly more calcified than the rest of the dentin.

Permanent teeth (dentes permanetes)   Final or lasting set of teeth that are typically of a very durable and lasting nature (opposite of deciduous).

Phenotype   External appearance or performance of an animal.

Phases of periodontal therapy   Include evaluation phase, preliminary phase, phase I (prophylaxis, minor work), phase II (periodontal surgery and endodontics), phase III (final restorations and prosthetics), and phase IV (maintenance)

Philtrum   Small depression at the midline of the upper lip.

Phoenix abscesses   Acute exacerbations of chronic apical periodontitis.

Physiologic mobility   Degree of tooth movement that can be considered normal, limited to the width of the periodontal ligament.

Physiologic movement   Movement in orthodontic treatment that occurs when a light-to-mild force is applied and acts as a stimulus to initiate cellular resorption on the pressure side and deposition of bone on the tension side.

Pica   An intense desire to ingest nonfood items.

Pier   Any abutment other than the terminal abutments.

Piezoelectric   Type of ultrasonic scaler, with a curved linear tip movement, that utilizes the expansion and contraction of quartz crystals to commonly provide frequencies of 20–45 kHz.

Pillars   Folds of tissue appearing in front of and behind the palatine tonsils.

Pin   A metal pin or wire cemented or threaded into the dentin at a preparation site to aid retaining a restoration.

Pin holes   Holes drilled into the dentin for a restorative to be packed into it—or for pins to be inserted into it—to provide retention or resistance for the restorative.

Pin ledging   Ledge on which the pin hole is placed on a tooth preparation.

Piston screw   Device used for the movement of a single tooth.

Piston spring screw   Form of piston screw that, when advanced, has a spring that can maintain a continuous pressure for a movement up to 0.5 mm before requiring readjustment.

Pit   A sharp, pointed depression usually located at the junction of two or more intersecting developmental grooves or at the termination of a single developmental groove.

Pit-and-fissure sealants   Sealants similar to composite resins and available with fluorides that are slowly released in small amounts. When placed on occlusal tables and other high-risk areas, they can provide a temporary barrier to cariogenic influences.

Planes   Reinforcements to the anchorage that allow a part of the resistance to be transferred from the teeth to paradental tissues, such as the palate.

Plaque   Collection of bacteria, salivary glycoproteins, and extracellular polysaccharides that adhere to the tooth surface.

Plasma cell   One of the cells that help produce antibodies.

Pledget   Small pellet of cotton used for carrying a medicament or material into the tooth preparation.

Pleurodont   The feature of having teeth that are not set in sockets but rather grow from pocket on the inside of the jaw. Most lizards and snakes, except agomid, are pleurodonts.

Pluggers   *See* condensers.

Point angle   Angle formed by the junction of three surfaces or walls at a point (eg, the mesiolabioincisal angle).

Polishing   Process of smoothing scaling defects in the enamel or cementum by using a pumice rubbed against the tooth.

Polyether   Rubber impression materials with a shorter working time, good dimensional stability, and less shrinkage compared with polysulfides.

Polyphyodont   The feature of having many sets of teeth that are continually replaced in either a horizontal or vertical manner.

Polysulfide   Rubber impression materials that have good accuracy and a tear resistance of about 700% tensile strain before tearing.

Pontic   Portion of a dental bridge that replaces a missing tooth.

Porcelain   Material used for dental restorations that is a combination of kaolinite, potash, feldspar, quartz, and glass modifiers.

Porcelain fused to metal (PFM)   Cast metal crown to which porcelain is bonded.

Porcelain jacket   Technique in which porcelain is used alone with a metal or glass ceramic substructure.

Position-indicating device (PID)   Cone of the radiographic unit to point the beam source.

Post   Cylindrical metal rod cemented or threaded into the root canal system as a retentive device for a core or post and crown. It can also be a prefabricated part of a post crown.

Post and core   Substructure for a crown that is retained by a post set into the root canal system. It can be a one-piece cast post and core or a post-and-core buildup made from a prefabricated post surrounded at its exposed part by a core built up of a restorative material (eg, amalgam, glass ionomer, composite).

Post crown   Crown retained with a metal post. *See also* dowel crown.

Posterior   Situated toward the back, such as premolars and molars.

Posterior cross-bite   Condition in which the cusps of a posterior tooth (premolar, molar) in one arch exceed the normal cusp relation of those in the opposing arch, buccally or lingually.

Posterior pillars   Folds of tissue behind the tonsil that contain the palatopharyngeus muscle.

Posterior teeth   Teeth of either jaw to the rear of the incisors and canines.

Posteruptive stage   Period of eruption from the time the teeth occlude until they are lost. It is characterized by occlusal wear of teeth and compensating eruption.

Preameloblast   Cell in the intermediate stage between an inner enamel epithelial cell and an ameloblast.

P-reamer   Endodontic instrument used to enlarge the root canal in the coronal third of the canal.

Precious metals   Silver and the seven noble metals.

Preemptive fracture repair   Process of strengthening a weak or thin bony structure to attempt to avoid future fracture.

Preeruptive stage   Period of time when the crown of the tooth is developing.

Prefunctional eruptive stage   *See* eruptive stage.

Preliminary phase therapy   Phase of periodontal treatment emergencies.

Premature contact area   Area where an upper and a lower tooth touch and hit each other before the rest of the teeth occlude together.

Premaxilla   Bony area of the upper jaw that includes the alveolar ridge for the incisors and the area immediately behind it in primates.

Premolars   Permanent teeth that replace the primary molars, designed to help hold and carry, like cuspids, and break food down into smaller pieces, like molars; also known as **bicuspids**.

Preparation margin   *See* cavosurface angle.

Preparation outline   *See* cavity outline.

Prepubertal periodontitis (PP)   Localized or generalized form of periodontitis seen in association with deciduous teeth that can be rapidly progressive.

Pressure side   Direction of tooth movement.

Preventive orthodontics   Evaluation and elimination of conditions that may lead to irregularities in the developing of mature occlusal complex.

Primary attachment epithelium   Remains of reduced enamel epithelium that provide initial attachment of mucosa at the base of gingival sulcus.

Primary cell layer   *See* odontoblastic cell layer.

Primary cleft   Cleft of the primary palate at the junction between the incisal bone and maxilla.

Primary dentin   Dentin formed from the beginning of calcification until tooth eruption.

Primary dentition   Deciduous teeth; also known as first set of teeth, baby teeth, milk teeth.

Primary enamel cuticle   Keratin-like covering on the surface of the enamel. It is the final product of the ameloblast.

Primary palate   Early developing part of the hard palate that comes from the medial nasal process and forms a "V"-shaped wedge of tissue that runs from the incisive foramen forward and laterally between the lateral incisors and canines of the maxilla.

Primary teeth   *See* deciduous teeth.

Primordial cyst   Cyst resulting from the degeneration of the stellate reticulum of the enamel organ, found in place of a tooth.

Procedural canal blockage   Obstruction of a once patent canal, preventing full instrument access to the apical stricture.

Prophylactic odontomy   Removal of disease-prone dental tissue that is then restored to a normal form, in the hope of preventing disease.

Prophylaxis (prophy) angles   Angles commonly used on slow-speed handpieces. The three main types of prophylaxis angles used for polishing are the contra-angle latch type, the right angle snap-on, and the right angle screw-on.

Protectants   Various topically applied medicaments that form a thin coating on the periodontal tissue.

Protrude   *See* protrusion.

Protrusion   Condition in which the teeth are thrust forward too far labially, such as protrusion of the anterior teeth. It also refers to the forward movement of the mandible.

Proximal   Nearest, next, immediately adjacent to distally or mesially.

Proximal contact areas   Proximal areas on a tooth that touch an adjacent tooth on the mesial or distal side.

Proximal surface   Surface of a tooth facing toward an adjoining tooth in the same arch (eg, both mesial and distal surfaces are proximal surfaces).

Pseudopockets   False gingival pockets in which gingival height is increased due to hyperplasia, resulting in deeper "pocket" readings but without attachment loss.

Ptyalism   Excessive salivation.

Pulpal exposure   Unnatural opening of the pulp chamber by pathologic or mechanical means.

Pulpal or pulp horns (horn of pulp)   Extensions of the pulp tissue into a thin point of the pulp chamber in the tooth crown. They contain the fibers of the dental pulp.

Pulpal necrosis   Partial or total pulpal death.

Pulpal wall   Internal wall of a cavity in the horizontal plane.

Pulp canal   Canal in the root of a tooth that leads from the apex to the pulp chamber. Under normal conditions, it contains dental pulp tissue.

Pulp capping   Treatment applied to the pulp to stimulate the formation of reparative dentin.

Pulp cavity   Entire cavity within the tooth, including the root canal, pulp chamber, and horns.

Pulp chamber   Cavity or chamber in the center of the crown of a tooth that normally contains the major portion of the dental pulp. The pulp canals lead into the pulp chambers.

Pulp, dental   Highly vascular and innervated connective tissue contained within the pulp cavity of the tooth. It is composed of arteries, veins, nerves, connective tissues and cells, lymph tissue, and odontoblasts.

Pulpectomy   Extirpation of the entire pulp.

Pulp fluid   Free tissue fluid in the pulp.

Pulpitis   Inflammation of the pulp that may be reversible or irreversible.

Pulpotomy   Surgical removal of a portion of the pulp in a vital tooth.

Pulp stones   Small dentin-like calcifications found in the pulp.

Pyogenic granuloma   Proliferation of the gingival margin that is red and friable, with a granulomatous component.

Quadrants   One-fourth of the dentition. The four quadrants are divided into right and left, maxillary and mandibular.

Rad   Radiation absorbed dose: 100 ergs of energy per gram of absorber; approximately one roentgen.

Radiation biology   Science dealing with the effects of radiation on living tissues.

Radiation exposure   Measurement of ionization in the air produced by gamma and x-radiation to which an individual is exposed.

Radiation fogging   Fogging of the radiographic image due to exposure of the film to radiation other than the useful primary beam, typically from scatter or backscatter.

Radicular ankylosis   Loss of part or all of the periodontal ligament, resulting in fusion of root cementum and socket bone.

Radicular hypsodont   Subdivision of hypsodont dentition, sometimes called closed-root, in which true roots erupt additional crown through most of life. These teeth eventually close their root apices and cease growth. As teeth are worn down, new crown emerges from the reserve or submerged crown of the teeth.

Radicular (root) movements   Occur when the apex of the tooth carries the primary or greatest distance of movement, in comparison with the crown.

Radiographic localization techniques   Three techniques for better distinguishing the position of objects in the image: definition evaluation, right-angle technique, and tube-shift technique.

Ramus of the mandible   Vertical portion of the mandible.

Ranula   Salivary retention cyst (sialocele) located under the tongue, caused by blockage of the sublingual duct or gland.

Rapidly progressive periodontitis (RPP)   A rapidly progressive form of periodontitis seen mostly in young adults, with cyclic episodes of acute infections and quiet periods.

Recession   Migration of the gingival crest in an apical direction, away from the crown of the tooth.

Recessive   An allele that produces an effect on the phenotype only when present in a double dose.

Reciprocal anchorage   When two teeth or tooth groups are moved to a similar extent, either away from or toward each other. To work properly, each group must provide a similar resistance.

Reduced enamel epithelium   Fusion of the ameloblast layer with the outer enamel epithelium.

Reduction angles   Special contra-angles that slow the rotational speed of the attached instrument; also known as **minimizers**.

Refractory rapidly progressive periodontitis (RRPP)   A therapy-resistant periodontitis that may be a subform of RPP. It may be localized or generalized.

Reinforced anchorage (planes and stationary)   Used on occasions when the action of an appliance with simple anchorage will be insufficient to resist the reaction of the movement target.

Releasing flaps   Gingival flaps raised to allow additional tooth root exposure for therapy.

Rem   Roentgen equivalents man: radiation dose expressed by taking into consideration that different types of radiation have different effects on tissue.

Removable appliances   Orthodontic devices designed to be easily and routinely removed, and then reinserted.

Reparative dentin (tertiary dentin)   Localized formation of dentin in response to local trauma, such as occlusal trauma or caries. This type of dentin forms at the tubule access once a dead tract is formed, as well as being formed by differentiated mesenchymal cells that migrate from the cell-rich zone.

Repositioned flap   Gingival flap that is sutured to a level that is different from its original position.

Resorption   Physiologic removal of tissues or body products, as of the roots of deciduous teeth or of some alveolar process after the loss of the permanent teeth.

Restorative margin   Restorative surface that abuts the cavosurface angle or preparation margin.

Restorative pins   Metal pins that can be an extension of a cast restorative or an independent entity that extends into both the tooth and the restoration.

Retainer   Portion of the bridge restoration that rebuilds the prepared abutment and pier teeth.

Retarded eruption   Delayed eruption of teeth from a variety of influences.

Retention stage   Stage of corrective orthodontics during which it is necessary to have the teeth stabilized in their new position to allow a harmonious state to develop.

Rete peg formation   Development of interdigitation between the epithelium and the underlying connective tissue.

Reticulation   Wrinkled appearance on a radiograph that occurs when the film is moved from warm developer to a cold water bath, causing shrinking of the emulsion.

Retroclination   Term sometimes used to describe the condition in which the anterior teeth are tilted lingually. *See also* lingual inclination.

Retromolar pad   Pad of tissue lingual and caudal to the mandibular molars in cats.

Retrusion   Act or process of retracting or moving back, as the mandible is placed in posterior relationship to the maxillae.

Reverse bevel gingivectomy   Procedure to reduce pocket depth by the removal of a portion of the inside layer of the sulcus and margin of the gingiva.

Reversible colloids (agar)   Impression material that, when heated, converts from a gel state to the sol state to obtain an impression and then back to the gel state on cooling, for a stable impression.

Reversible pulpitis   Inflammation of the pulp that can be resolved, returning the pulp to a healthy state.

Ribbon canals   Flat-shaped anomalous configuration of the root canal system.

Ridge   A linear elevation on the surface of a tooth. There are several common types:
    1. **Marginal ridges**   Elevated crests that form the mesial and distal margins of (a) the occlusal surfaces of posterior teeth and (b) the lingual surfaces of anterior teeth.

2. **Triangular ridges** Prominent elevations, triangular in cross-section, that extend from the tip of a cusp toward the central portion of the occlusal surface of a tooth.

3. **Cusp ridges** Elevations that extend in a mesial and distal direction from cusp tips. Cusp ridges form the buccal and lingual margins of the occlusal surfaces of posterior teeth.

4. **Incisal ridge** Incisal portion of a newly erupted anterior tooth.

5. **Oblique ridge** Elevated prominence on the occlusal surfaces of a maxillary molar extending obliquely between the tips of the distobuccal and mesiolingual cusps.

6. **Transverse ridge** Composed of the triangular ridges of a buccal and a lingual cusp that join to form a more or less continuous elevation extending transversely across the occlusal surface of a posterior tooth.

Ridge augmentation Process of strengthening the alveolar ridge with the use of osseo-conductive or -inductive materials.

Right angle technique Radiographic localization technique that uses two films in the occlusal plane: one exposed perpendicular to the film and one exposed at a 90° vertical angulation.

Risdon's interdental wiring technique Involves two sets of primary wires, right and left, that are anchored distally and then twisted as they extend to the symphysis, with secondary wires looped around additional teeth to secure the primary.

Rochette bridge Bridge in which the retainers are perforated at the areas where tooth contact is made, to enhance cementation. The retainers do not normally cover a cusp or incisal edge. These types of bridges generally result in the most conservative amount of natural tooth reduction for abutments and piers. At the same time, there is typically a tradeoff in lost retentive qualities.

Rod core Composed of hydroxyapatite crystals, surrounded by the rod sheath.

Rodent ulcer Ulcerated thickening of the upper lip at midline; a type of eosinophilic granuloma (indolent "not painful" ulcer).

Rod sheath Material surrounding the enamel rod. It is slightly more fibrous than the enamel rod.

Roentgen Unit of exposure dose needed to produce one electrostatic charge in one centimeter of air. It is the most commonly used unit for measuring radiation exposure.

Root That portion of a tooth normally embedded in the alveolar process and covered with cementum.

Root bifurcation That point at which a root trunk divides into two separate branches.

Root canal *See* pulp canal.

Root exposure Uncovering or exposing of root surfaces due to periodontal tissue loss.

Root planing Procedure for smoothing the cementum of the root of a tooth.

Root resection Cutting off of a root, but not its associated portion of crown.

Root trifurcation That point at which a root trunk divides into three separate branches.

Root trunk (base) That portion of a multirooted tooth between the cervical line and bifurcation or trifurcation of the separate roots.

Rotary bur Six-sided, noncutting soft steel bur that utilizes the high-speed handpiece on an air-driven unit and reaches a frequency of about 30 kHz.

Rotation movements Occur when the tooth is rotated on its long axis in one direction or the other.

Rotations Teeth that are turned or rotated; also known as **torsiversion** or **torsoversion**. The direction can be mesiolingual or distolingual.

"Rubber jaw" syndrome Condition in which the jaw structure is soft and flexible due to depletion or loss of calcium.

Rudimentary lobe   Small underdeveloped lobe of a tooth; less than a minor lobe.

Rugae   Small ridges of tissue extending laterally across the anterior of the hard palate.

Rule of dental succession   No successional and deciduous precursor should be erupted simultaneously or in competition for the same dental arcade space at the same time.

Salivary glands   Glandular system secreting saliva, a serous and mucous fluid that assists in the lubrication and digestion of food.

Same—lingual; opposite—buccal   *See* SLOB rule.

Sandwich technique   Technique in which glass ionomers are used as a laminate with composite resins.

Scissors bite   Normal relationship of the maxillary incisors overlapping the mandibular incisors whose incisal edges rest on or near the cingulum on the lingual surfaces on the maxillary incisors.

Sclerotic dentin (transparent dentin)   Condition in which the tubules have been filled in with mineral and material because of damage to the odontoblast.

Secodont   The feature of having cheek teeth with cutting tubercles or cusps arranged to provide a cutting or shearing interaction, such as premolars in most carnivores (eg, dogs, cats), especially the carnassial teeth.

Secondary attachment epithelium   Epithelium of free gingiva that produces mucosal attachment at the base of gingival sulcus.

Secondary cell zone   *See* cell-rich zone,

Secondary cleft   Palatal cleft of the secondary palate (ie, on the midline).

Secondary dentin   Normal physiologic dentin formed throughout the pulp cavity following eruption.

Secondary dentition   Permanent dentition.

Secondary enamel cuticle   Mucopolysaccharide cementing substance secreted by the reduced enamel epithelium that functions by cementing the base of the gingival sulcus to the tooth.

Secondary palate   The portion of the hard palate formed by the right and left palatine bones.

Secondary radiation   Radiation resulting from the primary beam reacting with objects, such as the plastic of a closed cone.

Second-order bends   Bends in orthodontic wire in the vertical plane.

Selenodont dentition   The feature of having cheek teeth with cusps that connect to form a crescentic outline, quarter-moon, or concavoconvex ridge pattern, as in the even-toed hoofed animals (order Artiodactyla), except swine.

Self-rectification   Pattern of a radiographic unit vacuum tube to produce x-radiation only when the filament is the cathode and the target is the anode in an alternating current.

Sensible dentin   Term used to imply that a tooth is vital.

Separating agent   Agent used when waxes, gypsums, or acrylics are to be worked on gypsum models, casts, or dies to prevent the materials from adhering or locking together.

Separation anxiety   Uncomfortable, uneasy, or panicky state of mind resulting from being separated from someone or something. It may result in improper behavior.

Shaft parallelism   Altered angulations of the shaft and handles of Gracey curettes in relation to the working surface of the tooth.

Sharpey's fibers   Part of the periodontal ligament, embedded in cementum or alveolar bone.

Shed   Term used for exfoliation of deciduous teeth.

Shell teeth   A hereditary and/or congenital disorder of teeth in which there is a a crown, but little to no root development.

Short bevel   Bevel involving no more than the external one-third of a cavity wall.

Short-cone technique   Reducing the focal–film distance to an "8-inch cone" to reduce linear distortion, particularly in the bisecting-angle technique.

Shortened teeth   Teeth that are lower in the occlusal plane than expected. This encompasses infraclusion, infraversion, and variations such as infralinguoclusion (base narrow and retarded height).

Short palate   Palate of insufficient length to meet the back wall of the throat.

Shoulder   Gingival wall of the extracoronal section of the cavity preparation placed at right angles to the long axis of the tooth.

Sialocele   Retention cyst of salivary fluids.

Sialolith   Salivary stone: calcifications found in salivary glands or ducts.

Sickle scaler   Instrument used for the removal of supragingival calculus.

Sight development   Development by observation, through the safe-light transparent top of a developer box, that the film image has emerged with no specific predetermined time.

Silicon carbide   Type of abrasive point that helps remove rough, bulky areas of a restorative; also known as green stones.

Silicone rubber   Elastomer with significant shrinkage, requiring special custom trays, a short working time, and a completely dry preparation area; otherwise, its physical properties will be altered.

Siloxane polymers   Used to provide accurate detailing for crown and bridge impressions. Lack of flowability of dental stone into the impression can be a problem.

Silver points   Cones of silver metal used as endodontic obturation core fill.

Simple anchorage   When a greater tooth resistance to movement is used in association with an appliance than that of the target of movement in the same dental arch.

Simplicidentata   Simple dentition.

Single-cone method   Obturation method performed in one of two ways: custom-instrument the canal to fit a specific size of prefabricated cone or custom-fabricate a cone to fit the canal.

Single root   Root with one main branch.

Sintering   The actual fusing of the porcelain powders into a single solid structure.

Sliding (pedicle) flap   Flap or graft of attached gingiva harvested from a site adjacent to the defect and rotated on its base to cover the defect.

SLOB rule   Same—lingual; opposite—buccal: tube-shift technique of taking a second radiograph with an adjustment in the horizontal angulation. If the angulation is adjusted caudally, the lingual object "shifts" in the same direction, toward the tube head.

Slot of Matzuri   Type of modified cavity preparation used in retrograde fillings.

Slow-speed handpieces   Dental handpieces with lower speed but high tactile sense. These handpieces are useful for finishing, polishing, certain pin placements, and laboratory procedures.

Smooth tongue   Genetic defect in some cattle breeds that results in a tongue without normal rough texture, which may cause difficulty in eating and resultant increased salivation.

Sodium monofluorophosphate (MFP)   Relatively stable inorganic salt that allows its combining with dentifrices and other compounds that have long shelf lives.

Soft palate   Unsupported soft tissue that extends back from the hard palate free of the support of the palatine bone.

Soft tissue   Noncalcified tissues, such as nerves, arteries, veins, and connective tissue.

Soft waves   One of the four basic categories of radiation wavelengths used for radiographs of thin tissue sections for research.

Sol   Form of hydrocolloid derived when water is first added to alginates or agars and heated and the material takes on a fluid state with low viscosity.

Sonic (subsonic) scalers   Scalers that operate by compressed gas or air pressure creating an oval–elliptical tip oscillation generally at much less than 20 kHz.

Space control   Includes treatment of traumatic, congenital, or hereditary anomalies, as well as dentally destructive diseases, and maintenance of dentally voided spaces.

Span   Portion of the bridge suspended between the abutments.

Specialized mucosa   Mucosa found on the top, or dorsum, of the tongue that includes the papillae and taste buds.

Specific plaque hypothesis   States that periodontitis is caused by specific strains of bacteria (only in certain forms of periodontitis).

Spillway   *See* embrasure.

Splint appliance   Orthodontic device used to stabilize mobile teeth in periodontal disease or fracture fragments.

Spreaders   Tapered metal instruments with a point, used to laterally condense filling material against the canal walls.

Spring bridge   *See* spring cantilever bridge.

Spring cantilever bridge   One-piece bridge in which the pontic is remotely attached to the retainer by a spring or bar; also known simply as a **spring bridge.**   This type of arrangement permits natural-appearing open contacts both mesially and distally to the pontic.

Squamous cell carcinoma (SCC)   Malignant tumor of the squamous epithelium. Most common malignancy in cats (second most common in dogs) having a variable presentation on the mucosa, gingiva (nontonsillar SCC), or tonsils (tonsillar SCC).

Stabilized chlorine dioxide   Chemical used in various products to reduce odor.

Standard type I gutta-percha points   Correspond to the sizes of standard endodontic instruments; also known as **primary** or **master points.**

Stannous fluoride   Tin–fluoride compound (SnF_2) with an acidic pH that exerts a mild antimicrobial effect.

Static occlusion   Relationship of the teeth when the jaws are closed in centric occlusion.

Stationary reinforcement   Use of fixed anchorage attachment that is designed so that only bodily movement of the anchorage teeth can occur.

Stellate reticulum   Ectodermal- and epithelial-derived middle layer of the enamel organ. It serves as a cushion for the developing enamel.

Stem-winding instrumentation   When an endodontic file is worked in a clockwise–counterclockwise rotation.

Sticky wax   Used to temporarily stick or fix various metallic, resin, or wax assembly parts of dental appliances to stone or plaster dental models.

Stillman cleft   Periodontal recession starting with the formation of a small groove.

Stipple   Pattern imprinted on the lead backing of an intraoral film.

Stippling   Image of the imprinted pattern on the lead backing of an intraoral film when the film has been placed incorrectly (lead toward tube head) in the mouth.

Stomatitis   Inflammation of the soft tissues of the oral cavity or mouth.

Stomodeum   Depression in the facial region of the embryo that is the beginning of the oral cavity; the primitive mouth.

Stout's multiple loop interdental wiring   Variation of the Ivy loop incorporating multiple teeth with a static wire that lays against the tooth and a working wire that is passed back and forth in the interdental spaces to secure the static wire.

Straight handpiece   Handpiece used in standard dental procedures that usually generates 6000 rpm.

Strategic teeth   Teeth that may be important to the animal's well-being, usually the cuspids and the carnassials.

Striae of Retzius   Incremental growth lines seen in microscopic sections of enamel.

Strict anaerobic bacteria   Live in a relatively oxygen-free environment.

Stripping, endodontic   Thinning of a lateral root canal wall, usually in the direction of the root tip curvature.

Stripping, operative   Process of reducing the interproximal contacts using various abrasive strips or thin-fluted burs.

Subgingival calculus scaling   Removal of subgingival deposits of calculus.

Subgingival curettage   Removal of diseased soft tissue within a periodontal pocket.

Subgingival debridement   Moderate scaling or gentle root planing and soft tissue debridement of subgingival areas.

Sublingual caruncle   Small elevation of soft tissue at the base of the lingual frenum that is the opening for the mandibular duct.

Sublingual fold   Fold of tissue extending backward on either side of the floor of the mouth. The duct of the mandibular gland lies below it.

Sublingual fossa   Depression for the sublingual gland on the medial surface of the mandible above the mylohyoid line in the canine region.

Sublingual salivary gland   Smaller of the major salivary gland pairs; monostomatic portion lies within the mandibular gland; major sublingual duct to sublingual caruncle (or near); polystomatic portion of 6–12 small scattered lobules of sublingual salivary tissue; several minor sublingual ducts into lateral sublingual recess.

Subluxation   Incomplete dislocation of a joint, such as the temporomandibular joint or a tooth.

Submandibular   Referring to the region below the mandible; a group of lymph nodes around the submandibular gland.

Submerged teeth   Teeth covered by bone.

Successional lamina   Lingual extensions developed during primary dentition from the dental lamina buds.

Successional (succedaneous) teeth   Permanent teeth that replace or succeed a deciduous counterpart, typically certain diphyodont incisors, cuspids, or premolars.

Sudden localized biting force   Force exerted on the few millimeters of tooth cusp contact with an abrupt closing or snapping of the jaws.

Sulcus   Elongated valley in the surface of a tooth formed by the inclines of adjacent cusps or ridges that meet at an angle.

Sulcus irrigation or lavage   Flushing debris from the sulcus or pocket with a liquid (eg, water, saline, 0.2% chlorhexidine, etc.).

Supereruption   Condition in which teeth have the cementoenamel junction erupted above normal. It may be be either supraclusion or supraversion.

Supernumerary roots   Those roots beyond the normal complement of a tooth.

Supernumerary teeth   Those beyond the normal complement (extra).

Supplemental canal   *See* accessory root canals.

Supplemental groove   Shallow linear groove in the enamel of a tooth. It differs from a developmental groove in that it does not mark the junction of lobes; it is a secondary, or smaller, groove.

Suprabony pocket   Periodontal pocket with its base, or bottom, coronal to the alveolar crestal bone.

Supraclusion Condition in which the teeth are above their appropriate occlusal level.

Supraeruption Eruption of a tooth beyond the occlusal plane.

Supraversion Condition in which a tooth is supererupted and in its proper position in the dental arch, but may have some degree of tilt, allowing passage beyond the teeth in the opposing dental arch.

Surfaces The sides and the top of a tooth.

Systemic lupus erythematosus (SLE) An autoimmune disease that may have oral painful lesions of shallow areas of ulceration with erythematous margins.

Taste buds Small pear-shaped structures in vallate, fungiform, and foliate papillae (gustatory) that detect taste.

Taurodontia Condition in which the crown and pulp chamber are enlarged and the root is typically small.

Telescoping hypocalcification Defect in teeth showing striated gradation of enamel hypocalcification lesions circling the tooth.

Temperament Personality of an individual.

Temporalis muscle Muscle of mastication arising from the temporal fossa and inserting on the coronoid process of the mandible to close the mandible.

Temporary bridge Bridge constructed and placed on the prepared site for protection of the preparation and/or for esthetics purposes, until the permanent bridge can be fabricated and placed.

Temporary Teeth Dentes temporaui, considered to be the first set of temporary teeth that are shed at some point and replaced by permanent teeth.

Temporomandibular joint Joint composed of the condylar process of the vertical ramus of the mandible and the mandibular fossa of the temporal bone of the skull.

Temporomandibular ligament Thickened part of the temporomandibular joint capsule on the lateral side.

Tension side Side away from the direction of tooth movement.

Tertiary dentin *See* reparative dentin.

Thecodont The feature of having teeth that are firmly set in sockets, typically using gomphosis, as in dogs, cats, and humans.

Theory of bone deposition in the alveolar crypt Eruption theory that bone deposition in the alveolar crypt forces the tooth to erupt.

Theory of growth of pulpal tissue Eruption theory that continued growth of the pulpal tissue propels the tooth.

Theory of periodontal ligament force Eruption theory that the periodontal ligament's force for occlusal maintenance also contributes to eruption.

Theory of root growth Eruption theory that root growth pushes the crown into the oral cavity.

Thermal tests Diagnostic means by which to assess the sensitivity or vitality of pulpal tissue in intact teeth.

Thermomechanical compaction Method of thermoplasticizing gutta-percha during obturation involving use of a compactor instrument on a slow-speed handpiece.

Thermoplasticizing Method involving the heating of gutta-percha to soften it and to improve the quality of obturation.

Third-order bends Bends in orthodontic wire that produce a torque force.

Thirds Imaginary divisions of a tooth crown or root as to length (eg, occlusal, middle, and gingival thirds) or mesiodistal breadth (eg, mesial, middle, and distal thirds).

Three-quarter crown *See* partial crown.

Three-wall defect   An infrabony pocket of one root in which the root forms one wall of the defect and three osseous surfaces.

Thunderstorm anxiety   Uncomfortable, uneasy, or panicky state of mind resulting from the proximity of thunderstorms.

Tight-lip syndrome   Condition in which the lower lip has a deficient vestibule, causing the lip to ride over the mandibular incisors and even canines. It is most commonly seen in the Shar-Pei dog.

Time/temperature development   Radiographic film-developing technique using the manufacturer's recommendations for a specific film and type of developer at time intervals based on the temperature of the solution.

Tipping   Condition in which the crown of a tooth is tipped or inclined; also called **inclinations** or **versions.**

Tipping movements   *See* tipping.

Tomes process (Tomes fibers)   *See* odontoblastic process.

Tongue   A mobile prehensile structure of the oral cavity used for grooming and intake of food and fluids.

Tongue-tie (tongue-tied)   Condition in which the lingual frenum is short and attached to the tip of the tongue. In animals with continually erupting or growing teeth, it is the condition in which the teeth pin the tongue to the roof or floor of the mouth.

Tonsillar squamous cell carcinoma (SCC)   Most aggressive form of SCC with high rate of early metastasis.

Tooth bud   *See* tooth germ.

Tooth discoloration   Can be caused by intrinsic or extrinsic effects, such as devitalization, tetracycline staining, or metal impregnation.

Tooth eruption   Emergence and movement of the crown of the tooth into the oral cavity.

Tooth germ   Soft tissue that develops into a tooth.

Tooth migration   Movement of a tooth through the bone and gum tissue.

Tooth resection   Cutting off of a portion of the crown with or without its associated root structure.

Torsiversion   *See* rotations.

Torsoversion   *See* rotations.

Toxic epidermal necrolysis   An extreme drug eruption with edema and massive tissue destruction and necrosis, including severe ulceration and hemorrhage.

Trabeculae   Interlacing meshwork that makes up the cancellous bony framework.

Tranquilize   To relax or decrease physical or emotional status.

Transcircumferential wiring   Single-wire technique that involves both a transosseous anchorage and circumferential placement around the rest of the bone.

Transillumination   Assessment of the reflectivity of the internal tooth structure to evaluate vitality of the pulp by placing a light behind a tooth and viewing it.

Translation or bodily movement   When the crown and apex of a tooth both travel in the same direction.

Transmissible veneral tumor (TVT)   Sexually transmitted lesion that can involve oral cavity, often appearing red with a raised hyperemic border. Most regress spontaneously.

Transosseous wiring   Placing wire(s) across a fracture line to incorporate the fragments for stabilization.

Transparent dentin   *See* sclerotic dentin.

Transposition   Condition in which two teeth have exchanged places during the development of the occlusion.

Transseptal fibers   Periodontal fibers that extend from the cementum of one tooth across the interproximal area to the cementum of the adjacent tooth.

Trench mouth   *See* Vincent's stomatitis

Trifurcation   Division of three tooth roots at their point of junction with the root trunk.

Trigeminal nerve   Cranial nerve V that innervates many of the muscles of mastication.

Trituration   Mixing or amalgamating of dry dental alloys and mercury into an amalgamated mass, or amalgam.

Trough   In reference to x-radiation waves, the depth of the wave.

True temporomandibular joint ankylosis   Inhibited jaw movement due to a bony union across the temporomandibular joint surface.

Tubercle   A slightly rounded elevation on the surface of a tooth (eg, lingual tubercle of the maxillary anterior teeth).

Tube-shift technique   Localization technique in which the horizontal angulation of a second radiographic film is taken to separate the images of two overlapping objects. *See also* SLOB rule.

Twinning disorder   Condition in which there has been a complete cleavage of the splitting gemination bud, with the extra tooth being a mirror image of the original, not a separate tooth bud.

Two-wall defect   An infrabony pocket that extends interdentally to communicate with the root of an adjacent tooth, with two osseous walls (facial and lingual).

Type II dental plaster   Produced by baking gypsum in open air to 110–120°C; also known as **beta-calcium sulfate hemihydrate.**

Type II gutta-percha points   Points with a taper similar to endodontic spreaders that are used as accessory points in lateral compaction; also called **conventional points.**

Type III unimproved dental stone   Developed by heating gypsum to 125°C under pressure and in the presence of water vapor; also known as **alpha-calcium sulfate hemihydrate.**

Type IV improved dental stone   Produced by removing the crystallization water with boiling in a 30% calcium chloride solution, with the chlorides then removed by washing in 100°C water. This is the most dense of the four types of dental gypsums and is usually referred to as high-strength dental stone.

Ulceromembranous stomatitis   Necrotizing ulcerative gingivitis.

Ultrasonic dental scalers   Dental scaling instruments functioning at greater than 20 kHz. These instruments work by two basic principles: mechanical kick and cavitation. Mechanical kick is the actual effect of the metal tip's contacting the calculus, while the water spray hitting the vibrating tip is energized to cavitate or clean the tooth surface.

Ultraviolet radiation   One of the wavelengths in the electromagnetic spectrum; found in sunlight and produced by sunlamps.

Underbite   A loose term generally applied to certain divisions of class I and III malocclusions, but most typically to class III malocclusions.

Undercut   A designed feature of a restorative preparation created by removing a portion of the dentin within the preparation to retentive qualities to a restoration.

Underextension   Too little filling in the vertical fill dimension of root canal obturation.

Underfilling   Too little filling in any dimension of root canal obturation.

Unfavorable fracture   Mandibular fracture running caudoventrally, with muscular forces being able to distract the segments.

United epithelium   Joining of the reduced enamel epithelium with the oral epithelium.

Universal curettes   Curettes that generally have two cutting blades and a 90° angulation to the shaft, although some have an 80° blade angle.

Universal system (universal code)   System of coding teeth using the numbers 1 to 32 for permanent teeth and the letters A to T for the deciduous teeth.

Utility wax   Wax having a variety of uses, most commonly used for increasing impression tray height.

Vallate papillae   A small number (3–6) of papillae found at the posterior border of the tongue where the conical papillae begin.

Varnish   Protective material that keeps chemical irritants from the pulp, as well as providing marginal seals to reduce microleakage.

Veneer   A thin restorative covering, generally used to conceal a discoloration, malformation, attritional wear, or other minor injury. It is typically made from acrylic, resin, glass, or porcelain but may be made from metal as either a restoration in itself or as an abutment for a bridge.

Venturi effect   Frictional vacuum effect caused by the rapid movement of a gas or liquid.

Vermillion zone   Red part of the lip, where the lip mucosa meets the skin.

Versions   Condition in which there is malposition of one or more teeth without bodily displacement.

Vertical angulation   Degree of angulation above or below the neutral line (a line perpendicular to the long axis of the tooth).

Vertical compaction   Root canal obturation using pluggers to press the fill material in an apical direction.

Vertical overlap   *See* overbite.

Vertical releasing incisions   Incisions made at the mesial and distal aspects of the horizontal releasing incision for a full releasing flap.

Vestibule   Space between the lips or cheeks and the teeth.

Vincent's stomatitis   Stomatitis that occurs when spirochetes and fusiform bacteria contribute to an opportunistic infection, often due to poor oral hygiene.

Viscosity   Characteristic of a fluid substance marked by variable degrees of thickness.

Vomer   Bone that forms the lower part of the nasal septum.

Von Willebrand's disease   Hereditary blood coagulation defect resulting in a bleeding disorder.

Wall   An enclosing side of a prepared cavity or of an infrabony defect.

Wavelength   In reference to x-radiation, the distance from the crest of one wave to the next, abbreviated with the Greek letter lambda (λ).

Wedge   Wedge-shaped device that pushes the matrix band tightly against the cervical part of the tooth.

Wedging   Placing and adapting of a small wedge-shaped object on the side of the matrix opposite the tooth with the cavity preparation to stabilize and adapt the matrix during the condensation of the plastic restorative material.

White stone   Type of abrasive point consisting of a dense, micrograined aluminum oxide bonded to a shape and then mounted on a mandrel.

Wolff's law of transformation of bone   "The law of transformation of bone is to be understood as that law under which, as a result of primary alteration in the form and function or of function alone of bone, there follow certain definite changes, determined by mathematical laws, in its inner architecture and as certainly according to the same laws of mathematics, secondary changes in its external form."

Woody tongue   Diffuse abscesses in the tongue in ruminants, caused by *Actinobacillus lignieresii*, in which there is proliferation of the connective tissue, making the tongue thick and stiff.

Wool sucking   An oral orientation to suck on certain types wool or wool-type materials. It is seen especially in cats.

Working time   Time from completion of mixing a material until its setting reaction begins.

Wry mouth   Condition in which one of the four jaw quadrants is grossly out of proportion to the other three, causing a facial deviation from the midline.

X-rays   A form of wave energy in the electromagnetic spectrum that can be directed and energized by frequency or wavelength to penetrate through opaque tissues or structures and effect a photographic emulsion on an acetate film.

Zinc ascorbate   Solutions that have been shown to support collagen synthesis and generally reduce bad breath for a short period of time.

Zinc oxide–eugenol (ZOE) materials   Used for obtaining impressions over large edentulous areas.

Zipping   Transportation or transposition of the apical portion of the canal; also called **elliptication.**

Zygomatic arch   Arch of bone on the side of the face or skull formed by the zygomatic bone and temporal bone.

Zygomatic bone   Bone that forms the cheek area.

Zygomatic salivary gland   Glands ventral to the rostral end of the zygomatic arch, of which there may be one major pair and up to four minor ducts to the zygomatic papilla; formerly known as the orbital gland.

Abbreviations, Dental and Oral Indices, International System of Units, Conversion Tables, and American National Standard and American Dental Association Specifications

ABBREVIATIONS

General Dental Abbreviations

A	Apical
B	Buccal
C	Coronal or cuspid (canine)
D	Distal
F	Facial
I	Incisal or incisor
L	Lingual
M	Mesial
M	Molar
O	Occlusal
OS	Occlusal survey
PM	Premolar
RAD	Radiograph
TMJ	Temporomandibular joint
TN	Treatment needed
TP	Treatment plan

Pathology

AB	Abrasion
AT	Attrition
BE	Biopsy, excisional
BI	Biopsy, incisional
BG	Buccal granuloma
CAL	Calculus
CI	Calculus index
CMO	Craniomandibular osteopathy
CWD	Crowding
2D	Secondary dentin
DLC	Dilacerated crown
DTC	Dentigerous Cyst
DR	Dilacerated root

ED		Enamel defect
EG		Eosinophilic granuloma
EGC		EG lip/cheilitis (lip)
EGL		EG lingual/tongue
EH		Enamel hypocalcification/hypoplasia
EP		Epulis
	EP/B	Epulis, basal cell carcinoma (acanthomatous)
	EP/F	Epulis, fibrous
	EP/G	Epulis, giant cell
	EP/O	Epulis, ossifying
FB		Foreign body
FEN		Fenestration
FX		Fracture (tooth, jaw, etc.)
GCF		Gingival crevicular fluid
GLS		Glossitis
GM		Glossal mass
HT		Hairy tongue
LFD		Lip-fold dermatitis
LG		Lingual granuloma
LUP		Lupus erythematosus
M0		Normal or no tooth mobility
M1		Slight tooth mobility
M2		Moderate tooth mobility
M3		Severe tooth mobility
MN/FX		Mandible fracture
MX/FX		Maxillary fracture
O		Circle around missing tooth on chart
OM		Oral mass
	OM/ADC	Oral mass, adenocarcinoma
	OM/FS	Oral mass, fibrosarcoma
	OM/LS	Oral mass, lymphosarcoma
	OM/MM	Oral mass, malignant melanoma
	OM/OSC	Oral mass osteosarcoma
	OM/SCC	Oral mass, squamous cell carcinoma
OST		Osteomyelitis
PAP		Papillomatosis
PD		Palatal defect
PEM		Pemphigus
	PEM/B	Bullous pemphigus
	PEM/V	Pemphigus vulgaris
PI		Plaque index
PLQ		Plaque
PT		Palatal trauma defect
RD		Retained deciduous
SAL		Salivary gland
	SM	Mandibular salivary gland
	SMo	Molar salivary gland
	SP	Parotid salivary gland
	SS	Sublingual salivary gland

	SZ	Zygomatic salivary gland
SL		Sublingual
SLG		Sublingual granuloma
SN		Supernumerary
STM		Stomatitis
SYM		Symphysis
SYM/S		Symphysis separation
TA		Tooth avulsed
TL		Tooth luxated
TMJ		Temporomandibular joint
	TMJ/DL	TMJ dislocation
	TMJ/DP	TMJ dysplasia
	TMJ/FX	TMJ fracture
	TMJ/L	TMJ luxation
VWD		von Willebrand disease

Periodontics

AL		Attachment loss
AP		Alveoloplasty
BG		Bone graft
BL		Bone recession (or bone loss, osseous recession, attachment recession)
CAL		Calculus
CI		Calculus index
	CI0	No calculus
	CI1	Supragingival calculus extending only slightly below free gingival margin
	CI2	Moderate amount of supra- and subgingival calculus or subgingival calculus only
	CI3	Abundance of supra- or subgingival calculus
CT		Citric acid treatment
CU		Contact ulcer ("kissing" ulcer)
FAR		Flap, apically repositioned
FCR		Flap, coronally repositioned
FE		Furcation exposure
	F1	Furcation exposed (eg, F1-F = Furcation exposure, exposed, facial entry)
	F2	Furcation undermined (eg, F2-M = Furcation exposure, undermined, mesial entry)
	F3	Furcation open through to other side
	Furcation subclass (vertical bone loss)	
	A	<25% (eg, F3FA: through exposure, facial, <25%)
	B	25–50%
	C	>50%
FG		Fluoride gel
FGG		Flap, free gingival graft
FLS		Flap, lateral sliding

FRB		Flap, reverse bevel
FRE		Frenectomy
FRN		Frenotomy
FV		Fluoride varnish
GCF		Gingival crevicular fluid
GH		Gingival hyperplasia/hypertrophy
GI		Gingivitis index
	GI0	Normal gingiva
	GI1	Mild inflammation, slight change in color, slight edema, no bleeding on probing
	GI2	Moderate inflammation; redness, edema and glazing; bleeding on probing
	GI3	Severe inflammation; marked redness, edema, ulceration; tendency to spontaneous bleeding
GM		Gingival margin
GP/GV		Gingivoplasty; gingivectomy
GR		Gingival recession
GTR		Guided tissue regeneration
IMP		Implant
LPS		Lymphocytic plasmocytic stomatitis
MGM		Mucogingival margin
MM		Mucous membrane
OAF		Oroantral fistula
ONF		Oronasal fistula
OP		Odontoplasty
P7		Periodontal pocket 7 mm deep, etc.
PDI		Periodontal disease index
	PD1	0% Attachment Loss (AL) (gingivitis only)
	PD2	<25% AL
	PD3	25–50% AL
	PD4	>50% AL
PDL		Periodontal ligament
PG		Periodonatl pocket, gingival (pseudopocket)
PI		Plaque index
	PI0	No plaque
	PI1	Thin film along gingival margin
	PI2	Moderate accumulation, plaque in sulcus
	PI3	Abundant soft material in sulcus
PLQ		Plaque
PP		Periodontal pocket
	PIB	Periodontal pocket, infrabony
	PSB	Periodontal pocket, suprabony
PRO		Complete prophylaxis, including scaling (supra- and subgingival), polishing, sulcus irrigation, and fluoride treatment
PS		Periodontal surgery
RE		Root exposure
RP		Root planing
RPC		root planing, closed
RPO		root planing, open

SBI	Sulcus bleeding index (0,1,2,3,4,5)
SC	Subgingival curettage
SPL	Splint
SUL	Sulcus
TP	Treatment planning
W1	Periodontal bony pocket, one wall
W2	Periodontal bony pocket, two wall
W3	Periodontal bony pocket, three wall
W4/CUP	Periodontal bony pocket, four wall; cup lesion

Restorative

BP	Bridge pontic
BR	Bridge
BRC	Bridge, cantilever
BRM	Bridge, Maryland
C1N	Class 1 pulp exposure, nonvital
C1V	Class 1 pulp exposure, vital
CA	Cavity, fracture, or defect
C1	Occlusal or pit and fissure; molars, premolars, cingulum, incisors, premolars, molars
C2	mesio-occlusodistal, mesio-occlusal, occlusodistal; molars premolars
C3	Mesial or distal; incisor no ridge
C4	Mesioincisodistal, mesioincisal, incisodistal; incisor with ridge
C5	Lingual or Facial, cementoenamel junction, no pit and fissure
C6	Cusp
C7	Root
C8	Root apex
CBU	Core buildup
CM	Crown, metal (CMG = gold; CMB = base metal, etc.)
C/MOD	Cavity, mesio-occlusodistal surface
CR	Crown (see also General above)
DB	Dentinal-bonding agent
IL	Inlay
OL	Onlay
P&F	Pit and fissure
P&FS	Pit and fissure sealer
PFM	Crown, porcelain fused to metal
R	Restoration
R/A	Restoration, amalgam
R/C	Restoration, composite
R/I	Restoration, glass ionomer
RL	Resorptive lesion (cervical line lesion)
	RL1	Into enamel only
	RL2	Into enamel and dentin

	RL3	Into root canal system
	RL4	Into root canal system, with extensive structural damage
	RL5	Crown lost, root tips remain
RR		Root resorption
SE		Staining, extrinsic (Metal, etc.)
SI		Staining, intrinsic (blood, tetracycline, etc.)
VBL/NVBL		Vital/nonvital bleaching
VER		Veneer

Endodontics

APG		Apexigenesis
APX		Apexification
AS		Apical sealer cement
CAM		Crown amputation, reduction
FX		Fractured tooth
GP		Gutta-percha
NE		Near exposure
NV		Nonvital
PC		Pulp capping
	PCD	pulp capping, direct
	PCI	pulp capping, indirect
PE		Pulp exposure
RC		Root canal therapy
RCS		Root canal, surgical (apicoectomy)
RGF		Retrograde filling (RGF/A = amalgam, etc.)
RRX		Root resection (hemisection)
TP		Treatment planning
TRX		Tooth resection (hemisection)
VP		Vital pulpotomy
VT		Vital tooth or pulp
ZOE		Zinc oxide–eugenol combination

Oral Surgery

ACY	Acrylic
BE	Biopsy, excisional
BFR	Buccal fold removal
BI	Biopsy, incisional
CFL	Cleft lip
CFP	Cleft palate
CFP/R	Cleft palate repair
DT/D	Deciduous tooth
EP	Epulis (see Oral above)
FR-P/PL/S	Fracture repair pin/ plate/ splint/ screw (SC)/ wire (W)
FX	Fractured tooth
IO	Interceptive orthodontics (see Orthodontics below)
OI	Osseous implant

OM		Oral mass (see Pathology above)
ONF		Oronasal fistula
ONF/R		Oronasal fistula, repair or restore
PLT		Palate
PT/P		Permanent tooth
RD		Retained deciduous tooth
RR		Retained root
SM		Surgery, mandibulectomy
SO		Surgical orthopedics
SP		Surgery, palate
SX		Surgery, maxillectomy
WIR		Wire, wiring
	CFW	Circumferential wiring
	IDW	Interdental wiring
	OSW	Osseus wiring
X		Simple extraction
XS		Extraction with sectioning of tooth
XSS		Surgical extraction

Orthodontics

AXB		Anterior cross-bite
BKT		Bracket
EC		Elastic chain (power chain)
EXT		Extrusion
IM		Impressions/models (orthodontic or restorative)
INT		Intrusion
IO		Interceptive orthodontics
	IOD	Interceptive orthodontics, deciduous tooth
	IOP	Interceptive orthodontics, permanent tooth
MAL		Malocclusion (modified Angle classification)
	MAL1	Cross-bite
	MAL2	Brachygnathism
	MAL3	Prognathism
OA		Orthodontic appliance
	OAA	OA, adjust
	OAI	OA, install
	OAR	OA, remove
OC		Orthodontic consultation (genetic counseling)
OR		Orthodontic recheck
PXB		Posterior cross-bite
ROT		Rotation
T		Bracket marked on chart
TIP		Tipping
TRANS		Body movement or translation
WRY		Wry mouth

Miscellaneous

CS	Culture/sensitivity
CUL	Culture

General Term Abbreviations (2)

AC, ac	Alternating current
ACS	American Chemical Society
ADA	American Dental Association
ANSC	American National Standards Committee
ASTM	American Society for Testing and Materials
AVD	Academy of Veterinary Dentistry
AVDC	American Veterinary Dental College
AVDS	American Veterinary Dental Society
Bis-GMA	Bisphenol A-glycidyl methacrylate
CDMIE	Council on Dental Materials, Instruments, and Equipment
CP	Chemically pure
DC, dc	Direct current
DMG	Dental materials group
EBA	Ethoxybenzoic acid
EDTA	Ethylenediaminetetraacetic acid
FDA	Food and Drug Administration
HEPA	High-efficiency particulate air
IADR	International Association for Dental Research
ISO	International Standardization Organization
JVD	Journal of Veterinary Dentistry
OSHA	Occupational Safety and Health Administration
RHN	Rockwell hardness number
UL	Underwriters Laboratories
USASI	United States of America Standards Institute
USP	United States Pharmacopoeia

Weights, Measurements, and Symbols Abbreviations (2)

Å	Angstrom unit (10^{-8} cm)
avdp	Avoirdupois
BW	Body weight
cm	Centimeter
dB	Decibel
º	Degree
ºC	Degrees centigrade (Celsius)
ºF	Degrees Fahrenheit
g	Gram
gal	Gallon
GHz	Gigahertz
h	Hour
Hz	Hertz

id	inside diameter
in	Inch
kg	Kilogram
kV	Kilovolt
kVp	Kilovolt peak
max	Maximum
m	Meter
mm	Micrometer
mg	Milligram
min	Minimum
MHz	Megahertz
mL	Milliliter
mm	Millimeter
MN	Meganewton
MPa	Megapascal
nm	Nanometer
od	Outside diameter
oz	Ounce
Pa	Pascal
ppm	Parts per million
psi	pounds per square inch
R	roentgen
rpm	revolutions per minute
rps	revolutions per second
s	second
SI	Systeme Internationale d'Unites (modern metric system)
sq	square
sq cm (cm2)	Square centimeter
V	Volt
wt	Weight

DENTAL AND ORAL INDICES

There are hundreds of indices described throughout dental literature, each having advantages and disadvantages. The following indices offer reasonable and practical tools for clinical assessment and treatment planning. However, they are not necessarily appropriate in all cases or for many research protocols.

Plaque Index (PI) (Silness and Loe) (3)

0	No plaque
1	Thin film along gingival margin
2	Moderate accumulation, plaque in sulcus
3	Abundant soft material in sulcus

Gingival Index (GI) (Loe and Silness) (4)

0	Normal gingiva
1	Mild inflammation, slight change in color, slight edema, no bleeding on probing
2	Moderate inflammation; redness, edema, and glazing; bleeding on probing
3	Severe inflammation

Sulcus Bleeding Index (SBI) (Muhlemann) (5)

0	Healthy appearance, no bleeding on sulcus probing
1	Apparently healthy, showing no change in color or swelling, but slight bleeding from sulcus on probing
2	Bleeding on probing; change of color due to inflammation; no swelling or macroscopic edema.
3	Bleeding on probing, change in color, slight edematous swelling
4	Bleeding on probing, change in color, obvious swelling
5	Bleeding on probing, spontaneous bleeding and change in color, marked swelling with or without ulceration

Calculus Index (CI) (Ramfjord) (6)

0	No calculus
1	Supragingival calculus extending only slightly below the free gingival margin
2	Moderate amount of supra- and subgingival calculus, or subgingival calculus only
3	Abundance of supra- or subgingival calculus

Periodontal Disease Index (1,7)

Probing depth (mm)[a]

Stage	Attachment loss	Dog	Cat
0: Normal	0%	<3	<0.5
1: Gingivitis	0%	<3	<0.5
2: Early	<25%	<5	<1.0
3: Moderate	<50%	<7	<2.0
4: Severe	>50%	>7	>2.0

[a]Probing depth is highly variable according to animal size, attachment loss is a more accurate measurement.

Radiographic Index (RI) Analysis for Periodontal Disease (PD) (8)

0	Normal
1	Early PD: crestal bone loss around teeth
2	Moderate PD: bone loss of <50% around tooth root(s)
3	Advance PD: bone loss of >50% around tooth root(s)

Furcation Exposure (FE) (9)

F1[a]	Soft tissue lesion extending to the furcation level with minimal osseous destruction
F2[a]	Soft tissue lesion combined with bone loss that permits a probe to enter the furcation from one aspect, but not to pass completely through the furcation
F3	Lesions with extensive osseous destruction that permits through and through passage of the probe with or without soft tissue obscuring the communication

[a]These two classifications are subdivided according to furcation position as facial (F), lingual (L), mesial (M), and distal (D). Example: F2-F, furcation exposure, undermined, on facial surface of tooth.

Tooth Mobility (M) (9)

0   None: normal
1   Slight: represents the first distinguishable sign of movement greater than normal
2   Moderate: movement of approximately 1 mm
3   Severe: movement >1 mm in any direction and/or is depressible

G.V. Black Modified Cavity Preparation Classification System (12)

Class	Tooth type	Characteristics
1	I,PM,M	Beginning in structural defects, such as pit or fissure, commonly found on occlusal surfaces
2	PM,M	Proximal surfaces; when a tooth with a class 2 lesion includes a class 1 lesion, it is still considered class 2
3	I,C	Proximal surfaces; incisal angle not included
4	I,C	Proximal surfaces; incisal angle included
5	I,C,PM,M	Facial or lingual, gingival third; excluding pit or fissure lesions
6	I,C,PM,M	Defect of incisal edge or cusp (not included in Black's original classification)

I, incisor; C, canine or cuspid; M, molar; PM, premolar.

Feline Dental Resorptive (FDR) Lesions[a] (1,10)

1   Into enamel only
2   Into dentin
3   Into pulp
4   Extensive structural damage
5   Crown lost, only roots remain

[a]These include cervical neck lesions (CNL), cervical line lesions (CLL), and resorptive lesion (RL). The types are generally referred to as stages and used in combination with Black's modified classification of tooth lesion locations.

Staging of Tooth Injuries (1,13,14)[a]

1   Simple fracture of the enamel
2   Fracture extends into the dentin
3   Fracture extends into the pulp chamber, pulp vital
4   Fracture extends into the pulp chamber, pulp nonvital
5   Tooth displaced
6   Tooth avulsed
7   Root fracture, no coronal involvement, tooth stable
8   Root fracture, combined with stage 1–2 coronal fracture, tooth stable
9   Root fracture, combined with stage 3 coronal fracture, tooth stable
10 Root fracture in combination with stage 1–4, unstable tooth

[a]The types are generally referred to as stages and used in combination with Black's modified classification of tooth lesion locations.

Mandibular Body Fractures Classification (15)

Region	Area of mandible affected
A	Symphyseal
B	From canine to 2nd premolar
C	From 2nd premolar to 1st molar
D	From 1st molar to 3rd molar
E	Vertical ramus
F	Coronoid process
G	Condylar process

Mandibular Symphyseal Injury Classification (15)

I	Separation with no break in soft tissues
II	Separation with break in soft tissues
III	Separation with break in soft tissues and comminution of bone; broken teeth not unusual.

Periodontic-Endodontic (Perio-Endo) Classification[a] (18)

Class O	Primary endodontic
Class I	Primarily endodontic with secondary periodontal
Class II	Primarily periodontal with secondary endodontic
Class III	True combined lesions

[a]Classification is based on physical and radiographic findings.

Classification of Root Resorption (16)

0	No loss
1	Slight blunting of apex
2	Moderate resorption, <25% root loss
3	Severe resorption, >25% root loss

Radiographic Staging of Cementomas (8)

1	Radiolucency around the root apex appears
2	Some radiopaque densities within the radiolucency
3	Entire lesion becomes radiopaque

Common Human Malocclusion Classification Comparisons (17)

Dr. Angle's classification		Dr. Lischen's classification
Class 0	Normal occlusion	Normal or orthoclusion
Class I	Malocclusion	Neutroclusion
Class II	Malocclusion	Distoclusion
Class III	Malocclusion	Mesioclusion
Class IV	Special malocclusions	Mesiodistoclusion

Basic Veterinary Carnivore Occlusal Classification[a]

Class 0 normal (orthoclusion)
>   Types:
>   1.   True normal
>   2.   Variant normal
>   3.   Normal class III occlusion (breed-normal prognathism)

Class I (neutroclusion)—both jaws of proper length and teeth in a normal mesiodistal location
>   Categories:
>   1.   Anterior cross-bite
>   2.   Posterior cross-bite
>   3.   Facial cuspids (base-wide canines)
>   4.   Lingual cuspids (base-narrow canines)
>   5.   Crowded or rotated teeth
>   6.   Certain partial level bites

Class II (distoclusion)
>   Categories:
>   1.   Short mandible
>   Brachygnathism (mandibular)
>   Mandibular retrognathism
>   Mandibular retrusion
>   Unilateral (wry bite)
>   2.   Long maxilla
>   Maxillary protrusion
>   Maxillary prognathism
>   Unilateral (wry bite)

Class III (mesioclusion)
>   Categories:
>   1.   Long mandible
>   Prognathism (mandibular)
>   Mandibular protrusion
>   Level bite
>   Unilateral (wry bite)
>   2.   Short maxilla
>   Brachycephalic
>   Maxillary retrusion
>   Maxillary retraction
>   Level bite
>   Unilateral (wry bite)

Class IV (mesiodistoclusion)—special classification of wry bite: one jaw in mesioclusion and the other in distoclusion.

---

[a]Adapted from Dr. Angle's and Dr. Lischen's classifications.

Approximate Tooth Root Surfaces (cm2) in Dogs

Tooth root	<10 lbs	<25 lbs	<50 lbs	<90 lbs
Maxillary				
1st incisor	0.7	1.0	1.3	1.7
2nd incisor	0.8	1.2	1.5	1.9
3rd incisor	1.2	1.6	2.25	2.6
Cuspid	3.4	5.4	7.8	9.5
4th premolar	2.5	4.15	5.25	6.75
1st molar	1.5	2.25	3.25	4.25
Mandibular				
1st incisor	0.6	0.9	1.2	1.6
2nd incisor	0.7	1.2	1.5	1.8
3rd incisor	0.9	1.4	1.7	2.0
Cuspid	3.3	5.25	7.65	9.25
4th premolar	1.3	1.9	3.25	3.75
1st molar	2.6	3.8	4.75	6.00

Orthodontic Wires Types and Uses (2)

Wire type	Use	Wire-diameter range (in.)
Round	Ligatures	0.007–0.012
	Fixed appliances	0.014–0.022
	Removal appliances	0.160–0.036
	Lingual arches	0.036
	Head gear	
	Inner arch	0.045–0.051
	Facial bow	0.060
Braided	Archwires	0.015–0.020
Rectangular	Edgewise-fixed appliances	0.022–0.028

Elastic Rings: Size and Strength

Size (in.)[a]	Strength (oz.)
1/8	Light (2)
3/16	Medium (3)
1/4	Heavy (4)
5/16	Extraheavy (6)
3/8	

[a]Size is based on approximate relaxed diameter.

Cranial Nerves

I	Olfactory	Sense of smell
II	Optic	Vision
III	Oculomotor	Eyelid and eye movement
IV	Trochlear	Oblique eyeball movements
V	Trigeminal	
	Ophthalmic	Eyeball, conjunctiva, lacrimal gland, nose, paranasal sinuses, dura mater
	Maxillary	Midface, upper lip, lower eyelid, maxillary teeth and gingiva, soft and hard palate, maxillary sinus, mucous membranes of the nasopharynx
	Mandibular	Muscles of mastication, lower face, mandibular teeth and gingiva, anterior two-thirds of tongue, temporomandibular joint
VI	Abducens	Eye movements
VII	Facial	Sensory of the anterior two-thirds of the tongue, soft palate and part of pharynx
VIII	Acoustic	Hearing
IX	Glossopharyngeal	Tongue, pharynx, palatine tonsil, and fauces
X	Vagus	Motor: laryngeal and pharyngeal muscles and to heart, lung, and alimentary canal
		Sensory: from heart, lungs, alimentary canal
XI	Accessory	Muscles of pharynx and larynx
XII	Hypoglossal	Muscles of tongue and floor of mouth

International System of Units (SI) (2)

Quantity	Unit	SI symbol	
Length	Meter	m	
Mass	Kilogram	kg	
Time	Second	s	
Electric current	Ampere	A	
Thermodynamic temperature	Degree Kelvin	°K	
Substance amount	Mole	mol	
Luminous intensity	Candela	cd	

Multiplication factor	Prefix	SI symbol	Decimal Number
10^{12}	tetra	T	1,000,000,000,000
10^{9}	giga	G	1,000,000,000
10^{6}	mega	M	1,000,000
10^{3}	kilo	k	1,000
10^{2}	hecto	h	100
10^{1}	deka	da	10
10^{0}			1.0
10^{-1}	deci	d	0.1
10^{-2}	centi	c	0.01
10^{-3}	milli	m	0.001
10^{-6}	micro	m	0.000001
10^{-9}	nano	n	0.000000001
10^{-12}	pico	p	0.000000000001
10^{-15}			0.000000000000001

CONVERSION TABLES

Length Conversion Tables

Meter	Millimeters	Inches	Feet
1.0000	1000.00	39.37	3.28
0.0010	1.00	0.03937	0.00328
0.0254	25.40	1.00	0.0833
0.3048	304.80	12.00	1.00

Millimeter	Micrometer	Nanometer	Angstrom
1	1,000	1,000,000	10,000,000

Liquid Capacity Conversion Tables

Minims	Fluid ounces	Milliliters
1.0000	0.002083	0.06161
480.0000	1.000000	29.5729
16.2311	0.033814	1.00000

1 milliliter	= 1 cubic centimeter	= 0.0021 pint
1 liter	= 1000 cubic centimeters	= 2.0 pints
2 pints	= 1 quart	= 0.25 US gallon
1 liter	= 1.057 quarts	= 0.2643 US gallon
3.7843 liters	= 4.0 quarts	= 1.0 US gallon

Weight Conversion Tables

1 milligram (mg)	= 0.001 gram	= 0.015 grain
1 gram	= 0.0022 pound	= 15.432 grains
1 gram	= 0.035 ounce	= 1,000 milligrams
1 kilogram	= 1000.0 grams	= 2.2046 pounds
1 ounce	= 28.35 grams	= 28,350 milligrams
1 pound	= 453.59 grams	= 16 ounces
1 grain	= 0.0648 gram	= 65 milligrams
1 Newton	= 0.2248 pounds	= 0.102 kilogram
1 Newton	= 100,000 dynes	
1 dyne	= 0.00102 gram	
1 pennyweight (dwt) (troy)	= 1.555 grams	= 24 grains

Area Conversion Table

Square centimeter	Square millimeter	Square feet	Square inch
1	100	0.0011	0.155
0.01	1	0.000011	0.00155
929.03	92,903	1.0	144
6.4516	645.16	0.00694	1

Volume Conversion Table

Cubic centimeter	Cubic millimeter	Cubic feet	Cubic inch
1	1000	0.0000353	0.0610
0.0001	1	0.0000000353	0.0000610
28,316.736	28,316,736	1	1728
16.387	16,387	0.0005787	1

Thermometer Conversion Tables

Celsius to Fahrenheit	$(°C \times 1.8) + 32° = °F$
Celsius to Kelvin	$°C + 273° = °K$
Fahrenheit to Celsius	$(°F - 32°)/1.8 = °C$

WORLD VETERINARY DENTAL COUNCIL/
WORLD VETERINARY DENTAL CONGRESS MEMBERSHIP LIST

United States
  American Veterinary Dental Society (AVDS)
  Academy of Veterinary Dentistry (AVD)
  American Veterinary Dental College (AVDC)
Australia
  Australian Veterinary Dental Society (AVDS)
Britain
  British Veterinary Dental Association (BVDA)
Canada
  Canadian Veterinary Dental Society (CVDS)
Europe
  European Veterinary Dental Society (EVDS)
France
  Groupe d'Etude Recherche en Odonto-Stomatologie (GEROS)
Japan
  Japanese Small Animal Dental Society (JSADS)

AMERICAN NATIONAL STANDARD AND AMERICAN DENTAL
ASSOCIATION SPECIFICATIONS (11)

ANSI/ADA Specification	Title
No.1	Alloy for Dental Amalgam and 1a Addendum
No.2	Gypsum-Bonded Casting Investment for Dental Gold Alloy
No.3	Dental Impression Compound
No.4	Dental Inlay Casting Wax
No.5	Dental Casting Alloy
No.6	Dental Mercury
No.7	Dental Wrought Gold Wire Alloy
No.8	Dental Zinc Phosphate Cement
No.9	Dental Silicate Cement
No.10	(Withdrawn)
No.11	Dental Agar Impression Material
No.12	Denture Base Resin
No.13	Denture Cold or Self-Curing Repair Resin
No.14	Denture Base Metal Casting Alloys
No.15	Acrylic Resin (Plastic) Teeth
No.16	Dental Impression Paste—Zinc Oxide–Eugenol Material
No.17	Denture Base Temporary Relining Resin
No.18	Dental Alginate Impression Material
No.19	Nonaqueous Elastomeric Dental Impression Material
No.20	Dental Duplicating Material
No.21	Dental Zinc Silico-Phosphate Cement
No.22	Intraoral Dental Radiographic Film

No.23	Dental Excavating Burs
No.24	Dental Baseplate Wax
No.25	Dental Gypsum Products
No.26	Dental X-Ray Equipment & Accessory Devices
No.27	Direct Filling Resins
No.28	Endodontic Files and Reamers (Type-K)
No.29	Dental Hand Instruments
No.30	Zinc Oxide–Eugenol and Non-Eugenol Cements
No.31	(Withdrawn)
No.32	Orthodontic Wires Not Containing Precious Metals
No.33	Dental Terminology and 33a Supplement
No.34	Aspirating Syringes and 34a Addendum
No.35	(Proposed) High-Speed Air-Driven Handpieces
No.36	(Proposed) Dental Diamond Rotary Cutting Instruments
No.37	Dental Abrasive Powders
No.38	Metal-Ceramic Systems
No.39	Pit and Fissure Sealants
No.40	A. Unalloyed Titanium for Dental Implants
	B. Cast Cobalt-Chromium-Molybdenum Alloys for Dental Implants
No.41	Recommended Standard Practices for Biological Evaluations of Dental Materials and 41a Addendum
No.42	(Proposed) Phosphate-Bonded Investments
No.43	Mechanical Amalgamators
No.44	Dental Electrosurgical Equipment
No.45	(Proposed) Porcelain Teeth
No.46	Dental Chairs
No.47	Dental Units
No.48	Ultraviolet Activator and Disclosing Lights
No.49	(Proposed) Analgesia Equipment
No.50	(Withdrawn)
No.51	(Withdrawn)
No.52	(Withdrawn) Uranium Content in Dental Porcelain and Porcelain Teeth
No.53	(Proposed) Crown and Bridge Plastics
No.54	Dental Needles
No.55	Dispensers of Alloy and Mercury for Dental Amalgam
No.56	(Withdrawn)
No.57	Endodontic Filling Materials
No.58	Endodontic Files (H-Type)
No.59	Portable Steam Autoclave Sterilizers
No.60	(Withdrawn)
No.61	Zinc Polycarboxylate Cement
No.62	Dental Abrasive Pastes
No.63	Rasps and Barbed Broaches
No.64	Dental Explorers
No.65	(Proposed) Low Speed Handpieces
No.66	Glass Ionomer Cements
No.67	(Withdrawn)
No.68	(Withdrawn)
No.69	Dental Ceramics

No.70	(Proposed) Dental X-Ray Protective Aprons and Accessory Devices
No.71	(Proposed) Endodontic Compactors (Condensers) and Spreaders
No.72	(Withdrawn)
No.73	Dental Absorbent Points
No.74	(Proposed) Dental Stools
No.75	(Proposed) Resilient Denture Liners
No.76	Non-Sterile Latex Gloves for Dentistry
No.77	(Proposed) Stiffness of Tufted Area of Toothbrushes
No.78	(Proposed) Dental Obturating Points
No.79	(Proposed) Dental Vacuum Pumps
No.80	Color Stability Test Procedure
No.81	(Proposed) Magnets and Keepers Used for Intraoral and Extraoral Retainers for Prosthetic Restorations
No.82	(Proposed) Combined Reversible/ Irreversible Hydrocolloid Impression Materials
No.83	(Withdrawn)
No.84	(Withdrawn)
No.85	(Proposed) Prophy Angles
No.86	(Withdrawn)
No.87	(Proposed) Impression Trays
No.88	(Proposed) Dental Brazing Alloys
No.89	(Proposed) Dental Operating Lights
No.90	(Proposed) Dental Dams
No.91	(Proposed) Ethyl Silicate Investments
No.92	(Proposed) Refractory Die Materials
No.93	(Proposed) Soldering Investments
No.94	(Proposed) Dental Compressed Air Quality
No.95	(Proposed) Root Canal Enlargers
No.96	(Proposed) Dental Water Base Cements

REFERENCES

1. Veterinary Dental Abbreviations. American Veterinary Dental College, Residency Tracking Committee, Suppl, 1994.
2. Dentist's Desk Reference: Materials, Instruments, and Equipment. 2nd ed. Chicago: American Dental Association; 1983:438.
3. Silness J, Loe H. Periodontal disease in pregnancy. II. Correlation between oral hygiene and periodontal conditions. Acta Odontol Scand 1964;22:121
4. Loe H, Silness J. Periodontal disease in pregnancy. I. Prevalence and severity. Acta Odontol Scand 1963;21:533
5. Muhlemann HR, Son S. Gingival sulcus bleeding: A leading symptom in initial gingivitis. Helv Odontol Acta 1971;15:107
6. Ramfjord SP. The periodontal disease index (PDI). J Periodontol II 1967;38:602
7. Wiggs RB, Lobprise HB. Oral disease. In: Norsworthy GD, ed: Feline Practice. Philadelphia: JB Lippincott Co; 1993:438
8. Frommer HH. Radiology for Dental Auxiliaries. 3rd ed. St. Louis, MO: CV Mosby Co; 1983:290
9. Diagnosis, prognosis and treatment planning. In: *Periodontic Syllabus*. Naval Graduate Dental School, Bureau of Medicine and Surgery; 1975:35.
10. Wiggs RB, Lobprise HB. Dental disease. In: Norsworthy GD, ed: Feline Practice. Philadelphia: JB Lippincott Co; 1993:290
11. Task Groups Report. Chicago: Department of Scientific Affairs, American Dental Association; 1994.
12. Howard WW, Moller RC. Atlas of Operative Dentistry. 3rd ed. St. Louis, MO: CV Mosby Co; 1981:4
13. Robinowich BZ. The fractured incisor. Pediatr Clin North Am 1956;3:979
14. Torres HO, Ehrlich A. Pedodontics. *Modern Dental Assisting.* Philadelphia, PA: 1980;725.

15. Weigel JP. Trauma to oral structures. In: Harvey CE, ed. Veterinary Dentistry. Philadelphia: WB Saunders Co; 1985:140
16. Kaley JD, Phillips C. Root resorption. Angle Orthod 1991;61:125
17. Angle EH. Treatment of Malocclusion of the Teeth and Fractures of the Maxillae, Angle's System. 6th ed. Philadelphia: SS White Dental Manufacturing Co; 1900.
18. Simon JHS, De Deus QD. Endodontic-periodontal relations. In: Cohen S, Burns RC, eds. Pathways to the Pulp. 5th ed. St. Louis, MO: Mosby-Year Book; 1991:548.

Index to Manufacturers and Distributors

This list of manufacturers has been compiled by the authors and is correct to the best of their knowledge. However, companies merge, dissociate, cease business, have area code changes, and change addresses and telephone numbers, and new companies come into existence on a regular basis. For these reasons, some information may not be correct at any one time, for which the authors apologize.

ADDISON BIOLOGICAL LABORATORY INC. (USA)
507 N. Cleveland Ave., Fayette, MO 65248; TEL: (816) 248-2215; (800) 311-2530. *Products or service:* Oral hygiene solutions and gels.

ALMORE INTERNATIONAL CO. (USA)
P.O. Box 25214 Portland, OR 97225; TEL: (503) 643-6633; (800) 547-1511; FAX: (503) 643-9748. *Products or service:* Restorative, endodontic, and prosthodontic instruments and equipment.

ALDRICH & CBI (USA)
3627 N. Andrews Ave., Ft. Lauderdale, FL 33309; TEL: (305) 561-8597; (800) 654-5705; FAX: (305) 563-1124. *Products or service:* Electric-, nitrogen-, and air-driven dental equipment.

AMERICAN STERILIZER CO. (USA)
2425 W. 23rd St., Erie, PA 16512; TEL: (814) 452-3100; FAX: (814) 870-8474. *Products or service:* Dental sterilizers.

AMADENT (USA) AMERICAN MEDICAL AND DENTAL CORP.
P.O. Box 733, 1236 Brace Rd., Bldg. B, Cherry Hill, NJ 08003; TEL: (609) 429-8297; (800) BUY-NEOS; FAX: (609) 429-2953. *Products or service:* Ultrasonic scalers, endodontic units, pulp testers, dental supplies.

AMPCO DENTAL EQUIPMENT (USA)
1101 Highland Way, Grover City, CA 93433; TEL: (805) 473-0660; (800) 444-3145. *Products or service:* Compressors, dental systems, handpieces, polishing instruments.

ANALYTIC TECHNOLOGY (USA)
15233 N.E. 90th St., Redmond, WA 98052-3561; TEL: (206) 883-2445; (800) 428-2808; FAX: (206) 882-3128. *Products or service:* Pulp testers, apex locators, gutta-percha heated plugger device.

ANAQUEST (USA) *See* OHMEDA.

ANDERSON DENTAL SERVICES (USA)
2054 Running Bridge Ct., Maryland Heights, MO 63043; TEL: (314) 878-8480. *Products or service:* Chairside and automatic film developers, development chemicals.

ARISTA SURGICAL SUPPLY (USA)
67 Lexington Ave., New York, NY 10010; TEL: (212) 679-3694; (800) 223-1984. *Products or service:* Dental and surgical instruments.

ARNOLDS VET PRODUCTS LTD. (UK)
Cartmel Drive, Harlescott, Shresbury, Shropshire, England SY1 3TB; TEL: 01743-231632; FAX: 01743-35211. *Products or service:* Veterinary and dental equipment and supplies.

ASEPTICO (USA)
P.O.Box 3209, Kirkland, WA 98083; TEL: (206) 487-3157; (800) 426-5913; Canada: (800) 543-4470; FAX: (206) 487-2608. *Products or service:* Dental units, magnification, lights.

ASH/DENTSPLY (USA)
P.O. Box 872, 570 West College Ave., York, PA 17405; TEL: (717) 845-7511; (800) 8770020; FAX: (717) 843-5951. *Products or service:* Restoratives, instruments, orthodontic appliances.

ASTRA INC. (USA)
50 Otis St., Westborough, MA 01581-4500; TEL: (617) 366-1100; (800) 225-2787; FAX: (508) 898-3570. *Products or service:* Local anesthetic materials.

ATRIX LABS INC. (USA)
2579 Midpoint Dr., Fort Collins, CO 80525; TEL: (970) 482-5868; FAX: (970) 482-9735. *Products or service:* Guided tissue regeneration materials, periodontitis medicaments.

AVLS (USA)
P.O. Box 67127, Lincoln, NE 68506; TEL: (800) 444-3634. *Products or service:* Client education aids.

AMERICAN VETERINARY MEDICAL ASSOCIATION (AVMA)/NETWORK OF ANIMAL HEALTH (NOAH) (USA)
1931 N. Meacham Rd., Suite 100, Schaumberg, IL 60173-4360; TEL: (708) 925-8070; (800) 248-2862; FAX: (708) 925-1329; E-mail: 72662.3435@Compuserve.Com. *Products or service:* Computer network.

BALDOR ELECTRIC (USA)
2520 West Barberry Pl., Denver, CO 80204; TEL: (303) 623-0127; (800) 888-0360; FAX: (303) 595-3772. *Product or service:* Laboratory and dental bench engines and associated equipment.

BECK & CO. (USA) *See* E.A. BECK & CO..

BELLE DE ST. CLAIRE (USA)
20600 Plummer St., Chatsworth, CA 91311; TEL: (818) 718-7000; (800) 322-6666; FAX: (818) 341-1142. *Products or service:* Alloys, waxes, prosthetic instruments.

BELL INTERNATIONAL (USA)
1313 North Carolan, Burlingame, CA 94010; TEL: (415) 348-2055; (800) 523-6640; FAX: (415) 348-3937. *Products or service:* Dental handpieces, instruments.

BIO-INTERFACES, INC. (USA)
11095 Flintkote Ave., San Diego, CA 92121-1202; TEL: (800) 231-1987; (619) 587-1806; FAX: (619) 587-0767. *Products or service:* Artificial bone replacement material.

BIOPLANT INC. (USA)
20 N. Main St., South Norwalk, CT 068541; TEL: (203) 899-0466; (800) 432-4487; FAX: (203) 899-0278. *Products or service:* Guided tissue regeneration materials, synthetic bone replacement.

BISCO (USA)
1500 W. Thomdale Ave., Itasca, IL 60143; TEL: (604) 276-8662; (800) BIS-DENT; FAX: (708) 773-6949. *Products or service:* Dentinal-bonding agents.

BOSWORTH (USA) *See* HARRY J. BOSWORTH CO.

BRASSELER USA INC. (USA)
800 King George Blvd., Savannah, GA 31419; TEL: (912) 925-8525; (800) 841-4522; FAX: (912) 927-8671. *Products or service:* 45-mm K-files, hand instruments, burs, diamonds, abrasives.

BUFFALO DENTAL MANUFACTURING CO. (USA)
575 Underhill Blvd., Syosset, NY 11791; TEL: (516) 496-7200; (800) 828-0203; FAX: (516) 496-7751. *Products or service:* Vibrators, waxing units, bench engines, flexible bowls.

BURNS VET SUPPLY INC. (USA)
1900 Diplomat Dr., Farmers Branch, TX 75234; TEL: (214) 620-9941 (800) 92-BURNS. *Products or service:* Veterinary and dental instruments, equipment, and supplies.

BUTLER CO. (USA)
5000 Braneton Ave., Dublin, OH 43017; TEL: (800) 848-5983; FAX: (614) 761-9096. *Products or service:* Veterinary and dental instruments, equipment, and supplies.

BUTLER J.O. *See* JOHN O. BUTLER CO.

CALCITEK (USA)
2320 Faraday Ave., Carlsbad, CA 92008; TEL: (800) 854-7019; (619) 431- 9515. *Products or service:* Artificial bone replacement material.

CAMERON-MILLER INC. (USA)
3949 S. Racine Ave., Chicago, IL 60609; TEL: (312) 523-6360; (800) 621-0142; FAX: (312) 523-9495. *Products or service:* Dental electrosurgical equipment, dental operatory equipment.

CAMPBELL ENTERPRISES (USA)
P.O. Box 122, Brush Prairie, WA 98606; TEL: (360) 892-9786; (800) 228-6364; FAX: (360) 944-9999. *Products or service:* Home care products, personalized toothbrushes, restraining devices.

CASTLE CO. (USA), DIVISION OF SYBRON CORP.
1777 E. Henriette Rd., Rochester, NY 14690. *Products or service:* Sterilizers.

CARLISLE LABS INC. (USA)
404 Doughty Blvd., Inwood, Long Island, NY 11696

CAULK CO. (USA) *See* L.D. CAULK CO.

C.D.M.V. INC. (CANADA)
C.P. 608.2999 Choquette St., Hyacinthe, Quebec, Canada J25 6H5; TEL: (514) 773-6073. *Products or service:* Veterinary and dental instruments, equipment, and supplies.

CENTRIX INC. (USA)
30 Stran Rd., Milford, CT 06460; TEL: (203) 878-7875; (800) 235-5862; FAX: (203) 877-6017. *Products or service:* Centrix syringes and tips.

CENVET (AUSTRALIA)
2 Healey Rd., Dandenong 3175, Victoria, Australia; TEL: (03) 9794-0422. *Products or service:* Dental equipment and instruments.

CISLAK MANUFACTURING (USA)
1866 Johns Dr., Glenview, IL 60025; TEL: (708) 729-2904; (800) 239-2904; FAX: (708) 729-2447. *Products or service:* Hand instruments, elevators, and sharpening equipment.

COE LABORATORIES INC. (USA) *See* GC AMERICA INC.

COLGATE-PALMOLIVE CO. (USA)
909 River Road, Piscataway, NJ 08854. *Products or service:* Dentifrice, brushes.

COLTENE (USA)
14 Cane Industrial Dr., Hudson, MA 01749; TEL: (508) 563-3881; (800) 882-3888. *Products or service:* Restorative products, impression materials, composite resins.

COLTENE AG (SWITZERLAND)
Feldwlesenstrasse 20, CH-9450 Altstatten, Switzerland; TEL: 011-41-71-75-41-21; FAX: 011-41-71-75-1695. *Products or service:* Restorative products, impression materials, composite resins.

COLTENE/WHALEDENT INC. (USA) *See* WHALEDENT/COLTENE INC.

COLUMBUS DENTAL *See* MILES INC.

COMMONWEALTH DENTAL SUPPLIES CO. (AUSTRALIA)
5-9 Elizabeth St., Richmond 3121, Victoria, Australia; TEL: (03) 9417-6688. *Products or service:* Dental equipment and supplies.

COOPER LABS
Cooper-Care: Division of Oral-B, Newark, NJ *See* ORAL-B LABS. *Products or service:* Bleaching aids, oral and dental care products.

CORE-VENT CORP. (USA)
15821 Ventura Blvd., Suite 410, Encino, CA 91436; TEL: (818) 783-0681; (800) 551-3838; FAX: (818) 783-0788. *Products or service:* Implants.

COSMEDENT INC. (USA)
5419 North Sheridan Rd., Chicago, IL 60640; TEL: (312) 989-6844; (800) 621-6729; FAX: (312) 989-1826. *Products or service:* Porcelains, prophy cups and pastes.

COTTRELL, LTD. (USA)
7399 S. Tucson Way, Englewood, CO 80112; TEL: (303) 799-9401; (800) 843-3343; FAX: (303) 799-9408. *Products or service:* Disposables and infection control products.

CRESCENT DENTAL MANUFACTURING CO. (USA)
7750 W. 47th St., Lyons, IL 60534; TEL: (312) 447-8050; (800) 433-6628; FAX: (708) 447-8190. *Products or service:* Restorative and prosthodontic instruments.

DARBY DENTAL SUPPLY CO. (USA)
100 Banks Ave., Rockville Centre, NY 11570; TEL: (516) 683-1800; (800) 448-7323; FAX: (516) 832-8771. *Products or service:* Dental instruments, equipment, and supplies.

DELMARVA LABS INC. (USA)
P.O.Box 525, Midlothian, VA 23113; TEL: (804) 794-7064; FAX: (804) 794-7835. *Products or service:* Ultrasonic dental scalers.

DEMENTRON RESEARCH CORP. (USA)
5 Ye Olde Rd., Danbury, CT 06810; TEL: (203) 748-0030; FAX: (203) 791-8284. *Products or service:* Visible light–curing lights, pulp testers, etc.

DEN-MAT CORP. (USA)
P.O. Box 1729, 631 S. College, Santa Maria, CA 93456-9967; TEL: (805) 922-8491; (800) 445-0345; FAX: (805) 922-6933. *Products or service: Restorative materials and products.*

DENTALAIRE INC. (USA)
1820 S. Grande Ave., Suite D, Santa Ana, CA 92705; TEL: (714) 540-9969; FAX: (714) 540-9945. *Products or service:* Air compressors and dental units.

DENTAL CONTROL PRODUCTS (USA)
590 Valley Rd., Upper Montclair, NJ 07043. *Products or service:* Mercury spill kits and vapor control.

DENTAL CORP. OF AMERICA (USA)
1592 Rockville Pike, Rockville, MD 20852. Products or service: Dental film duplicators, operatory equipment, dental X-ray film.

DENTAL ENTERPRISES INC. (USA)
1976 S. Bannock St., Denver, CO 80223; TEL: (303) 777-6717; (800) 466-1466. *Products or service:* Full service dental company.

DENTAL EXPRESS LTD. (UK)
Admail 335, Orpington, Kent BR5 2BR, England; TEL: 01689-89451; FAX: 01689-891179. *Products or service:* Dental disposables, materials, supplies, and equipment.

DEN-TAL-EZ INC.(USA) *See* STAR DENTAL MANUFACTURING CO.

DENTAL HEALTH PRODUCTS (USA)
P.O. Box 355, 4011 Creek Rd., Youngstown, NY 14174; TEL: (716) 745-9933; (800) 828-6868; FAX: (716) 745-4352. *Products or service:* Disposable paper supplies.

DENTSPLY INTERNATIONAL (USA)
P.O. Box 872, 570 W. College Ave., York, PA 17404-0872; TEL: (717) 845-7511; (800) 877-0020; FAX: (717) 854-2343. *Products or service:* Dental waxes, gypsum, handpieces, and instruments.

DENVET SALES (USA)
11897 Beckett Fall Rd., Florissant, MO 63033; TEL: (314) 653-0760; (800) 523-6640. *Products or service:* Electric handpieces.

DEPPEN ENTERPRISES INC./DOGGYDENT INTERNATIONAL (USA)
111 St. Matthews Ave., San Mateo, CA 94401; TEL: (415) 342-2976; FAX: (415) 342-7751. *Products or service:* Animal extraction and tarter removal forceps, home care products.

DIAMOND ROTARY AND CARBIDE INTERNATIONAL (CANADA)
P.O. Box 3092, Winnipeg, Manitoba, Canada R3C 4E5; TEL: (204) 452-9469; FAX: (204) 284-2433. *Product or service:* Dental burs and points.

DINE INC. (USA) *See* LESTER DINE.

DRI-CLAVE (USA) SUBSIDIARY OF COLUMBUS DENTAL (*See* MILES INC.)
634 Wager St., Columbus, OH 43206. *Products or service:* Sterilizers and evacuation systems.

DR. SHIPP'S LABORATORIES (USA)
351 N. Foothill Rd., Beverly Hills, CA 90210; TEL: (310) 550-0107; (800) 442-0107; FAX: (310) 550-1664. *Products or service:* Dental instruments, equipment and supplies.

DYNA-DENT (USA)
151 East Columbine Ave., Santa Ana, CA 92707; TEL: (800) 228-4298 (Calif); (800) 448-8882; (714) 546-4891; FAX: (714) 546-1109. *Products or service:* Dental equipment, handpieces.

E.A. BECK & CO. (USA)
P.O. Box 10859, 657 W. 19th St., Costa Mesa, CA 92627; TEL: (714) 645-4072; (800) 845-0153; FAX: (714) 645-4085. *Products or service:* Restorative and surgical instruments.

EASTMAN KODAK CO. (USA)
343 State St., Rochester, NY 14650; TEL: (716) 724-4000; (800) 242-2424; FAX: (716) 724-5797. *Products or service:* Dental x-ray and duplicating film, processing chemicals, radiographic accessories.

EASY VET EQUIPMENT (AUSTRALIA)
16 Foundry Rd., Seven Hills 2147, New South Wales, Australia; TEL: (02) 838-9200. *Products or service:* Dental equipment and instruments.

EDS (USA) ESSENTAL DENTAL SYSTEMS
89 Leuning St., Hackensack, NJ 07606; TEL: (201) 487-9090; (800) 22-FLEXI; FAX: (201) 487-5120. *Product or service:* Titanium-reinforced composite core and cement materials.

ELLMAN INTERNATIONAL (USA)
1135 Railroad Ave., Hewlett, NY 11557-2316; TEL: (516) 569-1482; (800) 835-5355; FAX: (516) 569-0054. *Products or service:* Electrosurgical equipment, dental products.

EMASDI S.A. (BELGIUM)
Avenue De l'Aulne 11, B-1180 Bruxelles, Belgium; TEL: (02) 376-44-89; FAX: (02) 376-44-29. *Products or service:* Endodontic equipment and supplies.

ENGLER ENGINEERING CORP. (USA)
1099 East 47th St., Hialeah, FL 33013; TEL: (305) 688-8581; (800) 445-8581; FAX: (305) 685-7671. *Products or service:* Scalers, polishers, dental materials.

EQUI-DENT TECHNOLOGIES, INC. (USA)
P.O. Box 5877, Sparks, NV 89432-5877. TEL: (702) 358-6695. *Products or service:* Equine dental instruments.

ESPE-PREMIER CORP. (USA)
P.O. Box 111, 1710 Romano Dr., Norristown, PA 19404; TEL: (215) 277-3800; (800) 344-8235; FAX: (215) 277-4270. *Products or service:* Restoratives, impression materials, curing lights.

ESPE AUSTRALIA PTY LTD.
24/566 Gradeners Rd., Alexandria NSW 2015, Australia; TEL: (02) 317-4800; (800) 257-042; FAX: (02) 317-4343.

ETHICON-DIVISION OF JOHNSON AND JOHNSON (USA)
Somerville, NJ 08876-0151; TEL (800) 255-2500. *Products or service:* Suture material.

FORT DODGE LABORATORIES (USA)
800 Fifth St., N.W., Fort Dodge, IA 50501; TEL: (515) 955-4600; (800) 477-1365; FAX: (515) 955-9183. *Products or service:* Animal oral rinsing solutions.

FRANKLIN DENTAL MANUFACTURING INC. (USA)
P.O. Box 93, 3670-B Parkway Ln., Hillard, OH 43206-0093. *Products or service:* Restorative dental instruments.

FRISKIES PETCARE CO. (USA)
800 N. Brand Blvd., Glendale, CA 91203; TEL: (818) 543-7749; FAX: (818) 549-6509. *Products or service:* Rawhide chews for dental care.

GC AMERICA INC. (USA)
3737 W. 127th St., Chicago, IL 60658; TEL: (708) 597-0900; (800) 323-7063; FAX: (708) 371-5103. *Products or service:* Restoratives, impression materials, gypsums, instruments.

GC INTERNATIONAL CORP. (JAPAN)
76-1 Hasunuma-cho, Itabashi-ku, Tokyo 174, Japan; TEL: 03-3558-5181; FAX: 03-3966-1470

GEL KAM INTERNATIONAL (USA)
P.O. Box 80004, Dallas, TX 75380; TEL: (214) 233-2800; (800) 527-0222; FAX: (214) 239-6859. *Products or service:* Stannous fluoride gels.

GENDEX CORP. (USA)
Box 21004, Milwaukee, WI 53221; TEL: (414) 769-2888; (800) 558-2900; FAX: (414) 769-2868. *Products or service:* Dental radiographic equipment and accessories

GEORGE TAUB PRODUCTS & FUSION (USA)
277 New York Ave., Jersey City, NJ 07307; TEL: (800) 828-2634; (201) 798-5353; FAX: (201) 659-7186. *Products or service:* Restorative casting materials, cyanoacrylic bonding adhesives.

G. HARTZELL & SON (USA)
2372 Stanwell Circle, P.O. Box 5988, Concord, CA 94520; TEL: (800) 950-2206; (510) 798-2206; FAX: (510) 798-2053. *Products or service:* Dental hand instruments and associated products.

GINGI-PAK (USA)

P.O. Box 240, Camarillo, CA 93011; TEL: (805) 484-1051; (800) 437-1514; FAX: (805) 484-5076. *Products or service:* Gingival packing instruments and cord, articulation sprays.

GIRARD INC. (USA)

1974 Ohio St., Lisle, IL 60532. *Products or service:* Periodontal instruments.

GOODWOOD DENTAL ARTS LABORATORY (USA)

647 E. Airport Ave., Baton Rouge, LA 70806; TEL: (504) 928-4239. *Products or service:* Veterinary dental laboratory.

GORE REGENERATIVE TECHNOLOGIES (USA) W.L. GORE & ASSOCIATES INC.

P.O. Box 2500, 1500 N. Fourth St., Flagstaff, AZ 86003; TEL: (602) 526-3030; (800) 528-1866; FAX: (602) 526-1822. *Products or service:* Guided tissue regeneration materials, synthetic membranes.

GRAY SUPPLY CO. (USA)

4415 Indianapolis Blvd., East Chicago, IN 46312; TEL: (800) 238-2244; FAX: (219) 398-0038. *Products or service:* Bulbs for curing lights, surgical lamps, columniators, projectors, etc.

GREAT LAKES ORTHODONTIC PRODUCTS (USA)

1550 Hertel Ave., Buffalo, NY 14216; TEL: (716) 695-6251; (800) 828-7626; FAX: (716) 695-0810. *Products or service:* Orthodontic equipment and supplies.

HAMPTON RESEARCH & ENGINEERING (USA)

2670 W. Interstate 40, Oklahoma City, OK 73108; TEL: (405) 232-5103; (800) 800-6369; FAX: (405) 232-5104. *Products or service:* Handpieces, dental units, endo and bur organizers, OSHA equipment.

HANAU ENGINEERING CO. (USA)

P.O. Box 203, Buffalo, NY 14225. *Products or service:* Articulators, amalgamators.

HANDLER MANUFACTURING CO. (USA)

P.O. Box 520, 612 North Ave., East Westfield, NJ 07090; TEL: (908) 233-7796; (800) 274-2635; FAX: (908) 233-7340. *Products or service:* Laboratory engines and model trimmers.

HARMON SMITH INC. (USA)

Suite 100 Park Plaza, 801 W. 47th St., Kansas City, MO 64112-1298; TEL: (816) 756-0756; FAX: (816) 756-0380. *Products or service:* Marketing and public relations.

HARRY J. BOSWORTH CO. (USA)

7227 N. Hamlin Ave., Skokie, IL 60076; TEL: (708) 679-3400; FAX: (708) 679-2080. *Products or service:* Oral hygiene products, cements, varnishes, dental instruments.

HARTZELL & SON (USA) *See* G. HARTZELL & SON.

HCC HYGENIC CORP. (CANADA)

Unit 3, 14 Northrup Crescent, St. Catharines, Ontario,Canada L2M 78N7; TEL: (800) 461-0574; FAX: (416) 937-7479. *Products or service:* Endodontic materials, waxes, acrylics, tray materials.

HEALTHCO INTERNATIONAL (USA)
6555 S. Kenton St., Englewood, CO 80111; TEL: (303) 799-4488; (800) 759-4488. *Products or service:* Impression materials, gypsum, dental instruments, and equipment.

HEINZ PET PRODUCTS (USA) AFFILIATE OF H.J. HEINZ CO.
P.O. Box 5700, Newport, KY 41071-4549; TEL: (800) 252-7022. *Products or service:* Dog biscuit chew treats.

HENRY SCHEIN INC. (USA)
5 Harbor Park Dr., Port Washington, NY 11050; TEL: (516) 367-9400; (800) 872-4346; FAX: (800) 483-8329; FAX: (516) 621-4300. *Products or service:* Veterinary and dental instruments, equipment, and supplies.

HENRY SCHEIN REXODENT (UK)
25-27 Merrick Road, Southall, Middlesex UB2 4AU, England; TEL: 0181-574-0335; FAX: 0181-843-9983. *Products or service:* Veterinary and dental instruments, equipment, and supplies.

HERAEUS KULZER (USA)
10005 Muirlands Blvd., Irvine, CA 92718-2595; TEL: (714) 770-0219; (800) 854-4003; FAX: (714) 770-5019. *Products or service:* Restoratives and general dental supplies and equipment.

H. KULZER LTD (AUSTRALIA)
P.O. Box 414, Northbridge NSW 2063, Australia; TEL: (02) 4178411; FAX: (02) 4175093.

HERAEUS KULZER GMBH (GERMANY)
Bereich Kulzer, Philipp-Res-Strasse 8/13, Postfach 12 42, D-61269 Wehrheim/Ts., Germany; TEL: (0 60 81) 9 95-0 415 863; FAX: (0 60 81) 9 59-3 04

HERAEUS LTD. (HONG KONG)
Kulzer Pacific Division, GPO Box 7926, Hong Kong; TEL: 3-890223; FAX: 3-436214

HILL'S PET NUTRITION (AUSTRALIA)
GPO Box 3964, Sidney NSW 2001, Australia; TEL: (1800) 800-733; New Zealand TEL: (04) 566-1614. *Products or service:* Prescription dental diet.

HILL'S PET NUTRITION (USA)
P.O. Box 148, Topeka, KS 66601; TEL: (913) 354-8523; (800) 255-0449. *Products or service:* Prescription dental diet.

HOWMEDICA INC. (USA)
Dental Division; 5101 South Keeler Ave., Chicago, IL 60632; TEL: (800) 438 1150; *Products or service:* Gypsum products, casting metals, porcelains, cements, solders.

HOYT LABS (DIVISION OF COLGATE PALMOLIVE) (USA)
633 Highland Ave., Needham, MA 02194; TEL: (800) 225-3756; (617) 821-2880; FAX: (617) 821-2644. *Products or service:* Dental restoratives, resins, oral hygiene aids.

HU-FRIEDY CO. (USA)
3232 N. Rockwell St., Chicago, IL 60618-5982; TEL: (312) 975-6100; (800) HU-FRIEDY; FAX: (800) 729-1299; (312) 975-1683. *Products or service:* Dental hand instruments.

HYGENIC CORP. (USA)
1245 Home Ave., Akron, OH 44310; TEL: (216) 633-8460; (800) 321-2135; FAX: (800) 633-7331; (216) 633-9359. *Products or service:* Endodontic materials, waxes, acrylics, tray materials.

ICN DOSIMETRY SERVICES (USA)
26201 Miles Rd., Cleveland, OH 44128. *Products or service:* Radiation monitoring service.

IDE (USA)INTERSTATE DENTAL & EQUIPMENT
1500 New Horizon Blvd., Amityville, NY 11701; TEL: (516) 957-8300; (800) 666-8100; FAX: (516) 957-1678. *Products or service:* Veterinary and dental instruments, equipment, and supplies.

IDEXX LABS (USA)
One IDEXX Dr., Westbrook, ME 04092; TEL: (207) 856-0300; (800) 548-6733; FAX: (207) 856-0625. *Products or service:* Blood chemistry and lab equipment.

IM3, INC. (USA)
12013 N.E. 99th St., Suite No. 1670, Vancouver, WA 98682; TEL: (360) 254-2981; FAX: (360) 254-2940. *Products or service:* Dental hygiene equipment, sonic and ultrasonic dental scalers.

IMMUNOVET CO. (USA) *See* VETOQUINOL INC..

INTERPORE INTERNATIONAL (USA)
P.O. Box 19369, 18008 Skypark Circle, Irvine, CA 92714; TEL: (714) 261-3100; (800) 722-4489; CA: (800) 722-4488; FAX: (714) 261-9409. *Products or service:* Guided tissue regeneration materials, synthetic bone.

IVOCLAR (AUSTRALIA)
1-5 Overseas Dr., Noble Park 3174, Victoria, Australia; TEL: (03) 9795-9188. *Products or service:* Dental equipment, instruments, supplies.

IVOCLAR (USA) *See* VIVADENT INC.

J.B. LIPPINCOTT CO. (USA) *(See* LIPPINCOTT–RAVEN PUBLISHERS)

J.F. JELENKO & CO. (USA) PENNWALT CORP.
99 Business Park Dr., Armonk, NY 10504; TEL: (914) 273-8600; (800) 431-1785; FAX: (914) 273-9379. *Products or service:* Casting alloys, gypsum and investments, polishing materials.

JENERIC/PENTRON INC. (USA)
P.O. Box 724, 53 N. Plains Industrial Rd., Wallingford, CT 06492; TEL: (203) 265-7397; (800) 551-0283; FAX: (203) 284-3310. *Products or service:* Composite resins, dentinal-bonding agents, impression materials.

J.M. NEY CO. (USA)
Ney Industrial Park, Bloomfield, CT 06002; TEL: (203) 242-2281; (800) 243-1942; FAX: (203) 242-5688. *Products or service:* Dental casting metals, gypsum, prosthodontic equipment.

J. MORITA USA INC. (USA)

14712 Bentley Circle, Tustin, CA 92680; TEL: (714) 544-2854; (800) 752-9729; FAX: (210) 608-9748. *Products or service:* Cements, bonding agents, restoratives, x-ray equipment.

J.S. DENTAL MANUFACTURING (USA)

P.O. Box 904, Ridgefield, CT 06877; TEL (800) 284-3368; (203) 483-8832; FAX: (203) 431-8485. *Products or service:* Endodontic materials.

JOHN O. BUTLER CO. (USA)

5635 W. Foster Ave., Chicago, IL 60630; TEL: (312) 777-4000; (800) 528-8537; FAX: (312) 777-5101. *Products or service:* Oral hygiene aids, guided tissue regeneration membranes.

JOHNSON & JOHNSON DENTAL PRODUCTS DIVISION (USA)

20 Lake Dr., East Windsor, NJ 08520; TEL: (908) 874-1000; (800) 526-3967; FAX: (908) 874-2545. *Products or service:* Instruments, equipment, restoratives, oral hygiene products.

JORGENSEN LABORATORIES (USA)

1450 N. Van Buren, Loveland, CO 80538; TEL: (303) 669-2500. *Products or service:* Dental and surgical hand instruments.

KAVO AMERICA (USA)

2200 W. Higgins Rd., Hoffman Estates, IL 60195. *Products or service:* Handpieces and surgical instruments.

KERR MANUFACTURING CO. (USA) SUBSIDIARY OF SYBRON CORP.

P.O. Box 455, 28200 Wick Rd., Romulus, MI 48174; TEL: (313) 946-7800; (800) 537-7123; FAX: (313) 946-8316. *Products or service:* Bonding agents, restoratives, endodontic instruments.

KODAK (USA) *See* EASTMAN KODAK CO.

KULZER *See* HERAEUS KULZER.

KYOCERA INTERNATIONAL (USA)

8611 Balboa Ave., San Diego, CA 92123; TEL: (619) 576-2600; (800) 421-5735; FAX: (619) 694-0157. *Products or service:* Dental implants.

LACTONA CORP. (USA)

1330 Industrial Rd., Hatfield, NJ 19440. *Products or service:* Oral hygiene aids, special purpose resins.

LANDAUER CO. (USA)

Glenwood Science Park, Glenwood, IL 60425-1586; TEL: (708) 755-7000; FAX: (708) 755-7016. *Products or service:* Radiation monitoring service.

LANG DENTAL MANUFACTURING CO. INC. (USA)

P.O. Box 969, 175 Messner Dr., Wheeling, IL 60090; TEL: (708) 215-6622; (800) 222-5264; FAX: (708) 215-6680. *Products or service:* Tooth shade, impression tray, orthodontic and other acrylics.

LARES RESEARCH INC. (USA)

1581 Industrial Rd., San Carlos, CA 94070; TEL: (916) 345-1767; (800) 347-3289; FAX: (916) 345-1870. *Products or service:* Dental handpieces, burs, restorative instruments, curing lights.

L.D. CAULK CO. (USA) DIVISION OF DENTSPLY INTERNATIONAL

P.O. Box 359, Lakeview and Clark Avenues, Milford, DE 19963; TEL: (302) 422-4511; (800) 532-2855; FAX: (800) 788-4110. *Products or service:* Restoratives, instruments, cements, impression materials, waxes.

LEE PHARMACEUTICALS (USA)

P.O. Box 3836, 1444 Santa Anita Ave., South El Monte, CA 91733; TEL: (818) 422-3141; (800) 423-4173; FAX: (818) 578-8607. *Products or service:* Restorative and endodontic materials, oral hygiene aids.

LESTER DINE (USA)

PGA Commerce Park, 351 Hiatt Dr., Palm Beach Gardens, FL 33418; TEL: (407) 624-9100; (800) 237-7226; FAX: (407) 624-9103. *Products or service:* Close-up cameras and accessories.

LIFELEARN INC. (CANADA)

MacNabb House, University of Guelph, Guelph, Ontario, Canada N1G 2W1; TEL: (519) 824-4120; FAX: (519) 767-1101. *Product or service:* Dental learning systems.

LIPPINCOTT–RAVEN PUBLISHERS (USA)

227 E. Washington Square, Philadelphia, PA 19106-3780; TEL: (215) 238-4205; FAX: (215) 238-4478. *Products or service:* Dental, medical and veterinary books.

LYPPARD PTY. LTD. (AUSTRALIA)

2 Searson Crescent, Mentone, Victoria 3194, Australia; TEL: (03) 9585-1600; FAX: (03) 9585-1611. *Products or service:* Complete dental supply distributor.

3M DENTAL PRODUCTS CO. (USA)

3M Building 225-4S-11, St. Paul, MN 55144-1000; TEL: (612) 733-8283; (800) 634-2249; FAX: (612) 733-2481. *Products or service:* Bonding agents, restoratives, impression materials.

MACAN ENGINEERING CO. (USA)

1564 N. Damen, Chicago, IL 60622; TEL: (312) 772-2000; FAX: (312) 722-2003. *Products or service:* Electrosurgical units, ultrasonic scalers.

MASEL ORTHODONTICS (USA)

2701 Bartrum Rd., Bristal, PA 19007-6892; TEL: (215) 785-1600; (800) 423-8227; FAX: (215) 785-1680. *Products or service:* Orthodontic supplies and equipment.

MATRIX MEDICAL INC. (USA)

145 Mid County Dr., Orchard Park, NY 14127; TEL: (716) 662-6650; (800) 847-1000. *Products or service:* Dental compressors, anesthetic equipment.

MEDICAL I.D. SYSTEMS (USA)

3954 44th St., S.E., Grand Rapids, MI 49512; TEL: (616) 698-0535; (800) 262-2399; FAX: (616) 698-0603. *Products or service:* X-ray identification labels.

MEDIFORCE (UK)
Carr House, Carrbottom Rd., Bradford BD5 9BJ, England; TEL: 01274-732328; FAX: 01274-391919. *Products or service:* Dental materials, instruments, and equipment.

MERCK MSD/AGVET DIVISION
Rahway, NJ 07065-0912; TEL: (215) 661-5000; (800) 637-2579; (908) 855-9366. *Products or service:* Periodontal medicaments.

MICROCOPY (USA)
P.O. Box 977, Newbury Park, CA 91320; TEL: (805) 498-3113; (800) 235-1863. *Products or service:* Dental x-ray identification numbers.

MICROLABS (USA)
6998 Sierra Ct., Dublin, CA 94568; TEL: (415) 829-3611; (800) 227-0936. *Products or service:* Full-service dental laboratory.

MICRO-MEGA–PRODONTA SA (SWITZERLAND)
Geneva and Zurich, Switzerland. *Products or service:* Handpieces.

MIDWEST DENTAL PRODUCTS (USA)
901 W. Oakton St., Des Plaines, IL 60018-1884; TEL: (708) 640-4800; FAX: (708) 640-6165. *Products or service:* Dental handpieces.

MILES INC. DENTAL PRODUCTS (USA)
4315 S. Lafayette Blvd., South Bend, IN 46614; TEL: (219) 291-0661; (800) 343-5336; FAX: (219) 291-0720. *Products or service:* Dental materials.

MILKBONE (USA) DIVISION OF NABISCO FOODS
East Hanover, NJ 07936; TEL: (800) 622-4726. *Products or service:* Dog biscuit chew treats.

MILLIPORE SA (FRANCE)
67 Molsheim, France. *Products or service:* Synthetic membranes (regenerative–periodontal).

MILTEX INSTRUMENT CO. (USA)
6 Ohio Dr., Lake Success, NY 11042; TEL: (516) 775-7100; (800) 645-8000; FAX: (516) 775-7185. *Products or service:* Dental burs and instruments.

MINIXRAY INC. (USA)
3611 Commercial Ave., Northbrook, IL 60062-1822; TEL: (708) 564-0323; (800) 221-2245; FAX: (708) 564-0323. *Products or service:* X-ray equipment and supplies.

MIZZY INC. (USA)
P.O. Box 632, Clifton Forge, VA 24422; TEL: (609) 663-4700; (800) 333-3131; FAX: (609) 633-0381. *Products or service:* Dental cements, cavity liners.

MODERN MATERIALS MANUFACTURING CO. (USA) SUBSIDIARY OF COLUMBUS DENTAL (*See* MILES INC.)
1021 S. Tenth St., St. Louis, MO 63104. *Products or service:* Dental gypsum, impression materials, dental waxes, resins.

MONOJECT (USA)
1831 Olive St., St. Louis, MO 63103. *Products or service:* Endodontic needles and syringes.

MORITA INC. (USA) *See* J. MORITA USA.

MOSBY-YEARBOOK INC. (USA)
11830 Westline Industrial Dr., St.Louis, MO 63146; TEL: (314) 872-8370; (800) 426-4545; FAX: (314) 432-1380. *Product or service:* Dental, medical, and veterinary books.

MOYCO/UNION BROACH INC. (USA)
2054 W. Clearfield St., Philadelphia, PA 19132-1516; TEL: (215) 229-0470; (800) 221-1344; FAX: (215) 229-3291. *Products or service:* Cements, cavity liners, amalgam, waxes, endodontic instruments.

MSD/AGVET (USA) *See* MERCK.

NEPHRON CORP. (USA)
321 E. 25th St., Tacoma, WA 98421; TEL: (206) 383-1002; (800) 426-3603; FAX: (206) 383-2751. *Products or service:* Dental units, handpieces, burs, instruments, and supplies.

NEY, J.M. CO. (USA) *See* J.M. NEY CO.

NOAH (USA) *See* American Veterinary Medical Association.

NPD DENTAL SERVICES (USA)
5 Jules Lane, New Brunswick, NJ 08901. *Products or service:* Endodontic and restorative materials.

NSK AMERICA CORP. (USA)
700 B Cooper Ct., Schumburg, IL 60173; TEL: (708) 843-7664; FAX: (708) 843-7622. *Products or service:* Dental handpieces.

NUTRAMAX LABS (USA)
5024 Campbell Blvd., Baltimore, MD 21236; TEL: (410) 931-4000; (800) 925-5187; FAX: (410) 931-4009; E-mail: Nutramax@AOL.COM. *Products or service:* Nutritional aids, diets, and dental implant material.

NYLABONE PRODUCTS (USA)
P.O. Box 427, One TFH Plaza, Third and Union Avenues, Neptune, NJ 07753; TEL: (908) 988-8400; (800) 631-2188; FAX: (908) 988-5466. *Products or serice:* Animal chewing products, animal related publications.

OFFICE OF OCCUPATIONAL SAFETY AND HEALTH (USA)
950 Upshur St., N.W, Washington, DC 20011; TEL: (202) 567-6339

OHMEDA (USA)
Ohmeda Dr., Madison, WI 53704; TEL: (608) 221-1551; (800) 345-2700; FAX: (608) 221-4384. *Products or service:* Anesthesia equipment and chemicals.

OMNI INTERNATIONAL (USA)
P.O. Box 100, Gravette, AR 72736; TEL: (501) 787-5232; (800) 643-3639; FAX: (501) 787-6507. *Products or service:* Fluoride gels.

ORAL-B LABS (USA)
1 Lagoon Dr., Redwood City, CA 94065; TEL: (415) 598-5000; (800) 446-7252; FAX: (415) 598-4059. *Product or service:* Oral hygiene care products.

ORASCOPTIC RESEARCH INC. (USA)
5225-3 Verona Rd., P.O. Box 44451, Madison, WI 53744-4451; TEL: (608) 256-0344; (800) 369-3698; (608) 256-1000. *Products or service:* Magnification, lighting, chairs.

OSE (USA) ORTHODONTIC SUPPLY AND EQUIPMENT.
7851 Airpark Rd., Unit #202, Gaithersburg, MD 20879-4123; TEL: (800) 634-7727; (800) 638-4003; FAX: (301) 869-3800. *Products or service:* Orthodontic equipment and supplies.

OSHA *See* Office of Occupational Safety and Health.

OSMED (USA) *See* THM BIOMEDICAL INC..

OXYFRESH USA INC. (USA)
P.O. Box 3723, E. 12928 Indiana, Spokane, WA 99220-3723; TEL: (509) 924-4999; (800) 333-7374; FAX: (509) 924-5285. *Products or service:* Oral hygiene and homecare products.

PACIFIC MEDICAL SUPPLIES CO. (AUSTRALIA)
484 Swan St., Richmond 3121, Victoria, Australia; TEL: (03) 9428-8118. *Products or service:* Guided tissue regeneration materials.

PARA-MEDICAL LABELS (USA)
P.O. Box 199000, 593 Short Rd., Diamond Springs, CA 95619-9725; TEL: (916) 626-5741; (800) 622-7009; FAX: (916) 626-1808. *Products or service:* Prescription labels, dental record stickers.

PARAVAX (USA)
1825 Sharp Point Dr., Fort Collins, CO 80525; TEL: (970) 493-7272; FAX: (970) 493-7333. *Products or service:* Periodontal medicaments.

PARKELL PRODUCTS INC. (USA)
155 Schmitt Blvd., Farmingdale, NY 11735; TEL: (516) 249-1134; (800) 243-7446; FAX: (516) 249-1134. *Products or service:* Electrosurgical units, ultrasonic scalers, endodontic equipment.

PASCAL CO. INC. (USA)
2929 N.E. Northrup Way, Bellevue, WA 98004; TEL: (206) 827-4694; (800) 426-8051; FAX: (206) 827-6893. *Products or service:* . Prosthodontic instruments and devices.

PATTERSON DENTAL CO. (USA)
1100 E. 80th St., Minneapolis, MN 55420-9938; TEL: (612) 854-2881; (800) 552-1260; FAX: (612) 854-8381. *Products or service:* Full-line dental distributor.

PELTON & CRANE (USA)
P.O. Box 241147, Charlotte, NC 28224; TEL: (704) 523-3212; (800) 659-6560; FAX: (704) 529-5523. *Products or service:* Sterilizers and accessories.

PERGAMON PRESS PLC (UK)
Headington Hill Hall, Oxford OX3 OBW, England; TEL: (0865) 74339; FAX: (0865) 60285. *Products or service:* Dental, medical, and veterinary books.

PERIOGIENE (USA) DIVISION OF CONNAISSANCE CORP.
P.O. Box 9, Fort Collins, CO 80522; TEL: (970) 493-8616; (800) 368-5776; FAX: (970) 498-0543. *Products or service:* Ultrasonic scalers, oral hygiene products.

PETCOM (USA) DIVISION OF AV LEARNING SYSTEMS (AVLS)
P.O. Box 67127, 4706 S. 48th, Lincoln, NE 68506; TEL: (402) 488-3338; (800) 444-3634; FAX: (402) 488-3267. *Products or service:* Dental reminder cards and marketing materials.

PETS VETERINARY DENTAL LABORATORY (USA)
P.O. Box 867, Waukesha, WI 53187-9986; TEL: (414) 542-9205; (800) 588-7734. *Product or service:* Veterinary dental laboratory.

PFIZER ANIMAL HEALTH (AUSTRALIA)
38-42 Wharf Rd., West Rhyde NSW 2114, Australia. *Products or service:* Antibiotics and home care products.

PFIZER ANIMAL HEALTH (USA)
235 E. 42nd St., New York, NY 10017; TEL: (212) 573-1298.

POH (USA) ORAL HEALTH PRODUCTS INC.
P.O. Box 470623, Tulsa, OK 74147; TEL: (918) 622-9412; (800) 331-4645. *Products or service:* Oral health care products and personalized toothbrushes.

PRECISION CERAMICS DENTAL LABORATORY (USA)
9591 Central Ave., Montclair, CA 91763; TEL: (714) 625-8787; (800) 223-6322; FAX: (714) 621-3125. *Product or service:* Veterinary dental laboratory.

PREMIER-ESPE SALES CORP. (USA) *See* ESPE-PREMIER CORP.

PREMIER DENTAL (CANADA)
480 Hood Rd., Unit 3, Markham, Ontario, Canada L3R 9Z3; TEL: (800) 465-8455. *Products or service:* Restoratives, cements, curing lights.

PROCTOR AND GAMBLE (USA)
1 Proctor and Gamble Plaza, Cincinnati, OH 45202; TEL: (513) 983-1100; (800) 447-4865; FAX: (513) 983-5593. *Products or service:* Dental supplies and materials.

PRODENTAL (AUSTRALIA)
37 Kensington St., East Perth 6004, Western Australia, Australia; TEL: (09) 325-2722. *Products or service:* Dental supplies and equipment.

PRO-DENTEC THERAPEUTICS (USA) PROFESSIONAL DENTAL TECHNOLOGY
P.O. Box 4129, Batesville, AR 72503-4129; TEL: (501) 698-2300; (800) 228-5595; FAX: (501) 793-5554. *Products or service:* Rotary electric toothbrush, dental diagnostic aids.

PULPDENT CORP. OF AMERICA (USA)
80 Oakland St., P.O. Box 780, Watertown, MA 02272; TEL: (617) 926-6666; (800) 343-4342; FAX: (617) 926-6262. *Products or service:* Cavity liners, dental cements, endodontic materials.

REGIONAL DENTAL CO. (AUSTRALIA)
68 Hanover St., Fitzroy, Victoria 3065, Australia; TEL: (03) 9419-5377; (1800) 33-3003; FAX: (03) 9417-6098. *Products or service:* Complete dental supply distributor.

RELIANCE DENTAL MANUFACTURING CO. (USA)
5805 W. 117th Pl., Worth, IL 60482; TEL: (708) 597-6694; FAX: (708) 597-7560. *Products or service:* Inlay pattern resins and acrylics.

RIBBOND INC. (USA)
1326 5th Ave., Suite 640, Seattle, WA 98101; TEL: (206) 340-8870; FAX: (800) 624-4554. *Products or service:* Dental splinting materials.

RINN CORP. (USA)
1212 Abbott Dr., Elgin, IL 60123-1819; TEL: (708) 742-1140; (800) 323-0970; FAX: (800) 544-0787; (708) 742-1122. *Products or service:* Film mounts, chairside developers, radiographic equipment.

ROCKY MOUNTAIN ORTHODONTICS (USA)
P.O. Box 1887, Denver, CO 80201; TEL: (303) 320-2868; (800) 346-6464. *Products or service:* Orthodontics equipment and supplies.

ROEKO (GERMANY/USA)
P.O. Box 1150, D-89122 Langenau, Germany; and 75 Union Ave., Sudbury, MA 01776; TEL: (800) 445-0572; (508) 443-7729; FAX: (508) 443-7730. *Products or service:* Cotton rolls.

ROTH DRUG (USA)
669 West Ohio St., Chicago, IL 60610; TEL: (800) 445-0572; (312) 733-1478; FAX: (312) 733-7398. *Products or service:* Endodontic materials.

RUGBY–DIVISION OF DARBY DRGUS (*See* DARBY)

SCHEIN INC. (USA) *See* HENRY SCHEIN INC.

SDI (USA) SENSOR DEVICES INC.
407 Pilot Ct., 400A, Waukesha, WI 53188; TEL: (414) 524-1000; FAX: (414) 524-1009. *Products or service:* Anesthetic monitoring devices.

SHIPP'S LABORATORIES (USA) *See* DR. SHIPP'S LABORATORIES.

SHOFU DENTAL CORP. (USA)
4025 Bohannon Dr., Menlo Park, CA 94025; TEL: (415) 324-0085; (800) 827-4638; FAX: (415) 323-3180. **SHOFU-RATINGEN (GERMANY)** TEL: 0 21 02 87 06 90. **SHOFU-KYOTO (JAPAN)** TEL: 075-525-0740. **SHOFU (SINGAPORE)** TEL: 65-339-7311. **SHOFU-TONBRIDGE (UK)** TEL: 01892-870800. *Products or service:* Glass ionomer cements and restoratives.

SHOR-LINE (USA) SCHROER MANUFACTURING CORP.
2221 Campbell St., Kansas City, MO 64108; TEL: (816) 471-0488; (800) 444-1579. *Products or service:* Manufacturers and suppliers of veterinary surgery and dental equipment.

SHOR-LINE LTD. (UK)
Llandow Industrial Estate, Cowbridge, South Glamorgan, Wales CF7 7YY UK; TEL: 0800-616770; FAX: 01446-773668.

SILENTAIRE TECHNOLOGY (USA) DIVISION OF WERTHER INTERNATIONAL INC.
711 Rutland, Houston, TX 77007; TEL: (713) 864-8996; (800) 972-7668; FAX: (713) 864-7314. *Products or service:* Compressors for dental use.

SMART PRACTICE (AUSTRALIA)/QUALITY PRACTICE INT. PTY LTD.
4/115 Hawthorn Rd., Caulfield 3161, Victoria, Australia; TEL: (1800) 817-103; FAX: (03) 538-8802. *Products or service:* Dental reminder cards, marketing materials, dental instruments.

SMART PRACTICE (USA)
3400 E. McDowell Phoenix, AZ 85008-7899; TEL: (602) 225-9090; (800) 522-0800; FAX: (800) 522-8329.

SONTEC INSTRUMENTS (USA)
6341 S. Troy Circle, Englewood, CO 80111; TEL: (303) 790-9411; (800) 821-7495. *Products or service:* Medical and dental hand instruments, instrument-sharpening service.

SOUTHWEST MEDICAL/DENTAL (USA)
1343 Manufacturing, Dallas, TX 75207; TEL: (214) 741-1266; FAX: (214) 741-1268. *Products or service:* Dental operatory equipment and x-ray equipment and accessories.

SPEEDENT DENTAL SUPPLIES (USA)
9591 Central Ave., Montclair, CA 91763; TEL: (909) 624-2351; FAX: (909) 621-3125. *Products or service:* Endodontic instruments, burs, prosthodontic supplies.

ST. JON LABORATORIES (USA) *See* VRx PRODUCTS.

ST. JON VRx LTD. (UK)
P.O. Box 57, Egham, Surrey TW20 9AE, England; TEL: (0800) 626409; FAX: (01932) 87496. *Products or service:* Oral hygiene and home care products.

STAR DENTAL MANUFACTURING CO. INC. (USA) DEN-TAL-EZ INC.
1816 Colonial Village Ln., Lancaster, PA 17601; TEL: (717) 291-1161; (800) 275-3320; FAX: (717) 291-5699. *Products or service:* Sonic scalers, handpieces.

STERLING WINTHROP (CANADA)
90 Allstate Pkwy, Markham, Ontario, Canada, L3R 6H3; TEL: (416) 513-4444; FAX: (416) 513-6137. *Products or service:* Synthetic bone replacement material.

S.S. WHITE BURS (USA)
1145 Towbin Ave., Lakewood, NJ 08701; TEL: (908) 905-1100; (800) 535-2877; Fax (908) 905-0987. *Products or service:* Rotary diamonds and dental burs.

SUBURBAN SURGICAL CO. (USA)
275 Twelfth St., Wheeling, IL 60090; TEL: (708) 537-9320; (800) 323-7366. *Products or service:* Dental units, tables, caging.

SULTAN CHEMICALS INC. (USA)
85 W. Forest Ave., Englewood, NJ 07631; TEL: (201) 871-1232; (800) 637-8582; FAX: (201) 871-0321. *Products or service:* Dental chemicals and sterilization aids.

SUMMIT HILL LABORATORIES (USA)
P.O. Box 535, Navesink, NJ 07752; TEL: (908) 933-0800; (800) 922-0722; FAX: (908) 933-0055. *Products or service:* Ultrasonic scalers, polishers, electrosurgical units, anesthetic machines, dental supplies.

TAUB, GEORGE PRODUCTS (USA) *See* GEORGE TAUB PRODUCTS & FUSION.

TELEDYNE-GETZ (USA)
1550 Greenleaf Ave., Elk Grove Village, IL 60007; TEL: (708) 593-3334; (800) 323-6650; FAX: (708) 593-0569. *Products or service:* Alginate, cements, cavity liners, resins.

TEXCEED CORP. (USA)
3001 Redhill Ave., Bldg 4 #104, Costa Mesa, CA 92626; TEL: (800) 344-1321; (714) 432-7083. *Products or service:* Endodontic equipment; thermoplastic gutta percha unit.

THERMAFIL (USA)
5001 E. 68th St., Tulsa, OK 74136; TEL: (918) 493-6598; (800) 662-1202; FAX: (918) 493-6599. *Products or service:* Endodontic supplies and materials, heated gutta-percha.

THOMAS PHARMACEUTICALS (USA)
Ronkonkoma, NY. *Products or service:* Oral topical medications.

THM BIOMEDICAL INC. (USA)
325 Lake Avenue So., Suite 608, Duluth, MN 55802; TEL: (218) 720-3628; (800) 327-6895; FAX: (218) 720-3715. *Products or service:* Polylactic acid surgical dressing.

TICONIUM CO., INC. (USA)
413 N. Pearl St., Albany, NY 12207; TEL: (518) 434-3147. *Products or service:* Polymers and casting alloys.

TLAR
PO Box 208, Pompano Beach, FL 33061. *Product or service:* Model finishing solutions.

TROPHY USA INC.
2252 N.W. Parkway, Suite F, Marietta, GA 30067; TEL: USA (404) 859-9033USA; (800) 642-1246; France (33-1) 49 57 37 37; Spain (34-1) 377 35 16; Germany (49) 78 51 25 81; Italy (39) 39 2300 131; UK (44) 81 291 99 09; FAX: USA (404) 859-0024; France (33-1) 43 28 43 84; Spain (34-1) 377 31 32; Germany (49) 78 5177 891; Italy (39) 39 2300 133; UK (44) 81 291 98 00. *Products or service:* Radiographic and imaging equipment and accessories.

TULSA DENTAL PRODUCTS (USA) *See* THERMAFIL.

ULTRADENT PRODUCTS INC. (USA)
1345 E. 3900 South, Salt Lake City, UT 84124; TEL: (801) 277-3203; (800) 552-5512; FAX: (801) 272-6716. *Products or service:* Hemostatic solutions, gingival packing cords, topical anesthetics.

ULTRASONIC SERVICES (USA)
7126 Mullins Dr., Houston, TX 77081; TEL: (800) 874-5332. *Products or service:* Ultrasonic scaler repairs.

UNION BROACH CO. (USA) *See* MOYCO/UNION BROACH INC.

UNITEK CORP. (USA)
2714 S. Peck Rd., Monrovia, CA 91016; TEL: (818) 445-7960; (800) 423-4588; FAX: (818) 547-4500. *Products or service:* Dental equipment and supplies, orthodontics materials.

UPJOHN CO. (USA)
Kalamazoo, MI 49001; TEL: (616) 323-4000; (800) 821-7000; FAX: (616) 323-4077. *Products or service:* Antibiotics, gelatin sponges.

US BIOMATERIALS CORP. (USA)
4940 Campbell Blvd., Suite 100, Baltimore, MD 21236; TEL: (410) 931-3800; (800) 797-9911; FAX: (410) 931-7363. *Products or service:* Guided tissue regeneration materials, demineralized freeze-dried bone, and synthetic bone.

VETERINARY DENTAL LAB OF AMERICA (USA)
7733 Main St., Fairview, PA 16415; TEL: (814) 474-5806. *Products or service:* Dental laboratory.

VETERINARY INSTRUMENTS (UK)
62 Cemetery Rd., Sheffield S11 8FP, England; TEL: (01142) 700078; FAX: (01142) 759471. *Products or service:* Veterinary surgical and dental instruments and equipment.

VETLAB (UK)
Unit 13, Broomers Hill Park, Broomers Hill Ln., Pulborough, West Sussex RH20 2RY, England; TEL: (01798) 874567; FAX: (01798) 874787. *Products or service:* Veterinary laboratory, dental instruments and equipment.

VETOQUINOL INC. (USA) IMMUNOVET CO.
5910-G Breckenridge Parkway, Tampa, FL 33610-4253; TEL: (800) 627-9447. *Products or service:* Oral hygiene bioadhesives.

VIDENT (USA)
3150 E. Birch St., P.O. Box 2340, Brea, CA 92621; TEL: (714) 961-6200; (800) 828-3839; FAX: (714) 961-6299. *Products or service:* . Prosthetic equipment and supplies, porcelains, and cast glass.

VIRBAC (USA)
P.O. Box 162059, Fort Worth, TX 76161; TEL: (817) 831-5030; (800) 338-3659; FAX: (817) 831-8327. *Products or service:* Home and professional dental hygiene products.

VITA (GERMANY)
VITA Zahnfabrik, H.Rauter GmbH & Co.KG, Postfach 1338, D-79704 Bad Sackingen, Germany; TEL: (0 77 61) 562-0; TELEX: 792 334 VITA D; FAX (0 77 61) 63 89. *Products or service:* Prosthetic equipment and supplies, porcelains, cast glass.

VIVADENT INC. (USA) DIVISION OF IVOCLAR INC.
P.O. Box 304, 182 Wales Ave., Tonowanda, NY 14150; TEL: USA (800)-5-DENTAL; Canada (800) 263-8182. *Products or service:* Restoratives, curing lights, cements, cavity liners.

VPL (USA) VETERINARY PRODUCTS LABS
P.O. Box 34820, Phoenix, AZ 85067-4820; TEL: (800) 825-2555. *Products or service:* Oral home care products, fluoride gels, chlorhexidine solutions.

VRx PRODUCTS (USA) VETERINARY PRESCRIPTION DIVISION OF ST. JON LABORATORIES
1656 W. 240th St., Harbor City, CA 90710; TEL: (213) 326-2720; (800) 969-7387; FAX: (310) 326-8026. *Products or service:* Oral home care products, toothbrushes, toothpastes, fluorides, chlorhexidine products.

WASHINGTON SCIENTIFIC (USA)
P.O. Box 88681, Tukwila, WA 98138; TEL: (206) 863-2854. *Products or service:* Close-up dental cameras, mirrors, flash attachments, accessories.

W.B. SAUNDERS CO. (USA)
625 Walnut St., Philadelphia, PA 19106-3399; TEL: (800) 545-2522; FAX: (800) 874-6418. *Products or service:* Dental, medical and veterinary books.

WESTERN INSTRUMENT CO. (USA) DIVISION OF COLORADO SERUM CO.
P.O. Box 16428, 4950 York St., Denver, CO 80216; TEL: (303) 295-7527; (800) 525-2065; FAX: (303) 295-1923. *Products or service:* Equine dental instruments.

WHALEDENT/COLTENE INC. (USA)
236 Fifth Ave., New York, NY 10001; TEL: (212) 696-8000; (800) 221-3046; FAX: (212) 532-1644. *Products or service:* Electrosurgical equipment, endodontic instruments, dental supplies.

WHIP MIX CORP. (USA)
361 Farmington Ave., P.O. Box 17183, Louisville, KY 40217; TEL: (502) 637-1451; (800) 626-5651; FAX: (502) 634-4512. *Products or service:* Dental gypsums, impression materials, and associated equipment.

WHITE, S.S. BURS (USA) *See* S.S. WHITE BURS.

X-RITE CO. (USA)
4101 Rodger Chaffee Dr., S.E., Grand Rapids, MI 49508; TEL: (616) 534-7663; FAX: (616) 534-9212. *Products or service:* Radiographic equipment.

YOUNG DENTAL (USA)
13705 Shorline Court East, Earth City, MO 63045; TEL: (314) 344-0010; (800) 325-1881; FAX: (314) 344-0021. *Products or service:* Prophy-angle lubricants, oral hygiene aids and equipment.

ZAHN DENTAL CO. INC. (USA)
5 Harbor Park Dr., Port Washington, NY 11050; TEL: (800) 225-8620; FAX: (508) 823-1821. *Products or service:* Dental laboratory equipment and supplies.

ZOLL DENTAL INC. (USA)
1866 Johns Dr., Glenview, IL 60025; TEL: (708) 729-2904; (800) 239-2904; FAX: (708) 729-2447. *Products or service:* Hand instruments, curettes, scalers, and elevators.

Subject Index

A

Abrasive materials, 27
  point shapes, 26–27
  strips, 27
Abscess
  equine, 569–571
  periodontal, 161, 206
Absorbent paper points
  endodontic therapy and, 298
Acanthomatous epulis, 132
Access site
  endodontic, 325–327
Acid-etching, 473
  tooth restoration and, 380–381
Acquired defects, surgical treatment of
  cheek, 250
  lips, 250
  palatal lesions, 243
  tongue, 251
Acquired disorders, 112–116
  dental resorptive lesions, 113
  dental tissue, 112–114
  G.V. Black classification system, 113, 114
  pulp, 114–116
  staging of tooth injuries, 114
Acral lick granuloma, 621
Acrylic splints
  oral fracture repair and, 274–275
Acrylics
  restorative use of, 33
Acute necrotizing ulcerative gingivitis
  feline, 499
Adjunct wiring
  oral fracture repair and, 274
Adult gingival cyst, 131
Adult periodontitis, 199. *See also* Periodontal
    disease; Periodontitis
Advanced endodontic therapy, 325–350. *See
    also* Endodontic therapy
  abnormal canals, 328–330
  access, 325–327
  immature deciduous teeth, 336–337
  immature permanent teeth, 337–341
  instrumentation errors, 331–335
  perforations, 327–328
  procedural blockage, 330–331
  root resectioning, 335–336
  surgical, 341–347. *See also* Surgical
    endodontics
  tooth resectioning, 335–336
Advertising issues, 583. *See also* Marketing issues
Aerobic bacteria
  periodontal disease and, 192

Aggression, 622–626
Aging signs
  radiographs and, 160
Air-driven units
  handpieces, 22
  power equipment and, 19–20
Alveolar ridge
  tooth retention and, 236
Amalgam
  insertion and finishing steps, 375–376
  instruments, 11
  restorative use of, 36–37
Amalgam restorations
  amalgam insertion and finishing,
    375–376
  bonding agents, 375
  cavity bases and liners, 374
  cavity preparations for, 371–376
  cavity varnishes, 375
  class I, II, III, and V, 372–373
  class IV and VI, 373–374
  history of, 370–371
  trituration, 374
American National standard coding
  endodontic instruments and, 291
Anaerobic bacteria
  periodontal disease and, 192
Anatomy and physiology
  endodontic, 280–283
  oral, 55–86. *See also* Oral anatomy and
    physiology
Anchorage
  tooth movement, 450–451
Anesthesia
  lagomorphs, 520–522
  rodents, 520–522
Ankylosis
  radiograph of, 161
Anomalies
  deciduous pathology, 171–176
  deciduous teeth and, 171. *See also*
    Deciduous teeth
  tooth eruption and, 170–171
Anterior cross-bites
  treatment of, 458
Antimicrobial therapy
  periodontal disease and, 211–212
Apex
  structure of, 72, 74
Apexification
  endodontic therapy and, 339–341
Apexigenesis
  endodontic therapy and, 337–339

Apical perforation
  endodontic instruments and, 332
Apical surgical endodontic procedures,
      343–347
  apical resection, 344–345
  apicoectomy, 344–345
  continually erupting teeth, 347
  indirect resection, 347
  periadicular drainage, 343–344
  periapical curettage, 344
  retrograde obturation/filling, 345–346
  retrograde root canal procedures, 347
Apicoectomy, 344–345
Appliance-associated trauma, 479
Appliances
  orthodontic, 452–456
Application of force
  orthodontics and, 451–452
Asymmetric palatal defect repair, 245–247
Atraumatic malocclusion
  Rodentia, 526–528
Attachment loss
  furcation exposure and, 92, 93
  periodontitis and, 201–203
  types of, 202–203
Autoimmune diseases
  feline, 509
Automated mechanical endodontic handpieces,
      302–303
Avulsion
  feline, 501. *See also* Feline oral trauma
Axial wall taper
  operative dentistry and, 417

B
Baboon
  dentition, 540
  gingival hyperplasia and, 550
Backup technique
  endodontic instruments and, 334
Bacteria
  periodontal disease and, 192
Barbed broach
  endodontic therapy and, 292–293
Bases
  restorative use of, 37–39
  tooth restoration and, 380
Basic endodontic therapy, 280–324. *See also*
      Endodontic therapy
Basic materials and supplies, 29–54
  cast materials, 42–45
  dental waxes, 44–45
  endodontic materials, 29–32. *See also*
      Endodontic instruments

impression materials, 39–42. *See also*
    Impression materials
  model materials, 42–45
  periodontal materials, 45–52. *See also*
    Periodontal materials
  restoratives, 33–39. *See also* Restoratives
Basrani's staging of teeth injuries, 355
Beaver
  dental formula, 523
Behavioral problems, 598–627
  acral lick granuloma, 621
  aggression, 622–626
  behavioral signs, 626
  in the clinic, 605–607
  coprophagia, 617–618
  dental injury and, 610–611
  destructive chewing, 612–614
  excessive chewing intensity, 621–622
  excessive oral grooming, 618–620
  feline, 607–609
  feline oral exam and, 609–610
  fence biting, 611–612
  grass ingestion and, 620–621
  kennel biting, 611–612
  mouth shyness, 615–616
  oral exam and, 616
  pica and, 614–615
  plant ingestion and, 620–621
  puppy oral tendencies, 602–604
  teeth brushing and, 604–605
  teething and, 600–602
  wool sucking and, 614–615
Bell stage
  enamel organ development and, 60, 61
Benign tumors
  acanthomatous epulis, 132
  adult gingival cyst, 131
  cementoma radiographic staging, 133
  odontogenic classification, 130
  soft tissue pathology and, 131–133
Benzoin
  tincture of myrrh and, 46
Beveling
  tooth restoration and, 379–380
Biology
  radiation, 145
Bird tongue, 176
Bisecting-angle technique
  intraoral radiology and, 151–152
Bites
  orthodontics and, 442
Bleaching
  nonvital teeth and, 389–392
  vital teeth and, 387–389

Blockage
  procedural canal, 330–331
Bobcat
  eruption times, 545
Bonding agents, 375
  dentinal, 381–382
  enamel, 381
  restorative use of, 35
Bovine eruption times, 576
Brachygnathism
  equine, 565–566
Bridges. *See also* Operative dentistry;
      Prosthodontics
  common types of, 410–412
  definition of, 410
  materials used for, 401–408
Broaches
  endodontic therapy and, 292–293
Buccal object rule, 152
Buccotomy
  equine, 575
Bud stage
  enamel organ development and, 58, 59
Bull terrier
  craniomandibular osteopathy and, 111
Burns
  feline, 502–503. *See also* Feline oral trauma
Burs, 23–26
  12-bladed finishing types and sizes, 25
  guide, 23
  shapes and sizes, 23
  standard types and sizes, 24

C

Cage-biter syndrome, 361, 548, 549
Calcifications
  radiographs and, 161
Calculus index, 196
Canine dental models
  marketing and, 592–595
Canines
  exodontia and, 237–238
Cantilever bridge
  components of, 411
Cap stage
  enamel organ development and, 59
Capybara
  dental formula, 523
Caries
  detection of, 369
  operating field and, 369
  radiographs and, 160
Carnivores
  dental abnormalities, 547–549

dentition, 540–546
Cast glass ceramic restorations
  operative dentistry and, 405–406
Cast materials, 42–45
  dental waxes, 44–45
Cat, 482–527
  acute necrotizing ulcerative gingivitis, 499
  advanced stomatitis, 497
  apicoectomy, 345
  autoimmune diseases, 509
  cervical line lesions, 487–496. *See also*
      Feline cervical line lesions
  congenital tooth disorders, 507–508
  dental chart, 100
  dental formula designations, 69
  dental models and, 592–595
  dental resorptive lesions, 355, 487–496. *See
      also* Feline dental resorptive lesions
  enamel organ development in, 58, 59, 60, 61
  eosinophilic granuloma complex, 511–512
  extrusion of cuspids, 486
  feline cuspid oronasal fistula, 241, 242
  gingival sulcus, 189
  juvenile gingivitis, 497
  juvenile-onset periodontitis, 496–497
  lingual molar salivary gland in, 84, 85
  lymphocytic plasmocytic stomatitis,
      496–499. *See also* Feline lymphocytic
      plasmocytic stomatitis
  malocclusions, 506–507
  mandibular trauma, 503–506. *See also* Feline
      mandibular trauma
  mucoperiosteal flap repair, 241, 242
  neoplasia, 509–511
  oral anatomy, 482–483
  oral behavioral concerns, 607–609
  oral disease, 483–499
  oral trauma, 499–503. *See also* Feline oral
      trauma
  osteodentin and, 488
  palatal defects, 508–509
  periodontal disease, 483–487. *See also*
      Periodontitis
  physical exam of, 482
  salivary gland disease, 512–513
  salivary glands of, 83
  salivary stones and, 126
  sialolith removal, 512
  sialoliths and, 126
  teeth eruption times, 97, 483
  tooth development of, 58
  tooth eruption in, 68
  tooth eruption sequences, 169
  vasodentin and, 488

Caudal hemimandibulectomy, 254–255
Cavities
    cavosurface angles, 363–364
    classification by location, 352
    classification by restored surface location, 354
    components created during preparation, 362–363
    G.V. Black classification system of, 352–354, 365
    line angles in, 363
    marginal finish lines, 363–364
    point angles in, 363
    preparation steps, 365–366
    wall surfaces of, 362
Cavity bases and liners, 374
Cavity preparations
    amalgam restoration and, 371–376. See also Amalgam restorations
    class I, II, III, and V restorations, 372–373
    class IV and VI restorations, 373–374
    components of, 400
    operative dentistry and, 398, 400, 401. See also Operative dentistry
Cavity varnishes, 375
Cavosurface angles
    preparation of, 363–364, 400–401
Cementation, 472–474
    procedure, 474
    selection of, 473–474
Cementoma
    radiographic staging of, 133
Cementomas
    radiographs and, 162
Cements
    endodontic, 312–314
    glass ionomer, 376–378. See also Glass ionomers
    restorative use of, 37–39
Central hemimandibulectomy, 254–255
Ceramometal restorations
    operative dentistry and, 407–408
Cervical line lesions
    feline, 487–496. See also Feline cervical line lesions
Cervical mucocele
    oral surgery and, 252
Charting
    oral and dental, 96–101
    periodontal disease and, 207–208
Cheek defects
    oral surgery and, 247–250. See also Lip and cheek defects

Cheek retractors, 367–368
Cheek teeth
    crown cusp terms of, 57
Chewing
    destructive, 612–614
Chimpanzee
    abscess and, 551
    eruption times, 552
Chinchilla
    baseline physiologic data, 521
    dental formula, 523
    incisor positioning, 525
Chinese Shar-Pei
    tight-lip syndrome and, 110, 248–249
Chisel, 8
Chow chow
    melanosarcoma, 134
Circumferential wiring
    symphyseal separation and, 267
Clark's rule, 152
Cleansing form
    cavity preparation and, 366
Cleft lip, 175
Cleft palate, 175
Clinical oral pathology, 104–139
    acquired disorders, 112–116. See also Acquired disorders
    developmental pathology, 105–112. See also Developmental pathology
    soft tissue pathology, 116–136. See also Soft tissue pathology
Col
    periodontal disease and, 188
Compactor
    McSpadden, 297
Composite resins, 378–384
    acid-etching, 380–381
    application of, 383–384
    bases, 380
    beveling considerations for, 379–380
    cavity preparation for, 383–384
    dentinal bonding, 381–382
    enamel bonding agents, 381
    indirect, 404–405
    liners, 380
    polymerization, 382–383
    restorative use of, 33–34
    shrinkage, 382–383
Compound bridge
    components of, 411
Concrescence
    radiographs and, 160
Condensers
    endodontic therapy and, 296

Congenital defects
palatal, 242–243
tongue, 250–251
Congenital tooth disorders
feline, 507–508
Conservation of teeth
operative dentistry and, 398. *See also*
Operative dentistry
restoration procedures and, 359. *See also*
Restorative dentistry
Contact points
teeth and, 72
Contacts
restoration procedures and, 360
Contours
restoration procedures and, 360
Convenience form
cavity preparation and, 366
Coprophagy
behavioral problems and, 617–618
lagomorphs and, 535
rodents and, 535
Corrective orthodontics, 445–446
Cotton rolls
sizes of, 367
Craniomandibular articulation
radiographs and, 162–163
Craniomandibular osteopathy, 111
radiographs and, 163
Crestal alveolar bone
orthodontic complications and, 476–477
Cross-bites
treatment of, 458, 464
Crown contours
operative dentistry and, 398
Crown cusp terms
cheek teeth and, 57
Crown line angles
teeth and, 71
Crowns, 395–434. *See also* Operative dentistry;
Prosthodontics
cementation of, 429
common abbreviations, 396–397
fitting of, 428–429
full metal crown in dog, 402
impressions and, 426–427
marginal finish of, 429
materials used, 401–408
models and, 427–428
partial, 408–409
preparation procedure, 424–431
restorative terms, 395–396
try-in of, 428–429
types of, 57

wax-pattern fabrication, 429
Curettage
periapical, 344
Curette, 3, 6–8
Gracey curette numbering nomenclature, 7
parts of, 1, 3
Currents
electrosurgical, 14–15
Curved scaler
parts of, 1, 2
Curved sickle scaler, 6
Cuspids
exodontia and, 237–238
Cyst
equine, 568
Cysts. *See* Tumors
odontogenic classification, 130
radiographs and, 163

D
Deciduous occlusion, 440
Deciduous teeth
anomalies, 171
endodontic therapy and, 336–337
endodontics, 171–172
eruption sequences of, 169
eruption times, 68, 97
extraction, 174–175
malocclusions, 172–174
oral cavity abnormalities and, 175–176
orthodontics, 172–174
pathology of, 171–176
periodontics and, 181–182
Defects. *See* Acquired defects; Congenital
defects;
Developmental defects
lip and cheek, 247–250. *See also* Lip and
cheek defects
palatal, 242–247. *See also* Palatal defects
Dens in dente
radiographs and, 160
Dens invaginatus
radiographs and, 160
Dental abbreviations, 100–101
Dental abnormalities
exotic animals and, 546–556
Dental abscess
equine, 569–571
Dental anatomy
diagram of, 73
lagomorphs, 522–526. *See also* Lagomorphs
rodent, 522–526. *See also* Rodents
Dental chart
for record, 100

Dental charting, 96–101
Dental defense mechanism, 357–359
  principles of, 397
Dental disease
  exotic animal, 538–558. *See also* Exotic
    animal dentistry
  feline, 482–517. *See also* Cat
  lagomorphs, 518–537. *See also* Lagomorphs
  large animal, 559–579. *See also* Equine
    dentistry; Porcine dentistry; Ruminant
    dentistry
  rodent, 518–537. *See also* Rodents
Dental equipment, 1–28
  hand equipment, 1–10. *See also* Hand
    equipment
  models and impressions, 11–12. *See also*
    Dental models
  operative hand instruments, 10
  orthodontics, 12–13
  periodontal equipment, 1–10. *See also*
    Periodontal equipment
  power equipment, 16–27. *See also* Power
    equipment
  power sources, 18–22
  restorative instruments and equipment,
    10–11
  surgical instruments, 13–15. *See also*
    Surgical instruments
Dental film, 146–150. *See also* Film;
    Radiology
  protective packet and, 146
  sizes, 148–149
  speeds, 149–150
  stipple pattern on, 147
  storage, 148
Dental formulas
  exotic animal, 541–544
  rodents and lagomorphs, 523
Dental injury
  behavioral problems and, 610–611
Dental laboratories
  orthodontics and, 472
Dental mirrors, 4
Dental models, 468–472
  identification, 472
  impression techniques, 469–470
  impression trays, 468–469
  marketing and, 591–596
  model techniques, 469–470
  pouring the cast, 471–472
  procedure for, 470–471
  storage, 472
  treatment of, 472
  trimming, 472

Dental prosthetic devices. *See also*
    Prosthodontics
Dental radiology, 140–166. *See also* Radiology
Dental resorptive lesions, 113
  feline, 487–496. *See also* Feline dental
    resorptive lesions
Dental restorative terminology
  common abbreviations of, 356. *See also*
    Restorative dentistry
Dental surgery
  periodontal disease and, 216–217
Dental tissue
  acquired disorders and, 112–114
  dental resorptive lesions, 113
  developmental pathology and, 105–108
  G.V. Black classification system, 113, 114
  peg tooth, 105
  staging of tooth injuries, 114
Dental waxes
  casts and, 44–45
Dentigerous cyst
  equine, 568
Dentin
  development of, 62–65
Dentinal tubules
  electron micrograph of, 63, 64
Dentofacial deformity, 437–438
Dermal papilla, 75
Destructive chewing
  behavioral problems and, 612–614
Developer solution
  film processing and, 154
Developmental defects
  cheek, 248–250
  lips, 248–250
Developmental pathology, 105–112
  craniomandibular osteopathy, 111
  dental tissues and, 105–108
  lips, 109–110
  oral cavity, 108
  palate, 108–109
  peg tooth, 105
  periodontal gingiva, 108
  periosteal proliferation, 111
  salivary gland, 109
  skeletal, 110–112
  soft tissue and, 108–112
  tight-lip syndrome, 110
  tongue, 109
Diagnostic procedures, 87–103. *See also* Oral
    diagnosis
Diagnostic tests
  oral, 94–96
  preanesthesia, 91

Diamond rotary instruments, 26–27
Dilaceration
 radiographs and, 160
Diphyodont tooth development
 common terms of, 56
Directional nomenclature
 line drawing of, 70
 teeth, 69–74. *See also* Teeth
Disclosing solution
 periodontal use of, 52
Discoloration, 387–392. *See also* Bleaching
Disorders
 acquired, 112–116. *See also* Acquired
  disorders
Displacements
 orthodontics and, 443–444
Distal inclination of maxillary cuspid
 treatment of, 466–467
Doberman pinscher
 peg tooth in, 105
Dog
 acanthomatous epulis, 132
 behavioral problems and, 600–604. *See also*
  Behavioral problems
 bird tongue, 176
 button brackets, 466
 craniomandibular osteopathy, 111
 dental formula designations, 69
 dental models and, 592–595
 distal inclination of maxillary cuspid,
  467
 elastic ligature placement, 459
 endodontic access, 305–309
 fading puppy syndrome, 176
 full metal crown in, 402
 gingival depth in, 92
 incisor movement, 459, 463
 mandibular brackets, 463
 mandibular premolar radiographs, 326
 melanosarcoma, 134
 peg tooth in, 105
 pemphigus vulgaris, 118
 pulp cavity size in, 326
 rostromesial inclination, 466
 rubber jaw syndrome, 121
 salivary glands of, 82
 teeth eruption times, 97
 tight-lip syndrome, 110, 168, 248–249
 tonsillar squamous cell carcinoma, 134,
  135
 tooth development of, 58
 tooth eruption in, 68
 tooth eruption sequences, 169
 tooth root surfaces, 448

Dowel crowns
 operative dentistry, 422–424
Dowels
 endodontic, 386–387
Drainage
 periadicular, 343–344
Drill
 Gates-Glidden, 297–298
Dry mouth
 periodontal disease and, 195
Dry socket
 exodontia and, 241

E
EDTA
 endodontic therapy and, 300, 301
Elastic impression materials, 40–42
 hydrocolloids, 40–41
 synthetic elastomers, 40–41
Elastic ligatures, 454, 459
Elastic rings
 sizes, 455
Elastic slippage
 orthodontic complications and, 479
Elastomers
 synthetic, 41–42
Elbow stricture
 endodontic instruments and, 332
Electric motor units
 power equipment and, 18–19
Electrocautery units, 14–15
Electrosurgery, 233
 currents, 14–15
 units, 14–15
Elementary cavity classification
 location and, 352
Elephant
 eruption times, 553, 554
 lophodont and, 555
Elliptication
 endodontic instruments and, 332
Embedded teeth
 exodontia and, 239
Embrasures
 teeth and, 72
Enamel
 development of, 62–65
Enamel bonding agents
 tooth restoration and, 381
Enamel coverage
 operative dentistry and, 417
Enamel organ development
 bell stage, 60, 61
 bud stage, 58

Enamel organ development (*contd.*)
  cap stage, 59
Enamel pearls
  radiographs and, 160
Enamelomas
  radiographs and, 160
Endodontic anatomy, 280–283
Endodontic cement, 312–314
Endodontic dowels, 386–387
Endodontic instruments, 29–32, 290–303. *See also* Endodontic therapy
  absorbent paper points, 298
  aids, 299–302
  American National standard coding, 291
  apexification, 339–341
  apexigenesis, 337–339
  apical perforation and, 332
  automated mechanical handpieces, 302–303
  backup technique and, 334
  broaches, 292–293
  classification of, 292–299
  color coding of, 291
  condensers, 296
  diameter of, 291
  elbow stricture and, 332
  elliptication and, 332
  endodontic stops, 303
  engine-driven root canal instruments, 297–298
  errors from, 331–335
  file variations/innovations, 295–296
  group I, 292–297
  group II, 297
  group III, 297–298
  group IV, 298–299
  gutta-percha points, 32, 298, 299
  H-type files, 293, 294–295, 296
  history, 290–292
  immature deciduous teeth and, 336–337
  immature permanent teeth and, 337–341
  irrigants, 299–302
  irrigation needles, 30
  K-type files and reamers, 293–294, 296
  lateral wall perforation and, 333
  ledging and, 331
  measurement aids, 302–303
  paper points, 30
  root resection and, 335–336
  silver points, 298–299
  sonics and, 302
  spreaders, 296
  stripping canal wall and, 333

  surgical, 341–347. *See also* Surgical endodontics
  terminology of, 291
  tooth resection and, 335–336
  ultrasonics and, 302
  zipping and, 332
Endodontic-periodontic lesions, 287–289
Endodontic stops, 303
Endodontic therapy. *See also* Obturation
  abnormal canals and, 328–330
  access of teeth for, 305–309
  access site, 325–327
  advanced, 325–350
  anatomy of, 280–283
  basic, 280–324
  deciduous, 171–172
  endodontic triad, 303–320
  equine, 569–571
  examination techniques, 289–290
  immature permanent teeth and, 180–181
  instrumentation errors and, 331–335
  instruments, 290–303. *See also* Endodontic instruments
  lesions, 287–289
  measurement aids, 302–303
  obturation, 311–320
  perforations and, 327–328
  periapical healing following, 320–321
  periapical pathology, 285–286
  periodontic-endodontic lesions, 287–289
  preparation for, 304
  procedural blockage and, 330–331
  pulp cavity size and, 326
  pulp tissue, 281
  pulpal pathology, 283–285
  root canal instrumentation, 309–310
  root canal procedure, 319–320
  root fractures, 286–287
  sealer cements, 312–314
  smear layer and, 282, 283
  sterilization techniques, 310–311
Endoliths
  radiographs and, 161
Engine-driven root canal instruments, 297–298
Eosinophilic granuloma complex
  feline, 511–512
Eosinophilic lesions, 119
Epithelial root sheath
  formation of, 65, 66
Equine dentistry, 559–575. *See also* Horses
  anatomy, 559
  buccotomy, 575
  dental abscess, 569–571

dental formula, 560
dental terminology, 560–561
dentigerous cyst and, 568
dentition, 559–561
ectopic eruption, 567
endodontic therapy, 569–571
endoscopy and, 565
eruption abnormalities, 567–568
eruption cyst and, 568
eruption sequence, 561
examination, 563–565
exodontia, 572–575
external observation and, 564
first premolar and, 568
incisors, 561–562
malocclusions, 565–567
mandibular brachygnathism, 565–566
maxillary brachygnathism, 566
molar hooks, 563
molars, 562–563
palpation and, 564
polydontia, 567
premolars, 562–563
radiography and, 564–565
retained deciduous teeth, 567–568
root canal therapy, 569–571
sinusotomy, 572, 574–575
soft tissue pathology, 575
supernumerary teeth, 567
teeth types, 561–563
tooth impaction, 568
tooth repulsion, 572–574
trephination, 572–574
wolf tooth and, 568
wry malocclusion, 566
Equipment
    dental, 1–28. *See also* Dental equipment
    power, 16–27. *See also* Power equipment
    restorative, 10–11
Eruption
    teeth, 169–171. *See also* Teeth
Eruption abnormalities
    equine, 567–568
Eruption cyst
    equine, 568
Eruption times, 97
Essig's wiring technique
    oral fracture repair and, 272–273
Esthetics
    operative dentistry and, 398
    restoration procedures and, 359–360
Examination procedures, 87–103. *See also* Oral
    diagnosis

Excessive oral grooming, 618–620
Exodontia, 234–242
    alveolar ridge for tooth retention, 236
    canines/cuspids, 237–238
    complications, 239–242
    dry socket and, 241
    embedded teeth, 239
    equine, 572–575
    fractured root tips and, 240
    indications, 234
    localized osteitis and, 241
    lower 1st molar, 238
    mucoperiosteal flap repair, 242
    oronasal fistula and, 241–242
    technique, 234–237
    upper 4th premolar, 238
Exotic animal dentistry, 538–558
    abscesses and, 551
    cage-biter syndrome, 548
    carnivore dentition, 540, 541–544
    carnivore disorders, 547–549
    dental abnormalities, 546–556
    dental formulas, 541–544
    dental variation, 540–546
    gingivitis and, 549
    herbivore dentition, 540–545
    herbivore disorders, 552–556
    lumpy jaw, 552, 553
    omnivore disorders, 549–552
    special considerations, 538–539
    zoonoses and, 538
Explorers
    periodontal, 5–6
Extraction
    deciduous tooth, 174–175
Extraoral radiology techniques, 152–153.
        See also Intraoral radiology;
        Radiology

F

Facultative anaerobes
    periodontal disease and, 192
Fading puppy syndrome, 176
Favorable fracture
    mandibular, 263
    transosseous wire and, 268
Feline cervical line lesions, 487–496. *See also*
        Feline dental resorptive lesions
    classification of, 492
    home care, 495–496
    professional aftercare, 495
Feline cuspid oronasal fistula
    exodontia and, 242

Feline dental chart. *See also* Cat
  for record, 100
Feline dental models
  marketing and, 595–596
Feline dental resorptive lesions, 487–496
  classification of, 492
  clinical signs, 490–491
  diagnosis, 491–494
  home care, 495–496
  prevalence studies, 487, 488
  professional aftercare, 495
  stage I, 489, 491, 492
  Stage II, 489, 491, 492–494
  stage III, 494
  stage IV, 494
  stage V, 491, 494
  staging of, 355
  treatment, 491–494
Feline juvenile gingivitis, 497
Feline lymphocytic plasmocytic stomatitis,
    496–499
  clinical signs, 497
  diagnosis of, 498
  home care, 499
  pathology, 496–497
  treatment of, 498–499
Feline mandibular trauma, 503–506
  clinical signs, 503
  horizontal ramus fractures, 504–505
  symphyseal separations/fractures, 503–504
  TMJ injuries, 505–506
Feline neoplasias, 509–511
Feline oral trauma, 499–503
  clinical signs, 500
  hard palate separations, 501–502
  labial avulsion, 501
  oral burns, 502–503
  tooth avulsion, 501
  tooth fractures, 500–501
Felines, 482–517. *See also* Cat
Fiberoptic handpieces, 22
Files
  H-type, 293, 294–295, 296
  Hedstrom, 293, 294–295, 296
  K-type, 293–294, 296
  periodontal, 8
  variation/innovations, 295–296
Filler
  lentula spiral, 297
Filling
  retrograde, 345–346
Film. *See also* Dental film; Radiology
  dental, 146–150
  developer solution and, 154

diagnostic quality of, 156–159
  fingerprints on, 158
  fixer solutions and, 154–155
  focal-film distance, 144–145
  identification of, 155
  mounting, 155–156
  object-film distance, 144–145
  processing faults, 156–158
  processing of, 153–156
  quality of, 156–159
  radiographic faults, 156–158
Finish line types
  operative dentistry and, 414
Fistula
  oronasal, 241–242
Fixation. *See also* Oral fracture repair
  external, 276
  interarcade, 274. *See also* Wiring
    techniques
  internal, 275–276
Fixed appliances, 452–453
Fixed-fixed bridge
  components of, 411
Fixed-movable bridge
  components of, 411
Fixer solutions
  film processing and, 154–155
Flap repair
  mucoperiosteal, 242
Fluoride
  topical application of, 182–183
  types of, 48–50
Focal–film distance, 144–145
Formulas
  dental designations, 69
Fractured root tips
  exodontia and, 240
Fractures
  favorable, 263
  mandibular body, 262–264
  mandibular body classification, 261
  maxilla, 265
  repair of, 759–779. *See also* Oral fracture
    repairs
  root, 286–287
  rostral mandibular, 261–262
  TMJ, 265
  unfavorable, 263–264. *See also* Unfavorable
    fracture
  vertical ramus, 264
  wiring techniques for, 266–274. *See also*
    Wiring techniques
Free gingival graft
  periodontal disease and, 215–216

Furcation exposure
  attachment loss and, 92, 93
  classification, 205
  periodontitis and, 204–205
Fusion teeth
  gemination vs., 160

G
Gates-Glidden drill
  endodontic therapy and, 297–298
Gemination
  fusion teeth vs., 160
Generators
  x-ray, 142–144
Gerbil
  baseline physiologic data, 521
  dental formula, 523
German shepherd
  tonsillar squamous cell carcinoma,
    135
Gingiva
  examination of, 89–90
  periodontal, 108
  soft tissue pathology and, 116–136. *See also*
    Oral mucosa
Gingival graft
  periodontal disease and, 215–216
Gingival hyperplasia, 550
Gingival index, 196
Gingival sulcus
  depth of, 92
  periodontal disease and, 188, 189
Gingivitis
  acute necrotizing ulcerative, 499
  definition, 186. *See also* Periodontal
    disease
  exotic animals and, 549
  feline juvenile, 497
Glands
  salivary, 81–85, 125–126, 251–252
Glass ionomers, 376–378
  application of, 377 378
  cavity prep for, 377–378
  classification of, 378
  restorative use of, 35–36
Glass restoratives. *See* Operative dentistry
Gorilla
  dentition, 545
Gracey curette, 6–8
  numbering nomenclature, 7
Graft
  gingival, 215–216
Grasps
  hand instruments and, 1-4

Grooves
  retentive, 420
Group I endodontic instruments, 292–297
  barbed broach, 292–293
  broaches, 292–293
  condensers, 296
  H-type file, 293, 294–295, 296
  K-type files and reamers, 293–294, 296
  spreaders, 296
Group II endodontic instruments, 297
Group III endodontic instruments, 297–298
Group IV endodontic instruments, 298–299
Guided tissue regeneration, 221–227
  barrier selection, 223
  bulk material and, 224–225
  discussion, 221–223
  membrane barriers and, 223–224
  objectives, 225–226
  osseous replacement barriers and,
    224–225
  postoperative care, 227
  procedure, 226
  site selection, 223
Guinea pig
  baseline physiologic data, 521
  cheek teeth overgrowth, 527
  dental formula, 523
Gutta-percha points
  endodontic therapy and, 298, 299
  type I and II, 32
G.V. Black classification system, 352–354, 396,
    401
  acquired disorders and, 114
  cavity preparation and, 365

H
Hamster
  baseline physiologic data, 521
  dental formula, 523
  isoflurane anesthesia induction, 521, 522
Hand equipment, 1–10
  chisels, 8
  curettes, 1, 3, 6–8
  curved scaler, 1, 2
  dental mirrors, 4
  files, 8
  hoe, 8
  instrument grasps, 1–4
  operative, 10
  oral irrigators, 9
  periodontal explorers, 5–6
  periodontal probes, 4–5
  scalers, 2, 6–8
  sharpening of, 8–9

Handpieces
  air-driven, 22
  classification by speeds, 21
  endodontic, 302–303
  fiberoptic, 22
  power equipment and, 20–22
Hard palate separations
  feline, 501–502. *See also* Feline oral trauma
Harmonic scalpels, 15
Hedstrom file
  endodontic therapy and, 293, 294–295
Hematologic abnormalities
  oral mucosa and, 120
Hemimandibulectomy, 254–255
Hemostatic solutions
  periodontal use, 47
Herbivores
  dental disorders, 552–556
  dentition, 540–545
  lumpy jaw and, 552–553
Hertwig's epithelial root sheath
  formation of, 65, 66
History gathering
  oral examination and, 87–88
Hoes, 8
Hole punch sizes
  rubber dam, 369
Home care
  preventive dentistry and, 183
Home care instructions
  orthodontics and, 475
Home prophylaxis (dental home care)
  frequency of, 219
  periodontal disease and, 217–219
  types of, 219
Horizontal ramus
  fractures of, 504–505. *See also* Feline
    mandibular trauma
Horses, 559–575. *See also* Equine dentistry
  brachygnathism, 565–566
  hypsodont cheek teeth, 560
  molar hooks, 563
Hot light
  radiographic viewing and, 159
Hydraulic scalers, 18
Hydrocolloid impression material, 40–41
Hygiene
  orthodontics and, 479
Hypercementosis
  radiographs and, 162

I

Identification of film, 155
Imaging. *See* Radiology

Immature deciduous teeth
  endodontic therapy and, 336–337
Immature permanent tooth pathology, 176–183
  endodontic therapy and, 337–341
  endodontics and, 180–181
  fluorides and, 182–183
  home care, 183
  operculum, 177
  orthodontics and, 179–180
  periodontics and, 181–182
  preventive dentistry, 182–183
Impacted teeth
  radiographs and, 160
Implant restorations, 431–432
Impression materials, 39–42
  elastic, 40–42
  hydrocolloids, 40–41
  nonelastic, 39–40
  synthetic elastomers, 41–42
Impression techniques, 469–470
Impression trays, 468–469
Impressions
  crowns and, 426–427
  equipment for, 11–12
Indirect composite resins techniques
  operative dentistry and, 404–405
Indirect resection, 347
Infrabony-pocket wall classification
  periodontitis and, 203–204
Infraversion
  treatment of, 457–458
Initial oral survey, 89–90
Injuries
  fractures, 162
  mandibular symphyseal classification, 262.
    See also Oral fracture repair
  traumatic, 162
Instrumentation aids
  endodontic therapy and, 299–302
Instruments
  endodontic, 290–303. *See also* Endodontic
    instruments
  grasps, 1–4
  operative hand–held, 10
  restorative, 10–11
  root canal, 309–310
  surgical, 13–15
Interarcade wiring/fixation
  oral fracture repair and, 274
Interceptive orthodontics, 445
Interdental wiring
  Essig's, 272–273
  ivy loop, 270–271
  oral fracture repair and, 270–274

Risdon's, 272–274
Stout's multiple loop, 271–272
Interfragmentary wiring
oral fracture repair and, 268
Internal fixation
oral fracture repair and, 275–276
Intraoral films
sizes of, 148
Intraoral radiology, 150–153
bisecting-angle technique, 151–152
extraoral techniques and, 152–153
film sizes, 148–149
localization techniques, 152
paralleling technique, 150, 151
SLOB rule, 152
Ionomers
glass, 35–36
Irrigants
endodontic therapy and, 299–302
Irrigation needles
endodontic use of, 30
Irrigators
oral, 9
Isoflurane induction, 521, 522
Isolation techniques
operating field and, 366–371
Ivy loop wiring technique
oral fracture repair and, 270–271

J

Jacquette scaler, 6
Jaguar
eruption times, 544
Jaw occlusal overlay
types of, 57–58
Juvenile-onset periodontitis
feline, 496–497

K

K-type files and reamers
endodontic therapy and, 293–294, 296
Klipspringer
lumpy jaw and, 553

L

Labial avulsion
feline, 501. *See also* Feline oral trauma
Labial maxillary arch bar with elastics,
461–462
Labrador retriever
rubber jaw syndrome, 121
Lagomorph malocclusion, 526–532
atraumatic, 526–527
traumatic, 528

treatment, 528–532
Lagomorphs, 518–537. *See also* Rabbits
anesthesia, 520–522
baseline physiologic data, 521
continually erupting teeth, 347
coprophagy, 535
dental anatomy, 522–526
dental chart, 518, 519
dental disease, 526–533
malocclusion, 526–532. *See also* Lagomorph
malocclusion
medications and, 534–535
oral assessment, 518–520
oral disease, 533–534
peg teeth incisors, 524
periodontal disease, 533
stomatitis, 533
Lateral root canal procedure, 319–320
Lateral wall perforation
endodontic instruments and, 333
Ledging
endodontic instruments and, 331
pin, 384, 420–421
Lentula spiral filler
endodontic therapy and, 297
Leopard
buccal erosive lesion, 548
eruption times, 544
Lesion
detection of, 369
endodontic-periodontic, 287–289
periapical, 161, 162
Lesion detection
operating field and, 369
Lesions
acquired defects, 243
dental resorptive, 113
eosinophilic, 119
feline dental resorptive, 355
G.V. Black classification system,
352–354
resorptive, 160
restorations and, 396
Line angles
cavities and, 363
teeth and, 71
Liners
restorative use of, 37–39
tooth restoration and, 380
Lingual maxillary arch bar with kick springs,
454, 459, 460
Lingual molar salivary gland, 84, 85
Linguoversion
treatment of, 458, 464

Lion
  eruption times, 544
Lip and cheek defects
  acquired, 250
  congenital/developmental, 248–250
  oral surgery and, 247–250
  tight-lip syndrome, 248–249
Lips
  cleft, 175
  developmental pathology and, 109
  soft tissue pathology and, 126–127
Localization techniques
  radiology and, 152. *See also* Intraoral
    radiology
Localized juvenile periodontitis, 199, 200
Localized osteitis
  exodontia and, 241
Lophodont, 555
Lower 1st molar
  exodontia and, 238
Lumpy jaw
  herbivores and, 552, 553
Lymphocytic plasmocytic stomatitis
  feline, 496–499. *See also* Feline lymphocytic
    plasmocytic stomatitis

M
Malar abscesses
  exotic animals and, 551
Malignant tumors
  fibrosarcoma, 134
  melanosarcoma, 134
  osteosarcoma, 135
  soft tissue pathology and, 133–136
  squamous cell carcinoma, 134
  tonsillar squamous cell carcinoma, 134, 135
Malocclusion, 442–443. *See also* Orthodontics
  classifications of, 440–444
  deciduous, 172–174
  divisions of, 440–444
  equine, 565–567. *See also* Equine dentistry
  feline, 506–507
  lagomorph, 526–532. *See also* Lagomorph
    malocclusion
  rodent, 526–532. *See also* Rodent
    malocclusion
  sequelae of, 436
  treatment of, 467–468
Mandibular anatomy, 78
Mandibular brachygnathism
  equine, 565–566
Mandibular brackets, 462, 463
Mandibular fractures
  body, 262–264

  favorable, 263
  rostral, 261–262
  treatment options for, 260
  unfavorable, 263–264
Mandibular labioversion
  treatment of, 458
Mandibular symphyseal injury
  classification of, 262
Mandibular trauma
  feline, 503–506. *See also* Feline mandibular
    trauma
Mandibulectomy, 253–255
  rostral hemimandibulectomy, 254
  rostral mandibulectomy, 253–254
  segmental hemimandibulectomy, 254–255
  total hemimandibulectomy, 255
Mann incline appliance, 456, 465
Marginal finish lines
  preparation of, 363–364, 400–401
Marketing issues, 580–597
  advertising, 583, 588
  cooperative direct advertising, 583
  definition of, 580
  dental models, 591–596
  dentistry reference chart, 589
  direct mail advertising, 583, 588
  getting started, 580–582
  handouts, 589–591
  hospital brochures, 588
  in-hospital displays, 588–589
  magazines and, 583, 584
  marketing to existing clients, 587–596
  newspapers and, 583, 584
  potential media questions, 584
  preoperative handout, 589–590
  product delivery, 582
  product development, 580–581
  product introduction, 581, 582
  protocol manual, 581, 582
  public relations, 583–585
  radio and, 583, 584
  special events, 585–587
  techniques, 582–583
  television and, 583, 585
  yellow-page advertising, 583
Maryland bridge
  components of, 411
Mass resection
  oral surgery and, 252–253
Mastication
  anatomy and physiology of, 79
Maxilla fractures, 265
Maxillary brachygnathism
  equine, 566

Maxillary expansion screw, 456, 460, 461
Maxillectomy, 255–256
   partial, 256
   premaxillectomy, 255
McSpadden compacter
   endodontic therapy and, 297
Mechanical endodontic handpieces
   automated, 302–303
Melanosarcoma
   tongue and, 134
Mesioclusion, 440, 441
Mesiodistoclusion, 440, 441
Metabolic disorders
   oral mucosa and, 119–120
Metal restoratives, 402–404
Mice
   dental formula, 523
Microglossia, 176
Midline palatal defect repair, 244–245
Mirrors
   dental, 4
Mixed occlusion, 440
Mobility
   periodontitis and, 205–206
Model materials, 42–45
Model techniques, 469–470
Models
   crowns and, 427–428
   dental, 468–472. *See also* Dental
      models
   equipment for, 11–12
Molar
   exodontia, 238
Molar salivary gland
   lingual, 84, 85
Mounting film, 155–156
Mounts
   types of, 155
Mouse
   baseline physiologic data, 521
Mouth
   anatomy and physiology of, 74–76
   dermal papilla, 75
   oral mucous membrane, 75–76
Mouth mirror
   suction and, 367
Mouth shyness
   behavioral problems and, 615–616
Mucocele
   cervical, 252
Mucoperiosteal flap
   periodontal disease and, 213, 214
Mucoperiosteal flap repair
   exodontia and, 242

Mucous membrane
   oral, 75–76
Myrrh
   tincture of benzoin and, 46

N
National Pet Dental Health Month
   marketing and, 585–587. *See also* Marketing
      issues
Needles
   irrigation, 30
Neoplasia
   feline, 509–511
   soft tissue pathology and, 128–136. *See also*
      Tumors
Neutroclusion, 440, 441
Nonelastic impression materials, 39–40
Nonspecific plaque hypothesis, 193
Nonvital teeth
   bleaching of, 389–392
Nutria
   dental formula, 523
Nutrition
   oral mucosa and, 120–122
   rubber jaw syndrome, 121
Nutritional deficiencies
   tongue and, 124

O
Object-film distance, 144–145
Obturation
   complication terms, 318–319
   endodontic therapy and, 311–320
   lateral root canal procedure, 319–320
   medicated sealer cements, 314
   retrograde, 345–346
   sealer cements, 312–314
   techniques, 314–318
Occlusal overlay
   jaw, 57–58
Occlusion
   classifications of, 440–444
   divisions of, 440–444
Odontogenic tumors/cysts
   classification of, 130
Omnivores
   dental abnormalities, 549–552
Operating fields
   amalgam restorations, 370–371
   caries detection, 369
   cheek retractors, 367–368
   cotton rolls and, 367
   isolation techniques for, 366–369

Operating fields (*contd.*)
  lesion detection, 369
  mouth mirror and suction, 367
  operative dentistry and, 401
  restorative materials, 370
  rubber dam and, 368–369
  tongue retractors and shields, 367–368
Operative dentistry, 351–394. *See also* Cavities;
      Restorative dentistry; Teeth
  armamentarium, 414–417
  axial wall taper, 417
  Basrani's staging of tooth injuries, 355
  bleaching teeth, 387–392
  bridge definition, 410
  caries detection and, 369
  cast glass ceramic and, 405–406
  cavity classifications, 352–354
  cavity preparation, 365–366, 398, 400, 401
  cavosurface angle preparation, 400–401
  ceramometal and, 407–408
  cheek retractors, 367–368
  common bridge types, 410–412
  components of prepared cavities, 362–363,
      400
  contacts and contours, 360
  core buildup, 421–422
  cotton rolls and, 367
  crown fitting, 428–429
  crown preparation procedure, 424–431
  crowns and, 395–434. *See also* Crowns
  dental defense mechanism, 357–359, 397
  dowel crowns, 422–424
  enamel coverage and, 417
  esthetics, 359–360, 398
  extension for prevention, 360, 398–399
  feline dental resorptive lesions, 355
  finish line types and uses of, 414
  identification and resolution of cause,
      360–361, 399
  implant restorations, 431–432
  impressions and, 426–427
  in-clinic composite crown restorations,
      409–410
  indirect composite resins techniques and,
      404–405
  indirect forms, 401
  lesion detection and, 369
  marginal finish lines preparation,
      400–401
  metal restoratives and, 402–404
  models and, 427–428
  mouth mirrors and suction, 367
  natural tooth structure conservation, 359, 398

  operating field and, 401
  operating field isolation techniques, 366–369
  partial crowns, 408–409
  pins, pin holes, pin ledging, 420–421
  polymer glass and, 406–407
  porcelain and, 407–408
  porcelain-fused-to-metal restorations,
      407–408
  post/core and crown, 422–424
  post crown, 422–424
  prosthodontics, 395–434. *See also*
      Prosthodontics
  reduction requirements for restoratives, 413
  resolution of cause, 360–361
  restoration rules, 359, 397–399
  restorative materials, 370–387. *See also*
      Amalgam restorations; Composite
      resins; Glass ionomers
  restorative terminology abbreviations, 356
  restorative terms, 395–397
  retention principles, 417–424
  retentive grooves and, 420
  rubber dam and, 368–369
  tongue retractors and shields, 367–368
  tooth coverage and, 417–420
  tooth crown contours and, 398
  tooth injury staging, 355
  tooth reduction, 413–414
  treatment planning, 361–365, 399
Operative hand instruments, 10
Operculum, 177
Oral anatomy and physiology, 55–86
  dental formula designations, 69
  equine, 559. *See also* Equine dentistry
  feline, 482–483. *See also* Cats
  lagomorphs, 522–526. *See also* Lagomorphs
  mastication, 79
  mouth, 74–76. *See also* Mouth
  oral cavity, 76–77. *See also* Oral cavity
  osseous tissue, 77–79
  rodent, 522–526. *See also* Rodents
  salivary glands, 81–85
  teeth, 55–74. *See also* Teeth
  tongue, 79–81
Oral burns
  feline, 502–503. *See also* Feline oral trauma
Oral cavity, 77
  abnormalities, 175–176
  anatomy and physiology of, 76–77
  behavioral problems and, 598–627. *See also*
      Behavioral problems
  developmental pathology and, 108
  feline autoimmune diseases, 509

soft palate, 77
vestibule, 76–77
Oral charting, 96–101
Oral diagnosis, 87–103
    dental abbreviations, 100–101
    dental chart for record, 100
    dental charting, 96–101
    diagnostic tests, 94–96
    furcation exposure, 92, 93
    gingiva examination, 89, 90
    gingival depth in dog, 92
    history gathering, 87–88
    in-depth oral examination, 91–94
    initial oral survey, 89–91
    oral charting, 96–101
    palate examination, 89–90
    physical examination, 88–89
    preanesthesia diagnostic tests, 91
    radiographs and, 93–94
    teeth eruption times, 97
    teeth examination, 89, 90
    tests and, 94–96
    tongue examination, 90–91
    transillumination, 95–96
Oral disease
    exotic animal, 538–558. *See also* Exotic
        animal dentistry
    feline, 482–517, 483–499. *See also* Cats
    lagomorphs, 518–537, 526–534. *See also*
        Lagomorphs
    large animals, 559–579. *See also* Equine
        dentistry; Porcine dentistry; Ruminant
        dentistry
    rodent, 518–537, 526–634. *See also* Rodents
Oral examination, 87–103. *See also* Oral
        diagnosis
    in depth, 91–94
    show dog and, 616
Oral fracture repair, 259–279
    acrylic splints, 274–275
    adjunct wiring, 274
    assessment, 259–261
    complications, 276–277
    favorable fracture, 263
    interarcade wiring/fixation, 274
    interdental wiring, 270–274
    internal fixation, 275–276
    mandibular body, 262–264
    mandibular body fractures classification, 261
    mandibular fracture line and, 260
    mandibular symphyseal injury classification,
        262
    maxilla, 265

    osseous wiring, 266–269
    rostral mandibular, 261–262
    tape muzzle, 265–266
    temporomandibular joint, 265
    treatment modalities, 265–276
    treatment planning, 261–265
    unfavorable fracture, 263–264
    vertical ramus, 264
    wiring techniques, 266–274. *See also* Wiring
        techniques
Oral irrigators, 9
Oral masses
    oral surgery and, 252–253
Oral mucosa
    eosinophilic lesions, 119
    hematologic abnormalities and, 120
    metabolic disorders and, 119–120
    nutrition and, 120–121
    pemphigus vulgaris, 118
    rubber jaw syndrome, 121
    soft tissue pathology and, 116–136
    trauma and, 122
    viral papillomatosis, 119
Oral mucous membrane
    anatomy and physiology of, 75–76
    dermal papilla, 75
Oral pathology
    clinical, 104–139. *See also* Clinical oral
        pathology
Oral radiology, 140–166. *See also* Radiology
Oral surgery, 232–258
    basic principles of, 232
    cervical mucocele, 252
    cheek defects and, 247–250. *See also* Lip
        and cheek defects
    electrosurgery, 233
    exodontia, 234–242. *See also* Exodontia
    hemimandibulectomy, 254–255
    lip defects and, 247–250. *See also* Lip and
        cheek defects
    mandibulectomy, 253–255. *See also*
        Mandibulectomy
    mass resection, 252–253
    maxillectomy, 255–256. *See also*
        Maxillectomy
    palatal defects and, 242–247. *See also* Palatal
        defects
    radiosurgery, 233
    repair techniques for the palate, 243–247
    salivary gland resection, 252
    salivary glands and, 251–252
    tight-lip syndrome and, 248–249
    TMJ and, 256

Oral surgery (*contd.*)
tongue and, 250–251. *See also* Tongue
tonsils and, 251
Oral syndromes
periodontitis and, 200–201
Oral tendencies
feline, 607–609
puppies, 602–604
Oral trauma
feline, 499–503. *See also* Feline oral trauma
Oral tumors
feline, 509–511
soft tissue pathology and, 128–136. *See also* Tumors
Oronasal fistula
exodontia and, 241–242
Orthoclusion, 436, 440, 441
Orthodontics. *See also* Malocclusion
acid-etching, 473
age and, 446–447
anchorage and, 450–451
appliance-associated trauma, 479
appliance prescriptions, 472
appliance removal, 476
appliance types, 452–456
application of force, 451–452
band and bracket placement, 472–474
basics of, 435–481
bites, 442
cementation, 472–474. *See also* Cementation
complications, 476
crestal alveolar bone and, 476–477
deciduous, 172–174
dental models, 468–472. *See also* Dental models
dentofacial deformity, 437–438
diagnostic aids, 446
displacements and, 443–444
elastic rings, 454–455
elastic slippage and, 479
equipment for, 12–13
ethical standards of, 436–437
etiology, 437–439
fixed appliances, 452–453
heredity and, 438–439
history of, 436
home care instructions, 475
hygiene and, 479
immature permanent teeth and, 179–180
inclinations and, 443
laboratories and, 472
local influences, 439
malpositioning of teeth and, 442–443

materials, 453–454
occlusions, 441
origin of, 435
periodontal ligament and, 476, 477–478
pulp and, 476, 478
removable appliances, 452
retainers, 475–476
retention period, 475–476
root structure and, 476, 477
site selection, 472–473
systemic influences, 439
tipping and, 443
tooth discoloration and, 478–479
tooth movement and, 447–450
treatable conditions, 457–468
treatment categories, 445–446
treatment goals, 444
treatment release form, 437, 438
treatment timing, 446–447
versions and, 443, 444
wire types, 453
Osseous tissue
anatomy and physiology of, 77–79
Osseous wiring
oral fracture repair and, 266–269
Osteitis
localized, 241
Osteodentin
cats and, 488
Osteomyelitis
soft tissue pathology and, 128
Osteomyelitis of the jaw
radiographs and, 163
Osteopathy
craniomandibular, 111
Outline form
cavity preparation and, 365

P
Palatal defects
acquired, 243
asymmetric defect repair, 245–247
congenital, 242–243
deep palatal troughs and, 247, 248
feline, 508–509
midline defect repair, 244–245
oral surgery and, 242–247
osseous defect, 244
palatal trauma, 243, 244
repair techniques, 243–247
split U-flap palatal repair, 246–247

Palatal troughs
    periodontal disease and, 247, 248
Palate
    cleft, 175
    developmental pathology and, 108–109
    examination of, 89–90
    soft, 77
Paper points
    absorbent, 298
    endodontic use of, 30
Papilla
    dermal, 75
Papillomatosis
    viral, 119
Paradental anatomy
    diagram of, 73
Paralleling technique
    intraoral radiology and, 150, 151
Parrot mouth
    equine, 565
Partial crowns, 408–409
Partial maxillectomy, 256
Pathology
    clinical oral, 104–139. *See also* Clinical oral
        pathology
Pathology removal form
    cavity preparation and, 366
Pedicle flaps
    periodontal disease and, 215
Pedodontics, 167–185
    bird tongue, 176
    deciduous tooth pathology, 171–176. *See
        also* Deciduous teeth
    endodontics, 180–181
    eruption anomalies, 170–171
    eruption of teeth, 169–171
    eruption sequences, 169
    fading puppy syndrome, 176
    fluoride use, 182–183
    home care, 183
    immature permanent tooth pathology, 176–183
    microglossia, 176
    operculum, 177
    oral cavity abnormalities, 175–176
    oral structural development, 168
    orthodontics, 179–180
    periodontics, 181–182
    preventive dentistry, 182–183
    primary palate cleft, 175
    Shar-Pei tight lip syndrome, 168
    tooth development, 167–168
Peeso reamer
    endodontic therapy and, 297–298

Peg tooth
    Doberman pinscher and, 105
Pemphigus vulgaris, 118
Percentage attachment loss index, 196
Perforation
    apical, 332
    endodontic therapy and, 327–328
    lateral wall, 333
Periadicular drainage, 343–344
Periapical curettage, 344
Periapical healing
    endodontic therapy and, 320–321
Periapical lesion
    radiograph of, 162
Periapical pathology
    etiology of, 285–286
Periapical surgical endodontic procedures,
        343–347. *See also* Apical surgical
        endodontic procedures
Periodontal abscess
    periodontitis and, 206
Periodontal abscesses
    radiographs and, 161
Periodontal disease. *See also* Periodontitis;
        Periodontology
    anatomy, 187–191
    antimicrobial therapy, 211–212
    bacteria and, 192
    causative factors, 191–199
    charting, 207–208
    col and, 188
    definition, 186
    dental surgery, 216–217
    dry mouth and, 195
    evaluation for, 207
    feline, 483–487. *See also* Cat
    free gingival graft, 215–216
    general health and, 186–187
    gingival sulcus, 188, 189
    guided tissue regeneration, 221–227. *See
        also* Guided tissue regeneration
    histologic changes in, 197
    home prophylaxis, 217–219
    indices for, 196–197
    lagomorphs, 533. *See also* Lagomorphs
    periodontal surgery for, 212–215
    periodontal therapy, 210–211
    periodontitis, 199–206. *See also*
        Periodontitis
    plaque hypotheses and, 193
    professional prophylaxis, 208–211
    prognosis by stage, 220
    radiographs and, 160

Periodontal disease (*contd.*)
  rodents, 533. *See also* Rodents
  signs and symptoms, 187
  staging of, 197–199
  therapy, 208–219
  treatment plan for, 220–221
Periodontal disease index
  veterinary, 198
Periodontal-endodontic lesions, 287–289
Periodontal equipment, 1–10
  chisels, 8
  curettes, 3, 6–8
  dental mirrors, 4
  explorers, 5–6
  files, 8
  hand equipment, 1-10. *See also* Hand
    equipment
  hoe, 8
  instrument grasps, 1–4
  oral irrigators, 9
  probes, 4–5
  scalers, 2, 6–8
  sharpening of, 8–9
Periodontal explorers, 5–6
Periodontal file, 8
Periodontal gingiva
  developmental pathology and, 108
Periodontal ligament
  orthodontic complications and, 476, 477–478
Periodontal materials, 45–52
  disclosing solution and, 51
  fluoride and, 48–50
  hemol sol, 47
  retraction cord, 47
  tincture of myrrh and benzoin, 46
Periodontal probes, 4–5
Periodontal surgery
  periodontal disease and, 212–215
Periodontal therapy
  periodontal disease and, 210–211
Periodontics
  deciduous and immature permanent teeth
    and, 181–182
  endodontic-periodontic lesions, 287–289
Periodontitis
  adult, 199
  attachment loss and, 201–203
  definition, 186. *See also* Periodontal disease
  endodontic-periodontic relationship and, 206
  feline juvenile-onset, 496–497
  feline treatment, 485–487. *See also* Cat
  feline types, 484–485
  furcation exposure and, 204–205
  histologic changes in, 197

  infrabony-pocket wall classification and,
    203–204
  localized juvenile, 199, 200
  mobility and, 205–206
  oral syndromes and, 200–201
  pathobiologic classification of, 199–206
  periodontal abscess and, 206
  prepubertal, 199, 200
  rapidly progressive, 199–200
  recession and, 202–203
  refractory rapidly progressive, 199,
    200
Periodontology, 186–231. *See also* Periodontal
    disease
  definition, 186
Periosteal proliferation
  radiograph of, 111
Permanent occlusion, 440
Permanent teeth
  endodontic therapy and, 337–341
  eruption sequences of, 169
  eruption times, 68, 97
  immature, 176–183. *See also* Immature
    permanent tooth pathology
Permanent tooth pathology
  immature, 176–183
Physical examination, 88–89
Physiology and anatomy
  oral, 55–86. *See also* Oral anatomy and
    physiology
Pica
  behavioral problems and, 614–615
Pin holes, 384, 420–421
Pin ledging, 384, 420–421
Pins
  operative dentistry and, 420–421
  restoration, 384–386
Plaque hypothesis, 193
Plaque index, 196
Plastics/resins
  acrylics, 33
  bonding agents, 35
  composite resins, 33–34
  restorative use of, 33–35
Point angles
  cavities and, 363
  teeth and, 71
Points
  absorbent paper, 298
  gutta-percha, 32, 298, 299
  paper, 30
  silver, 298–299
Polydontia
  equine, 567

Polymer glass
  operative dentistry and, 406–407
Porcelain-fused-to-metal restoration
  operative dentistry and, 407–408
Porcelain restorations
  operative dentistry and, 407–408
Porcine dentistry, 578–579
  eruption times, 576
Porcupine
  dental formula, 523
Post/core and crown, 422–424
Post crown
  operative dentistry, 422–424
Posterior cross-bites
  treatment of, 464
Posts
  root canal, 386–387
Power equipment, 16–27
  abrasive materials and, 27
  abrasive points, 26–27
  abrasive strips and, 27
  air-driven units, 19–20, 19–22
  burs, 23–26. *See also* Burs
  diamond abrasive points, 26–27
  electric motor units, 18–19
  handpieces, 20–22
  scalers, 16–18. *See also* Scalers
  sources of power, 18–22
Preanesthesia diagnostic tests, 91
Premaxillectomy, 255
Premolar
  exodontia and, 238
Preoperative handout form, 589–590
Preparation cleansing form
  cavity preparation and, 366
Prepubertal periodontitis, 199, 200
Preventive dentistry
  fluoride topical application and, 182–183
  home care, 183
Preventive orthodontics, 445
Probes
  periodontal, 4–5
Procedural canal blockage
  endodontic therapy and, 330–331
Professional prophylaxis
  periodontal disease and, 208–211
Prophylaxis
  periodontal disease and, 208–211, 217–219
Prosthodontics, 395–434. *See also* Crowns;
    Operative dentistry
  abbreviations, 396–397
  bridge definition, 410
  common bridge types, 410–412
  restorative terms, 395–396

Pulp
  acquired disorders and, 114–116
  cavity size, 326
  development of, 62–65
  endodontic anatomy of, 280–324. *See also*
    Endodontic therapy
  orthodontic complications and, 476, 478
  pathology of, 283–285
  smear layer and, 282, 283
  tissue, 281
Pulp stones
  radiographs and, 161
Pulpal pathology
  etiology of, 283–285
Pulpitis
  radiographs and, 161
Puma
  eruption times, 544

R

Rabbits. *See also* Lagomorphs
  baseline physiologic data, 521
  dental chart, 518, 519
  incisor positioning, 525
  peg teeth incisors, 524
Radiographic film speeds, 149–150
Radiographic index, 197
Radiographic interpretation, 159–163
  ankylosis, 160, 161
  periapical lesion, 161, 162
Radiographic viewing, 159
Radiology, 140–166
  buccal object rule, 152
  Clark's rule, 152
  dental film, 146–150. *See also* Dental film
  extraoral techniques, 152–153
  film processing, 153–156
  film quality, 156–159
  focal-film distance, 144–145
  history, 141–142
  hot light and, 159
  interpretation, 159–163
  intraoral techniques, 150–153. *See also*
    Intraoral radiography
  object-film distance, 144–145
  oral diagnosis and, 93–94
  personal safety and protection, 145–146
  radiation biology, 145
  review questions, 163–165
  SLOB rule, 152
  viewing procedures, 159
  x-radiation, 140–141
  x-ray generators, 142–144
  x-ray machines, 142–144

Radiology (*contd.*)
    x-ray wavelengths and use, 141
Radiosurgery, 233
Radiosurgery units, 14–15
Ramus
    fractures of, 504–505. *See also* Feline
        mandibular trauma
Rapidly progressive periodontitis, 199–200
Rats. *See also* Rodents
    baseline physiologic data, 521
    dental formula, 523
    intraoral dental film usage, 520
Reamer
    K-type, 293–294
    Peeso, 297–298
Reduction requirements
    restoratives and, 413
Refractory rapidly progressive periodontitis,
    199, 200
Removable appliances, 452
Repair
    oral fracture, 259–279. *See also* Oral fracture
        repair
Resection
    apical, 344–345
    indirect, 347
    mass, 252–253
    salivary glands, 252
    tooth/root, 335–336
Resins
    indirect composite, 404–405
    restorative use of, 33–35. *See also*
        Plastics/resins
Resistance form
    cavity preparation and, 366
Resorptive lesions
    dental, 113
    radiographs and, 160
    staging of, 355
Restorations
    lesions and, 396
    rules of, 396–399. *See also* Operative
        dentistry
Restorative dentistry, 351–394. *See also*
        Cavities; Operative dentistry; Teeth
    bleaching teeth, 387–392
    caries detection, 369
    cavity classification systems, 352–354
    cavity preparation, 365-366
    cheek retractors, 367–368
    classifications of, 352–354
    common abbreviations of, 356
    components of prepared cavities, 362–363

    contacts and contours, 360
    cotton rolls and, 367
    dental defense mechanism, 357–359
    esthetics and, 359–360
    extension for prevention, 360
    feline dental resorptive lesions, 355
    identification and resolution of cause,
        360–361
    lesion detection, 369
    materials used in, 370–387. *See also*
        Amalgam restorations; Composite
        resins; Glass ionomers
    mouth mirror and suction, 367
    natural tooth structure conservation, 359
    operating field isolation techniques, 366–369
    rubber dam and, 368–369
    rules of, 359–361
    terms of, 351–352
    tongue retractors and shields, 367–368
    tooth injury staging, 355
    treatment planning, 361–365
Restorative instruments and equipment, 10–11
Restorative materials, 370–387. *See also*
        Amalgam restorations; Composite
        resins; Glass ionomers
    amalgam, 371–376
    composite resins, 378–384
    endodontic dowels, 386–387
    glass ionomers, 376–378
    pin holes, 384
    pin ledging, 384
    pins, 384–386
    root canal posts, 386–387
Restorative procedures
    basic concepts of, 359–361
    esthetics, 359–360
    extension for prevention, 360
    identification and resolution of cause,
        360–361
    natural tooth structure conservation, 359
Restorative terminology
    abbreviations, 395–397
Restoratives, 33–39
    acrylics, 33
    amalgam, 36–37
    bases, 37–39
    bonding agents, 35
    cast glass ceramic, 405–406
    cements, 37–39
    ceramometal, 407–408
    composite resins, 33–34
    glass ionomers, 35–36
    in-clinic composite crown, 409–410

indirect composite resins techniques, 404–405
liners, 37–39
metals, 402–404
partial crowns, 408–409
plastics/resins, 33–35
polymer glass, 406–407
porcelain, 407–408
porcelain fused to metal, 407–408
reduction requirements for, 413
retention principles and, 417–424
tooth reduction and, 413–414
varnishes, 37–39
Restored surfaces
cavity classification and, 354
Retainers
orthodontics and, 475–476
Retention
principles of, 417–424
Retention form
cavity preparation and, 366
Retentive grooves
operative dentistry and, 420
Retraction cord
periodontal use, 47
Retractors
cheek and tongue, 367–368
Retrograde obturation/filling, 345–346
Retrograde root canal procedures, 347
Ridge nomenclature, 69–74. *See also* Teeth
Risdon's wiring technique
oral fracture repair and, 272–274
Rodent malocclusion, 526–532
atraumatic, 526–527
traumatic, 528
treatment, 528–532
Rodents, 518–537. *See also* Rats
anesthesia, 520–522
baseline physiologic data, 521
continually erupting teeth, 347
coprophagy, 535
dental anatomy, 522–526
dental disease, 526–533
intraoral dental film usage, 520
malocclusion, 526–532. *See also* Rodent
malocclusion
medications and, 534–535
oral assessment, 518–520
oral disease, 533–534
periodontal disease, 533
stomatitis, 533
Root canal
abnormal, 328–330

Root canal instruments
endodontic therapy and, 309–310
engine driven, 297–298
Root canal posts, 386–387
Root canal procedure. *See also* Endodontic
therapy
retrograde, 347
Root canal sealer cement, 312–314
Root canal therapy
equine, 569–571
Root formation
anatomy and physiology of, 65–68
Root fractures
endodontic therapy and, 286–287
Root resection
endodontic therapy and, 335–336
Root resorption
classification of, 477
Root structure
orthodontic complications and, 476, 477
Root tips
fractured, 240
Rostral hemimandibulectomy, 254
Rostral mandibular fractures, 261–262
Rostral mandibulectomy, 253–254
Rostral maxillectomy, 255
Rostromesial inclination
treatment of, 466
Rotary instruments, 26–27. *See also* Power
equipment
Rotary scalers, 18
Rotation
treatment of, 457
Rubber dam, 368–369
hole punch sizes, 369
Rubber jaw syndrome
radiograph of, 121
Ruminant dentistry, 576–578
acquired diseases, 577–578
dentition, 576–577
developmental abnormalities, 577

S
Salivary gland disease
feline, 512–513
Salivary glands
anatomy and physiology of, 81–85
cat, 83
developmental pathology and, 109
dog, 82
lingual molar, 84, 85
oral surgery and, 251–252
resection, 252

Salivary glands (*contd.*)
    soft tissue pathology and, 125–126
Salivary stones, 126
    radiographs and, 162
Scalers, 2, 6–8
    curved, 1, 2
    hydraulic, 18
    magnetostrictive ultrasonic scaler stacks, 17
    powered, 16–18
    rotary, 18
    sonic, 17
    ultrasonic, 16–17
Scalpels
    harmonic, 15
Sealer cements
    endodontic, 312–314
Segmental hemimandibulectomy,
        254–255
Shar–Pei
    tight–lip syndrome and, 110, 168,
        248–249
Sharpening
    hand instruments and, 8–9
Sheltie
    pemphigus vulgaris, 118
Shepherd
    German. *See* German shepherd
Shields
    tongue, 367–368
Show dogs
    oral examination and, 616
Sialoliths, 126
    radiographs and, 162
    surgical removal of, 512
Silver points
    endodontic therapy and, 298–299
Sinusotomy
    equine, 572, 574–575
Skeletal problems
    developmental, 110–112
Skeletomuscular disorders
    soft tissue pathology and, 127–128
Skull anatomy, 78
Sliding flaps
    periodontal disease and, 215
SLOB rule, 152
Smear layer
    endodontic therapy and, 282, 283
Sodium hypochlorite
    endodontic therapy and, 300, 301
Soft palate, 77
    soft tissue pathology and, 122–123
Soft tissue
    craniomandibular osteopathy, 111

developmental pathology and, 108–112
    lips, 109–110
    oral cavity, 108
    palate, 108–109
    periodontal gingiva, 108
    periosteal proliferation, 111
    salivary gland, 109
    skeletal, 110–112
    tight–lip syndrome, 110
    tongue, 109
Soft tissue pathology, 116–136
    adult gingival cyst, 131
    benign tumors, 130–133. *See also* Benign
        tumors
    cysts. *See* Tumors
    eosinophilic lesions, 119
    equine, 575
    gingiva, 116–122
    hematologic abnormalities and, 120
    lips, 126–127
    malignant tumors, 133–136. *See also*
        Malignant tumors
    metabolic disorders and, 119–120
    neoplasia, 128–136
    nutrition and, 120–122
    oral mucosa, 116–122
    osteomyelitis and, 128
    pemphigus vulgaris, 118
    rubber jaw syndrome, 121
    salivary glands, 125–126
    salivary stones, 126
    sialoliths, 126
    skeletomuscular disorders, 127–128
    soft palate, 122–123
    temporomandibular joint, 127–128
    tongue, 123–125
    trauma and, 122
    tumors, 128–136
    viral papillomatosis, 119
Sonic handpieces
    endodontic therapy and, 302
Sonic scalers, 17
Specific plaque hypothesis, 193
Splints
    acrylic, 274–275
Split U-flap palatal repair, 246–247
Spreaders
    endodontic therapy and, 296
Spring cantilever bridge
    components of, 411
Springer spaniel
    acanthomatous epulis, 132
Squamous cell carcinoma
    female, 510

Squirrel
  dental formula, 523
  incisor extraction, 531
  incisor overgrowth, 526
  malocclusion, 526
  traumatic avulsion of incisors, 531
Standard Gracey curette, 6–8
Sterilization
  endodontic therapy and, 310–311
Stipple pattern
  dental film and, 147
Stones
  pulp, 161
  salivary, 126, 162
Stops
  endodontic, 303
Stout's multiple loop wiring technique
  oral fracture repair and, 271–272
Straight sickle scaler, 6
Strict anaerobes
  periodontal disease and, 192
Stricture
  elbow, 332
Stripping
  canal wall, 333
Suction
  mouth mirror and, 367
Sulcus bleeding index, 196
Supernumerary teeth and roots
  radiographs and, 160
Surface nomenclature, 69–74. *See also* Teeth
Surgery
  dental, 216–217. *See also* Operative dentistry
  oral, 232–258. *See also* Oral surgery
  periodontal, 212–215
  TMJ, 256
Surgical endodontics. *See also* Advanced
      endodontic therapy; Endodontic therapy
  apical resection, 344–345
  apical surgical procedures, 343–347. *See
      also* Apical surgical endodontic
      procedures
  apicoectomy, 344–345
  classical, 341–347
  continually erupting teeth, 347
  contraindications, 342
  indirect resection, 347
  periadicular drainage, 343–344
  periapical curettage, 344
  periapical surgical procedures, 343–347. *See
      also* Apical surgical endodontic
      procedures
  retrograde obturation/filling, 345–346
  retrograde root canal procedures, 347

selection criteria, 341–342
Surgical instruments, 13–15
  electrosurgery, electrocautery, radiosurgery
      units, 14–15
  harmonic scalpels, 15
Symphyseal injury
  classification of, 262, 504
Symphyseal separation
  circumferential wiring and, 267
Symphyseal separation/fracture
  feline, 503–504. *See also* Feline mandibular
      trauma
  radiograph of, 504
Synthetic elastomers
  impressions and, 41–42

T

Tape muzzle
  oral fracture repairs and, 265–266
Taper
  axial wall, 417
Taurodontia
  radiographs and, 160
Teeth. *See also* Cavities; Operative dentistry;
      Restorative dentistry
  anatomy and, 55–74
  apex structure, 74
  Basrani's staging of injuries, 355
  bell stage, 60, 61
  bleaching of, 387–392
  bud stage, 58
  cap stage, 59
  cat oral anatomy, 58
  cavity preparation, 365–366
  cheek teeth, 57
  contact points, 72
  continually erupting, 347
  crown cusp terms, 57
  crown line angles, 71
  crown types, 57
  dental anatomy, 73
  dental formulas, 69
  dentin, 62–65
  dentinal tubules, 63, 64
  development of, 58–69, 167–168
  development types, 55–56
  diphyodont development, 56
  directional nomenclature, 69–74
  dog oral anatomy, 58
  embedded, 239
  embrasures, 72
  enamel, 62–65
  enamel organ development, 58, 59, 60, 61
  endodontic access site, 325–327

Teeth (*contd.*)
    endodontic anatomy, 280–283. *See also* Endodontic therapy
    eruption anomalies, 170–171
    eruption of, 68–69, 169–171
    eruption sequences, 169
    eruption times, 97
    examination of, 89, 90
    feline eruption times, 483. *See also* Cat
    function of, 72–74
    fusion, 160
    Hertwig's epithelial root sheath, 65, 66
    immature deciduous, 336–337
    immature permanent, 337–341
    immature permanent tooth pathology, 176–183. *See also* Immature permanent tooth pathology
    impacted, 160
    jaw occlusal overlay types, 57–58
    natural structure conservation, 359
    operating field, 366–371
    operculum and, 177
    oral fracture repair, 259–279. *See also* Oral fracture repair
    paradental anatomy, 73
    pedodontics, 167–185. *See also* Pedodontics
    peg, 105
    physiology of, 55–74
    point angles, 71
    pulp, 62–65
    restorative materials, 370–387. *See also* Amalgam restorations; Composite resins; Glass ionomers
    ridge nomenclature, 69–74
    root formation, 65–68
    shapes of, 56
    staging of injuries, 355
    staging of tooth injuries, 114
    supernumerary, 160
    surface nomenclature, 69–74
    transillumination and, 95–96
    types of, 56
    vertebrate anchorage types, 56–57
Teeth cleaning
    periodontal disease and, 208–211
Teeth endodontic access, 305–309
Teething
    behavioral problems and, 600–602. *See also* Behavioral problems
Temporomandibular joint
    fractures, 265
    radiographs and, 162–163
    soft tissue pathology and, 127–128

Temporomandibular joint injuries
    feline, 505–506. *See also* Feline mandibular trauma
Temporomandibular joint surgery, 256
Terrier
    craniomandibular osteopathy and, 111
Tiger
    eruption times, 544
    metal crown placement, 549
Tight-lip syndrome, 110
    oral surgery and, 248–249
    Shar-Pei and, 168
Tincture of myrrh and benzoin
    periodontal use of, 46
Tissue
    dental. *See* Dental tissue
    osseous, 77–79
Tissue pathology
    soft, 116–136. *See also* Soft tissue pathology
Tissue regeneration
    guided, 221–227. *See also* Guided tissue regeneration
Tongue
    acquired defects, 251
    anatomy and physiology of, 79–81
    congenital defects, 250–251
    developmental pathology and, 109
    examination of, 90–91
    melanosarcoma on, 134
    oral surgery and, 250–251
    soft tissue pathology and, 123–125
Tongue retractors and shields, 367–368
Tonsillar squamous cell carcinoma, 134, 135
Tonsils
    oral surgery and, 251
Tooth avulsion
    feline, 501. *See also* Feline oral trauma
Tooth coverage
    operative dentistry and, 417–420
Tooth crown contours
    operative dentistry and, 398
Tooth discoloration
    orthodontic complications and, 478–479
Tooth fractures
    feline, 500–501. *See also* Feline oral trauma
Tooth mobility
    periodontitis and, 205–206
Tooth mobility index, 205
Tooth movement
    anchorage and, 450–451
    histologic aspects of, 447–449
    physiologic aspects of, 447–449
    tissue changes, 449

types of, 449–450
Wolff's law, 447
Tooth reduction
  restoratives and, 413–414
Tooth repulsion
  equine, 572–574
Tooth resection
  endodontic therapy and, 335–336
Tooth retention
  alveolar ridge and, 236
Tooth root surfaces
  dog, 448
Toothbrushes
  basic requirements of, 218
Torsion movements
  treatment of, 457
Total hemimandibulectomy, 255
Transcircumferential wiring
  unfavorable fracture and, 269
Transillumination
  tooth vitality and, 95–96
Transosseous wiring
  favorable fracture and, 268
  unfavorable fracture and, 268–269
Trauma
  behavioral problems and, 610–611
  oral mucosa and, 122
  orthodontic appliance-associated, 479
  palatal, 243, 244
Traumatic injuries
  radiographs and, 162
Trephination
  equine, 572–574
Triangular configuration wiring pattern
  unfavorable fracture and, 269
Trituration, 374
Tumors
  benign, 130–133. *See also* Benign tumors
  general finding of, 129
  malignant, 133–136. *See also* Malignant
    tumors
  radiographs and, 163
  soft tissue pathology and, 128–136
  tongue and, 124
Turgeon modified Gracey curette, 6, 8

U
Ultrasonic handpieces
  endodontic therapy and, 302
Ultrasonic scalers, 16–17
Unfavorable fracture
  mandibular, 263–264
  transcircumferential wiring around, 269

transosseous wiring and, 268–269
triangular configuration wiring pattern, 269
Universal curette, 6, 7
Upper 4th premolar
  exodontia and, 238

V
Varnishes
  restorative use of, 37–39
Vasodentin
  cats and, 488
Versions
  orthodontics and, 443, 444
Vertebrate tooth anchorage
  common types of, 56–57
Vertical ramus
  fractures of, 505. *See also* Feline mandibular
    trauma
Vertical ramus fractures, 264
Vestibule
  oral cavity, 76–77
Veterinary periodontal disease index, 198
Viewing procedures
  radiographic, 159
Viral papillomatosis, 119
Vital teeth
  bleaching of, 387–389

W
Wall form
  cavity preparation and, 366
Wall perforation
  lateral, 333
Wall surfaces
  cavities and, 362
Wall taper
  axial, 417
Wavelengths
  x-ray, 141
Waxes
  dental, 44–45
Wires
  orthodontic, 453
Wiring techniques
  adjunct, 274
  circumferential wiring, 267
  Essig's, 272–273
  interarcade, 274
  interdental wiring, 270–274
  interfragmentary wiring, 268–269
  ivy loop, 270–271
  oral fracture repair and, 266–274
  osseous wiring, 266–269

Wiring techniques (*contd.*)
   Risdon's, 272–274
   Stout's multiple loop, 271–272
   transcircumferential wiring, 269
   transosseous wiring, 268–269
Wolf tooth
   horses and, 568
Wolff's law of transformation of bone, 447
Wry malocclusion
   equine, 566

X

X-radiation, 140–141. *See also* Radiology
X-ray generators, 142–144
X-ray machines, 142–144
X-ray wavelengths
   uses for, 141

Z

Zipping
   endodontic instruments and, 332

ISBN 0-397-51385-2

9 780397 513857